TEXTBOOK OF
DIAGNOSTIC ULTRASONOGRAPHY

TEXTBOOK OF
DIAGNOSTIC
ULTRASONOGRAPHY

SANDRA L. HAGEN-ANSERT, B.A., R.D.M.S.

Division of Non-Invasive Cardiology, Echocardiology Section,
Toronto General Hospital, Toronto, Ontario; formerly Educational
Coordinator, University of Wisconsin Clinical Science Center,
Department of Radiology, Section of Diagnostic Ultrasound,
Madison, Wisconsin

SECOND EDITION
with 1460 illustrations

THE C. V. MOSBY COMPANY

ST. LOUIS · TORONTO · LONDON   1983

MOSBY

A TRADITION OF PUBLISHING EXCELLENCE

Editor: Don Ladig

Assistant editor: Rosa Kasper

Manuscript editor: George B. Stericker, Jr.

Design: Nancy Steinmeyer

Production: Margaret B. Bridenbaugh, Judy England, Jeanne A. Gulledge

SECOND EDITION

Previous edition copyrighted 1978

Printed in the United States of America

The C.V. Mosby Company
11830 Westline Industrial Drive, St. Louis, Missouri 63141

Library of Congress Cataloging in Publication Data

Hagen-Ansert, Sandra L.
    Textbook of diagnostic ultrasonography.

    Bibliography: p.
    Includes index.
    1. Diagnosis, Ultrasonic. I. Title. [DNLM:
1. Echocardiography. 2. Ultrasonics—Diagnostic
use. WB 289 H143t]
RC78.7.U4H33 1983   616.07'543   82-8190
ISBN 0-8016-2016-3

GW/CB/B 9 8 7 6 5 4 3 2 1   01/D/064

Contributors

KEVIN E. APPARETI, B.S., R.D.M.S.
Educational Coordinator, University of Colorado Medical Center,
Department of Radiology, Section of Ultrasound, Denver, Colorado

A. ABIGAIL BROGDEN, B.A. R.D.M.S.
Department of Pediatrics, Division of Pediatric Cardiology,
University of Wisconsin Clinical Science Center, Madison, Wisconsin

JAN EWENKO, R.D.M.S.
Department of Pediatrics, Division of Pediatric Cardiology,
University of Wisconsin Clinical Science Center, Madison, Wisconsin

MELANIE G. EZO, R.T., R.D.M.S.
Educational Director, Breast Training Center, Technicare Corporation,
Denver, Colorado

MICHAEL L. JOHNSON, M.D.
Associate Professor of Medicine and Radiology, Division of Radiology,
Ultrasound and Body Computed Tomography, University of Colorado
Medical Center, Denver, Colorado

BECKY LEVZOW, R.T., R.D.M.S.
Department of Radiology, Section of Ultrasound, University of
Wisconsin Clinical Science Center, Madison, Wisconsin

LINDA LONDON, M.S., R.D.M.S.
Chief Sonographer, University of California, San Francisco, Moffitt
Medical Center, Department of Radiology, Section of Ultrasound,
San Francisco, California

RICHARD E. RAE II, R.T., R.D.M.S.
Staff Sonographer, Goethe Link Centenary Vascular Doppler Laboratory,
St. Vincent Hospital and Health Care Center, Indianapolis, Indiana

CAROL RUMACK, M.D.
Associate Professor of Medicine and Radiology, University of Colorado
Medical Center, Denver, Colorado

LAURA SCHORZMAN, R.T., R.D.M.S.
Chief Sonographer, Department of Radiology, Division of Ultrasound,
University of California Medical Center, San Diego, California

JAMES A. ZAGZEBSKI, Ph.D.
Associate Professor, Departments of Medical Physics, Radiology,
and Human Oncology, University of Wisconsin Medical School,
Madison, Wisconsin

WILLIAM J. ZWIEBEL, M.D.
Assistant Professor of Radiology, University of Wisconsin Clinical
Science Center, Madison, Wisconsin

For their love and understanding,
ARTHUR, REBECCA, AND ALYSSA

Foreword

It is a distinct pleasure for me to write the foreword for this important textbook of diagnostic ultrasonography. Since the introduction of the first edition in 1978, it has become widely acclaimed by professionals in the field for the high quality of its images and the clarity of the accompanying text. It is only natural that a second edition should be produced to incorporate the rapid changes in technology that have occurred in the interval.

The second edition contains important new sections on pediatric echocardiography, breast sonography, and the evolving field of superficial organ scanning. The physics and biologic effects sections have been dramatically revised to better meet the needs of practicing ultrasonographers.

I believe that I am in a unique position to preface this text since it was my good fortune to introduce the author to the field 13 years ago. The science or art of ultrasonography in those days was quite limited when compared to modern practice. Nevertheless, it was always exciting, and each new day seemed to bring forth an interesting finding that would at least temporarily perplex us. The close collaboration that existed between us has become typical of this important field. There is no question that today's ultrasonographers command considerable respect for their dedication and advancement of the profession. Sandra Hagen-Ansert is directly responsible for much of this development, since upon leaving our laboratory she has worked tirelessly in educating both physicians and ultrasonographers.

I am sure that she has learned (as have I) that the greatest professional joy results from stimulating others to ever increasing achievement and better patient care. It is to that goal that this text is directed.

George R. Leopold, M.D.

Preface
TO THE SECOND EDITION

At the completion of this revised edition I no longer wonder why there are not more complete textbooks on diagnostic ultrasonography available. The task of compiling all the material necessary to complete such a feat is enormous and one that could not be done without the cooperation of excellent contributors, enthusiastic students, and a supportive departmental staff.

The primary goal of preparing such a textbook was to have information on all areas of sonography available in one source textbook. A number of areas have been updated to include real time and automation techniques as they apply to current diagnostic practice. New chapters have been added to cover applications to the breast, neonates, and superficial structures.

Since there are so many excellent atlas textbooks available on ultrasonography, emphasis is placed on information that the sonographer needs to know and understand in order to be a quality diagnostic ultrasonographer. In an effort to help the sonographer understand the total clinical picture that the patient presents prior to the sonographic examination, anatomy, physiology, laboratory data, clinical signs and symptoms, pathology, and sonographic findings are found in each specific chapter.

I would like to extend my sincere appreciation to the following individuals who helped to make this edition possible: William Zwiebel, M.D., for his help on the liver chapter and in finding interesting cases; Chris Labinski, Rhonda Aborgast, and Jackie Cassidy for their continued support; Barbara VanderWerff, Becky Levzow, and Susan Yourd, for their comments and critiques; Tom Yourke, Jeannie McFadden, Lorrie Stadtmueller, Judy McClellan, John Mayer, Marty Gebhart, and Earl Bell, for their review of the manuscript; Robert Vennie, for his photographic assistance; Jeffrey Allyn Slade, for his medical illustrations; Shirley Wikum and Cindy Johnson, for their secretarial assistance; Jeff Brown, M.D., and Charlie Austin, M.D., for their encouragement and support; Tom Lawson, M.D., and Vicki Vieaux, for their Octoson images from Milwaukee County Medical Center; Marcia Lavery, for her real time images and protocol from the New England Deaconess Hospital; Jean Corneil, for her photographic support to portions of the echocardiography chapters; Harry Rakowski, M.D., and Bob Howard, M.D., for their support and contributions to chapters in adult and congenital heart disease; and Don Ladig, Rosa Kasper, Karen Edwards, and especially George Stericker at C.V. Mosby, for their endless hours and support in completing this textbook.

Sandra L. Hagen-Ansert

Preface
TO THE FIRST EDITION

Medicine has always been a fascinating field. I was introduced to it by Dr. Charles Henkelmann, who provided me with the opportunity to learn radiography. Although x-ray technology was interesting, it was not challenging enough. It did not provide the opportunity to evaluate patient history or to follow through interesting cases, which seemed to be the most intriguing aspect of medicine and my primary concern.

Shortly after I finished my training, I was assigned to the radiation therapy department, where I was introduced to a very quiet and young, dedicated radiologist, whom I would later grow to admire and respect as one of the foremost authorities in diagnostic ultrasound. Convincing George Leopold that he needed another hand to assist him was difficult in the beginning, and it was through the efforts of his resident, Dan MacDonald, that I was able to learn what has eventually developed into a most challenging and exciting new medical modality.

Utilizing high-frequency sound waves, diagnostic ultrasound provides a unique method for visualization of soft tissue anatomic structures. The challenge of identifying such structures and correlating the results with clinical symptoms and patient data offered an ongoing challenge to the sonographer. The state of the art demands expertise in scanning techniques and maneuvers to demonstrate the internal structures; without quality scans, no diagnostic information can be rendered to the physician.

Out initial experience in ultrasound took us through the era of A-mode techniques, identifying aortic aneurysms through pulsatile reflections, trying to separate splenic reflections from upper-pole left renal masses, and, in general, trying to echo every patient with a probable abdominal or pelvic mass. Of course, the one-dimensional A-mode techniques were difficult for me to conceptualize, let alone believe in. However, with repeated success and experience from mistakes, I began to believe in this method. The conviction that Dr. Leopold had about this technique was a strong indicator of its success in our laboratory.

It was when Picker brought our first two-dimensional ultrasound unit to the laboratory that the "skeptics" started to believe a little more in this modality. I must admit that those early images were weather maps to me for a number of months. The repeated times I asked, "What is that?" were enough to try anyone's patience.

I can recall when Siemens installed our real-time unit and we saw our first obstetric case. Such a thrill for us to see the fetus move, wave its hand, and show us fetal heart pulsations.

By this time we were scouting the clinics and various departments in the hospital for interesting cases to scan. With our success rate surpassing our failures, the case load increased so that soon we were involved in all aspects of ultrasound. There was not enough material or reprints for us to read to see the new developments. It was for this reason that excitement in clinical research soared, attracting young physicians throughout the country to develop techniques in diagnostic ultrasound.

Because Dr. Leopold was so intensely interested in ultrasound, it became the diagnostic method of choice for our patients. It was not long before conferences were incomplete without the mention of the technique. Later, local medical meetings and eventually national meetings grew to include discussion of this new modality. A number of visitors were attracted to our laboratory to learn the technique, and thus we became swamped with a continual flow of new physicians, some eager to work with ultrasound and others skeptical at first but believers in the end.

Education progressed slowly at first, with many laboratories offering a one-to-one teaching experience. Commercial companies thought the only way to push the field was to develop their own national training programs, and thus several of the leading manufacturers were the first to put a dedicated effort into the development of ultrasound.

It was through the combined efforts of our laboratory and commercial interests that I became interested in furthering ultrasound education. Seminars, weekly sessions, local and national meetings, and consultations became a vital part of the growth of ultrasound.

Thus, as ultrasound grew in popularity, more intensified training was desperately needed to maintain its initial quality that its pioneers strived for.

Through working with one of the commercial ultrasound companies conducting national short-term training programs, I became acquainted with Barry Goldberg and his enthusiasm for quality education in ultrasound. His organizational efforts and pioneer spirit led me to the east coast to further develop more intensive educational programs in ultrasound.

Through these experiences the need for a diverse ultrasound textbook was shown. Thus this text was written for the sonographer involved in clinical ultrasound, with emphasis on anatomy, physiology, pathology, and ultrasonic techniques and patterns. Clinical medicine and patient evaluation are important parts of the ultrasonic examination and as such are discussed as relevant to pathology demonstrated by ultrasound.

It is my hope that this textbook will not only introduce the reader to the field of ultrasound but also go a step beyond to what I have found to be a very stimulating and challenging experience in diagnostic patient care.

I would like to acknowledge the individual who contributed most to my early interest in diagnostic ultrasound, George R. Leopold, M.D., for his personal perseverance and instruction, as well as for his outstanding clinical research. My thanks also to Dr. Sam Halpern for the encouragement to publish; to Dr. Barry Goldberg for the opportunity to develop training programs in an independent fashion and for his encouragement to stay with it; to Drs. Barbara Gosink, Robert O'Rourke, Mike Crawford, and David Sahn for their encouragement throughout the years at U.C.S.D.; to Drs. Jagdish Patel and Carl Rubin for their continued interest in developing ultrasonic techniques; to Dr. Daniel Yellon for his early hours of anatomy dissection and instruction in clinical cardiology; to Dr. Carson Schneck for his excellent instruction in gross anatomy and sections of "Geraldine"; to Dr. Harvey Watts for his help in the preparation of the gross anatomy pathology photographs from Episcopal Hospital; to Dr. Jacob Zatuchni for the interest, enthusiasm, and understanding he showed me while at Episcopal Hospital; to Drs. Paul Walinski and Edward Sacks for their enthusiastic support in echocardiology; to Reuben Mezrich, David Vilkomberson, Ray Wood, Joe Geck, and Nate Pinkney for their continued support and participation in the physics chapter; to Marcia Lavery for her support with the liver chapter; to John Dietz for the photography of the equipment and patient positions; to Bill Burke, medical illustrator, for his aid in the preparation of the photographs and cardiac illustrations; to Arthur J. Ansert, Jr., who provided the atmosphere of productivity to complete such a book.

The students in diagnostic ultrasound from Episcopal Hospital and Thomas Jefferson University Medical Center continually work toward the development of finer ultrasound techniques and instruction, and for their support I would like to thank them.

A special acknowledgment is made to the many contributors of various chapters within the textbook. Much of this information was accumulated as part of their student participation in the Ultrasound Program at Episcopal Hospital and Thomas Jefferson University Medical Center.

Sandra L. Hagen-Ansert

Contents

TEXTBOOK OF
DIAGNOSTIC ULTRASONOGRAPHY

1

Physics of diagnostic ultrasound

JAMES A. ZAGZEBSKI

NATURE OF SOUND WAVES

The passage of sound through a medium involves wave propagation, in which particles within the medium are caused to vibrate about their *rest* position. This disturbance propagates through the medium at a speed determined by the properties of the medium itself. Passage of the wave results in the transfer of *energy* through the medium. However, there is no net transfer of particles (i.e., after a sound wave has passed through the medium the particles return to their normal, equilibrium position; we are assuming that the strength of the wave is low enough to allow this latter statement to be made). Sound waves can be transmitted through many materials, such as air, water, wood, plastic, and biologic tissues. They can-

not be transmitted through a vacuum because they require some form of matter for their propagation.

Sound waves are produced by vibrating sources. One of the simplest examples of a source of sound is a tuning fork vibrating in air (Fig. 1-1, *A*). The vibrations of the tuning fork cause adjacent molecules in the air to be compressed together and drawn apart, depending on the direction of movement of the arm of the tuning fork. Molecules that are compressed together push other molecules closer together, which push other farther molecules closer together, etc.; thus the acoustic disturbance propagates outward.

A tuning fork vibrates back and forth in a regular fashion, sometimes referred to as *simple harmonic motion*. The resultant air compressions are accompanied by increases in the pressure. If it were possible to measure the pressure at different points near the tuning fork at any instant of time, the measurement results would appear as in Fig. 1-1, *B*. The pressure varies with distance, tracing out a *sine wave*, as shown. Here *0* pressure refers to equilibrium, ambient conditions, usually the atmospheric pressure if we are considering a sound wave in air. Places where particles are squeezed together are referred to as regions of *compression* and the pressure here is greater than 0. The maximum pressure swing occurring during passage of the wave is called the *pressure amplitude*, also defined in the figure. Places where the particles are drawn apart are referred to as regions of *rarefaction* and the pressure here is less than 0. The distance over which the curve repeats itself is called the acoustic *wavelength*, given by the symbol λ in the figure.

Just as the vibrating tuning fork does not remain stationary, so a plot of pressure versus distance also varies from one instant to

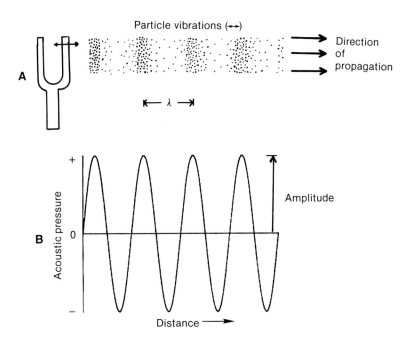

Fig. 1-1. Generation of a sound wave in air by a vibrating tuning fork. The graph shows the acoustic pressure versus distance at some instant of time.

the next (Fig. 1-2). This is because the sound wave is propagating outward from the source. A useful way of expressing the temporal behavior of a sound wave is to plot the pressure versus time at a single point in the medium. The resultant curve also traces out a *sine wave* (Fig. 1-3). The number of times per second the disturbance is repeated at any point is called the *frequency*. The time it takes for the disturbance to repeat itself is the *period*, labeled T in Fig. 1-3. Frequency, f, and period, T, are inversely related; that is,

$$T = \frac{1}{f} \qquad (1\text{-}1)$$

Example: Suppose the period of a waveform is 0.5 second. Calculate the frequency.

Solution: You can rearrange Equation 1-1 by multiplying both sides of the equation by f and dividing both sides by T. The result is

$$f = \frac{1}{T}$$

Substituting gives

$$f = \frac{1}{0.5 \text{ sec}} = 2/\text{sec}$$

In other words, if the period is 0.5 second, the frequency is 2 times per second.

Fig. 1-4 shows that as the period decreases, the frequency increases, and vice versa.

TYPES OF SOUND WAVES

Sound waves are mechanical vibrations that propagate in a medium. In response to the sound wave, particles in the medium are displaced from their rest position and vibrate back and forth. In the example in Fig. 1-1 the particle displacement is in the same direction as the wave propagates. This mode of vibration is referred to as *longitudinal wave* propagation. Other types of vibrations are possible, depending on the type of medium. For example, transverse vibrations or shear waves may be transmitted through solid materials. These are characterized by particle vibrations perpendicular to the direction of vibration (Fig. 1-5). In this textbook we are concerned mainly with propagation of sound in the soft tissues of the body. Only longitudinal waves are of interest here because this is the only mode of vibration that can be transmitted through soft tissue.

FREQUENCY

It was mentioned earlier that the sound frequency is the number of oscillations per second that the source or the particles in the medium make as they vibrate about their rest position. The unit for frequency is *cycles per second* or *hertz*. Commonly used multiples of 1 hertz are as follows:

1 cycle per second = 1 hertz = 1 Hz

1000 cycles per second = 1000 hertz = 1 kilohertz = 1 kHz

1,000,000 cycles per second = 1,000,000 hertz = 1 megahertz = 1 MHz

The metric notation will be used consistently in this book. Appendix F gives the more common metric prefixes and their decimal equivalents.

A classification scheme for acoustic waves according to their frequency is given in Fig. 1-6. Most humans can hear sound if it has a frequency in the range of 15 Hz to approximately 15 to 18 kHz. This is referred to as the *audible frequency* range. Frequencies greater than 20 kHz are referred to as *ultrasonic*. Vibrations whose frequencies are below the audible range are termed *infrasonic*. Examples of infrasonic transmissions include vibrations introduced by air ducts, ocean waves, and seismic waves.

The ultrasonic frequency range is used extensively, both by humans and by animals. Except for therapy ultrasound, most medical applications utilize frequencies that lie in the 1-to-20-MHz range.

SPEED OF SOUND

The speed with which acoustic waves propagate through a medium is determined by the *characteristics of the medium* itself. (There are slight dependences on other factors, such as the ultrasonic frequency, but these are so small that they can be ignored completely in our discussion.) Specifically, for longitudinal sound waves in either liquids or body tissues an expression for the speed of sound, c, is

$$c = \sqrt{\frac{B}{\rho}} \qquad (1\text{-}2)$$

In this equation B refers to the elastic properties of the medium and is called the *bulk modulus*. The symbol ρ is the density, given in g/cm^3 (grams per cubic centimeter) or kg/m^3 (kilograms per cubic meter). Thus we see that the speed of sound in a medium depends on the elastic properties, or "stiffness," of the medium and on the density. Appropriate units for speed are m/sec (meters per second). The speeds of sound in some nonbiologic materials are as follows[1,6]:

	m/sec
Air	330
Silastic materials	950
Ethyl alcohol	1177
Water	1480
Lead	2400
Crown glass	6120
Aluminum	6400

The speed of sound in biologic tissues is an important parameter in imaging applications.[4] Values that have been measured in different human tissues are as follows[6]:

	m/sec
Lung	600
Fat	1460
Aqueous humor	1510
Liver	1555
Blood	1560
Kidney	1565
Muscle	1600
Lens	1620
Skull bone	4080

The lowest speed shown is that for lung tissue, due to the presence of air-filled alveoli in this tissue. Most tissues of concern to us, that is, those through which sound can be readily propagated in the megahertz frequency range, have speeds of sound in the neighborhood of 1500 to 1600 m/sec. Fat is seen to come out on the low end of this chart whereas muscle tissue and the lens of the eye come out on the high-speed end. Measurements of the speed of sound in bone tissue result in values two to three times those recorded in most soft tissues.

The average speed of sound in soft tissues (excluding the lung) is 1540 m/sec, and range-measuring circuits on many diagnostic ultrasound instruments are calibrated on this basis. Close inspection of the biologic tissue list above reveals that the propagation speed in every soft tissue of concern to us in diagnostic ultrasound is within a few percentage points of 1540 m/sec.

WAVELENGTH

The acoustic wavelength (λ), as defined above and illustrated in Fig. 1-1, depends on the speed of sound in the medium, c, and the frequency, f, according to the following relationship:

$$\lambda = \frac{c}{f} \qquad (1\text{-}3)$$

Thus the wavelength is simply the speed of sound divided by the ultrasonic frequency. The speeds of sound in soft tissues vary by only a few percentage points. We can see from Equation 1-3 that the higher the ultrasonic frequency the smaller will be the wavelength.

Example: Calculate the wavelength for a 2-MHz ultrasound beam in soft tissue. Assume the speed of sound is 1540 m/sec.

Solution: The wavelength can be calculated directly using Equation 1-3, with $c = 1540$ m/sec and $f = 2$ MHz $= 2 \times 10^6$ cycles/sec.

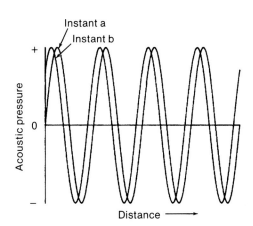

Fig. 1-2. Acoustic pressure versus distance at two different times. Same setup as in Fig. 1-1. The two curves are identical except for being slightly out of phase.

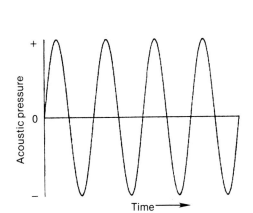

Fig. 1-3. Pressure versus time measured at a single point.

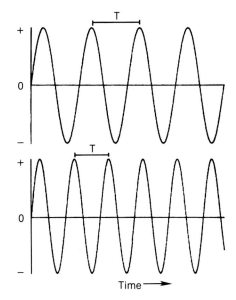

Fig. 1-4. Sine waves of two different frequencies.

Thus $\lambda = \dfrac{1540 \text{ m/sec}}{2 \times 10^6 \text{ cycles/sec}}$

$= 0.0077 \text{ m/cycle}$

$= 0.77 \text{ mm/cycle}$

We always drop the /cycle since it is obviously included in our designation *wavelength*.

So $\lambda = 0.77$ mm is the correct answer.

You may wish to study the material in Appendix F at this stage to review metric conversions. Appendix E also contains examples of addition, subtraction, multiplication, and division in which numbers are expressed as exponentials (i.e., 2,000,000 cycles/sec = 2×10^6 cycles/sec). Although to be a successful sonographer may not require mastering problems of this type, nevertheless, we will continue to explore examples such as this throughout the first few chapters of this book in an effort to improve our understanding of the physical factors involved in sound transmission through soft tissue.

The wavelength concept is important in ultrasound physics because it is related to imaging factors such as *spatial resolution*. In addition, the physical size of an object (e.g., a reflecting surface or a transducer surface) is significant only when we compare it to the ultrasonic wavelength. It might be said then that the wavelength is our "acoustic yard-

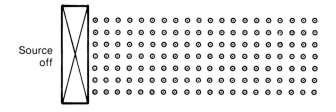

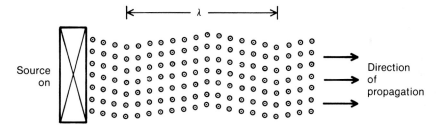

Fig. 1-5. Characteristics of transverse waves, for which the particles in the medium vibrate perpendicular to the direction of propagation of the wave.

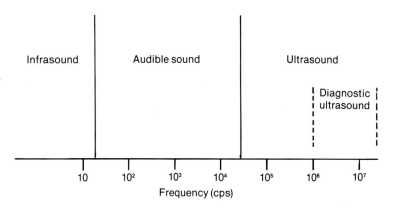

Fig. 1-6. Division of sound into different frequency ranges. *Ultrasound* refers to a sound wave whose frequency is greater than 20 kHz.

stick" (Fig. 1-7). Objects are large or small depending on their size relative to it. In soft tissue, wavelengths for diagnostic ultrasound are on the order of 1 mm or less, with 0.77-mm wavelengths for 2-MHz beams and proportionally smaller ones for higher frequencies.

AMPLITUDE AND INTENSITY

When discussing reflection, attenuation, and scatter, we often must make a quantitative statement regarding the magnitude of a sound wave. One variable that can be used here is the *pressure amplitude*. The acoustic pressure amplitude was illustrated in Fig. 1-1 and was defined as the maximum increase (or decrease) in the pressure relative to ambient conditions in the absence of the sound wave. Other parameters that could have been used in an analogous fashion include the maximum *particle displacement* in the wave and the maximum *particle velocity*.

In some applications, particularly when discussing biologic effects of ultrasound (Chapter 6), it is useful to specify the acoustic intensity. The intensity, I, is related to the square of the pressure amplitude, P, according to the relationship:

$$I = \frac{P^2}{2 \rho c} \qquad (1\text{-}4)$$

where, again, ρ is the density of the medium and c the speed of sound.

Acoustic intensity will be discussed in greater detail in Chapter 6.

ACOUSTIC IMPEDANCE

The product of the density of a material and the speed of sound in that material is a quantity called the characteristic acoustic impedance or, for our purposes, simply the *acoustic impedance* of a medium. The significance of this quantity is its role in determining the amplitude of reflected and transmitted waves at an interface. This is discussed in the next section.

Except for the fact that we must concern ourselves with some fairly large numbers and some units that may be difficult to relate to, determining the impedance for materials is just a case of carrying out the simple multiplication involved, or

$$Z = \rho c \qquad (1\text{-}5)$$

where Z is the impedance and ρ and c are as already defined.

Following is a compilation of acoustic impedance values for both nonbiologic and biologic tissues. The units for expressing these are kg/m²/sec (kilograms per square meter per second), which result after multiplying

density times speed. Sometimes we find impedance given in *rayls*. One rayl is the same as 1 kg/m²/sec:

	rayls
Air	0.0004×10^6
Lung	0.18×10^6
Fat	1.34×10^6
Water	1.48×10^6
Liver	1.65×10^6
Blood	1.65×10^6
Kidney	1.63×10^6
Muscle	1.71×10^6
Skull bone	7.8×10^6

REFLECTION

Whenever an ultrasound beam is incident on an interface formed by two materials having different acoustic impedances, in general, some of the energy in the beam will be reflected and the remainder transmitted. The amplitude of the reflected wave depends on the difference between the acoustic impedances of the two materials forming the interface.

Consider, first, the case of normal or perpendicular beam incidence on a large flat interface (Fig. 1-8). A large smooth interface such as depicted here is termed a *specular interface*—with dimensions that are much greater than the ultrasonic wavelength. The ratio of the reflected pressure amplitude, P_r, to the incident pressure amplitude, P_i, is called the *amplitude reflection coefficient*—given by R. This ratio depends on the acoustic impedances at the interface according to the expression:

$$R = \frac{P_r}{P_i} = \frac{Z_2 - Z_1}{Z_2 + Z_1} \qquad (1\text{-}6)$$

where Z_2 is the acoustic impedance on the distal side of the interface and Z_1 is the impedance on the proximal side.

Example: Using the values for acoustic impedance just given, calculate the amplitude reflection coefficient for a fat-liver interface.

Solution: The acoustic impedance of fat is 1.34×10^6 rayls, that of liver 1.65×10^6 rayls. From Equation 1-6

$$R =$$
$$\frac{1.65 \times 10^6 \text{ rayls} - 1.34 \times 10^6 \text{ rayls}}{1.65 \times 10^6 \text{ rayls} + 1.34 \times 10^6 \text{ rayls}}$$

Factoring out 10^6 rayls gives

$$R = \frac{(1.65 - 1.34) \times 10^6 \text{ rayls}}{(1.65 + 1.34) \times 10^6 \text{ rayls}}$$
$$= \frac{(1.65 - 1.34)}{(1.65 + 1.34)} = \frac{0.31}{2.99} = 0.10$$

We see from the example that the ratio of the reflected to the incident amplitude is quite small. In fact, at most soft tissue–soft tissue interfaces in the body the reflection coefficient is fairly small and most of the sound

is *transmitted* through the interface. If this were not the case, it would be difficult to use diagnostic ultrasound for examining anatomic structures at significant tissue depths.

Example: Calculate the reflection coefficient for a muscle-air interface.

Solution: From the acoustic impedances given in the list, calculate

$$R = \frac{0.0004 \times 10^6 - 1.7 \times 10^6}{0.0004 \times 10^6 + 1.7 \times 10^6}$$
$$= \frac{0.0004 - 1.7}{0.0004 + 1.7}$$
$$= -0.99$$

(Notice that several of the mathematical steps illustrated in the previous example were combined into one step.) In this case the beam is almost completely reflected. This example illustrates the difficulty in transmitting ultrasound beyond any tissue-to-air interface. Nearly total reflection results in virtually no sound beyond the interface (Fig. 1-9). The complete reflection at air interfaces also explains the need for a coupling medium, such as gel or oil, between the ultrasound transducer (discussed in Chapter 2) and the patient during ultrasound examinations. The coupling material ensures that no air is trapped between the transducer and the skin surface, thereby providing good sound transmission into the patient.

Other examples of reflection coefficients (P_r/P_i) calculated for specular reflecting interfaces are as follows:

Muscle-air	−0.99
Fat-liver	0.10
Kidney-liver	0.006
Liver-muscle	0.018
Muscle-bone	0.64

The data presented here show that a soft tissue–to–bone interface also is a fairly strong reflector. In the majority of ultrasound examinations discussed in this text, bone is avoided because of this and other difficulties associated with propagation through it. Most soft tissue interfaces of importance are fairly weakly reflecting, just as we calculated in the first example.

In summary, reflection of a sound beam occurs whenever the beam is incident on an interface formed by two tissues having different acoustic impedances. The acoustic impedance difference could be caused by a change in speeds of sound, a change in densities, or both. The magnitude of the reflected wave, expressed here as the ratio of the reflected wave amplitude to the incident amplitude, is mainly dependent on the acoustic impedance *difference* at the interface. Interfaces characterized by a large difference in acoustic impedances reflect more of the inci-

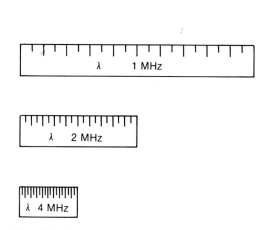

Fig. 1-7. The wavelength is often used as an acoustic yardstick.

REFLECTION

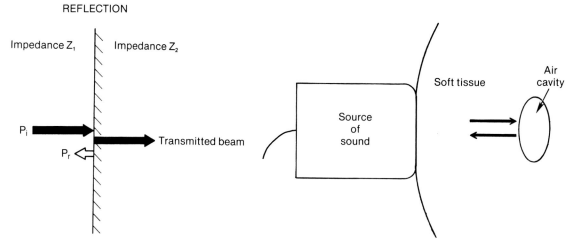

Fig. 1-8. Reflection for perpendicular beam incidence on a specular reflector. P_i is the pressure amplitude of the incident beam, and P_r the amplitude for the reflected beam.

Fig. 1-9. Reflection at a tissue-air interface. Essentially all the sound energy is reflected.

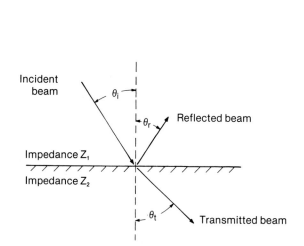

Fig. 1-10. Reflection and refraction for nonperpendicular beam incidence. The incident beam angle, θ_i, reflected beam angle, θ_r, and transmitted beam angle, θ_t, are illustrated.

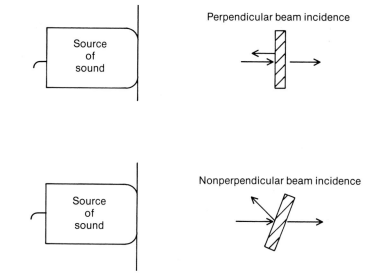

Fig. 1-11. For perpendicular beam incidence the echo returns from a specular reflector toward the source. For nonperpendicular incidence the echo travels in a direction that may miss the source.

dent beam energy than do interfaces where the acoustic impedance difference (*mismatch*) is small.

One additional note: some authors utilize the intensity reflection coefficient rather than the amplitude reflection coefficient to quantify the reflection process. The expression for the size of the reflection looks similar to Equation 1-6, except that the quantity involving the acoustic impedances is squared. In other words, if I_r is the reflected intensity and I_i is the incident intensity, then

$$\frac{I_r}{I_i} = \left[\frac{Z_2 - Z_1}{Z_2 + Z_1}\right]^2 \qquad (1\text{-}7)$$

The two expressions (Equations 1-7 and 1-6) are not contradictory. Recall from our earlier discussion that the intensity is *proportional* to the square of the amplitude. Therefore the ratio of the reflected intensity to the incident intensity at an interface is *equal* to the square of the ratio of the reflected amplitude to the incident amplitude.

NONPERPENDICULAR SOUND BEAM INCIDENCE

For nonperpendicular beam incidence on a specular reflector the situation changes somewhat.

First, the reflected beam does not travel back toward the source (Fig. 1-10) but instead travels off at an angle, θ_r, that is equal to the incident angle, θ_i, only in the opposite direction. This has an effect on echo detection from interfaces. As we shall see in Chapter 3, in many diagnostic applications of ultrasound the sound beam source is also used to detect echoes from reflectors in the beam. The amplitude of an echo that is detected depends on the orientation of the interface relative to the incident beam (Fig. 1-11). Because of this significant angular dependence on the detection of an echo, specular reflectors are sometimes difficult to pick up by a single pulse-echo transducer.

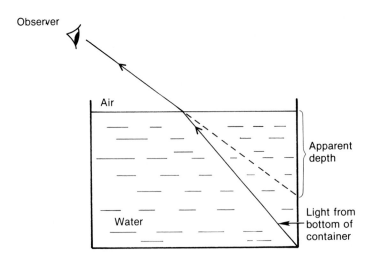

Fig. 1-12. Refraction of light at a water-air interface. To the observer the container of water seems to be shallower than it actually is.

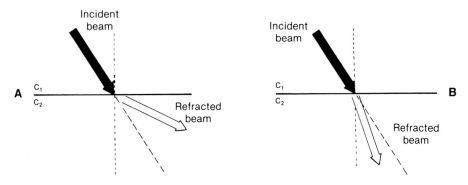

Fig. 1-13. Refraction. **A,** c_2 greater than c_1. **B,** c_2 less than c_1.

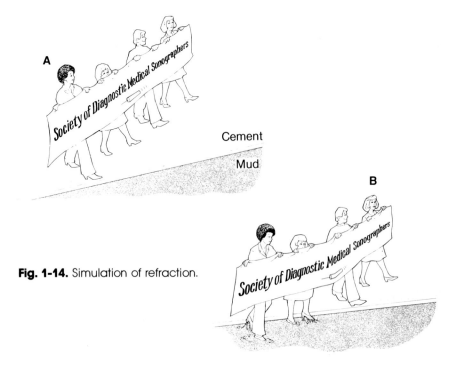

Fig. 1-14. Simulation of refraction.

A second factor that arises when the incident beam is not perpendicular to an interface is the possibility of refraction of the transmitted beam. *Refraction* refers to a bending of the sound beam at the interface, causing the transmitted beam to emerge in a different direction from the incident beam (Fig. 1-10). Most of us are familiar with the effects of refraction of light waves; for example, due to refraction a swimming pool appears shallower than it actually is (Fig. 1-12).

Two conditions are required for refraction of a sound wave to occur:

1. The sound beam must be incident on the interface at an angle that is not perpendicular.
2. The speeds of sound must be different on the two sides of the interface.

Notice what the second condition is saying: it is not sufficient simply to have a reflecting interface to produce refraction; there *also* must be a speed of sound change at the interface for refraction to occur.

The direction of the transmitted (not reflected) beam is governed by Snell's law. The direction is related to the speed of sound on the incident beam side of the interface, c_1, to the speed of sound on the transmitted beam side of the interface, c_2, and to the incident beam direction, θ_i (Fig. 1-10), according to the following relationship:

$$\sin \theta_t = \frac{c_2}{c_1} \sin \theta_i \qquad (1\text{-}8)$$

The angle θ_t is also shown in Fig. 1-10. Equation 1-8 is a statement of Snell's law.

The relationship between an angle and its trigonometric sine ("sin") is discussed in Appendix D. It is possible to calculate θ_t, given the incident beam direction and the speeds of sound at the interface. We will not do calculations here using Equation 1-8; suffice to say that the sine of any angle between 0 and 90 degrees increases as the angle itself increases. Therefore, if c_2 is greater than c_1, the angle θ_t will be greater than θ_i; and vice versa (Fig. 1-13). Notice, if c_2 equals c_1, θ_t equals θ_i (i.e., there is no refraction).

To help understand the process of refraction, consider the situation of a row of sonographers carrying a long banner (Fig. 1-14, A). Suppose the sonographers are all walking at the same speed on a concrete pavement as shown. At the end of the pavement is a field of mud, which significantly slows the pace each sonographer can run upon entering it. Then, at some later time, the different speeds that can be maintained on either side of the concrete-mud interface result in the situation of Fig. 1-14, *B*. When all sonographers have entered the mud, their direction of travel will have altered.

Refraction results in a change in sound beam direction. Situations in which refraction may occur are those for which a sound beam is incident nonperpendicularly on an interface and the speed of sound changes across the interface. The degree of refraction depends on the difference between the speeds of sound; the greater the difference, the larger the effect. If we reexamine the acoustic impedance values of soft tissues only, it appears that interfaces involving fat (i.e., fat-muscle) offer the best chances for significant (measured) beam refraction. Investigators believe that both fat-nonfat interfaces and sharply curved interfaces (e.g., walls of vessels) provide the best surfaces for refraction to occur.

GRAZING INCIDENCE

Additional complexity may be introduced if the sound beam is incident on a reflector at nearly grazing incident angles. The situations to be described occur only if the speeds of sound on the two sides of the interface are different. Such conditions appear to arise in some diagnostic situations involving, for example, small cysts and vessels. Therefore we will consider them briefly.

If the speed of sound in the material on the transmitted beam side of the interface, c_2, is greater than that in the material on the incident beam side, c_1, the possibility of *critical angle* refraction exists. This occurs when refraction causes the angle of the transmitted beam, θ_t, to equal 90 degrees (Fig. 1-15). The critical angle is the incident beam angle, θ_i, when this situation occurs. If θ_i is greater than the critical angle, all the energy is reflected and none is transmitted.

If c_2 is less than c_1, no critical angle exists. However, for grazing incident beam angles the reflected amplitude still increases above the value obtained for perpendicular beam incidence. The reflection coefficient approaches 1 (all the sound reflected and none transmitted) as the incident beam angle approaches 90 degrees.

Both these situations are illustrated by the graphs in Fig. 1-16. In *A*, in which the speed of sound through fat is greater than that through liver, a critical angle exists. For these tissues we see that with a perpendicular beam incidence, or with modest angles, the reflected wave is of a relatively low amplitude and most of the sound energy is transmitted through the interface. However, at a grazing incidence, as illustrated in *B*, the

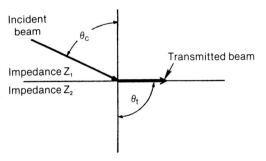

Fig. 1-15. Demonstration of the critical angle, or the incident beam angle, corresponding to a 90-degree transmitted beam angle. It can occur when c_2 is greater than c_1. All the incident sound is reflected for incident angles greater than the critical angle.

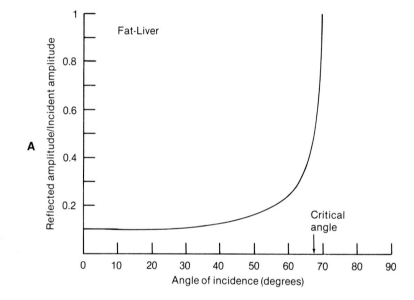

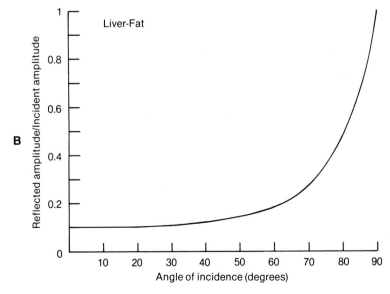

Fig. 1-16. Variation of the amplitude reflection coefficient versus the angle of incidence of the sound beam, **A,** A fat-liver interface. **B,** A liver-fat interface.

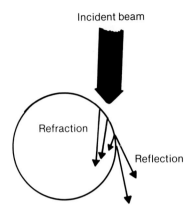

Incident beam

Refraction

Reflection

Fig. 1-17. Sound transmission and reflection near the edge of a circular or tubular structure.

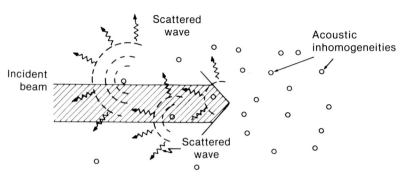

Fig. 1-18. Scattering of sound at small interfaces.

interface becomes a near perfect reflector and does not allow any of the sound energy to pass through.

Small vessels, ducts, and cysts are examples in which the processes just mentioned could have a significant effect (Fig. 1-17). Considerable disruption of the sound beam at the edge of such a structure leads to a shadow appearance beyond the structure.[4] An example is presented in Chapter 4.

SCATTER

In our discussion of specular reflectors we were considering reflections from smooth interfaces that are much larger than the ultrasonic wavelength. Other types of inhomogeneities exist in the body that can give rise to echoes. For structures that are smaller than the wavelength, a process referred to as ultrasonic *scatter* takes place (Fig. 1-18). In this figure, scatterers are represented as small objects distributed at random locations in the volume of interest. Waves that are scattered tend to travel off in all directions, as suggested in the diagram.*

Since the scattered waves spread in all directions, echo signals detected from a volume containing small scatterers are not highly dependent on the orientation of individual scatterers. This is in contrast to the strong orientation dependence seen for specular reflectors. For very small scatterers, echo signals do depend on

1. The number of scatterers per unit volume
2. The acoustic impedance changes at the scatterer interfaces
3. The size of the scatterer; scattering usu-

---

*There may be some directional patterns depending on the nature of the scatterer, but we do not need to discuss them here.

Table 1-1. Amplitude and intensity ratios and their equivalent values expressed in decibels

Amplitude ratio A_2/A_1	Log A_2/A_1	dB	Intensity ratio I_2/I_1	Log I_2/I_1
1	0	0	1	0
1.414	0.15	3	2	0.3
2	0.3	6	4	0.6
4	0.6	12	16	1.2
10	1	20	100	2
100	2	40	10,000	4
1000	3	60	1,000,000	6
$\frac{1}{2}$	−0.3	−6	$\frac{1}{4}$	−0.6
$\frac{1}{10}$	−1	−20	$\frac{1}{100}$	−2
$\frac{1}{100}$	−2	−40	$\frac{1}{10,000}$	−4

ally increases with increasing radius for very small scatterers
4. The ultrasonic frequency; scattering usually increases with increasing frequency for very small scatterers

The dependence on frequency can sometimes be used to an advantage in ultrasound imaging. Since specular reflection is frequency independent and scattering increases with frequency, it is often possible to enhance scattered signals over specular echo signals by utilizing higher ultrasonic frequencies. Examples of small scatterers include red blood cells and small structures distributed throughout the parenchyma of most organs.

DECIBEL NOTATION

Let us digress briefly and discuss a fairly standard method for quantifying amplitudes, intensities, or power levels in ultrasound. The *decibel notation* provides a comparison of two signal levels, such as two amplitudes or two intensities. It is used primarily to ex-

press changes in these quantities resulting, for example, from attenuation, signal amplification, or instrument power control variations.

Consider two wave amplitudes, A_1 and A_2. We could compare these two amplitudes directly, for example, by simply taking the ratio of one to the other; or, using decibels, we could express the relationship between A_1 and A_2 as follows:

$$\text{Signal level (dB)} = 20 \log \frac{A_2}{A_1} \quad (1\text{-}9)$$

If the power or intensity is used rather than the amplitude, the expression appears on the surface to be somewhat different:

$$\text{Signal level (dB)} = 10 \log \frac{I_2}{I_1} \quad (1\text{-}10)$$

where I refers to an intensity.

In fact, Equation 1-9 can be shown to be equivalent to Equation 1-10. To do this we make use of the fact that the logarithm of a number raised to any power (e.g., log 10^2) is equal to that power *times* the logarithm of the number alone:

$$\log 10^2 = 2 \times \log 10$$

If we use the expression for decibels employing the intensities (Equation 1-10)

$$\text{Signal level (dB)} = 10 \log \frac{I_2}{I_1}$$

and note from Equation 1-4 that the intensity is proportional to the amplitude squared

$$\frac{I_2}{I_1} = \left[\frac{A_2}{A_1} \right]^2$$

(the other terms in Equation 1-4 divide out), we can write

$$\text{Signal level (dB)} = 10 \log \left[\frac{A_2}{A_1} \right]^2$$
$$= 20 \log \frac{A_2}{A_1}$$

which is identical to Equation 1-9. Different authors usually present the decibel notation in either of these two forms. The purpose of this exercise is to show that both forms are essentially the same.

The amplitude and intensity ratios corresponding to a given decibel level can be calculated fairly easily. Some examples are presented in Table 1-1. The first column in this table presents selected amplitude ratios, and the second column gives the computed logarithm for each ratio. Multiplying the logarithm of the ratio by 20 yields the decibel relation between the two amplitudes, shown in column 3.

If we square the amplitude ratio in column 1, we wind up with the intensity ratio (column 4). The logarithm of each intensity ratio is given in column 5. Multiplying the logarithm of the intensity ratio by 10, we get back the decibel level; in each case it is identical to the value given in column 3.

It often happens that when we are comparing signal amplitudes or intensities the ratio (column 1 or column 4) is a fraction. This is generally the case when considering effects of attenuation, discussed in the next section. The decibel notation allows us to account for such changes conveniently—simply by using the fact that if n is any number then

$$\log \frac{1}{n} = -\log n$$

So, for an amplitude ratio of $^1/_{10}$, $\log ^1/_{10}$ is equal to $-\log 10$. Therefore this amplitude ratio corresponds to a -20 dB signal change. For convenience, Table 1-1 is expanded in the lower rows to provide decibel levels corresponding to fractional amplitude and intensity ratios.

An interesting feature that may be helpful in attempting to relate to decibels is discernible in Table 1-1. Whenever the amplitude doubles (A_2/A_1 goes from 1 to 2, 2 to 4, etc.), this corresponds to a 6-dB change. Whenever the intensity doubles, this corresponds to a 3-dB change.

One of the conveniences of the decibel notation is that it compresses the range of numbers that must be used when large differences in amplitude or intensity are found. This compression of the number scale should be apparent in Table 1-1.

In summary, decibels do not represent absolute signal levels but quantitatively describe the *ratio* of two amplitudes or intensities. The decibel notation is used to express the amplification or gain of an amplifier. The amplification is the ratio of the output amplitude of the amplifier to the input amplitude. Thus this ratio is conveniently expressed in decibels.

• • •

Decibels are also used to calibrate output power controls on instruments and to express ultrasonic attenuation in tissue.

ATTENUATION OF ULTRASOUND BEAMS IN TISSUE

As a sound beam traverses tissue, its amplitude and intensity are reduced as a function of distance. If we have a parallel beam of sound waves, the amplitude at different distances as the beam progresses farther and farther through the tissue will trace out a curve such as the one in Fig. 1-19. This reduction in amplitude (or intensity) with distance is referred to as *attenuation*.

Several sources of sound beam attenuation have been found to exist in body tissues.

First, *reflection and scatter* of sound at tissue interfaces can contribute to the attenuation process. In some situations (e.g., in the presence of small calcifications or stones) reflective losses may contribute substantially to the attenuation. For large organs, however, reflection and scatter apparently contribute less significantly although their exact contribution to the total attenuation has not yet been determined exactly.

Another source of attenuation is *absorption*, whereby acoustic energy is converted to heat energy. (Under ordinary circumstances with diagnostic ultrasound, the amount of heat produced is too small to cause a measurable temperature change.)

The degree of sound beam attenuation in a

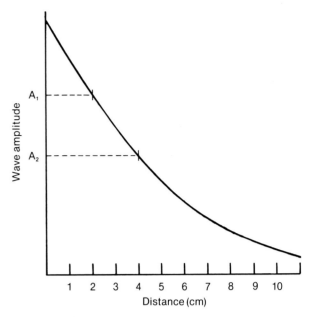

Fig. 1-19. Reduction in sound beam amplitude with increasing distance due to attenuation.

tissue is usually given in decibels per centimeter (dB/cm). In Fig. 1-19, let A_1 be the amplitude at some spot in the beam and let A_2 be the (reduced) amplitude, say, 2 cm farther into the medium. If the reduction in amplitude is due only to attenuation, we can compute the attenuation coefficient for that medium using

$$\text{Signal change (dB)} = 20 \log \frac{A_2}{A_1}$$

This gives the amplitude change in decibels. Since the amplitude change is assumed to occur over a 2-cm distance, dividing this value by 2 cm will yield the attenuation for that tissue in dB/cm.

Typical values reported for the ultrasonic attenuation coefficient in soft tissues are as follows:

Water	0.0002
Blood	0.18
Liver	0.65
Muscle	1.2

(More complete compilations are provided, for example, by Goss et al.[2] and by Parry and Chivers.[3] These values presented are for a frequency of 1 MHz. At this frequency the attenuation coefficient of water is very low, that of organ parenchyma (e.g., the liver) is intermediate, and that of muscle is somewhat higher.

Much of the present information on attenuation in tissues is based on measurements of excised organs. Techniques are being developed to allow measurements in vivo. Results

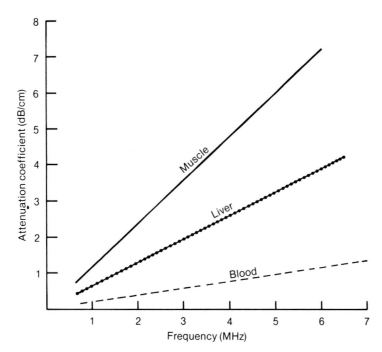

Fig. 1-20. Dependence of attenuation on the ultrasonic frequency for typical soft tissues.

obtained with these techniques suggest that in vivo attenuation coefficients may be somewhat lower than the above values.[3]

As a rough guide, we find that for most soft tissues the attenuation coefficient is in the neighborhood of 0.5 to 1 dB/cm at 1 MHz.

Attenuation in soft tissues is highly dependent on the ultrasonic frequency. In most cases attenuation is *nearly proportional* to the frequency, tracing out a curve as shown in Fig. 1-20. Thus, if the attenuation coefficient for a tissue is given at a frequency of 1 MHz, it would be doubled at 2 MHz, quintupled at 5 MHz, and so forth. This dependence of ultrasonic attenuation on frequency represents one of the limitations imposed on diagnostic ultrasound. We shall see in Chapter 2 that the best spatial detail (spatial resolution) is obtained when imaging is done at high ultrasound frequencies. However, it has just been pointed out that high ultrasound frequencies are accompanied by high attenuation losses. This prohibits their use at anything but very superficial tissue levels. The frequency range used in most scanning applications is a compromise between attenuation losses in tissue and spatial resolution requirements.

To determine the amount of attenuation occurring when a sound beam passes through a given thickness of tissue, simply multiply the attenuation coefficient (in dB/cm) by the distance traveled (cm). Thus

$$\text{Attenuation (dB)} = \alpha \times d \qquad \text{(1-11)}$$

where α is the attenuation coefficient and d the distance.

Example: Calculate the attenuation for a 1-MHz beam traversing 10 cm of water.

Solution: $\alpha = 0.002$ dB/cm $\times$ 10 cm
$= 0.02$ dB (a very small attenuation)

Example: Calculate the attenuation for a 1-MHz beam traversing 10 cm of muscle.

Solution: $\alpha = 1.2$ dB/cm $\times$ 10 cm
$= 12$ dB

Example: If the frequency were raised to 5 MHz, what would the attenuation in the previous example be?

Solution: The attenuation coefficient at 5 MHz is 5 times that at 1 MHz, so
$\alpha = (1.2$ dB/cm$) \times 5 \times 10$ cm
$= 60$ dB

It is left as an exercise for you to use Table 1-1 to compare the amplitude ratios for the two circumstances. The problem of beam penetration at higher frequencies should be apparent when considering the last two examples.

WAVE INTERFERENCE

When waves are produced by more than one source, they may overlap and produce *interference.* The effect at any point may be greater or less than that for either wave alone, depending on the relative *phase* of the two waves.

To see how this applies, consider the two sine waves of the same frequency depicted in Fig. 1-21. In *A* the waves are exactly in phase although their amplitudes are slightly different. Their net effect at the point shown is just the sum of the individual waves, added point by point. In *B* the waves are completely out of phase. The positive-going part of one wave occurs exactly during the negative-going part of the other. Although the amplitudes of the waves from both sources are greater than in the first example, the net effect at the point considered is notably smaller. This method by which waves add together is termed *interference.* Interference may be *constructive* or *destructive* depending on the relative phase of the individual waves. We can conceive of a situation in which completely destructive interference might occur (Fig. 1-22), wherein two waves of equal amplitude but exactly out of phase are summed up.

DOPPLER EFFECT

For any sound beam, whenever there is relative motion between the source and the listener, the frequency heard by the listener will differ from that produced by the source. The perceived frequency will be either greater or less than that transmitted by the source depending on whether the source and the listener are moving toward or away from one another. Such a shift in the perceived frequency relative to the transmitted frequency is called a Doppler shift. A Doppler frequency shift can occur for a moving source and stationary listener, a moving listener and stationary source, or a moving source and moving listener.

The origin of a Doppler shift is depicted in Fig. 1-23. In *A* a stationary sound source is shown transmitting diverging waves with a particular frequency. The circles can be taken as individual cycles of the sound wave each separated by one wavelength. The number of cycles per second heard by the listener, f_o, is the same as that transmitted. (It is assumed that no movement of the medium occurs, such as caused by wind, etc.) If the source is moving toward the listener (*B*), the appearance of the wavefronts changes somewhat.

The motion causes wavefronts between the source and the listener to be squeezed together somewhat. Likewise, if the movement is away from the listener, the wavefronts will be pulled apart somewhat. For movement toward the listener a greater number of cycles is heard per second than for the stationary source and listener. Hence there is an increase in the perceived sound

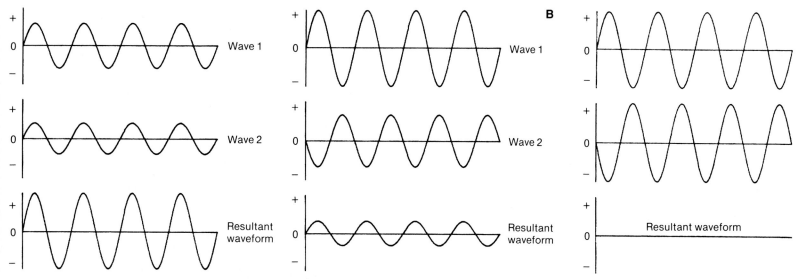

Fig. 1-21. Interference of two sine waves of equal frequency. **A,** When the two waves are in phase. **B,** When the two waves are of opposite phase.

Fig. 1-22. Complete destructive interference. The two waves are of equal amplitude and exactly opposite phases.

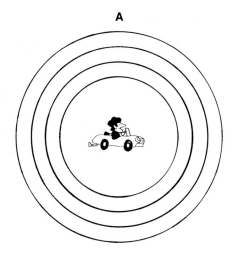

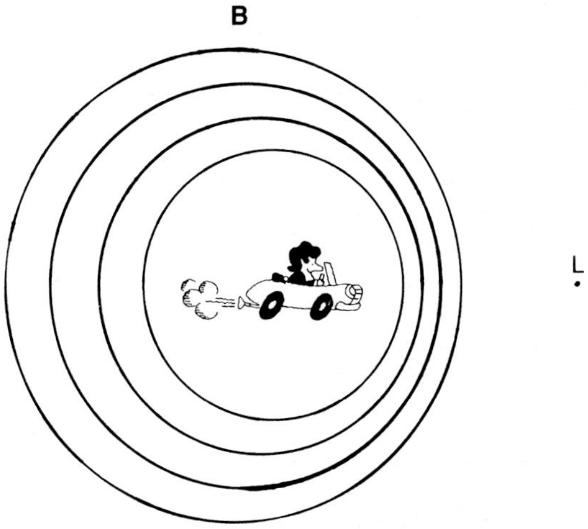

Fig. 1-23. Origin of the Doppler shift. **A,** Stationary sound source and stationary listener, *L.* **B,** Moving sound source and stationary listener.

frequency relative to the transmitted frequency. The opposite is true for movement away from the listener.

The ultrasound Doppler effect is employed in diagnosis following the scheme shown in Fig. 1-24. A stationary sound source produces a sound beam whose frequency is f_o. A reflected beam from the moving interface is shown directed back toward the sound source. The frequency of the reflected signal is given by f_r in the figure. The Doppler shift frequency, f_D, is the difference between the transmitted and the received frequencies and is given by

$$f_D = f_o - f_r$$
$$= 2\frac{f_o V}{c} \qquad (1\text{-}12)$$

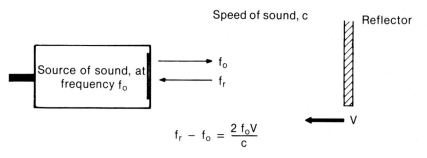

$$f_r - f_o = \frac{2 f_o V}{c}$$

Fig. 1-24. Doppler frequency shift for a moving reflector. The reflector is moving toward the source. (From Zagzebski, J.: Semin. Ultrasound **2:**246, 1981.)

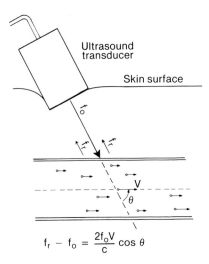

$$f_r - f_o = \frac{2f_o V}{c} \cos \theta$$

Fig. 1-25. Doppler frequency shift for a moving reflector. The direction of the reflector's movement is at an angle to the sound beam. (From Zagzebski, J.: Semin. Ultrasound **2**:246, 1981.)

where V is the velocity of the reflector and c is the speed of sound in the medium.

Example: Suppose $f_o = 2$ MHz and $V = 5$ cm/sec. What is the Doppler frequency? Assume the speed of sound is 1540 m/sec.

Solution: Simply substitute the given values into Equation 1-2. Notice that 2 MHz $= 2 \times 10^6$ cycles/sec.

$$f_D = \frac{2 \times 2 \times 10^6 \text{ cycles/sec} \times 0.05 \text{ m/sec}}{1.54 \times 10^3 \text{ m/sec}}$$

The units *m/sec* in the numerator and denominator cancel each other. Simplifying gives

$$f_D = \frac{0.2 \times 10^6 \text{ cycles/sec}}{1.54 \times 10^3}$$
$$= 1.3 \times 10^2 \text{ cycles/sec}$$

or

$$f_D = 130 \text{ Hz}$$

The Doppler frequency shift is directly proportional to the reflector velocity. In other words, the shift in frequency can be used to measure the speed of a reflector.

For many practical applications the sound beam and the direction of motion do not fall on the same line. For example, in Chapter 23 we consider Doppler signals resulting from red blood cells moving in an artery. The situation is usually as shown in Fig. 1-25. The sound beam is incident at an angle, θ, relative to the velocity of the moving scatterers. The Doppler frequency shift in this case is given by

$$f_D = f_o - f_r$$
$$= 2 \frac{f_o V}{c} \cos \theta \qquad (1\text{-}13)$$

This is identical to Equation 1-12 except for the cos θ term. The behavior of the cosine function is discussed in Appendix 1-1. Notice that if θ is 0 degrees then cos $\theta = 1$ and the situation returns to that described in the previous example. Notice further that if the sound beam direction and the reflector motion are at a right angle then $\theta = 90$ degrees and cos $\theta = 0$. In this case there would be no detected Doppler shift frequency.

REFERENCES

1. Eggleton, R.C., and Whitcomb, J.: Tissue simulators for diagnostic ultrasound. In Proceedings of the 2nd International Symposium on Ultrasonic Imaging and Tissue Characterization, NBS special publication 525, 1977.
2. Goss, S., Johnston, R., and Dunn, F.: Comprehensive compilation of empirical ultrasonic properties of mammalian tissue, J. Acoust. Soc. Am. 64:423, 1978.
3. Kuc, R., and Taylor, K. Repeatability of attenuation slope estimates for diffuse liver disease. Proceedings and abstracts, 25th meeting of the American Institute of Ultrasound in Medicine, New Orleans, 1980.
4. Parry, R., and Chivers, R.: Data on the velocity and attenuation of ultrasound in mammalian tissues—a survey. In Proceedings of the 2nd International Symposium on Ultrasonic Imaging and Tissue Characterization, NBS special publication 525, 1977.
5. Robinson, D., Wilson, L., and Kossoff, G.: Shadowing and enhancement in ultrasonic echograms by reflection and refraction, J. Clin. Ultrasound 9:181, 1981.
6. Wells, P.N.T.: Biomedical ultrasonics, New York, 1977, Academic Press, Inc.
7. Zagzebski, J.: Physics and instrumentation in Doppler ultrasonography, Semin. Ultrasound 2:246, 1981.

2

Properties of ultrasound transducers

JAMES A. ZAGZEBSKI

The general term *transducer* refers to any device that is used to convert energy from one form to another. Even in medicine many different types of transducers are used to measure patient or laboratory data. Most of these respond to the parameter of interest (e.g., pressure, electrolyte levels, or movement) by converting energy into electric signals, which can be applied to electronic instruments for processing and display. *Ultrasonic transducers* convert acoustic energy to electric signals and electric energy to acoustic energy. Thus these transducers can be used both as detectors and transmitters of ultrasonic waves.

PIEZOELECTRIC EFFECT

There are several types of devices that can be used to generate and detect ultrasonic waves. The most common type of transducer used in medical ultrasound employs the *piezoelectric effect*.

The word piezoelectric originates from the Greek *piezein*, to press. The piezoelectric effect was discovered in the 1880s by Pierre and Jacques Curie. They discovered that when a force is applied perpendicular to the faces of a quartz crystal an electric charge will result (Fig. 2-1). This charge can be detected and amplified, producing a useful electric signal. Conversely, if an electric signal is applied to the crystal, expansion or contraction of the crystal will take place depending on the polarity of the signal (Fig. 2-2). Oscillating signals cause the crystal to vibrate, resulting in propagation of sound waves into the medium with which the crystal is in contact.

A number of substances, including quartz and tourmaline, are naturally piezoelectric and have been used for medical ultrasound transducers. Quartz is still used, especially for precision acoustic measurements in the laboratory and occasionally for high-power applications. However, it has been superseded for the most part by *piezoelectric ceramic* transducer elements.

Ceramic elements, such as *lead zirconate titanate* (PZT), consist of mixtures of microscopic crystals randomly oriented throughout the volume of the element (Fig. 2-3). To be useful as medical transducers, these ceramics must first be *polarized*—which is done by heating the material above the Curie temperature (365° C for PZT) and applying a very high voltage across its face. This results in partial alignment, or *polarization*, of the microscopic crystals. The element is then cooled with the voltage still applied. It will now remain polarized with the voltage removed and exhibit piezoelectric properties. The element can lose its piezoelectric properties (become depolarized) if it is inadvertently heated above the Curie temperature.

A piezoelectric transducer element has a natural resonance frequency. At this frequency it is most efficient in converting electric energy to acoustic energy and vice versa. The resonance frequency is determined mainly by the thickness of the piezoelectric element: thin elements have high resonance frequencies, and thick elements have lower resonance frequencies (Fig. 2-4). Piezoelectric elements of various shapes and sizes are employed in ultrasound transducers.

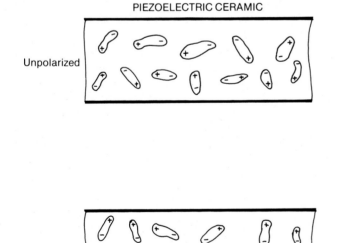

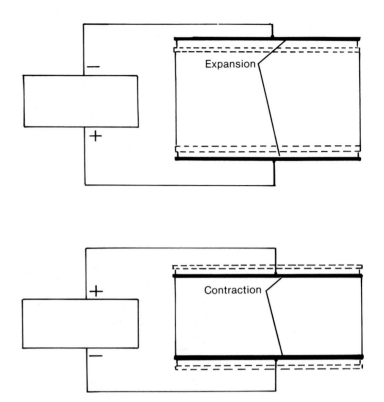

Fig. 2-1. The piezoelectric effect. A force applied to the opposite faces of certain materials results in an electric signal.

Fig. 2-2. The reverse piezoelectric effect. Application of an electric signal causes the element to contract or expand.

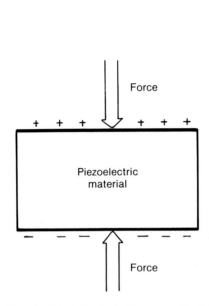

Fig. 2-3. Rough schematic of a piezoelectric ceramic element. *top,* Before polarization; *bottom,* after polarization. The dark lines are electrodes adhered to the element.

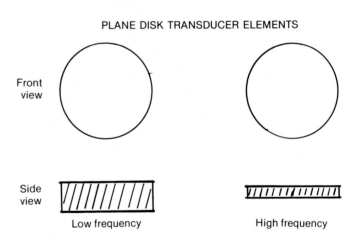

Fig. 2-4. The thickness of a piezoelectric element determines the element's resonance frequency.

TRANSDUCER CONSTRUCTION

Different diagnostic ultrasound instruments require different transducer designs. Some general properties of transducer design and performance will be illustrated by considering a specific type of transducer used in pulse-echo work, a plane disk nonfocused probe. In later sections focusing techniques, transducer arrays, and transducer designs for continuous wave applications (e.g., Doppler work) will be brought out.

A diagram of a single-element nonfocused transducer is presented in Fig. 2-5. Such a transducer is used both to produce brief pulses (or bursts) of ultrasound and to detect echoes resulting from reflections of the sound pulses as they travel through the medium. The piezoelectric element for this application consists of a flat circular disk. The thickness of the element is selected in accordance with the desired operating frequency of the transducer. The element is mounted coaxially in a cylindrical case. Acoustic insulation such as rubber or cork is necessary to avoid coupling ultrasonic energy to the case. A metal electric shield prevents pickup of extraneous electric noise signals by the transducer leads. Such signals are undesirable because they contribute to excessive noise on a display during echo detection. Wires that connect to a tuning coil and then to the external connectors provide electric contact between the transducer element and the instrument.

Pulsed transducers are excited by a short burst of electric energy from a pulser. In response to this excitation pulse the transducer element "rings," vibrating at its resonance frequency. The vibrations are damped quickly, producing a short-duration acoustic pulse that propagates into the medium.

The backing material of some transducers plays a major role in *damping out* the transducer vibrations. This material needs to have two properties to facilitate this role. First, its acoustic impedance must be comparable to the impedance of the piezoelectric element (Table 2-1). This reduces reflections at the transducer–to–backing material interface so that any energy propagated in the backward direction is transmitted out of the element. Second, it is filled with a special preparation so that sound waves transmitted into it are completely absorbed. A heavy sound-absorbing backing material serves to damp the vibrations of the piezoelectric element, and this results in the transmission of short-duration acoustic impulses into the medium.

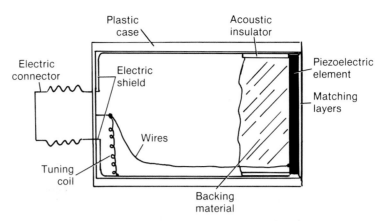

Fig. 2-5. Schematic of a single-element nonfocused transducer used in pulse-echo applications.

Table 2-1. Acoustic impedances of materials relevant to transducer design

Material	Impedance (rayls)
Piezoelectric ceramic (lead zirconate titanate)	30×10^6
Backing material (without impedance-matching layers on transducer face)	Matched to that of ceramic element
Matching layers*	7×10^6
Typical soft tissue	1.7×10^6

*Actual values used may differ depending on state-of-the-art manufacturing techniques.

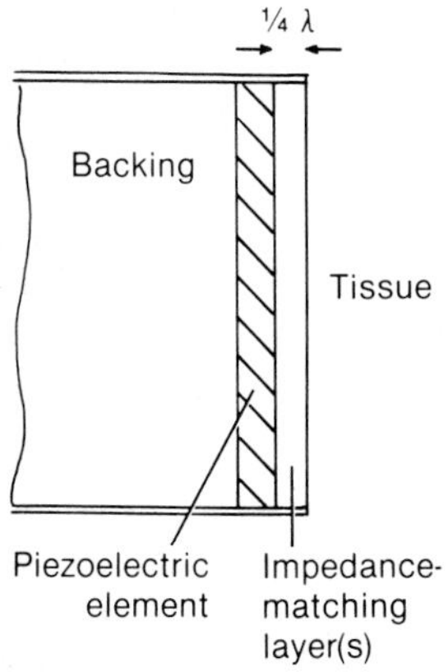

QUARTER-WAVE AND MULTIPLE MATCHING LAYERS

Many modern transducers use *impedance-matching layers*, which both improve the sensitivity of the transducer (the ability to detect very weak echoes) and change the requirements for the backing material. Impedance-matching layers provide efficient transmission of sound waves from the transducer element to soft tissue and vice versa.

Inspection of Table 2-1 shows that the acoustic impedance of piezoelectric ceramics, such as PZT, is about 20 times the impedance of soft tissue. This is a significant mismatch, producing a reflection coefficient of 0.82 if an element is used in contact with the skin surface. (It never is, but let's continue the discussion anyway.) The presence of a plastic wear face between the element and the skin surface improves the situation somewhat but does not provide the best results possible.

Transmission of sound into soft tissue is

Fig. 2-6. Attachment of impedance-matching layers to the front face of the transducer provides more efficient transmission of sound from the transducer into the patient.

improved when matching layers are attached to the transducer element. These layers make it "appear" to the transducer that the tissue has the same impedance as the piezoelectric element. (Hence the term *impedance matching* is used.) A single quarter-wave matching layer has the following properties:

1. Its acoustic impedance, Z_m, is intermediate between the impedance of the transducer element, Z_t, and the impedance of soft tissue, Z_s. (Actually $Z_m = \sqrt{Z_s \times Z_t}$ is the appropriate value.)

2. Its thickness exactly equals one fourth of the ultrasonic wavelength in the layer.

If these properties are achieved, there is no reflection at a soft tissue–transducer interface; hence sound transmission is very efficient (Fig. 2-6).

As will be seen later in this chapter, a pulsed transducer emits not a single ultra-

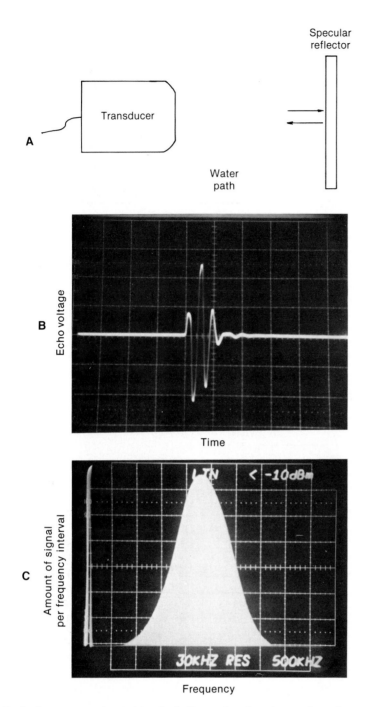

Fig. 2-7. A, Arrangement used to study the echo signal waveform for a pulse-echo transducer. **B,** Echo signal waveform obtained from a planar reflector. **C,** Frequency spectrum of the waveform in **B.**

matching layers can improve the sensitivity of ultrasound transducers.

TRANSDUCER FREQUENCY CHARACTERISTICS

In pulse-echo ultrasound the transducer is excited with a brief electric signal, after which it oscillates near its *resonance* frequency. As has been pointed out, the resonance frequency of a transducer is determined for the most part by the thickness of the piezoelectric element. Other factors—including the mounting of the transducer element in the assembly, the precise thickness of the front surface matching layers, and the electric components within the transducer assembly (e.g., the tuning coil in Fig. 2-5) and the ultrasound instrument—also can affect the frequency characteristics.

A pulse of sound emitted by a transducer contains ultrasonic energy at the resonance frequency of the transducer. It also contains ultrasonic energy at frequencies above and below the resonance frequency, covering a fairly wide spectrum. The frequency range represented in the pulse is described in terms of the *frequency bandwidth* of the ultrasound transducer. The bandwidth may be determined by *spectral analysis* of an echo signal obtained from a plane smooth reflector.

For an illustration of how this works, consider the experimental arrangement shown in Fig. 2-7. The beam from a pulsed transducer is directed toward a large smooth reflector. The reflector is so oriented that the largest possible echo signal amplitude is obtained at the transducer. A typical signal is shown in Fig. 2-7, *B*. Instruments are available that can be used to measure the relative amount of signal at different frequencies in a pulsed waveform of this type. They are called *spectrum analyzers*. If the signal shown in Fig. 2-7, *B*, is applied to a spectrum analyzer, an envelope (Fig. 2-7, *C*) is obtained.

The spectral display represents a plot of the fraction of signal within a given frequency increment versus the frequency (Fig. 2-8). The curve usually peaks out at or near the resonance frequency of the transducer, with a gradual falloff on either side of the maximum value. Occasionally secondary peaks are found in the frequency spectrum. Depending on the application, these may or may not be desirable. A frequency plot of this type is one performance measurement applied to transducers by the manufacturer.

The frequency bandwidth is a measure of the spread of frequencies in the plots of Figs. 2-7 and 2-8. It turns out that, for a given resonance frequency, the shorter the pulse

sonic frequency but rather a *spectrum* of frequencies. A single quarter-wave matching layer is exactly one quarter wavelength *only for one frequency.* Thus all frequencies in a pulsed waveform are not efficiently transmitted with a single matching layer. Transducer manufacturers overcome this problem by designing transducers with *multiple* matching layers adhered to the face of the element. Multiple matching layers provide efficient sound transmission between the piezoelectric element and soft tissue for a range, or *spectrum,* of ultrasonic frequencies.

We saw that a short-duration pulse is produced by quick damping of the vibrations of the piezoelectric element after it is pulsed. Damping can be achieved by using a heavy absorbing material in contact with the back of the element. This reduces the transducer efficiency somewhat because energy is lost in the backing material. With matching layers, however, it is not necessary to couple energy out of the back of the transducer to damp the vibrations because the ultrasonic energy is very efficiently transmitted into the patient. This is another way in which duration the wider is the frequency bandwidth; and, vice versa, the longer the pulse duration the narrower the frequency bandwidth.* Pulse duration and frequency bandwidth are illustrated for three hypothetical waveforms in Fig. 2-9.

AXIAL RESOLUTION

The transducer frequency characteristics are closely related to the spatial resolution of a pulse-echo system. The *spatial resolution* refers to how close two reflectors can be to one another and still be seen as separate reflectors. It can be thought of as consisting of two components: axial or range resolution and lateral or azimuthal resolution.

Axial resolution refers to the minimum reflector spacing along the axis of a sound beam that results in separate echoes from the two reflectors. The axial resolution is limited by the duration of the ultrasonic pulse transmitted into the medium. The *longer* the pulse duration, the *worse* will be the axial resolution; and, in general, the shorter the pulse duration the better will be the axial resolution.

Axial resolution is illustrated schematically in Fig. 2-10, wherein an ultrasound transducer is positioned to obtain echo signals from a walled tube. In the top waveform the pulse duration is depicted as extremely long, so that it extends simultaneously over the entire tube. A single echo signal is detectable from the tube. In the middle waveform the pulse duration is depicted as short enough that each wall is insonified by the beam at different times. Now separate echo signals are detectable from the two walls of the tube. Finally, the bottom waveform depicts a situation in which the pulse duration is extremely short compared to the other two. The very closely spaced inner and outer margins of the walls are resolved with the short-duration pulse in this schematic representation.

Short pulse durations are obtained by using high-frequency transducers. For a given resonance frequency, short pulses are obtained by rapidly damping the "ringing" of the transducer after it is excited. This is done by means of heavy absorbing backing material and/or matching layers attached to the front of the element. The relationship between pulse duration, axial resolution, and frequency bandwidth is illustrated on p. 18.

---

*Occasionally one sees mention of a parameter called the transducer *Q*. The *Q* factor is inversely related to the bandwidth: a narrow bandwidth means a higher *Q* factor. It is preferable to employ the bandwidth, however, since this parameter is more commonly used when describing transducer performance.

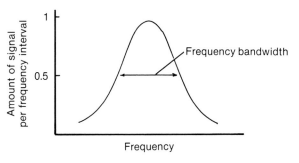

Fig. 2-8. Frequency spectrum and bandwidth of an ultrasound signal.

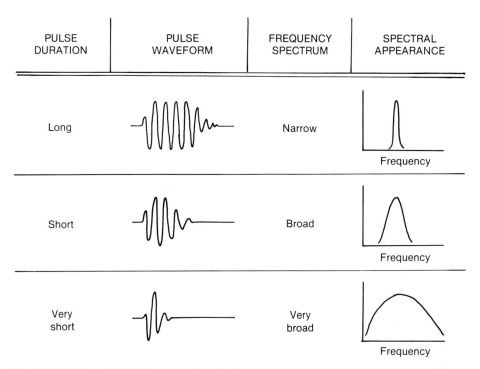

Fig. 2-9. Relationship between pulse duration and frequency bandwidth for a pulsed waveform.

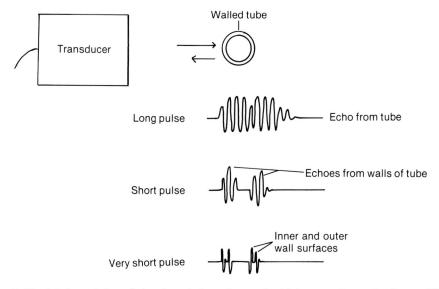

Fig. 2-10. Axial resolution. Echo signals from the walled tube are shown for three different pulse durations. The shorter the pulse duration, the better is the detail (i.e., the better the axial resolution).

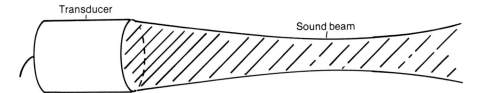

Fig. 2-11. An ultrasound beam produced by a medical transducer is very directional, somewhat like a flashlight beam.

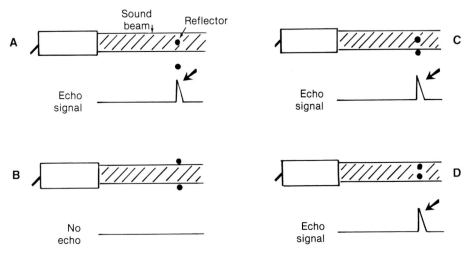

Fig. 2-12. Relationship between transducer beam width and lateral resolution. In **A** and **B** the reflector spacing is greater than the displayed beam width. This is sufficient to enable the two reflectors to be resolved. In **C** and **D** the reflectors are too closely spaced to be detected as separate individual echo sources.

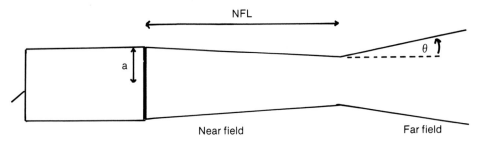

Fig. 2-13. Schematic of the beam from an unfocused circular transducer, showing the near field length (NFL) and the angle of beam divergence, θ, in the far field.

Pulse duration	Axial resolution	Frequency bandwidth
Long	Poorer	Narrow
Short	Better	Wide

TRANSDUCER BEAMS; LATERAL RESOLUTION

Many sources of audible sound appear as *point sources* in that the sound energy emitted radiates outward in all directions. An ultrasound beam produced by a medical transducer, on the other hand, is very *directional*. Most of the acoustic energy in the beam is confined to a region close to the axis of the transducer (Fig. 2-11). This directionality is a result of the fact that the dimensions of the transducer face are large compared to our "acoustic yardstick," the ultrasound wavelength. Typically the diameter of the face is 20 or more wavelengths at the frequencies used.

The *lateral resolution* of an ultrasound imaging system refers to the ability of the instrument to distinguish two closely spaced reflectors that are positioned perpendicular to the axis of a sound beam. For pulse-echo ultrasound the lateral resolution is most closely related to the transducer beam width at the depth of interest. This is illustrated in Fig. 2-12. Panels A and B depict relatively widely spaced reflectors, with an echo obtained from one of the reflectors in A. Translation of the transducer results in no detectable echo signal when the beam is positioned between the reflectors. Thus the translation enables the presence of two separate reflectors to be determined. However, from this orientation it is impossible to view the two very closely spaced reflectors (panels C and D) separately. They cannot be resolved because their spacing is less than the ultrasound beam width.

In this section we will examine the sound beam pattern for single-element transducers and study how the width of the beam at different depths changes with the frequency and diameter of the ultrasound transducer.

Let us start by considering the beam produced by an unfocused circular transducer. It may be modeled as shown in Fig. 2-13, wherein two distinct regions are identified. The *near field*, or Fresnel zone, extends from the transducer face outward approximately to the distance:

$$\text{NFL} = \frac{a^2}{\lambda} \qquad (2\text{-}1)$$

where *NFL* stands for near field length, *a* is the transducer radius, and λ is the ultrasonic wavelength. For a single ultrasound frequency the near field is characterized by point-to-point fluctuations in the amplitude and intensity of the beam both along and perpendicular to the axis of the beam (Fig. 2-14).

Example: What is the near field length for a 2.25-MHz 13-mm diameter transducer?

Solution: You are given the diameter and hence the transducer radius, *a*, which is 6.5 mm. You need to know the wavelength, λ, before computing the NFL. From Chapter 1

$$\lambda = \frac{c}{f}$$

where *c* is the speed of sound and *f* the frequency. First, find

$$\lambda = \frac{1540 \text{ m/sec}}{2.25 \times 10^6/\text{sec}}$$
$$= 6.8 \times 10^{-4} \text{ m}$$
$$= 0.68 \text{ mm}$$

Then, from Equation 2-1,

$$\text{NFL} = \frac{a^2}{\lambda}.$$
$$= \frac{(6.5 \text{ mm})^2}{0.68 \text{ mm}}$$
$$= 62 \text{ mm}$$
$$= 6.2 \text{ cm}$$

The near field for this transducer extends out to a distance of 6.2 cm. Now consider a similar situation, only one in which the ultrasound frequency is greater.

Example: What is the near field length for a 5-MHz 13-mm diameter transducer?

Solution: First, compute the wavelength.

$$\lambda = \frac{1540 \text{ m/sec}}{5.0 \times 10^6/\text{sec}}$$
$$= 3 \times 10^{-4} \text{ m}$$
$$= 0.3 \text{ mm}$$

Again, from Equation 2-1,

$$\text{NFL} = \frac{(6.5 \text{ mm})^2}{0.3 \text{ mm}}$$
$$= 140 \text{ mm}$$
$$= 14 \text{ cm}$$

From these two examples we see that the NFL increases with increasing frequency. It also increases with increasing transducer size. This is discussed in more detail below.

The region of the beam beyond the NFL is called the *far field* of the ultrasound transducer. A beam profile obtained in this region exhibits a smooth curve, as illustrated in Fig. 2-14. In the far field the beam gets weaker and begins to diverge with increasing distance from the transducer. The divergence angle, θ in Fig. 2-13, depends on the wavelength and transducer size via the relationship

$$\sin \theta = \frac{0.61 \lambda}{a} \qquad (2\text{-}2)$$

where λ and a are the same as in Equation 2-1.

Trigonometric functions are reviewed in Appendix D. The sine of an angle is a function that increases with increasing angle (if the angle is between 0 and 90 degrees), as shown in Fig. 1-1, *B*. Thus, as sine θ increases, the divergence angle (θ) also increases. Equation 2-2 tells us exactly how the sine of θ (and hence θ) behaves with changes in the wavelength or changes in the radius.

We can modify Equations 2-1 and 2-2 slightly to show how the NFL and the angle of divergence are dependent on the transducer radius, a, and the frequency, f. We utilize the fact that the wavelength, λ, is given by the speed of sound, c, divided by the frequency, f:

$$\lambda = c/f$$

Then, inserting this value for λ in the two equations,

$$\text{NFL} = \frac{a^2}{\lambda} \quad \frac{a^2}{c/f} \quad \frac{a^2 f}{c}$$

and

$$\sin \theta = \frac{0.61\lambda}{a} = \frac{0.61}{a} \quad \frac{c}{f}$$

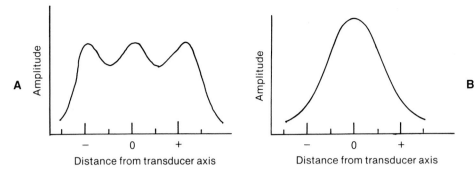

Fig. 2-14. Typical transducer beam profiles, obtained by detecting the amplitude in the beam at different points, moving perpendicular to the axis of the transducer. **A,** In the near field. **B,** In the far field.

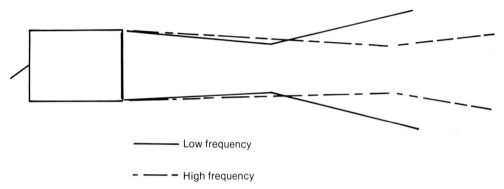

Low frequency
High frequency

Fig. 2-15. Changes in the near field length and the far field divergence angle with changes in frequency.

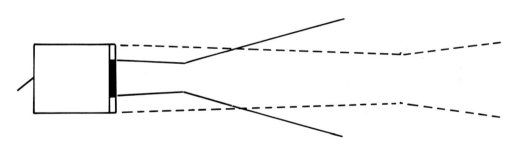

Fig. 2-16. Changes in the near field length and the far field divergence angle with changes in the radius or diameter of a transducer (same frequency).

So, if the sound beam is propagating into water or soft tissue (c is nearly always a constant), we see that for a given transducer size

1. The NFL increases with increasing frequency.
2. Beam divergence is less for higher frequencies.

The dependence of these two beam characteristics on transducer frequency is illustrated in Fig. 2-15.

The dependence on transducer diameter is also illustrated by the equations and may be summarized as follows:

1. For a given frequency the NFL extends farther for larger-diameter transducers.
2. For a given frequency beam divergence in the far field *decreases* with *increasing* transducer size.

The beam patterns shown in Figs. 2-15 and 2-16 give some hints as to how the lateral resolution behaves with frequency and transducer size. The smaller divergence angle with higher frequencies indicates that lateral resolution would generally be improved if higher frequencies were used. Also, at large distances from the transducer (Fig. 2-16) a larger-diameter transducer results in better lateral resolution than does a smaller-diameter transducer.

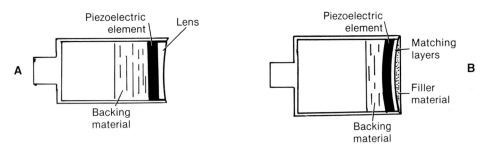

Fig. 2-17. Single-element transducer focusing. **A,** With a concave lens. **B,** With a curved transducer element.

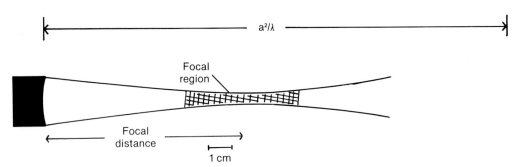

Fig. 2-18. Schematic of a focused transducer beam. The sketch is taken from data for a 3.5-MHz 19-mm diameter transducer with a focal distance of 8 cm (Zagzebski, 1982). The lines actually delineate the regions where an echo signal from a 6-mm diameter rod reflector is within 25% (−12 dB) of the echo signal obtained along the beam axis at the same depth. The focal distance and the focal region (crosshatched area) are illustrated.

FOCUSED TRANSDUCERS

Single-element transducers may be focused by using an acoustic lens along with a planar piezoelectric element or by using an element that is curved. Both techniques are illustrated in Fig. 2-17. The curved element is the more common approach employed with single-element pulse-echo transducers. As shown in the figure, both the transducer element and the matching layers are curved. The latter is done so the correct matching layer thickness can be maintained over the face of the transducer. Usually the concave center is filled in with material to help maintain transducer contact with the skin.

Focusing has the effect of narrowing the beam profile and increasing the amplitude of echoes from reflectors over a limited axial range in comparison to an equivalent unfocused transducer (here *equivalent* refers to one having the same diameter and frequency).

The beam margins* for a focused trans-

*The beam, of course, does not end abruptly at the sketched boundaries in any of these diagrams; but the amplitude varies with distance from the axis, as the beam profiles in Fig. 2-14 indicate. The sketched boundaries in Figs. 2-13, 2-15, 2-16, and 2-18 are useful for indicating the general beam shape, however. See also Appendix E.

ducer are illustrated schematically in Fig. 2-18. Also shown is the distance, a^2/λ, for this transducer; it would be the NFL if the beam were not focused. The *focal distance* corresponds to the plane where the beam width is narrowest. The *focal zone* corresponds to the region over which the width of the beam is less than 2 times the width at the focal distance.

The lens or the element curvature plays a major role in aiming the focal distance to a particular depth. However, most focused transducers used for scanning are "weakly focused."[2] This means that their beam patterns depend on the transducer diameter and frequency as well as the curvature of the element. The following general principles apply to weakly focused transducers:

1. Focusing, or beam narrowing, always occurs in the near field of an equivalent unfocused transducer. If the curvature of the element or lens were such as to aim the focal distance into the far field, focusing would still take place in the near field.

2. The actual focal distance falls short of the aimed-at focus, the latter determined by the element or the lens curvature.

3. Identical transducers (same diameter, same curvature) but of different frequencies have slightly different focusing properties. Higher frequencies tend to focus closer to the aimed-at focus; lower frequencies tend to focus at a point falling farther short of the aimed-at focus.

TRANSDUCER SELECTION

The label printed on most transducers or transducer assemblies provides information relevant to their suitability for specific diagnostic applications.

Important information included in most cases is the following:

1. Transducer frequency (sometimes referred to as the center frequency)
2. Element dimensions
3. Focal distance
4. Focal region

For instruments having interchangeable transducers, significant improvements in image quality and diagnostic information can be realized by optimizing the transducer for the study at hand. When spatial resolution requirements are of prime concern, beam profiles supplied with transducers (Appendix E) often will aid in optimization. It should go without saying that a transducer whose focal region encompasses the region of interest in the patient is the best one to use for any study. Notice that this usually requires a narrow-diameter high-frequency transducer for structures located close to the probe and a large-diameter probe for deep-lying structures. (The general principles illustrated in Fig. 2-16 do, of course, apply to some extent for focused transducers.) Although lateral resolution is better at higher frequencies, due to attenuation a deeper-lying structure will sometimes be difficult to pick up with high frequencies.

Since the focal region of single-element transducers is fixed, it is sometimes necessary to interchange transducers during the course of a single study to optimize the transducer choice. (However, in Chapter 3 it will be shown that some instruments have transducer assemblies with variable focal regions. These are found on many automatic scanning systems.)

Experience has shown that the detail obtained regarding contrast between different reflectors (differences in echo amplitude) can sometimes be improved by using higher frequencies. Scattering from many structures increases with frequency while reflections from specular interfaces usually do not change with frequency. Thus one effect of using higher-frequency transducers may be to enhance signals from scatterers over echo signals from specular interfaces.

ULTRASOUND TRANSDUCER BEAM FORMATION*

The beam of an ultrasound transducer is somewhat complicated—with minima and maxima in the near field, a near field length depending on factors such as the transducer radius and the wavelength, and a far field in which the beam gradually diverges with distance. These characteristics are part of the normal diffraction pattern of an ultrasound transducer. *Diffraction* refers to the pattern obtained when waves from different regions of an obstacle or source add up at different points in the beam.

A rather simple source of sound from the point of view of the beam pattern is a point source. This source has dimensions that are small compared to the wavelength. We can simulate a point source by dropping a small stone into a quiet pond of water. Waves that are produced by this disturbance in the water radiate in all directions, somewhat like the situation shown schematically in Fig. 2-19.

The radiating surface of most diagnostic ultrasound transducers is large compared to the ultrasonic wavelength. Engineers and physicists sometimes describe the sound beam mathematically by conceptually dividing the transducer face into an array of small point sources (Fig. 2-20). A diverging wave, analogous to that shown in Fig. 2-19, emanates from each source. The strength of the beam at any position in the transducer field can be found by adding together the contributions from each point source on the transducer surface. The point sources are sometimes referred to as Huygen sources, and the individual diverging waves as Huygen wavelets.

In Chapter 1 the phenomenon of interference of waves produced by two different sources was discussed. It was mentioned that when both waves reach a spot in space in phase the resultant amplitude at that spot is the sum of the individual wave amplitude. If the waves are out of phase, destructive interference occurs, with the signals partially or totally canceling each other depending on their relative amplitudes and phases.

We have just seen an ultrasound transducer model described as a distribution of point sources. The amplitude of the beam at any spot in the field is equal to the total effect (or superposition) of waves emitted from all the point sources. Although the diverging

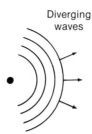

Fig. 2-19. Waves emanating from a point source spread in all directions.

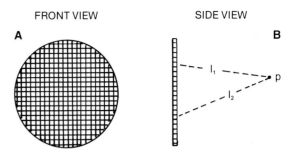

Fig. 2-20. A, A transducer may be thought of as a large number of point sources distributed over the surface. **B,** Side view of the transducer. The distances l_1 and l_2 could be such that the waves from the two point sources indicated arrive at point P out of phase.

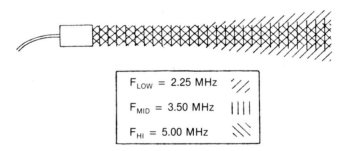

$$F_{LOW} = 2.25 \text{ MHz}$$
$$F_{MID} = 3.50 \text{ MHz}$$
$$F_{HI} = 5.00 \text{ MHz}$$

Fig. 2-21. Schematic of a 13-mm diameter broad-band transducer beam. The relative directionality of the 2.25, 3.5, and 5 MHz frequency components is shown, wherein Equations 2-1 and 2-2 were used for modeling.

waves start from all the point sources in phase, any given spot *close to the ultrasound transducer* is usually an unequal distance from the various point sources. Therefore the individual wavelets do not necessarily arrive at that spot in phase (Fig. 2-20). When we sum up the contributions from the entire transducer, we find that the amplitude in the near field of the beam is very strongly dependent on the position. At some spots the summation yields a large amplitude whereas at others a smaller net amplitude is obtained. The minima and maxima in the near field of an ultrasound transducer are a result of constructive and destructive interference among waves emanating from different points on the surface of the transducer.

In the far field the beam pattern is smooth, exhibiting none of the minima and maxima found in the near field. This is because the phase differences due to the different paths from the field pointing to separate regions of the transducer face are never very great. The far field of a transducer is sometimes characterized as a region where the transducer itself begins to look like a point source as we get farther and farther away.

EFFECTS OF THE FREQUENCY SPECTRUM

For pulsed transducers a spectrum of frequencies is emitted, and this adds some complexity to our simple beam models. The different components of the frequency spectrum of a pulsed transducer (Fig. 2-8) have slightly different beam-forming characteristics. This follows from reasoning presented for single frequencies. The resultant beam in this case is the net effect of all frequencies available in each pulse—illustrated schematically in Fig. 2-21 for a hypothetical 3.5-MHz center-frequency transducer. Fig. 2-21 illustrates the fact that in the far field the higher-frequency components of a pulsed beam are more directional; that is, they lie closer to the central axis of the beam than do the lower-frequency components. Although the illustration is presented for an unfocused transducer, the same principle applies to focused transducers. During clinical scanning, attenuation in soft tissues modifies the frequency spectrum since higher frequencies in the pulse are attenuated to a greater degree than are lower frequencies. This leads to some loss of resolution in tissue during clinical scanning.[4]

DAMAGE TO TRANSDUCERS

Ultrasound transducers should not be heat sterilized, since this can damage the probe severely. One manifestation of heat damage is depolarization if the transducer is heated above its Curie temperature. (See Fig. 2-3.) Actually transducer damage due to heat occurs at elevated temperatures that are lower than the Curie temperature, for the different bonding joints and cements in the probe are susceptible to thermal damage.

If a transducer is dropped or sustains an impact, damage to the interior of the probe may occur. A cracked transducer surface can lead to a dangerous situation involving electric shock. This is especially true with the use of acoustic coupling materials since they also tend to be good conductors. A transducer that has a cracked face should be replaced immediately.

A frequent source of transducer malfunction, especially probes having built-in cables, is damage to the cable assembly. Twisting and bending that take place quite naturally during handling may cause cable damage and lead to loss of sensitivity, intermittent operation, and/or excessive electric noise on the display.

Damage to the transducer can also result from excessive wear when it is being attached to an ultrasonic scanner arm, particularly when it is heavily "torqued" to assure good electric contact. Besides damaging the transducer itself, excessive force can damage the connections in the scanner arm. When attaching transducers to threaded connectors, try to obtain a firm snug fit; but avoid excessive force when tightening the probe.

REFERENCES

1. Banjavic, R., Zagzebski, J., Madsen, E., and Goodsitt, M.: Distortion of ultrasound beams in attenuating media, Acoust. Imag. Holog. 1:165, 1979.
2. Kossoff, G.: Analysis of focusing action of spherically curved transducers. Ultrasound Med. Biol. 5:359, 1979.
3. Wells, P.N.T.: Biomedical ultrasonics. New York, 1977, Academic Press, Inc.
4. Zagzebski, J., Banjavic, R., Madsen, E., and Schwabe, M.: Focused transducer beams in tissue-mimicking material, J. Clin. Utrasound. 10:159, 1982.

3 Pulse-echo ultrasound instrumentation

JAMES A. ZAGZEBSKI

PULSE-ECHO ULTRASOUND

This chapter describes instrumentation that utilizes pulse-echo ultrasound to localize and image structures in the body. In these techniques an ultrasound transducer transmits a short-duration acoustic pulse that propagates in a direction determined by the orientation of the transducer and at a speed determined by the properties of the medium. Echo signals resulting from scatter and reflections at interfaces in the medium are detected, usually by the same transducer. The time delay between pulse propagation and echo signal detection is used to determine the transducer-to-reflector distance.

The principle is illustrated in Fig. 3-1. A reflector is positioned a distance, d, from the transducer. The time, t_1, it takes for a pulse of sound to travel to the interface is given by

$$t_1 = \frac{d}{c} \qquad (3\text{-}1)$$

where c is the speed of sound in the medium. If the interface reflects part of the incident pulse, it also takes time t_1 for an echo to return to the transducer. The total delay time between pulse transmission and echo detection, t, is therefore

$$t = \frac{2d}{c} \qquad (3\text{-}2)$$

So, if the speed of sound, c, and the reflector distance, d, are known, the delay time can be determined.

Example: If the speed of sound is 1540 m/sec and a reflector is positioned 1 cm from the transducer, how long does it take a pulse of sound to propagate 1 cm, be reflected, and return to the transducer?

Solution: The time required is that needed for the pulse to propagate to and from the interface. From Equation 3-2

$$t = \frac{2d}{c}$$
$$= \frac{2 \times 1\,\text{cm}}{1.54 \times 10^5\,\text{cm/sec}}$$
$$= 1.3 \times 10^{-5}\,\text{sec}$$
$$= 13\,\mu\text{sec}$$

It is also possible to compute the reflector distance if the delay time, t, and the speed of sound, c, are known.

Example: If the delay time is 130 μsec and the speed of sound is 1540 m/sec (1.54×10^5 cm/sec), what is the reflector distance?

Solution: First, isolate d on one side of Equation 3-2.

$$t = \frac{2d}{c}$$
$$2d = ct$$
$$d = \frac{ct}{2}$$

Then

$$d = \frac{1.54 \times 10^5\,\text{cm/sec} \times 130 \times 10^{-6}\,\text{sec}}{2}$$
$$= 10\,\text{cm}$$

The expression given by Equation 3-2 is sometimes referred to as the *range equation*.

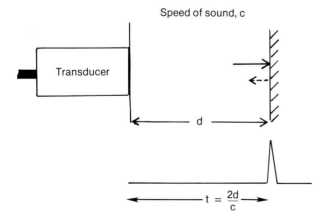

Speed of sound, c

Transducer

$t = \frac{2d}{c}$

Fig. 3-1. Demonstration of pulse-echo ultrasound for determining reflector distances.

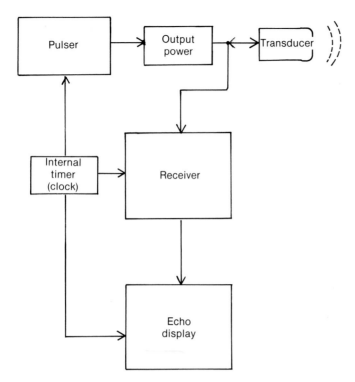

Fig. 3-2. Simplified block diagram of a pulse-echo instrument, omitting scanning electronics and/or M-mode display system.

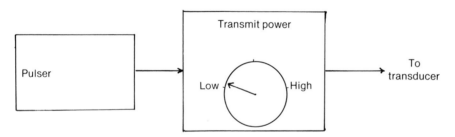

Fig. 3-3. Power output controls; on different instruments they may be labeled transmit, output, power, or damping.

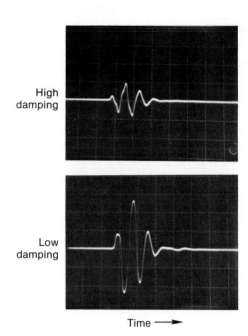

Fig. 3-4. Echo waveform shown for different damping control settings.

This relationship between echo transit time, t, and reflector depth is implicitly built into pulse-echo imaging instruments.

A simplified block diagram showing principal components of the echo acquisition and display chain of a pulse-echo instrument is presented in Fig. 3-2. Later in this chapter additional components for scanning and for M-mode displays will be discussed.

INSTRUMENTATION
Pulser

The function of the pulser is to provide signals for driving the piezoelectric transducer. This is done at a fixed rate, called the pulse-repetition frequency (prf), as determined by the instrument. The prf is usually set high enough that the display of echo signals appears to be continuous. (There is an upper limit to the prf, which will be discussed below in conjunction with rapid scanning instruments.)

The amplitude of the electric signal applied to the transducer is a factor in determining the acoustic power emitted by the instrument. Output power controls are available on some instruments and are used mainly to vary the sensitivity of the unit. (*Sensitivity* refers to the weakest echo signals that the instrument is capable of detecting and displaying.) By increasing the output power to the transducer we produce higher-intensity transmit pulses and large-amplitude echo signals, and in so doing allow weaker echoes to be visualized on the display.

The output power control may take the form of a variable electric attenuator connected between the pulser and the trans-

ducer. The settings on the attenuator are under the control of the operator (Fig. 3-3). Some instruments employ a damping control, which produces results similar to those of an attenuator. Damping has already been discussed in terms of its effect on the pulse duration and the axial resolution of a pulse-echo transducer. Reference was made to mechanical damping, which is inherent in the design of the transducer. However, electronic damping controls on instruments that provide this feature affect both the amplitude and the duration of the transmit pulse (as suggested in Fig. 3-4). Thus these controls also vary the acoustic power emitted by the transducer.

The product of the prf (number of pulses/sec) and the time duration of each pulse (sec/pulse) is a dimensionless quantity called the *duty factor*. The duty factor is the fraction of time that the transducer is actually emitting sound. In a typical single-element transducer system the prf is 500/sec and the pulse duration is 1.0 μsec or less (1×10^{-6} sec). The duty factor here is (5.00×10^2/sec) $\times$ (1×10^{-6} sec) = 0.5×10^{-3}. Expressed as a percentage, this is 0.05%, which means that the transducer is transmitting less than 0.05% of the time; most of the time it is "listening" for echo signals reflected from interfaces.

Receiver

Echo signals detected by the transducer are applied to the receiver, where they are processed for display. The first part of this processing involves echo signal amplification and compensation for attenuation losses.

Signal amplification is necessary since the amplitudes of echo signals at the transducer are generally too low to allow visualization on a display. The degree of amplification is called the *gain* of the receiver, which is merely the ratio of the output signal amplitude to the input signal amplitude (Fig. 3-5). The gain may be expressed as a simple ratio (say, 100). More commonly it is expressed in decibels, whereby a gain of 100 is equivalent to a gain of 40 dB. (See Table 1-1.) Depending on the instrument, the maximum gain available in the receiver of a pulse-echo instrument may exceed 80 dB. A significant fraction of this range is taken up by swept gain or compensation circuitry, discussed below.

For most clinical ultrasound applications echoes returning to the transducer from structures situated at large distances generally are weaker than echoes returning from nearby structures. This is a result of sound beam attenuation in the medium. (The situation is depicted schematically in Fig. 3-6, *A*.) If the reflection coefficients of the interfaces giving rise to the echo signals shown were all the same and if there were no source of amplitude change other than attenuation (e.g., transducer beam focusing), a gradual weakening of the echo signals with increasing reflector distance would result from attenuation.

Sound beam attenuation is compensated for using swept gain (also called *TGC*, for time gain compensation, and *DGC*, for depth gain compensation) in the receiver. *Swept gain* refers to a process whereby the receiver amplification is increased with time following the transmit pulse so that echo signals originating from distal reflectors are amplified more than echo signals originating close to the transducer. Fig. 3-6, *B* and *C*, illustrates this process. In *C* the receiver gain is graphically portrayed as it might be adjusted to increase gradually with time after each transmit pulse. Before the transmit pulse the gain is reduced as shown. Proper application of the swept gain function has the effect of equalizing echo signals from similar reflectors, as shown in *B*.

Swept gain controls are available on nearly every pulse-echo instrument, although the form these controls take may differ considerably among instruments. Two commonly followed approaches are shown in Figs. 3-7 and 3-8. In 3-7 the principal operator controls are labeled *initial*, *slope*, and *far* and their actions on the receiver gain are illustrated with the aid of the swept gain curves. The initial

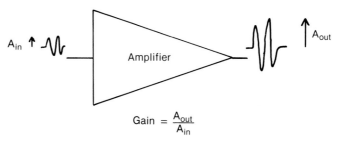

$$\text{Gain} = \frac{A_{out}}{A_{in}}$$

Fig. 3-5. Receiver gain function.

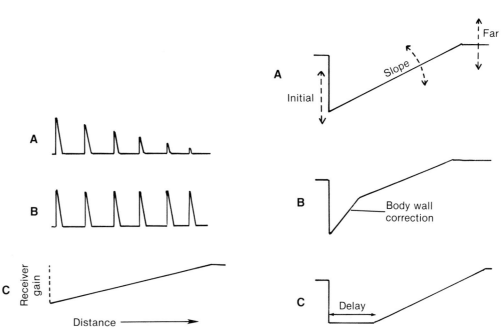

Fig. 3-6. Demonstration of swept gain. **A,** Echo signal versus distance (time) in the presence of attenuation, with no swept gain. **B,** Echo signals after application of swept gain. **C,** Display of swept gain function.

Fig. 3-7. A, Function of principal swept gain controls. **B,** Swept gain with body wall correction. **C,** Function of the slope delay.

setting adjusts the receiver gain at the time of pulse transmission by the transducer. The slope control adjusts the rate of compensation. Ordinarily the slope is adjusted to reflect the rate of sound beam attenuation in soft tissue. Thus, as the ultrasonic frequency is increased by, for example, switching to a higher-frequency transducer, the slope should also be increased. The far gain control adjusts the height of the knee of the curve, and thus the maximum receiver gain applied following each ultrasound transducer pulse.

As mentioned, the slope sensitivity control should reflect the rate of attenuation of the sound beam in tissues. For many imaging situations the ultrasound beam undergoes a hefty amount of attenuation just while traversing the body wall (i.e., the skin, connective tissue, fat, and muscle interfaces over-

lying internal organs). Some instrument manufacturers have found it useful to add additional controls for the swept gain curve to compensate for these losses. The addition of a body wall correction (Fig. 3-7, *B*) facilitates use of a gradual slope for the compensation through the organ parenchymal path while a steeper slope, compensating for the more highly attenuating body wall, is utilized for the first few centimeters of tissue. Additional controls are available to adjust the slope of the body wall compensation and the distance over which this compensation takes place.

Some instruments provide a control to vary the depth at which the increase in swept gain begins. This variable delay (Fig. 3-7, *C*) may be positioned at different depths to further control the swept gain function.

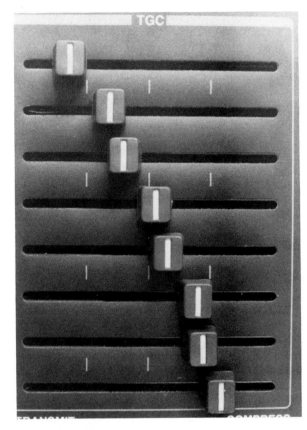

Fig. 3-8. Multicontrol swept gain function.

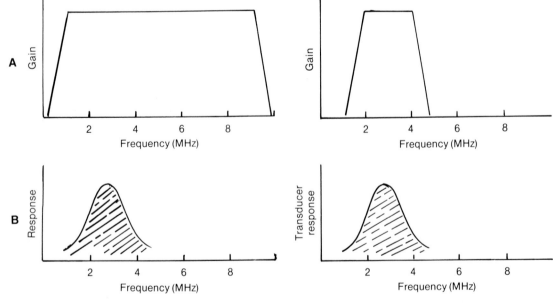

Fig. 3-9. A, Amplifier gain versus signal frequency for a wide-band amplifier. Signal frequencies from all transducers used with the instrument are amplified. **B,** Typical range of frequencies for a pulse-echo transducer.

Fig. 3-10. Narrow-band amplifier frequency response characteristic. A switch is usually provided to tune for different-frequency transducers.

Another form of swept gain control is illustrated in Fig. 3-8. Individual gain control knobs adjust the sensitivity, each controlling the gain over a specific depth range. The advantage of this system is that virtually any swept gain function, including compensation for body wall attenuation, can be achieved if fine enough control (sufficient number of control knobs) is provided.

Individual gain controls (Fig. 3-8) are especially handy in echocardiographic examinations in which slightly different use of the TGC control is sometimes necessary. In echocardiography it occasionally is useful to enhance the sensitivity over a given depth range only, for example, to detect echo signals from a weakly reflecting valve in the presence of strongly reflecting specular interfaces.

Narrow-band versus wide-band amplifiers

The frequency bandwidth of an ultrasonic transducer has been discussed in Chapter 2. Just as the response of a transducer is not equal at all frequencies so the gain of the amplifier in a receiver may not be the same at all frequencies. The *frequency bandwidth* of a receiver refers to the range of ultrasound signal frequencies that the receiver can amplify with maximum or nearly maximum gain.

Two types of amplifiers are in common use in pulse-echo work, and they are referred to as *wide-band* or *narrow-band* depending on their frequency characteristics.

A wide-band amplifier's frequency characteristics are illustrated in Fig. 3-9. The amplifier is designed to respond to all ultrasonic echo signals over a large frequency range. It is often designed to amplify signals from approximately 1 to 8 MHz. This range is shifted upward for instruments utilizing higher-frequency transducers. Fig. 3-9, *B*, illustrates a typical pulsed transducer frequency response curve along with the receiver's characteristics. A wide-band amplifier will usually respond equally to all frequencies produced by the different transducers that can be used with the system.

A narrow-band amplifier (Fig. 3-10) amplifies a narrower frequency range of signals than does the wide-band amplifier. To accommodate transducers of different frequencies, it is necessary to adjust a frequency control switch on some instruments. The response is designed to amplify only frequencies available from the transducer being employed, discriminating against other frequencies. This often is advantageous for reducing effects of spurious electronic noise signals on the echo display.

Signal processing

Echo signal processing is amplification and other operations that are applied to echo signals to condition them effectively for display. One of the signal-processing operations applied to echo signals is referred to as *compression*.

Echo signal compression may be employed if the range of signal amplitudes is too large for display devices as well as for further stages of signal processing. The total range of signal amplitudes available at some stage of an instrument is referred to as the *dynamic range* at that stage. One function of compression amplifiers is to reduce the difference between amplified echo signals from large-amplitude and those from small-amplitude echoes. This enables later stages of signal processing and display to accommodate all echo signals of interest. For example, in a logarithmic amplifier (Fig. 3-11) weak echo signals are amplified more than large-amplitude signals. Logarithmic compression is frequently employed since it enables variations in signal amplitude of both weakly reflecting and strongly reflecting interfaces to be visualized on the same display. Signal compression and compression curves are discussed in more detail below in connection with scan converters.

Rectification and rejection

The oscillating type of echo signal waveforms (Fig. 3-12, *A*) are referred to as radiofrequency or rf signal waveforms. Echo signals are seldom displayed in this format except in ophthalmologic instruments used for accurate distance measurements (biometry). The rf display offers the best precision possible in such applications. For display purposes the rf waveform is first rectified (Fig. 3-12, *B*), resulting in oscillations in one direction only with respect to the *0 volts* line. Additional electronic smoothing, or envelope detection, applied to this signal produces a single spike (Fig. 3-12, *C*) for each echo signal.

Some instruments also provide *rejection* controls at this stage of signal processing. This control and the associated circuitry eliminate low-level (very small-amplitude) signals from being displayed (as shown in Fig. 3-13). Reject controls are sometimes used to keep electronic noise from being visualized. The circuitry eliminates all signals (echo signals and noise) below a threshold signal level determined by the reject con-

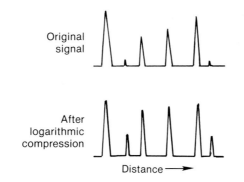

Original signal

After logarithmic compression

Distance ⟶

Fig. 3-11. Logarithmic compression of signals.

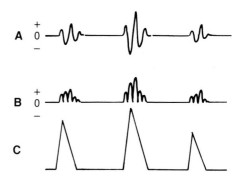

Fig. 3-12. Echo signal rectification and detection. **A,** Original signal waveform. **B,** Rectified signal. **C,** Smoothed signal.

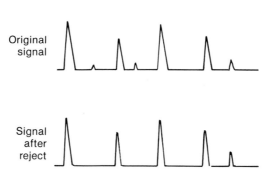

Original signal

Signal after reject

Fig. 3-13. Effect of reject controls on the echo display.

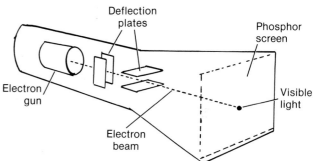

Deflection plates

Phosphor screen

Electron gun

Visible light

Electron beam

Fig. 3-14. Diagram of an oscilloscope.

trol setting. Caution should be exercised because if a reject control exists on an instrument it can also reduce the number of distinct echo levels available on the display.

OSCILLOSCOPE DISPLAYS

An oscilloscope is an effective instrument for displaying echo signals with any of several display modes or formats. The operation of a standard *cathode ray tube* (CRT) oscilloscope is illustrated with the aid of Fig. 3-14. Electrons (or "cathode rays") are produced in an electron gun by heating a filament. The electrons are focused into a well-defined beam and accelerated toward a phosphor screen. Upon striking the phosphor they cause the phosphor to emit light, which is visible to anyone observing the screen from the outside.

The usefulness of the device lies in the fact that the electron beam can be swept or steered across the screen by applying electric signals to the deflection plates. For example, it may be swept from left to right on the screen, tracing out a straight line. If a sinusoidally oscillating signal waveform of sufficient amplitude is applied to the vertical deflection plates at the same time that the

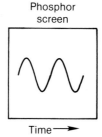

Phosphor screen

Time ⟶

Fig. 3-15. Application of a signal to the vertical deflection plates. Such a signal varies sinusoidally with time whereas a sweep signal is applied to the horizontal plates.

left to right sweep is applied, this waveform will be traced out in time (as shown in Fig. 3-15).

A-MODE, B-MODE, AND M-MODE

An *A-mode*, or amplitude mode, echo display may be produced by synchronizing the oscilloscope sweep to the transmit pulse applied to the ultrasound transducer and applying the echo signal waveform from Fig. 3-12, *C*, to the vertical axis. Thus echo signals are represented as deflections on the display,

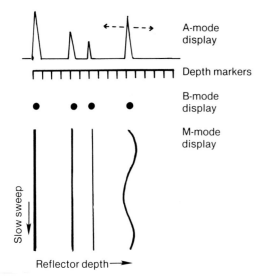

Fig. 3-16. A-mode, B-mode, and M-mode displays.

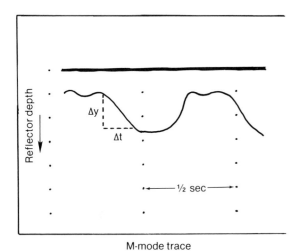

Fig. 3-17. Computing the velocity of a moving reflector. Here Δy is the distance moved per unit time, represented by Δt. The velocity is equal to $\Delta y / \Delta t$.

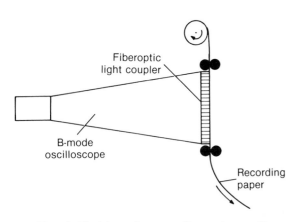

Fig. 3-18. M-mode recording using a fiberoptic recorder and light-sensitive paper.

the actual deflections (or height of the spike) being related to the amplitude of individual echo signals.

Through precise adjustment of the sweep speed it is possible to relate reflector distances to the position of an echo signal on the A-mode trace. This is done by assuming that all transmitted ultrasonic pulses and echo signals propagate with the same speed. The speed usually assumed is 1540 m/sec, a reasonable average for soft tissues. Thus the horizontal axis in Fig. 3-16 represents both the pulse-echo delay time and the echo-source distance. On most A-mode display screens suitable calibration markers are also presented so the distance to a reflector may be read out directly. Calibration depth markers are produced from a precision crystal oscillator.

B-mode refers simply to brightness modulation of the echo display screen. Echo signals are presented as brightened dots on the display screen, the distance of a given dot from the origin of the trace still representing the distance from the transducer to a particular reflecting surface. The B-mode display is used for displaying echo signals in nearly every pulse-echo scanning system, including manual scanners, slow automatic scanners, and rapid scanning or real time systems. The brightness mode display is also employed in M-mode instruments for viewing moving reflectors.

Several choices are available regarding the nature of the brightness modulations that form the B-mode display. In older ultrasound scanning instruments and in certain special-purpose scanners and M-mode units, a *leading-edge* display scheme is employed. Any echo signal above some threshold level established internally in the instrument appears as a dot on the display. All dots are of the same brightness, regardless of the amplitude of the echo signal that they represent. The leading edge processing results in a very contrasty echo signal presentation on the display.

Gray scale refers to modulating the brightness of the B-mode display, usually according to the amplitude of the individual echo signals. Many M-mode and most scanning instruments employ gray scale processing and displays.

The *M-mode* (motion mode; also called the T-M mode for time-motion) display is obtained by sweeping the B-mode trace across the display (as shown in Fig. 3-16). Stationary echo sources produce straight lines on this display. Moving interfaces, on the other hand, yield a curved line from which char-

acteristics of the movement pattern can be studied.

The M-mode trace represents the distance to a reflector along one axis and time along a perpendicular axis. Most instruments have a variable sweep speed, allowing the time representation to be magnified or compressed. The time calibration is usually achieved by internal markers multiplexed on the echo display line at prescribed time intervals, such as every ½ second. The markers also can be made to provide echo depth information by being produced to correspond to 1-cm distance intervals. Since the velocity is the displacement per unit time, the velocity component of a reflector along the line of site of the transducer can be computed from the slope of the M-mode trace. The slope is given by $\Delta y / \Delta t$, where Δy and Δt are as shown in Fig. 3-17.

At the present time the most practical M-mode display instruments are those employing a fiberoptic CRT face along with movement of the recording paper across the stationary B-mode display (Fig. 3-18). One process uses ultraviolet light to expose the paper, forming a latent image. The paper is developed by exposure to visible light. Another type of recorder uses dry silver paper as the recording medium. The latent image is developed in a thermal processor housed in the recorder. The chief advantage of the latter technique is that better gray scale can be obtained on hard-copy records.

ULTRASOUND B-MODE SCANNING

Both manual and automatic B-mode scanning instruments are in common use in ultrasound clinics. Manual scanners are discussed first. Automatic scanning instruments will be described in a later section (p. 35).

Ultrasound B-mode scans are obtained by scanning the sound beam over the region of interest while causing the B-mode trace to track the position and orientation of the ultrasonic beam (Fig. 3-19). No matter where the transducer is placed (in this example), the B-mode sweep is set to start in a position on the display corresponding to the transducer position. The orientation of the B-mode sweep is forced to correspond to the sound beam orientation in the patient. Thus, in building up an ultrasound B-scan image, the instrument makes two assumptions to position echo signals on the display:

1. Echo signals originate from along the axis of the transducer.
2. The time between sound pulse transmission and echo reception is propor-

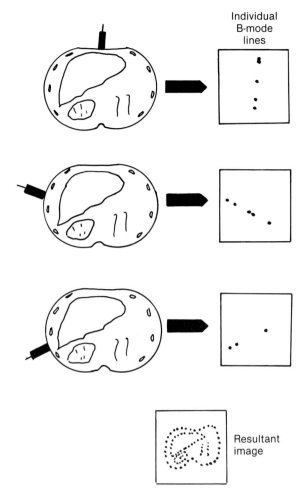

Fig. 3-19. Production of a B-mode scan by a manual scanner.

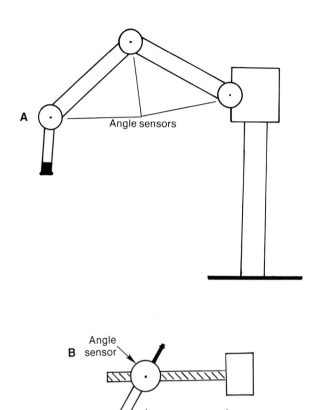

Fig. 3-20. Manual scanners. **A,** Arm commonly used for abdominal scanning. **B,** Arm used for ophthalmologic scanning.

tional to the distance between reflector and transducer.

If these two assumptions are met to a reasonable degree and if the B-mode display is integrated during the scan, the resultant echogram image provides a representation of the anatomic positions of reflectors in a plane in the body.

Manual scanners

Manual scanning instruments employ a scanning arm (as shown in Fig. 3-20) to facilitate image formation. The scanning arm carries out two functions:

1. It provides signals that enable the instrument to track the position and orientation of the ultrasonic transducer. This information, along with the echo return time, is required to place echo signals in their proper position on the display.
2. It constrains the transducer to a single plane during scan operations. This enables definition of the image scanning plane to be made in the patient.

Function 1 above is performed by sensors at the various arm joints that track the relative angle each arm section makes with other sections. In the case of the three-section scanning arm (Fig. 3-20, A) the angles along with the arm section lengths are all that is required for the instrument to keep track of the transducer coordinates. In Fig. 3-20, B, the single arm angle and the position 1 are required. The accuracy with which the transducer coordinates are determined forms one part of the compound registration accuracy of scanning instruments. This is discussed in detail in Chapter 5.

Types of scan motions

Common transducer or sound beam scanning motions employed in B-mode imaging are illustrated in Fig. 3-21. If the transducer is swept in a straight line, the operation is referred to as a linear scan. A scan obtained by pivoting the transducer about its face is called a sector scan. A compound scan is obtained by combining two more of the basic motion patterns. In some applications the

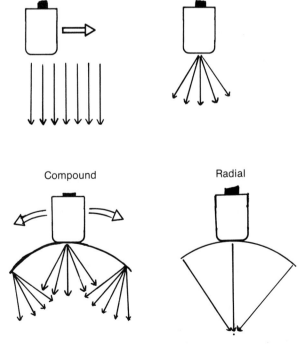

Fig. 3-21. Common scan motions.

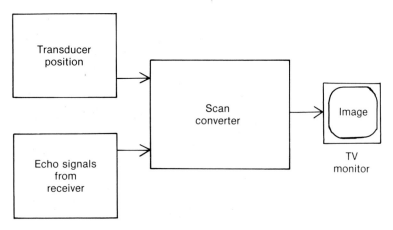

Fig. 3-22. A scan converter provides intermediate image storage, for viewing and photographing.

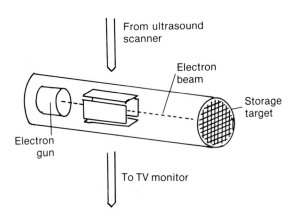

Fig. 3-23. Operation of an analog scan converter.

sound beam is always directed toward a point in the patient while the transducer is swept around—and the setup is referred to as a *radial scan*. This list is not by any means exhaustive, and different scan patterns may be identified according to the imagination, needs, and whims of the inventor.

B-MODE SCAN DISPLAY TECHNOLOGY

In early ultrasound scanners the primary device for displaying ultrasound images was an oscilloscope, whose operation has been described. An oscilloscope is useful in this application because its electron beam can be deflected in any direction and brightened at any spot on the phosphor screen; this permits actual tracking of the sound pulse position as it is reflected from interfaces at different depths. The sweep of the electron beam on the screen can be made to follow the sound beam for any of the scan motions outlined in Fig. 3-21. A special-purpose memory oscilloscope, or *storage* oscilloscope, can also be employed, allowing the image to be viewed directly during and after image buildup. Ultrasound images built up on storage oscilloscopes most often employ leading-edge signal processing along with a bistable storage screen. This produces a very contrasty scan on which each section of the display is either white or black depending upon whether an echo signal happens to be detected from the corresponding point in the patient. Leading-edge signal processing and storage oscilloscope displays are still employed in some special-purpose scanners.

In gray scale processing echo signal amplitudes are encoded in display intensity. Early gray scale scanning consisted of building up the image on photographic film, which was continuously exposed by the oscilloscope

screen during scanning.[4] The method is especially suitable for motor-driven scanning units, which can uniformly sample all areas of the scanned region. This method is difficult to employ with manual scanners because of the dependence of image brightness on scan speed and scan uniformity. The most successful manual gray scale scanners employ a scan converter for intermediate storage of images during scan buildup and image photography.

Analog scan converters

The scan converter accepts B-mode echo signal amplitude and position information from the ultrasonic scanner (Fig. 3-22), stores these signals in an internal memory, and reads out the resultant scan information to a TV monitor, on which the image is displayed and photographed.

The operation of an analog scan converter is similar to that of an ordinary CRT oscilloscope, except the scan converter does not have a phosphor screen for viewing signals. Instead of a screen, it contains a high-resolution target on which electric charge can be deposited with an interrogating electron beam (Fig. 3-23).

Electrons are produced by an electron gun and are collimated, forming a well-focused beam that is accelerated toward the target. Just as in an oscilloscope, the electron beam can be swept across the target along a line that corresponds to the direction of the sound beam emitted by the transducer. Echo signals cause electric charge to be stored at a spot on the target corresponding to the reflector position. The echo return time and the position and orientation of the ultrasound transducer are used to place echo signals in their proper position on the target.

The electric charge deposited on any spot on the target is made proportional to the processed echo signal amplitude, enabling gray scale images to be built up. For manual scanners this operation is done without overwriting by operating the target in *peak detection mode* (sketched in Fig. 3-24). Suppose an echo signal, S_1, has been detected and stored in a particular position on the target. Now suppose that another echo signal, S_2, is obtained and directed toward this same target position. The peak detection logic keeps S_1 if it is greater than S_2. On the other hand, if S_2 is greater than S_1, then S_2 is written on the target. Peak detection mode enables gray scale scans to be produced by manual scanners, without significant overwriting if the transducer beam dwells over one area for a long time. The brightness of the display is not dependent on the amount of time spent over a particular area or on whether a given region in the patient is scanned several different times in forming a single image.

Television monitors

The output of the scan converter is channeled to a television monitor for display and hard-copy recording. Television monitors are advantageous in that they can produce a large number of distinct brightness levels or gray levels and are capable of excellent spatial resolution.

TV monitors also function somewhat like oscilloscopes, having an electron beam that is accelerated and directed toward a phosphor screen. The screen emits light in response to the electron beam, the brightness of the light being controlled by the intensity of the electron current. In contrast to an oscilloscope display, the electron beam scanning arrange-

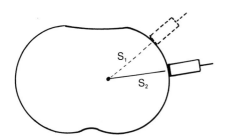

Fig. 3-24. Peak detection mode of storing echo signals in a scan converter.

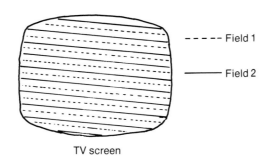

TV screen

Fig. 3-25. Sweep operation of a 512-line 2-field television monitor.

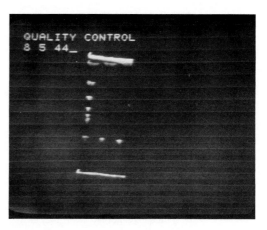

Fig. 3-26. Venetian blind effect, resulting when the electron beam in an analog scan converter is switched rapidly between the read mode and the write mode during image buildup.

ment of most TV monitors is fixed in a repeating raster format (Fig. 3-25). Ordinary 512-line monitors sweep the electron beam over the screen in two passes, referred to as *fields*. In the first field the raster scan arrangement traces out 256 lines on the screen, the process taking $1/60$ of a second. In the second field the electron beam is swept so that it fills in between the lines of the first field, again taking $1/60$ of a second. (A completed frame consists of both fields and requires $1/30$ of a second.)

The scan converter therefore must operate in two distinct sweep modes during ultrasound scanning. The target is written with sweep controls dictated by the ultrasound scanner. These, in turn, follow the position and orientation of the transducer beam. The target is read by sweeping a beam across it synchronously with the internal sweeps on the TV monitor. Stored charge on the target resulting from detected echo signals is converted to a brightness variation on the TV display screen. During image buildup the analog scan converter must alternate rapidly between writing and reading if the operator is to be able to view the echogram while scanning. Consequently a venetian blind effect (Fig. 3-26) is seen on the display.

Analog versus digital scan converters

Digital scan converters have, for the most part, replaced analog scan converters in ultrasound instruments. Distinct advantages of digital over analog systems include the following:
1. Improved stability. Analog scan converters are subject to electronic drift

in the gray scale output signal. Digital electronics is much less susceptible to drift problems.
2. Focus and image sharpness. When an analog scan converter is finely tuned, it possesses excellent spatial resolution characteristics. However, this requires sharp focusing of its electron beam, also subject to drift. Digital systems are not subject to focus problems since they do not employ internal electron beams.
3. Image uniformity. Slight variations in gray scale level from one part of the image to another can occur with analog scan converters because of nonuniformities in electron beam target sampling.
4. Improved peak detection capability and less dependence of image brightness on the scan speed. Analog scan converters do not function perfectly as peak detectors, usually resulting in some dependence of the image on scan speed and uniformity. This is not the case with digital systems.

Digital representations of values

Parameters such as signal amplitude, time, and temperature may be represented and displayed in either an analog or a digital format. In an analog format the represented values of a quantity vary continuously between a minimum and a maximum level. In digital format the values are represented using distinct levels, with discrete steps between the levels.

Digital systems offer advantages in terms of stability and immunity to electronic noise. These properties stem from the fact that all

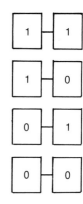

Fig. 3-27. A two-bit word can represent any of four signal levels. Each bit can be in either the 0 state or the 1 state. The four possible combinations are illustrated.

digital systems employ as a basic unit a stable electronic circuit, referred to as a *bit*. The circuit comprising a single bit can exist in either of two states, with the output terminals being either high (at some positive voltage level) or low (near zero volts). These states may be used to represent the numbers 1 and 0 respectively. Thus a single bit could represent a quantity as being either of two different levels.

Additional signal level representations for a quantity are obtained by stringing a number of bits together to form a multibit word. Consider the very simple situation of a word that consists of two bits. How many discrete values could that word represent? If we allow each bit to be in its *0* or its *1* state (Fig. 3-27), there are four different possibilities or four signal levels that can be represented. If we add an additional bit, it can be seen quite readily that now eight different combina-

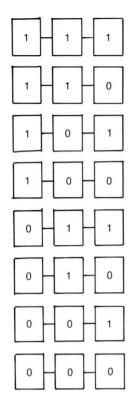

Fig. 3-28. A three-bit word can represent eight different values of a quantity. The eight possible states are illustrated.

tions are possible (Fig. 3-28). In fact, we can generalize by saying that the number of discrete levels, N, possible from a word consisting of n bits is equal to 2 raised to the power of the number of bits ($N = 2^n$). The following list gives the number of discrete signal levels that can be represented for different word configurations. This information is useful in comparing the memory size of the different digital scan converters commonly used.

Bits	Discrete levels
1	2
2	4
3	8
4	16
5	32
6	64

Appropriate coding applied to the string of bits allows these digital words to represent numbers. Computers employ the binary number system as a basis for mathematical computations. Analogous to the decimal number system, employing 10 as a base and using the digits 0 through 9 to represent numbers, the binary number system employs 2 as a base and uses only the digits 0 and 1 to represent numbers. The more bits available in a single word, the larger is the integer number that can be represented. It is beyond the scope of this text, however, to treat the binary number system further.

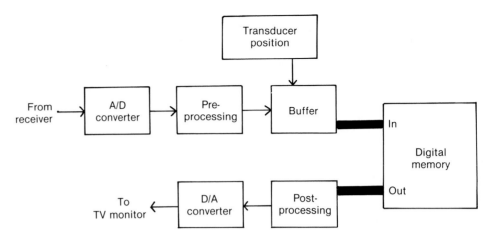

Fig. 3-29. Schematic of a digital scan converter and its relationship to other components of an ultrasound scanning instrument.

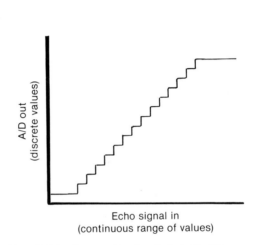

Fig. 3-30. An analog-to-digital (A/D) converter is used to transfer echo signals, whose levels may vary continuously, to digital signals, in which only discrete levels are possible.

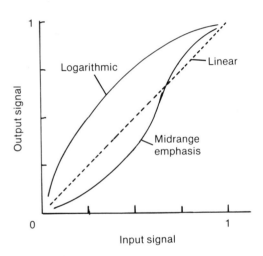

Fig. 3-31. Signal compression curves.

Digital scan converters

A functional block diagram listing essential components of a digital scan converter and their relationships to the scanning instrument and display electronics are shown in Fig. 3-29. The scan converter accepts echo signals from the receiver of the instrument and stores these in a digital memory at an "address" that corresponds to the location of the echo source. The contents of the memory are read out on a TV monitor, forming an image. Echo signals are in analog format as they emerge from the receiver; they are transferred to a digital format by an *analog-to-digital (A/D) converter*. Here continuously varying analog signals are transferred into discrete digital levels (Fig. 3-30). Once in digital format, echo signals may undergo further preprocessing prior to their entry into memory.

More on signal processing

It was mentioned earlier that one of the steps involved in signal processing consists of *compression* of the echo amplitudes. At that point only reduction of the amplified echo signal amplitude range corresponding to a given echo level range was discussed. Whereas echo signals spanning a 40-dB dynamic range might have amplitudes of 0.01 to 1 V in the receiver before compression, this same echo range might have a signal amplitude range of 0.1 to 1 V after compression.

Different formats can be followed in signal compression, but it appears that none is universally acceptable by all instrument users for all applications. Three possibilities are presented in Fig. 3-31. Logarithmic compression amplifies low-amplitude echo signals more than high-amplitude signals. Thus amplitude variations among the low signal

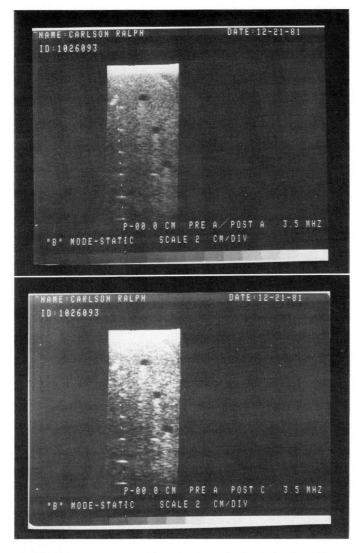

Fig. 3-32. These two scans of a phantom that mimics liver tissue are identical except that different postprocessing functions were used when the images were recorded.

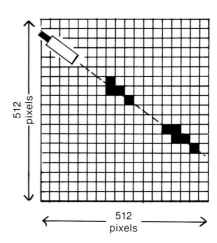

Fig. 3-33. A digital memory for a manual scanner may consist of a matrix of 512 × 512 pixels.

levels are emphasized on the display. Other formats provide emphasis to different regions of the echo dynamic range. For example, the S-shaped curve emphasizes variations over the middle of the echo signal range, as shown.

Some instruments allow selection of signal compression schemes through choice of preprocessing controls. *Preprocessing* here refers to manipulation of digitized echo signals prior to their storage in the memory. Preprocessing functions are normally stored in a read-only memory (ROM) in this section of the system. A user-selected switch provides any of several schemes, perhaps one of those sketched in Fig. 3-31. Another interesting function that can be performed during preprocessing is compensation for the variation in sensitivity of a transducer with reflector distance. (See, for example, the pulse-echo

beam profiles in Figs. E-2 to E-5.) Beam profile corrections may be done by selectively decreasing the digital echo values that correspond to the transducer focal region. A means of "recognizing" the transducer must be provided in the instrument, since different transducers require different beam profile corrections.

Operation of the digital scan converter

Echo signals can be inserted into the memory in a position corresponding to the reflector location by using the echo delay time and the transducer beam coordinates to compute the correct address. Peak detection capability is provided, analogous to that discussed earlier with regard to analog scan converters (Fig. 3-24). Besides peak detection, the digital memory allows for other

choices in updating echo information, such as insertion of the *last value* directed to any particular address location, and the choice is sometimes available through an operator switch. The latter function has been found useful for survey scanning; when used, it appears that the memory is being erased and written simultaneously.

No matter what function is adopted, there is no apparent interruption of operator viewing during scan buildup as was the case with analog scan converters (no venetian blind effect). Buffer registers allow transfer of data in and out of the memory at a rate not visible on the display.

The digital memory is read by transference of pixel values to a digital-to-analog (D/A) converter, providing signals for intensity modulating a screen or a TV monitor. The assignment of stored digital echo values to brightness levels on the TV monitor can be varied if postprocessing control options are provided (Fig. 3-32). In contrast to preprocessing, postprocessing does not require rescanning of the patient to study the effects of a particular setting on the resultant image.

The digital scan converter memory is divided into discrete and separately addressable elements, referred to as *picture elements* or *pixels* (Fig. 3-33). For compound scanners the memory size typically is 500 to 600 pixels wide by 500 pixels high. Currently most instruments use either a four-bit or a five-bit word to represent the echo value in each pixel location. Examination of the list on p. 32 shows that this bit representation provides respectively either 16 or 32 distinct echo levels.

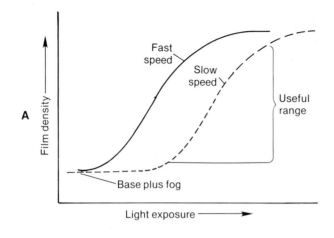

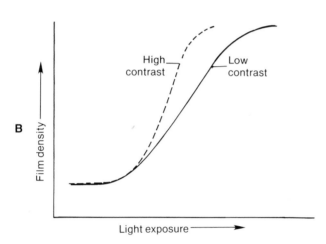

Fig. 3-34. A, Characteristic curves for two films having different speeds. **B,** Characteristic curves for two films having different contrast.

IMAGE PHOTOGRAPHY

The most common method of obtaining hard copy of ultrasound images is to photograph a monitor that is continuously viewing the image stored in the scan converter. This can be done with any type of photographic negative film, Polaroid positive film, or image-recording transparency film. In addition, special copying techniques such as thermal printing and ultraviolet-sensitive paper are sometimes used; these are especially handy in systems designed for M-mode recording because they can provide long continuous records. No matter what the image-recording process, the hard-copy materials and camera settings all require proper matching to optimize the end results. A basic comprehension of the principles of these recording techniques is especially useful in understanding the tradeoffs in this matching process and helping to pinpoint problems in image recording when they exist.

The ensuing discussion deals with the principles underlying recording images on photographic film, since many of these also apply in the other recording medium mentioned. Photographic film contains small grains of silver bromide crystals suspended in a gelatin and supported on a cellulose acetate sheet. When light strikes the crystals, they form a *latent image* and are very susceptible to chemical change upon development. During the development process the crystals that absorbed light are converted to silver grains. Any unexposed crystals are removed from the film during the fixing stage, leaving behind the exposed silver grains, which form an image.

Several types of film are used in medical image recording. Their properties can be compared with the aid of characteristic curves (examples shown in Fig. 3-34). These curves are obtained by exposing patches of a film, and then determining the *optical density*, a measurement of the opacity of the exposed part of the film. The density is plotted against the relative exposure, the latter being the product of the intensity of the light and the exposure time.

The *base plus fog* refers to a slight opacity of the film, found upon developing without any exposure. There is a threshold exposure required before any additional film darkening occurs, this threshold level varying for different films. There also is a maximum exposure, above which no additional exposure can cause film darkening. The useful exposure range is situated between these extremes, wherein a change in the light level will be recorded as a change in the developed film density.

The curves in Fig. 3-34, *A*, are for two films having different speeds. The higher-speed film requires less light exposure to cause film darkening than does the low-speed film. The two curves in Fig. 3-34, *B*, are for films with different contrast. The steeper curve is for a high-contrast film, which takes only a small exposure variation to go from minimum to maximum optical density. Low-contrast film has a wider latitude, accommodating a much wider light exposure range.

For optimal results the monitors used for exposing film must be matched in terms of brightness, contrast, and exposure time; so the particular film used is exposed to a level corresponding to its useful range on its characteristic curve. Ideally exposure settings should be such that variations in image brightness caused by amplitude changes among high-level echo signals are successfully recorded at the same time that the weakest echo signals (e.g., recorded from organ parenchyma) are detected on the film image. This can usually be achieved with proper exposure and camera monitor control settings. It often requires an experienced serviceman or sonographer to determine the correct settings.

The results of the developing process are highly dependent on the developing time and the temperature of the processor and the condition of the processing chemicals. Most medical imaging facilities regularly test the photography performance and maintain quality assurance notebooks in which important processing parameters are logged on a daily basis. In addition, it is important to keep in mind that photographic films can be adversely affected by storage conditions of high temperature and humidity. To assure consistent clinical results, one should always follow the film manufacturer's instructions for film handling and processing.

SPATIAL RESOLUTION LIMITATIONS INTRODUCED BY IMAGE STORAGE AND DISPLAY DEVICES

In Chapter 2 there is a discussion of ways in which the spatial resolution of an ultrasound instrument is limited by the transducer. It is not always appreciated that the spatial resolution may be limited instead by the image memory or the image display device, or both. These components usually are limiting factors when small image magnifications (i.e., large fields of view) are employed.

In the following discussion we will consider spatial resolution limitations introduced by the digital memory of an ultrasound imaging system. The general principles also apply to other devices (e.g., television monitors).

Consider an image stored in a digital scan converter memory in which a large field of view (say, 40 cm) is used (Fig. 3-35). Assume that the memory consists of 500 rows of pixels, with 500 pixels in each row—a reasonable size. If there are 500 pixels shared over a 40-cm field of view, each centimeter increment in the patient is represented by

$$\frac{500}{40 \text{ cm}} \sim 12 \text{ pixels/cm}$$

Recall that when we first considered spatial resolution it was described as the ability to resolve closely spaced reflectors into individual echo sources. Suppose we have reflectors so close to each other that their imaged positions overlap (as shown by the insert in Fig. 3-35). Whether or not these reflectors are distinguishable by the transducer, they cannot be resolved by the imaging system because they fill adjacent pixels in the scan converter. There is no way for the observer to distinguish one reflector from another.

On the other hand, if there is a gap between pixels storing echo signals from two separate reflectors, the reflectors can be distinguished on the image. This gives us a rough idea of the spatial resolution limitations introduced by the scan converter. Assume now that the closest that two reflectors can be and still be "resolved" is a separation corresponding to a 2-pixel spacing in the scan converter. What does this spacing translate into as far as patient dimensions if a 40-cm field of view is used?

As mentioned above, if there are 500 pixels representing a 40-cm range, this means there are 12 pixels for every 1 centimeter in the patient. If the minimum resolved reflector spacing is that corresponding to a 2-pixel separation, this translates into

$$\frac{2 \text{ pixels}}{12 \text{ pixels/cm}} = 0.16 \text{ cm}$$

or a 1.6-mm spacing, which is worse than the axial resolution limitation introduced by a typical ultrasonic transducer.

We can improve the situation by using a large image magnification (and smaller field of view) when scanning. For small fields of view we usually find the transducer to be the limiting factor in the spatial resolution.

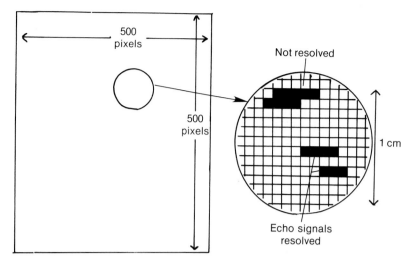

Fig. 3-35. Spatial resolution limitations introduced by the scan converter.

REAL TIME AUTOSCAN INSTRUMENTS

Instruments that scan with sufficient speed to allow rapidly moving interfaces in the body to be visualized without significant blurring are called real time scanners. These scanners are a subset of a general class of instruments referred to as autoscanners (or automatic scanners). Autoscan instruments employ mechanical or electronic steering of the ultrasound beam to produce ultrasonic B-scans. Their development and use provide certain performance capabilities not easily attainable with manual scanners—including the ability to visualize the chambers and valves of the heart in echocardiography studies, the ability to relate very readily the scanning plane to the three-dimensional anatomic structure of the patient, and for some units the relatively low cost and portability of the instrument.

Scanning speed limitations

Scanning speed, or image frame rate, is an important performance characteristic in some applications of rapid scanners. The maximum speed with which a real time as well as many slower autoscan instruments can build up images is limited by the finite travel time of sound pulses in tissue. The basic principle behind this limitation is quite simple: the separate transducer beam lines used to form an image each require a small time interval to detect all echoes emerging from that line. This introduces the requirement for a time delay between sound pulses transmitted along separate lines. The time delay required between pulses depends on the speed of sound in the medium and the maximum visualization depth.

Consider the sector scan arrangement in

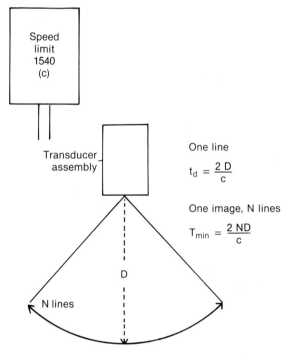

Fig. 3-36. Relationship between the time required for a simple scan, T_{min}, and the number of lines in the image, N, the maximum depth imaged, D, and the speed of sound, c.

Fig. 3-36. The transducer assembly could be one of several types that will be discussed later. An image is produced by separate ultrasound beams distributed evenly throughout the sector angle. The number of separate beam lines needed is dictated by factors such as image quality requirements and size of the sector. For simple scanning arrangements such as shown here it might be useful to employ 120 or more individual lines to form an image covering a 90-degree sector angle. Fewer lines could be used, but only at the cost of larger gaps between individual lines, which might be undesirable.

If the field of view setting in Fig. 3-36 results in a maximum visualization depth of D, the delay time, t_d, needed to collect all echoes from any single line is given by

$$t_d = \frac{2D}{c} \qquad (3\text{-}3)$$

where c is the speed of sound in the medium. Notice that this equation is nearly identical to the pulse-echo range equation (3-2) above. The minimum time required to produce a complete image consisting of N such lines is simply $N \times t_d$ or

$$T_{min} = Nt_d = \frac{2 \times N \times D}{c} \qquad (3\text{-}4)$$

Example: Suppose the field of view of a sector scanner was set for a maximum echo depth of 20 cm. Furthermore, N is 120 lines. Calculate T_{min}; also the maximum frame rate.

Solution: Using Equation 3-4

$$T_{min} = \frac{2 \times 120 \times 20 \text{ cm}}{1.54 \times 105 \text{ cm/sec}}$$

$$= 0.031 \text{ sec}$$

Note that the minimum allowable time to produce a single image is 0.03 second. (In practice slightly longer times are allowed so the chances of producing an artifact by overlapping of pulses will be minimized.) The maximum frame rate possible (R) is simply the inverse of the minimum scan time

$$R = \frac{1}{T_{min}} \qquad (3\text{-}5)$$

For the present example

$$R = \frac{1}{0.031 \text{ sec}} = 32/\text{sec}$$

Consider one more example. The purpose is not to dazzle the less mathematically inclined reader with algebra but to demonstrate that some practical consequences of a simple although very important concept can be approached through reasoning.

Example: Show that if the distance, D, in Equation 3-3 is expressed in centimeters (i.e., $D = d$cm) then the maximum frame rate can also be expressed as

$$R = \frac{77,000/\text{sec}}{N\ d} \qquad (3\text{-}6)$$

where N is the number of acoustic lines per frame and d is the centimeters of distance.

Solution: As stated earlier, the maximum frame rate, R, may be expressed as

$$R = \frac{1}{T_{min}}$$

Now plug in the expression for T_{min} (Equation 3-4) to get

$$R = \frac{c}{2\ ND}$$

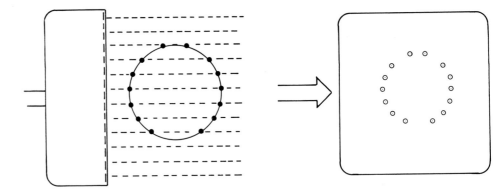

Fig. 3-37. Schematic of a sequential–linear-array scanner.

The expression then pops right out after substituting for c and letting D be d cm:

$$R = \frac{1.54 \times 10^5 \text{ cm/sec}}{2\ N\ d \text{ cm}}$$

$$= \frac{77,000}{Nd}/\text{sec}$$

It is not necessary (nor is it very desirable) to memorize expressions such as Equation 3-6 to grasp the principles being discussed. If you understand that the scan speed is limited by the time required for echo signals to return from the maximum image depth along each acoustic line, then it is fairly easy to reason out some important design tradeoffs in rapid-scanning instruments. Scanners employing a large field of view (e.g., 21 × 21 cm) are somewhat limited in frame rate if a sufficient line density is employed for reasonable image quality. Reduced fields of view, such as employed in some high-frequency small parts scanners, allow significantly higher frame rates. Instruments with variable magnification sometimes decrease the frame rate or decrease the number of lines in the image when the field of view is increased.

Sequential-array scanners

Sequential–linear-array scanners produce images by transmitting sound beams parallel with one another, beginning at one end of the array and continuing along to the opposite end (Fig. 3-37), after which the sequence is repeated.[1] The scan is produced by using a stationary transducer assembly and electronically switching from one group of transducer elements to another to generate pulsed beams. Echoes obtained from reflectors in the beam are presented on the B-mode display. In each case the B-mode display line is so positioned that it corresponds to the central axis of the pulsed sound beam.

Typical sequential arrays utilize 60 to 120 or more rectangular piezoelectric elements

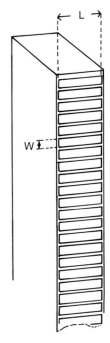

Fig. 3-38. Transducer assembly arrangement in a sequential-array scanner.

arranged side by side (as shown in Fig. 3-38). The element width, W, is usually one or two wavelengths and the length, L, sufficient to provide a reasonably collimated sound beam in a direction perpendicular to the scan plane. The choice of a small element width provides the ability to produce closely spaced ultrasound beams; this is necessary so that fine spatial detail of anatomic structures will be obtained.

Individual ultrasound beams are produced by exciting a cluster of elements in the array, after which the same element grouping is used to detect echo signals. Received signals from individual elements are added together electronically, forming a net echo signal that is amplified and processed for display. After this occurs, a new cluster is formed by

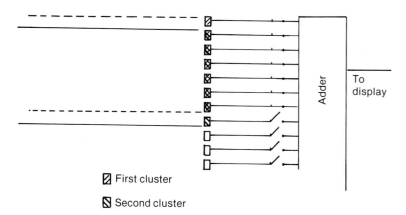

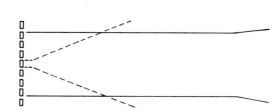

Fig. 3-39. Method of scanning a sequential-array transducer assembly.

Fig. 3-40. Schematic of a sound beam from a single element in an array compared to the beam from a cluster of elements.

switching over one element in the array and the process repeated (Fig. 3-39).

The use of a cluster of perhaps seven elements rather than a single element is dictated both by sensitivity and by lateral resolution requirements. The sound beam from a single very narrow transducer element (on the order of the wavelength in size) is quite broad (Fig. 3-40). Consequently the lateral resolution from such a device is very poor, especially beyond the first few millimeters of tissue. However, the beam pattern emerging from the cluster of elements possesses much more desirable properties in terms of lateral resolution. The wider aperture formed by the cluster produces a narrower sound beam in the patient. The general properties of transducer beams discussed in Chapter 2 for circular disk transducers apply in the present case. (Note the similarity between Figs. 3-40 and 2-16.)

Equations similar to 2-1, for the near field length, and 2-2, for the divergence of the beam in the far field, can be written down for rectangularly shaped sources. Rather than do this, it is sufficient to say that the previous expressions for circular elements will serve as a useful guide for estimating the foregoing transducer beam parameters if half the aperture size is substituted for the radius in Equations 2-1 and 2-2. The interested reader is referred to Dick and Carson[2] for further details and more exact expressions.

Even-odd element firing. The center of the sound beam produced from the element cluster should lie along the central element in the cluster (as shown in Fig. 3-39). Subsequent beams are produced by dropping the top element and picking up the next lower element and exciting this new cluster. The effect is to move the central region of the beam down one element. The process con-

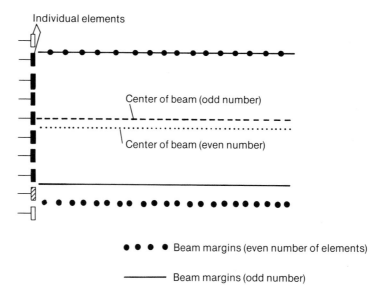

Fig. 3-41. Even-odd element firing to provide beam spacing of one half rather than one element.

tinues down the entire array, producing a single ultrasonic B-scan.

Finer spacing of the ultrasound beams can be obtained if a process referred to as *even-odd* element firing is employed. With an odd number of elements the center of the beam corresponds to the middle of the central element (Fig. 3-41). With an even number the center of the beam is situated along a line that cuts between the central two elements in the cluster. If a beam is formed of an odd number of elements, followed by another formed of an even number, followed by another of an odd number, etc., there are half-element spacings between individual scan lines forming the image.

Other schemes involving electronic beam deflections are employed in some instruments to increase the number of independent acoustic lines forming the image.[3] This

technique is not discussed in this book; however, actual electronic beam steering is taken up later in this chapter.

Electronic focusing of arrays. The elements making up individual clusters for beam formation can be pulsed individually. This allows the beams in the array to be focused in the scanning plane. Although the necessary electronics can add complexity and cost to a sequential array, focusing has proved to be advantageous in improving the lateral resolution.

When all elements in an array cluster are excited precisely at the same time, the effect is analogous to the situation in which a planar unfocused transducer element is pulsed. The resultant beam is directional but unfocused. Electronic focusing can be achieved by introducing time delays in the application of the excitation pulses to the separate ele-

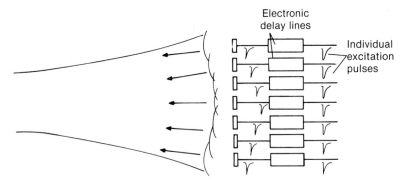

Fig. 3-42. Electronic focusing of a sequential array. Focusing may be achieved by means of time delays in the pulsing circuitry.

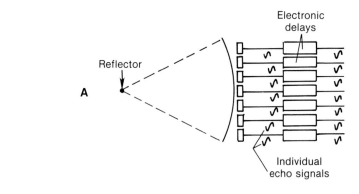

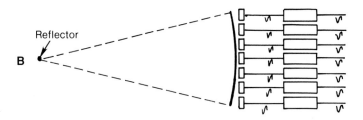

Fig. 3-43. A, Electronic focusing of the received echoes. The time delay is introduced in the receiver circuit, before echo signals are added. **B,** The electronic delay settings necessary to focus during reception vary with the depth of the reflector.

ments (Fig. 3-42). In this case the wavefronts emerging from the transducer converge toward the focal position, producing a narrower sound beam over a fixed region than exists when a planar element is used.

Time delays are produced by *electronic delay lines,* which hold an electric signal for a fixed time, depending on the delay line setting, before passing the signal on. If the delays are such that the outer elements of a cluster are excited before the inner ones in the sequence suggested in Fig. 3-42 the beam emerging from the transducer will converge toward a focal position. Electronic focusing can also be employed during echo reception. The echo signal from a reflector positioned on the axis of a sound beam will

arrive at the central element of the cluster slightly before it arrives at the outer elements (Fig. 3-43). This is due merely to the greater distance between the reflector and the outer elements of the active cluster. The echo signals detected by individual elements would be slightly out of phase. Focusing during reception involves introducing time delays in the received echo signals before all echoes are summed up, so the echoes from a single reflector will all be in phase.

Instruments that provide electronic focusing may differ in whether the focusing occurs during transmission, during echo reception, or both. Also, in some instruments, focusing can be selective for each transducer assembly, thereby allowing for optimization of the

lateral resolution and the sensitivity at the depth of interest. Selective focus is varied by means of front panel controls.

Dynamic focusing. The focal distance for a beam transmitted by an array is fixed and depends on electronic delay control settings at the time of pulse transmission. In the foregoing discussion, focusing upon reception was treated as if this function were also fixed in a similar manner. Just as for focusing the transmitted beam, the electronic delay settings required to focus the received echo signals vary with distance. In Fig. 3-43, *A,* the delay needed between the middle element and the outer elements of the array is greater than in Fig. 3-43, *B,* wherein the reflector is depicted further from the transducer assembly. It is possible to vary the focus control dynamically so the focal distance tracks the depth of the received echo. This can be done in real time as echo signals are being received by the array. The process of varying the focal distance so it keeps up with the position of the transmitted acoustic pulse is referred to as *dynamic focusing* and is provided on some instruments.

Focusing perpendicular to the scan plane. Original sequential arrays provided no focusing perpendicular to the scanning plane; the beam shape was determined by the transducer element size and the ultrasonic frequency. Performance of sequential arrays was improved by providing mechanical focusing in this plane, using shaped transducer elements analogous to those described for single-element transducer construction (Fig. 3-44). More commonly acoustic lenses, such as the planoconvex lens system in Fig. 3-44, *C,* are used.

Electronic (phased-array) sector scanners

The sound beam produced by an array of transducer elements can be steered off at an angle with respect to a line perpendicular to the array surface. This can be done by introducing appropriate time delays in the excitation pulses applied to individual elements in the array. The direction in which the sound beam is steered is dependent on the exact time delay settings and can be varied from one transmit pulse to the next.

If the widths of individual elements in the array are small enough (i.e., smaller, or not much bigger, than the ultrasonic wavelength) the sound radiation pattern from each of these elements is quite broad (Fig. 3-45, *A*). This is analogous to the situation discussed earlier for sequential arrays. Each element emits a diverging beam, as shown.

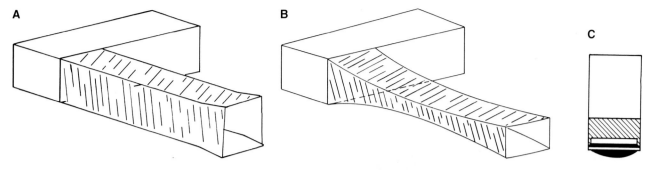

Fig. 3-44. Sequential array focusing perpendicular to the scanning plane. **A,** Schematic, unfocused beam. **B,** Schematic, focused beam. **C,** Method of focusing employing a convex lens. In this lens the speed of sound is lower than it is in tissues; therefore it focuses the beam.

The net sound beam produced by the entire array travels in a direction perpendicular to a line connecting points of equal phase in the beams from individual elements. This direction is given by the angle A in Fig. 3-45, B. The method is employed for scanning the transmit beam in phased-array transducer assemblies. In a similar manner the received signals from individual elements in the array are delayed before being added together. Thus *steering* occurs during both transmission and echo reception.

Electronic focusing may be done by programming delay settings for focusing, similar to those described for sequential-array focusing, along with the beam-steering delays. Both fixed focusing and dynamic focusing have been used in phased arrays.

The region of a transducer assembly through which sound is coupled to the patient is sometimes referred to as the entrance window. An advantage of electronically sectored arrays is their relatively small entrance window, permitting coupling through the intercostal space. Electronically sectored arrays may have 30 to 60 or more individual piezoelectric elements packed into a 1-to-2-cm row. Thus they may be used effectively in adult cardiac imaging.

Another advantage of electronic sector scanners is the flexibility introduced in the scanning format. It is quite easy to share a scanning beam with one or more static M-mode lines, for example, enabling multiple-trace M-mode displays to be produced along with a two-dimensional image. Also, since there are no mechanical movements involved in producing the scan, it is quite easy to synchronize scanning movements to external triggers, such as derived from ECG signals. Both these features have been employed in some electronic sector scanning instruments.

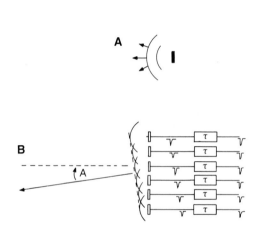

Fig. 3-45. Electron sector scanner operation. A sound beam of an array is steered by time delays in the pulsing and receiving circuits. **A,** Sound beam pattern from an individual element in the array. **B,** Beam from the array in which electronic delays are adjusted to steer at the angle A.

Off-axis radiation from arrays

In pulse-echo imaging it is desirable to have a well-defined narrow sound beam when the clinical application requires high spatial resolution. Beam-forming principles using arrays have been described wherein element clusters are employed to provide a large transducer size and mechanical as well as electronic focusing is used to narrow the beam. One additional difficulty that must be overcome with arrays is their strong tendency to produce significant sound radiation in directions other than that of the central beam.[2]

Most transducers produce *side lobes* as part of their normal radiation pattern. These are recognized as small off-axis peaks in the lateral beam profile in the far field. For sin-

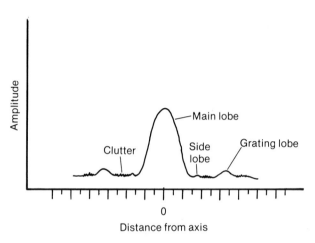

Fig. 3-46. Schematic beam profile in the far field of a transducer array, illustrating side lobes, grating lobes, and clutter.

gle-element weakly focused transducers (discussed in detail in Chapter 2) the side lobes usually are suppressed as a result of the transducer design and the pulsing characteristics. Thus, under normal circumstances, they are probably inconsequential to the image. With arrays additional off-axis radiation, resulting from the presence of *grating lobes* and to some extent *interelement coupling*, is present and can be demonstrated quite readily on an image.

A schematic representation of a far field sound beam pattern from a multielement array is presented in Fig. 3-46. The side lobe is a natural part of any pattern, whether the beam is produced by a circular or a rectangular element. (The relative contributions of the beam pattern components shown are not meant to be representative for any particular array; they are critically dependent on the specific array design.) The grating lobes re-

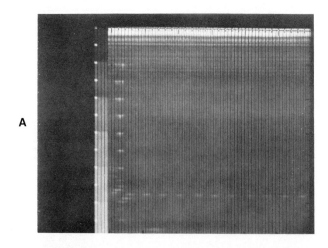

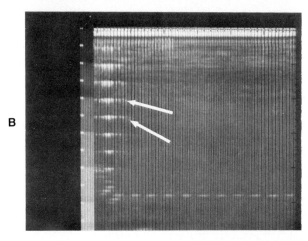

Fig. 3-47. Image of line targets when a sequential array is used. **A,** At low sensitivity settings. **B,** At high sensitivity settings. Grating lobes are indicated with arrows.

sult from the division of the transducer into small individual elements that are regularly spaced across the aperture. They are quite well understood and predictable. Grating lobes may be reduced in amplitude and directed further away from the main beam axis (where their effects would be less important) if narrow closely spaced elements are used. The additional *clutter* level in the beam pattern apparently arises from a number of factors, including failure to isolate completely the various elements in the array from one another and other modes of oscillation of the elements besides their thickness mode.

The effects of off-axis insonification may be demonstrated by imaging an isolated reflector immersed in a water bath or a tissue phantom. At low receiver gain settings such targets produce a line image (as shown in Fig. 3-47, *A*). Higher sensitivity settings result in broadening of the line image since the reflector can be detected even though it may be considerable distances from the axis of the beam. Part of the broadening stems from grating lobes.

The degree to which grating lobe and off-axis sonification exist varies considerably among different transducer assembly designs. Substantial improvements in array design in the past few years have resulted in B-scan image quality using arrays that favorably competes with image quality from manual scanners that use single-element transducers.

Rapid mechanical scanners

Conceptually the simplest types of rapid autoscanners are mechanical systems. These usually employ one or more single-element transducers to transmit and receive ultrasound signals. They have been designed in many different scanning arrangements. Several examples are shown in Fig. 3-48.

In Fig. 3-48, *A*, a single-element transducer is shown oscillating about a pivot point. Some systems employing this arrangement provide transducer interchangeability in the scanning assembly. Others employ a servodrive, which helps reduce effects of mechanical vibration.

The multiple transducer rotating wheel has proved to be very effective in mechanical sector scanners. This arrangement employs from two to four separate transducers on the rim of the wheel (Fig. 3-48, *B*). Transducers are pulsed only during the time they sweep past the scanning window, as shown. The transducer assembly housing must be filled with a fluid to assure acoustic coupling between the transducer element and the window. (The type of fluid used and whether it is user replenishable if, for example, air bubbles are formed should be explained in the accompanying owner's manual.)

The mechanical scanning arrangement shown in Fig. 3-48, *C*, consists of three separate rotating wheels each having two transducers.

The fourth system (shown in Fig. 3-48, *D*) uses a stationary element to generate sound beams. Beam deflection is done with an oscillating acoustic mirror housed in the transducer assembly.

Unlike sequenced linear arrays and electronically sectored arrays, mechanical scanners contain moving parts to generate the scan. The parts may consist of gears, pulleys, wheels, or oscillating shafts depending on the design. Normal wear and tear on the drive mechanism can be reduced by placing the transducer assembly in a nonscanning mode when not in use. Again, consult the owner's manual for the recommended transducer assembly standby mode between patient scans.

Freeze frame

The intermediate image storage function on a rapid scanner is called a *freeze frame memory.* On state-of-the-art systems the memory functions similarly to that in a scan converter, discussed earlier in this chapter. It accepts digitized A-mode signals and stores them in a position (address) that corresponds both to the sound beam orientation relative to the transducer assembly and to the echo transit time. Output is in TV format, suitable for input to a monitor, a multiformat camera, or a videotape recorder.

Digital memory for most rapid scanners is more limited than the memory used in digital scan converters of manual scanners. Since the imaged field is also more limited, however, this does not constitute a serious disadvantage. For a sector scanner a typical memory size is 256×150 pixels, with anywhere from 2 to 6 bits representing echo amplitudes. (Review the list on p. 32 to see the number of discrete signal amplitudes possible with different bit representations.)

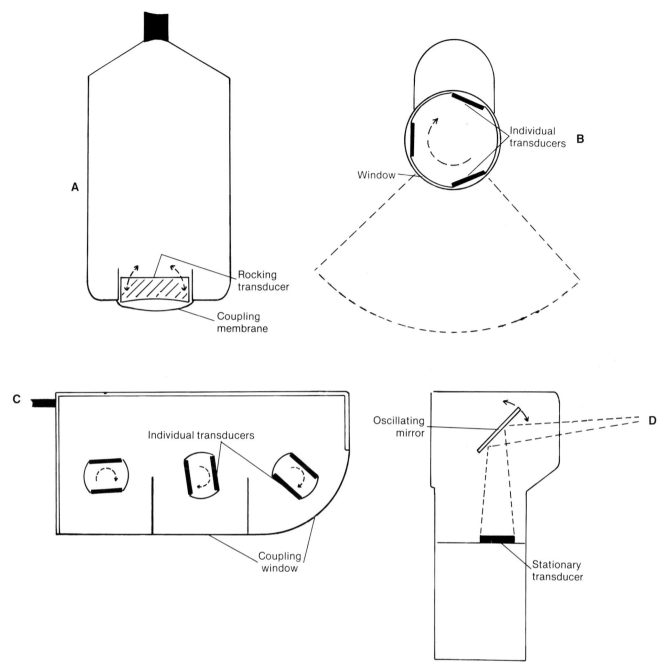

Fig. 3-48. Four different scanning arrangements employed with small hand-held mechanical autoscanners.

Another method of converting from the ultrasound scan format to the TV format is to use a television camera trained on a B-mode oscilloscope. The camera signal is then available for direct viewing on a TV monitor or for tape recording.

One operation not necessary with the scan conversion process used with rapid scanners is peak detection. Since the automatic scanning mechanism sweeps the ultrasound beam evenly, there is no dependence of the gray scale scan on the operator's ability to uniformly scan all regions of the imaged field.

A few rapid scanners transfer signals di-rectly from the receiver to a videotape re-corder. In one such system the scans are pro-duced at a rate of 60 Hz; thus the scanning mechanism is synchronized to the television sweeps.

LARGER WATER PATH AUTOMATIC SCANNERS

For some B-mode scanning applications it has been found advantageous to use large transducer aperture, water path scanners. Performance capabilities obtained with this type of scanner include the following:

1. Automation of the scanning operation.

This allows rapid production of serial plane echograms. In some systems automation also provides accurate cor-relation of scans from different sets of image planes (e.g., transverse and lon-gitudinal sets).

2. Uniform scanning of the entire imaged field.

3. Extended transducer focal region. This has been achieved by using single-ele-ment transducers with a fixed focus, multiple transducers with different focal regions, and annular-array trans-ducers.

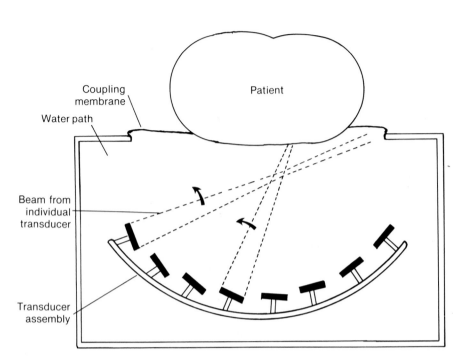

Fig. 3-49. Water path scanner employing eight large-aperture (large-diameter) transducers. (Based on schematics courtesy the Ausonics Corporation, New Berlin, Wisconsin.)

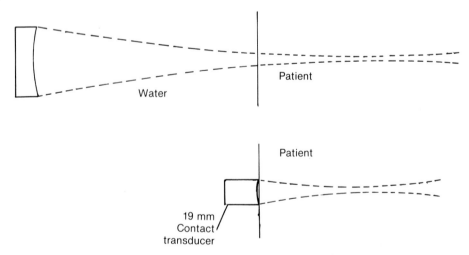

Fig. 3-50. With a large-aperture transducer and moderate focusing an extended focal region is produced. The transducer is backed away from the skin surface, placing the patient in the focal region. For comparison a 19-mm contact transducer beam is also illustrated.

Three different water path scanners will be described here, illustrating the approaches just mentioned to obtain an extended focal region.

The eight-transducer water path scanner system illustrated in Fig. 3-49 is an example of the first of these systems. Each transducer has a large diameter and is *moderately focused* so an extended focal region is produced (Fig. 3-50). The intervening water path between the transducer surface and the patient's skin enables the patient to be situated in the transducer focal region. The beam width and the lateral resolution do not change as much with increasing depth into the patient as they do when, for example, a contact transducer is used.

To form an image, each transducer carries out a single sector scan. The system can be programmed to accept pulse-echo data from any combination of transducers. Multiple transducers are used in this instrument primarily to increase the scanning speed over that which can be achieved with a single transducer. The instrument outlined in Fig. 3-49 has been used for general-purpose scanning as well as for more specialized applications (e.g., breast scanning).

Because of the irregularity of breast anatomy and the ease with which breast tissue can be compressed and distorted by contact transducers, water path scanners have been used for ultrasonic breast scanning in some institutions. Special-purpose scanners have been developed for this application. In one such system, shown schematically in Fig. 3-51, scanning is achieved by rotating each wheel transducer assembly as well as by translating the assembly laterally. Individual transducers in the assembly are sharply focused, each at a different depth (Fig. 3-51, *B*). An extended focal region is obtained in the image by accepting echo signals only when they originate within a given transducer's focal region. As the first transducer scans the breast, the receiver is *gated* to allow only echo signals from the focal region of this probe to be displayed; the gate is adjusted to pass echo signals from the focal region of the next probe in the assembly when it scans the breast, etc. Thus an image is produced by using multiple transducers that are sharply focused at different depths and accepting echo signals only from within the focal zone of each transducer.

Different focal distances from a single transducer aperture can also be obtained by using an annular-array transducer (Fig. 3-52). Its focusing operation is analogous to the electronic focusing characteristics of linear arrays. The annular array consists of either a flat or a spherical transducer surface cut in annular rings with a central disk. The sound beam may be focused by exciting the different elements of the array at slightly different times. Varying the excitation sequence timing allows the focal distance to be changed. The annular array can be focused during transmission (focal distance fixed for each transmit pulse) or reception, during which dynamic focusing is possible. Some annular-array transducer assemblies use an oscillating mirror to scan the sound beam. The water path standoff allows the beam from a large array to be focused even at the skin surface.

REFERENCES

1. Bom, N., Lancee, C., Honkoop, J., et al.: Ultrasonic viewer for cross-sectional analysis of moving cardiac structures, Biomed. Eng. **6:**500, 1971.
2. Dick, D., and Carson, P.: Principles of auto scan ultrasound instrumentation. In Fullerton, G., and Zagzebski, J., editors: Medical physics of CT and ultrasound, New York, 1980, American Association of Physicists in Medicine.
3. Iinuma, K., Kidokora, T., Ogura, I., et al.: High resolution electronic-linear-scanning ultrasonic diagnostic equipment, Ultrasound Med. Biol. **5:**51, 1979.
4. Kossoff, G., Garrett, W., Carpenter, D., et al.: Principles and classification of soft tissues by grey scale echography, Ultrasound Med. Biol. **2:**89, 1976.

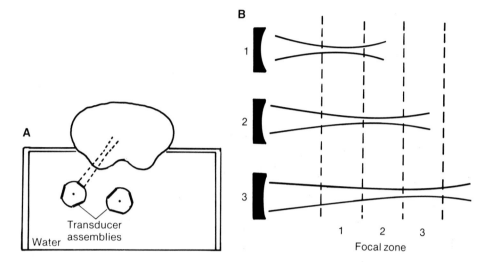

Fig. 3-51. A, Schematic of a special-purpose breast scanner employing two separate transducer assemblies to scan the breast immersed in water. **B,** Each transducer assembly contains three sharply focused transducers. The focal distance is different for each of the transducers, providing an extended focal region in the image. (Courtesy Life Instruments, Inc., Boulder, Colorado.)

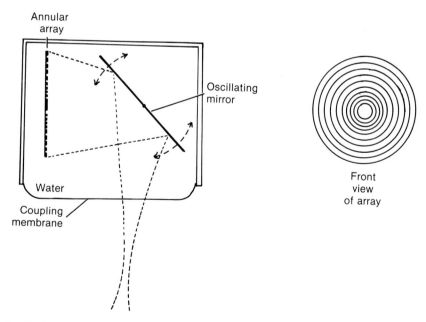

Fig. 3-52. Annular-array transducer assembly, with an oscillating mirror to scan the sound beam.

4

Images and artifacts

JAMES A. ZAGZEBSKI

An ultrasound B-scan image is produced by exciting a transducer that is in acoustic contact with a patient, detecting echo signals, and displaying these signals on the B-mode display. The displayed echo position corresponds to its anatomic origin in the body. The separate aspects of this imaging process have been discussed in Chapters 1 to 3. The interactions between acoustic waves and tissues, including the speed of sound, ultrasonic attenuation, and reflection and scatter, are patient-based factors contributing to the process. Communication between the anatomic region of interest and an instrument that can process echo information and display this information in a fashion that may be understood by human observers is the function of the ultrasound transducer. The transducer adds its own "signature" to the echo information in the form of beam width effects, axial resolution limitations, and frequency characteristics. Finally, the options available for amplification signal processing and echo signal display as well as the number of operator choices available for control of the related instrumentation can lead to significant differences in the displayed appearance of otherwise similar echo data.

Our overall task in this chapter is to examine ultrasound pulse-echo images in more detail than we did in previous examples, by studying the information that the images convey and the artifacts they contain. Those who understand the physical basis for production of signals displayed on ultrasound images are in a better position to judge the adequacy of a clinical scan, avoid or minimize artifacts on images, and interpret the results of studies.

SPECULAR VERSUS DIFFUSE REFLECTIONS

Longitudinal scans of the liver contain many practical examples of the tissue–sound beam interactions that were considered earlier from a conceptual point of view. Proper scanning techniques for imaging the liver with B-mode ultrasonography are discussed in Chapter 10.

With a manual scanner a single-pass scanning motion of the transducer obtains images of the liver from an anterior subcostal window. This approach is optimal for clinical demonstration of image features that are useful in a diagnosis of liver disease. It is not necessarily optimal for outlining organ boundaries, where specular reflectors are involved. A case in point is the upper pole of the right kidney (Fig. 4-1). Although a segment of the interface between the kidney and liver is seen quite vividly, other sections are barely perceptible because this interface behaves, for the most part, like a specular reflector. At such interfaces a large-amplitude echo signal can often be obtained for perpendicular beam incidence; however, a significantly weaker signal is obtained when the interface is tilted with respect to the incident beam direction (Fig. 1-11) because the reflected beam travels in a different direction rather than back toward the ultrasound transducer. The scanning technique used results in only perpendicular beam incidence over a limited region of the liver-kidney interface, which produces a large-amplitude echo signal.

Interfaces that reflect sound in all directions are sometimes referred to as *diffuse reflectors*. Very small reflectors are usually referred to as *scatterers*. The parenchyma of most organs, including the liver and kidneys, contains a large number of acoustic scatterers. Echo signals from scattering regions are much less dependent on the transducer beam orientation* than are echoes from specular reflectors. Thus the echo amplitude from different regions of the liver does not vary greatly, no matter what transducer angle is needed to visualize that region.

Regional variations in the scattered signal amplitude sometimes provide diagnostic in-

---

*We are ignoring *anisotropic* behavior in scattering that may exist in some tissue.

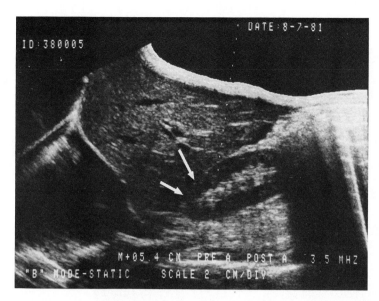

Fig. 4-1. B-mode scan of the liver. The interface between the liver and the upper pole of the right kidney *(arrows)* is not well delineated because it is a specular reflector that is tilted with respect to the incident beam.

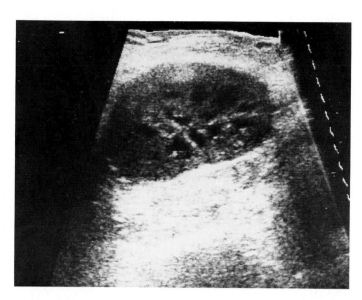

Fig. 4-2. B-mode scan of a kidney. The renal pyramids are visualized due to variations in scattered echo signal amplitudes detected from these regions.

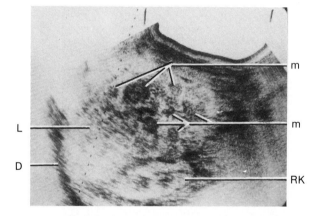

Fig. 4-3. Scan of the liver showing focal lesions, *m,* visualized mainly because of differences in ultrasonic scatter level. *L,* Liver; *D,* diaphragm; *RK,* right kidney.

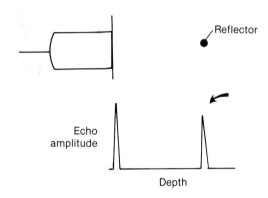

Fig. 4-4. Echo signal from a single scatterer.

formation or added anatomic detail. With a gray scale display these amplitude variations are transformed into changes in displayed echo brightness. An example is the visualization of the kidney pyramids (Fig. 4-2) as a result of scatter level changes. Focal lesions in the liver (Fig. 4-3) are often partly diagnosed by either an increased or a subdued ultrasound scatter level in comparison to the normal surrounding parenchyma.

TEXTURE IN AN ULTRASOUND B-SCAN IMAGE

The arrangement of dots or B-mode marks on an ultrasound image of an organ or tissue site is sometimes referred to as *image texture.* Texture in an ultrasound image results from scattered and reflected waves from sites distributed throughout an organ. At present the interfaces and scattering sites giving rise to these scattered signals are not precisely known for many anatomic regions that are imaged. This is the subject of ongoing research studies in a number of laboratories. In most cases, however, the displayed echo pattern referred to as "texture" is due to *interference* of waves originating from multiple scatterers in the sound beam.

Interference between waves was discussed in Chapter 1, and it may be useful to review

that material here. It was indicated there that when sound waves are received simultaneously from two separate sources the waves can partially or completely cancel, or partially or completely reinforce, one another depending on the relative *phase* of the waves from the two sources.

A single reflector in the beam of a pulse-echo transducer will yield an echo signal whose magnitude depends on the position of the reflector in the beam (Fig. 4-4). If a group of reflectors is positioned in the beam, the *average* signal* obtained depends on factors

---

*Purists will say "the average intensity of the signal."

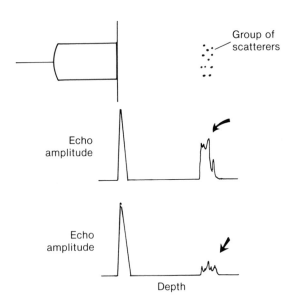

Fig. 4-5. The net echo from a group of scatterers can be of any magnitude, depending on the number and arrangement of the scatterers contributing to the signal at any one time. Two possible A-mode signals from the situation schematically illustrated at the top of the figure are presented.

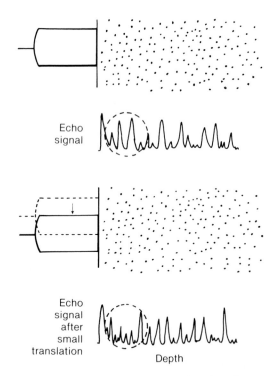

Fig. 4-6. Fluctuations in the echo signal as a transducer beam is moved laterally through a volume of closely spaced scatterers. On a B-scan image the fluctuations produce gray scale texture.

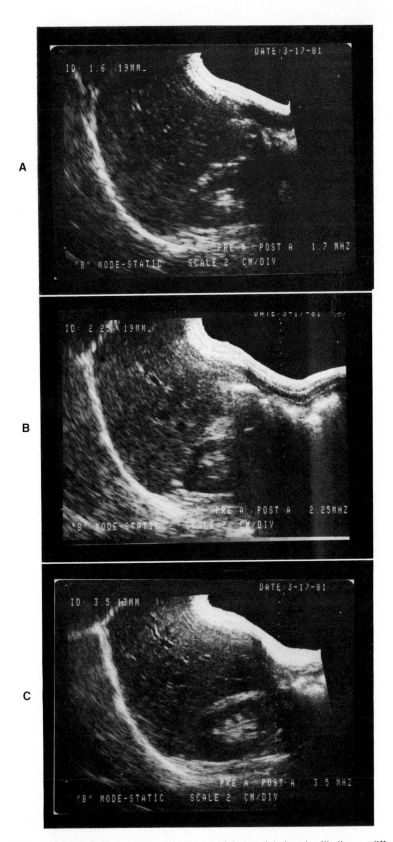

Fig. 4-7. Longitudinal scans of the liver and kidney obtained with three different contact transducers. **A,** 1.7 MHz; **B,** 2.2 MHz; **C,** 3.5 MHz. All transducers were 19-mm diameter. The subject assumed the same degree of inspiration for each scan; thus all scans depict nearly the same structures. The variation in the spatial characteristics of the texture pattern resulting from use of different-frequency transducers is illustrated.

discussed in Chapter 1 (viz., the scatterer size, number of scatterers per unit volume, scatterer interface characteristics, and frequency). However, an echo signal originating from this group could be of any magnitude, depending on the relative spatial distribution of the reflectors. The reflectors could be so arranged (by chance) that a relatively large amplitude echo signal would be obtained; or they also could be so arranged that *destructive interference* of the scattered waves would occur, resulting in a low amplitude echo from the group (Fig. 4-5). When a pulsed sound beam is scanned over a volume of tissue that contains a fairly large number of closely spaced scatterers, the echo signal amplitude at any depth will fluctuate from one beam position to another (Fig. 4-6). The fluctuations result from random variations in the number and positions of scatterers contributing to the echo signal at any instant of time. Fluctuations in the echo signals as the sound beam is scanned produce a texture pattern on a B-mode display. Although individual B-scan marks resemble those from individual discrete reflectors, in fact, collections of scatterers contribute to each dot on the displayed image.

The spatial characteristics of the texture pattern, including the size of individual B-scan marks and the number of marks or dots per unit area on the image, turn out to be strongly dependent on the ultrasonic transducer and the depth of the reflectors. Usually the texture pattern is quite fine for positions near the transducer face, less so near the focal region, and smeared out beyond the focal region. Transducers of different nominal frequency result in different texture patterns for the same scatterers, as shown by the longitudinal liver scans in Fig. 4-7. To facilitate comparisons of the results for the three cases, the scans were all obtained in the same image plane.

Notice in Fig. 4-7 how the texture from any one region varies when different transducers are used. The very fine-grained texture pattern close to the anterior skin surface for the 3.5-MHz transducer is a good example of the fact that multiple reflectors contribute to each element of the pattern. Of the three transducers used, the probe has the widest beam width in this region of the sound beam. Yet in this region the texture pattern appears with the finest spacing.

Several conclusions regarding this aspect of image texture can be made:

1. The pattern results from groups of scatterers rather than from individual reflectors imaged separately.

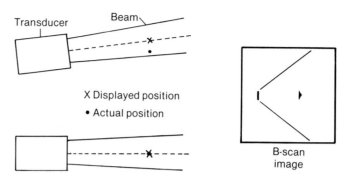

Fig. 4-8. Origination of a displayed beam width artifact. No matter where a reflector is positioned in the beam, a properly calibrated scanner displays the echo signal in a position corresponding to the central axis of the beam.

2. For a given anatomic site the pattern obtained is dependent on the transducer frequency, diameter, and focusing properties and on the distance from the transducer.
3. Differences in texture have also been noted to be due to anatomic variations.
4. Individual dot sizes on images from such scatterers are not indicators of spatial resolution. In fact, as in the lower image of Fig. 4-7, the texture pattern is finest in the near field of the transducer, where the spatial resolution is worse.

IMAGE ARTIFACTS

When an ultrasound pulse-echo image is produced, two assumptions are implicitly built into the instrument to place echo signals in their proper position on the display:

1. The echo source is assumed to lie along the axis of the ultrasonic transducer beam.
2. The delay time between transmission of an acoustic pulse by the transducer and reception of an echo signal is assumed to be directly proportional to the distance from the transducer to the echo source.

We have seen in Chapter 3 (Fig. 3-19) how utilization of these assumptions leads to production of a B-mode image. Significant deviations from the assumed conditions can give rise to image artifacts on a display.

An artifact is any echo signal whose displayed position does not correspond to the position of a reflector in the body. It could also refer to displayed signal amplitude variations that are not due to properties of reflectors being displayed but to properties, for example, of intermediate tissues. The first type of artifact we will consider is related to the width of ultrasound transducer beams used for scanning.

BEAM WIDTH EFFECTS; LATERAL RESOLUTION

When an ultrasound beam is scanned over a small reflector, the resultant B-scan image of the reflector consists of a line. The generation of this line is rather straightforward. Consider the mechanical scanner arrangement shown in Fig. 4-8. A transducer beam is oriented in two directions relative to a small stationary reflector. If the instrument's sensitivity is set high enough, an echo signal may be detected from the reflector, even when it is near the periphery of the beam. A properly calibrated B-mode scanning instrument positions detected echo signals along the assumed axis of the ultrasound beam. If we fill in the figure by adding the sound beam orientations that are between the extreme positions shown, the resultant image from the reflector forms a line. The breadth of this line may be called the *displayed beam width* for this target and the imaging conditions employed.

The displayed beam width can be studied by scanning line reflectors in a test object or phantom. (We will talk more about specific test object configurations in Chapter 5.) An

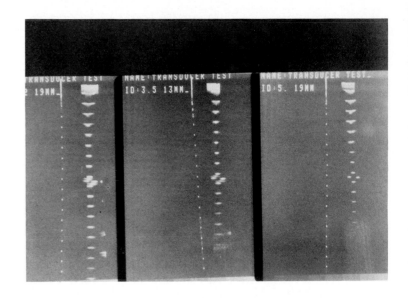

Fig. 4-9. Scan of small line reflectors, each separated by 1 cm, showing displayed beam width for a 2.2-MHz 19-mm diameter transducer *(left)*, a 3.5-MHz 13-mm diameter transducer *(center)*, and a 5.0-MHz 19-mm diameter transducer *(right)*.

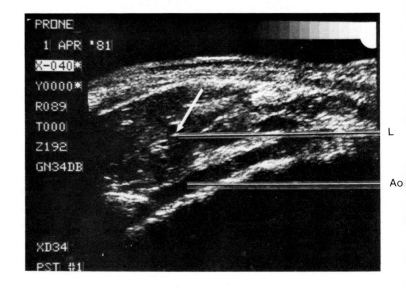

Fig. 4-10. Evidence of beam width effect from an apparently discrete reflector *(arrow)*, presenting an echo signal above that of the background texture.

example of this is shown in Fig. 4-9, wherein the image of a column of thin nylon fibers each separated by a distance of 1 cm is presented for three transducers. The displayed beam width varies with distance from the transducer; in fact, the transducer beam pattern strongly affects the overall pattern observed. The region where the displayed beam width is narrowest corresponds approximately to the pulse-echo focal region of the transducer. The *displayed* beam width depends on numerous factors in addition to the transducer beam pattern, however. These include the attenuation in the medium; the dimensions, orientation, and reflection coefficient of the reflector; the instrument's pulser power; the gain and signal processing of the receiver; and the characteristics of the echo display.

The beam width contributes to spreading of the image pattern obtained from discrete reflectors. This may sometimes be observed in large organs, such as shown in Fig. 4-10; however, it is difficult to distinguish actual beam spreading in cases such as this from actual breadth of the reflecting interface. Small discrete reflectors such as stones and calcifications will yield a discrete pattern whose extent is due mainly to the beam width.

The effects of displayed beam width can also be seen at times in M-mode records of heart structures. In Fig. 4-11 the double echo complex obtained from the anterior surface of the mitral valve can often be avoided by using a transducer with a narrower beam at the depth of this structure.

Beam width effects and poor lateral resolution can contribute to artifactual fill-in of echo-free structures on B-scan images, for example, small cysts or small blood vessels. The situation is depicted schematically in Fig. 4-12. The circular structure is characterized as having no echo signals originating within its borders. However, if the edge of the sound beam intercepts reflecting interfaces at the same time that the axis of the beam projects through the echo-free volume, echo signals will be detected. On a B-mode display these signals would be displayed in a position corresponding to the interior of the volume. When this occurs, artifactual *echo fill-in* of the image of the echo-free volume takes place. The situation can be optimized, of course, by choosing an ultrasound transducer that has a narrow beam at the depth of greatest interest.

Fill-in of cystlike structures is demonstrated in Fig. 4-13 with a tissue-mimicking phantom and simulated cysts. The diameters

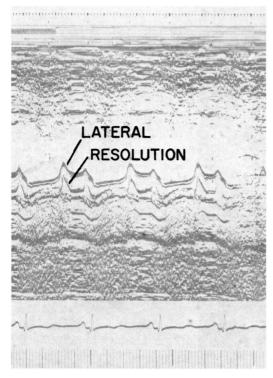

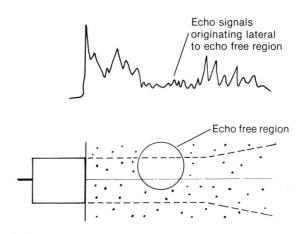

Echo signals originating lateral to echo free region

Echo free region

Fig. 4-11. Double echo obtained from the area of the mitral valve. The two distinct echoes originate from different surfaces of the mitral valve structure, each in a slightly different part of the beam.

Fig. 4-12. Schematic fill-in of the echo-free area due to beam width effects.

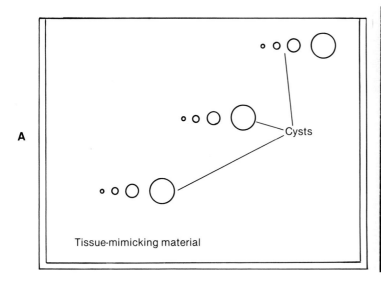

A

Cysts

Tissue-mimicking material

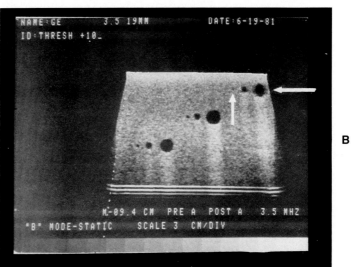

B

Fig. 4-13. A, Tissue-mimicking phantom with simulated cysts of 2 and 1 cm and 5 and 2 mm diameters. **B,** Image of this phantom. At 3 cm below the surface of the phantom the large cyst appears oval shaped *(horizontal arrow)* from fill-in of the lateral margins due to beam width effects. The 5-mm diameter *(upward arrow)* cyst cannot be detected. Notice that at a depth of 6 cm, which is near the focal region of the transducer, much better delineation of the stimulated cysts is possible.

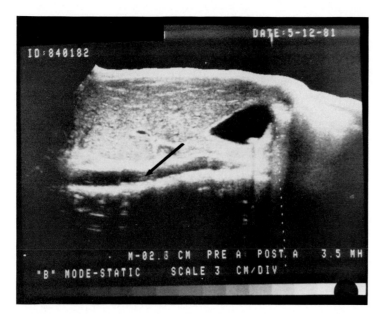

Fig. 4-14. Partial echo fill-in *(arrow)* of the aorta due to transducer beam width effects extending out of the image plane.

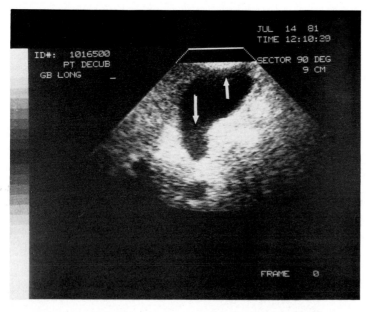

Fig. 4-15. Gallbladder image showing real *(downward arrow)* and artifactual *(upward arrow)* fill-in of echoes.

of the cysts are 2 and 1 cm and 5 and 2 mm. Sets of cysts are shown at depths of 3, 6, and 10 cm below the phantom surface. With a 3.5-MHz 19-mm diameter transducer excessive fill-in due to beam width effects occurs at 3 cm. The large cyst appears oval shaped due to fill-in of the lateral margins. The smaller-diameter structures cannot be distinguished from the background. Conditions are more favorable for the 6-cm deep set, which are near the focal distance of this transducer. Much sharper delineation of the structures is possible at this depth.

Structures contributing to beam width artifacts do not necessarily have to be located in the plane of the scan, as in the previous examples. In the longitudinal scan shown in Fig. 4-14 partial fill-in of the aorta can be seen. In this case fill-in was probably due to echo signals arising from structures lateral to the vessel, out of the indicated plane of the image. This manifestation of the effects of the displayed beam width has been termed *slice thickness artifact.*[1]

A task in each of the foregoing situations is differentiating artifactual echo signals from

signals due to actual ultrasonic scatterers in the region of concern. We see that not every apparent echo signal on a display corresponds to an actual reflector. Conversely, we must exercise caution to avoid judging actual reflectors and scatterers as simple artifacts. The gallbladder image in Fig. 4-15 shows partial fill-in of echo signals that are not due to beam width effects in this case but are due to sludge debris in the neck region (downward arrow). On the other hand, the upward-extending arrow in the same image points to artifactual echo signals due to reverberations in overlying structures. (Reverberations are discussed in more detail below.) It would be difficult to differentiate real echo signals from artifact signals on the basis of the echo pattern as such. It is necessary to consider all possible sources of signals, both artifactual and actual, when attempting to determine the acoustic properties of a particular region. A knowledge of the physical principles underlying the imaging process and experience with one's own equipment certainly aid in this differentiation process.

REVERBERATION ARTIFACTS

Many tissue interfaces in the body can produce a relatively large-amplitude echo. This could, in turn, lead to reverberation artifacts on an A-mode, M-mode, or B-mode display.

Consider the situation shown schematically in Fig. 4-16. The reflector could be, for example, a fat-muscle interface just below the skin surface. In the figure a reflected wave (solid arrow) from this interface is shown directed back toward the transducer, where it is detected, amplified, and displayed. If the echo is of significant magnitude, it will be partially reflected at the transducer surface and redirected back toward the interface. Reflection of this reverberation pulse back to the transducer produces a reverberation echo signal. The reverberation echo results from a pulse that has traveled the round trip distance between the transducer and interface *twice*. Thus it is displayed in a position corresponding to twice the reflecting interface distance (echo 2 in Fig. 4-16). Additional reverberations, such as echo 3 in Fig. 4-16, corresponding to three round trips of the sound pulse between the transducer and the interface, are sometimes observed. Reverberations produce artifactual echo signals that can partially mask actual echo signals on a display.

Examples of reverberation artifacts appearing on a B-mode display appear in Figs. 4-17 and 4-18. In the case of the urine-filled bladder (Fig. 4-17) ghost images of superficial structures are easily identifiable be-

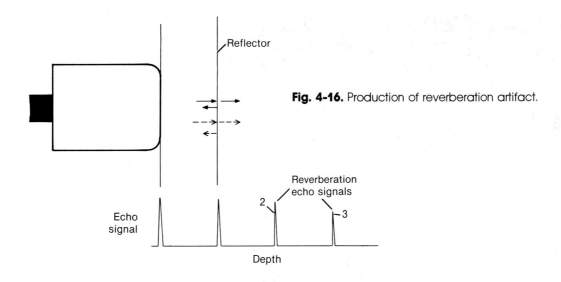

Fig. 4-16. Production of reverberation artifact.

Reflector

Reverberation
echo signals

2

3

Echo
signal

Depth

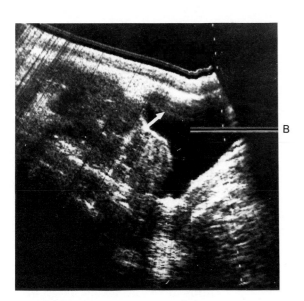

Fig. 4-17. Reverberation artifact *(arrow)* in the urine-filled bladder, *B.*

B

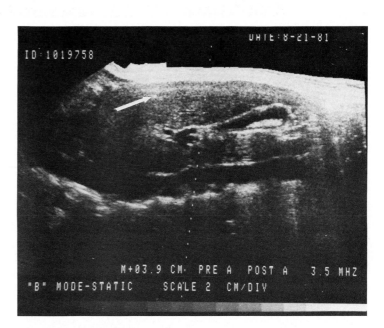

Fig. 4-18. Reverberation artifact *(arrow)* in an image of the liver.

cause of the echo-free void usually obtained during scanning of fluid filled volumes. The ghost images are produced by sound pulse reverberations as the transducer beam is scanned over the anatomic regions shown. Reverberations and similar ghost images occur in the liver scan in Fig. 4-18. Here the artifact pattern is more difficult to distinguish than in the previous case because it mixes with the real echo signal pattern. A double reverberation originates from the gas-filled bowel loop in Fig. 4-19.

Reverberation artifacts can contribute to artifactual echo fill-in of small echo-free cysts, abscesses, and vessels. This often leads to difficulties in identifying and/or diagnosing such structures echographically.

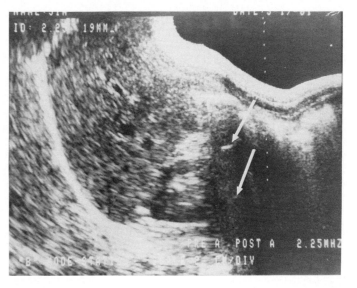

Fig. 4-19. Double reverberation *(arrows)* from the loop of bowel gas in the upper abdomen.

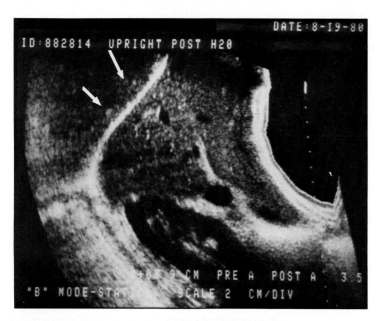

Fig. 4-20. Echoes originating beyond the diaphragm, resulting from a reverberation path.

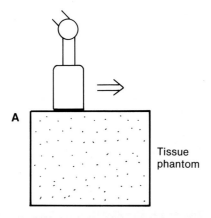

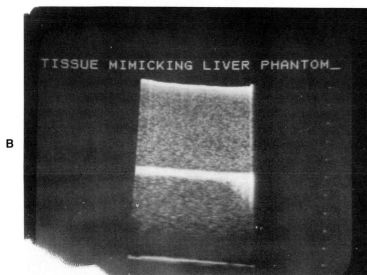

Fig. 4-21. A, Scan of a liver-mimicking phantom. **B,** Echoes apparently originating beyond the margin of the phantom in **A.** They are due to secondary reflection from the parenchymal scatterers in the phantom.

A more subtle reverberation artifact results in the detection of scattered echo signals that appear to originate beyond the diaphragm or beyond other highly reflecting surfaces enclosing reflectors and scatterers (Fig. 4-20). This artifact is also easily demonstrated with a tissue phantom. For example, Fig. 4-21 shows a similar result that occurs during scanning of a homogeneous tissue-mimicking phantom. Echo signals appear to originate beyond the end of the phantom, although the sound beam is completely reflected at this interface.

The origin of this artifactual pattern is as follows: As the incident beam traverses the medium, scattering occurs, producing the texture echoes seen on the display (Fig. 4-22, *A*). The beam is shown striking the bottom surface of the phantom, where a large fraction of the energy is reflected. Analogous to scattering of the incident beam, scattering of the reflected beam may also occur (Fig. 4-22, *B*). Scattered waves from the reflected beam path may themselves reflect off the bottom surface and trail the main reflection back toward the transducer (Fig. 4-22, *C*). Since these latter echo signals return to the transducer *after* the echo from the bottom surface is detected, they appear to originate from beyond this surface.

In Fig. 4-20 the tissue-air interface of the diaphragm of a normal adult represents a highly reflective surface, analogous to the bottom of the phantom in the example above. Sound waves reflected from the diaphragm can be partially scattered by reflections in the liver. A portion of these scattered waves returns to the diaphragm (Fig. 4-23) and are reflected back to the transducer. The longer echo transit time, of course, results in their position on the display beyond the echo from the diaphragm.

SHADOWING AND ENHANCEMENT

If output power controls and receiver sensitivity controls are properly adjusted, a uniform echo signal brightness level can be obtained on ultrasound scans of reasonably homogeneous tissue volumes. In particular, adequate setting of the swept gain controls on the receiver can result in a uniformly displayed echo level versus depth, even when sound beam attenuation takes place in the medium. The requirement for this condition is that the attenuation rate not vary significantly from one area to another. Variations in the ultrasonic attenuation are detected on pulse-echo scans because of *partial* or *total acoustic shadowing* or because of distal *echo enhancement*. The resultant artifacts actually provide useful diagnostic information.

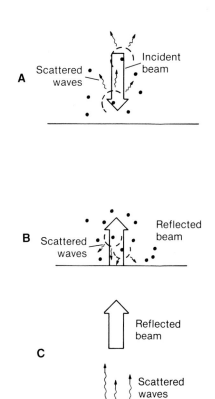

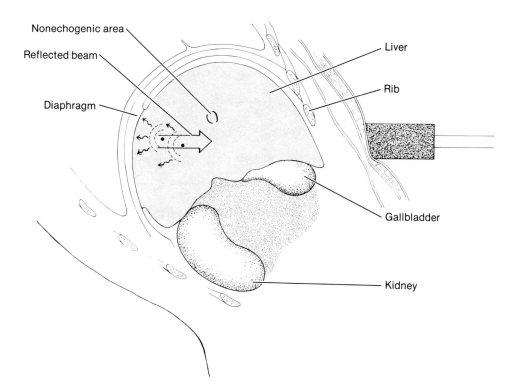

Fig. 4-22. Steps in the production of the artifactual echo signals displayed beyond the imaged margin of the phantom in Fig. 4-21.

Fig. 4-23. Production of artifactual echoes beyond the diaphragm.

Partial shadowing is a reduction in the amplitude of echo signals detected from regions distal to a mass whose attenuation is greater than that of the surrounding region. This is illustrated in Fig. 4-24. In *A* an A-mode display corresponds to transducer placement over a volume of tissue assumed to have uniform scattering and attenuation properties. Here the swept gain, or TGC, is adjusted to compensate for the sound beam attenuation in the tissue path, yielding an A-mode display that, on average, does not vary significantly with distance. Now consider what would happen if the transducer were moved to an adjacent region with a mass whose attenuation coefficient is greater than that of the background *(B)*. The added attenuation in this mass is not compensated for in the instrument, since the swept gain rate is assumed to be the same as for *A*. Therefore all echo signals originating distal to this mass are displayed as having lower amplitudes, even though the scatter properties of the region are identical to those of the corresponding distance in *A*. This situation is known as a partial acoustic shadow.

The opposite effect takes place when a low-attenuating mass, such as a cyst, is encountered in a similar situation (Fig. 4-24, *C*). Here the reduction of ultrasonic attenuation in the mass results in overcompensation by

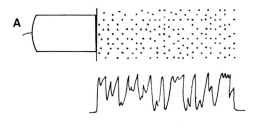

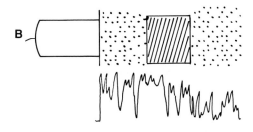

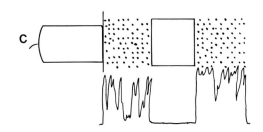

Fig. 4-24. Origin of partial acoustic shadowing and echo enhancement, showing A-mode echo signals. **A,** From a volume having uniform attenuation, with the swept gain set adequately to compensate for the attenuation. **B,** From a path that is uniform except for a mass in which the attenuation is greater than in the surrounding medium, **C,** From a path that is uniform except for a cystic region.

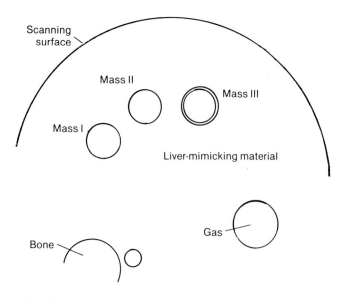

Fig. 4-25. Phantom used for demonstrating partial shadowing and echo enhancement due to differences in ultrasonic attenuation between masses and background material.

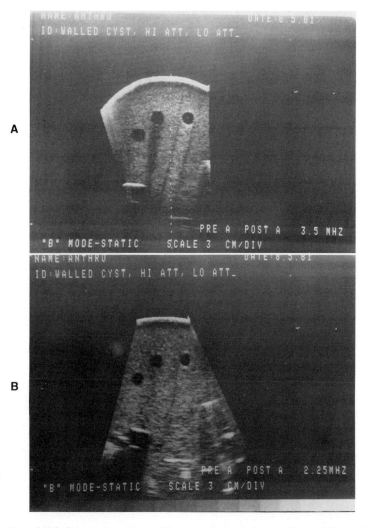

Fig. 4-26. B-scan images of the phantoms in Fig. 4-25. **A,** With a 3.5-MHz transducer. **B,** With a 2.25-MHz transducer.

Table 4-1. Ultrasonic properties of masses in Fig. 4-25 (compared to the background)

Mass	Scatter level	Attenuation level
I	Lower	Slightly lower
II	Lower	Higher
III	Lower	Lower

the swept gain (TGC) circuitry, still assumed to be adjusted for the situation in *A*. Echo signal *enhancement* is said to take place because of the increased amplitude of the displayed signals beyond the cyst. Occasionally we say that the mass has good *through-transmission* properties. As the diagram suggests, echo enhancement is exhibited by all echoes detected distal to the low attenuating mass.

The presence of either of these features provides clues regarding the nature of masses visualized on an ultrasound scan. To see how this occurs, consider the phantom diagramed in Fig. 4-25. This is a section of a larger teaching phantom for sonographers.[8] It contains three spherical masses, whose acoustic properties compared to the background material are described in Table 4-1. Mass *III* mimics a walled cyst, whereas the other two mimic structures with acoustic properties as shown in the table.

Ultrasound B-scan images of these masses are presented in Fig. 4-26. Both images were obtained with a single scan motion of the manual scanner, a technique that helps emphasize the partial shadowing and enhancement features of an image. (A compound scan motion would fairly well camouflage these features. Why?)

The walled cyst yields typical image features of a cystic structure, including an echo-free interior and excellent through-transmission properties, the latter being indicated by the echo enhancement distal to the margins of the mass. Partial shadowing is seen in Fig. 4-26, *A*, for the highly attenuating mass. It is difficult to visualize any enhancement distal to mass *I;* apparently its attenuation coefficient is too close to that of the background material.

How would enhancement and partial shadowing be affected by changes in the ultrasonic frequency? In Chapter 1 it was stated that ultrasonic attenuation in soft tissues is proportional to the frequency. Therefore differences in the attenuation between two regions are also frequency dependent. If we reduce the ultrasonic frequency (by using a lower-frequency transducer), adjust the sensitivity controls to provide a uniform display of the background, and scan the phantom section again, the image shown in Fig.

4-26, *B*, results. Echo enhancement and partial shadowing are much less pronounced in this case.

The situation is described further in Fig. 4-27. Here plots of the echo amplitude versus distance, obtained through a homogeneous section of the phantom and through a path containing a highly attenuating mass, are shown for two ultrasonic frequencies (referred to as *low* and *high*). Without TGC (swept gain) the echo amplitude decreases gradually with distance, the decrease being more rapid for the higher-frequency beam. When swept gain controls are properly set, the echo amplitude stays approximately the same at all distances. When the beam passes through the mass with greater ultrasonic attenuation (dashed lines), the amplitude of echo signals detected distal to this mass is lowered, as shown. TGC, of course, does not compensate for the added attenuation.

The degree of partial shadowing is portrayed by the *separation* of the curves representing echo signal amplitudes through the mass and signal amplitudes through the adjacent homogeneous region. The increased rate of attenuation for higher-frequency sound beams results in a greater separation of these curves for the latter case. If we had considered transmissions through the simulated cyst, the argument would be similar. The only difference would be that the dashed curves representing echo signals detected through the cyst would be placed *above* the solid lines, representing transmission through the homogeneous medium.

In essence, we see that partial acoustic shadowing and echo enhancement distal to masses are more pronounced for higher-frequency sound beams.

Some interfaces in the body produce nearly complete acoustic shadowing on an image. Tissue-air interfaces (e.g., loops of gas-filled bowel or airways) are completely impenetrable because of the large impedance mismatch associated with them. In the above image (Fig. 4-19) reverberation echo signals are displayed distal to the air interface. In some situations a shadow could occur without the obvious echo signal from the interface if the interface were tilted with respect to the direction of the incident sound beam. Such a situation could mimic an attenuating mass, and the unwary sonographer might be fooled into a wrong interpretation unless all the acoustic signs were considered.

Nearly complete shadowing is also obtained from gallstones and other calcified objects (Fig. 4-28). Manifestation of such shadowing from small objects is significantly dependent on the objects' positions in the

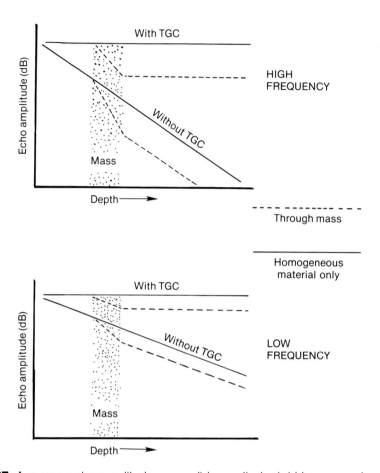

Fig. 4-27. Average echo amplitude versus distance that might be encountered in the situation shown in Fig. 4-26, when a mass whose attenuation is greater than the background is included in a scan. A high-frequency case and a low-frequency case are shown. *Solid line,* Average signal through the background only; *dashed line,* average echo signal when the beam passes through the mass. The difference between these two lines indicates the degree of partial shadowing.

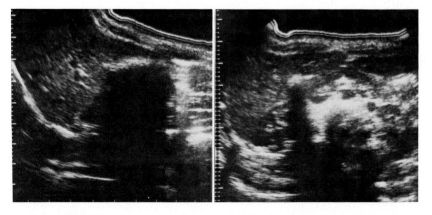

Fig. 4-28. Complete shadowing of an ultrasound beam by gallstones.

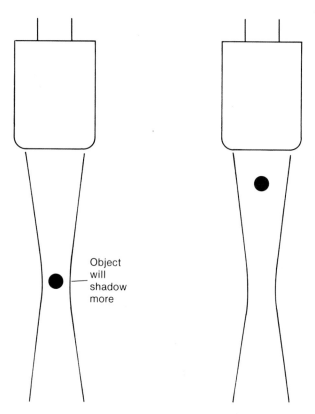

Fig. 4-29. The degree of shadowing by a small object depends on where the object is with respect to the ultrasound beam. Maximum shadowing is, of course, obtained when the object is in the focal region of the transducer.

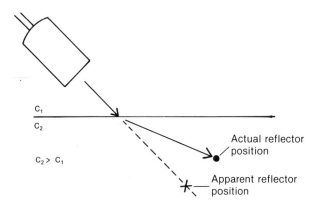

Fig. 4-30. If sound beam deflection or refraction occurs, echo signals are displayed as though they originated along the axis of the transducer.

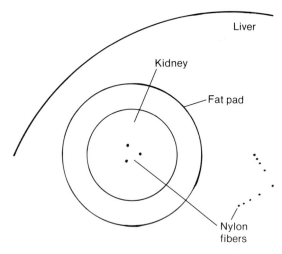

Fig. 4-31. Section of a torso phantom containing a simulated kidney and fat pad. Also shown is an L-shaped set of line reflectors.

ultrasound beam. If a small shadowing object is nearly in the focal region of the transducer, it stands a better chance of interrupting a significant fraction of the sound beam than if it is placed in other regions of the beam (Fig. 4-29). Thus, when stones or other small calcifications are being diagnosed, the choice of transducer diameter and focal length should be dictated by the depth of the region of interest.

SOUND BEAM DEFLECTION

Occasionally all or part of the energy within the sound beam will be deflected at a significant angle relative to the original sound beam axis. Sources of beam deflection include refraction and reflections at specular interfaces. The apparent echo position (Fig. 4-30) is along the line of sight of the undeflected transducer beam axis. Thus echo signals could appear on a B-scan image in a

position quite remote from their actual anatomic origin.

Refraction of a sound beam takes place when the beam strikes an interface at an angle and the speed of sound is different on each side of the interface. The larger the difference in the speeds of sound, the greater the refraction effect will be. The greatest speed-of-sound difference where refraction can occur is at a soft tissue–bone interface. However, refraction here is usually of little practical consequence because in most instances we do not image through bone interfaces. (In fact, the significant refraction effect contributes to the problem of transmission through bone.) The major exception of clinical interest is imaging through the skull.

Soft tissue interfaces that can cause significant refraction artifacts include those formed with the lens of the eye plus those formed with fat.

Due to the relatively high speed of sound in the lens and the curvature of the tissue surfaces, this structure can significantly distort and deflect a sound beam. Excellent demonstrations of this effect using Schlieren photography have been published.[2] For this reason imaging the eye with ultrasound usually involves the use of windows that exclude the lens, unless one is specifically interested in this structure in the examination.

Fat can also result in substantial refraction artifacts. The speed of sound through fat is significantly lower than that through most soft tissues. Moreover, fat is often found in abundance in planes throughout the body. These planes could be imaged with sharp angles of the incident sound beam.

Refraction and beam deflection artifacts

involving fat have been demonstrated by Madsen et al.[4] using an abdominal tissue phantom. The phantom contains various structures embedded in a liver-mimicking material. Included in this phantom is a simulated kidney with a surrounding fat pad (Fig. 4-31) in turn surrounded by liver-mimicking material. The speed of sound through the fat pad material is 1450 m/sec whereas through the simulated liver and kidney it is 1560 m/sec; this is sufficient difference to produce refraction for the curvature of the interfaces involved.

Images through a section of this phantom are shown in Fig. 4-32. The structures seen to the right of the kidney and fat pad are images of a set of thin nylon fibers whose axes are perpendicular to the plane of the image. Several fibers forming a backward L make up the set. The scan in Fig. 4-32, *A*, was obtained with a simple scan technique, no compound scan motion being employed. That in Fig. 4-32, *B*, from the same region of the phantom, shows significant distortion of the fiber images, due to transmission through the kidney and fat pad. It was produced by sectoring the transducer beam from several positions on the surface, including positions above the fat pad region. The effects on the fiber images are quite dramatic. With a simple phantom as this, it was possible to account for the reflections and refraction that make up the distorted image. The case presented shows the effects that beam deflection and refraction can have on a B-scan image. Under most clinical circumstances the geometry and complexity of the patient's anatomy make it difficult to recognize such artifacts, if indeed they exist, in clinical scans.

ADDITIONAL EXAMPLES OF BEAM DEFLECTION, SHADOWING, AND ENHANCEMENT

An intriguing artifact is frequently observed distal to the lateral margins of some cysts and vessels, including the gallbladder (Fig. 4-33). It is a shadowing effect below these areas. This also is a useful artifact since it sometimes aids in characterizing these structures.

Depending on the characteristics of the medium, the artifact may be related to attenuation of the sound beam through beam deflection and refraction at the vessel interface; it may also be partially due to attenuation in the vessel walls.

If the speed of sound through a circular object is lower than through the surrounding material, a sound beam incident on the edge

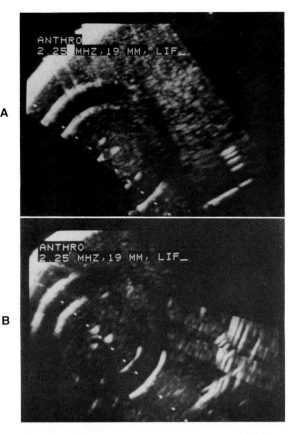

Fig. 4-32. B-scan images of a simulated kidney with surrounding fat pad in a tissue mimicking liver material. **A,** Simple single-pass scan. **B,** Compound scan. The nylon fibers were imaged with beams passing through the kidney and fat pad region, where they were severely deflected. (From Madsen, E., et al.: Med. Phys. **7:**43, 1980.)

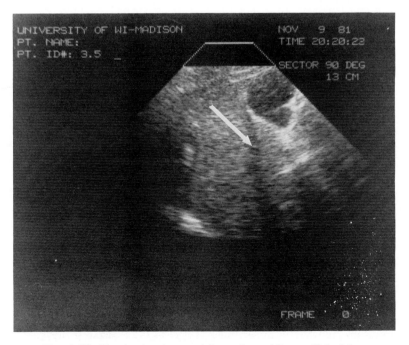

Fig. 4-33. Shadowing beyond the edge of the gallbladder.

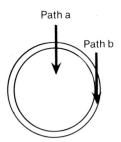

Fig. 4-34. If the walls of a structure are highly attenuating compared to the background, greater attenuation will occur for a sound beam that passes through the edge (path *b*) of the structure than through the middle (path *a*).

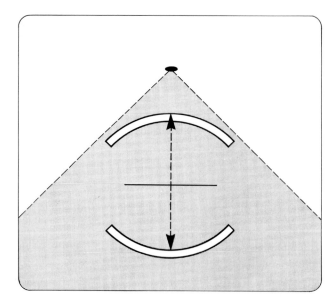

Fig. 4-35. Arrows illustrate the best choice of echo signal reference spots for distance measurements on echograms. The leading edge (with respect to the transducer position) of the echo signal is preferred.

of the object will be deflected in the manner shown in Fig. 1-17.[6] Beam spreading of this type is accompanied by significant attenuation. Reflectors situated distal to regions where beam spreading occurs will yield lower-level echo signals than if the beam is unperturbed. Thus the apparent partial shadow occurs.

Robinson et al.[6] and Madsen et al.[3] have both demonstrated that circular objects through which the speed of sound is lower than through the surrounding material also focus the acoustic energy transmitted directly through the object. This focusing contributes to echo enhancement beyond these structures. An important clinical example is the bile ducts distributed in the liver, which result in significant echo enhancement distal to them.

Another source of beam attenuation along the margins of cystic regions may be the walls of these structures. It is easy to see from Fig. 4-34 that the thickness of the wall material that must be traversed by the beam is greater at the periphery of the structure. If the attenuation coefficient of the wall is greater than that of the surrounding tissues, the increased path length will result in greater attenuation at the periphery.

In any case the edges of many cysts and vessels produce a so-called lateral shadow sign. A combination of the lateral shadow sign and the echo enhancement accompanying the transmission of sound through low-attenuating masses has come to be called the tadpole tail sign. This is evident in the image of the simulated walled cyst in Fig. 4-26, *A*.

SPEED OF SOUND ARTIFACTS

If the sound propagation path to a reflector is partially through bone, wherein the speed of sound is greater than in the average soft tissue (assumed in the calibration of an instrument), echo position registration artifacts will be produced. Reflectors appear *closer* to the transducer than their actual distance because of this greater speed of sound, resulting in a shorter echo transit time than for paths not containing bone.

The opposite effect is seen in Figs. 19-32 and 35-5. Here the sound propagation path is through silicone (breast implant) or a Silastic material (artificial heart valve), wherein the speed of sound is lower than in soft tissue. All structures distal to either of these two materials will appear *distal* with respect to their anatomic position because of this longer echo transit time.

DISTANCE, AREA, AND VOLUME COMPUTATIONS
Distance

Accurate measurements of organ and structure dimensions are possible in diagnostic ultrasound because the speed of sound in most soft tissues is known to within about 1%. By using an instrument's internal depth markers whose spacing corresponds to a known distance in tissue when a speed of sound of 1540 m/sec is assumed, a measurement accuracy to within 1% or 2% can usually be achieved. Even greater measurement accuracy can be obtained in ophthalmologic applications because of the use of high frequencies, careful scanning, and well-known speeds of sound in the media traversed.

Careful choice of measurement reference positions is necessary to realize maximum accuracy for distance measurements. On A-mode or B-mode displays the leading edge of the reflector echo signal is usually the best choice (Fig. 4-35). This point is least affected by variations in echo signal amplitude stemming from the reflectors themselves or the settings and characteristics of the instrument.

Of course, distance measurements are always more accurate if the direction over which the measurement extends corresponds to an ultrasonic beam axis orientation at the time the scan was done (Fig. 4-36). This is because the reflector position can be pinpointed more accurately since the axial resolution of a pulse-echo imaging system is generally better than the lateral resolution. In addition, any errors due to simple or compound scan position registration accuracy (discussed in Chapter 5) will not contribute to the distance measurement error if distances are measured along a sound beam axis.

Utilization of depth markers can be done reliably since these are produced by stable electronic circuitry and usually correspond to 1-cm depth intervals in tissue. Care required in proper utilization of depth markers requires that their calibration be checked routinely. This can be done as part of a normal quality assurance program for ultrasound equipment (Chapter 5). Also, primarily for manual scanners in which the depth markers can be produced at different orientations on the screen, caution must be exercised to avoid measurement inaccuracies due to TV monitor distortion. A common source of distortion is unequal display magnification in the horizontal and vertical directions. The distance on hard copy between two reflectors may appear different when measurements are obtained by means of depth markers produced in the vertical and the horizontal directions. Errors resulting from possible TV monitor distortion can be minimized if the depth markers are generated as closely as possible and in the same orientation as the line segment connecting the points to be measured. Proper and improper depth marker positioning is illustrated in Fig. 4-37.

Measurements can also be done with digital calipers on units having this feature. Operationally the digital calipers in many instruments determine the pixel separation between two specified points on the image and convert this to a distance. The user merely places the cursors on the two points between which a measurement is desired. The instrument determines the number of pixels separating the two cursors, multiplies this number by an appropriate magnification factor depending on the field of view, and provides a numerical readout of the distance in the patient (Fig. 4-38).

Digital caliper circuitry is also subject to error, and its calibration should be assessed routinely (Chapter 5).

Areas

In certain situations the cross-sectional area of a structure viewed on an echogram provides diagnostic information. For an object such as a rectangle the area is simple to compute. In some situations the area can be estimated by assuming a shape and applying appropriate formulas to the area measurement. For circles and ellipses the areas are presented in Fig. 4-39.

When a simple shape cannot be assumed for the object of interest, the area can be determined by using a *planimeter*. These devices are available from cartographers. By tracing the region of interest using the planimeter and then applying an appropriate conversion factor to change from unit area on the image to unit area in the patient, the operator can obtain a reasonable estimate of the area.

It is also quite simple to provide area analysis software in ultrasound imaging instruments so the area measurements can be made directly from the echogram. These schemes usually require the operator to trace the region of interest using a joystick or cursor; once this is carried out, the system can be programmed to first count the number of pixels enclosed by the outlined region. Each pixel can be thought of as a tiny piece of the area of the entire contour (Fig. 4-40); that

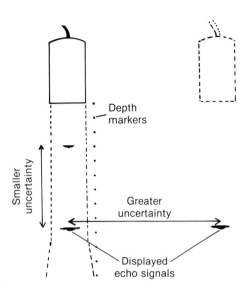

Fig. 4-36. From the standpoint of ultrasound beam width considerations, distance measurements along a transducer beam line of site are more accurate than measurements at an angle to the ultrasound beam.

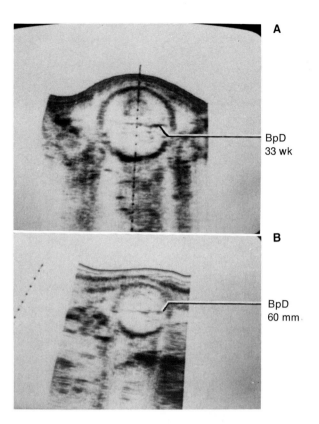

Fig. 4-37. Proper, **A,** and improper, **B,** positioning of depth markers on an image for biparietal diameter measurements.

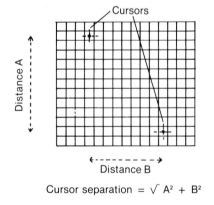

Cursor separation = $\sqrt{A^2 + B^2}$

Fig. 4-38. Operation of one type of digital caliper circuitry.

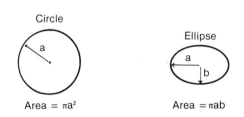

Circle

Area = πa^2

Ellipse

Area = πab

Fig. 4-39. Formulas for computing the area of a circle and an ellipse.

Fig. 4-40. Area algorithm by a digital instrument. The operator traces out the region of interest. A microprocessor in the instrument computes the number of pixels enclosed by the contour and multiplies by the area per pixel to obtain the contour area.

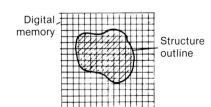

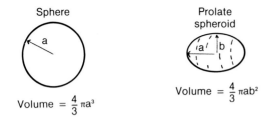

Fig. 4-41. Formulas for computing the volume of a sphere and a prolate spheroid.

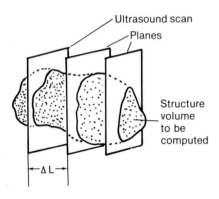

Fig. 4-42. Bread-slice approach to computing the volume of a structure from serial scans.

is, when the number of pixels within the contour is multiplied by an *area* magnification factor, the area enclosed by the contour may be estimated. Software such as this is available in some digital instruments.

Volumes

Ultrasound images can also be used to estimate the volumes of structures and organs. Such measurements may provide more sensitive indications of changes in structure dimensions than simple distance or area measurements.

Volume estimates are sometimes made by assuming a simple shape and using ultrasound scans to obtain the necessary dimensions to plug into equations for the volumes. In certain cases, for example, it is reasonable to estimate the volume by assuming that the shape is a sphere (Fig. 4-41). In this case the volume is that shown in the figure. Another common shape is a prolate spheroid, also shown in the figure.

For irregularly shaped structures in which a sphere or spheroid is not appropriate for estimating the volume, a serial scan approach can be followed. This technique, outlined in Fig. 4-42, is sometimes referred to as the *bread-slice* approach. Serial scans a known separation apart, ΔL, are obtained through the region of interest. Then the area of the structure in question is estimated for each echogram on which the structure is included. The area can be estimated by any of the methods just outlined.

The area multiplied by the distance between echograms represents a section of the volume, or one slice of the loaf of bread. Summing all the volume sections corresponding to each scan that cuts through the structure provides an estimate of the volume.

REFERENCES

1. Goldstein, A., and Madrazo, B.: Slice thickness artifact in gray-scale ultrasound, J. Clin. Ultrasound **9**:365, 1981.
2. Lizzi, F., Burt, W., and Coleman, D.: Effects of ocular structures on the propagation of ultrasound in the eye, Arch. Ophthalmol. **84**:635, 1970.
3. Madsen, E., Zagzebski, J., Frank, G., et al.: Three anthropomorphic breast phantoms for assessing ultrasonic imaging system performance, J. Clin. Ultrasound **10**:91, 1982.
4. Madsen, E., Zagzebski, J., and Ghilardi-Netto, T.: An anthropomorphic torso phantom for ultrasonic imaging, Med. Phys. **7**:43, 1980.
5. Robinson, D., Kossoff, G., and Garrett, W.: Artifacts in ultrasonic echoscope examinations, Ultrasonics **4**:186, 1966.
6. Robinson, D., Wilson, L., and Kossoff, G.: Shadowing and enhancement in ultrasonic echograms by reflection and refraction, J. Clin. Ultrasound **9**:181, 1981.
7. Skolnick, M., Meire, H., and Lecky, J.: Common artifacts in ultrasound scanning, J. Clin. Ultrasound **3**:273, 1975.
8. Zagzebski, J., Madsen, E., Frank, G., et al.: A teaching phantom for ultrasonographers. Program and abstracts, 26th annual meeting of the American Institute of Ultrasound in Medicine, San Francisco, August, 1981.

5 Instrument quality assurance

JAMES A. ZAGZEBSKI

In diagnostic ultrasound the term *quality assurance* refers to steps that are taken to satisfy ourselves that an instrument is operating consistently at its expected level of performance. In a general sense quality assurance encompasses an entire gamut of checks and measures that are part of the routine operation of an ultrasound department. In this chapter one aspect of a quality assurance program will be discussed: *objective tests* for evaluating the performance of ultrasound instruments. When done routinely, such tests help document gradual deterioration of instrument performance and provide a more objective means of assessing operating consistency than can be obtained, for example, from impressions of image quality on clinical scans. A quality assurance program requires initial planning, routine performance measurements, careful analysis of results and record keeping, and follow-through on corrective action.

TEST OBJECTS AND PHANTOMS

Phantoms and test objects have been developed that facilitate performance measurements of ultrasound systems. Such devices are useful insofar as they provide stable sources of echo signals in known geometric configurations. A *test object* is a device used to measure some aspect of ultrasound system performance. Included are the AIUM 100 mm test object[1]; the sensitivity, uniformity, and axial resolution (SUAR) test object[5]; and the electronic burst generator.[4] A *tissue-mimicking phantom* is a device that closely simulates actual tissues in the transmission of ultrasound. Both anthropomorphic phantoms[11] and phantoms for specific quality assurance testing of instruments[3] have been described.

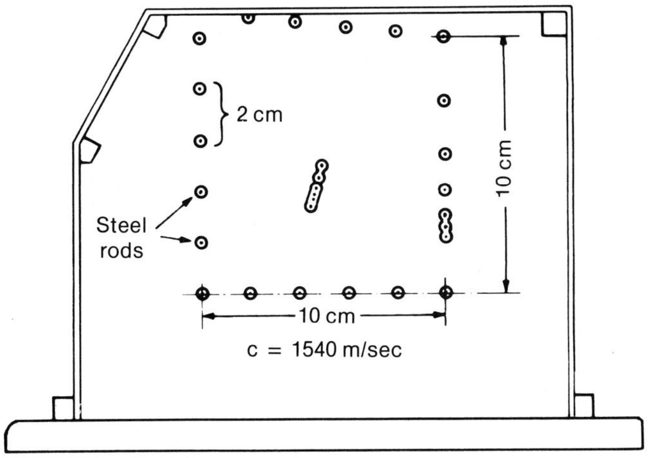

AIUM 100-mm test object

A diagram of the standard AIUM 100-mm test object is presented in Fig. 5-1. It consists of a series of stainless steel reflectors arranged as targets for geometric tests of ultrasound pulse-echo instruments. The reflectors are immersed in a liquid medium in which the speed of sound is 1540 m/sec. Both an open and an enclosed version of the test object are available.

The important features of the AIUM 100 mm standard test object are summarized as follows:

Standardized reflectors (0.75-mm diameter stainless steel rods)

Standard geometric arrangement for reflectors

Speed of sound, 1540 m/sec

The speed of sound of 1540 m/sec is obtained using water *plus* an additive. For example, 8% ethyl alcohol (by volume) added to ordinary water at 22° C (approximately room temperature) results in the correct speed of sound.[1] Plain tap water alone will not do and should not be used to fill the test object. The speed of sound in water is only 1480 m/sec, a value that is 3% too low. On some tests this could lead to significant errors. Small temperature variations should not pose a major problem with the test object's use since speed of sound variations of only about 0.1% per degree Celsius are typical. If a test object is purchased that is already

Fig. 5-1. Enclosed version of the standard AIUM 100-mm test object.

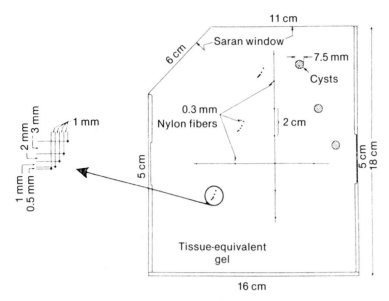

Fig. 5-2. One version of a tissue-mimicking phantom. (Courtesy Radiation Measurements, Inc., Middleton, Wisconsin.)

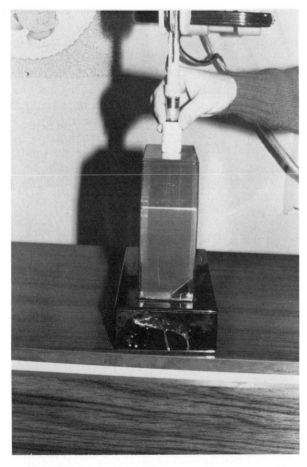

Fig. 5-3. Phantom/test object setup for performance checking of large manual scanners. In this position the tilt is adjusted so the transducer beam is perpendicular to the phantom surface.

filled with an appropriate liquid, one need only verify that the speed of sound in the liquid is indeed 1540 m/sec. Test objects that require filling can be filled following a formula supplied with the test object or available in the references.[5,7]

A 100-mm test object built according to the American Institute of Ultrasound in Medicine standard specifications consists of stainless steel rods, 0.75 mm in diameter, as reflectors. The extreme rods on each side of the test object are separated by 100 mm. This should be verified with a ruler.

Tissue-mimicking phantoms

The utilization of a tissue-mimicking material in a test object or phantom provides the capability of testing equipment performance under conditions that more closely simulate clinical conditions than do simple liquid-filled test objects. Several types of tissue phantoms, including those with anthropomorphic shapes[10,11] and with fixed geometry targets[3] have been developed.

Ideally materials for use in ultrasound phantoms should have the same density, speed of sound, ultrasonic attenuation properties and acoustic scattering characteristics as the tissues they represent. Acoustic properties of specific soft tissues were discussed in Chapter 1. A number of different types of materials have been described for use in phantoms.[13] In these materials the speeds of sound, attenuation properties, and to some extent ultrasonic scattering can be varied to match those properties in tissues.

The phantom shown in Fig. 5-2 has been developed for quality assurance testing of ultrasound instruments. The tissue-mimicking material consists of a water-based gelatin in which microscopic graphite particles are mixed uniformly throughout its volume. The ultrasonic properties of the material are as follows:

Speed of sound, 1540 m/sec
Ultrasonic attenuation, 0.65 dB/cm/MHz
Attenuation proportional to frequency
0.3-mm nylon fiber reflectors
Parenchyma-like ultrasonic scatter

An important characteristic of the material is that its ultrasonic attenuation coefficient is controllable; thus specific tissues can be mimicked. Very significantly the *ultrasonic attenuation* in the material has nearly the *same frequency dependence as that in most soft tissues*. This is not the case for all materials being employed in tissue phantoms. Having the same frequency dependence allows a phantom to be used effectively with different-frequency transducers. Moreover, it distorts ultrasonic pulses and sound beams similarly to soft tissues.[12]

The simulated cysts are low-attenuating scatter-free cylinders. Discrete reflectors consisting of nylon fibers are distributed in arrangements for checking distance calibration, resolution, and registration accuracy.

Some tissue phantoms provide image contrast from one region to another. This can be done fairly easily by varying the scatter level, the ultrasonic attenuation, or both.

Phantom setup for equipment performance tests

In assessing performance of large manual scanners the first step is to position the phantom properly. This requires a flat rigid surface that can be placed in the same position as the patient would be during routine clinical scans. It is best to avoid using soft patient couches since some tests require that the phantom remain perfectly stationary while being scanned. Proper positioning also requires the phantom and the instrument scanning arm be oriented so the transducer face can be placed flush with all windows. Start with the top window and adjust the scan plane tilt so the transducer face can be placed flush with the surface (Fig. 5-3). Then orient the phantom so the transducer face is flush with one side window (Fig. 5-4, A). Finally, be sure the transducer face can also be placed flush with the opposite side without moving the phantom (Fig. 5-4, B).

For hand-held automatic scanners, simply place the phantom on a rigid table.

CHOICE OF TRANSDUCER

For scanners that employ interchangeable transducers or transducer assemblies, choose a transducer that will become a *standard* for all test procedures. In general, 3.5-MHz and higher frequencies are preferred for tests using tissue phantoms. Be sure to record all necessary transducer assembly identification information so future tests will be conducted with the same transducer.

INSTRUMENT SENSITIVITY CONTROLS

If a liquid-filled test object (e.g., the AIUM 100-mm) is used, sensitivity controls, including those adjusting the output power and the receiver gain, should be set fairly low. Usually no swept gain (TGC) is applied because there is very little sound beam attenuation in the test object liquid. Also the stainless steel rod reflectors produce very large-amplitude echo signals, requiring little if any amplification for their visualization on a display. (Some authors[5] have recommended

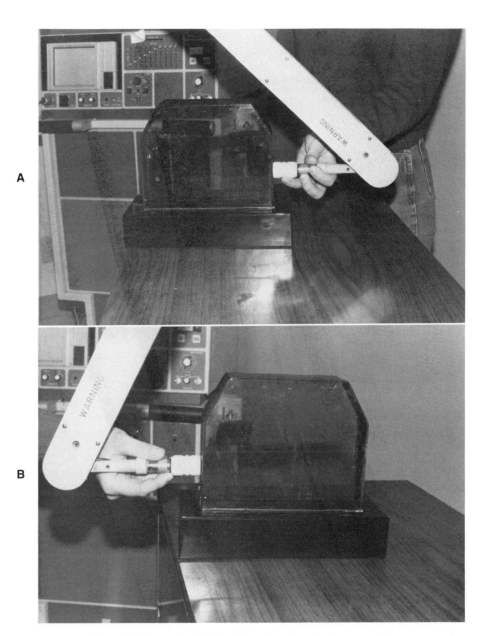

Fig. 5-4. Steps in orienting the phantom before scanning.

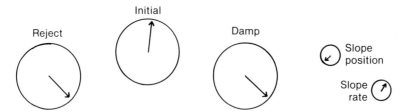

Fig. 5-5. Chart documenting equipment sensitivity controls for performance tests (ATL 600 B pulse-echo instrument; RMI 412 phantom). When optimal control settings are determined for an instrument, these should be used for future performance tests.

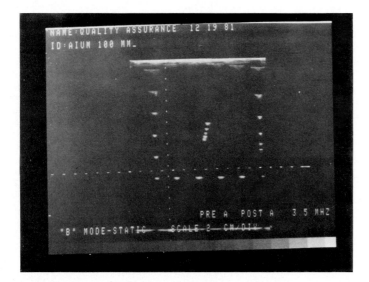

Fig. 5-6. Image of the AIUM 100-mm test object, along with horizontal and vertical depth markers, for checking distance calibration accuracy and image distortion. The image includes a column of reflectors spaced in 2-cm increments.

a procedure for sensitivity control determination involving a sensitivity threshold for displaying the reflectors.) If a tissue phantom is employed, sensitivity control settings similar to those employed during patient scans will be necessary, including swept gain to compensate for attenuation. It is convenient to keep a record of the sensitivity control settings used for performance tests to help assure reproducibility of results (Fig. 5-5).

DISTANCE CALIBRATION ACCURACY; IMAGE DISTORTION

Instruments that are used for measuring structure dimensions should be tested periodically for accuracy of distance indicators. These usually include 1-cm depth markers on A-mode, M-mode, and B-mode scanning displays and digital calipers on some B-mode scanning systems.

A column or row of reflectors with known spacing is used for this test. Both the AIUM 100-mm test object and some tissue phantoms contain appropriate reflectors. A single-pass linear scan of the phantom is obtained and depth markers are positioned vertically and, if possible, horizontally on the image (Fig. 5-6). A set of dividers may be used to compare the image distance between reflectors spaced 10 cm apart with the depth markers positioned along the same direction (Fig. 5-7, A and B). The distances should agree to within 1 or 2 mm.

If a discrepancy exists in this comparison, it may be due to either of two sources:
1. The speed of sound in the medium in the test object or phantom may not be close enough to 1540 m/sec. Allowable tolerance is about 1%. Also the reflectors may not be positioned properly.
2. An error exists in the depth marker circuitry of the instrument.

The first source of error listed might be suspected if a new test object or phantom is being used for the first time, especially one that requires filling by the user prior to its employment. Comparisons of the same test by different ultrasound instruments and intercomparison of different test objects may pinpoint the fault as most likely originating from source 1 or 2 above. Normal temperature variations in the speed of sound (0.1% per degree Celsius) ordinarily are not a factor.

Distortion on video monitors used for photographing images can cause slight differences between the magnification scale factors in the horizontal and vertical directions. (Of course, we would expect these magnification factors to be exactly the same.) One way to test for distortion is to use the target spacing employed above and compare it with distances as indicated by orthogonally positioned depth markers (Fig. 5-7, C). Differences in the indicated distances greater than 3% should be noted.

For precise distance measurements on B-scan images, the depth markers should always be positioned on the image as closely as possible and in the same orientation as the line joining the two points being measured (Fig. 4-37, A). Then, even if there is significant distortion, accurate distance measurements are still possible because the depth marker image will suffer the same distortion as the B-scan image itself.

DIGITAL CALIPER CHECKS

Digital caliper circuitry provides a readout of the distance between two cursors that may be positioned anywhere on a B-scan display. The readout accuracy is assessed by the same scan just produced. Position the cursors to measure the distance between reflectors just utilized for depth calibration checks (Fig. 5-8). When positioning the cursors, be sure that the center of the cross hairs is placed in the same relative position on the two rod images being used, as shown in the figure. The best policy is to place them on the *leading edge* (with respect to the transducer position when the scan was done) of the rod images, since this point will be least susceptible to variations introduced by echo amplitude changes, gain variations, etc. (In Fig. 5-8, A, note a 2% error in the caliper readout, 10.2 cm for a 10 cm spacing.)

It may be useful to assess the accuracy of digital calipers placed in an orthogonal direction as well. Here the cursors should be placed so they read out the distance between centers of the imaged rods situated at the extreme ends of a row of targets (Fig. 5-8, B). The center of a rod image corresponds to the displayed echo position when the axis of the transducer beam is directly over a reflector.

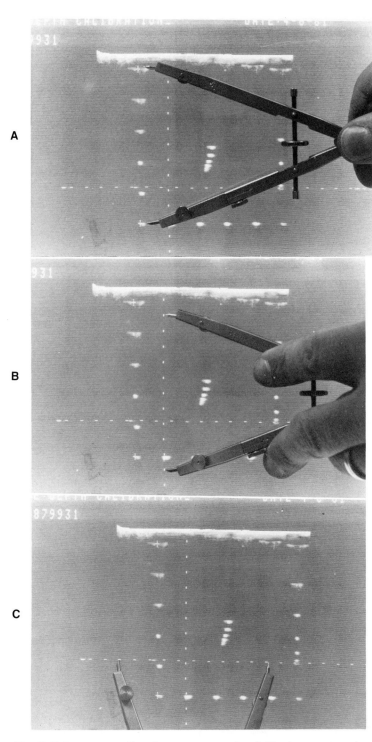

Fig. 5-7. Distance calibration accuracy check. The image spacing for the 10-cm reflector separation, **A,** is checked with the vertical depth markers, **B.** Checking the same image spacing using the horizontal depth markers, **C,** allows image distortion to be detected.

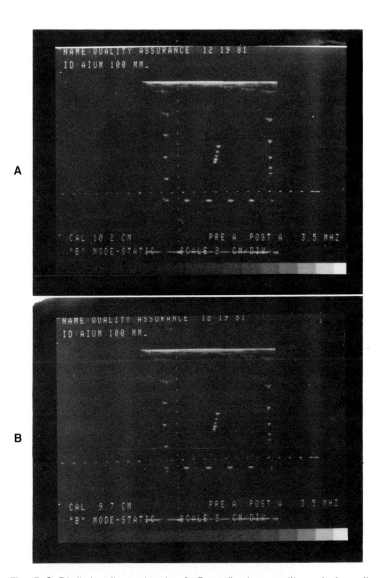

Fig. 5-8. Digital caliper checks. **A,** For reflectors positioned along the axis of the transducer. **B,** For reflectors perpendicular to the transducer axis.

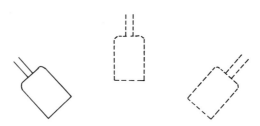

Fig. 5-9. Compound-position registration accuracy.

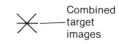

Combined target images

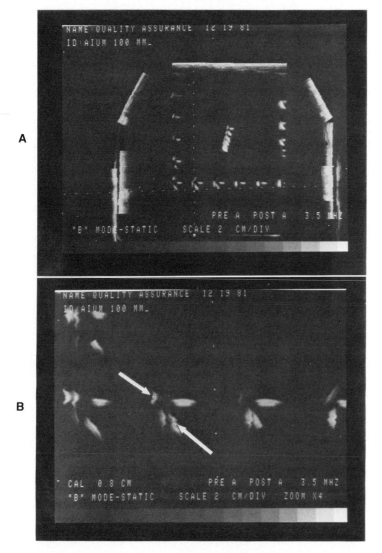

Fig. 5-10. Measurement of compound-position registration accuracy. **A,** Large field of view. **B,** Magnified image. The error to quote in this example is 8 mm, corresponding to the maximum separation of centers of the target images from a single reflector *(arrows).*

(There is a 3% error in the digital caliper readout in the example shown, 9.7 cm for a 10 cm reflector separation.) Even when the centers of the B-scan marks from the reflectors are being used, it is difficult to provide a measurement to within 3 mm for a reflector spacing of 100 mm on the image. The best results for any distance measurement on a clinical scan are obtained when the measurement line is along the axis of the transducer beam.

COMPOUND SCAN POSITION REGISTRATION ACCURACY

When a small point or line target is scanned from different directions with a manual scanner, the resultant B-mode image should consist of a series of crossing lines (Fig. 5-9). When the instrument is performing properly, the *centers* of individual images of a given reflector will coincide, forming an asterisk, as shown in the figure. The accuracy with which an instrument positions echo signals from a single reflector on the display, when the reflector is scanned from different transducer orientations in a fixed scanning plane, is referred to as the *compound position registration accuracy.*

Compound position registration accuracy is determined by scanning test object targets from several windows. Caution should be exercised to ensure that the test object remains perfectly stationary during the scan. On the resultant scan, pick out the reflector for which individual image lines appear farthest apart. Measure the distance between the *centers* of the individual lines and report the registration error as the largest distance between rod image centers (Fig. 5-10).

Any error in the speed of sound in the test object medium would contribute to apparent compound-position registration errors.[7] Therefore it is necessary to be sure that the acoustic properties of the test object are within specification.

SIMPLE SCAN REGISTRATION ACCURACY

There is an analogous position registration measurement for hand-held automatic scanners. With these instruments individual reflectors are not imaged from different orientations; however, echo position computation circuitry still comes into play during image buildup. *Simple scan registration accuracy* refers to the accuracy with which reflectors a known distance apart are positioned on the display for sector and sequential-array scanners (Fig. 5-11). Depending on the measurement options available on the instrument,

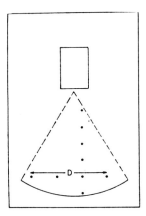

Fig. 5-11. Simple scan registration accuracy for hand-held automatic scanners.

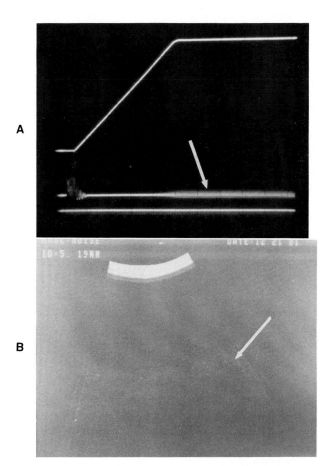

Fig. 5-12. Electric noise. **A,** On an A-mode display. **B,** On a B-mode display.

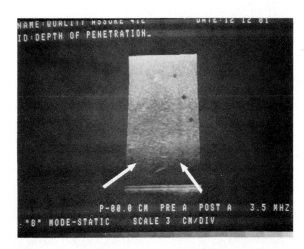

Fig. 5-13. Scan to assess the maximum depth of penetration *(arrows)* for detection of parenchymal echos from a tissue phantom.

this parameter may be included during digital caliper checks. The test and analysis are rather straightforward, involving a simple image and measurement of the separation of reflectors positioned perpendicular to the central beam axis.

VARIATIONS IN THE MAXIMUM SENSITIVITY

The *sensitivity* of an instrument refers to the weakest echo signal level that can be detected and displayed clearly enough to be discernible. Most instruments have controls that vary the receiver amplification and the output power. These are used to adjust the sensitivity during clinical examinations. When the controls are positioned for their maximum sensitivity settings, we refer to the *maximum sensitivity* of an instrument. Often the maximum sensitivity is limited by electric noise on the display (Fig. 5-12). The noise may be generated externally, for example, by electronic communication networks or computer terminals. It may also arise from within the instrument itself.

To allow use of higher-frequency ultrasound transducers for imaging large structures and organs, various steps have been taken to improve the maximum sensitivity on instruments. For example, in Chapter 2 it was pointed out that the use of quarter-wave matching layers on the transducer assembly improves the sensitivity. Other instrument components for establishing the maximum sensitivity include the pulser, the receiver, and the echo display chain. In addition to these, a frequent source of reduction in the maximum sensitivity is frail cables, especially those connecting the transducer assembly to the instrument. They may be damaged by twisting and bending when the transducer assembly is being handled.

During routine performance tests *varia-* *tions* in the maximum sensitivity of an instrument are most easily monitored (as opposed to measuring the *absolute* maximum sensitivity). One way of detecting variations in maximum sensitivity is to measure the depth of penetration for parenchymal echoes obtained from a tissue-mimicking phantom such as the one shown in Fig. 5-2. Receiver sensitivity controls are adjusted so the echo signals will be obtained from as deep as possible into the phantom. (Experience helps in establishing these control settings; they should be recorded as in Fig. 5-5.) The phantom is scanned and the maximum depth of penetration estimated (Fig. 5-13). In addition to doing this measurement using the standard transducer, it may be useful to perform the test occasionally using different

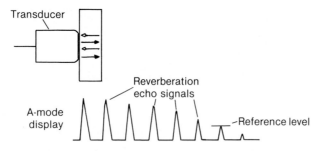

Fig. 5-14. A-mode display of echo signals from an acrylic block. This monitors changes in system sensitivity.

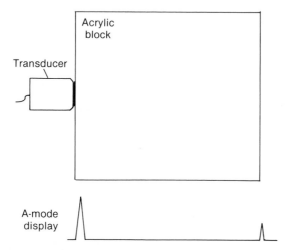

Fig. 5-15. Thick attenuating block for detecting changes in the sensitivity of an instrument.

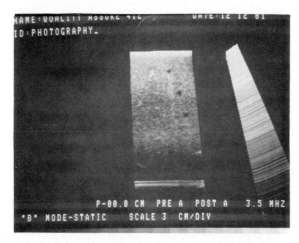

Fig. 5-16. Gray scale photography testing. This is done by determining whether both large-amplitude echo level variations and weak parenchymal echoes are successfully recorded on the image.

transducers. This would then help to pinpoint the source of any decrease in the maximum sensitivity or at least determine whether the standard transducer was at fault.

Alternative methods for monitoring variations in maximum sensitivity involve displaying echo signals from a reflecting surface, such as the side of a plastic block. One implementation of this technique involves coupling the transducer to a 2-to-4-cm thick block of acrylic and displaying the resultant A-mode waveform. Standard gain and power settings are used from one test date to another. Although the block attenuates the sound beam to a degree, it is thin enough to let multiple echo signals resulting from reverberations be detected (Fig. 5-14). Reduction in the echo signal amplitudes during routine monitoring means a reduction in the overall sensitivity of the instrument. Perhaps a better approach, although very similar, is to utilize a thick acrylic block and note the sensitivity control settings required to display an echo signal at some reference level from the distal end of the block (Fig. 5-15). Variation in the required settings indicates a change in the sensitivity of the instrument.

GRAY SCALE PHOTOGRAPHY

Gray scale photography is usually evaluated critically during routine patient scans. Again, slow deterioration can be documented if routine quality assurance tests are carried out and the results recorded.

In the discussion of film and recording media characteristics in Chapter 3, it was pointed out that camera or strip chart recorder exposure controls should be adjusted in a way that all brightness variations on the monitor due to echo amplitude changes are successfully recorded on the hard-copy image. Images of a tissue-mimicking phantom, along with the gray bar pattern appearing on the edge of most monitors, can be used for assessing photography.

On an image of a tissue phantom, check to see whether weak echo signals (e.g., those appearing near the maximum depth of detection of parenchymal echoes) are successfully recorded. It is useful to compare the hard-copy image directly with the same image left displayed on the instrument monitor. (This will have to be done in minutes if an analog scan converter is used because the analog scan converter's image fades with time.) When the photography controls are properly adjusted, the weak echo signals will be visible above the background at the same time that brightness changes produced by variations of large-amplitude echoes are de-

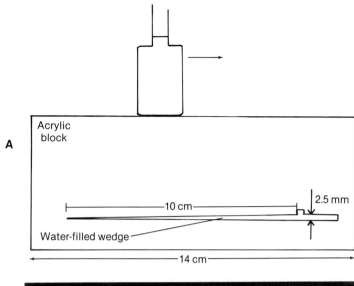

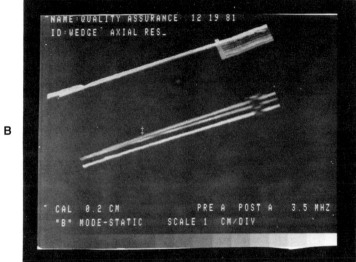

Fig. 5-17. A, SUAR test object for measuring axial resolution. **B,** Image of the SUAR test object.

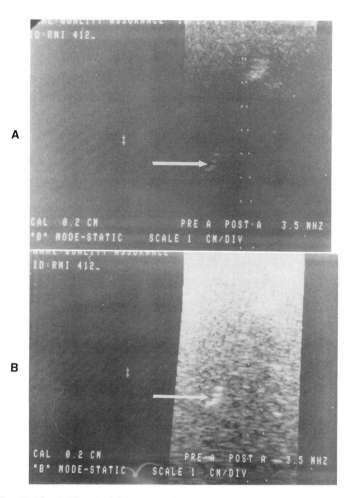

Fig. 5-18. A, Threshold image of axial resolution fibers in the tissue-mimicking phantom shown in Fig. 5-2. **B,** Image of the same reflectors after the sensitivity is increased 20 dB. This yields a measure of the −20-dB axial resolution.

tectable. On systems with a built-in gray bar test pattern the large-amplitude echo signal variations can be assumed to be successfully recorded if contrast between the corresponding high-level section of the gray bar pattern is easily visible (Fig. 5-16). Additional high-level echo signals can be obtained by coupling a small metallic object such as a coin to the transducer surface and arcing the transducer, producing the additional echo patch shown.

SPATIAL RESOLUTION TESTS

The quality assurance tests outlined above form a useful battery of procedures that can be done and the results analyzed fairly quickly. Meaningful tests of both axial and lateral resolution require more exacting procedures, since measurement results are a function of the sensitivity control settings of the instrument.

One approach that has been used for resolution tests is to define the resolution with respect to a threshold level on the B-scan display. This will be described for *axial* resolution tests in this section. Similar procedures can be followed for lateral resolution measurements, but they will not be described here.

One requirement for quantitative resolution tests is a calibrated sensitivity control on the instrument. If this is not available, you should consult the instrument manufacturer or a physicist or engineer who may be able to provide such a calibration. The axial resolution fibers in the phantom shown in Fig. 5-2, or a planar wedge[5] may be used. The latter test object, (shown in Fig. 5-17) is advan-

tageous because it provides a continuous reflector spacing. The discrete targets, of course, are only steps in the distance between reflectors. Reflectors are imaged at a sensitivity level for which they are just barely discernible on the display (Fig. 5-18). Then a calibrated control is adjusted to increase the sensitivity by a fixed amount (e.g., 20 dB) and the scan is repeated. On the resultant image the reflector spacing that can be resolved is quoted as the axial resolution at the level below threshold corresponding to the sensitivity control increase above.

OTHER HINTS

During routine performance testing it is a good idea to perform other equipment-related chores that require occasional attention. These include cleaning air filters on instruments requiring this service, checking for loose and frayed electric cables, noting any loose handles or control arms on the scanner, and performing recommended preventive maintenance of photography equipment. The last may include dusting or cleaning of photographic monitors and cleaning the developing rollers in Polaroid cameras.

THE QUALITY ASSURANCE NOTEBOOK

To complete the procedure on a given day, it is necessary to document the results of the performance checks. This is best done by using a *quality control notebook*, in which a log of the test results, along with appropriate images, can be kept. It may be desirable to develop a *worksheet*, such as the one shown in Appendix G, to serve as a reminder of the data that should be recorded, provide guidance on fields of view (display magnifications) and sensitivity controls appropriate for a given test, and furnish space for recording of results.

It is also useful to maintain a log of equipment malfunctions and equipment service calls in the quality control data book for each instrument. This information provides fairly complete documentation of the operating and performance characteristics of an instrument over a time.

REFERENCES

1. AIUM standard 100 mm test object, and recommendations for its use, Reflections 1:74, 1975.
2. AIUM standard specification of echoscope sensitivity and signal to noise level, including recommended practice for such measurements, Reflections 5:41, 1979.
3. Burlew, M., Madsen, E., Zagzebski, J., et al.: A new ultrasound tissue-equivalent material with a high melting point and extended speed of sound range, Radiology 134:517, 1980.
4. Carson, P.: Rapid evaluation of many pulse echo system characteristics by use of a triggered pulse burst generator with exponential decay, J. Clin. Ultrasound 4:259, 1976.
5. Carson, P., and Dubuque, G.: Ultrasound equipment quality control procedures, CRP Report no. A3, 1979.
6. Carson, P., and Zagzebski, J.: Pulse echo ultrasound imaging systems: performance tests and criteria, AAPM Report no. 8, 1980.
7. Goldstein, A.: Quality assurance in diagnostic ultrasound, Washington, D.C., 1980, AIUM.
8. Lopez, H., and Smith, S.: Implementation of a quality assurance program for ultrasound B-scanners, HEW Publication no. 80-8100, 1979.
9. Madsen, E., Zagzebski, J., Banjavic, R., and Jutila, R.: Tissue mimicking material for ultrasound phantoms, Med. Phys. 5:391, 1978.
10. Madsen, E., Zagzebski, J., Frank, G., et al.: Three anthropomorphic breast phantoms for assessing ultrasonic imaging systems performance for training ultrasonographers, J. Clin. Ultrasound 10:91, 1982.
11. Madsen, E., Zagzebski, J., and Ghilardi-Netto, T.: An anthropomorphic torso phantom for ultrasonic imaging, Med. Phys. 7:43, 1980.
12. Zagzebski, J., Banjavic, R., Madsen, E., and Schwabe, M.: Focused transducer beams in tissue-mimicking material, J. Clin. Ultrasound. 10:159, 1982.
13. Zagzebski, J., and Madsen, E.: Tissue equivalent materials and phantoms. In Wells, P., and Ziskin, M., editors: New techniques and instrumentation in ultrasonography, vol. 5, New York, 1979, Churchill Livingstone, Inc.

6

Bioeffects and safety considerations

JAMES A. ZAGZEBSKI

The passage of sound through a medium involves acceleration and displacement of particles in the medium as well as localized forces and stresses. When sound wave transmission is through tissues, the possibilities of biologic effects, no matter how remote, come into question. It is well known that ultrasound beams of sufficient intensity can modify and even damage biologic tissues. It is not known, however, whether *diagnostic ultrasound beams* produced during clinical studies can cause harmful effects. The vast experience that has been gained with clinical ultrasound equipment has been accompanied by no known tissue damage.[11] Thus we are led to believe that diagnostic ultrasound is "safe" or, at least, is accompanied by a low risk of producing biologic effects. Unfortu-

nately insufficient experimental data exist at present to satisfactorily define this risk factor. Research laboratories continue therefore to investigate effects of low-level ultrasound on biologic tissues.

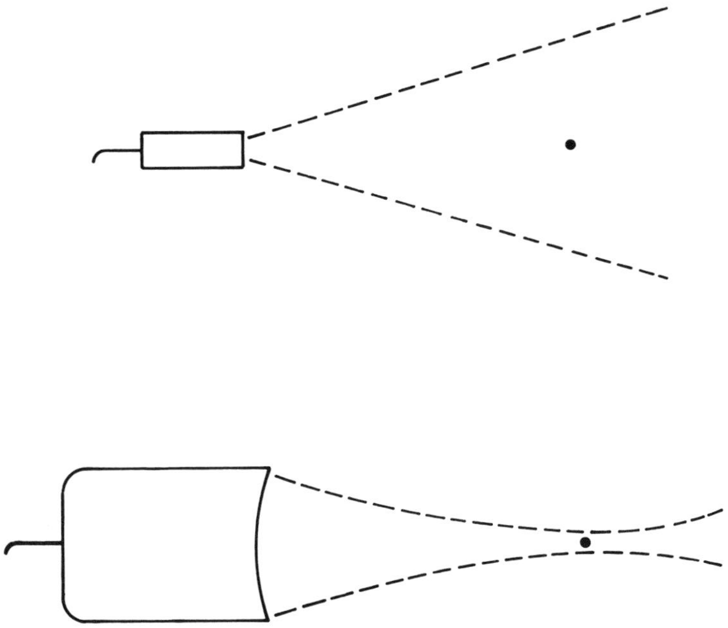

In this chapter important acoustic exposure quantities for diagnostic instruments are outlined briefly, with discussion of the methods used to measure these parameters. The topic of ultrasound bioeffects also is considered, especially as it relates to the operation of clinical ultrasound scanning equipment.

ACOUSTIC POWER; ACOUSTIC INTENSITY

An ultrasound source transmits energy into the medium with which it is in contact. To quantify the amount of acoustic energy transmitted and describe how this energy is distributed, physicists and engineers measure the *acoustic power* and the *acoustic intensity* in the beam.

Power is the *rate* at which energy is transmitted from the transducer into the medium. Appropriate units for power are watts (W) or milliwatts (mW). (Not surprisingly, these are the same units [watts] that are used to specify the rate of energy consumption by electric appliances.) The acoustic power emitted by a diagnostic ultrasound transducer transmitting into tissue is typically on the order of 1 to 10 mW.

Simply specifying the power results in a very incomplete description of the situation, because the distribution of this ultrasonic energy also needs to be taken into account. For example, suppose the acoustic power for each of the two transducers shown in Fig. 6-1 is the same. Our own intuition tells us that the two cases shown could result in substantially different effects. In one case the ultrasonic energy is distributed over a fairly broad region whereas in the other it is concentrated through focusing. Variations in the spatial

Fig. 6-1. Even if the acoustic power from these two transducers were the same, the intensity of the beam at the point marked on each beam axis could be significantly different.

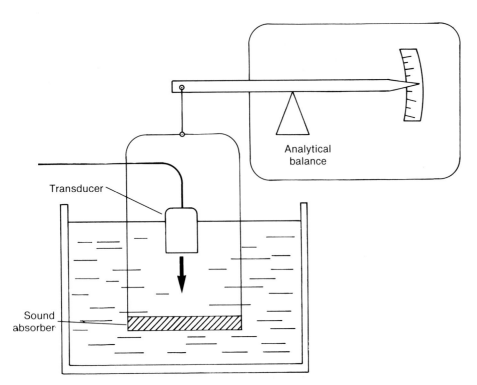

Fig. 6-2. Schematic of the measurement of ultrasonic power by a radiation force balance.

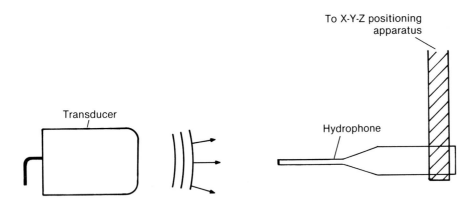

Fig. 6-3. Miniature hydrophone in position to measure the acoustic intensity at a point in the beam of an ultrasound transducer.

An alternative, although less commonly used, technique for measuring total acoustic power from diagnostic ultrasound instruments is *calorimetry*. Here the ultrasound beam is transmitted into a liquid. Sensitive thermal monitoring apparatus is used to determine a temperature elevation in the liquid caused by absorption of the ultrasonic energy. The temperature change can be related directly to the acoustic power.

For dosimetric purposes the shape of the ultrasound beam and the intensity distribution within the beam are measured by a miniature hydrophone (Fig. 6-3). Such a device consists of a small-diameter probe with a piezoelectric element, usually 0.5 to 1 mm in diameter, at one end. When placed in an ultrasound beam, the hydrophone produces an electric signal whose amplitude is proportional to the acoustic pressure amplitude. If this signal is squared, the resultant signal is proportional to the instantaneous intensity at the position of the hydrophone face. Thus hydrophones may be used to map the *relative* intensity distributions of ultrasound beams. For some applications hydrophones are calibrated by measuring their response in an acoustic beam whose intensity is known. When this is done, the hydrophone will measure the absolute intensity at points in a sound beam.

PEAKS AND AVERAGES

The intensity of a diagnostic ultrasound beam turns out to be a complicated quantity to specify and measure.

One reason for this is the point-to-point variation in intensity within the ultrasound beam. To avoid the need to describe the complete beam point by point, acceptable parameterization schemes for sound fields have been defined.

For diagnostic instruments both the *spatial average intensity*, I(SA), at a specified distance from the transducer and the *spatial peak intensity*, I(SP), are used frequently. The I(SA) is equal to the acoustic power, P, contained within the beam, divided by the beam area, A:

$$I(SA) = \frac{P}{A} \qquad (6\text{-}1)$$

Example: If the ultrasonic power emitted by a 2-cm diameter transducer is 10 mW, what is the spatial average intensity at the transducer surface? (See Fig. 6-4.)

Solution: The intensity averaged over the area of the sound beam at the transducer surface is equal to the acoustic power divided by the beam area. Very close to the transducer surface, take the

distribution of the ultrasonic power are described by specifying the *intensity* at different points in a beam. Intensity is the ultrasonic power per unit area, given in watts per square meter (W/m²) or, more commonly, milliwatts per square centimeter (mW/cm²).

MEASUREMENTS OF POWER AND INTENSITY

Several methods are available for measuring the two dosimetric quantities listed.

Practical measurements of the very low ultrasonic power levels produced by diagnostic instruments can be carried out by measuring the *radiation force*, a small steady force that is produced when a sound beam strikes a reflecting or an absorbing interface.

It may be measured by a laboratory force balance (Fig. 6-2). If the acoustic power is 10 mW, the resultant force is roughly equal to the weight of a stationary drop of water 1 mm in diameter.* (Anyone who may have tried to weigh a drop of water this size knows that this is a very small force indeed!) Although of very low magnitude, the force can be measured by using sensitive analytical balances. The radiation force is directly related to the ultrasonic power through a simple conversion factor.*

---

*For an absorbing target (e.g., that in Fig. 6-2) the radiation force produced by a 1-mW beam is equal to the weight of a 68-μg mass. This assumes ultrasonic transmission into water and no reflection at the water-absorbing target interface.

beam area, A, as being equal to the area of the transducer.

$$A = \pi r^2 \quad (6\text{-}2)$$

where r is the transducer radius and π is 3.14. Thus

$$A = 3.14 \times (1 \text{ cm})^2$$
$$= 3.14 \text{ cm}^2$$

Solving for the spatial average intensity, $I(SA)$, gives

$$\frac{P}{A} = \frac{10 \text{ mW}}{3.14 \text{ cm}^2} \simeq 3 \text{ mW/cm}^2$$

The spatial average intensity is approximately equal to 3 mW/cm² at the transducer surface.

The I(SP) is the maximum intensity in the sound field. For the single-element transducer illustrated in Fig. 6-4 it is usually along the axis, near the focal distance. The spatial peak intensity is usually 3 to 4 times greater than the spatial average intensity at the transducer surface for unfocused transducers. For focused probes the I(SP) may exceed the I(SA) at the transducer surface by a factor of 10 or more.

A second reason contributing to the complexity of measuring the acoustic intensity for many ultrasound beams is the temporal variation in intensity when pulsed ultrasound is used. If the intensity is averaged over the time between pulses, a relatively low value is obtained, called the *time average intensity*, I(TA). However, the instantaneous peak intensity, I(IP), during the time of the pulse may exceed the I(TA) by a factor of 1000 or more.

The situation is illustrated schematically in Fig. 6-5. The top waveform in this figure might correspond to the signal detected when a hydrophone is positioned in the beam of a pulsed transducer. (We are assuming a somewhat idealized pulse, ignoring variations in amplitude during the pulse itself.) This waveform is a brief steadily repeating signal. The number of signals produced in a second is the pulse-repetition frequency (prf). The time interval from the beginning of one pulse to the beginning of the next is called the pulse repetition period (τ), given by

$$\tau = \frac{1}{\text{prf}} \quad (6\text{-}3)$$

It is possible to compute the relationship between the I(TA) and the I(IP). To do this, we must also know the *duty factor*, the fraction of time that the transducer is emitting sound. If the pulse duration (illustrated in Fig. 6-5) is *pd*, then the duty factor, *DF*, is simply

$$DF = \frac{pd}{\tau} \quad (6\text{-}4)$$

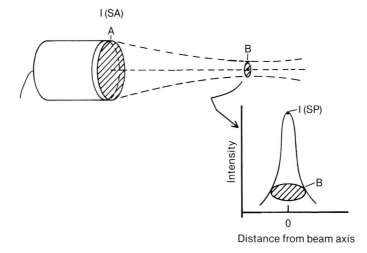

Fig. 6-4. The spatial average intensity, *I(SA)*, may be specified anywhere in the beam. It is commonly given at the transducer surface and is obtained by averaging the intensity over the shaded area, *A*. The spatial peak intensity, *I(SP)*, is shown by the point on the intensity profile in the focal region.

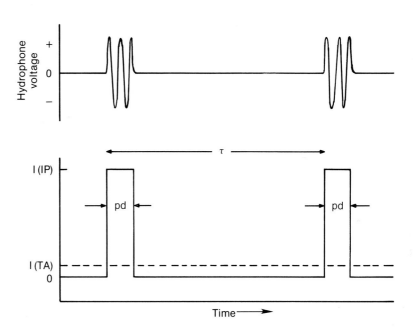

Fig. 6-5. Schematic of a waveform *(top)* obtained by a hydrophone placed in the beam of a pulsed transducer and the instantaneous intensity *(bottom)* as well as the time average corresponding to this waveform. The instantaneous intensity is shown varying from *0* to *I(IP)*, the instantaneous peak intensity. In addition, the time average intensity, *I(TA)* (dashed line), is shown. τ, Pulse-repetition period; *pd*, pulse duration.

In words, the duty factor is equal to the pulse duration divided by the pulse-repetition period. Careful study of Fig. 6-5 will show that this equation follows directly from the definition for duty factor.

Example: Suppose a diagnostic instrument has a pulse repetition frequency of 500/sec and a pulse duration of 1 μsec. What is the duty factor?

Solution: First, compute the pulse repetition period, given by Equation 6-3.

$$\tau = \frac{1}{\text{prf}} = \frac{1}{500/\text{sec}} = 0.002 \text{ sec}$$

Then, using Equation 6-4, find the duty factor.

$$DF = \frac{pd}{\tau} = \frac{1 \mu\text{sec}}{0.002 \text{ sec}} =$$
$$\frac{1 \times 10^{-6} \text{ sec}}{2 \times 10^{-3} \text{ sec}} = 0.0005$$

(Notice that this is similar to an example worked out in Chapter 3. Also, notice that duty factor has no units.)

In Fig. 6-5 the beam intensity is schematically illustrated for the waveform at the top of the diagram. The instantaneous peak intensity, $I(IP)$, is the maximum intensity attained during the pulse. The instantaneous intensity oscillates between 0 and $I(IP)$, as shown. The time-averaged intensity, $I(TA)$, is equal to the instantaneous peak intensity multiplied by the duty factor.

$$I(TA) = I(IP) \times DF \qquad (6\text{-}5)$$

Example: Suppose the instantaneous peak intensity for a diagnostic instrument is 1000 mW/cm² . If the duty factor is 0.001, what is the time averaged intensity?

Solution: Use Equation 6-5.
$$I(TA) = 1000 \text{ mW/cm}^2 \times 0.001$$
$$= 1 \text{ mW/cm}^2$$

Example: If the time-averaged intensity is 10 mW/cm² and the duty factor is 0.0005, estimate the instantaneous peak intensity.

Solution: Since you are interested in $I(IP)$, you must first isolate this parameter on one side of Equation 6-5.
$$I(IP) = \frac{I(TA)}{DF}$$
Inserting the values given leads to
$$I(IP) = \frac{10 \text{ mW/cm}^2}{0.0005} =$$
$$2000 \text{ mW/cm}^2 = 20 \text{ W/cm}^2$$

The point should be apparent from the two examples: For pulsed sound beams low values for the time-averaged intensity are quite usual, as long as the duty factor is low. Low time-averaged intensities for these beams are accompanied by large values for the instantaneous peak intensity. Instantaneous intensities of several hundred watts per square centimeter have been estimated for some instruments.[4]

In the discussions until now, spatial and temporal aspects of the sound beam intensity have been considered separately. In fact, both designations must be provided simultaneously to indicate which measure of intensity is being referred to. Intensity values commonly measured for diagnostic instruments are as follows:

I(SATA): Spatial average–time average intensity; often it is specified at the transducer surface or at the surface of a transducer assembly where the sound beam enters the patient
I(SPTA): Spatial peak–time average intensity
I(SPIP): Spatial peak–instantaneous peak intensity

Values for the acoustic power and intensities measured for diagnostic ultrasound instruments are presented in Table G-1.

MODES OF PRODUCTION OF BIOLOGIC EFFECTS

At sufficiently high intensities and long enough exposure times, ultrasound is capable of producing a measurable effect on tissues. The effect may be a small temperature elevation or complete destruction of tissue depending on the acoustic exposure. We shall consider briefly some of the modes whereby a sound beam can produce a biologic effect.

Heating. As a sound beam propagates through tissue, it undergoes attenuation. A significant fraction of this attenuation is due to *absorption* or, essentially, conversion of the ultrasonic energy into heat. For very low ultrasonic power levels any heat that is deposited by the sound beam is quickly dissipated. Therefore no measurable temperature increase occurs. On the other hand, ultrasound therapy devices operating at spatial average–time average intensities of nearly 1000 mW/cm² with a duty factor of 1 (continuous wave excitation of the transducer) can cause significant temperature elevations in tissue. In fact, deep heating is one of the beneficial effects of this mode of therapy.

Cavitation. Intense ultrasound beams in a fluid can generate tiny bubbles from dissolved gases in the fluid. In the presence of the sound beam the bubbles can grow in size and produce an effect on the medium. The cavitation bubbles expand and contract synchronously with pressure oscillations in the sound field. This, in turn, causes particle displacements and stresses in excess of those resulting from the sound beam alone. Some experimentally induced biologic effects have been attributed to this cavitation process.

Two types of cavitation may exist. *Stable cavitation* refers to the creation of bubbles that oscillate with the sound beam, as mentioned. *Transient cavitation*, in which the oscillations grow so intense that the bubbles collapse, has been detected at time average intensity levels substantially greater than those measured for diagnostic ultrasound beams. Whether either form of cavitation can be produced in tissue by *diagnostic* ultrasound beams has not been demonstrated.

Direct mechanical effects. Sound transmission is associated with displacements, accelerations, and stresses on particles in the medium. Thus it is possible that the perturbations caused by passage of sound waves will lead directly to "bioeffects." Biologic effects have been produced in some experimental studies on plants and cells in which no temperature rise could have occurred and cavitation was known to be absent. When

these two mechanisms are ruled out, direct mechanical effects of the ultrasound beam are usually thought to have occurred.

IS THERE A RISK?

Nearly every clinical study and therapeutic action involves some calculated risk to patients. In many of these cases the level of risk is quite well known. In making a decision as whether to do any procedure on a patient, clinicians must weigh the risk against the expected benefit.

For diagnostic ultrasound we must presume that there is some element of risk to ultrasound exposures, no matter how low it may be. What researchers are attempting to obtain, and will probably be seeking for a long time, are data that will enable them to better quantify the risk level for different ultrasound exposure conditions. Out of perhaps hundreds of thousands of individuals already insonified during diagnostic ultrasound examinations, no known ill effects have been suffered from these exposures. This information, though certainly very comforting, also indicates that the task of determining a *risk factor* for diagnostic ultrasound is a very difficult one.

A number of different approaches are being followed in these investigations. Epidemiologic studies are aimed at determining whether previous diagnostic ultrasound examinations of fetuses (in utero) may have resulted in any ill effect. Such investigations involve comparisons of medical records and present physical condition of groups of individuals insonified in utero and presumably identical groups of individuals who were not insonified. The work is very time consuming, because to obtain valid results investigators must study large numbers of patients.

In addition to epidemiologic investigations, numerous studies have been and continue to be performed on animals in vivo and on mammalian cells in vitro. Excellent reviews of the recent literature on bioeffects[7,8] have been published. When diagnostic ultrasound instruments are used in these studies, equivocal results often appear. A positive finding of an effect in one laboratory may be impossible to duplicate in another laboratory (and sometimes in the same laboratory). Experiments have been done in which small animals were insonified for an extensive time (hours) by diagnostic instruments and no effects were observed.[9] Recently, however, several studies using ultrasound at diagnostic intensities have produced positive effects. For example, Liebeskind et al.[5] used a diagnostic instrument and demonstrated that ultrasound appeared to cause detectable effects on DNA and growth patterns of animal cells exposed in vitro. Perhaps as biologic indicators and assay techniques become more sensitive, it will be possible to obtain a quantifiable indication of risk factors associated with diagnostic ultrasound exposures.

Definitive evidence for biologic effects has been obtained in investigations in which small animals were insonified, usually at average intensities and exposure times that in most cases could not be obtained with diagnostic equipment.[8] At such intensity levels fetal weight reductions in rats, death of rat fetuses, and altered mitotic rates were observed. For these effects to be produced, it was usually necessary to expose the animal to some minimal intensity for a given time. If the intensity was reduced, the exposure time had to be increased to compensate for the reduced acoustic energy.

This last statement is illustrated in Fig. 6-6 for mammalian tissues exposed to high-intensity ultrasound. Curves such as the one shown have been produced by researchers in an attempt to place the vast amount of experimental data on bioeffects research into perspective. The line divides the data into a region where exposure conditions were sufficient to produce an effect (above the line) and a region where no effect could be demonstrated (below the line). At high spatial peak intensities only a brief exposure resulted in an effect. To produce an effect at lower intensity levels, it was necessary to expose the animal for a longer time. For spatial peak–time average intensities greater than 100 mW/cm², the demarcation line follows a curve in which the product of the intensity, I, and the exposure time, T, is given by

$$I \times T = 50 \ (W/cm^2) \ \text{sec} \qquad (6\text{-}6)$$
$$= 50 \ \text{joules/cm}^2*$$

Below 100 mW/cm² these data indicate that none of the effects for which the researchers were looking could be produced—no matter how long the exposure.

To help clarify these data, a committee of the American Institute of Ultrasound in Medicine issued the following statement:

In the low megahertz frequency range there have been no independently confirmed significant

biological effects in mammalian tissues exposed to intensities* below 100 mW/cm². Furthermore, for ultrasonic exposure times† less than 500 seconds and greater than one second, such effects have not been demonstrated even at higher intensities, when the product of intensity* and exposure time† is less than 50 joules/cm².

This statement was carefully prepared by the AIUM Bioeffects Committee after careful examination of all pertinent literature. Based upon the biologic effects data available to the committee at the time it was made, it provides some information relative to the current knowledge of risk factors for diagnostic ultrasound. If the acoustic intensities (spatial peak, time average) can be kept substantially below 100 mW/cm², it would appear from the statement that the risk factor is low. For situations in which the spatial peak–time average intensity approaches or even exceeds 100 mW/cm², we may be dealing with ultrasonic exposures that carry a higher risk of producing some effect on tissues.

It should be pointed out, once again, that the data upon which the 1978 statement was based were for ultrasonic exposures in small animals. The statement does not offer absolute safe levels, or even state-permissible levels; nor does it suggest upper intensity limits for ultrasound equipment.

The data in Fig. 6-6 also suggest that if the exposure time is kept low the possibility of biologic effects will be minimized. The in-

sonification schemes (e.g., the duty factor and the pulse duration) used by the researchers in generating the data summarized in Fig. 6-6 are not the same as those used in pulsed ultrasound. Nevertheless, the principle would seem to apply to all modes of diagnostic ultrasound.

A RATIONAL APPROACH

No matter what the outcome of bioeffects studies, prudence dictates that the lowest possible acoustic exposures be used during ultrasound examinations. The following points are offered in accordance with this philosophy:

1. One should not hesitate to use diagnostic ultrasound when the situation warrants. However, diagnostic ultrasound should be used only when there is a valid medical reason. For example, it seems difficult to justify ultrasound exposures of individuals during commercial demonstrations.

    Responsible individuals will not treat ultrasound as a novel plaything but will utilize it to obtain an anticipated benefit such as diagnostic information or research results.

2. Users should familiarize themselves with their equipment so they can recognize which operating modes and which control settings result in high or low acoustic intensities. Thus they can avoid using high acoustic intensities, except when the examination warrants. They should avoid using an instrument for purposes for which it may not have been designed. Appendix H shows that

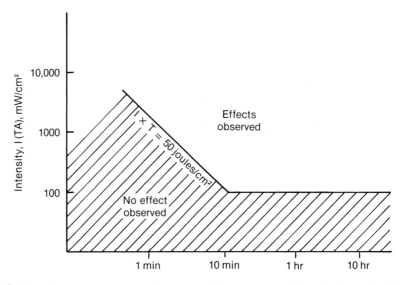

Fig. 6-6. Intensity versus exposure time curve. Exposure conditions that resulted in positive biologic effects are separated from conditions in which no effects were observed for animal studies. (From Nyborg, W.: HEW Publication no. [FDA] 78-8062, 1978.)

---

*Recall that power is the rate at which energy is applied and may be expressed in watts. Energy may be expressed in joules. A *watt* is the same as a *joule per second*. If power (watts or joules/second) is multiplied by exposure time (seconds), the resultant quantity is in joules.

*Spatial peak, temporal average, as measured in a free field of water.
†Total time; this includes off-time as well as on-time for a repeated-pulse regimen.[2]

the spatial peak–temporal average intensity for different classes of instruments may vary significantly.

Information on acoustic exposure from ultrasound instruments is beginning to be provided by ultrasound equipment manufacturers. In most cases this information is available in the operator's manual.

3. Many instruments have controls that vary the acoustic power. On such instruments as a general rule, USE A HIGH RECEIVER GAIN SETTING AND A LOW POWER SETTING, NOT VICE VERSA!

Start an examination with power settings initially adjusted for low power output. Increase the power only when adequate sensitivity cannot be attained with the receiver gains peaking out at their maximum values. Be aware that a 10-dB reduction in the output power means a factor of 10 reduction in the acoustic intensity; a 20-dB reduction in the power output means a factor of 100 reduction in the intensity! (See Table 1-1.)

4. Reduce the exposure time by avoiding repeat scans if possible and avoiding holding the transducer stationary in contact with the patient unless the examination warrants this.

Ultrasound instrument manufacturers are expected to design their equipment so it will deliver the lowest possible acoustic exposures consistent with the diagnostic expectations of that equipment.[1] However, as the foregoing points indicate, user awareness and responsibility are major elements in assuring patient safety during an ultrasound examination.

REFERENCES

1. AIUM/NEMA ultrasound safety standard, Washington, D.C., 1981, AIUM. (Also available from National Electrical Manufacturers Association, 2101 L Street, N.W., Washington, D.C. 20037.)
2. Bioeffects Committee, AIUM: Who's afraid of a hundred milliwatts per square centimeter (100 mW/cm²) SPTA? Washington, D.C., 1979, AIUM.
3. Carson, P.: Diagnostic ultrasound emissions and their measurement. In Fullerton, G., and Zagzebski, J., editors: Medical physics of CT and ultrasound, New York, 1980, AAPM.
4. Carson, P., Fischella, P., and Oughton, T.: Ultrasound power and intensities produced by diagnostic ultrasound equipment, Ultrasound Med. Biol. 3:341, 1978.
5. Liebeskind, D., Bases, R., Elequin, F., et al.: Diagnostic ultrasound: effects on the DNA and growth patterns of animal cells, Radiology **131:**177, 1979.
6. Nyborg, W.: Physical mechanisms for biological effects of ultrasound (Evelyn Byers Surles, editor), HEW Publication no. (FDA) 78-8062, 1978.
7. O'Brien, W.: Safety of ultrasound. In de Vleger, M., et al., editors: Handbook of clinical ultrasound, New York, 1978, John Wiley & Sons, Inc.
8. O'Brien, W.: Biological effects of ultrasound. In Fullerton, G., and Zagzebski, J., editors: Medical physics of CT and ultrasound, New York, 1980, AAPM.
9. Smythe, M.: Animal toxicity studies with ultrasound at diagnostic power levels. In Grossman, C.C., et al., editors: Diagnostic ultrasound, New York, 1966, Plenum Press.
10. Statement on mammalian in vivo ultrasonic biological effects, Reflections **4:**311, 1978.
11. Taylor, K.J.W.: Current status of toxicity investigations, J. Clin. Ultrasound **2:**149, 1974.

7

Cross-sectional anatomy

The embryologic development of all abdominal organs occurs retroperitoneally. The kidneys and ureters remain retroperitoneal, whereas the other organs protrude into the peritoneum or become surrounded by it (Fig. 7-1).

Abdominopelvic cavity

The peritoneum is a thin, translucent, serous membrane. To understand its complexities, one must appreciate certain fundamental facts about it:

1. It lines the walls of the abdominal cavity.

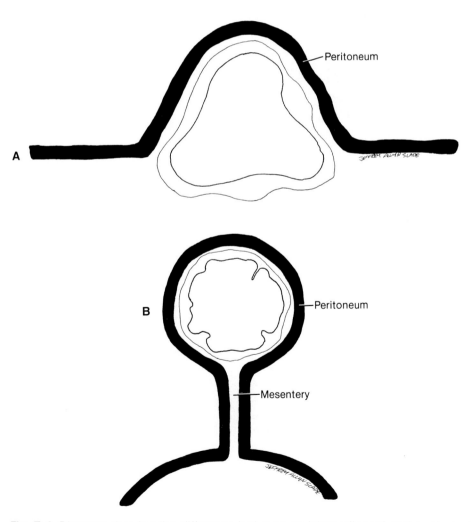

Fig. 7-1. Diagram showing the difference between an intraperitoneal and a retroperitoneal organ. Both organs are actually outside the peritoneal sac. **A,** Retroperitoneal. **B,** Intraperitoneal.

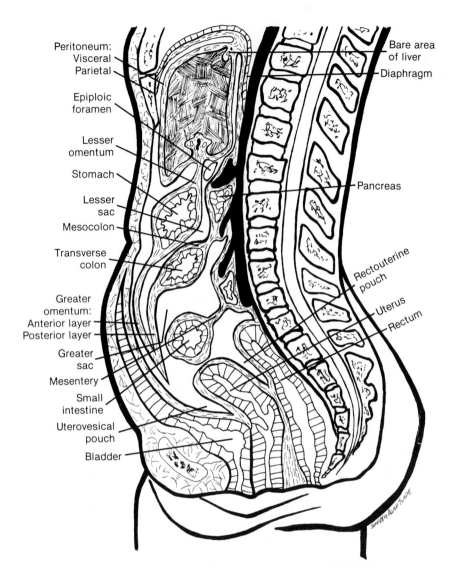

Fig. 7-2. Reflections of the peritoneum. Sagittal section of the abdominal cavity in the female. The layers of the greater omentum are fused; and the anterior layers are attached to the transverse colon, thus forming the gastrocolic ligament.

2. It forms a completely closed sac or cavity—except in the female where the mouths of the uterine tubes (fallopian tubes) open into it (Fig. 7-2).

3. Immediately outside it is an extraperitoneal (subperitoneal) fatty layer. In this layer the organs and their vessels develop and lie.

4. Retroperitoneal organs remain behind the sac (retro) and are merely covered in front with peritoneum. This generally applies to the urinary system.

5. An organ that invaginates the sac is invested in peritoneum. The layer closest to the invaginating organ is the serous coat of the organ. In general, this applies to the gastrointestinal system.

6. The mobility of an organ depends to a great extent on its peritoneal covering.

7. Two layers of peritoneum are attached to each of the two curvatures of the stomach. They are the omenta. The lesser omentum is attached to the lesser curvature, and the greater omentum to the greater curvature (Figs. 7-3 and 7-4).

8. Mesenteries are two layers of peritoneum that "sling" the intestine from the posterior abdominal wall. Vessels and nerves travel to and from the intestine between the two layers.

9. All other double layers and folds of peritoneum are called peritoneal ligaments.

10. Everywhere within the peritoneal cavity the peritoneum is in contact with peritoneum. The cavity is merely a potential space containing a small amount of lubricating serous fluid. It

helps the intraabdominal organs move upon one another without friction. Under certain pathologic conditions the potential space of the peritoneal cavity may be distended into an actual space containing several liters of fluid. This accumulation of serous fluid in the peritoneal cavity is known as ascites. Other substances (blood from a ruptured spleen, bile from a rupture bile duct, fecal matter from a ruptured intestine) also may accumulate in the abdominal cavity.

The abdominal cavity (excluding the retroperitoneum and pelvis) is bounded superiorly by the diaphragm, anteriorly by the abdominal wall muscles, posteriorly by the vertebral column, ribs, and iliac fossa, and inferiorly by the pelvis.

Liver

The diaphragmatic surface of the liver consists of the right and left lobes, with the falciform ligament separating each lobe. Within this ligament is a round fibrous cord, the *ligamentum teres*, which represents the old umbilical vein. The left lobe reaches to approximately 2 cm below the nipple. The visceral surface of the liver is subdivided into four lobes: right, left, anterior quadrate, and posterior caudate.

Vascular access to the liver is through the porta hepatis via the portal vein and hepatic artery. The portal triad that contains these two vessels also contains the common bile duct.

The *bare area* of the liver is where the peritoneal reflections from the liver onto the diaphragm leave an irregular triangle of liver without peritoneal covering. The peritoneal reflections around the bare area are called the coronary ligament. The caudal part of the coronary ligament is reflected onto the diaphragm and the right kidney and is called the *hepatorenal ligament*. Below this is a potential peritoneal space, the hepatorenal pouch or *recess of Morison*, bounded by the liver, kidney, colon, and duodenum.

Gallbladder

The gallbladder projects to the lateral margin of the right rectus abdominis. It is attached to the inferior surface of the liver. Its duct system is composed of the cystic duct, the common bile duct, and the right and left hepatic ducts.

Vessels

The major great vessels are related to the posterior abdominal wall, with branches to the visceral organs. The blood supply for the gonads is near the renal artery throughout development. The left gonadal vein drains into the left renal vein.

Pancreas

The pancreas is a retroperitoneal gland that is bounded anteriorly by the stomach and duodenum and posteriorly by the pre-vertebral vessels.

Spleen

The spleen has a smooth convex diaphragmatic surface that fits under the diaphragm in the left upper quadrant. The hilum of the spleen contains the splenic artery and vein. The spleen also has gastric, renal, and colic surface relationships.

Digestive tract

The esophagus descends from the thorax to enter the upper abdomen through the diaphragm and becomes continuous with the stomach. The stomach is a J-shaped structure anteriorly related to the thoracic cavity and muscles of the abdominal wall. It contacts the left lobe of the liver (the gastric area on the visceral hepatic surface). Posterior to the bed of the stomach lies the pancreas, with a layer of peritoneum separating the two structures. The greater curvature contacts the transverse colon. The stomach is divided into fundus, body, antrum, and pyloric region. The last turns into the duodenum. The duodenum remains retroperitoneal throughout development.

The intestine is suspended by the mesentery to give it greater mobility. The junction between the ileum and the cecum occurs on the right side of the abdomen. Much of the large ascending colon is retroperitoneal to the hepatic flexure. The transverse colon is a free structure, suspended by mesentery, whereas the splenic flexure to the descending colon is retroperitoneal to the sigmoid mesocolon, surrounded by mesentery.

Peritoneal gutters

The mesentery of the small intestine, ascending colon, and descending colon is attached to the posterior abdominal wall. As a result four gutters exists that can conveniently conduct materials (ascites, inflammatory products, blood, bile) from one point of the peritoneal cavity to another.

1. Right lateral (*paracolic*) gutter, to the right of the ascending colon; it may conduct fluid from the omental bursa via the hepatorenal pouch into the pelvis

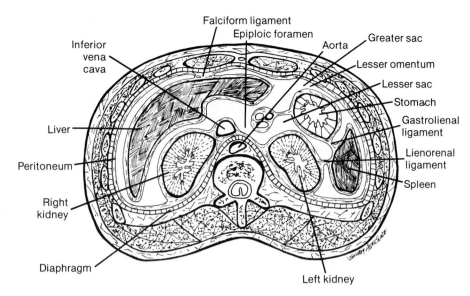

Fig. 7-3. Reflections of the peritoneum. Transverse section of the abdominal cavity through the epiploic foramen.

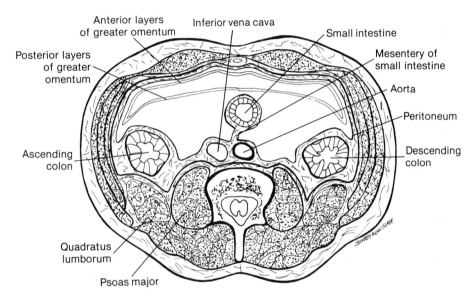

Fig. 7-4. Reflections of the peritoneum. Transverse section of the abdominal cavity at the fourth lumbar vertebra. In reality there is no space between the anterior and posterior layers of the greater omentum; they are almost always fused.

2. Left lateral (*paracolic*) gutter, to the left of the descending colon
3. Gutter to the right of the mesentery
4. Gutter to the left of the mesentery; it opens widely into the pelvis

Kidneys

The kidneys rest on the psoas and quadratus lumborum in the retroperitoneal cavity. The left kidney contacts the spleen, pancreas, colon, and jejunum, and its superomedial pole holds the adrenal gland. The right kidney contacts the liver, colon, and adrenal gland.

The kidneys are protected posteriorly by the eleventh and twelfth ribs. The inferior poles are not well protected except for the quadratus lumborum. On the medial surface of the kidney is the hilum, the point of exit of the renal vein and entrance of the renal artery. The renal pelvis is also at the hilum and forms the ureter, which narrows to flow posteriorly into the bladder. The kidneys develop in the true pelvis and ascend into the abdomen. Occasionally the inferior poles will fuse, and the upper poles will ascend into the mesentery at the site of the inferior mesenteric artery to form a *horseshoe* kidney.

Pelvic cavity

The pelvis is divided into the greater and lesser pelves. The pelvic brim is the circumference of a plane dividing these two portions. The greater or *false* pelvis is superior to the pelvic brim and is bounded on each side by the ilium. The lesser or *true* pelvis is situated caudal to the pelvic brim. The walls of the pelvic cavity are lined with muscles. The floor of the pelvis is formed by muscles collectively called the pelvic diaphragm.

The peritoneal cavity extends into the lesser pelvis and invests several pelvic organs—the rectum, bladder, and uterus. In the female the peritoneum descends from the anterior abdominal wall to the level of the pubic bone onto the superior surface of the bladder. It then passes from the bladder to the uterus to form the *vesicouterine pouch*. It covers the fundus and body of the uterus and extends over the posterior fornix and the wall of the vagina. Between the uterus and the rectum the peritoneum forms the deep *rectouterine pouch*.

The sonographer must have a solid knowledge of gross anatomy, including cross-sectional and sagittal planes. Although "normal" anatomy is often illustrated throughout this book, the student must keep in mind the numerous variations that can occur in the anatomic structure. Thus organ and vessel relationships to neighboring structures should be carefully evaluated rather than a memorization made of where in the abdomen a particular structure ought to be. For example, it is better to recall the location of the gallbladder as anterior to the right kidney and medial to the liver than to remember that it is usually found 6 to 8 cm above the umbilicus.

TRANSVERSE CROSS-SECTIONAL ANATOMY

The guide below should aid the reader in reviewing the illustrations throughout the abdominal chapters:

In Figs. 7-5 to 7-18 transverse anatomic cross sections were obtained from an elderly woman with a number of pathologic disorders. Rheumatic disease of the heart left calcification on her aortic and mitral valves. The left atrial cavity was enlarged, and the left ventricular cavity demonstrated increased wall thickening. Her pancreas was in an oblique lie and was huge, extending throughout several transverse sections yet maintaining its relationship to the prevertebral vessels. Her gallbladder likewise was distended on several sections. The bowel was somewhat redundant, extending into the upper abdomen to the lower extent of the pelvis.

Transverse cross sections were made at 2-cm increments. X = xyphoid; I = inferior; S = superior. *Text continued on p. 95.*

AscAo	Ascending aorta	**IVS**	Interventricular septum	**TL**	Teres ligament
DscAo	Descending aorta	**D**	Diaphragm	**SMA**	Superior mesenteric artery
SVC	Superior vena cava	**L**	Liver	**SMV**	Superior mesenteric vein
MSB	Main bronchus	**FL**	Falciform ligament	**RK**	Right kidney
E	Esophagus	**PC**	Peritoneal cavity	**LK**	Left kidney
OF	Oblique fissure	**CL**	Caudate lobe	**LRV**	Left renal vein
RL	Right lung	**RLL**	Right lobe of liver	**LRA**	Left renal artery
PA	Pulmonary artery	**LLL**	Left lobe of liver	**RRV**	Right renal vein
Br	Bronchus	**VL**	Venous ligament	**RRA**	Right renal artery
LowLL	Lower lobe of left lung	**St**	Stomach	**I**	Ileum
PT	Pulmonary trunk	**LS**	Lesser sac	**Du**	Duodenum
PB	Pulmonary branch	**S**	Spleen	**Gb**	Gallbladder
Stn	Sternum	**LGA**	Left gastric artery	**Py**	Pylorus
LA	Left atrium	**P**	Pancreas	**Ps**	Psoas
RA	Right atrium	**PV**	Portal vein	**DuJ**	Duodenojejunal flexure
PV	Pulmonary vein	**CBD**	Common bile duct	**GDA**	Gastroduodenal artery
PS	Pericardiac sac	**HA**	Hepatic artery	**SFC**	Splenic flexure colon
POT	Pulmonary outflow tract	**CT**	Celiac trunk	**DscC**	Descending colon
RCA	Right coronary artery	**SA**	Splenic artery	**Sml**	Small intestine
MV	Mitral valve	**SV**	Splenic vein	**IMA**	Inferior mesenteric artery
RV	Right ventricle	**RAG**	Right adrenal gland	**HF**	Hepatic flexure
TV	Tricuspid valve	**LAG**	Left adrenal gland	**CA**	Celiac artery
		RF	Retroperitoneal fat	**Ad**	Adrenal gland

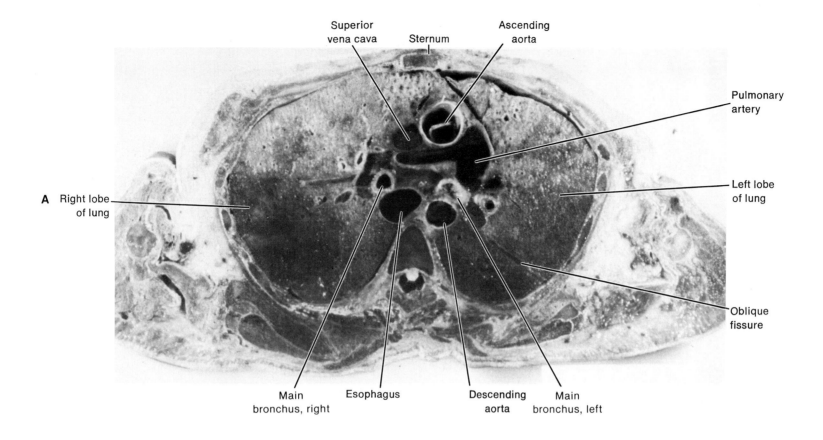

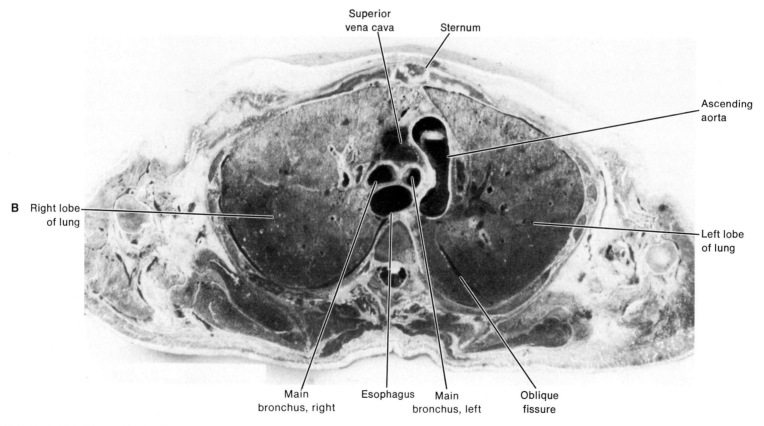

Fig. 7-5. A, X + 10 cm. **B,** X + 9 cm.

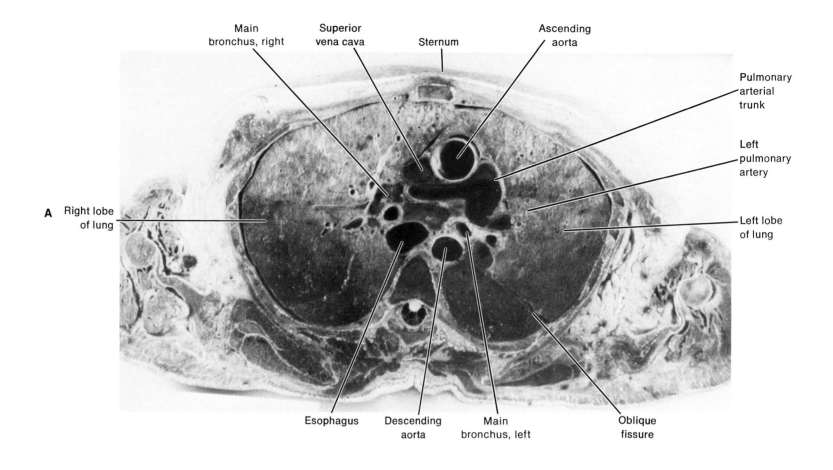

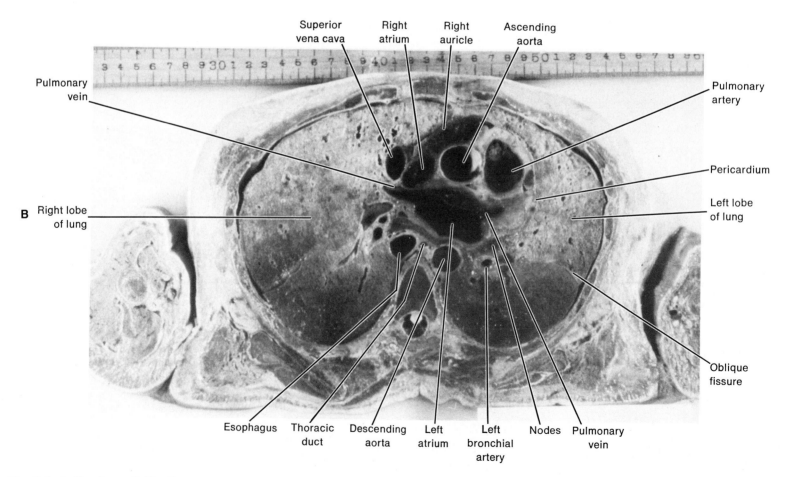

Fig. 7-6. **A,** X + 8 cm. **B,** X + 7 cm.

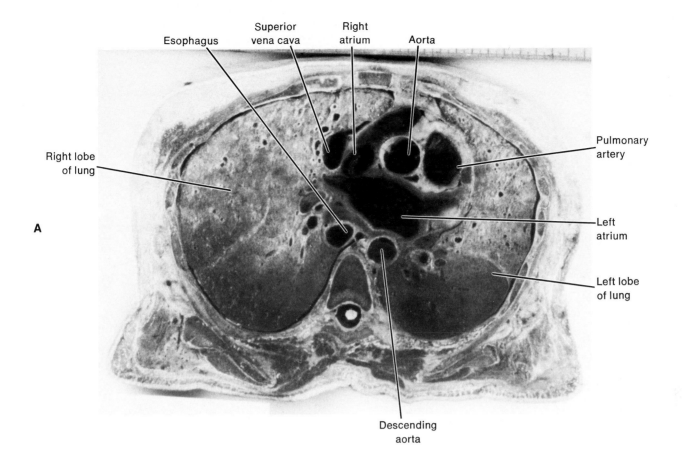

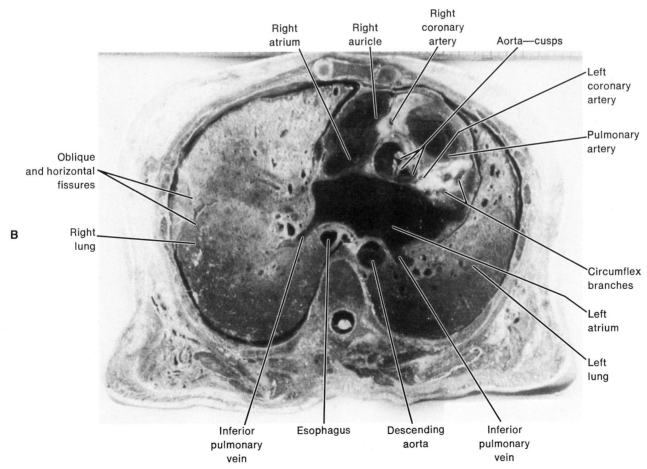

Fig. 7-7. A, X + 6 cm. **B,** X + 5 cm.

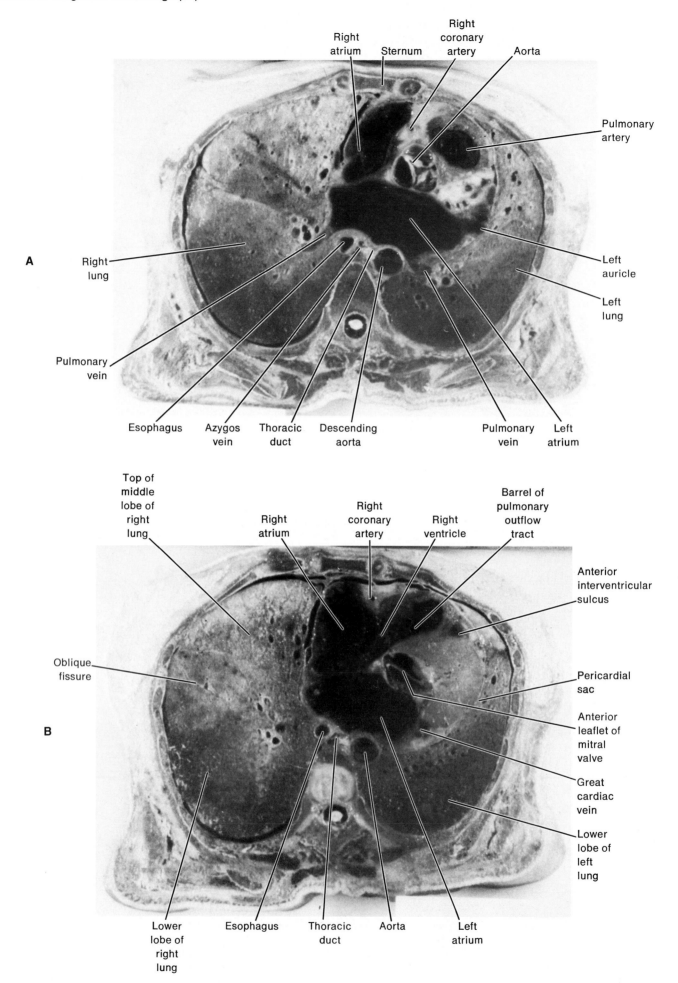

Fig. 7-8. A, X + 4 cm. **B,** X + 3 cm.

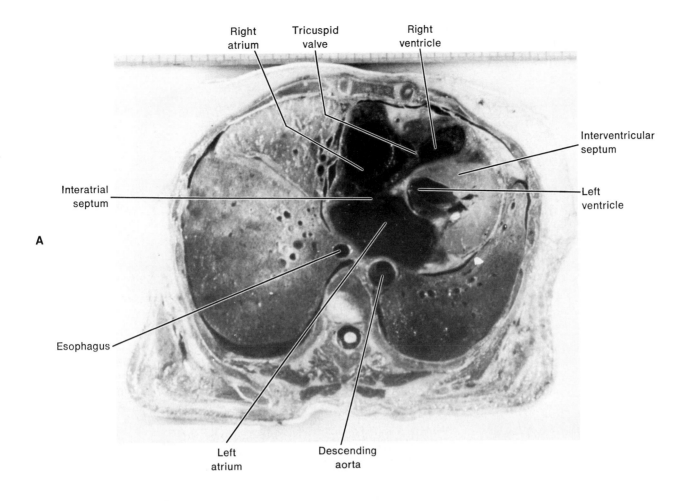

A

Right atrium | Tricuspid valve | Right ventricle

Interventricular septum

Interatrial septum

Left ventricle

Esophagus

Left atrium | Descending aorta

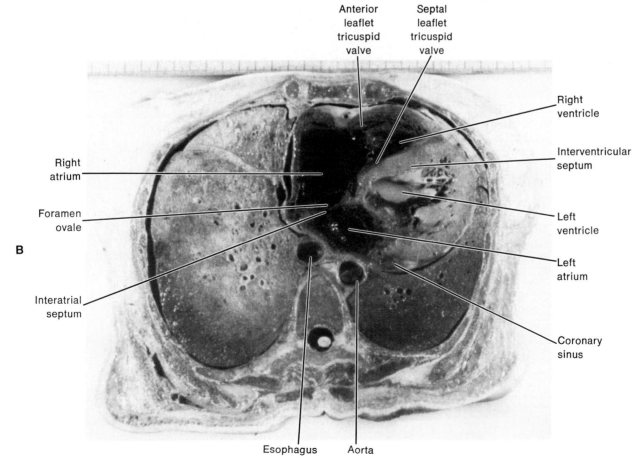

B

Anterior leaflet tricuspid valve | Septal leaflet tricuspid valve

Right ventricle

Interventricular septum

Right atrium

Foramen ovale

Left ventricle

Interatrial septum

Left atrium

Coronary sinus

Esophagus | Aorta

Fig. 7-9. A, X + 2 cm. **B,** X + 1 cm.

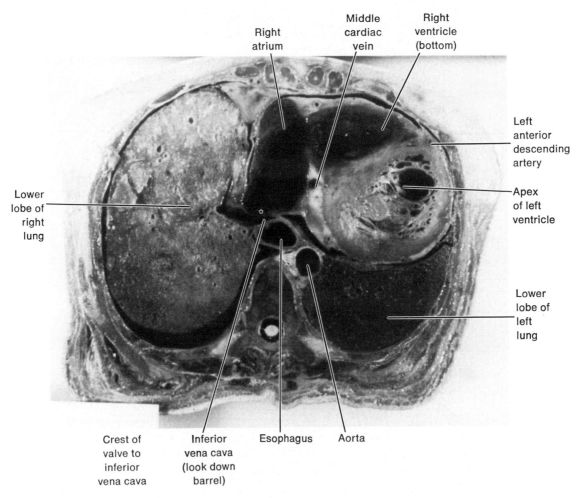

Fig. 7-10. Xyphoid.

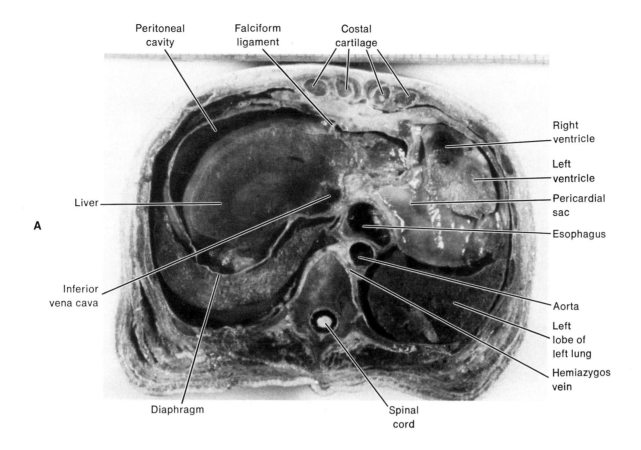

Peritoneal cavity — Falciform ligament — Costal cartilage

Right ventricle

Left ventricle

Liver —

Pericardial sac

A

Esophagus

Inferior vena cava —

Aorta

Left lobe of left lung

Hemiazygos vein

Diaphragm

Spinal cord

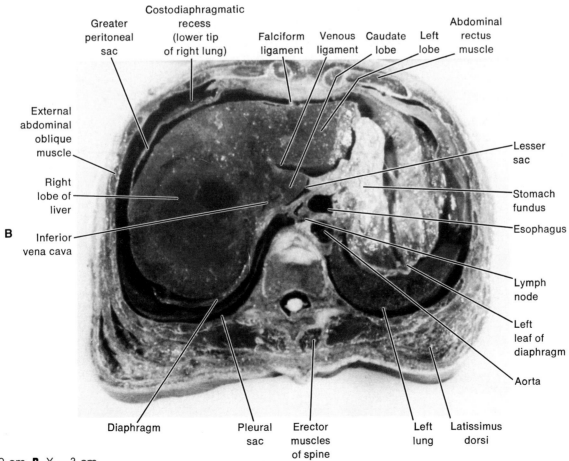

Costodiaphragmatic recess (lower tip of right lung)

Greater peritoneal sac — Falciform ligament — Venous ligament — Caudate lobe — Left lobe — Abdominal rectus muscle

External abdominal oblique muscle —

Lesser sac

Right lobe of liver —

Stomach fundus

B

Esophagus

Inferior vena cava —

Lymph node

Left leaf of diaphragm

Aorta

Diaphragm — Pleural sac — Erector muscles of spine — Left lung — Latissimus dorsi

Fig. 7-11. A, X — 2 cm. **B,** X — 3 cm.

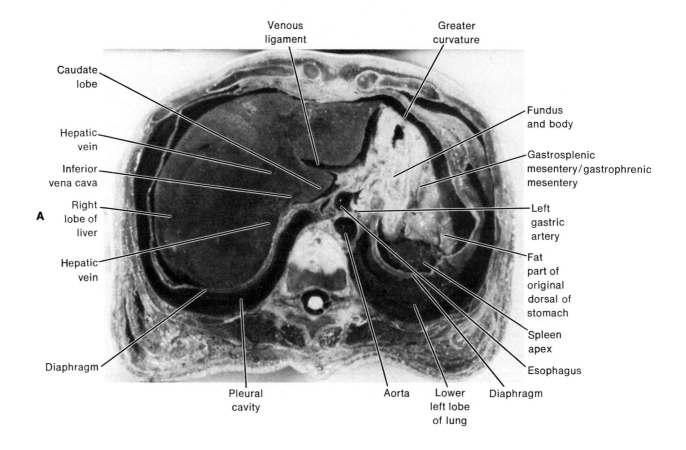

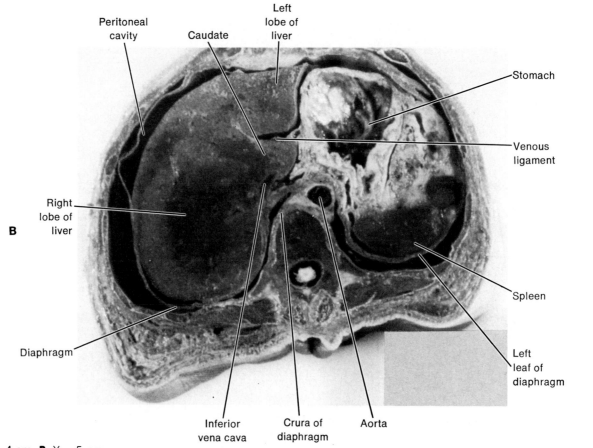

Fig. 7-12. A, X − 4 cm. **B,** X − 5 cm.

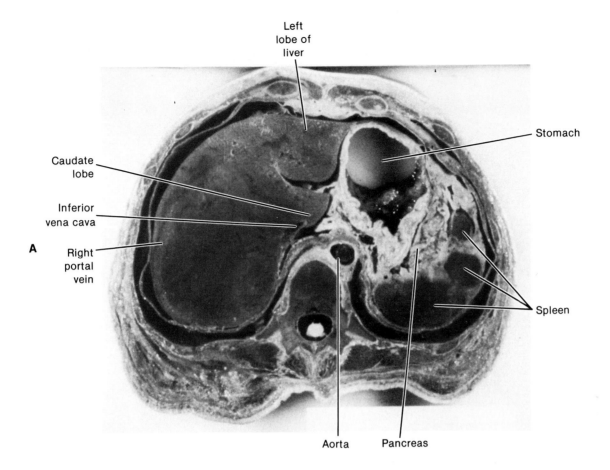

A

Left lobe of liver

Stomach

Caudate lobe

Inferior vena cava

Right portal vein

Spleen

Aorta

Pancreas

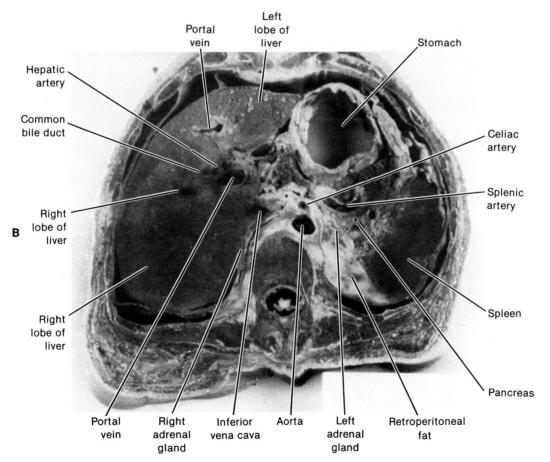

B

Portal vein

Left lobe of liver

Stomach

Hepatic artery

Common bile duct

Right lobe of liver

Celiac artery

Splenic artery

Right lobe of liver

Spleen

Portal vein

Right adrenal gland

Inferior vena cava

Aorta

Left adrenal gland

Retroperitoneal fat

Pancreas

Fig. 7-13. A, X − 6 cm. **B,** X − 7 cm.

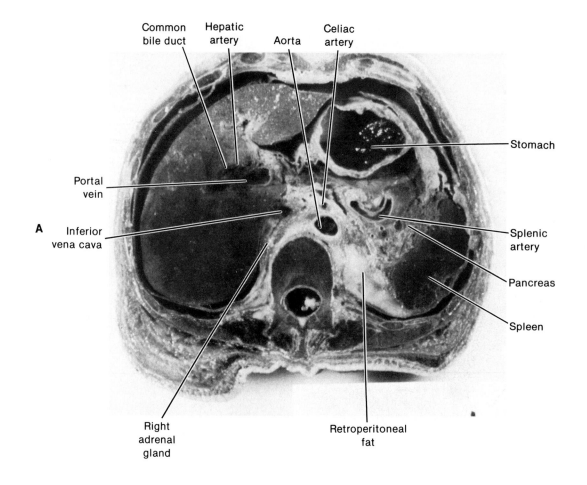

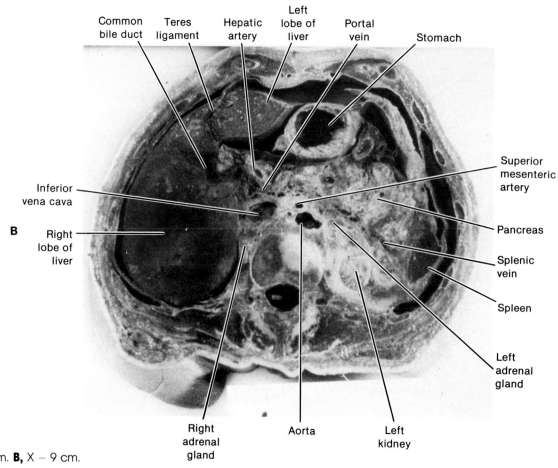

Fig. 7-14. A, X − 8 cm. **B,** X − 9 cm.

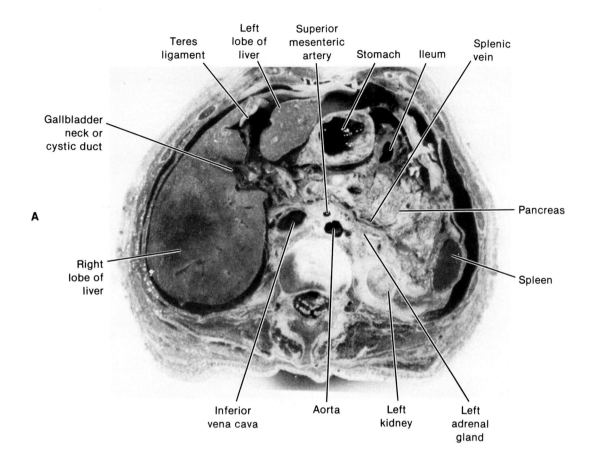

Teres ligament — Left lobe of liver — Superior mesenteric artery — Stomach — Ileum — Splenic vein

Gallbladder neck or cystic duct

A

Pancreas

Right lobe of liver

Spleen

Inferior vena cava — Aorta — Left kidney — Left adrenal gland

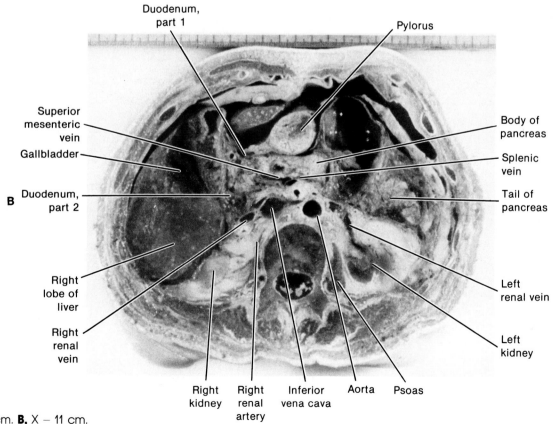

Duodenum, part 1 — Pylorus

Superior mesenteric vein

Body of pancreas

Gallbladder

Splenic vein

B Duodenum, part 2

Tail of pancreas

Right lobe of liver

Left renal vein

Right renal vein

Left kidney

Right kidney — Right renal artery — Inferior vena cava — Aorta — Psoas

Fig. 7-15. A, X − 10 cm. **B,** X − 11 cm.

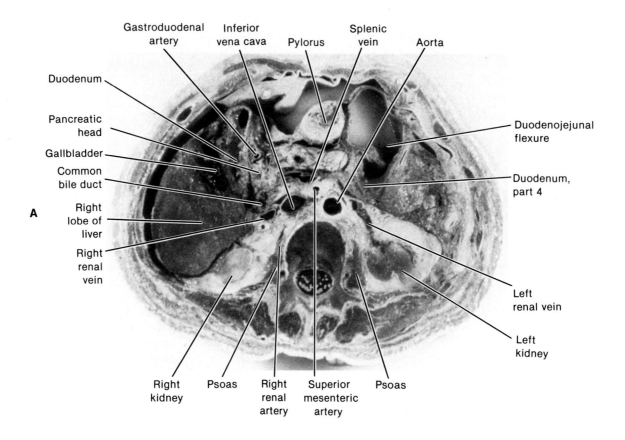

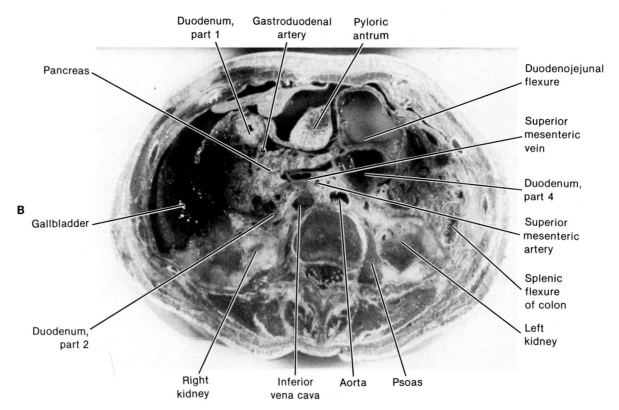

Fig. 7-16. A, X − 12 cm. **B,** X − 13 cm.

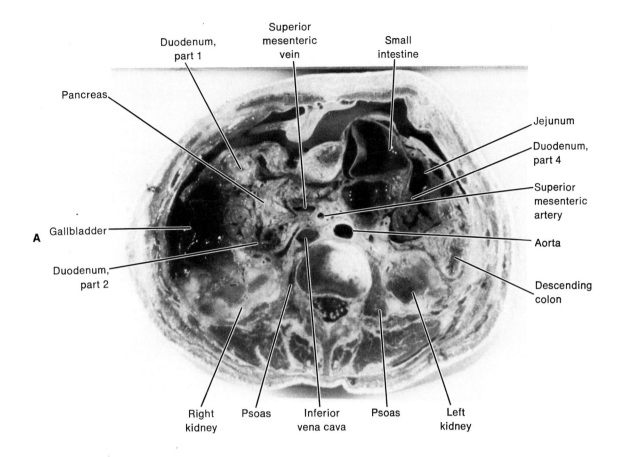

Pancreas

Duodenum, part 1

Superior mesenteric vein

Small intestine

Jejunum

Duodenum, part 4

Superior mesenteric artery

Aorta

A Gallbladder

Duodenum, part 2

Descending colon

Right kidney

Psoas

Inferior vena cava

Psoas

Left kidney

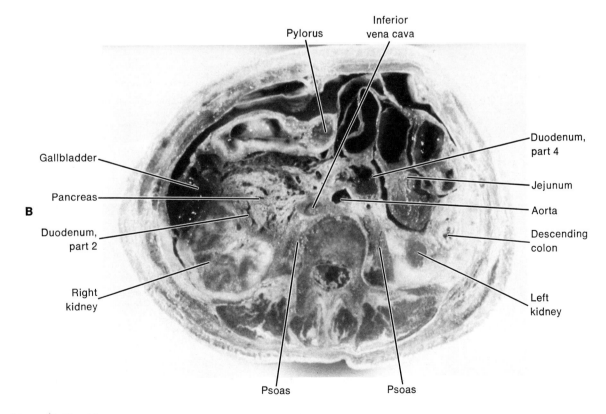

Pylorus

Inferior vena cava

Gallbladder

Pancreas

B

Duodenum, part 2

Right kidney

Duodenum, part 4

Jejunum

Aorta

Descending colon

Left kidney

Psoas

Psoas

Fig. 7-17. A, X − 14 cm. **B,** X − 15 cm.

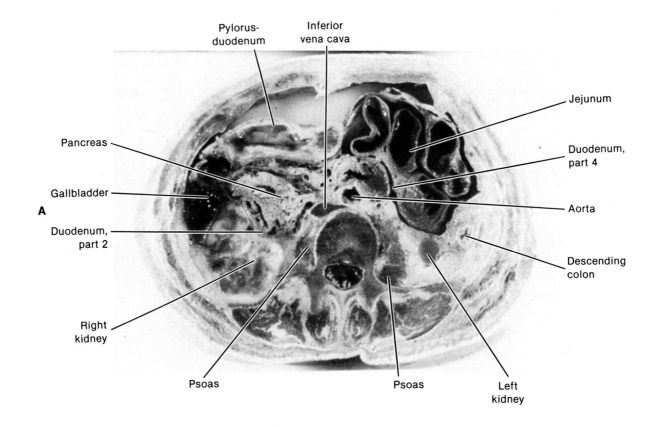

Pylorus-duodenum

Inferior vena cava

Jejunum

Pancreas

Duodenum, part 4

Gallbladder

Aorta

A

Duodenum, part 2

Descending colon

Right kidney

Psoas

Psoas

Left kidney

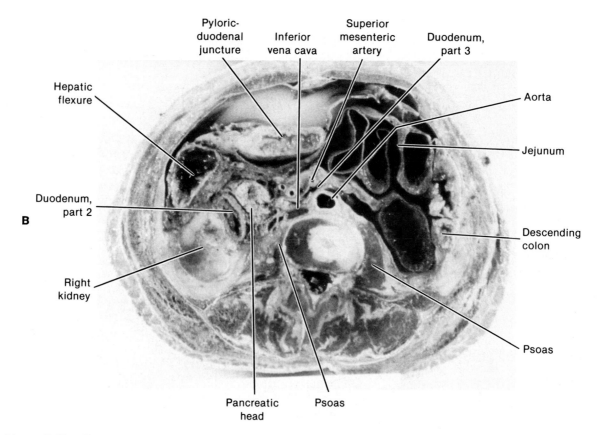

Pyloric-duodenal juncture

Inferior vena cava

Superior mesenteric artery

Duodenum, part 3

Hepatic flexure

Aorta

Jejunum

B

Duodenum, part 2

Descending colon

Right kidney

Psoas

Pancreatic head

Psoas

Fig. 7-18. A, X − 16 cm. **B,** X − 17 cm.

SAGITTAL CROSS-SECTIONAL ANATOMY

Figs. 7-19 to 7-28 are sagittal cross sections obtained from another patient. The abbreviations in the adjacent box apply and should be used to interpret the ultrasonic scans.

S	Spleen	**RA**	Right atrium
C	Colon	**SB**	Small bowel
Ps	Psoas	**U**	Uterus
LK	Left kidney	**PV**	Portal vein
RK	Right kidney	**B**	Bladder
L	Liver	**R**	Rectum
H	Heart	**Lg**	Lung
IVC	Inferior vena cava	**St**	Stomach

The longitudinal gross anatomic sections were obtained from an elderly woman who had undergone a right thoracotomy. As a result of this surgery the heart shifted its normal position to lie in the right thoracic cavity. She also had slight scoliosis, which shifted her spine to the right.

Fig. 7-19 begins at the right lateral border of the abdominal cavity. Figs. 7-20 to 7-28 are slices made approximately 2 cm apart. R = right; L = left.

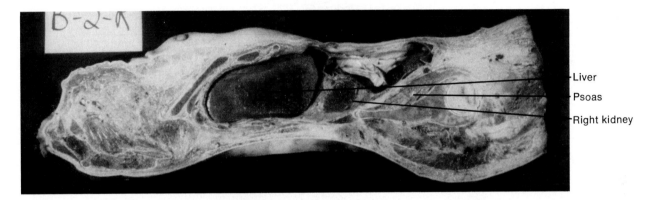

Liver
Psoas
Right kidney

Fig. 7-19. R + 9 cm.

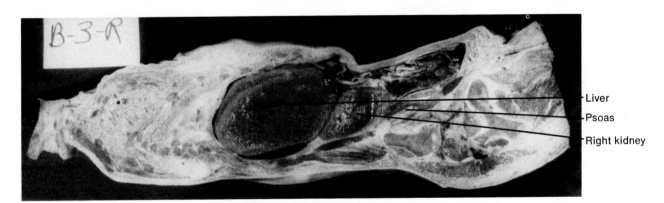

Liver
Psoas
Right kidney

Fig. 7-20. R + 7 cm.

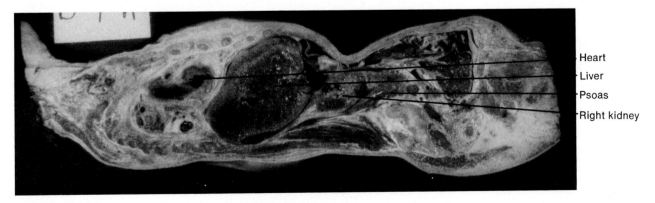

Heart
Liver
Psoas
Right kidney

Fig. 7-21. R + 5 cm.

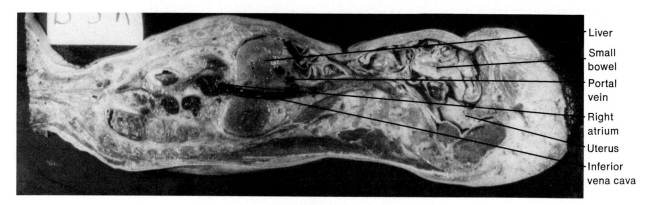

Liver

Small
bowel

Portal
vein

Right
atrium

Uterus

Inferior
vena cava

Fig. 7-22. R + 3 cm.

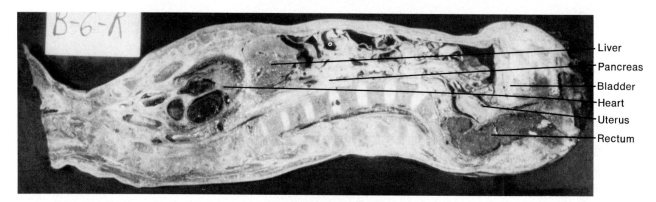

Liver

Pancreas

Bladder

Heart

Uterus

Rectum

Fig. 7-23. R + 1 cm.

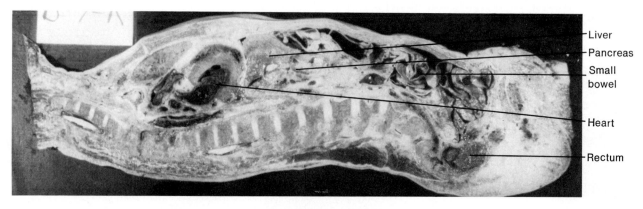

Liver

Pancreas

Small
bowel

Heart

Rectum

Fig. 7-24. L − 1 cm.

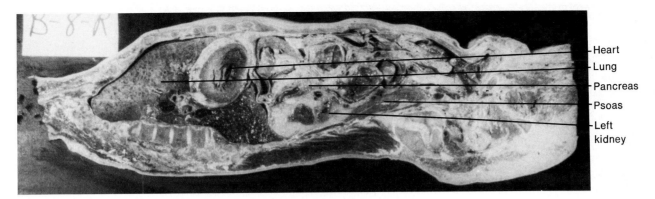

Fig. 7-25. L − 3 cm.

Heart
Lung
Pancreas
Psoas
Left kidney

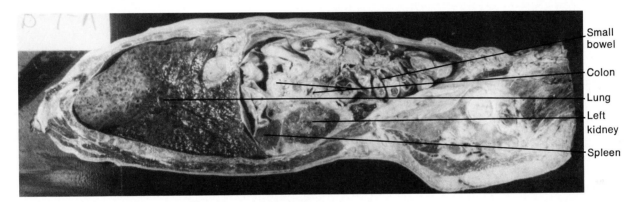

Fig. 7-26. L − 5 cm.

Small bowel
Colon
Lung
Left kidney
Spleen

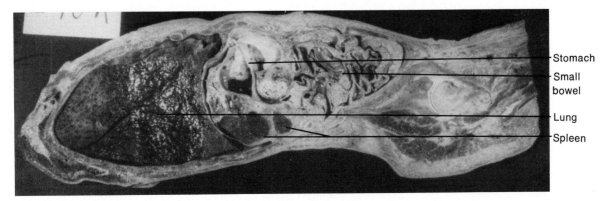

Fig. 7-27. L − 7 cm.

Stomach
Small bowel
Lung
Spleen

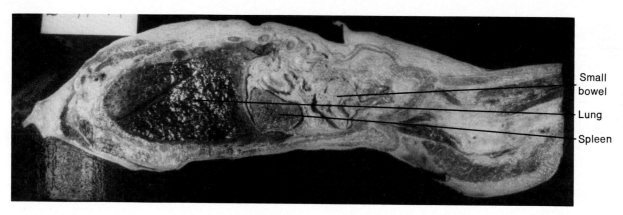

Small bowel

Lung

Spleen

Fig. 7-28. L − 9 cm.

8 Introduction to scanning techniques and protocol

The state of the art of ultrasound demands a high degree of manual dexterity and hand-eye coordination. This applies to all specialties currently making use of ultrasonic interpretation (i.e., neurology, cardiology, abdominal studies, obstetrics, and gynecology). Specific applications of B-scanning will be further discussed in this chapter, and other applications are discussed in later chapters.

To obtain expertise in scanning technique, the sonographer must be thoroughly familiar with anatomy, pathology, patient contours, machine capabilities, and transducer characteristics. Although it is difficult to appreciate scanning technique from a book, individual training in diagnostic ultrasound is part of the sonographer's experience in producing high-quality scans. The sonographer must be familiar with special scanning techniques, artifacts, and equipment malfunction to be able to produce consistently high-quality scans. Automated ultrasound equipment is currently being evaluated clinically for more efficient diagnostic results. Such units would replace the "art" in most of the scanning, in turn allowing the sonographer to fully concentrate on anatomy and pathology.

With the advent of scan convertors for gray scale, some of the "art" in performing an adequate scan has been removed. By performing single scans with very slight sectoring motion, high-quality ultrasonograms can be made.

Ultrasound has the capability of distinguishing interfaces among soft tissue structures of different acoustic densities. The strength of the echoes reflected is dependent on the acoustic interface and the angle at which the sound beam strikes the interface. It is for this reason that a compound sector-scanning motion is used to record a maximum number of interfaces. If too much sectoring is used, the scan will lose much of its detail; therefore the sonographer must judge during the performance of the scan when the scan is completed.

ORIENTATION TO LABELING AND PATIENT POSITION
Labeling

An orderly procedure should be used to identify the anatomic position where the transverse and longitudinal scans have been taken. The illustrations in this book use the umbilicus or the symphysis pubis in the transverse supine position; in the sagittal supine position the xyphoid and umbilicus are used; for the prone position the iliac crest is used as a landmark (Fig. 8-1).

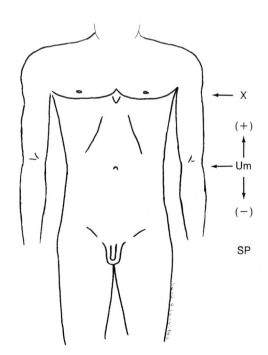

Fig. 8-1. Transverse labeling. *Um,* Umbilicus; *SP,* symphysis pubis; *X,* xyphoid.

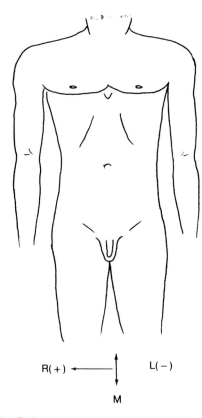

Fig. 8-2. Longitudinal labeling. *M*, Midline.

R(+) ← | → L(−)

M

All transverse supine scans are oriented with the liver to the left of the scan. Prone transverse scans orient the liver to the right. Longitudinal scans present the patient's head to the left and feet to the right of the scan.

The umbilicus or iliac crest is usually considered zero point for the upper abdomen. Scans cephalad from this point are labeled "+"; scans caudad are labeled "−."

Longitudinal scans utilize the xyphoid, umbilicus, and symphysis to denote the midline of the scan. Right of the midline is designated "+," and a "−" is used for the left. For example, a scan made 2 cm to the right is R + 2 cm; a scan made 1.5 cm to the left is L − 1.5 cm (Fig. 8-2).

All scans should be appropriately labeled for future reference. This includes the patient's name, date, and anatomic position.

Patient position

The position of the patient should be described in relation to the table (i.e., a right decubitus would mean the right side down, a left decubitus the left side down). If the scanning plane is oblique, we merely state that it is an oblique view without specifying the exact degree of obliquity.

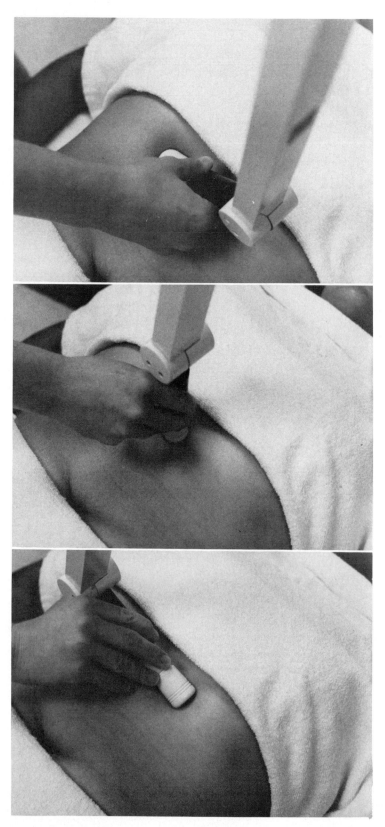

Fig. 8-3. Articulated arm single pie-sweep technique. The transducer face is angled sharply to the far right side of the abdomen and then slowly arced toward the far left. The patient is in full inspiration.

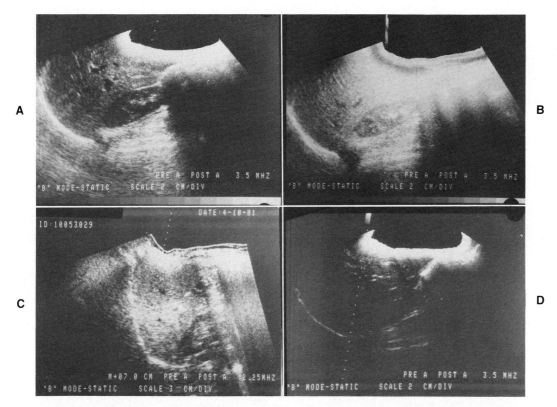

Fig. 8-4. A, Sagittal scan of the liver and right kidney with the correct balance of TGC and sensitivity settings. **B,** Sagittal scan of the liver and right kidney with incorrect TGC settings. The near gain is too high and obliterates the anterior detail of the liver parenchyma. **C,** Sagittal scan of the liver and right kidney with the TBC set incorrectly. The white band of echoes in the middle of the liver indicates that the TGC is broken at this point; to balance the echoes, the TGC should be broken further back, closer to the posterior border of the liver. **D,** Sagittal scan of the liver with incorrect TGC and sensitivity settings. The sensitivity setting is too low and the TGC set too steep.

CRITERIA FOR AN ADEQUATE SCAN

Transverse scans

1. The horseshoe-shaped contour of the vertebral column should be well delineated to ensure that the sound is penetrating through the abdomen without obstruction from gas interference.

2. The prevertebral vessels should be well delineated anterior to the vertebral column. These are usually best demonstrated with a single "pie" sweep technique (Fig. 8-3).

3. The posterior surface of the liver edge should be seen as the transducer is arced across the anterior abdominal wall. This ensures that the time gain compensation (TGC) is set correctly. If this posterior surface is not seen, the TGC may have to be broken earlier and the overall gain increased to allow adequate penetration. If there are too many echoes posterior to the liver, the overall gain should be decreased (Fig. 8-4).

4. The individual organs should be well delineated with their specific echo patterns within their peripheral borders.

Sagittal scans

1. The diaphragmatic surface of the liver should be outlined to ascertain that the dome of the liver has been evaluated.

2. The posterior aspect of the liver should project the same fine echo pattern as the anterior surface. Gain adjustments should be made for overall penetration, or a lower-frequency transducer could be used for increased penetration to the posterior surface.

3. The prevertebral vessels should be outlined with a single sweep technique.

Abdominal scans are probably the most difficult to produce because of the multiple interfaces and curved surfaces within the abdominal cavity. Some laboratories will require the complete abdominal contour on each scan. Precise scanning technique is required to be able to demonstrate the vessels in the midline with a single "pie" sweep. Careful sector scanning along the lateral margin is necessary to outline the liver, the lateral and medial margins of both kidneys, and the spleen. Avoidance of the ribs is important to eliminate rib artifacts that may destroy necessary information. Quick sector scans over their borders usually work well to avoid these ring-down artifacts.

Automated equipment and real time devices provide uniformity in scans for the unskilled sonographer. However, most of these complex machines provide so much detail and resolution that the sonographer must be well qualified in the areas of anatomy and pathology to produce optimum scans.

REAL TIME PROTOCOL

The inclusion of real time examination as an integral part of the ultrasound evaluation can be a very useful contribution to the diagnostic decision if a standard protocol is fol-

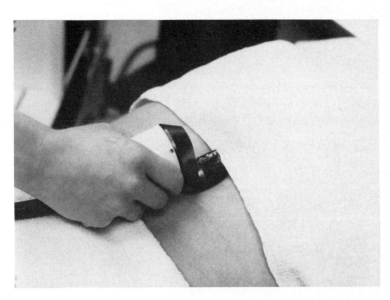

Fig. 8-5. Transverse scan of the upper abdomen with a real time sector scanner.

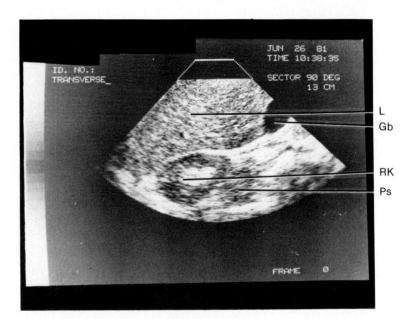

Fig. 8-6. Transverse scan of the liver, *L*, gallbladder, *Gb*, right kidney, *RK*, and psoas, *Ps.*

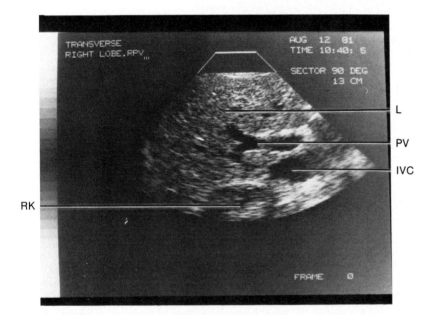

Fig. 8-7. Transverse scan of the liver, *L*, portal vein, *PV*, inferior vena cava, *IVC*, and right kidney, *RK.*

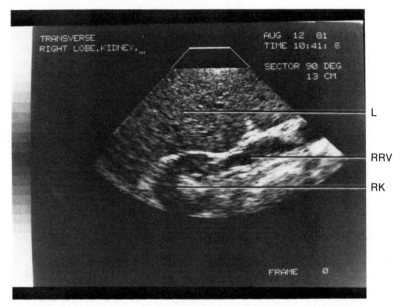

Fig. 8-8. Transverse scan of the liver, *L*, right kidney, *RK*, and right renal vein, *RRV.*

lowed. Unlike articulated arm scans, which allow a panoramic view of the anatomic structures, real time provides a limited-view sector of specific areas of the body. To make the scans easier to interpret, we mark the area of interest on each scan and closely follow a standard protocol for evaluating the upper abdomen. For example, if we are looking at the gallbladder and common bile duct, the scan will be marked *Gb and CBD.*

To avoid getting carried away with a particular piece of anatomy, it is important to adhere to a standard protocol when performing the real time examination. Many times

we have found, for example, the gallbladder to appear normal on the supine view only to contain stones on the decubitus view or upright view.

It has been extremely useful to administer fluid (either by mouth or by water enema) to follow the pattern on real time and distinguish normal anatomy from fluid-filled loops of bowel.

The protocol is as follows:

1. Transverse scans of liver, gallbladder, and right kidney—with special attention to left and right portal veins; look for duct dilation (Figs. 8-5 to 8-8)

2. Transverse scans of
   a. Celiac axis (Fig. 8-9)
   b. Tail of pancreas (Fig. 8-10)
   c. Splenic-portal vein to include body of pancreas; look for pancreatic duct (Fig. 8-11)
   d. SMA-SMV to show uncinate and head of pancreas (Fig. 8-12)
   e. If possible, gastroduodenal artery and CBD for lateral margin of head of pancreas; water may be administered to separate lateral margin from duodenum (Fig. 8-13)

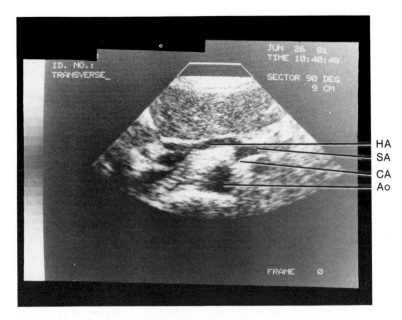

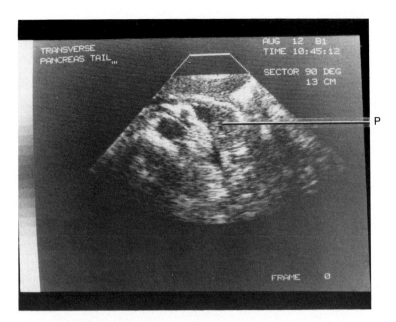

Fig. 8-9. Transverse scan of the celiac axis, *CA*, splenic artery, *SA*, hepatic artery, *HA*, and aorta, *Ao*.

Fig. 8-10. Transverse scan of the tail of the pancreas, *P*.

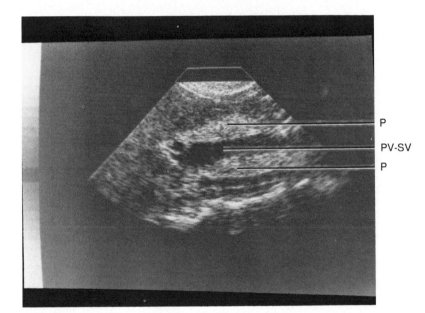

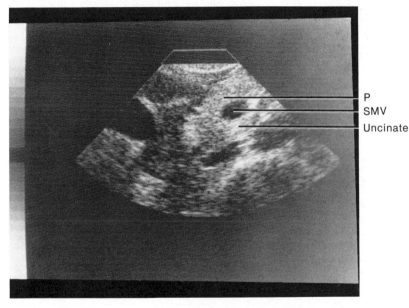

Fig. 8-11. Transverse scan of the splenic-portal vein, *PV-SV*, to include the body of the pancreas.

Fig. 8-12. Transverse scan of the superior mesenteric vein, *SMV*, to show the uncinate and head of the pancreas, *P*.

f. Aorta; look for aneurysm or lymphadenopathy (Fig. 8-14)

3. Longitudinal scans (Fig. 8-15) to include
   a. Left lobe of liver (Fig. 8-16)
   b. Tail of pancreas (Fig. 8-17)
   c. Aorta, celiac axis, SMA, body of pancreas (Fig. 8-18)
   d. SMV, body and uncinate of pancreas (Fig. 8-19)
   e. Head of pancreas, GDA, CBD (Fig. 8-20)
   f. Right lobe of liver (Fig. 8-21)

g. Right kidney (Fig. 8-22)
h. Gallbladder (Fig. 8-23)

4. Left decubitus views to include
   a. Gallbladder (Fig. 8-24)
   b. CBD (Fig. 8-25)
   c. Head of pancreas; if possible, gallbladder (Fig. 8-26)
   d. Right kidney (Fig. 8-27)
   e. Right lobe of liver; this view is best for part of right lobe that is lateral, or that is near dome of liver (Fig. 8-28)
   f. Tail of pancreas

5. Right decubitus views to include
   a. Spleen (Fig. 8-29)
   b. Tail of pancreas (Fig. 8-30)
   c. Transverse and sagittal scans of left kidney (Figs. 8-31 and 8-32)

ARTICULATED ARM PROTOCOL

Prior to the sonographic examination, the sonographer should review the patient's chart, previous radiographic films, and/or other diagnostic tests. Pertinent questions should be asked in regard to the patient's current illness. If a mass is suspected, gentle

Text continued on p. 109.

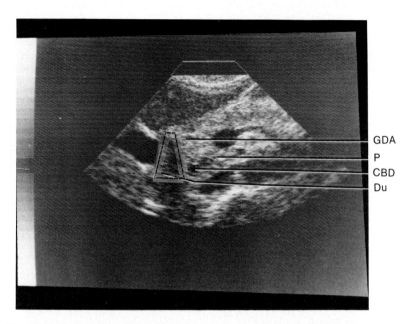

Fig. 8-13. Transverse scan of the pancreas, *P*, gastroduodenal artery, *GDA*, common bile duct, *CBD*, and duodenum, *Du*.

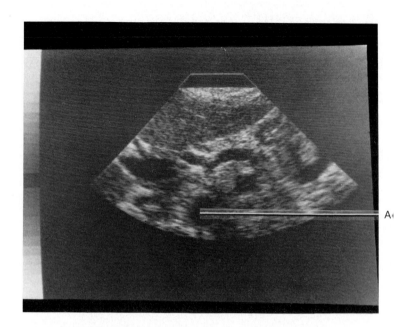

Fig. 8-14. Transverse scan of the aorta, *Ao*.

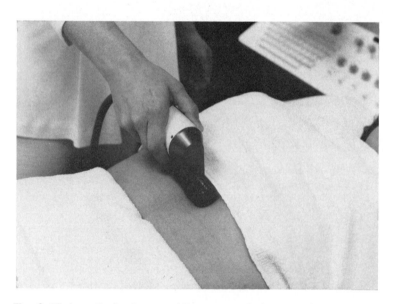

Fig. 8-15. Longitudinal scan of the upper abdomen with a real time sector scanner.

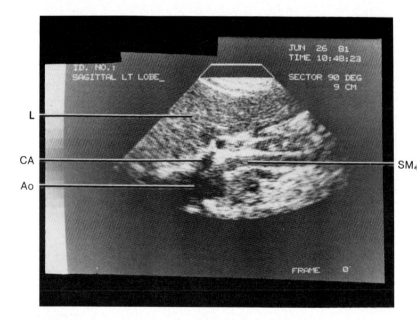

Fig. 8-16. Longitudinal scan of the left lobe of the liver, *L*, aorta, *Ao*, celiac axis, *CA*, and superior mesenteric artery, *SMA*.

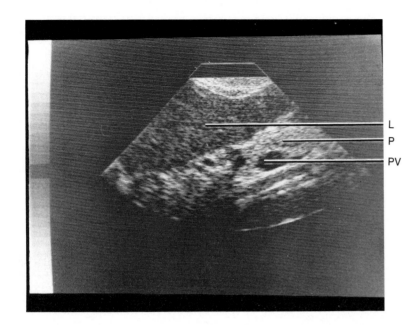

Fig. 8-17. Longitudinal scan of the tail of the pancreas, *P*, liver, *L*, and portal-splenic vein, *PV*.

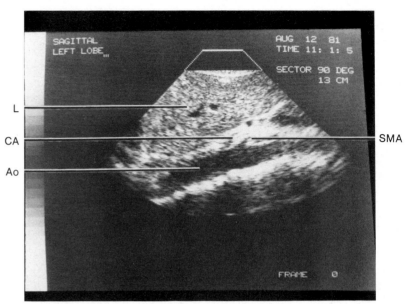

Fig. 8-18. Longitudinal scan of the aorta, *Ao*, celiac axis, *CA*, superior mesenteric artery, *SMA*, and liver, *L*.

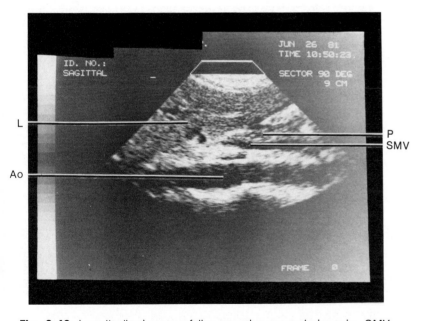

Fig. 8-19. Longitudinal scan of the superior mesenteric vein, *SMV*, pancreas, *P*, aorta, *Ao*, and liver, *L*.

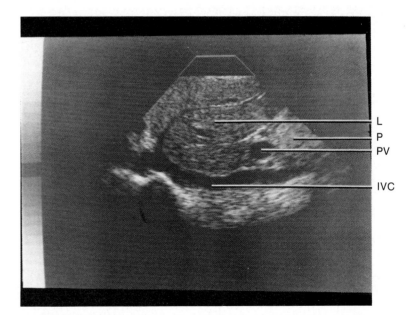

Fig. 8-20. Longitudinal scan of the head of the pancreas, *P*, portal vein, *PV*, inferior vena cava, *IVC*, and liver, *L*.

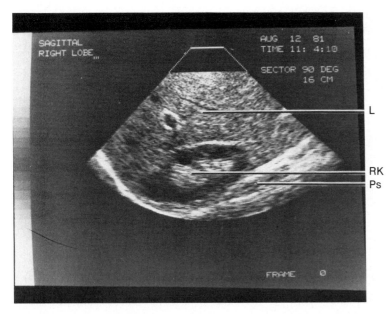

Fig. 8-21. Longitudinal scan of the right lobe of the liver, *L*, right kidney, *RK*, and psoas, *Ps*.

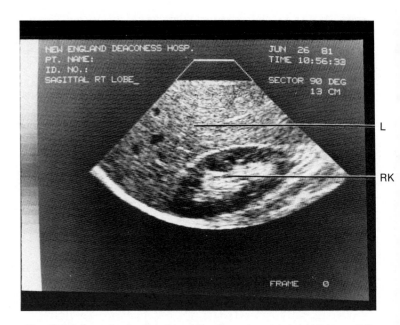

Fig. 8-22. Longitudinal scan of the liver, *L*, and right kidney, *RK*.

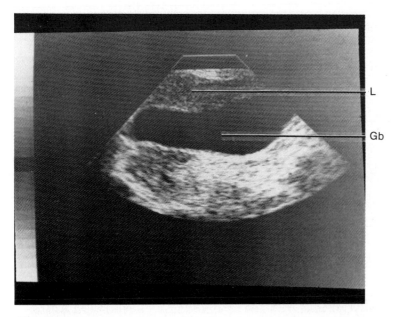

Fig. 8-23. Longitudinal scan of the liver, *L*, and gallbladder, *Gb*.

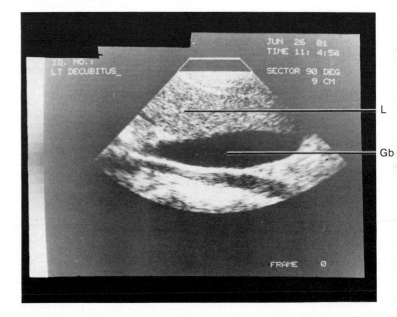

Fig. 8-24. Left decubitus view of the liver, *L*, and gallbladder, *Gb*.

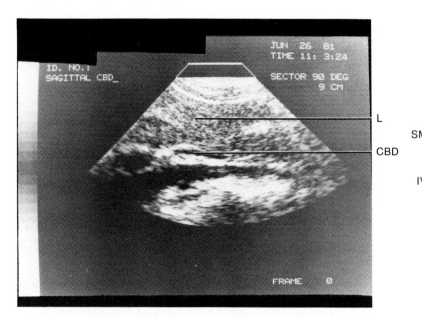

Fig. 8-25. Left decubitus view of the liver, *L*, and common bile duct, *CBD*.

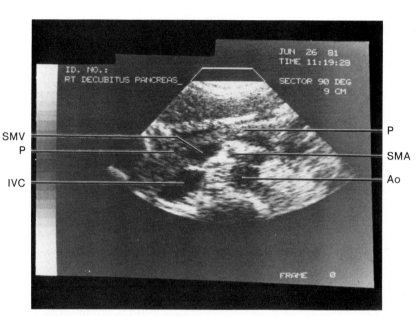

Fig. 8-26. Left decubitus view of the head of the pancreas, *P*, superior mesenteric vein and artery, *SMV* and *SMA*, inferior vena cava, *IVC*, and aorta, *Ao*.

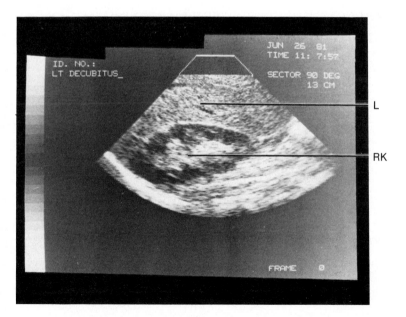

Fig. 8-27. Left decubitus view of the right kidney, *RK*.

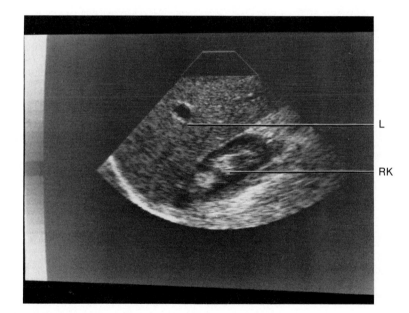

Fig. 8-28. Left decubitus view of the right lobe of the liver, *L*, and right kidney, *RK*.

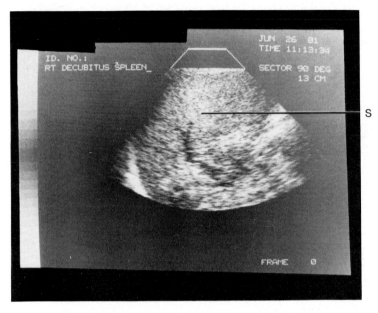

Fig. 8-29. Right decubitus view of the spleen, *S*.

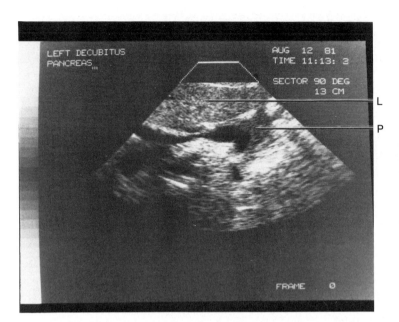

Fig. 8-30. Right decubitus view of the tail of the pancreas, *P*, and liver, *L*.

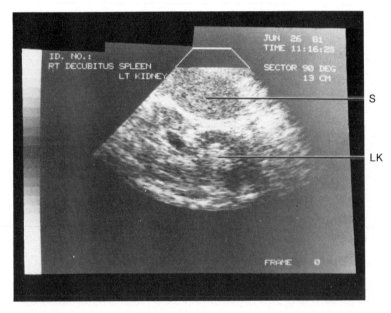

Fig. 8-31. Transverse right decubitus view of the spleen, *S*, and left kidney, *LK*.

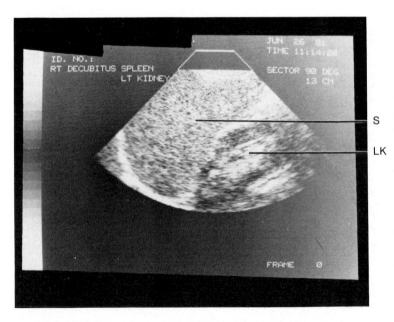

Fig. 8-32. Longitudinal right decubitus view of the spleen, *S*, and left kidney, *LK*.

palpation over the area of interest may be done prior to the coating of a contact substance (mineral oil, Aquasonic gel, etc.) over the patient's abdomen. If real time is available, it may be used for the initial examination as a survey of the upper abdomen. The protocol for the real time examination has been previously described and illustrated. The articulated arm (AA) protocol for individual organs is described below. It may vary slightly according to patient needs and particular problems, but it is presented as a starting point for the novice sonographer. Illustrations are found in the specific organ chapters.

Baseline upper abdomen

1. Transverse scan, 1-cm intervals, from xyphoid to lower right lobe of liver; pie sweep of pancreas and prevertebral vessels
2. Longitudinal scan, 1-cm intervals, to show
   a. Aorta, SMA, CA
   b. SMV
   c. IVC and portal-splenic vein
   d. CBD
   e. Gb (slight decubitus)
   f. Right kidney (slight decubitus)

Liver

1. Major area: liver
2. Ancillary areas: spleen, right kidney, head of pancreas, gallbladder, diaphragm
3. Essential scans
   a. Survey longitudinal and transverse RUQ at 1-cm intervals
   b. Coronal views of left decubitus views if necessary
4. Procedure
   a. Patient supine, real time survey RUQ followed by RUQ survey AA contact scans in deep inspiration to demonstrate uniform texture of liver parenchyma
   b. Left decubitus views of lateral portion of right lobe or subphrenic space as needed

Jaundice

If the patient has jaundice, obtain information from
- Chart (bilirubin level, known primary, etc.)
- Other diagnostic tests (CT, nuclear medicine, etc.)

Decide whether the jaundice is obstructive or nonobstructive
1. Intrahepatic ducts

   a. Look for intrahepatic duct enlargement
   b. Subcostal views of RUQ every 2 cm
   c. Longitudinal views important over area of right kidney (because that is where the intrahepatic ducts are located)
2. Extrahepatic ducts
   a. Longitudinal to see proximal duct anterior to portal vein
   b. Look for distal duct draining into head of pancreas
   c. If everything is normal in proximal duct and intrahepatic duct, probably no obstruction
3. Obstructive: look for dilated ducts (intrahepatic and extrahepatic); if intrahepatic ducts are dilated and extrahepatic ducts are normal, then it most likely is from a metastasis
4. Nonobstructive: if all ducts are normal, evaluate liver closely for
   a. Metastases (primary tumor?)
   b. Cirrhosis (alcoholic history, laboratory data)
   c. Ascites
5. Increased CBD-gallbladder: stones and size; cause of dilation (stones, tumors, or strictures); whether patient is acutely or chronically ill (acute, most likely is stones)
6. Distal duct (posterior to head of pancreas); if gassy, give water or scan upright or right side–down decubitus; follow duct to see whether increased in size; look for stone in duct or enlarged pancreas

Gallbladder and biliary system

1. Major areas: gallbladder and biliary system
2. Ancillary areas: right kidney, head of pancreas, liver, portal vein
3. Essential scans
   a. Continuous survey or at 0.5-cm intervals, transverse and longitudinal to gallbladder with the patient supine or in left decubitus or upright position
   b. Longitudinal or oblique image of common bile duct
   c. Transverse (Mickey Mouse) image of common bile duct
   d. RUQ survey to include liver and head of pancreas at 2-cm intervals
4. Procedure
   a. Patient supine, real time survey RUQ in deep inspiration
   b. Real time scans of gallbladder and biliary system

   c. Patient left decubitus or upright, real time scans of gallbladder and CBD

Gallstones. If there is a question of gallstones, first obtain
- Chart (laboratory values, bilirubin)
- Previous radiographs (was there a recent nonviscous contrast study?)
- Previous surgery (was gallbladder removed?)

Then proceed with a real time survey to demonstrate
1. Gallbladder and biliary system
2. Wall thickness
3. Echogenic bile
4. Stones or polyps (change position of patient)
5. "Packed bag"

Spleen

1. Major area: spleen
2. Ancillary areas: left kidney, tail of pancreas, stomach, diaphragm
3. Essential scans
   a. Transverse LUQ, 1-to-2-cm intervals
   b. Right decubitus, longitudinal and transverse to spleen, at 1-to-2-cm intervals
   c. Prone or upright longitudinal and transverse spleen and LUQ
4. Procedure
   a. Patient supine, real time survey followed by transverse AA images
   b. Longitudinal right decubitus images through intercostal margins
   c. Prone scan if necessary
   d. Upright longitudinal scan to separate left upper pole kidney, stomach, and tail of pancreas from spleen

Pancreas

1. Major areas: pancreas, abdominal vessels (aorta, IVC, SMA, SMV, splenic-portal vein, left renal vein), CBD
2. Ancillary areas: liver, gallbladder, and intrahepatic bile ducts
3. Essential scans
   a. Longitudinal and transverse survey, RUQ at 1-cm intervals
   b. Pie sweep longitudinal and transverse to pancreas
   c. Fluid in stomach to define head or tail of pancreas
   d. Longitudinal and transverse of common bile duct
4. Procedure
   a. Patient supine, real time survey RUQ followed by survey AA scans in full inspiration with specific views of pancreas and biliary ducts

b. Upright or decubitus scans to delineate pancreas from stomach and bowel
c. Fluid-filled stomach views as needed to see tail of pancreas or to separate pancreatic head from duodenum

Aorta

1. Major areas: aorta, common iliacs
2. Ancillary areas: SMA, celiac axis, kidneys, renal arteries
3. Essential scans
   a. Longitudinal and transverse, 1-cm intervals, from xyphoid to bifurcation of aorta
   b. Iliacs, longitudinal to each vessel and transverse to patient's body
   c. Transverse, both kidneys (compare size)
4. Procedure
   a. Patient supine, real time survey followed by AA images
   b. Determine relationship of aneurysm when possible to SMA and to celiac or renal arteries
   c. Visualize thrombus; dissection or flap if present.

Kidneys

1. Major area: kidneys
2. Ancillary areas: perirenal structures, pelvis (if obstructed), ureters (if enlarged), psoas, true pelvis (in cases of obstruction)
3. Essential scans
   a. Decubitus, longitudinal and transverse to the kidneys, at 1-cm intervals
   b. Supine of right kidney through the long axis of the liver

4. Procedure
   a. Real time survey followed by AA images in full inspiration
   b. Upright longitudinal view if necessary to see left upper pole of kidney

Renal transplant. A baseline study is acquired 2 to 7 days after the transplant. Scan the pelvis and transplant site preliminarily with real time to
a. Determine axis of transplant
b. Exclude abnormal fluid collections
c. Rule out ureteral obstruction

Then scan the transplant along its longitudinal and transverse axes, obtaining sections at 0.5-cm intervals longitudinally and 1-cm intervals transversely.

Pelvis

1. Major areas: (female) bladder, uterus, ovaries, cervix; (male) bladder, prostate, seminal vesicle
2. Ancillary areas: (female) iliopsoas, obturator internus, pubococcygeus, rectum; (male) iliopsoas, rectum
3. Essential scans
   a. (female), patient supine:
      (1) Real time survey followed by AA images, longitudinal and transverse
      (2) Right or slight left decubitus to outline ovaries or adnexal area
      (3) Water enema if adnexal mass is present
   b. (male), patient supine:
      (1) Real time survey followed by longitudinal and transverse AA scans of bladder
      (2) Longitudinal and transverse scans of prostate and seminal vesicle if needed with steep caudad angle of transducer to image prostate

9   Vascular structures

The recognition of vascular structures within the upper abdomen becomes very useful to the sonographer in identifying specific organ structures. It is important to understand the origin and anatomic variation of the major arterial and venous structures to be able to identify the anatomy correctly on the sonographic image.

GENERAL COMPOSITION OF VESSELS

Blood is carried away from the heart by the arteries, and it is returned from the tissues to the heart by the veins. Arteries divide into smaller and smaller branches, the smallest of which are the *arterioles*. These lead into the *capillaries*, which are minute-sized vessels that branch and form a network where the exchange of materials between blood and tissue fluid takes place. After the blood passes through the capillaries, it is collected in the small veins or *venules*. These small vessels unite to form larger vessels that eventually return the blood to the heart for recirculation.

A typical artery in cross section consists of three layers (Fig. 9-1):

1. *Tunica intima* (inner layer), which itself consists of three layers: a layer of endothelial cells lining the arterial passage (lumen), a layer of delicate connective tissue, and an elastic layer made up of a network of elastic fibers
2. *Tunica media* (middle layer), which consists of smooth muscle fibers with elastic and collagenous tissue

3. *Tunica adventitia* (external layer), which is composed of loose connective tissue with bundles of smooth muscle fibers and elastic tissue

Smaller arteries will contain less elastic tissue and more smooth muscle. The elasticity of the large arteries is important to the maintenance of a steady blood flow.

The veins have the same three layers as do the arteries, but they are different in their thinner tunica media layer. They appear collapsed due to the little elastic tissue or muscle in their walls.

Veins have special valves within them that permit blood to flow only in one direction, toward the heart. They have a larger total diameter than do arteries, and the blood moves toward the heart slowly as compared to the arterial circulation.

MAIN SYSTEMIC VEINS
Inferior vena cava

The inferior vena cava (IVC) is formed by the union of the common iliac veins behind the right common iliac artery. It ascends vertically through the retroperitoneal space on the right side of the aorta posterior to the liver, piercing the central tendon of the diaphragm at the level of the eighth thoracic vertebra and entering the right atrium of the heart. Its entrance into the lesser sac separates it from the portal vein.

The tributaries of the IVC are the hepatic veins, the right adrenal vein, the renal veins, the right testicular or ovarian vein, the inferior phrenic vein, the four lumbar veins, the two common iliac veins, and the median sacral vein.

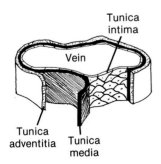
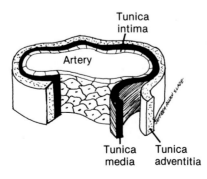

Fig. 9-1. Cross section of an artery and vein showing the distinction between tunica intima, tunica media, and tunica adventitia.

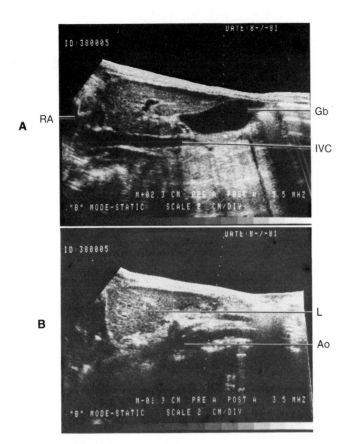

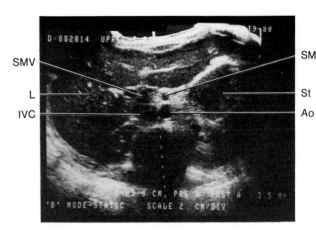

Fig. 9-3. Transverse scan of the great vessels, *Ao* and *IVC*, the superior mesenteric artery and vein, *SMA* and *SMV*, the fluid-filled stomach, *St*, and the liver, *L*.

Fig. 9-2. A, Sagittal scan of the inferior vena cava, *IVC*, as it courses posterior to the liver to empty into the right atrial chamber, *RA*. Gallbladder, *Gb*. **B,** Sagittal scan of the abdominal aorta, *Ao*, as it follows the curvature of the spine. Liver, *L*.

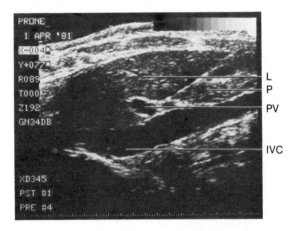

Fig. 9-4. The portal vein, *PV*, serves as a useful landmark on the sagittal scan since the pancreas, *P*, is found just inferior to its margin and anterior to the inferior vena cava, *IVC*.

On most scans the IVC can be seen from the diaphragm to its bifurcation. Differentiation from the aorta is easily made. The IVC has a horizontal course with the proximal portion curving slightly anterior, whereas the aorta follows the curvature of the spine with the distal portion going more posterior (Fig. 9-2). The proximal portion can often be seen to enter the right atrium on longitudinal scans. The IVC serves as a landmark for many other structures in the abdomen and should be routinely visualized on all abdominal scans. On transverse scans its almond-shaped structure serves as a landmark for localization of the superior mesenteric vein, which is generally found anterior and slightly to the right of or just medial to the IVC (Fig. 9-3). On longitudinal scans it serves as a landmark for the portal vein, which is located just anterior to and midway down the IVC. It is also useful in locating the pancreas, which is found just inferior to the portal vein and anterior to the IVC, making a slight impression or indentation on the anterior wall of the IVC (Fig. 9-4).

Transverse scans should be made beginning at the xyphoid and moving toward the umbilicus at 1-cm increments. Longitudinal scans should begin at the midline and proceed in small intervals to the right until the entire vessel is visualized (Fig. 9-5). Again a single sweep of the transducer should be used to image the vessels clearly. If patients are instructed to hold their breath, most likely they will perform a slight Valsalva maneuver toward the end of the breath holding. This maneuver allows normal veins to increase in size with inspiration and decrease in size with expiration. The IVC may expand as much as 3 to 4 cm in diameter with this maneuver.

Real time will allow one to visualize the normal respiratory variation in caliber of the IVC. It is not unusual for the IVC to expand considerably in younger patients during a Valsalva maneuver.

Dilation of the IVC is noted in several pathologic conditions: right ventricular failure, constrictive pericarditis, tricuspid disease, and right atrial myxoma. Dilation of the IVC is also seen in patients with hepatomegaly. The hepatic veins are dilated with increased pressure transmitted through the sinusoids, resulting in portal vein distention.

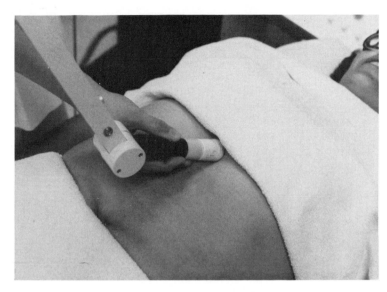

Fig. 9-5. Longitudinal scan technique to outline the venous structures. To record maximum information, the transducer should follow a course perpendicular to the vessel.

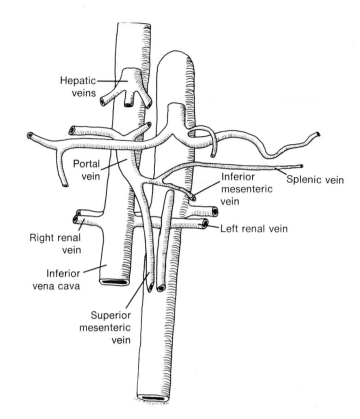

Fig. 9-6. Superior and inferior mesenteric veins joining the splenic vein to form the portal vein.

If cirrhosis is present, the sinusoids may be unable to transmit pressure and then the portal veins will not distend.

The presence of thrombus within the vessel should be evaluated especially in patients with a renal tumor. Other distortions of the inferior vena cava may be due to an extrinsic retroperitoneal mass, hepatic neoplasm, or pancreatic mass.

Portal vein

The portal vein (PV) is formed posterior to the pancreas by the union of the superior mesenteric and splenic veins (Fig. 9-6). Its trunk is 5 to 7 cm in length. It runs upward and to the right, posterior to the first part of the duodenum, and enters the lesser omentum. It then ascends in front of the opening into the lesser sac to the porta hepatis, where it divides into right and left terminal branches. It drains blood out of the gastrointestinal tract from the lower end of the esophagus to the upper end of the anal canal, from the pancreas, gallbladder, and bile ducts, and from the spleen. It has an important anastomosis with the esophageal veins, rectal venous plexus, and superficial abdominal veins. The portal venous blood traverses the liver and drains into the inferior vena cava via the hepatic veins.

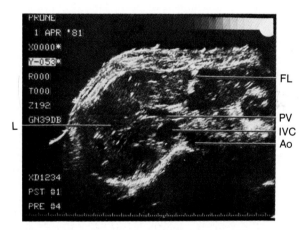

Fig. 9-7. Transverse scan of the portal vein lying anterior to the inferior vena cava. *FL,* Falciform ligament.

The PV is clearly seen on both transverse and longitudinal scans. On transverse scans it is a thin-walled circular structure, generally lateral and somewhat anterior to the inferior vena cava (Fig. 9-7). With the single-sweep technique, it is often possible to record the splenic vein crossing the midline of the abdomen to join the portal trunk. Thus a long section of the vein can be visualized. Often the right or left PV can be seen coming off the portal trunk and entering the hilum of the liver. In the longitudinal plane, slightly to the right of midline, the PV is situated between the inferior vena cava and the liver (Fig. 9-8). It is anterior to the IVC and posterior to the liver. A landmark for locating the pancreas can be established with the demonstration of these vessels. The pancreas is anterior to the IVC and caudal to the portal vein.

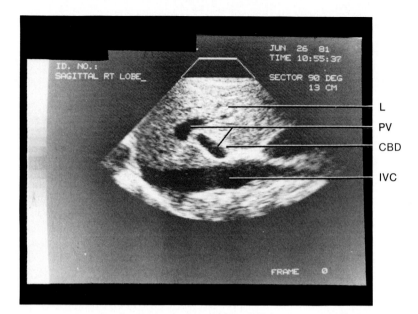

Fig. 9-8. Sagittal scan of the portal vein anterior to the inferior vena cava. It may serve as a useful landmark to the common bile duct, which is seen to lie along its anterior margin.

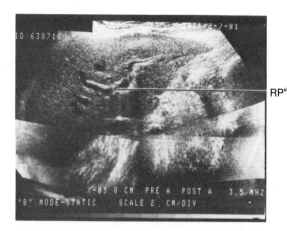

Fig. 9-9. Transverse view of the right portal vein as it courses throughout the right lobe of the liver.

Portal vein dilation can be seen with many forms of hepatic disease, especially cirrhosis.

Portal veins become smaller as they progress from the porta hepatis. Large radicles situated near or approaching the porta hepatis are portal veins, not hepatic veins. They are characterized by high-amplitude acoustic reflections that presumably arise from the fibrous tissues surrounding the portal triad as it courses through the liver substance.

The right and left portal veins course transversely through the liver. Thus transverse scans will display their longest extent. The right PV is most consistently demonstrated on the sonogram (Fig. 9-9). Anatomically any intraparenchymal segment of the portal venous system lying to the right of the lateral aspect of the inferior vena cava is a branch of the right portal system. The left PV has a narrow-caliber trunk and may be seen coursing transversely through the left hepatic lobe from a posterior to an anterior position (Fig. 9-10).

The caudate lobe of the liver lies just cranial to the bifurcation of the main PV (Fig. 9-11) and may separate the cava from the portal vein; usually, however, it does not occur throughout the entire course of the vein. This relationship is best seen on the longitudinal scan.

Since the portal radicle may have many different variations, it is important to become familiar with their patterns to be able to distinguish them from dilated biliary radicles.

Splenic vein

The splenic vein (SV) is a tributary of the portal circulation. It begins at the hilum of the spleen as the union of several veins and is then joined by the short gastric and left gastroepiploic veins. It passes to the right within the lienorenal ligament and runs posterior to the pancreas below the splenic artery (SA). It then joins the superior mesenteric vein behind the neck of the pancreas to form the portal vein. It is joined by veins from the pancreas and the inferior mesenteric vein.

The SV is best visualized in the transverse plane as it crosses the abdomen from the hilum of the spleen to join the portal vein slightly to the right of midline (Fig. 9-12). Single-sweep technique should be used, with the patient performing a Valsalva maneuver or in suspended respiration. The SV crosses anteriorly to the aorta and the IVC and generally relates to the medial and posterior borders of the pancreatic body and tail. Its course is variable, so small degrees of obliquity may be necessary. It is usually smaller than the SMV and the main portal vein.

On longitudinal scans the splenic vein can be visualized posterior to the left lobe of the liver and anterior to the major vascular structures (Fig. 9-13), and the pancreas may be seen inferior and slightly anterior to the vein.

The larger diameter of the PV is the result of the influx of blood from the SMV. An obvious widening is demonstrated at the junction of the portal and splenic veins.

When splenomegaly is present, it is often

possible to identify the origin of the SV at the splenic hilum.

Superior mesenteric vein

The superior mesenteric vein (SMV) is also a tributary of the portal circulation. It begins at the ileocolic junction and runs upward along the posterior abdominal wall within the root of the mesentery of the small intestine and on the right side of the superior mesenteric artery (SMA). It passes anterior to the third part of the duodenum and posterior to the neck of the pancreas, where it joins the splenic vein to form the portal vein. It also receives tributaries that correspond to the branches of the SMA, joined by the inferior pancreaticoduodenal vein to the right and the right gastroepiploic vein from the right aspect of the greater curvature of the stomach to the left.

The SMV is somewhat variable in its anatomic location. Generally it is related to the inferior vena cava in an anterior position. Often on ultrasound it is seen slightly to the right or to the left of the IVC and to the right of the SMA (Fig. 9-14). Since the SMV drains into the portal vein (with the splenic vein), the sonographer should not be able to demonstrate these three structures together on a single transverse scan. Thus the SMV doubles as the posterior border of the neck of the pancreas and as the anterior border where it crosses over the uncinate process of the pancreatic head. On longitudinal scans the SMV appears as a long tubular structure generally anterior to the inferior vena cava

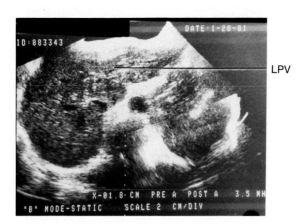

Fig. 9-10. The left portal vein has a narrow-caliber trunk and may be seen to course transversely through the left lobe of the liver.

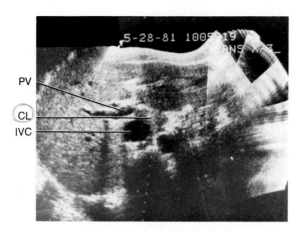

Fig. 9-11. The caudate lobe is the tonguelike projection of the liver lying between the portal vein and inferior vena cava. This may look more pronounced as the cephalic angle is increased.

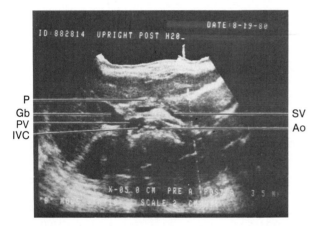

Fig. 9-12. Transverse scan of the splenic vein as it courses from the hilum of the spleen and flows posterior to the body of the pancreas to form the portal vein.

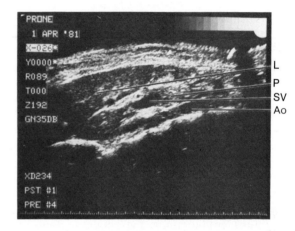

Fig. 9-13. Sagittal view of the splenic vein with the body of the pancreas inferior. This is near the junction of the splenic-portal confluence.

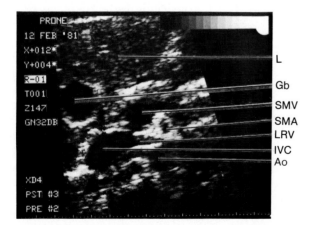

Fig. 9-14. Transverse scan of the superior mesenteric vein and artery. These vessels serve as the posterior border of the body of the pancreas. The left renal vein, *LRV*, is seen to flow anterior to the aorta and posterior to the SMA to enter the IVC.

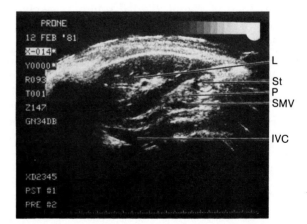

Fig. 9-15. Sagittal scan of the superior mesenteric vein as it courses anterior to the uncinate process of the pancreas and posterior to the neck of the pancreas.

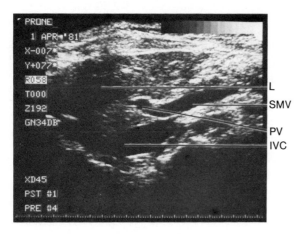

Fig. 9-16. Sagittal scan of the superior mesenteric vein as it joins the portal vein.

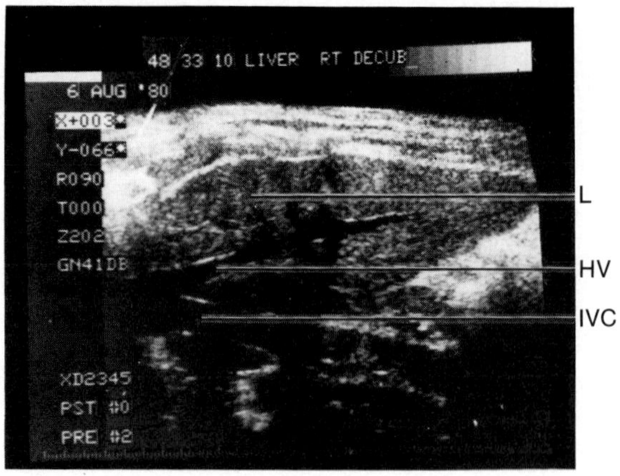

Fig. 9-17. Sagittal scan of the hepatic veins as they empty into the inferior vena cava at the level of the diaphragm. Their naked borders are well demonstrated, which is in part due to the transducer approach (not perpendicular to the borders of the vessel).

(Fig. 9-15). Often with correct oblique angulation of the transducer, the path of the SMV can be traced into the portal system (Fig. 9-16).

The following points help to distinguish the SMA from the SMV:

1. The SMV is of larger caliber than the SMA.
2. Respiratory variations are seen in the SMV.
3. On sagittal scans the SMA angles away from the aorta whereas the SMV tends to parallel the aorta or course anteriorly away from the aorta near the portal-splenic confluence.
4. Real time identification of the confluence of SMV-SV-PV or SMA is possible as the SMA originates from the aorta.

Inferior mesenteric vein

This vein is a tributary of the portal circulation. It begins midway down the anal canal as the superior rectal vein. It runs up the posterior abdominal wall on the left side of the inferior mesenteric artery and duodeno-jejunal junction and joins the splenic vein behind the pancreas. It receives many tributaries along its way, including the left colic vein.

The IMV is difficult to recognize on ultrasound because of its anatomic location and small diameter. It is generally covered by small bowel tissue and has no major vascular structures posterior to it.

Hepatic veins

The hepatic veins are the largest visceral tributaries of the IVC. They originate in the liver and drain into the IVC, returning blood from the liver that was brought to it by the

hepatic artery and the portal vein. Their minor tributaries—right hepatic vein in the right lobe, middle hepatic vein in the caudate lobe, and left hepatic vein in the left lobe—empty into the IVC at the level of the diaphragm.

The hepatic veins are frequently visualized on longitudinal sections of the liver (Fig. 9-17). Transverse scans obtained with a cephalic tilt of the transducer at the level of the xyphoid often show at least two of the three veins draining into the IVC. The two veins resemble the *Playboy* bunny emblem on the sonogram (Fig. 9-18).

The ability to distinguish hepatic veins from other vascular structures depends on recognition of their anatomic patterns. Hepatic veins drain cephalad toward the diaphragm and then dorsomedially toward the inferior vena cava. Hepatic veins increase in caliber as they approach the diaphragm. Unlike portal veins, they are not surrounded by bright acoustic reflections although a slight amount of acoustic enhancement may be seen along their posterior border.

Renal veins

The right renal vein (RV) is seen best on the transverse sonogram with a single-sweep technique. It can be seen to flow directly from the renal sinus into the posterolateral aspect of the inferior vena cava (Fig. 9-19).

The left RV may not be seen so easily. However, when it is seen, it exits the renal sinus and takes a course anterior to the abdominal aorta and posterior to the superior mesenteric artery to enter the medial aspect of the inferior vena cava (Fig. 9-20).

Above the entry of the renal veins the inferior vena cava enlarges. The increased vol-

ume of blood returning from the kidneys to the IVC accounts for this enlargement.

MAIN SYSTEMIC ARTERIES
Aorta

The systemic circulation leaves the left ventricle of the heart by way of the aorta. The aorta is the largest artery in the body. After it arises a short distance from the left ventricle, it ascends behind the pulmonary artery. It then arches to the left and curves downward to form the descending or thoracic aorta. The descending aorta enters the abdomen through the aortic opening of the diaphragm in front of the twelfth thoracic vertebra in the retroperitoneal space. It descends anteriorly to the bodies of the lumbar vertebrae. At the level of the fourth lumbar vertebra it divides into the two common iliac arteries. The aorta is usually 2 to 4 cm in diameter. Although its diameter may vary slightly along the aortic contour as it branches to the visceral organs, the diameter is generally believed to be fairly uniform. The aorta has four main branches that supply other visceral organs and the mesentery—the celiac trunk, the superior and inferior mesenteric arteries, and the renal arteries (Fig. 9-21).

The common iliac arteries arise at the bifurcation of the aorta and run downward and laterally along the medial border of the right and the left psoas. At the level of the sacroiliac joint each iliac artery bifurcates into an external and an internal iliac artery.

The external iliac artery runs along the medial border of the psoas, following the pelvic brim. It gives off the inferior epigastric and deep circumflex iliac branches before passing under the inguinal ligament to be-

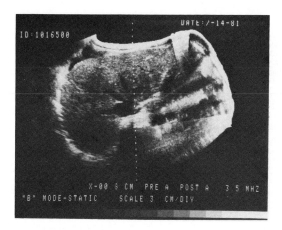

Fig. 9-18. Transverse scan of the hepatic veins as they drain into the inferior vena cava and resemble the *Playboy* bunny sign.

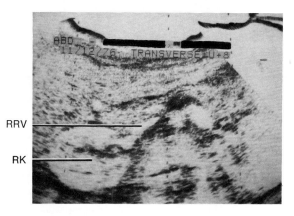

Fig. 9-19. The right renal vein can be seen to flow from the right kidney directly into the inferior vena cava.

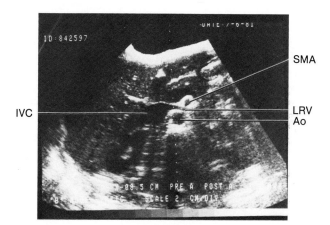

Fig. 9-20. Transverse scan of the left renal vein as it flows posterior to the SMA and anterior to the aorta to enter the inferior vena cava.

come the femoral artery. The internal iliac artery enters the pelvis in front of the sacroiliac joint, at which point it is crossed anteriorly by the ureter. It also divides into anterior and posterior branches to supply the pelvic viscera, peritoneum, buttocks, and sacral canal.

The abdominal aorta is ordinarily one of the easiest abdominal structures to visualize by ultrasound because of the marked change in acoustic impedance between its elastic walls and its blood-filled lumen. Early detection of the abdominal aorta was made by A-mode techniques. The aorta was located approximately by manual palpation, and the transducer was placed over the area suspected to be aneurysmal. On the A-mode trace the aorta appeared as parallel pulsatile movements, reflected from its anterior and posterior walls. Increased echoes within the aortic walls represented thrombus or clot. Patients with arteriosclerotic disease demonstrated decreased motion in the aortic walls, and thus the vessel became more difficult to recognize on the A-mode trace. Calcification of the aorta produced denser echoes than did a noncalcified aorta.

Gray scale sonography provides the diagnostic information needed to visualize the entire abdominal aorta, to assess its diameter, and to visualize the presence of thrombus, calcification, or dissection. The visualization of abdominal vessels is made with an articulated arm or real time B-scanner. In many patients it will be more expedient to follow the course of the vessel with a real time scanner than to try to "plot" its course with an articulated arm scanner. Real time also allows visualization of arterial pulsations, which may help to distinguish an artery from a vein.

The patient's abdomen should be palpated

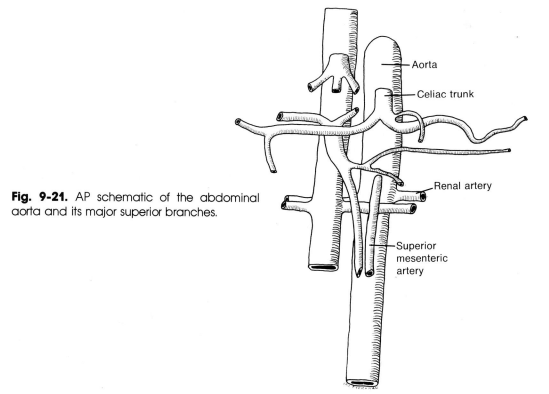

Fig. 9-21. AP schematic of the abdominal aorta and its major superior branches.

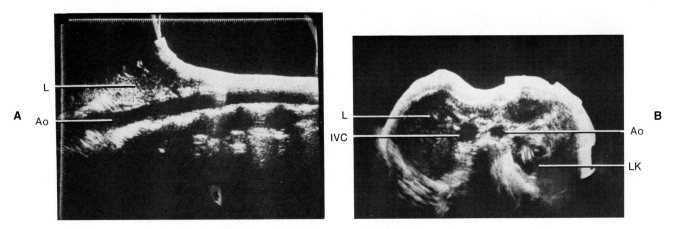

Fig. 9-22. Longitudinal, **A,** and transverse, **B,** scans of the abdominal aorta.

prior to scanning so the course of the abdominal aorta can be predetermined and its extent into the iliac arteries noted. The patient is routinely scanned in the supine position. Gas-filled or barium-filled loops of bowel may prevent adequate visualization of the aorta, but this can be overcome by applying gentle pressure with the transducer to the area of interest or by changing the angle of the transducer or the patient. To outline the course of the vessel, initial scans should be made in the longitudinal plane (Fig. 9-22). Each longitudinal scan should include the area from the xyphoid to well below the level of the bifurcation. In the normal individual the aorta shows a gradual tapering of its luminal dimension as it proceeds distally in the abdomen. Goldberg's ultrasound study of the aortic lumen measured 23 mm at the eleventh rib, 20 mm above the renal arteries, 18 mm below the renal arteries, and 15 mm at the bifurcation. Longitudinal scans are made beginning at the midline with successive scans at 0.5-to-1-cm intervals out in each direction for several centimeters. A low to medium gain should be used with the single-sweep technique to demonstrate the aorta without internal artifactual echoes.

Weak echoes may appear within the echo-free lumen of the vessel. These are artifactual, due to reverberations and not to clot formation (Fig. 9-23). Usually clot will produce echoes of a greater intensity than reverberation echoes. By reduction of the sensitivity or adjustment of the time gain compensation (TGC), the electronic noise can be eliminated and thus a "cleaner" lumen obtained. Lateral resolution can also account for these spurious echoes. Poor lateral resolution results in echoes that are recorded at the same level as those from soft tissues that surround the vessel lumen. This is particular-

ly true of the vessels are smaller in diameter than the transducer.

Since the aorta follows the anterior course of the vertebral column, it is important that the transducer also follow a perpendicular path along the entire curvature of the aorta. A very slight sectoring motion may be needed if the echoes are not recorded from all borders. As the sectoring motion is begun, the sensitivity should be decreased to avoid overwriting the walls of the aorta. The anterior and posterior walls should be easily seen as a thin line for accuracy in measuring the diameter of the lumen. This facilitates measuring the anteroposterior diameter of the aorta, which in most institutions is done from the leading edge of the anterior to the leading edge of the posterior aortic wall (Fig. 9-24).

In an effort to measure the anteroposterior width of the abdominal aorta, transverse scans are usually made every 1 to 2 cm from the xyphoid to the bifurcation. The normal aorta is visualized as a circular structure anterior to the spine and slightly to the left of midline. In some cases the transverse diameter of the aorta differs from the longitudinal measurements; thus it is important to identify the vessel in two dimensions. If the patient has a very tortuous aorta, scans may be difficult to obtain in a single plane (Fig. 9-25). As one scans in the longitudinal plane, the upper portion of the abdominal aorta may be well visualized but the lower portion may be out of the plane of view. In this case the examiner should obtain a complete scan of the upper segment and then concentrate fully on the lower segment. Sometimes it is helpful to mark the areas of the aorta on the abdomen with a wax pencil so that proper alignment can be obtained with the transducer and an oblique scan made. However, if it is difficult

to outline the aorta in the longitudinal plane, transverse scans may be used. We have seen the abdominal aorta stretch from the far right of the abdomen to the far left in certain patients.

To better visualize the aortic bifurcation, one may employ the lateral decubitus position. The patient should be examined in deep inspiration, which projects the liver and diaphragm into the abdominal cavity and creates an acoustic window for visualizing the vascular structures. If splenomegaly or a transonic left-sided mass is present, the right lateral decubitus position may be used. The patient should be rotated 5 to 10 degrees posteriorly from the true lateral position. Longitudinal scans along the axis of the abdominal aorta from the level of the xyphoid to the bifurcation should be made. Slight medial or lateral angulation (10 to 15 degrees) may be needed to obtain the bifurcation. The inferior vena cava may also be visualized anterior to the aorta in this plane.

Celiac trunk

The celiac trunk, originating within the first 2 cm of the abdominal aorta, is surrounded by the liver, spleen, inferior vena cava, and pancreas (Fig. 9-26). It immediately branches into the left gastric, splenic, and common hepatic arteries.

The splenic artery is the largest of the three branches of the celiac trunk. From its origin it takes a somewhat tortuous course horizontally to the left, usually along the upper margin of the pancreas. At a variable distance from the spleen it divides into two branches. One of these runs caudally into the greater omentum toward the right gastroepiploic artery. This branch is the left gastroepiploic artery. The other runs cephalically and divides into the short gastric artery,

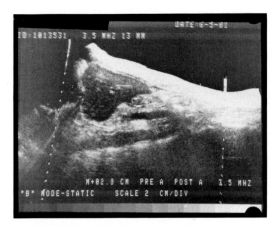

Fig. 9-23. The abdominal aorta can appear to have low-level echoes within its lumen if the sensitivity is too high. These are artifactual echoes and should not be confused with thrombus.

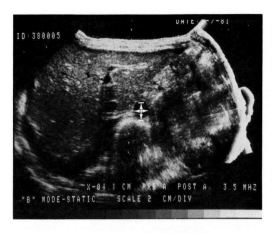

Fig. 9-24. The exact measurements of the aorta should be made on the ultrasound image to provide accurate follow-up for aneurysm patients.

which supplies the fundus of the stomach, and a number of splenic branches that supply the spleen. Several small branches originate at the splenic artery as it runs along the upper border of the pancreas. The dorsal pancreatic, great pancreatic, and caudal pancreatic arteries are pertinent. The dorsal pancreatic (also known as the superior pancreatic) artery usually originates from the beginning of the splenic artery but may also arise from the hepatic artery, celiac trunk, or aorta. It runs down behind and in the substance of the pancreas, dividing into right and left branches. The left branch comprises the transverse pancreatic artery. The right branch constitutes an anastomotic vessel to the anterior pancreatic arch and also a branch to the uncinate process. The great pancreatic artery originates from the splenic artery further to the left and passes downward, dividing into branches that anastomose with the transverse or inferior pancreatic artery. The caudal pancreatic artery supplies the tail of the pancreas and divides into branches that anastomose with terminal branches of the transverse pancreatic artery. The transverse pancreatic artery courses behind the body and tail of the pancreas close to the lower pancreatic border. It may originate from or communicate with the superior mesenteric artery.

The common hepatic artery comes off the celiac trunk and courses to the right of the aorta at almost a 90-degree angle. It courses along the upper border of the head of the pancreas, behind the posterior layer of the peritoneal omental bursa, to the upper margin of the superior part of the duodenum, which forms the lower boundary of the epiploic foramen. It ascends into the liver with

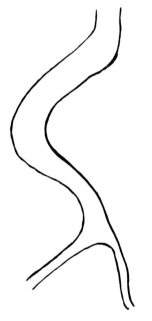

Fig. 9-25. Schematic of a tortuous aorta. The correct obliquity must be found with real time so the long segment of the vessel can be assessed.

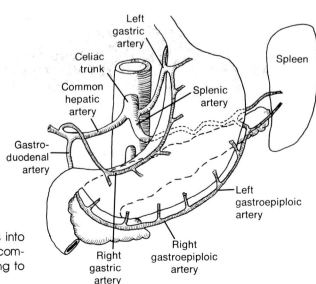

Fig. 9-26. Celiac trunk and its branches into the left gastric artery, splenic artery, and common hepatic artery, with further branching to the stomach and pancreatic area.

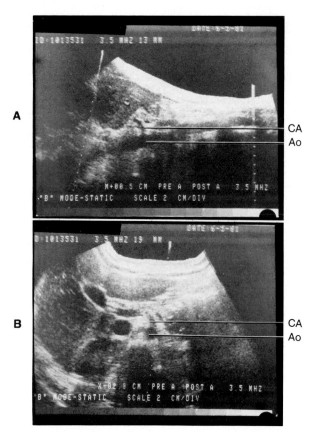

Fig. 9-27. A, Sagittal scan of the abdominal aorta with the celiac axis, *CA,* arising from its anterior border. **B,** Transverse scan of the celiac axis arising from the aorta.

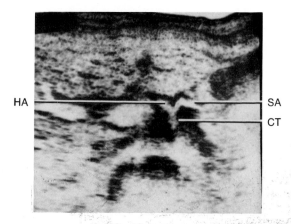

Fig. 9-28. Transverse scan of the celiac trunk, *CT,* with a branch to the right representing the common hepatic artery and a branch to the left the splenic artery.

the hepatic duct, which lies to the right, and the portal vein, which is posterior. It then divides into two major branches at the portal fissure that subdivide as they enter the liver to supply the right and left lobes:

1. The right hepatic branch, serving the gallbladder via the cystic artery

2. The smaller left branch, serving both the caudate and the left lobes of the liver

Within the liver parenchyma the hepatic arterial branches further divide repeatedly into progressively smaller vessels that eventually supply the portal triad.

The head of the pancreas, the duodenum, and parts of the stomach are supplied by the gastroduodenal artery, which arises from the common hepatic artery.

The celiac trunk is best visualized ultrasonically on the longitudinal scan as the aorta pierces the diaphragm and extends into the abdominal cavity (Fig. 9-27). It is usually seen as a small vascular structure arising anteriorly from the abdominal aorta. Since it is only 1 to 2 cm long, it is sometimes difficult to record unless careful evaluation near the midline of the aorta is made. Sometimes the celiac trunk can be seen to extend in a cephalic rather than a caudal presentation. The superior mesenteric artery is usually just inferior to the origin of the celiac trunk and may be used as a landmark in locating the celiac trunk. Transversely, one can differentiate the celiac trunk as the wings of a seagull arising directly anterior from the abdominal aorta (Fig. 9-28). The splenic artery may be seen to flow from the celiac trunk toward the spleen. Since it is so tortuous, it is difficult to follow routinely on the transverse scan. Generally small pieces of the splenic artery are visible as the artery weaves in and out of the left upper quadrant. The hepatic artery can be seen to flow anterior and to the right of the celiac trunk, where it then divides into the right and left hepatic arteries.

The left gastric artery is of very small diameter and often difficult to visualize by ultrasound. It becomes difficult to separate from the splenic artery unless distinct structures are seen in the area of the celiac trunk branching to the left of the abdominal aorta.

Superior mesenteric artery

The superior mesenteric artery (SMA) arises anteriorly from the abdominal aorta approximately 1 cm below the celiac trunk. It runs posterior to the neck of the pancreas, passing over the uncinate process of the pancreatic head anterior to the third part of the duodenum, where it enters the root of the mesentery and colon. It has five main branches: the inferior pancreatic, duodenal, colic, ileocolic, and intestinal arteries (Fig. 9-29). These branch arteries to the small bowel themselves consist of 10 to 16 branches arising from the left side of the superior mesenteric trunk. They extend into

the mesentery, where adjacent arteries unite with them to form loops or arcades. Their distribution is to the proximal half of the colon and small intestine.

The SMA is well seen on both transverse and longitudinal scans. A single-sweep technique should demonstrate it arising from the anterior aortic wall. It may follow a parallel course along the abdominal aorta or branch off at a slight angle to the anterior wall of the aorta and then follow a parallel course (Fig. 9-30). If the angle is severe, adenopathy should be considered. The SMA generally arises from the aorta and takes an anterior course as it moves inferiorly to branch to the mesentery and colon. Transversely it can be seen as a separate small circular structure anterior to the abdominal aorta and posterior to the pancreas (Fig. 9-31). Characteristically, it is surrounded by highly reflective echoes from the retroperitoneal fascia.

As it courses caudally, the SMA exits from its position posterior to the pancreatic body and lies medial to the head of the pancreas. The origin of the SMA can be found by locating the left renal vein, where it enters the IVC at the origin of the SMA.

Inferior mesenteric artery

The inferior mesenteric artery (IMA) arises from the anterior abdominal aorta approximately at the level of the third or fourth lumbar vertebra. It proceeds to the left to distribute arterial blood to the descending colon, sigmoid colon, and rectum. It has three main branches: the left colic, sigmoid, and superior rectal arteries.

The IMA is more difficult to visualize by ultrasound; but when it is seen, it generally is on a longitudinal scan. It is a small structure inferior to the SMA and celiac trunk. On transverse scans it is difficult to separate from small loops of bowel within the abdomen.

Renal arteries

The right and left renal arteries arise anterior to the first lumbar vertebra and inferior to the SMA from the posterolateral or lateral walls of the aorta. They divide into anterior and inferior suprarenal branches.

Both renal arteries are best seen on transverse sonograms. The right artery passes posterior to the IVC and anterior to the vertebral column in a posterior and slightly caudal direction (Fig. 9-32). Occasionally on longitudinal scans a segment of the right renal artery is seen as a circular structure posterior to the IVC. The left renal artery has a direct course from the aorta anterior to the psoas and enters the renal sinus (Fig. 9-33).

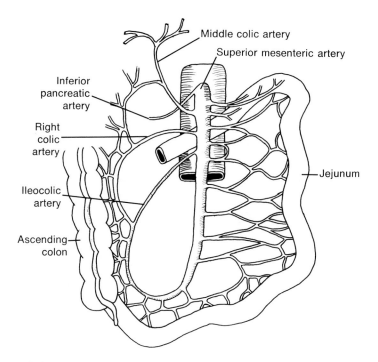

Fig. 9-29. Superior mesenteric artery and its branches to the small bowel and colon.

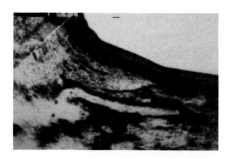

Fig. 9-30. Longitudinal scan of the superior mesenteric artery as it courses from the anterior aortic wall just inferior to the celiac trunk.

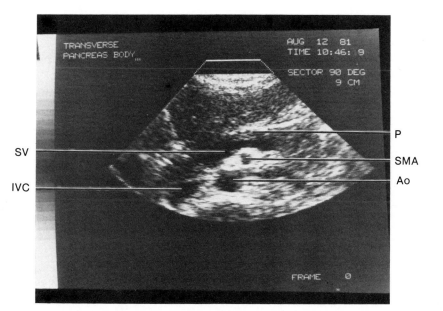

Fig. 9-31. Transverse scan of the superior mesenteric artery with its echogenic border from the retroperitoneal fascia.

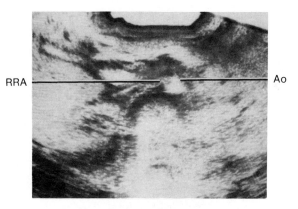

Fig. 9-32. The right renal artery can be seen to flow from the lateral margin of the aorta, posterior to the inferior vena cava.

Fig. 9-33. The left renal artery takes a direct course from the lateral wall of the aorta to the left kidney.

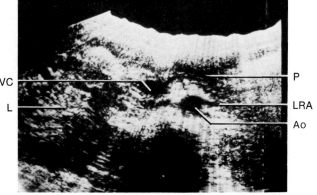

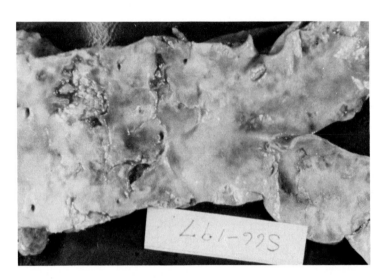

Fig. 9-34. Gross specimen of arteriosclerotic disease of the aorta and iliac vessels.

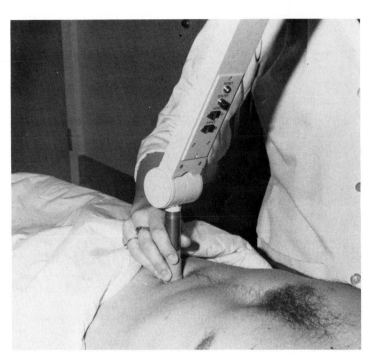

Fig. 9-35. Longitudinal scan technique to outline the abdominal aorta. To record maximum information, the transducer should follow a perpendicular course to the aortic wall.

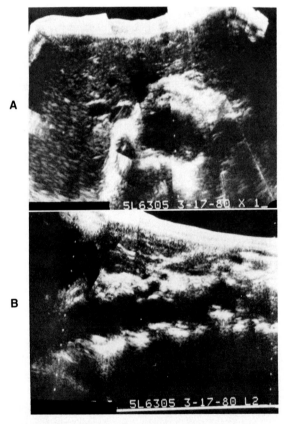

Fig. 9-36. A, Transverse scan of an abdominal aortic aneurysm with clot along its anterior wall. The aneurysm is larger in the transverse than the anteroposterior direction. **B,** Sagittal scan of the aneurysm showing a fusiform dilation of the vessel.

PATHOLOGY OF VASCULAR STRUCTURES
Aneurysms

The greatest value of ultrasound in visualizing the abdominal aorta is the assessment of its luminal diameter for the purpose of ruling out aneurysm. Aneurysms usually are caused by atherosclerotic changes in the arterial wall. Less frequently they are due to mycotic or dissecting lesions.

The most common presentation of an atherosclerotic aneurysm is a fusiform dilation of the distal aorta (at the level of the bifurcation) (Fig. 9-34). Atherosclerosis will also cause decreased pulsations of the aortic walls with bright echoes reflecting the degree of thickening and calcification.

Saccular aneurysms that show only a small connection to the aorta have also been found by ultrasound. Often these are mistaken for a retroperitoneal mass or lymphadenopathy if the examiner does not carefully follow their extent and note their relationship to the aorta. Pulsations are usually diminished due to clot formation or they may appear within the aneurysm due to transmission from the aorta.

Long-term clinical evaluations of patients with an aneurysm have been conducted to determine whether the size of an aneurysm changes (Fig. 9-35). Aneurysms of less than 5 cm maximum diameter (transverse-AP, width, and longitudinal measurements) rup-

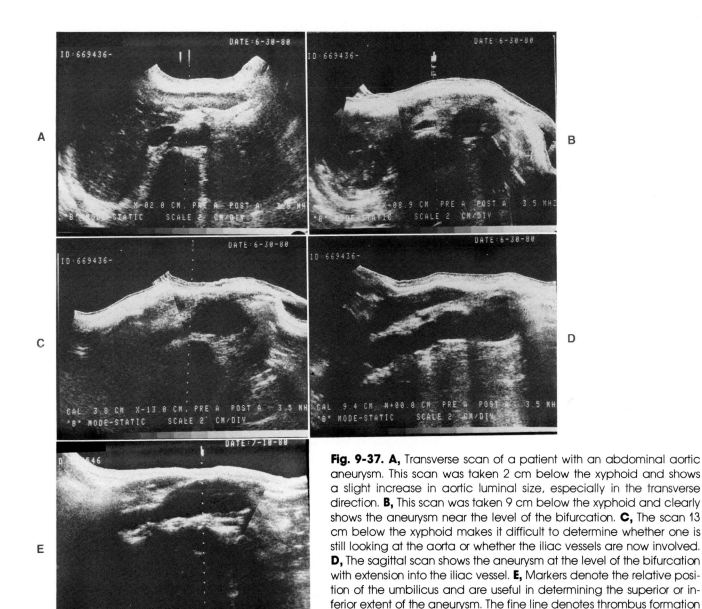

Fig. 9-37. A, Transverse scan of a patient with an abdominal aortic aneurysm. This scan was taken 2 cm below the xyphoid and shows a slight increase in aortic luminal size, especially in the transverse direction. **B,** This scan was taken 9 cm below the xyphoid and clearly shows the aneurysm near the level of the bifurcation. **C,** The scan 13 cm below the xyphoid makes it difficult to determine whether one is still looking at the aorta or whether the iliac vessels are now involved. **D,** The sagittal scan shows the aneurysm at the level of the bifurcation with extension into the iliac vessel. **E,** Markers denote the relative position of the umbilicus and are useful in determining the superior or inferior extent of the aneurysm. The fine line denotes thrombus formation along the anterior border.

ture in 1% of cases whereas those that exceed 6 cm show a 40% chance of rupture. Aneurysms that exceed 7 cm are more likely to rupture (60% to 80% of cases). The patient who presents with an aneurysm probably has a number of other medical problems as well. Thus it becomes important for the clinician to be able to evaluate the size of the aneurysm noninvasively and to follow it sequentially over a 3-to-6-month period by ultrasound. It is also important in these cases to mark on the films the exact location of the aneurysm, with the measurement given in the report so follow-up information will be accurate. It has been found that most aneurysms under 6 cm show little (less than 0.5 cm) or no change in growth over several years. Aneurysms over 6 cm may show dramatic increases in diameter (0.5 cm or more) over a 3-to-6-month interval (Figs. 9-36 and 9-37).

Another important consideration is the relationship of the aneurysm to the renal arteries. Thus not only the diameter should be expressed but also the longitudinal extent of the aneurysm as it relates to the origin of the renal vessels. Often bowel gas impairs adequate visualization of the renal arteries and an indirect method must be used to locate the origin of the superior mesenteric artery. The renal arteries usually originate about the same level as the SMA.

If an aneurysm extends beyond the diaphragm into the thoracic aorta, it may be difficult to trace with ultrasound due to lung interference in the beam (Fig. 9-38). Several attempts may be necessary to demonstrate this thoracic aneurysm. The transducer can be sharply angled from the xyphoid toward the sternal notch to visualize the lower extent of the aorta. In another technique the transducer may execute a longitudinal parasternal scan over the long axis of the heart. The thoracic aorta should be seen posterior to the cardiac structures. A third alternative is to scan the patient's back with the patient upright or prone. The transducer should be angled slightly medial and placed in a sagittal plane along the left intercostal space. This is very effective if the thoracic aorta is deviated slightly to the left of the spine. Scal-

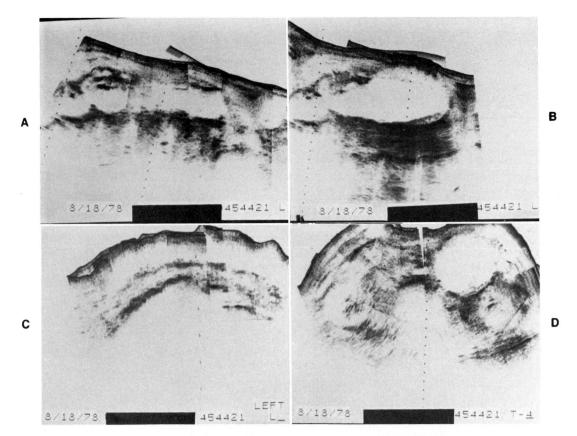

Fig. 9-38. A, Sagittal scan of a fusiform dilation of the abdominal aorta. **B,** Extension into the left iliac vessel is well seen. **C,** Further extension of the aneurysm in the thoracic aorta. **D,** Transverse scan of the aneurysm and its relationship to the renal arteries.

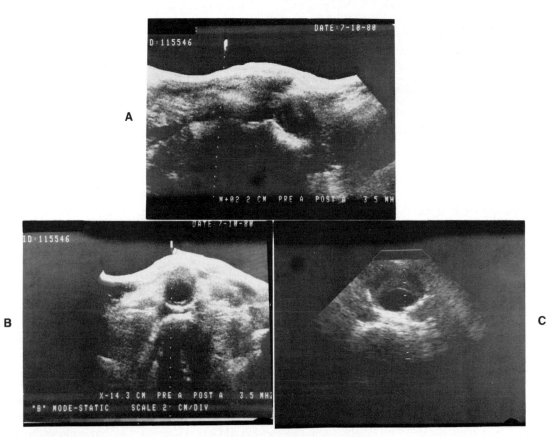

Fig. 9-39. A, Sagittal scan of an iliac artery aneurysm. **B,** Transverse scan of the aneurysm with low-level thrombus along the anterolateral border. **C,** Real time often allows a better appreciation of the amount and extent of thrombus material since the transducer is able to be more perpendicular to thrombus interfaces.

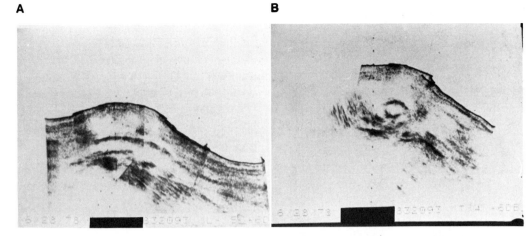

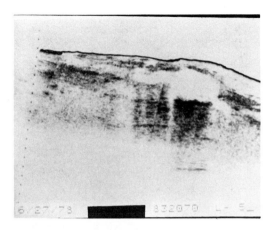

Fig. 9-40. A, Longitudinal and, **B,** transverse scans of a femoral artery graft. There is a mild dilation of the femoral artery, along with a large collection at the junction of the graft with the femoral artery. This could represent a graft abscess or hematoma, and clinical correlation is needed.

Fig. 9-41. Longitudinal scan of an aneurysm of the femoral artery. It measured 3.5 cm in anteroposterior and transverse dimensions and was 5.5 cm long.

loped reverberations from the ribs will be recorded, with the luminal echoes directly posterior.

Thrombus within an aneurysm is shown ultrasonically as medium-to-low-level echoes. Generally increased sensitivity is likely to highlight the thrombus echoes. The echoes should be seen in both planes on more than one scan to be separated from low-level reverberation echoes. Thrombus formation is usually more frequent along the anterior and lateral walls than along the posterior wall of the aorta (Fig. 9-39).

Filly et al. state that three characteristics of thrombus are seen by ultrasound:

1. A fresh clot that is completely jelled and uniform tends to be anechoic.
2. A clot with fissures or irregularities results in interfaces with many reflections.
3. An organized thrombus that is vascularized tends to generate many internal echoes.

An aneurysm that reaches the bifurcation may well extend into the iliac vessels. Real time allows the sonographer rapidly to assess the lumina of these vessels and to trace their course into the pelvic cavity (Figs. 9-40 and 9-41).

Aortic grafts

An abdominal aortic aneurysm may be surgically repaired with a flexible graft material attached to the end of the remaining aorta (Fig. 9-42). The synthetic material used for a graft produces bright echo reflections as com-

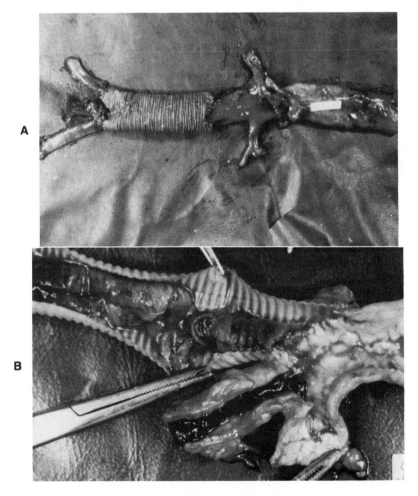

Fig. 9-42. A, Gross specimen of the abdominal aorta with a graft attached below the renal arteries and above the iliac arteries. **B,** Thrombus and clot within the vessel at dissection.

A

B

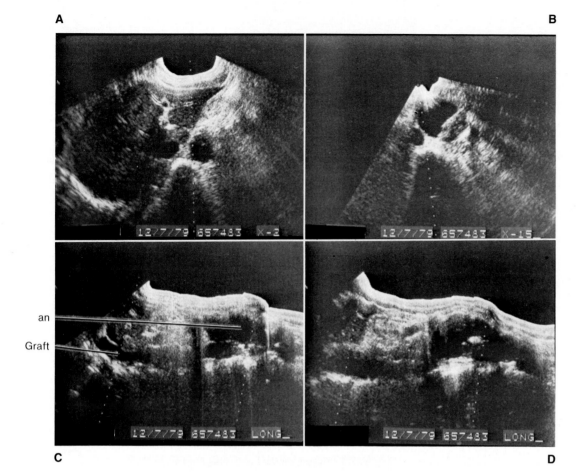

an

Graft

C

D

Fig. 9-43. A, Transverse scan near the level of the xyphoid on a patient with an aorto-femoral graft who presented with a 4-cm aneurysm. **B,** Transverse scan at the level of the bifurcation showing the aneurysm with echogenic clot along its lateral border. **C,** Sagittal scan of the aneurysm and graft. **D,** Sagittal scan of the aneurysm as it extends into the iliac vessel. Echogenic thrombus is seen within the aneurysm.

pared with those from the normal aortic walls. Postsurgically the attached walls may swell at the site of the attachment and form another aneurysm (pseudoaneurysm). Ultrasound is useful for postsurgical aneurysm studies as well as follow-up studies to visualize the graft and the normal aortic attachment.

Dissecting aneurysms

A dissecting aneurysm may be detected by ultrasound and usually displays one or more of the following characteristic signs (Fig. 9-43):

1. Generally the patient is known to have an abdominal aneurysm, and sudden back pain may develop due to a dissection.
2. Since most aneurysms enlarge fairly symmetrically in the anteroposterior and lateral dimensions, an irregular enlargement with scattered internal echoes may represent an aneurysm with clot.
3. A double lumen may also represent a tear in the aortic wall.

Real time techniques may be used to detect the intimal flap or site of the dissection along the abdominal wall. If real time is not available, the A-mode or M-mode may be held over the site of dissection for observation of the irregular movement of the flap of the abdominal aortic wall.

10 Liver

SANDRA L. HAGEN-ANSERT
WILLIAM J. ZWIEBEL

The liver is the largest organ in the body and is quite accessible to sonographic evaluation. The parenchyma of the normal liver is utilized to evaluate other organs and glands in the body (e.g., the kidneys, spleen, and pancreas). The size and shape of the liver determine the quality of the sonographic examination performed; that is, a prominent left lobe of the liver will facilitate visualization of the pancreas, which is situated just inferior to the border of the left lobe, whereas if the right lobe extends just below the costal margin it may facilitate visualization of the gallbladder and right kidney.

GROSS ANATOMY

Liver parenchymal pattern changes—as seen in hepatocellular, cystic, or metastatic disease—reveal a distinct pattern on the ultrasound examination.

The liver occupies almost all of the right hypochondrium, the greater part of the epigastrium, and usually the left hypochondrium as far as the mammillary line. The contour and shape of the liver vary according to patient habitus and lie. Its shape is also influenced by the lateral segment of the left lobe and the length of the right lobe. The liver lies close to the diaphragm. The ribs cover the greater part of the right lobe (usually a small part of the right lobe is in contact with the abdominal wall). In the epigastric region the liver extends several centimeters below the xyphoid process. Most of the left lobe is covered by the rib cage.

Projections of the liver may be altered by some disease states. Downward displacement is often caused by tumor infiltration, cirrhosis, or a subphrenic abscess whereas ascites, excessive dilation of the colon, or abdominal tumors can elevate the liver. Retroperitoneal tumors may move the liver slightly forward.

Lobes

Right lobe. The right lobe is the largest of the four lobes of the liver (Fig. 10-1). It exceeds the left lobe by a ratio of 6:1. It occupies the right hypochondrium and is bordered on its upper surface by the falciform ligament, on its posterior by the left sagittal fossa, and in front by the umbilical notch. Its inferior and posterior surfaces are marked by three fossae: the porta hepatis, the gallbladder fossa, and the inferior vena cava fossa. A congenital anomaly, Riedel's lobe, can sometimes be seen as an anterior projection of the liver and may extend to the iliac crest.

Left lobe. This lobe lies in the epigastric and left hypochrondriac regions. Its upper surface is convex and molded onto the diaphragm. Its undersurface includes the gastric impression and omental tuberosity.

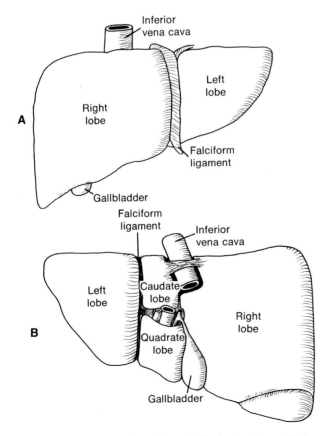

Fig. 10-1. A, Anterior view of the liver. **B,** Posterior view with the medial attachment of the gallbladder.

127

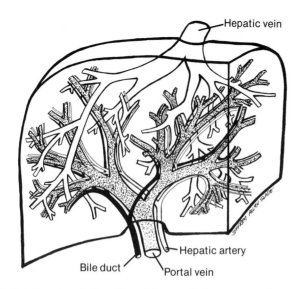

Fig. 10-2. Intimate relationship of the portal venous system, hepatic venous system, biliary system, and hepatic artery.

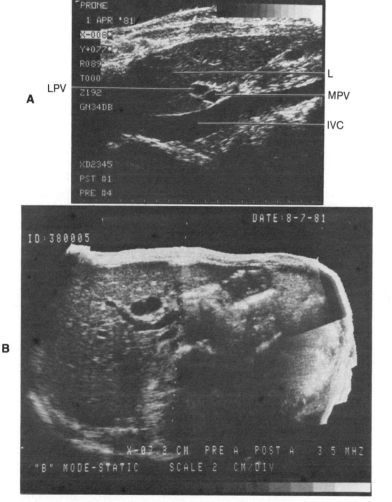

Fig. 10-3. A, Sagittal view of the main and left portal veins as they lie anterior to the inferior vena cava. **B,** Transverse view of the main portal vein.

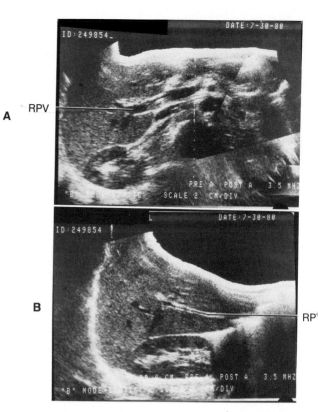

Fig. 10-4. A, Transverse view of the right portal vein. **B,** Sagittal view of the right portal vein in the right lobe of the liver.

Caudate lobe. This small lobe is situated on the posterosuperior surface of the right lobe opposite the tenth and eleventh thoracic vertebrae. It is bounded below by the porta hepatis, on the right by the fossa for the inferior vena cava, and on the left by the fossa for the venous duct.

Quadrate lobe. This lobe is oblong and situated on the posteroinferior surface of the right lobe. In front it is bounded by the anterior margin of the liver, behind by the porta hepatis, on the right by the fossa for the gallbladder, and on the left by the fossa for the umbilical vein.

Portal and hepatic venous anatomy

As described by Marks et al., the portal venous system is a reliable indicator of various ultrasonic tomographic planes throughout the liver (Fig. 10-2).

Main portal vein. This vessel approaches the porta hepatis in a rightward, cephalic, and slightly posterior direction within the hepatoduodenal ligament. It comes in contact with the anterior surface of the inferior vena cava near the porta hepatis and serves to locate the liver hilum (Fig. 10-3). It then divides into two branches, the right and left portal veins.

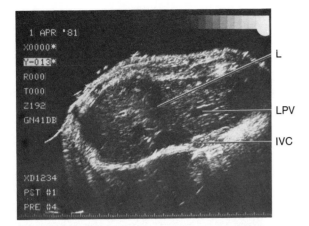

Fig. 10-5. Transverse view of the left portal vein.

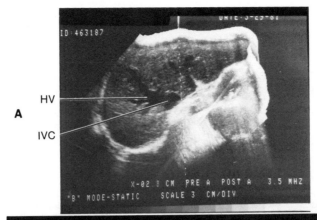

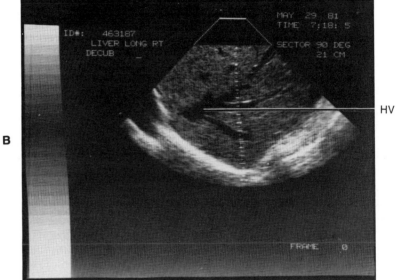

Fig. 10-6. A, Transverse and, **B,** sagittal views of the hepatic veins as they drain into the inferior vena cava at the level of the diaphragm.

Right portal vein. This branch is the larger of the two and requires a more posterior and more caudal approach (Fig. 10-4). It usually is possible to identify the anterior and posterior divisions of the right portal vein on sonography. The anterior division closely parallels the anterior abdominal wall.

Left portal vein. This branch lies more anterior and cranial than the right portal vein. The main portal vein is seen to elongate at the origin of the left portal vein (Fig. 10-5). The vessel lies within a canal containing large amounts of connective tissue, which results in the visualization of an echogenic linear band coursing through the central portion of the lateral segment of the left lobe.

Hepatic veins. The hepatic veins are divided into three components: right, middle, and left (Fig. 10-6). The right hepatic is the largest and enters the right lateral aspect of the inferior vena cava. The middle hepatic enters the anterior or right anterior surface of the IVC. The left hepatic, which is the smallest, enters the left anterior surface of the IVC.

Often it is possible to identify a long horizontal branch of the right hepatic vein coursing between the anterior and posterior divisions of the right portal vein.

Distinguishing characteristics of hepatic and portal veins. The best way to distinguish the hepatic from the portal vessels is to trace their points of origin. The hepatic vessels flow into the inferior vena cava (Fig. 10-7) whereas the portal system arises from the main portal vein. Real time sector allows the sonographer to make this assessment within a few seconds.

Two other characteristics help distinguish the vessels:

1. Hepatic veins course between the he-

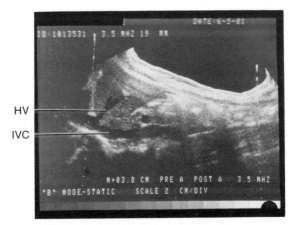

Fig. 10-7. Sagittal scan of the hepatic veins flowing into the inferior vena cava at the level of the diaphragm. The hepatic veins increase caliber as they approach the IVC.

Table 10-1. Anatomic structures useful for dividing and identifying the hepatic segments

Structure	Location	Usefulness
RHV	Right intersegmental fissure	Divides cephalic aspect of anterior and posterior segments of right hepatic lobe and courses between anterior and posterior branches of RPV
MHV	Main lobar fissure	Separates right and left lobes
LHV	Left intersegmental fissure	Divides cephalic aspects of medial and lateral segments of left lobe
RPV (anterior)	Intrasegmental in anterior segment of right hepatic lobe	Courses centrally in anterior segment of right hepatic lobe
RPV (posterior)	Intrasegmental in posterior segment of right hepatic lobe	Courses centrally in posterior segment of right hepatic lobe
LPV (initial)	Courses anterior to caudate lobe	Separates caudate lobe posteriorly from medial segment of left lobe anteriorly
LPV (ascending)	Turns anteriorly in left intersegmental fissure	Divides medial and lateral segments of left lobe
IVC fossa	Posterior aspect of main lobar fissure	Separates right and left hepatic lobes
Gb fossa	Main lobar fissure	Separates right and left hepatic lobes
Ligamentum teres	Left intersegmental fissure	Divides caudal aspect of left hepatic lobe into medial and lateral segments
Fissure of ligamentum venosum	Left anterior margin of caudate lobe	Separates caudate lobe from medial and lateral segments of left lobe

From Callen, P.W.: [Letter], J. Clin. Ultrasound **7**(2):81, 1979.

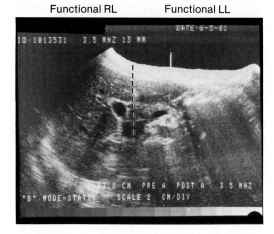

Functional RL   Functional LL

Fig. 10-8. Transverse scan of the functional right and left lobes of the liver. The functional right lobe includes everything to the right of a plane through the gallbladder fossa and inferior vena cava. The functional left lobe includes everything to the left of that plane.

patic lobes and segments; the major portal branches course within the lobar segments.

2. Hepatic veins drain toward the right atrium; the portal veins emanate from the porta hepatis (i.e., hepatic veins are larger near the diaphragm whereas portal veins are larger nearer the porta hepatis).

Segmental liver anatomy

The liver is divided essentially into two lobes, each of which has two segments. The right lobe is divided into anterior and posterior segments, and the left lobe into medial and lateral segments. The quadrate lobe is a portion of the medial segment. The caudate lobe is the posterior portion of the liver lying between the fossa of the inferior vena cava and the fissure of the ligamentum venosum. The caudate lobe receives portal venous and hepatic arterial blood from both the right and the left systems. The anatomic features that assist in determining the positions of the various hepatic segments are listed in Table 10-1.

Functional division of the liver

The purpose of a functional division of the liver is to separate the liver into component parts according the blood supply and biliary drainage so one component can be removed in the event of tumor invasion or trauma. There are two functional divisions, a right and a left. The right functional lobe includes everything to the right of a plane through the

gallbladder fossa and inferior vena cava (which corresponds to the anatomic right lobe) (Fig. 10-8). The left functional lobe includes everything to the left of the above plane (which corresponds to the left lobe, caudate lobe, and quadrate lobe).

Ligaments and fissures

There are three important ligaments and fissures to remember in the liver. The falciform ligament extends from the umbilicus to the diaphragm in a parasagittal plane, containing the ligamentum teres (Fig. 10-9). In the anteroposterior axis the ligament extends from the right rectus muscle to the bare area of the liver, where its reflections separate to contribute to the hepatic coronary ligament and attach to the undersurface of the diaphragm. The ligamentum teres appears as a bright echogenic focus on the sonogram and is seen as the rounded termination of the falciform ligament (Fig. 10-10). Both the ligamentum falciforme and the ligamentum teres divide the medial segments of the left lobe of the liver. The fissure for the ligamentum venosum separates the left lobe from the caudate lobe (Fig. 10-11).

Relational anatomy

The fundus of the stomach lies posterior and lateral to the left lobe of the liver and may frequently be seen on transverse sonograms. The remainder of the stomach lies inferior to the liver and is best visualized on sagittal sonograms. The duodenum lies adjacent to the right and quadrate lobes of the

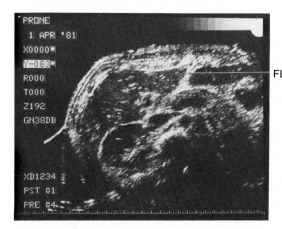

Fig. 10-9. Transverse scan showing the echogenic falciform ligament, which divides the left lobe from the quadrate lobe.

liver. The pancreas is usually seen just inferior to the liver. The posterior border of the liver contains the right kidney, IVC, and aorta. The diaphragm covers the superior border of the liver. The liver is suspended from the diaphragm and anterior abdominal wall by the falciform ligament and from the diaphragm by the reflections of the peritoneum. Most of the liver is covered by peritoneum, but a large area rests directly on the diaphragm and this is called the bare area (Fig. 10-12). The subphrenic space between the liver (or spleen) and the diaphragm is a common site for abscess formation. The lesser sac is an enclosed portion of the peritoneal space posterior to the liver and the stomach (Fig. 10-13). This sac communicates with the

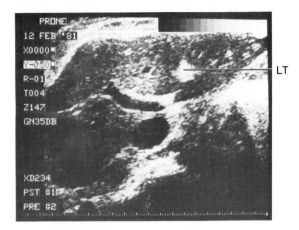

LT

Fig. 10-10. The ligamentum teres appears as a very echogenic circular structure at the termination of the falciform ligament. Care should be taken not to confuse this with metastases to the liver.

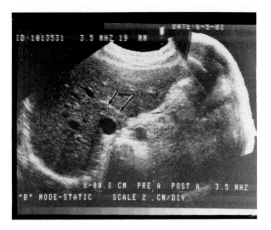

Fig. 10-11. Transverse scan of the fissure for the ligamentum venosum, which separates the left lobe from the caudate lobe *(arrows)*.

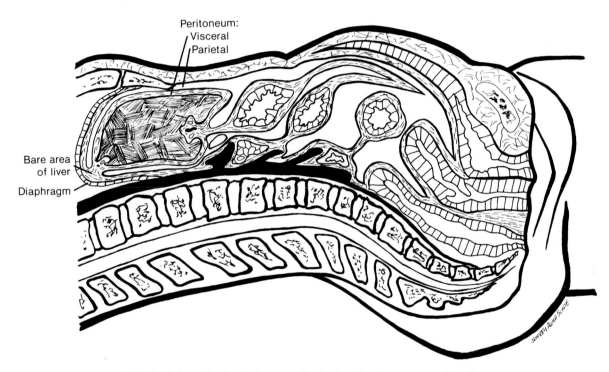

Peritoneum:
Visceral
Parietal

Bare area
of liver

Diaphragm

Fig. 10-12. Longitudinal diagram illustrating the bare area of the liver.

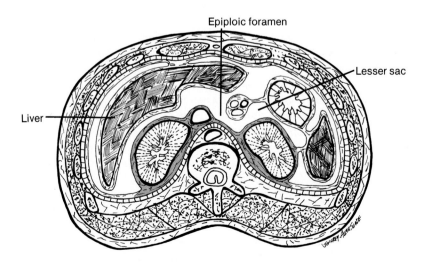

Epiploic foramen

Lesser sac

Liver

Fig. 10-13. Transverse section of the lesser sac, which is found posterior to the liver and the stomach and may be a site for abscess formation.

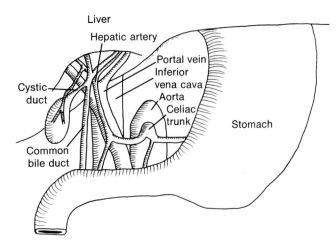

Fig. 10-14. Formation of the porta hepatis by the hepatic artery, portal vein, and common bile duct.

rest of the peritoneal space at a point near the head of the pancreas. It also may be a site for abscess formation.

Intrahepatic vessels and ducts

The portal veins carry blood from the bowel to the liver whereas the hepatic veins drain the blood from the liver into the IVC. The hepatic arteries carry oxygenated blood from the aorta to the liver. The bile ducts transport bile, manufactured in the liver, to the duodenum (Fig. 10-14).

HEPATOBILIARY PHYSIOLOGY AND LABORATORY DATA

The liver, bile ducts, and gallbladder constitute the hepatobiliary system, which performs metabolic and excretory functions essential to physical well-being. Ultrasonography is an important method for detecting anatomic changes associated with hepatobiliary disease; but accurate ultrasound evaluation can be accomplished only when other diagnostic information, including signs, symptoms, and laboratory results, are considered with the ultrasound findings. The task of correlating these clinical and ultrasound data falls primarily to the sonologist. However, the sonographer must also understand the entire clinical picture to be able to plan and properly perform the ultrasound examination. It is necessary therefore that the sonographer be aware of the normal and abnormal physiology of the hepatobiliary system. This section is intended as a primer of hepatobiliary physiology with particular attention to physiologic alterations that commonly occur in hepatobiliary disease.

The liver

The liver is a major center of *metabolism,* which may be defined as the physical and chemical process whereby food stuffs are synthesized into complex elements, complex substances are transformed into simple ones, and energy is made available for use by the organism. The liver is also a center for *detoxification* of the waste products of metabolism accumulated from other sources in the body and foreign chemicals (usually drugs) that enter the body. The liver expels these waste products from the body via its excretory product, bile, which also plays an important role in fat absorption. Finally, the liver is a *storage* site for several compounds used in a variety of physiologic activities throughout the body. In hepatobiliary disease each of these functions may be altered, leading to abnormal physical, laboratory, and sonographic findings.

Hepatocellular versus obstructive disease. Diseases affecting the liver may be classified as hepatocellular, when the liver cells or hepatocytes are the immediate problem, or obstructive.

Viral hepatitis is an example in which the virus attacks the liver cells and damages or destroys them, resulting in an alteration of liver function. In obstructive disorders the flow of bile from the liver is blocked at some point and secondarily results in liver malfunction.

The differentiation between hepatocellular and obstructive diseases is of considerable importance clinically. Hepatocellular diseases are treated medically with supportive measures and drugs; obstructive disorders are usually relieved by surgery. In some cases the distinction between hepatocellular and obstructive disease can be made through clinical laboratory tests, but often the laboratory findings are equivocal. Ultrasonography has been of great benefit since it allows for the first time the physician to accu-

rately separate hepatocellular and obstructive causes of liver disease.

Hepatic metabolic functions. Raw materials in the form of carbohydrates (sugars), fats, and amino acids (the basic components of proteins) are absorbed from the intestine and transported to the liver via the circulatory system. In the liver these substances are converted chemically to other compounds or are processed for storage or energy production. The following is a brief discussion of the metabolic functions of the liver and basic disturbances in these functions that result from liver disease.

Carbohydrates. Sugars may be absorbed from the blood in several forms, but only glucose can be used by cells throughout the body as a source of energy.

The liver functions as a major site for conversion of dietary sugars into glucose, which is released into the bloodstream for general use. The body requires only a certain amount of glucose at any one time, however, and excess sugar is converted by the liver to glycogen (a starch), which may be stored in the liver cells or transported in the blood to distant storage sites. When dietary sugar is unavailable, the liver converts glycogen released from stores into glucose; it can also manufacture glucose directly from other compounds, including proteins or fats, when other sources of glucose have been depleted. Thus the liver helps to maintain a steady state of glucose in the bloodstream. In very severe liver disease, unless glucose is administered intravenously, the body may become glucose deficient (hypoglycemic) with profound effects on the function of the brain and other organs. Alternately, uncontrolled increases in blood glucose (hyperglycemia) may occur in severe liver disease if large doses of glucose are administered since the liver fails to convert the excess glucose to glycogen.

Fats. The liver is also a principal site for metabolism of fats, which are absorbed from the small intestine in the form of mono- and diglycerides.

Dietary fats are converted in the hepatocytes to lipoproteins, in which form fats are transported throughout the body to sites where they are used by other organs or stored. Conversely, stored fats may be transported to the liver and converted into energy, yielding glucose or other substances such as cholesterol which have important and widespread uses.

In severe liver disease abnormally low blood levels of cholesterol may be noted since the liver is the principal site for cholesterol synthesis. Furthermore, failure of hepatic conversion of fat to glucose in liver disease may contribute to hypoglycemia. A striking histologic manifestation of many forms of hepatocellular disease is the so-called fatty liver. On gross pathologic examination the fatty liver has a yellow color and a greasy feel; on microscopic study globules of fat (primarily triglycerides) crowd the hepatocytes. The cause of fat accumulation in the liver cells is poorly understood but is believed to result from failure of the hepatocytes to manufacture special proteins, called lipoproteins, that coat small quantities of fat making the fat soluble in plasma and allowing for its release into the bloodstream. Fatty liver is a nonspecific finding that may be seen in a variety of illnesses including viral hepatitis, alcoholic liver disease, and exposure to toxic chemicals.

Proteins. The liver produces a wide variety of proteins either indirectly from amino acids absorbed from the gut or directly from raw materials stored within the body.

Albumin, in particular, is produced in great quantities. In the bloodstream it functions as a transport medium for a wide variety of molecules. Since it is nonionic, it also functions to draw water into the vascular system from tissue spaces; stated more technically, it helps to maintain oncotic pressure within the vascular system. When the liver is chronically diseased, clinical laboratory results may reveal a significant lowering of the serum albumin (hypoalbuminemia). The accompanying loss of oncotic pressure in the vascular system allows fluid to migrate into the interstitial space, resulting in edema (swelling) in dependent areas such as the lower extremities. In patients with severe liver disease, especially advanced cirrhosis, ascites also develops. Hypoalbuminemia may account in part for the ascites, but the development of ascites is not well understood. Other factors, including portal hypertension (elevated pressure in the portal venous system), may be involved.

In addition to being the primary source of albumin synthesis, the liver is the principal source of proteins necessary for blood coagulation, including fibrinogen (Factor I), prothrombin (Factor II), and Factors V, VII, IX, and X. In liver disease, decreased production of these proteins may lead to inadequate blood coagulation and uncontrollable hemorrhage. Commonly such hemorrhages occur into the bowel following rupture of a dilated vein or development of ulcer disease and are often the immediate or contributing cause of death. Deficiencies of clotting Factors I, VII, IX, and X also may result from failure of intestinal absorption of vitamin K,

Table 10-2. Comparison of laboratory abnormalities in hepatocellular disease and biliary obstruction

	Bilirubin	Serum albumin	SGOT	SGPT	Alkaline phosphatase
Hepatocellular disease	↑ ↑↑ ↑↑↑	↓ ↓↓		↑↑ ↑↑↑	↑ ↑↑
Obstruction	↑ ↑↑	→	↑ ↑↑	↑ ↑↑	↑↑↑

↑ Minimal; ↑↑ moderate; ↑↑↑ severe increase; → normal.

which is a precursor (raw material) required for synthesis of these factors. Vitamin K is a fat-soluble vitamin (so are vitamins D, A, and E) and is absorbed only from the intestine in solution with fat. Fat absorption is severely limited in cases of bile duct obstruction because of the absence of bile salts (discussed later), and absorption of fat-soluble vitamins is therefore severely reduced. Ultimately the deficiency of vitamin K lowers the amount of the above-mentioned factors and coagulation is retarded. Deficiency of prothrombin and other vitamin K–dependent factors can be corrected in cases of obstruction through parenteral administration of vitamin K. In hepatocellular disease, administration of vitamin K may improve the coagulopathy but frequently will not restore normal clotting function since the primary problem is hepatocyte dysfunction.

Clotting deficiencies related to liver disease may be detected with several laboratory tests. Of particular interest are the prothrombin time (pro time) and partial thromboplastin time (PTT). The results of these tests are presented as percentages of the time required for certain coagulation steps to occur in the patient's blood as compared with normal blood. Longer periods (lower percentages) indicate greater degrees of abnormality in each of these tests.

Hepatic enzymes. Enzymes are protein catalysts utilized throughout the body in all metabolic processes. Since the liver is a major center of metabolism, large quantities of enzymes are present in hepatocytes and these leak into the bloodstream when the liver cells are damaged or destroyed by disease. The presence of increased quantities of enzymes in the blood is a very sensitive indicator of hepatocellular disorder. In hepatobiliary disease the enzymes SGOT (serum glutamic oxaloacetic transaminase), SGPT (serum glutamic pyruvate transaminase), and alkaline phosphatase are of particular interest. Serum levels of all three of these enzymes are increased both in hepatocellular disease and in biliary obstruction, but the patterns of elevation may help differentiate between hepatocellular and obstructive causes (Table 10-2). In biliary obstruction, elevation of SGOT and SGPT is usually mild

(serum levels typically do not exceed 300 units). However, in severe hepatocellular destruction such as acute viral or toxic hepatitis, striking elevation of SGOT and SGPT may be seen (levels frequently exceed 1000 units). Marked elevation of alkaline phosphatase, on the other hand, is typically associated with biliary obstruction or the presence of mass lesions in the liver (e.g., metastatic disease or abscesses). Low levels of alkaline phosphatase are very unusual in obstruction and high levels (greater than 15 Bodansky units) are uncommon in hepatocellular disorders. Alkaline phosphatase is such a sensitive indicator of obstruction that it may become elevated before the serum bilirubin in cases of acute obstruction. Hence disproportional increase of alkaline phosphatase relative to bilirubin always suggests obstruction. Elevation of serum alkaline phosphatase may be the only abnormal laboratory finding in metastatic disease.

Whereas the pattern of enzyme abnormality may strongly suggest hepatocellular disease or obstruction in some cases, it may not allow this distinction to be made in others since obstruction may be superimposed on preexisting hepatocellular disease or unrelieved obstruction may cause hepatocellular damage. Confusion in interpretation of serum enzyme abnormalities may also occur when SGOT, SGPT, or alkaline phosphatase is released from diseased tissues other than the liver. For instance, SGOT and SGPT are increased with damage to heart and skeletal muscle and alkaline phosphatase is elevated in bone disease and in normal pregnancies. Since SGPT is somewhat more specific for liver disease than SGOT, elevation of SGPT above SGOT suggests a hepatic cause.

Hepatic detoxification functions. The liver is a major location for detoxification of waste products of energy production and other metabolic activities occurring throughout the body. It is also the principal site of breakdown of foreign chemicals such as drugs. Although these functions fall under the general definition of metabolism and could therefore be grouped in the preceding section, it is useful for instructional purposes to think of these functions as separate categories of hepatic activity.

Table 10-3. Bilirubin metabolism

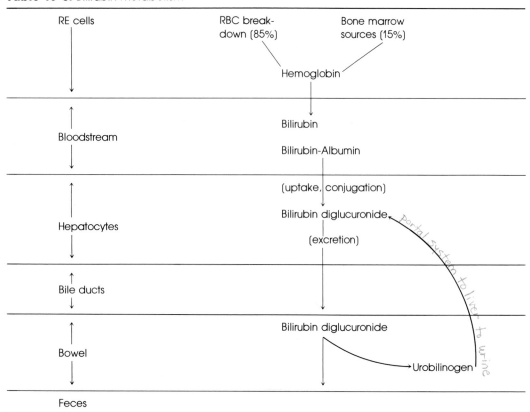

Ammonium, a toxic product of nitrogen metabolism, is converted to nontoxic urea in the liver, which is practically the only site where this conversion occurs. Urea is subsequently eliminated from the body by the kidneys. The level of urea in the blood is measured as the blood urea nitrogen (BUN), and in severe liver disease (acute or chronic) the BUN may be abnormally low due to fall-off of urea production. The exhaled breath of patients with severe liver disease may have a fruity or pungent odor (known as fetor hepaticus) because of ammonium (NH_4) accumulation. More important, the concentration of NH_4 in the blood may rise to toxic levels and cause brain dysfunction (including confusion, coordination disturbances, tremor, and coma). Gastrointestinal hemorrhage frequently leads to the accumulation of toxic levels of NH_4 in the blood. Blood lost into the intestine is broken down by bacteria into nitrogen-containing substances, which are absorbed into the bloodstream. The failing liver may therefore be presented with a large amount of NH_4 that it cannot detoxify; coma may result and is frequently a precursor to death if the patient does not succumb to the direct effects of blood loss. Thus failure of ammonium detoxification is a serious consequence of liver failure.

Bilirubin detoxification. Bilirubin, the breakdown product of hemoglobin, is also an important substance detoxified in the liver. Besides detoxification, the liver also excretes bilirubin into the gut via the biliary tree (Table 10-3).

Red blood cells survive an average of 120 days in the circulatory system; they are then trapped and broken down by reticuloendothelial (RE) cells, primarily within the spleen. Hemoglobin released from the red cells is converted to bilirubin within the RE system and is then released into the bloodstream. The bilirubin molecules become attached to albumin in the blood and are transported to the liver, where the following metabolic steps take place in the hepatocytes:

1. Uptake. The bilirubin is separated from albumin, probably at the cell membrane, and is taken with the hepatocytes.
2. Conjugation. The bilirubin molecule is combined with two glucuronide molecules, forming bilirubin diglucuronide.
3. Excretion. The bilirubin molecule is actively transported across the cell membrane into the bile canaliculi, which are the microscopic headwaters of the biliary system. Bilirubin released

from the hepatocytes passes through the bile ducts with other components of bile and is delivered to the bowel, where most bilirubin diglucuronide is excreted into the feces (a small portion is broken down into urobilinogen by intestinal bacteria, absorbed into the portal system, and reexcreted by the liver).

Measurement of the concentration of bilirubin in the blood is a standard laboratory test for hepatocellular disease. Two fractions of bilirubin are measured: the direct-acting fraction, which reacts chemically in an aqueous medium and consists of conjugated bilirubin, and the indirect-acting fraction, which consists of unconjugated bilirubin released from the RE system. Indirect bilirubin reacts only in a nonaqueous (alcohol) medium. The total bilirubin is the sum of the direct-acting and the indirect-acting fractions and normally does not exceed 1 mg/100 ml of serum. In hematologic diseases associated with abrupt breakdown of large numbers of red blood cells (hemolytic anemias, transfusion reactions), the liver may receive more bilirubin from the RE system than it can detoxify. The level of indirect or unconjugated bilirubin will therefore be elevated in hematologic diseases associated with abrupt breakdown of large numbers of red blood cells (hemolytic anemias, transfusion reactions), and the liver may receive more bilirubin from the RE system than it can detoxify. The level of indirect or unconjugated bilirubin is thus elevated in such hematologic disorders as the following:

	Direct bilirubin predominates	Indirect bilirubin predominates
Hemolysis		X
Hepatocellular disease	X	
Biliary obstruction	X	

In biliary obstruction the hepatocytes pick up bilirubin and conjugate it with glucuronide molecules but cannot dispose of it. The conjugated form is then regurgitated into the bloodstream, with resultant elevation of the direct-acting bilirubin fraction. The indirect-acting bilirubin may also rise slightly in biliary obstruction, but the direct bilirubin predominates.

The direct or conjugated form also predominates in hepatocellular disease. Excretion of bilirubin is the step most readily affected when the hepatocytes are damaged; therefore the diseased hepatocytes continue to take in and conjugate bilirubin but are unable to excrete it. As in biliary obstruction, the accumulated conjugated bilirubin is regurgitated into the blood.

Elevation of serum bilirubin results in jaundice, which is a yellow coloration of the skin, sclerae, and body secretions. Jaundice is a nonspecific finding seen in massive blood breakdown, hepatocellular disease, or biliary obstruction. Chemical separation of bilirubin into direct and indirect fractions helps to specify a hepatocellular or hematologic cause for jaundice. Furthermore, if jaundice is due to liver disease, the level of bilirubin may help to separate hepatocellular disease from obstruction since it is uncommon for the total bilirubin to rise above 35 mg/100 ml of serum with obstruction.

Hormone and drug detoxification. The liver breaks down several hormones that otherwise would accumulate in the body. For example, failure to metabolize estrogen in men with chronic hepatocellular disease such as cirrhosis causes gynecomastia (breast enlargement), testicular atrophy, and changes in body hair patterns. Reduced detoxification of the hormone glucagon, which is an insulin antagonist, occurs in liver disease and may contribute to the fluctuations in blood sugar levels seen in severe hepatic disorders. The liver is also the primary location for breakdown of medications and other foreign chemicals administered orally or parenterally. It is of particular concern that doses of medications be reduced to compensate for the loss of this function in patients with severe liver disease; otherwise accumulation of drugs may lead to overdosage.

Storage. The final category of hepatic function to be considered is storage. The liver stores glycogen (a starch), fats, vitamins, iron, and copper. Storage is probably the least important function of the liver; consequently relatively little adverse effects arise from this category of liver disease. The most important consequence is loss of glycogen storage, which may contribute to wide fluctuations of serum glucose levels seen in hepatocellular disease.

Bile

Bile is the excretory product of the liver. It is formed continuously by the hepatocytes, collects in the bile canaliculi adjacent to these cells, and is transported to the gut via the bile ducts. The principal components of bile are water, bile salts, and bile pigments (primarily bilirubin diglucuronide). Other components include cholesterol, lecithin, and protein. The primary functions of bile are the emulsification of intestinal fat and the removal of waste products excreted by the liver.

Fats are absorbed into the portal blood and intestinal lymphatics in the form of monoglycerides and triglycerides by the action of the intestinal mucosa, but efficient absorption occurs only when the fat molecules are suspended in solution through the emulsifying action of bile salts. As emulsifiers, bile salts act like nonionic detergents to suspend fats in solution within the watery medium of the intestinal contents. Both hepatocellular disease and biliary obstruction affect the amount of bile salts available for fat absorption, but obstruction generally has the more profound effect. Absence of bile salts may lead to steatorrhea (fatty stools), but a more important effect is failure of absorption of the fat-soluble vitamins (D, A, K, and E). As previously noted, vitamin K is an essential precursor for hepatic production of several clotting factors; the absence of this vitamin leads to bleeding tendencies in patients with hepatobiliary disease.

Bile pigments. According to Filly et al., bile pigments are the principal cause of ultrasonic scattering in echogenic bile although cholesterol crystals may also contribute to this finding. The presence of echogenic bile indicates stasis, but this stasis is not always pathologic and may simply result from prolonged fasting.

Portal hypertension

The majority of blood passing through the small and large bowel is collected in the portal venous system and transported to the liver. In the liver it passes through an intricate system of vascular channels, which allows maximum contact of the blood with hepatocytes. Many hepatocellular diseases, and particularly those associated with chronic inflammation (i.e., cirrhosis), result in scarring of the hepatic parenchyma and distortion of the hepatic architecture. The narrow passageways through which the portal blood travels are obstructed by the scarring process, interfering with the flow of portal blood through the hepatic parenchyma. When restriction to flow is advanced, portal hypertension (increased venous pressure) occurs and portal blood is forced to bypass the liver via collateral channels. Many of these collateral pathways include small veins in submucosal locations in the stomach and esophagus. These vessels are not equipped to accept the pressure and flow associated with portal hypertension and they are therefore subject to rupture. Major blood loss into the gastrointestinal tract may ensue, especial-

ly in the presence of coagulation disorders, which are commonly associated with severe liver disease. The combination of anatomic and metabolic abnormalities produces a dangerous situation that, as noted previously, is often the direct or indirect cause of death.

SONOGRAPHIC EVALUATION

Since it is so important to visualize the liver adequately for comparison of parenchymal patterns with those in surrounding structures (i.e., kidney and pancreas), more attention will be devoted here to proper technique and equipment settings than is found in subsequent chapters.

The time gain compensation (TGC) should be set according to normal soft tissue attenuation. Generally this means that the slope of the gain curve should be elevated so the "knee" of the slope occurs about 15 cm from the initial main bang reflection. Most patients, front to back, measure approximately 15 cm to the posterior edge of their liver, which allows this technique to work quite consistently. Taylor suggests using the A-mode to adjust the TGC curve. When set correctly, the internal parenchymal echoes from the liver should be about a third to a half the size of the echo returning from the diaphragm. This method allows quick visualization of inadequate gain settings, which will be displayed as an uneven distribution of echoes throughout the liver. Too much anterior gain wipes out the abdominal musculature and the anterior edge of the liver; too little far gain leaves the far posterior border of the liver sonolucent. The principal sensitivity control should then be adjusted to permit visualization of uniform low-level parenchymal echoes throughout the liver (Fig. 10-15).

Various transducers may be needed to obtain the optimum balance of echoes throughout the liver. Most patients can be scanned with a 3.5-MHz 19-mm diameter transducer, which provides a long focus. Smaller patients may require a higher-frequency smaller-diameter transducer with a medium focus for better visualization of the liver parenchyma.

A

B

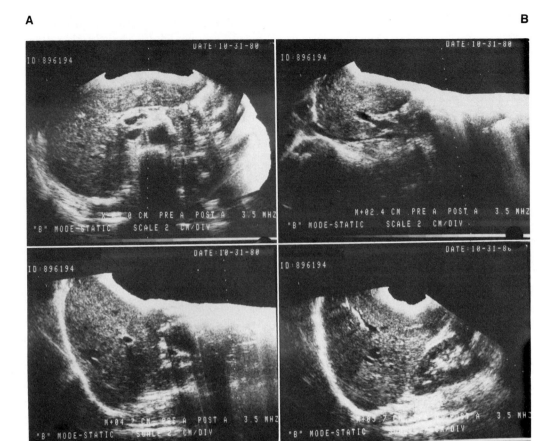

C

D

Fig. 10-15. A, Transverse and, **B** to **D,** sagittal scans of normal liver parenchyma. The diaphragm is well shown posterior to the uniform medium-level echo reflections. Multiple hepatic and portal structures are seen throughout the liver parenchyma. The right kidney is the posteroinferior border of the right lobe of the liver.

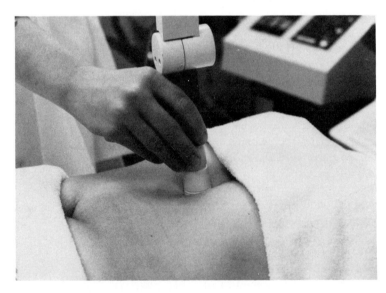

Fig. 10-16. Supine transverse scans of the abdomen should begin at the level of the xyphoid. The transducer arm is angled 10 to 12 degrees cephalad for visualizing the dome of the liver. A 19-mm diameter transducer will allow a deeper focus and thus provide better penetration in the average patient.

Supine transverse scans

The patient is generally supine for the initial transverse upper abdomen scan. To obtain a perpendicular axis with the dome of the liver and the transducer face, the transducer arm should be angled 10 to 15 degrees cephalad (Fig. 10-16). Begin at the level of the xyphoid and move caudally by 1-cm intervals until the lower margin of the right lobe of the liver is shown. The patient should be examined in full inspiration so maximum detail of the liver parenchyma, vascular architecture, and ductal structures will be recorded.

In transverse scans two separate techniques should be used to record maximum information. One is a compound scanning technique in which the transducer is sectored perpendicular to multiple interfaces to record the entire abdominal outline. To do this scan, the sonographer should pie-sweep the midline area and then sector along the sides of the abdomen, always angling the transducer back toward the spine. Often this technique can be done rapidly with the patient in suspended respiration, which allows a panoramic view of the liver and splenic parenchyma and often helps in orientation.

Single scans are also very useful and often give maximum resolution when performed correctly. Such scans are "pie" single sweeps, so called because the actual face of the transducer moves very little across the abdomen. With the patient in full inspiration, the transducer is severely angled to one side of the abdomen and slowly arced across to a severe angle on the other side. It is important not to move the transducer across the abdomen; rather the beam should be arced severely enough to record a large area in the sweep. This generally gives excellent visualization of the smaller vessels and ducts within the liver.

Supine longitudinal scans

Generally the longitudinal or sagittal scan offers a better outline of the liver parenchyma than does the transverse scan because the transducer can be swept under the patient's costal margin perpendicular to the diaphragm and the dome of the liver (Fig. 10-17). In the transverse scan the overlying lung and costal margin tend to interfere with adequate visualization in the dome of the liver, and thus the longitudinal scan becomes the scan of choice for liver detail.

Usually the scan is centered midway between the umbilicus and xyphoid in the midline of the patient. Smaller increments of 0.5 or 1 cm are made in the prevertebral

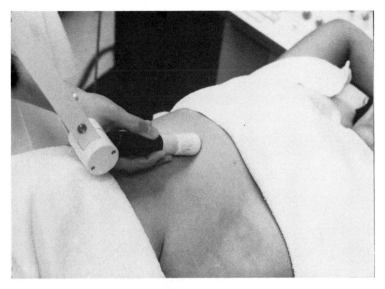

Fig. 10-18. Sagittal supine oblique subcostal scan with the patient rolled to a slight left decubitus in an effort to visualize the liver better.

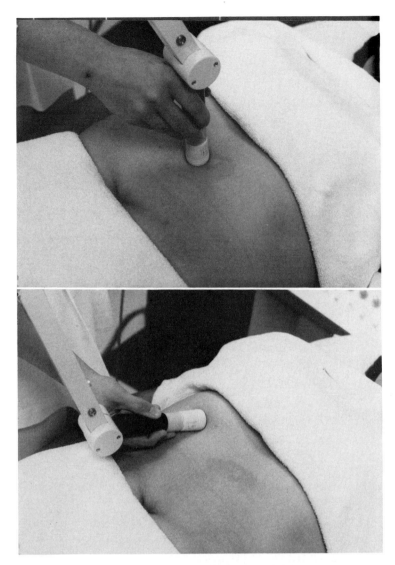

Fig. 10-17. The sagittal scan is an excellent way to visualize the liver parenchyma. The transducer is directed in a perpendicular path along the anterior abdominal wall until the costal margin is reached. At that point a sharp angulation of the transducer face should be directed toward the diaphragm in an effort to record the dome of the liver from a perpendicular angle. Often a slight amount of pressure is necessary to obtain this angle.

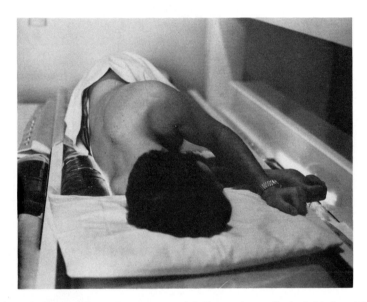

Fig. 10-19. An alternative approach is the water path straight decubitus position for visualizing the liver between the costal margins.

area to outline the smaller vessels posterior to the liver. As the sweep moves out of this area, larger increments of 1 to 2 cm complete the series. The transducer should be directed under the rib cage and angled cephalad as much as possible with the patient in full inspiration. With a continuous sweep the beam should slowly be angled caudally to record the lower segment of the right lobe.

Supine oblique subcostal scans

For a supine oblique scan the transducer is placed just beneath and parallel with the right costal margin using a 10-to-15-degree cephalad angle of the transducer head. This technique usually enables examination of serial sections of the liver to be done with greater ease than in the straight transverse plane. The beam can be directed under the costal margin to avoid reflections and reverberations from the rib interfaces (Fig. 10-18).

Another technique that works well with dehydrated patients is to ask the patient to expand the abdomen to make the path of the anterior abdominal wall smooth in relation to the costal margin.

Right anterior oblique scans

Right anterior oblique scans require that the patient roll slightly to the right; a 45-degree sponge is placed under the left hip for support. This allows better visualization of the lower liver segment, usually displacing the duodenum and transverse colon out of the field of view (Fig. 10-19).

PATHOLOGIC PATTERNS OF LIVER DISEASE

The evaluation of the liver parenchyma includes assessment of its size, configuration, and contour. The determination of liver volume can be made from serial scans in an effort to detect subtle increases in size or hepatomegaly. As in other organ systems, the hepatic parenchymal pattern changes with disease processes. The detection of cirrhosis, ascites, or the cause of jaundice may be ac-

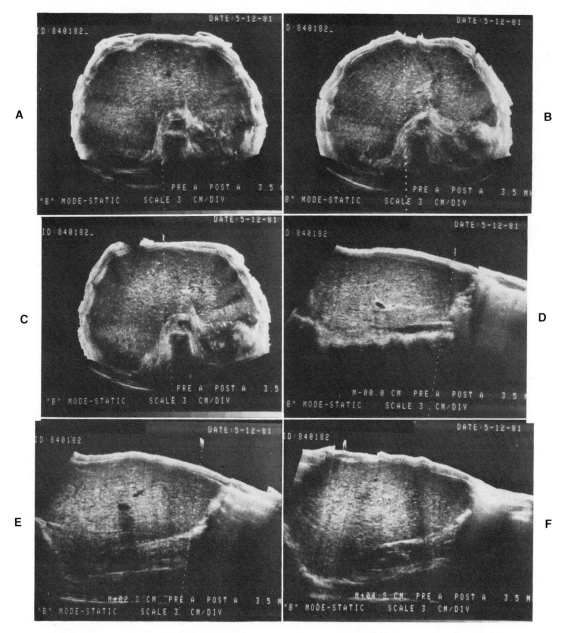

Fig. 10-20. A to **C,** Transverse and, **D** to **F,** sagittal scans of an alcoholic patient with hepatocellular disease. Gross hepatomegaly is shown. There is decreased transmission in the liver due to the absorption of sound by the infiltrative disease. The parenchymal echoes are brighter than those from normal liver.

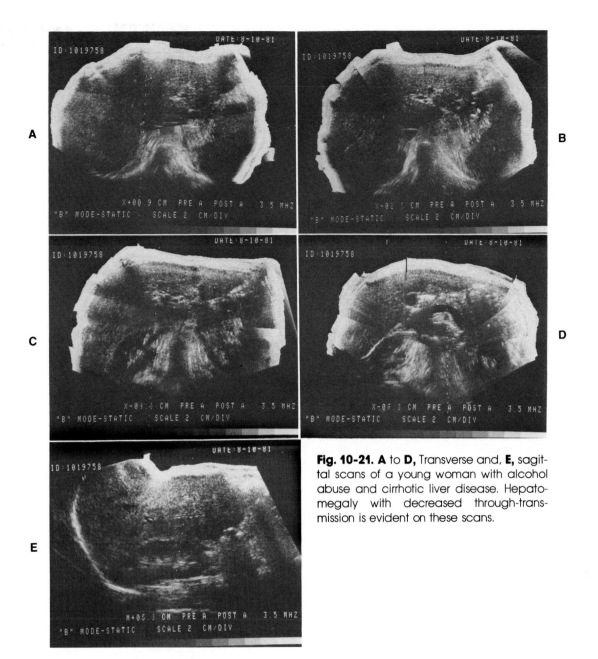

Fig. 10-21. A to **D,** Transverse and, **E,** sagittal scans of a young woman with alcohol abuse and cirrhotic liver disease. Hepatomegaly with decreased through-transmission is evident on these scans.

complished by sonography. Intrahepatic, extrahepatic, subhepatic, and subdiaphragmatic masses can be outlined and their internal composition recognized by specific echo patterns in efforts to provide a differential diagnosis for the clinician.

Hepatitis

The most common liver disease is viral hepatitis. The liver becomes inflamed, and hepatocellular function is diminished. Clinically the liver is enlarged and tender. Sonography may disclose hepatomegaly.

Fatty infiltration

Fatty infiltration can be produced secondary to congestive cardiac failure, obesity, or (more commonly) alcoholic liver disease. Cirrhosis is the result of prolonged and excessive alcohol ingestion. At first, the damage to the hepatocytes causes fat to accumulate within the liver cells (fatty liver). Later (perhaps even years later) as the hepatocytes die, scarring causes liver shrinkage, interference with the flow of portal blood (portal hypertension), and regeneration of liver cells in an abnormal pattern; the abnormal regeneration leads to the development of regener-

ative nodules. The hepatocellular dysfunction, in both the fatty liver and the scarring stages, causes a loss of processing and production as well as of storage and detoxification. The first and last of these losses lead eventually to death.

The ultrasound manifestations of the fatty infiltrative stage are hepatomegaly, increased number of echoes in liver, increased brightness of echoes, decreased number of vascular structures, and decreased through-transmission due to increased attenuation and reflection of sound (Figs. 10-20 and 10-21).

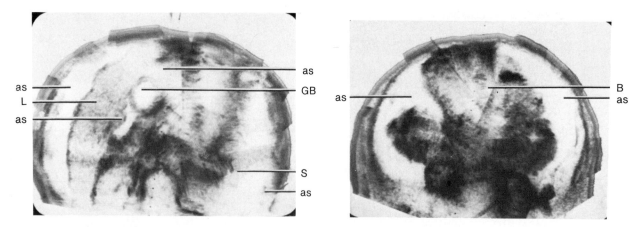

Fig. 10-22. Transverse scans of a cirrhotic liver (shrunken), massive ascites, thick-walled gallbladder, and multiple loops of bowel. Ascites, *as.*

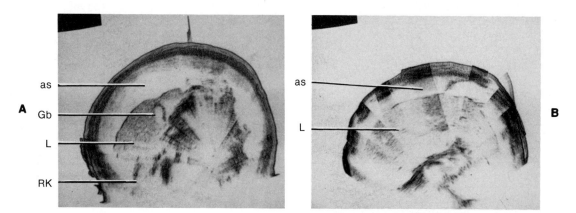

Fig. 10-23. Transverse scans of advanced cirrhosis with massive ascites. The falciform ligament is well seen in **B,** with ascitic fluid separating the liver from the anterior abdominal wall.

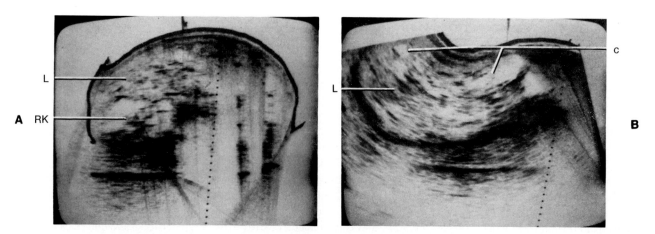

Fig. 10-24. A, Transverse scan of a polycystic kidney and liver disease. **B,** Sagittal scan of the multiple cysts within both organs.

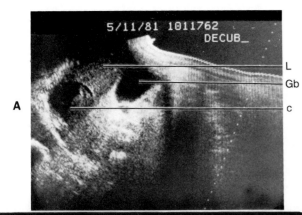

A

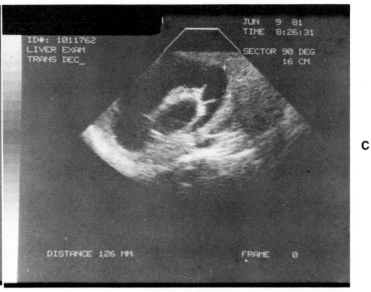

C

Fig. 10-25. This middle-aged man presented with hepatomegaly and low-grade fever. He had been experiencing mild back pain. The sonogram showed a complex mass in the right lobe of the liver just below the diaphragm. Multiple internal reflections were seen within the mass. An ultrasound-guided biopsy was performed and a septated cyst diagnosed. **A,** Sagittal scan of the gallbladder, liver, and cyst. **B,** Sagittal scan taken 1 month after the aspiration. The fluid collection remained very complex in nature. A catheter had been left in for drainage but had become blocked due to the viscous debris. **C,** Transverse scan of the cyst with septations.

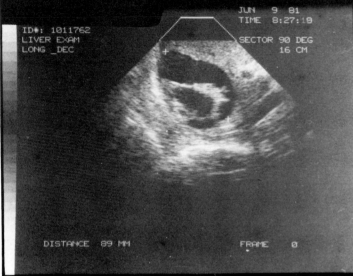

The ultrasound findings of a fibrotic stage of liver disease are small liver, increased number and brightness of echoes, decreased number of vascular structures, inhomogeneity due to focal areas of regenerative nodules (may be difficult to distinguish from metastases), and ascites (Figs. 10-22 and 10-23).

Thus diffuse liver disease produces a sonogram with increased number and brightness of echoes and decreased vascular structures and transmission. These findings are not specific but may be seen in any patient with diffuse liver disease regardless of its cause.

Hepatic cysts

Cystic disease in the liver may be congenital or acquired. Generally the cysts are solitary although they may be multiple, especially in polycystic liver disease. Patients are usually asymptomatic, except in polycystic disease (wherein occasionally a large cyst interferes with liver function and causes jaundice) (Fig. 10-24). Usually the liver cysts are small and are found incidentally. Occa-

sionally they become large and the patient presents with hepatomegaly. Sonographically they appear sonolucent with sharp well-defined borders and posterior enhancement. They are usually round, lobular, or ovoid. Occasionally the walls appear minimally irregular by ultrasound and the through-transmission is somewhat variable. In these patients the cyst should be aspirated for a diagnostic evaluation of the contents of the fluid. Septations may also be seen within cystic structures (Fig. 10-25).

Cystic-type lesions may also be seen in necrotic masses within a tumor. Care must be taken to examine the entire liver parenchyma thoroughly and to separate the normal liver texture patterns from the abnormal. Usually necrosis will present with low-level debris and irregular walls. These help differentiate it from a simple cyst.

Hepatic abscess

There are three basic types of abscess formation: intrahepatic, subhepatic, and subphrenic. Generally the patient will present

with fever, elevated white cell count, and right upper quadrant pain. Frequently the patient has undergone surgery. The search must be made for solitary or multiple collections of abscess material, which may be intrahepatic or extrahepatic.

Intrahepatic abscess. Its origin is usually blood-borne bacteria, or it is the result of penetrating trauma to the liver. Symptoms are chills, spiking fever, elevated white cell count, and tender liver. Although sonographic findings are variable (some abscesses look like cysts; others look like solid tumors), generally the collection will be a round intrahepatic lesion with scattered internal echoes due to septa and debris (Fig. 10-26). Through-transmission is usually good, although it depends on the amount of debris (Fig. 10-27). The walls are shaggy and thick as compared to those of a simple cyst.

Subhepatic abscess. This collection of fluid is found inferior to the liver, anterior to the right kidney. It usually can be differentiated from ascites since ascites is generally echo free and bilateral. A common site for

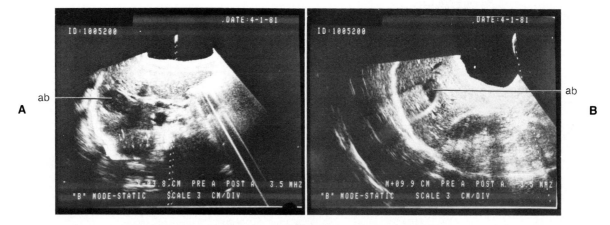

Fig. 10-26. A, Transverse and, **B,** sagittal scans of a young patient who presented with abdominal pain, elevated white cell count, spiking fever, and chills. Two abscess formations were found within the liver. The collections of fluid were well defined with low-level echoes from debris within their borders.

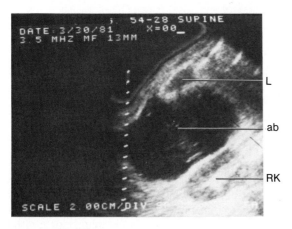

Fig. 10-27. Transverse scan over the right upper quadrant showing a huge collection anterior to the right kidney. This was an intrahepatic abscess formation.

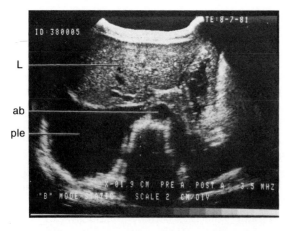

Fig. 10-28. Transverse scan of a patient with a huge pleural effusion, *ple.*

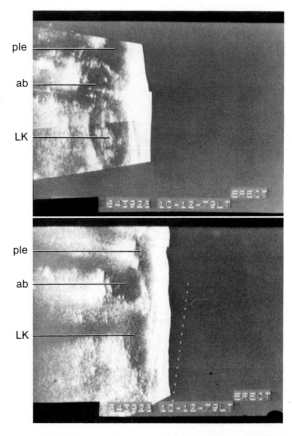

Fig. 10-29. Upright sagittal scans over the LUQ were performed in a 53-year-old woman status post–gastrectomy, splenectomy, hemipancreatectomy, and partial cholectomy for gastric carcinoma. She had a left pleural effusion with signs and symptoms suggesting a subphrenic abscess. The scans show a complex fluid collection posterior to the diaphragm and pleural effusion, *ple*, superior to the left kidney, *LK*.

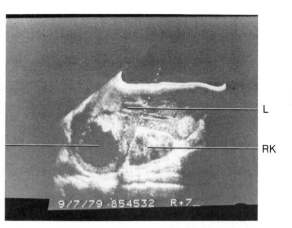

Fig. 10-30. Sagittal scan of a patient with a huge necrotic tumor metastasis to the liver, *m.* There are other echogenic metastases within the liver parenchyma.

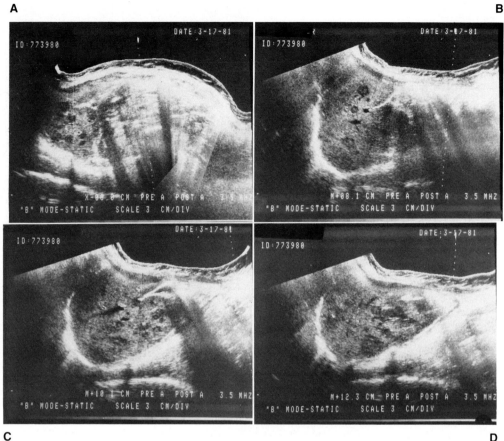

Fig. 10-31. A, Transverse and, **B** to **D,** sagittal scans in a patient with multiple liver metastases. The liver parenchyma is quite inhomogeneous with marked areas of well-defined hypoechoic areas.

collection is the bed of the gallbladder (after cholecystectomy) or Morison's pouch.

Subphrenic abscess. Its origin is usually bacteria that have spilled into the peritoneum at surgery, a bowel rupture, a peptic ulcer perforation, or trauma. The motion of the diaphragm causes a vacuum in the subphrenic space, drawing the material upward. Patient symptoms are fever, elevated white cell count, and right upper quadrant pain and tenderness. There may be fluid in the chest on the side of the abscess (Fig. 10-28). The ultrasound findings are a sonolucent collection above the liver, inferior to the diaphragm. The collection may have low-level echoes due to debris. The collection usually spreads out beneath the diaphragm whereas in intrahepatic abscesses near the dome of the liver it indents the liver parenchyma. If the collection is small, alterations in patient position may be necessary (i.e., steep decubitus or upright) in efforts to move the fluid into a better sonographic window (Fig. 10-29).

Hepatic hematoma

A hematoma is usually iatrogenic or traumatic. It may be deep within the parenchyma or subcapsular. The sonographic findings are a sonolucent collection within the parenchyma or beneath the capsule if it is a recent hematoma. Later, as the hematoma organizes, the collection becomes more echogenic. It may become sonolucent again as a hygroma is formed.

Hepatic neoplasms

A neoplasm is any new growth or development of an abnormal tissue; it may be either malignant or benign. A malignant mass is uncontrolled and prone to metastasize to nearby or distant structures. The degree of malignancy varies among tumors. A benign growth occurs locally but does not spread or invade surrounding structures. It may push surrounding structures aside or adhere to them. Its surgical resection leads to a complete cure.

Benign hepatic tumors. Three benign tumors are relatively common: hamartoma, adenoma, and hemangioma. The hamartoma and adenoma are associated with oral contraceptives. All types of liver cells are present in the hepatic hamartomas, whereas only the hepatocyte-like cells are present in adenomas. The hepatic hemangioma is a vascular tumor composed of blood vessel cells and small blood vessels. The sonographic findings are very nonspecific. Any of the tumors may consist of increased or decreased echogenic foci. Generally adenomas and hamartomas occur along the inferior margin of the liver and are quite large.

Malignant hepatic tumors. The primary hepatic tumor that is malignant in adults is the hepatoma; in children it is the hepatoblastoma. The hepatoma arises from liver cells and is usually poorly defined since it tends to infiltrate the hepatic architecture. Hepatomas are usually more or less echogenic than normal liver. The borders are poorly defined. The tumor may be solitary or may occur simultaneously in several portions of the liver. Solitary lesions are often quite large.

Metastases. Metastatic liver disease represents the most common intrahepatic neoplasm. The echogenic metastases are common with certain bowel tumors, but their appearance is not specific for the tumor origin. Target-type metastases occur due to edema around the tumor or to necrosis or hemorrhage within the tumor and have been called the bulls-eye effect.

Three patterns most commonly encountered in metastic disease are

1. Well-defined hypoechoic mass—contains fewer echoes than the adjacent surrounding parenchyma (Figs. 10-30 to 10-32)
2. Well-defined echogenic mass—con-

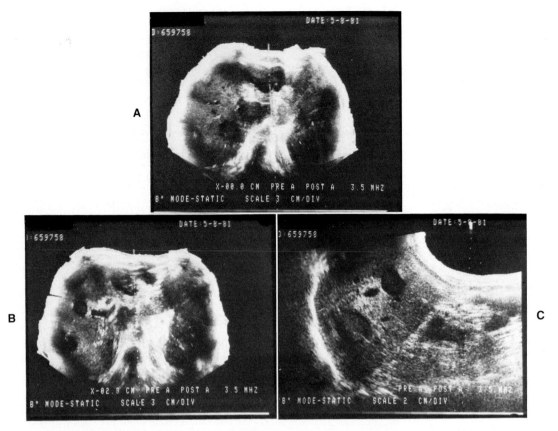

Fig. 10-32. A and **B,** Transverse scans of liver metastases with splenomegaly in a patient with lung carcinoma. **C,** Sagittal scan of the hypoechoic areas within the liver parenchyma.

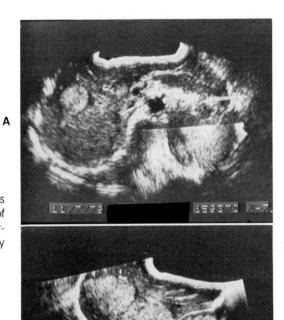

Fig. 10-33. A, Transverse and, **B,** sagittal scans of a 53-year-old man status post-resection of distal colonic carcinoma. Extensive hyperechoic masses and paraaortic adenopathy were seen.

tains higher-amplitude echoes than the surrounding parenchyma (Fig. 10-33)
3. Diffuse distortion of normal homogeneous parenchymal pattern without focal masses—contains multiple echogenic and hypoechoic areas without dominant focal lesions (Figs. 10-34 to 10-36)

Various combinations of these patterns can be seen simultaneously in a patient with metastatic liver disease. Generally the first abnormality seen will be hepatomegaly or alterations in contour, evident especially on the lateral segment of the left lobe. The lesions may be solitary or multiple, variable in size and shape, and may have sharp or ill-defined margins. Some metastases are totally sonolucent with central liquefaction necrosis and irregular inner margins. A calcified liver metastasis would be highly echogenic with an acoustic shadow posterior. Metastases may be extensive or localized to produce a dishomogeneity of hepatic architecture. Such changes may be very subtle and require close attention to scanning technique.

Lymphoma. Generally patients with lymphoma have hepatic involvement that shows sonographically as hepatomegaly with a nor-

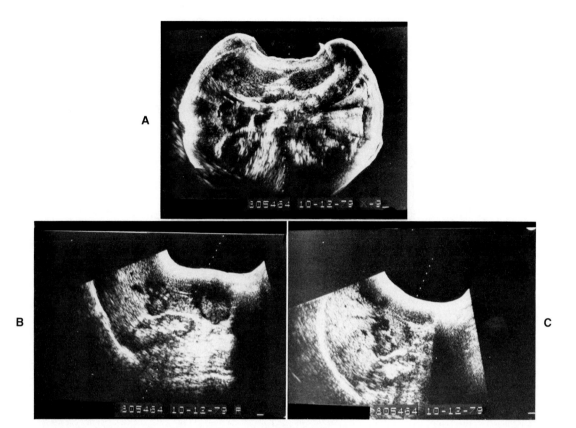

Fig. 10-34. A, Transverse and, **B** and **C,** sagittal scans of liver metastases showing diffuse distortion of the normal homogeneous parenchymal pattern.

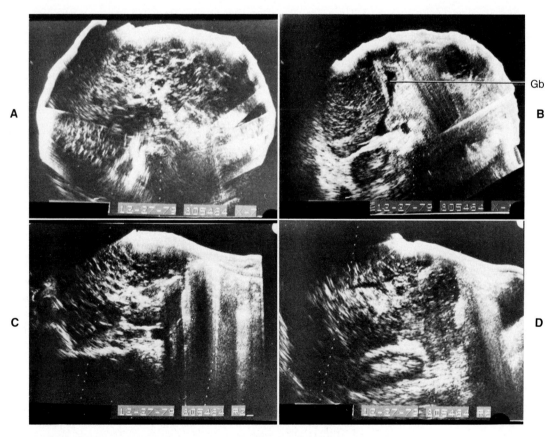

Fig. 10-35. A and **B,** Transverse and, **C** and **D,** sagittal scans of a patient with diffuse liver metastases. A thickened gallbladder wall is also seen in **B.**

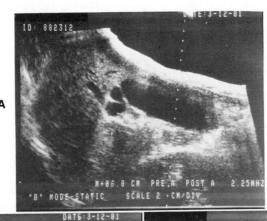

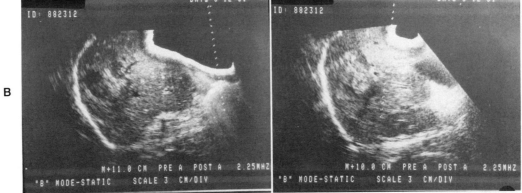

Fig. 10-36. Sagittal scans of a young patient with oat cell carcinoma who now presents with jaundice, hepatomegaly, and anorexia. The ultrasound showed a mass in the pancreatic head causing duct obstruction and a distended gallbladder, **A,** and multiple liver metastases. The areas of inhomogeneity in the right lobe of the liver are evident in **B** and **C.**

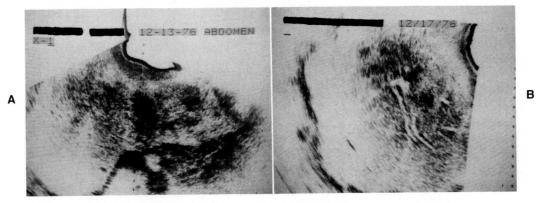

Fig. 10-37. A, Transverse scan of a patient with dense liver metastases. **B,** Sagittal scan of the porta hepatic mass causing duct dilation and jaundice.

mal liver pattern or a diffuse alteration of echo architecture with no evidence of a focal mass. Occasionally a focal echogenic or sonolucent mass is seen in a lymphoma patient. The presence of splenomegaly or retroperitoneal nodes may help to confirm the diagnosis of lymphadenopathy.

Diffuse abnormalities. Diffuse abnormalities of the liver may be seen sonographically as inhomogeneities within the liver parenchyma. Such abnormalities as biliary obstruction, hepatic metastases, common duct stones and stricture, extrahepatic masses, and passive hepatic congestion will be discussed as they present sonographically.

Biliary obstruction proximal to the cystic duct can be carcinoma of the common bile duct or hepatic metastases in the porta hepatis. In the former, jaundice and pruritus are the clinical signs. Laboratory data show an increase in direct bilirubin and alkaline phosphatase. The echo appearance of carcinoma of the common bile duct is tubular branching with fluid-filled structures (dilated hepatic ducts) that are best seen in the periphery of the liver on longitudinal scans. No mass is visualized. The gallbladder is of normal size, even after a fatty meal.

Hepatic metastases in the porta hepatis present the same clinical signs and laboratory data, except that there is abnormal hepatocellular function. The echo appearance is of an intrahepatic mass in the area of the porta hepatis that may be more or less echo producing than the normal parenchyma (Fig. 10-37). The dilated hepatic bile ducts are best seen on the longitudinal scans. Intrahepatic masses are usually associated with other hepatic metastases in other areas of the liver. The gallbladder is of normal size, even after a fatty meal.

Biliary obstruction distal to the cystic duct may be caused by common duct stones, extrahepatic masses in the porta hepatis, or common duct stricture.

1. Common duct stones cause right upper quadrant pain, jaundice, and pruritus as well as an increase in direct bilirubin and alkaline phosphatase. The echo appearance, best seen on sagittal scans, shows the dilated hepatic bile ducts in the periphery of the liver. The gallbladder size is variable, usually small. Gallstones are often present and appear as dense echoes along the bed of the gallbladder with an acoustic shadow posterior. The stones within the duct may be seen if they are large enough; a shadow may also be present.

2. Clinical signs of the extrahepatic masses at the porta hepatis include jaundice and symptoms referable to primary disease, and laboratory data are the same as for a stone in the common duct. The echo appearance shows an extrahepatic mass in the area of the porta hepatis, which could be lymph node enlargement, pancreatitis, a pseudocyst, or carcinoma in the head of the pancreas. The tubular branching and fluid-filled, dilated hepatic ducts are seen on longitudinal and transverse scans. The gallbladder is dilated, with no change in size after a fatty meal.

3. Common duct stricture can be diagnosed by jaundice and past history of cholecystectomy. Direct bilirubin is increased, as is alkaline phosphatase. The echo appearance is dilated hepatic ducts with no porta hepatic mass.

Passive hepatic congestion is another diffuse hepatic abnormality. Generally it develops secondary to congestive heart failure, showing clinical signs of hepatomegaly. Laboratory data indicate normal or slightly abnormal hepatocellular function. The echo appearance shows dilated hepatic and portal veins that are more prominent centrally than peripherally. These structures are usually nonbranching (as the hepatic ducts are) and may decrease in size with expiration or increase with inspiration. The inferior vena cava is usually dilated, as are the superior mesenteric and splenic veins.

11

Gallbladder and the biliary system

Ultrasonic evaluation of the gallbladder and biliary system has been very effective in the diagnosis of disease. Furthermore, real time evaluation of the patient with gallbladder disease has proved to be an efficient method of diagnosing such diseases as cholelithiasis, cholecystitis, or duct dilation.

ANATOMY OF THE EXTRAHEPATIC BILIARY APPARATUS

The extrahepatic biliary apparatus consists of the right and left hepatic ducts, the common hepatic duct, the common bile duct, the gallbladder, and the cystic duct (Fig. 11-1).

Hepatic ducts

The right and left hepatic ducts emerge from the right lobe of the liver in the porta hepatis and unite to form the common hepatic duct, which then passes caudally and medially. The hepatic duct runs parallel with the portal vein. Each duct is formed by the union of bile canaliculi from the liver lobules.

The common hepatic duct is approximately 4 mm in diameter and descends within the edge of the lesser omentum. It is joined by the cystic duct to form the common bile duct.

Common bile duct

(.16 cm)

The normal common bile duct has a diameter of up to 6 mm. In the first part of its course it lies in the right free edge of the lesser omentum (Fig. 11-2). In the second part it is situated posterior to the first part of the duodenum. In the third part it lies in a groove on the posterior surface of the head of the pancreas. It ends by piercing the medial wall of the second part of the duodenum about halfway down the duodenal length. There it is joined by the main pancreatic duct; and together through a small ampulla (the ampulla of Vater) they open into the duodenal wall. The end parts of both ducts and the ampulla are surrounded by circular muscle fibers known as the sphincter of Oddi.

The proximal portion of the common bile duct is lateral to the hepatic artery and anterior to the portal vein. The duct moves more posterior after it descends behind the duodenal bulb and enters the pancreas. The distal duct lies parallel with the anterior wall of the vena cava.

Within the liver parenchyma the bile ducts follow the same course as the portal venous and hepatic arterial branches. All the structures are encased in a common collagenous sheath forming the *portal triad.*

Gallbladder

The gallbladder is a pear-shaped sac in the anterior aspect of the right upper quadrant closely related to the visceral surface of the liver (Fig. 11-3). It is divided into the fundus, body, and neck (Fig. 11-4). The rounded fundus usually projects below the inferior margin of the liver, where it comes into contact with the anterior abdominal wall at the level of the ninth right costal cartilage. The body generally lies in contact with the visceral surface of the liver and is directed upward, backward, and to the left. The neck becomes continuous with the cystic duct, which turns into the lesser omentum to join the right side of the common hepatic duct to form the common bile duct.

The neck of the gallbladder is oriented posteromedially toward the porta hepatis; and the fundus is situated lateral, caudal, and anterior to the neck. Occasionally the gallbladder lies in an intrahepatic or other anomalous location, and it may be difficult to detect by sonography if the entire upper abdomen is not examined.

The size and shape of the gallbladder are variable. Generally most normal gallbladders are about 3 cm in diameter and 7 to 10 cm long. The walls are less than 2 mm thick.

There are several anatomic variations that may occur in the gallbladder to give rise to

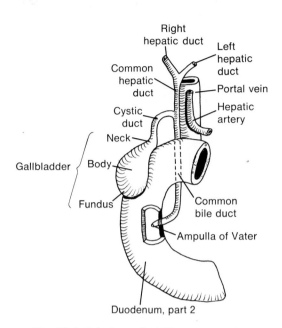

Fig. 11-1. Extrahepatic biliary apparatus.

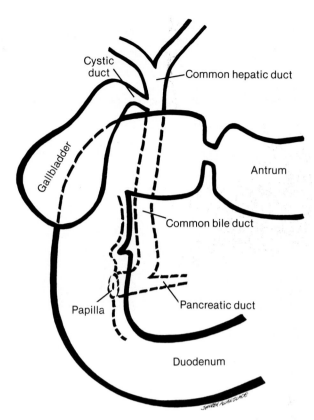

Fig. 11-2. The posteroinferior surface of the body of the gallbladder usually lies against the anterolateral aspect of the upper ascending duodenum.

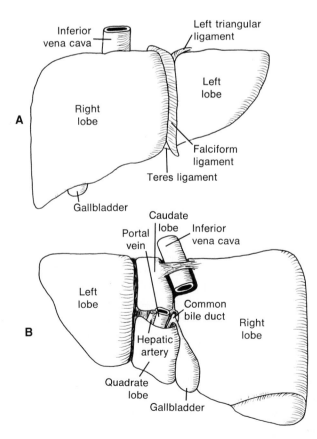

Fig. 11-3. Anterior, **A,** and posterior, **B,** projections of the liver and gallbladder.

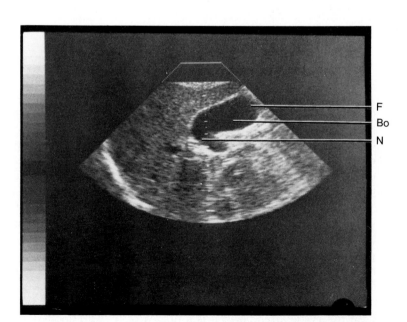

Fig. 11-4. Sagittal scan of the normal gallbladder. Fundus, *F;* body, *Bo;* neck, *N.*

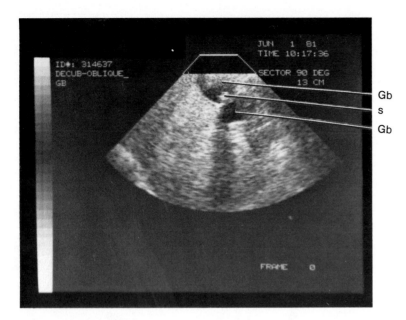

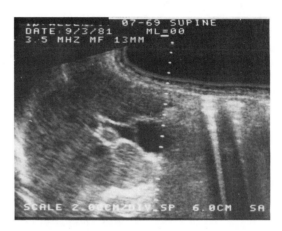

Fig. 11-5. Oblique decubitus scan of a patient with a double gall-bladder. A stone is in the more anterior sac. The acoustic shadow is posterior. Gallbladder, *Gb*; stone, *s*.

Fig. 11-6. One anatomic variation of the normal gallbladder includes a folding of the fundus (Phrygian cap).

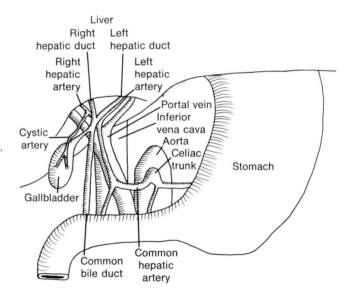

Fig. 11-7. Structures entering and leaving the porta hepatis.

its internal echoes. The gallbladder may fold back on itself at the neck, forming Hartmann's pouch. Other anomalies include partial septation, complete septation (double gallbladder), and folding of the fundus (Phrygian cap) (Figs. 11-5 and 11-6).

With a capacity of 50 ml, the gallbladder serves as a reservoir for bile. It also has the ability to concentrate the bile. To aid this process, its mucous membrane contains folds that unite with each other, giving the surface a honeycomb appearance.

The arterial supply of the gallbladder is from the cystic artery, which is a branch of the right hepatic artery. The cystic vein drains directly into the portal vein. A number of smaller arteries and veins run between the liver and the gallbladder (Fig. 11-7).

Function. Bile is produced continuously, but digestion is an intermittent process; the gallbladder therefore functions to store bile for intermittent release in conjunction with eating.

To facilitate storage, the gallbladder mucosa concentrates bile by active transport of water; and as a result gallbladder bile may be twice as concentrated as hepatic bile. Filling of the gallbladder is passive and occurs during fasting, when the sphincter of Oddi (located at the junction of the common bile duct and the duodenum) is closed. The valves of Heister in the neck of the gallblad-

der are not really valves and do not affect flow into or out of the gallbladder. Instead, they probably function to prevent kinking of the duct. Release of bile from the gallbladder appears to result from combined hormonal and neuronal activity, including simultaneous contraction of the gallbladder and relaxation of the sphincter of Oddi. The mechanism is not well established, however. Contraction of the gallbladder against a closed outlet is reported to cause pressures of 100 to 200 mm of water, a factor no doubt accounting for the severe pain that occurs when a stone obstructs the cystic duct.

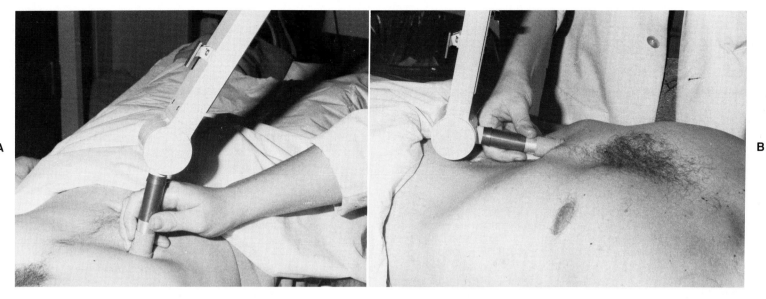

Fig. 11-8. A, Transverse oblique scan technique used for better visualizing the gallbladder under the costal margin. **B,** Longitudinal oblique scans of the gallbladder area are performed with the patient in deep inspiration. The transducer is arced under the costal margin to record the interface of the gallbladder and liver.

Cystic duct

The cystic duct is about 4 cm long and connects the neck of the gallbladder with the common hepatic duct to form the common bile duct. It is usually somewhat S shaped and descends for a variable distance in the right free edge of the lesser omentum.

SONOGRAPHIC EVALUATION OF THE GALLBLADDER AND BILIARY SYSTEM
Gallbladder

To ensure maximum dilation of the gallbladder, the patient should be NPO at least 8 to 12 hours prior to the ultrasound examination. The patient is initially examined in the supine position with a real time sector scanner. Transverse, oblique, and sagittal scans are made over the upper abdomen to identify the gallbladder, biliary system, liver, right kidney, and head of the pancreas (Fig. 11-8). The patient should also be rolled into a steep decubitus or upright position in an attempt to separate small stones from the gallbladder wall or cystic duct (Fig. 11-9).

The gallbladder may be identified as a sonolucent oblong structure located anterior to the right kidney, lateral to the head of the pancreas and duodenum, indenting the inferior to medial aspect of the right lobe of the liver. The sagittal scans show the right kidney posterior to the gallbladder. The fundus is generally oriented slightly more anterior and on sagittal scans often reaches the anterior abdominal wall.

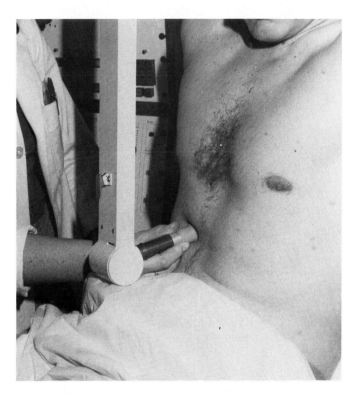

Fig. 11-9. Upright scan performed to evaluate the internal echoes within the gallbladder. Normally the bile should be sonolucent, but with disease low-level to bright-reflector echoes appear. A change in position should alter these echoes to prove that they are stones or real structures within the gallbladder parenchyma.

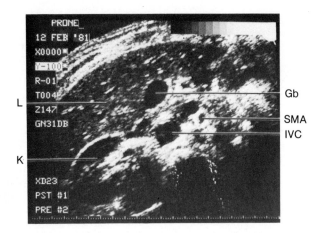

Fig. 11-10. Transverse scan of the right upper abdomen showing the normal anatomy. The gallbladder, *Gb*, is a sonolucent structure anterior to the right kidney, *RK*, and medial to the liver, *L*.

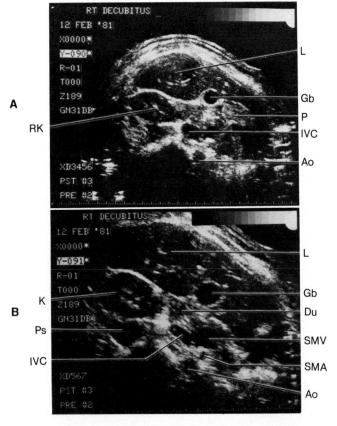

Fig. 11-11. A, Right decubitus of the normal gallbladder. Pancreas, *P*; inferior vena cava, *IVC*; aorta, *Ao*. **B,** Right decubitus of the normal gallbladder as it rests anterior to the great vessels, duodenum, and right kidney. Psoas muscle, *Ps*.

If real time equipment is not available, the patient may be examined with an articulated arm scanner. Scanning is begun in the supine transverse position at the level of the xyphoid and moves caudad by 1 cm increments (Fig. 11-10). When the area of the gallbladder is seen, the increments are reduced to 0.5 cm. Difficulties may be encountered if the costal margin is obstructing the field of view by casting a shadow as the transducer moves across the abdominal wall. To avoid such interference, several technique variations may be employed. The patient may be rolled into a semidecubitus position and subsequent scans made in an oblique manner along the costal margin, thus projecting the gallbladder slightly more anterior (Fig. 11-11). The angle of the transducer arm may be increased 5 to 15 degrees in a cephalic direction to avoid the costal margin interference; or, conversely, the angle may be directed 5 to 15 degrees caudad to utilize the liver as an acoustic window for visualizing the gallbladder. The patient may also be scanned in an upright position, thus causing the gallbladder to fall to a more inferior position.

Carter et al.[2] have reported seeing on sagittal scans a bright linear echo within the liver connecting the gallbladder and the right or main portal vein in a high percentage of patients (Fig. 11-12). They stated that the neck of the gallbladder usually comes into contact with the main segment of the portal vein near the origin of the left portal vein. The gallbladder commonly resides in a fossa on the medial aspect of the liver. Due to fat or fibrous tissue within the main lobar fissure of the liver (which lies between the gallbladder and the right portal vein), this bright linear reflector was a reliable indicator of the location of the gallbladder. The gallbladder lies in the posterior and caudal aspect of the fissure. The caudal aspect of the linear echo "pointed" directly to or touched the gallbladder.

A small echogenic fold has been reported to occur along the posterior wall of the gallbladder at the junction of the body and infundibulum. It may be very small (3 to 5 mm) but may give rise to an acoustic shadow in the supine position. It is not duplicated in the oblique position (Fig. 11-13). The causes for such a junctional fold are the incisurae between the body and infundibulum or the Heister valves, which are spiral folds beginning in the neck of the gallbladder and lining the cystic duct.

A prominent gallbladder may be normal in some individuals because of their fasting state (Fig. 11-14). A large gallbladder has been detected in patients with diabetes, patients who are bedridden with protracted illness or pancreatitis, and those who are taking anticholinergic drugs. Such a gallbladder may even fail to contract following a fatty meal, or intravenous cholecystokinin and other studies may be needed to make the diagnosis of obstruction.

If a gallbladder appears too large, a fatty meal may be administered and further sonographic evaluation made to detect whether the enlargement is abnormal or normal. If the gallbladder fails to contract during the examination, further investigation of the pancreatic area should be made. Courvoisier's sign indicates an extrahepatic mass com-

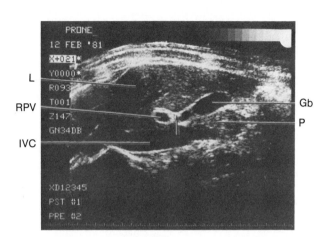

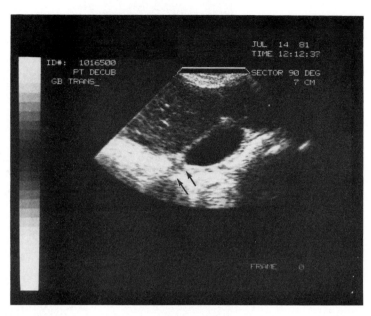

Fig. 11-12. Sagittal scan of the gallbladder, right portal vein, and linear bright reflector of the main lobar fissure of the liver *(arrow)*.

Fig. 11-13. The neck of the gallbladder may project soft shadowing due to the folds at the junction of the body and infundibulum *(arrow)*.

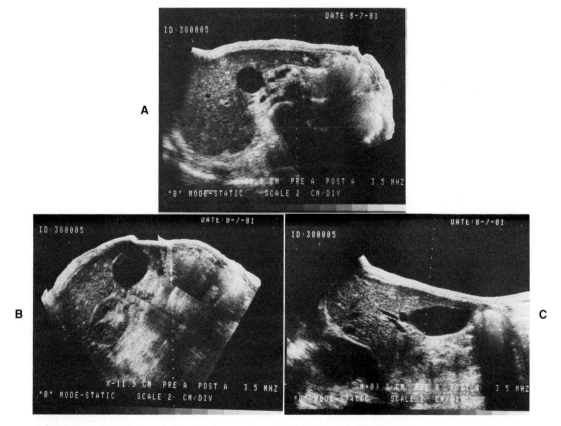

Fig. 11-14. A and **B,** Supine transverse scans of a prominent gallbladder. The AP dimension is 4.3 cm, chunky for a normal gallbladder. This patient should be given a fatty meal and rescanned in 40 minutes to see whether the gallbladder will contract. **C,** Sagittal scan of the gallbladder. The portal veins are shown superior to the neck.

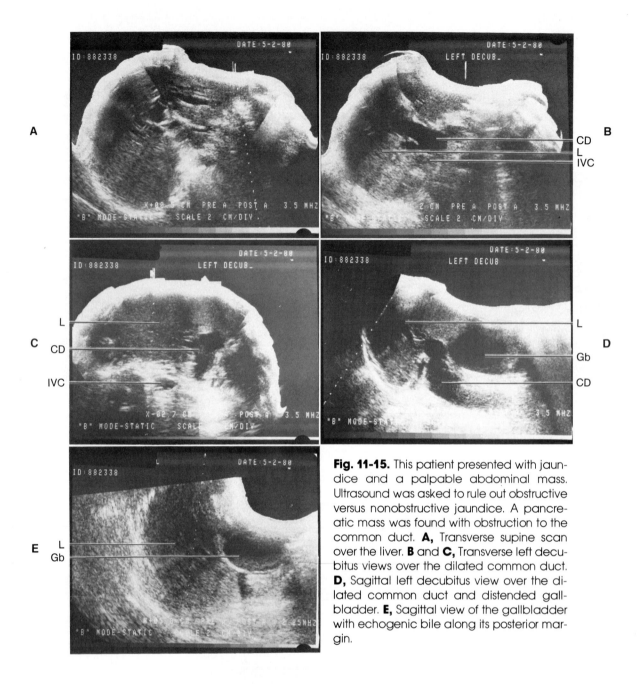

Fig. 11-15. This patient presented with jaundice and a palpable abdominal mass. Ultrasound was asked to rule out obstructive versus nonobstructive jaundice. A pancreatic mass was found with obstruction to the common duct. **A,** Transverse supine scan over the liver. **B** and **C,** Transverse left decubitus views over the dilated common duct. **D,** Sagittal left decubitus view over the dilated common duct and distended gallbladder. **E,** Sagittal view of the gallbladder with echogenic bile along its posterior margin.

pressing the common bile duct, which can produce an enlarged gallbladder (Fig. 11-15). In addition, the liver should be carefully examined for the presence of dilated bile ducts.

In a well-contracted gallbladder the wall changes from a single to a double concentric structure with three components recognized as reported by Marchal et al.[13]: (1) a strongly reflective outer contour, (2) a poorly reflective inner contour, and (3) a sonolucent area between both reflecting structures.

Bile ducts

Sonographically the common duct lies anterior and to the right of the portal vein in the region of the porta hepatis and gastrohepatic ligament (Fig. 11-16). The hepatic artery lies anterior and to the left of the portal vein. On a transverse scan the common duct, hepatic artery, and portal vein have been referred to as the Mickey Mouse sign by Bartrum and Crow[1] (Fig. 11-17). The portal vein serves as Mickey's face, with the right ear the common duct and the left ear the hepatic artery. To obtain such a cross section, the transducer must be directed in a slightly oblique path from the left shoulder to the right hip (Fig. 11-18).

On sagittal scans the right branch of the hepatic artery usually passes posterior to the common duct. The common duct is seen just anterior to the portal vein before it dips posteriorly to enter the head of the pancreas

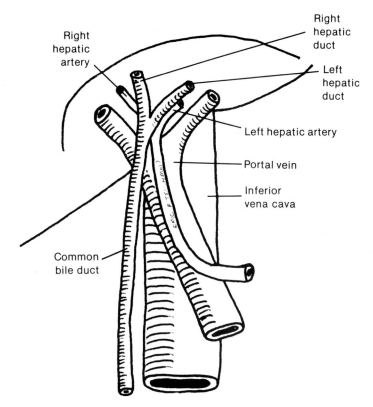

Fig. 11-16. AP of the biliary apparatus as it enters the porta hepatis.

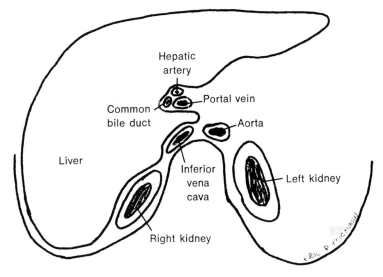

Fig. 11-17. Transverse view of the upper abdomen to show the Mickey Mouse sign of the portal vein. Common bile duct to the right, hepatic artery to the left.

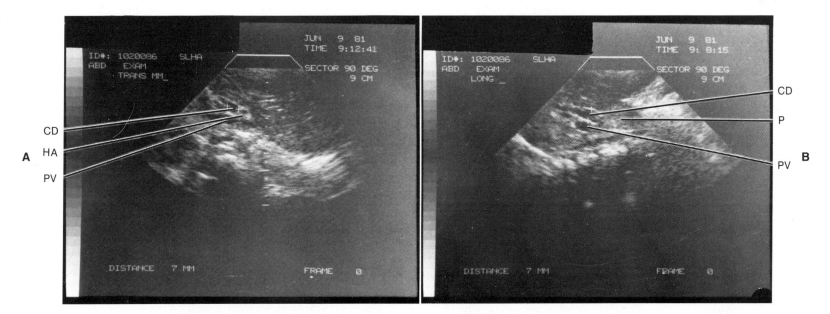

Fig. 11-18. A, Transverse of the portal vein, *PV*, common bile duct, *CD*, and hepatic artery, *HA*. The calipers measure the common bile duct at 7 mm. **B,** Sagittal of the common duct, *CD*, as it lies anterior to the portal vein, *PV*, before dipping posteriorly into the pancreas, *P*.

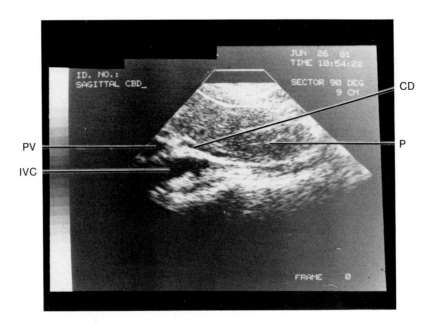

Fig. 11-19. Sagittal scan of the common bile duct.

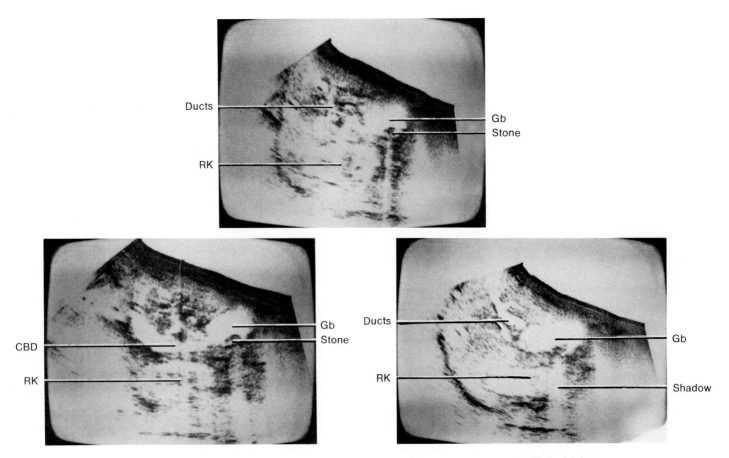

Fig. 11-20. Longitudinal view of a dilated gallbladder with stones and dilated intra-hepatic ducts.

(Fig. 11-19). The patient may be rotated into a slight (45-degree) or steep (90-degree) right anterior oblique position with the beam directed posteromedially to visualize the duct. This enables the examiner to avoid cumbersome bowel gas and to utilize the liver as an acoustic window.

When the right subcostal approach is used, the main portal vein may be seen as it bifurcates into the right and left branches. As the right branch continues into the right lobe of the liver, the right branch can be followed laterally in a longitudinal plane. The portal vein appears as an almond-shaped sonolucent structure anterior to the inferior vena cava. The common hepatic duct is seen as a tubular structure anterior to the portal vein. The right branch of the hepatic artery can be seen between the duct and the portal vein as a small circular structure.

The small cystic duct is generally not identified; and since this landmark is needed to distinguish the common hepatic from the common bile duct, a more general term of common duct is used to refer to these structures.

In an excellent study Laing, London, and Filly[11] give five characteristics that distinguish bile ducts from other intrahepatic structures (parasagittal scans provided the best visualization of the ducts):

1. Alteration in the anatomic pattern adjacent to the main (right) portal vein segment and the bifurcation. This was more pronounced in individuals who displayed greater degrees of dilation of the intrahepatic bile ducts (Fig. 11-20).
2. Irregular walls of dilated bile ducts. As the intrahepatic biliary system dilates, the course and caliber of ducts become increasingly tortuous and irregular (Fig. 11-21).
3. Stellate confluence of dilated ducts. This was noted at the points where the ducts converge. Dilated ducts look like spokes of a wheel (Fig. 11-22).
4. Acoustic enhancement by dilated bile ducts. Both portal veins and ducts have high-amplitude reflections surrounding them (Fig. 11-23).
5. Peripheral duct dilation. It is normally unusual to visualize hepatic ducts in the liver periphery whereas dilated bile ducts may be observed (Fig. 11-24).

Dilated ducts

The common hepatic duct has an internal diameter of less than 4 mm.[9,10] A duct diameter of 5 mm is borderline, and 6 mm requires further investigation. A patient may have a normal-sized hepatic duct and still have distal obstruction. The distal duct is often obscured by gas in the duodenal loop.

The common bile duct has an internal diameter slightly greater than that of the hepatic duct. Generally a duct over 6 mm is considered borderline, and over 10 mm is dilated (Fig. 11-25). Minimal dilation (7 to 11 mm) may be seen in nonjaundiced patients with gallstones or pancreatitis or in jaundiced patients with a common duct stone or tumor (Fig. 11-26). However, a diameter of more than 11 mm suggests obstruction by stone or tumor of the duct or pancreas or some other source. Parulekar[14] measured the common duct at 7.7 mm in nonjaundiced patients who had undergone cholecystectomy.

Dilated ducts may also be found in the absence of jaundice. The patient may have biliary obstruction involving one hepatic duct, an early obstruction secondary to carcinoma, or gallstones causing intermittent obstruction due to a ball-valve effect.

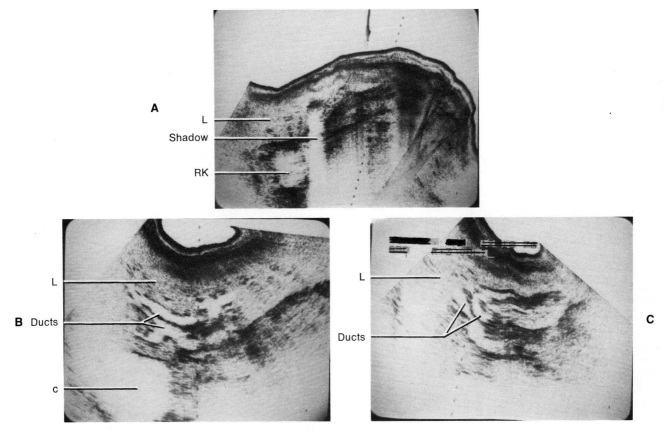

Fig. 11-21. A, Transverse supine scan of a "packed bag." The acoustic shadow is posterior. **B,** Transverse scan of dilated ducts. A large renal cyst is shown posterior to the dilated ducts. **C,** Transverse scan of the stellate pattern of the dilated ducts.

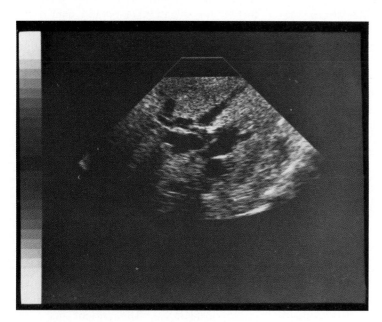

Fig. 11-22. Sagittal scan of the stellate confluence of dilated ducts at the points where the ducts converge.

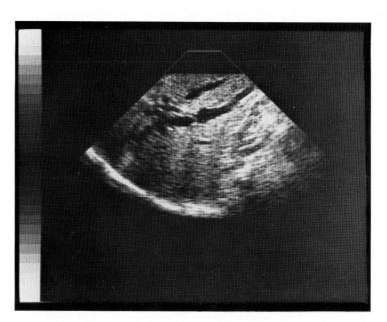

Fig. 11-23. As ducts dilate, acoustic enhancement may be seen due to the high-amplitude reflections that surround their borders.

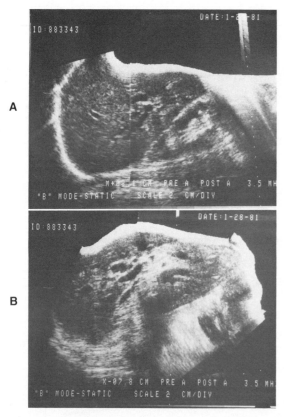

Fig. 11-24. A, This patient underwent cholecystectomy 1 year prior to the onset of jaundice and RUQ tenderness. Pancreatic carcinoma with involvement to the lymph nodes caused intrahepatic duct dilation. **B,** Transverse scan of the dilated ducts.

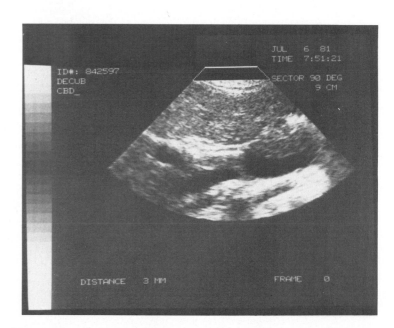

Fig. 11-25. Sagittal of a normal common bile duct. This duct measures 3 mm, which is far below the normal 6 mm measurement.

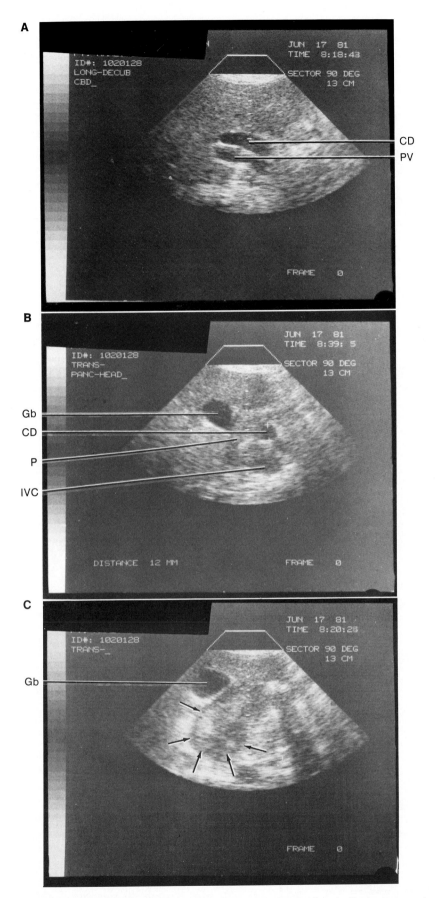

Fig. 11-26. This patient presented with recurrent abdominal pain that worsened upon eating. The sonogram showed a dilated common duct with a large irregular mass in the head of the pancreas. **A,** Sagittal of the common duct, *CD,* which measures 12 mm. **B,** Transverse of the common duct. Pancreas, *P;* gallbladder, *Gb;* inferior vena cava, *IVC.* **C,** Transverse of the gallbladder and pancreatic mass in the head of the gland *(arrow).*

CLINICAL SYMPTOMS OF GALLBLADDER DISEASE

The most classic symptom of gallbladder disease is right upper quadrant abdominal pain, usually occurring after ingestion of greasy foods. Nausea and vomiting may occur and may indicate the presence of a stone in the common bile duct. A gallbladder attack may cause pain in the right shoulder, with inflammation of the gallbladder often causing referred pain in the right shoulder blade.

Gallstones

After a fatty meal the gallbladder contracts to release bile; and if the outflow tract is blocked by gallstones, pain results. As the bile is being stored in the gallbladder, small crystals of bile salts precipitate and may form gallstones varying from pinhead size to the size of the organ itself. There may be a single large gallstone or hundreds of tiny ones. The tiny stones are the most dangerous, since they can enter the bile ducts and obstruct the outflow of bile.

Jaundice

Jaundice is characterized by the presence of bile in the tissues with resulting yellow-green color of the skin. It may develop when a tiny gallstone blocks the bile ducts between the gallbladder and the intestines, producing pressure on the liver and forcing bile into the blood.

Cholecystitis

Inflammation of the gallbladder usually is a chronic illness punctuated by intermittent acute episodes, which occur when the cystic duct is obstructed by a calculus. Calculi (gallstones) are almost always associated with cholecystitis although rare cases of "acalculus cholecystitis" are believed to occur. About 85% of gallstones are composed entirely of cholesterol; 10% are bile pigment stones, and 5% are a combination of bile pigments and cholesterol. Varying degrees of calcification may be superimposed, with the result that some stones are visible radiographically. Gallstones occur commonly in whites (more than 25% of persons over age 40) and occur with even higher incidence in specific populations such as Swedes and American Indians.

The relationship of gallstones to the pathogenesis of cholecystitis has long been a point of debate. Which comes first, the stone or the inflammation? The current tendency is to regard cholecystitis as a result of gallstone formation rather than a cause of it. This view is supported by the discovery of *lithogenic*

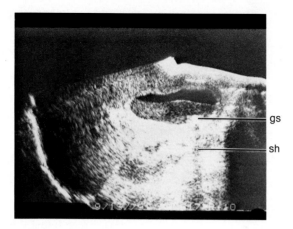

Fig. 11-27. Sagittal of a prominent gallbladder with echogenic bile layering along the posterior border. In addition, a bright reflector from a gallstone is seen along the posterior border with a shadow posteriorly. Gallstone, *gs;* shadow, *sh.*

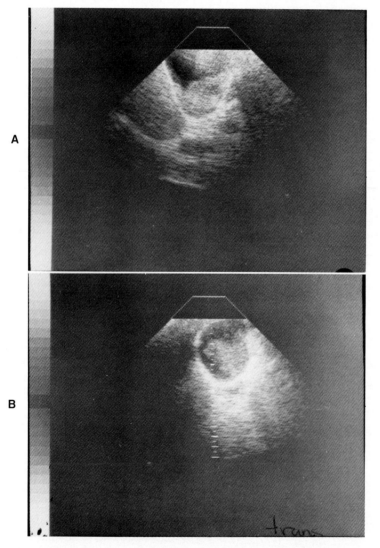

Fig. 11-28. A, Sagittal scan of a gallbladder with inspissated bile. **B,** Transverse scan with echogenic bile appearing very irregular and not layering out as would be expected. A tumor was questioned but ruled out because the echoes were not reflective as one would expect tumor echoes to be.

bile, a form of bile supersaturated with cholesterol that is found in some individuals but not in others. *Lecithin* and bile salts keep cholesterol in *solution* in bile; hence the relative concentration of these elements may determine whether cholesterol precipitates and forms stones. In patients with lithogenic bile the liver secretes too much cholesterol relative to the amount of lecithin and bile salts present. It is believed that precipitated cholesterol crystals in such patients aggregate and grow, forming stones. Gallstones may result in inflammation of the gallbladder mucosa through direct contact or by intermittent obstruction of the cystic duct. In the latter case, overdistension is believed to stretch the gallbladder wall excessively and produce ischemia. Obstruction also causes stasis, which promotes bacterial growth in the bile. Both ischemia and stasis are believed to account for the inflammation and scarring that occur in cholecystitis.

The gallbladder is not an essential organ, and certain mammals such as deer are not equipped with one. When the gallbladder is removed surgically, the common duct is believed to distend in some cases and take over the reservoir function. Recent sonographic results, however, suggest that this may not be as frequent an occurrence as previously suspected.

PATHOLOGIC PATTERNS OF GALLBLADDER DISEASE
Gallbladder sludge

Occasionally a patient presents sonographically with a prominent gallbladder containing low-level internal echoes that may be attributed to thick or inspissated bile (Fig. 11-27). Filly et al.[5] state that the source of echoes in biliary sludge is particulate matter (predominantly pigment granules with lesser amounts of cholesterol crystals). They report that the viscosity does not appear to be important in the generation of internal echoes in fluids. The particles can be very small and still produce perceptible echoes.

Some gallbladders may be so packed with inspissated bile that it becomes difficult to separate the gallbladder from the liver parenchyma (Fig. 11-28). Occasionally the thick bile is also found in the common duct due to obstruction.[4] Sludge is gravity dependent; thus with alterations in patient position, one may be able to separate sludge from occasional artifactual echoes found in the gallbladder. Filly et al.[5] state that sludge should be considered an abnormal finding, because either a functional or a pathologic abnormality exists when calcium bilirubin or choles-

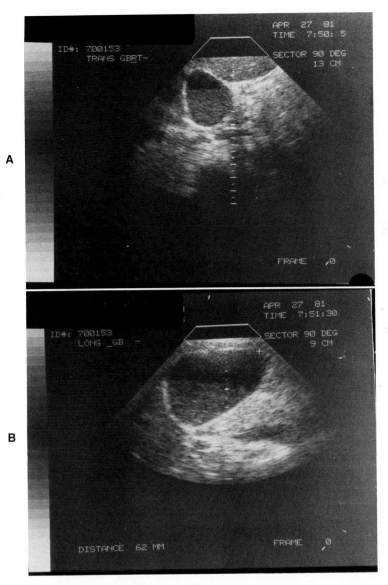

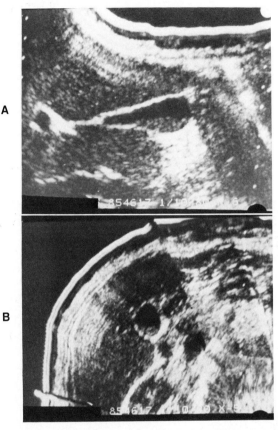

Fig. 11-29. A, Transverse scan of a gallbladder with echogenic bile. **B,** Sagittal scan showing some distension with layering of echogenic bile.

Fig. 11-30. A, Sagittal scan of a gallbladder with echogenic bile. **B,** Transverse scan with a small amount of echogenic bile.

terol precipitates in bile (Figs. 11-29 and 11-30).

Wall thickness

The normal wall thickness of the gallbladder is 1 to 2 mm. Sonographically it may be underestimated when the wall has extensive fibrosis or is surrounded by fat[7] (Fig. 11-31).

The sonographic appearance of acute cholecystitis has been identified as a gallbladder with an irregular outline of a thickened wall. In addition, Marchal et al.[12,13] have found a sonolucent area within the thickened wall probably due to edema (Fig. 11-32). A study by Engel et al.[4a] of wall thickness indicated that 98% of patients whose gallbladder walls were over 3.5 mm thick had disease

whereas 50% with gallbladder disease had a wall thickness of less than 3 mm.

Sanders[15] states that the wall is not always thick in acute cholecystitis. Some walls will be thicker due to pericholecystic abscess. Occasionally a thickened gallbladder wall is seen in normal individuals. It seems to be related to the degree of contraction of a normal gallbladder. Sanders found the gallbladder wall thickened symmetrically with smooth outlines in patients with acute cholecystitis without abscess or ascites. If the thickened wall is localized and irregular, one should consider cholecystosis or carcinoma of the gallbladder.

Another condition wherein the gallbladder wall may be thickened is gangrenous chole-

cystitis. The wall is also edematous with focal areas of exudate, hemorrhage, and necrosis. In addition, there may be ulcerations and perforations resulting in pericholecystic abscesses or peritonitis. Gallstones or fine gravel occur in 80% to 95% of the patients. Kane[10a] states that the common echo features of gangrene are the presence of diffuse medium to coarse echogenic densities filling the gallbladder lumen in the absence of bile duct obstruction. This echogenic material has three characteristics: (1) it does not cause shadowing, (2) it is not gravity dependent, and (3) it does not show a layering effect. The lack of layering is attributed to increased viscosity of the bile.

Fiski et al.[8] have stated that a thickened

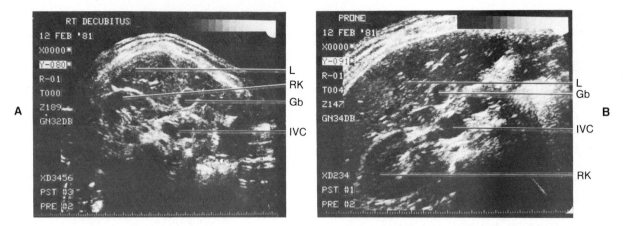

Fig. 11-31. A, Right decubitus of a normal gallbladder. Generally the wall is measured from the anterior border so artifacts and reverberation echoes from the posterior border will be avoided. **B,** The gallbladder wall thickness may be underestimated if the wall has extensive fibrosis or is surrounded by fat. A high-frequency transducer will help in distinguishing normal wall thickness from artifact.

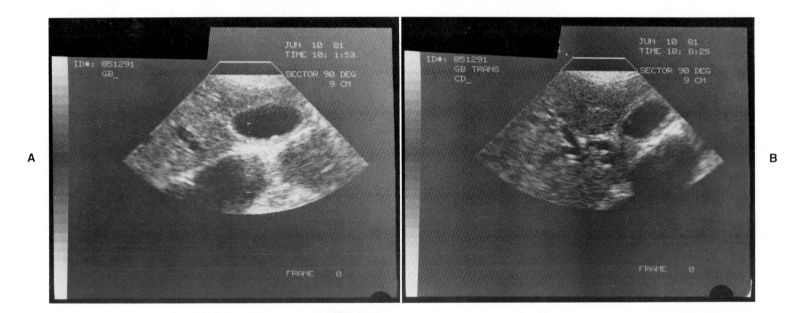

Fig. 11-32. This patient presented with jaundice and increased alkaline phosphatase values. **A,** Sagittal view demonstrating the gallbladder to be of normal size but increased thickness in the walls. **B,** Transverse view showing the thickened walls with too many tubes.

wall is a nonspecific sign and is not necessarily related to gallbladder disease. It may be found in the following conditions besides those previously discussed: hepatitis, adenomyomatosis, gallbladder tumor, or severe hypoalbuminemic states (Figs. 11-33 to 11-35).

Cholelithiasis

The evaluation of gallstones with real time has proved to be an extremely useful procedure in patients who present with symptoms of cholelithiasis (Fig. 11-36). The gallbladder is evaluated for increased size, wall thickness, presence of internal reflections within the lumen, and posterior acoustic shadowing. Frequently patients with gallstones will have a dilated gallbladder. Stones that are less than 1 to 2 mm may be difficult to separate from one another by ultrasound evaluation and thus are reported as gallstones without comment on the specific number that may have been seen on the scan.

If an articulated arm scanner is used, care must be exercised in evaluating the gallbladder by use of a single-sweep technique and remaining perpendicular to the gallbladder and the stone. Slight sectoring will almost certainly fill in the shadow posterior to the stone and thus cause the stone to be overlooked (Fig. 11-37).

Regardless of the equipment used, the patient's position should be shifted during the procedure to demonstrate further the presence of the stones. Patients should be scanned in the right-side-up decubitus, right lateral, or upright position. The stones should shift to the most dependent area of the gallbladder. In some cases the bile has a

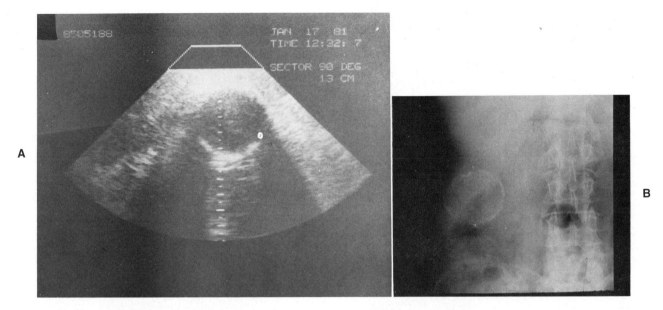

Fig. 11-33. A, If the gallbladder walls are calcified, wall thickness may be difficult to assess. The walls are very bright reflectors, and decreased through-transmission with shadow is noted posteriorly. **B,** Radiography of the calcified "porcelain" gallbladder.

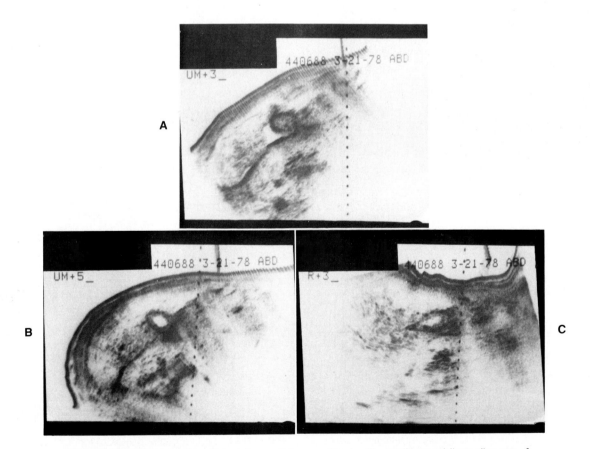

Fig. 11-34. Thickened gallbladder wall in a patient with ascites and liver disease. **A,** Transverse scan showing the gallbladder surrounded by ascitic fluid. **B,** Transverse scan. **C,** Sagittal scan of the shrunken thick-walled gallbladder.

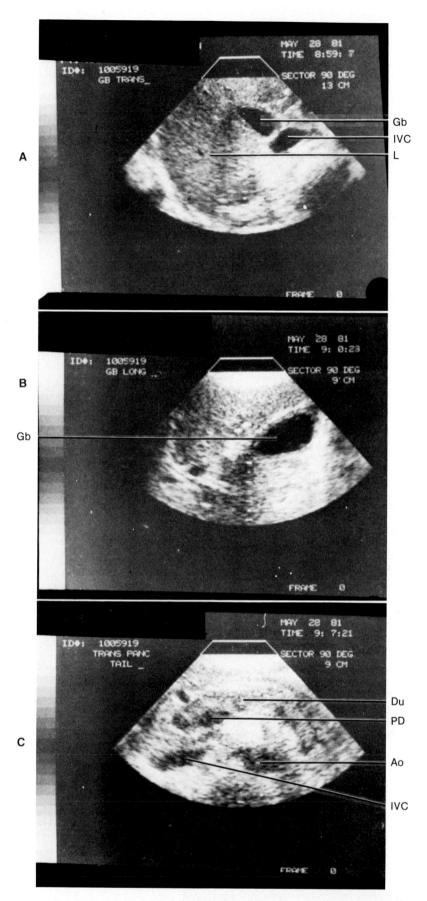

Fig. 11-35. A patient presented with chronic pancreatitis and epigastric pain. **A,** Transverse scan of the thick-walled gallbladder anterior to the inferior vena cava. **B,** Sagittal scan of the gallbladder. **C,** Transverse scan of the echogenic pancreas with a dilated pancreatic duct.

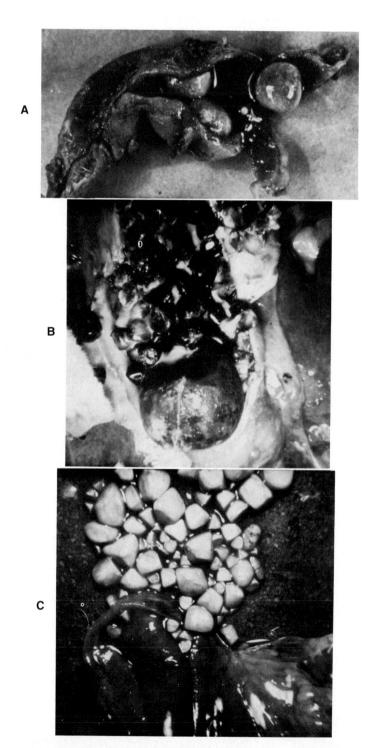

Fig. 11-36. A, Diseased gallbladder with multiple large stones. **B,** Gallbladder with multiple small stones. **C,** Gross specimen of gallstones.

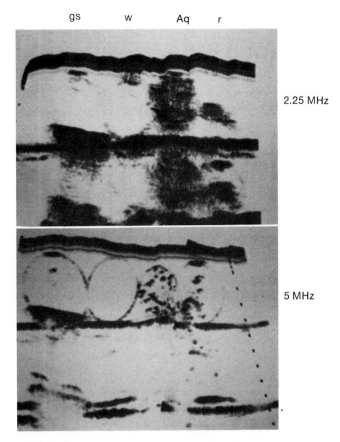

Fig. 11-37. An experimental study was performed with a simulated gallbladder (a balloon) filled with sand to represent gallstones, *gs*, water to represent bile, *w*, Aquasonic to represent thickened bile, *Aq*, and an actual gallstone, *r*. Scans were performed with a 2.25- and a 5.0-MHz transducer to evaluate resolution capabilities of the equipment. Low and high sensitivities were used to evaluate transmission quality.

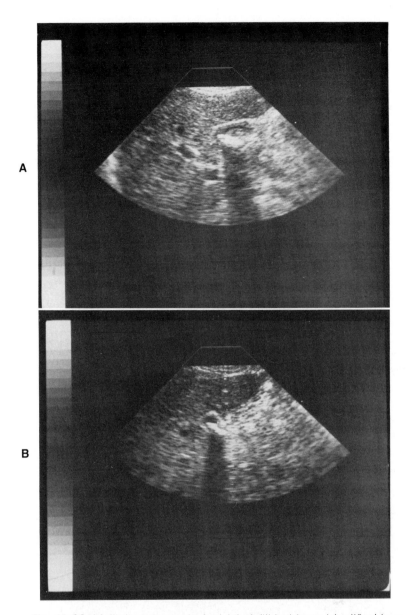

Fig. 11-38. Multiple echogenic foci (cholelithiasis) are identified in a gallbladder with posterior acoustic shadowing.

thick consistency and the stones remain near the top of the gallbladder. Thus the density of the stones and the shadow posterior will be the sonographic evidence for stones (Figs. 11-38 to 11-43).

Gonzalez and MacIntyre[9] have evaluated the theory for acoustic shadowing formed from gallstones and discovered that scattered reflections do not affect shadowing as much as specular reflections do. The factors that produced a shadow were attributed to acoustic impedance of the gallstones; refraction through them or diffraction around them; their size, central or peripheral location, and position in relation to the focus of the beam; and the intensity of the beam.

Filly et al.[5,6] found in their in vitro phantom studies that all stones cast acoustic shadows regardless of the specific properties of the stones. The size of the stone was important, with stones greater than 3 mm always casting a shadow and those smaller than 3 mm sometimes not casting one. They found that any stone scanned two or more times

with the same transducer and machine settings might or might not generate a shadow even though the scans were taken within seconds of each other. The shadow was highly dependent on the relationship between the stone and the acoustic beam. If the central beam was at or near the stone, a shadow would be seen. Thus some critical ratio between the stone diameter and the beam width must be achieved before shadowing is seen.

Floating gallstones

Some stones are seen to float when contrast material from an oral cholecystogram is present. This is due to the higher specific gravity of the contrast material than of the

bile. The gallstones seek a level where their specific gravity equals that of the mixture of bile and contrast material[16] (Fig. 11-44).

Gas in the biliary tree shadow

Another cause for shadowing in the right upper quadrant is gas in the biliary tree. This is a spontaneous occurrence due to the formation of a biliary enteric fistula in chronic gallbladder disease.[7] The sonogram demonstrates the liver parenchyma to be disrupted by narrow bands of acoustic shadows lying behind well-defined discrete high-amplitude echoes deep within the liver parenchyma (Fig. 11-45).

Text continued on p. 172.

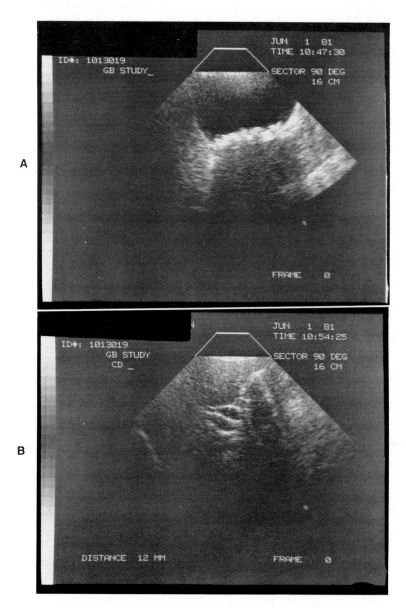

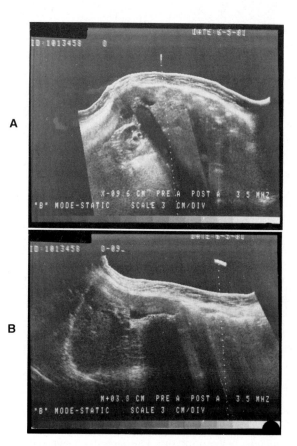

Fig. 11-39. Nonviscous oral cholecystogram. **A,** Sagittal scan demonstrating a large gallbladder with multiple reflective stones along the posterior wall. An acoustic shadow is present. **B,** The common duct measures 12 mm.

Fig. 11-40. This patient presented with liver metastases and a "packed bag." **A,** Transverse scan showing the anterior border of the gallbladder with a strong acoustic shadow posteriorly. **B,** Sagittal scan showing the sharply marginated shadow from the packed bag.

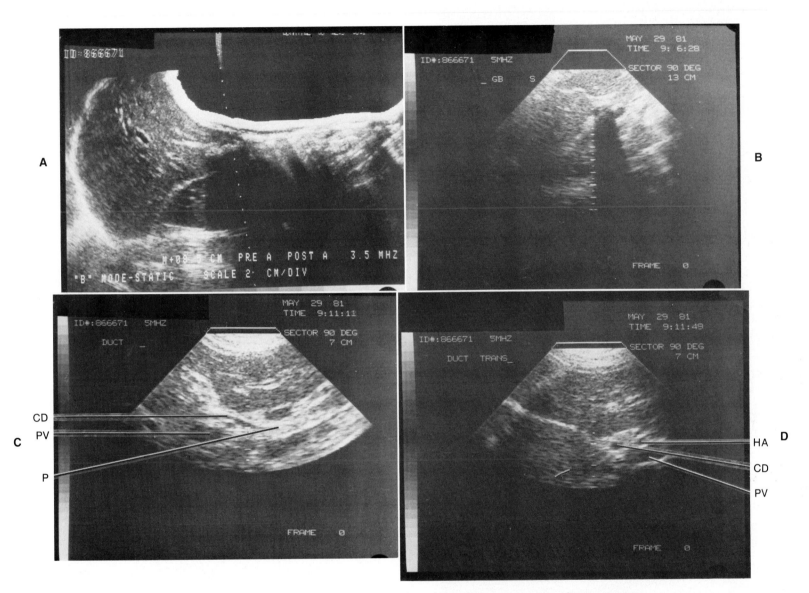

Fig. 11-41. This patient presented with abdominal pain. **A,** Sagittal scan of the packed bag with acoustic shadow preventing the lower pole of the right kidney from being imaged. **B,** Transverse scan of the packed bag. **C,** Sagittal scan of the common duct as it passes anterior to the portal vein before entering the posterior margin of the pancreatic head. **D,** Transverse view of the common duct, hepatic artery, and portal vein.

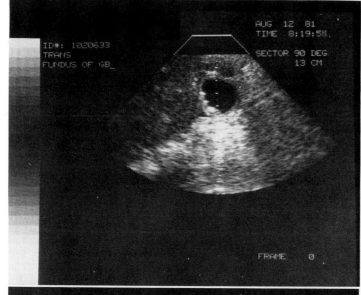

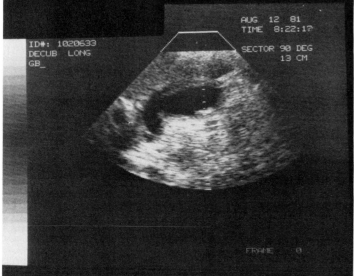

Fig. 11-42. A, Transverse view of a patient with cholelithiasis and thickened gallbladder walls. The stones are very bright reflectors along the lateral wall. There is no shadow because the transducer was not perpendicular to the interface of the stone. **B,** Sagittal view of the gallbladder. The stones are near the fundus.

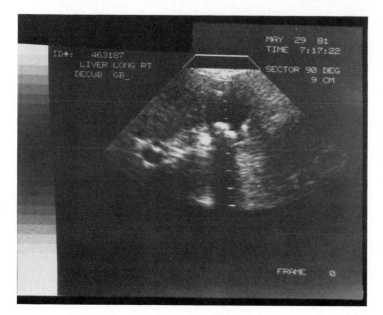

Fig. 11-43. Decubitus sagittal view showing multiple large gallstones, which cast an acoustic shadow.

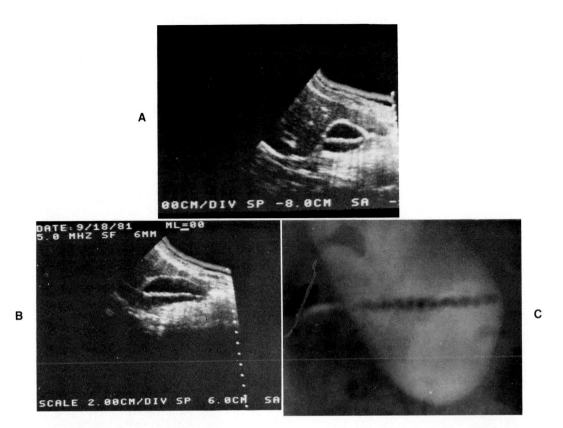

Fig. 11-44. Floating gallstones. **A,** Transverse view; **B,** sagittal view; **C,** radiograph. (Courtesy VA Hospital, Madison, Wis.)

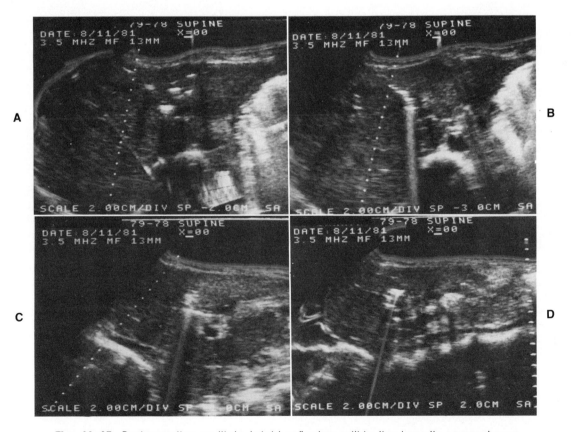

Fig. 11-45. Postoperative multiple bright reflectors within the hepatic parenchyma. There is acoustic shadowing beyond. This represented gas in the biliary tree. **A** and **B,** Transverse supine scans; **C** and **D,** sagittal scans. (Courtesy VA Hospital, Madison, Wis.)

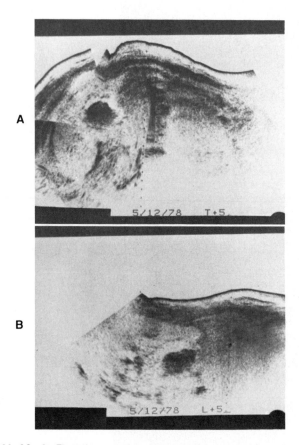

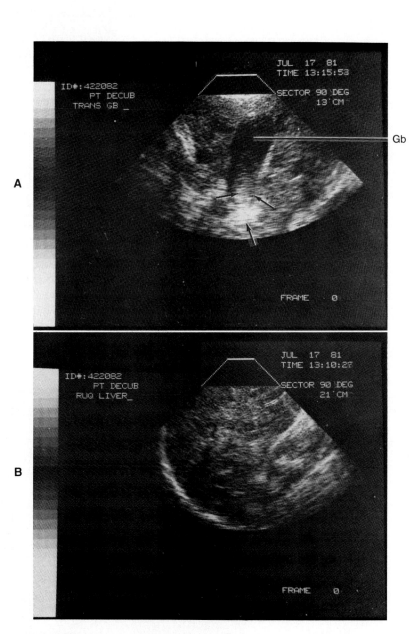

Fig. 11-46. A, The dense echogenic mass within the gallbladder is much brighter than one would expect to see with echogenic bile. This patient had carcinoma of the gallbladder as well as of the mesenteric structures in the vicinity of the porta hepatis. He did not become jaundiced until after surgery was performed. **B,** Sagittal scan of the tumor within the gallbladder.

Fig. 11-47. A, This patient had liver metastases and a polypoid mass within the gallbladder. **B,** Sagittal scan of the liver with multiple focal defects.

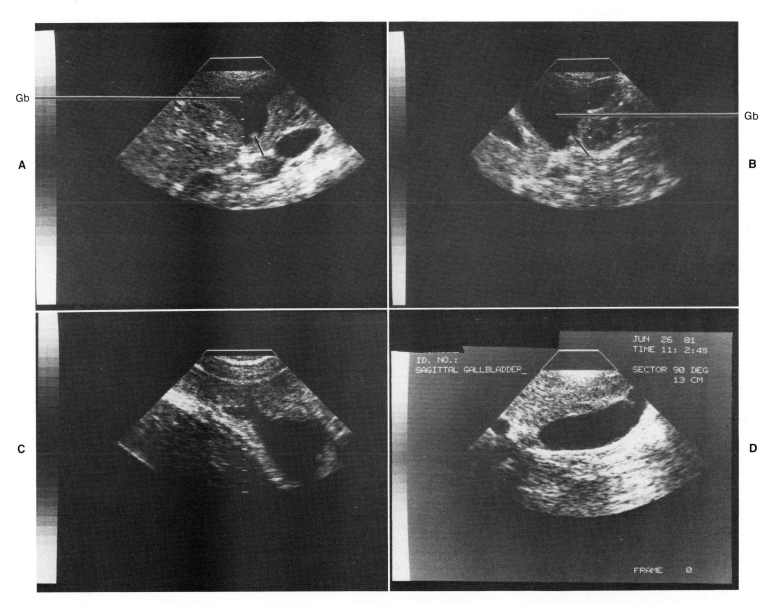

Fig. 11-48. A, Transverse scan of a distended gallbladder with low-level irregularity attached to the wall *(arrow)*. **B,** The small mass represented a polyp and did not change position. **C,** Decubitus of the gallbladder and polyp. **D,** Sagittal of the distended gallbladder with a fold near the fundus.

— tumor resembling a granuloma or xanthoma

Primary carcinoma of the gallbladder

Carcinoma of the gallbladder is very rare. A small tumor in the neck may not even be seen by sonography if secondary signs of obstruction and dilation are absent. The most frequent sonographic sign is a large, irregular, fungating mass that contains low-intensity echoes within the gallbladder (Fig. 11-46). Sometimes the mass will completely fill the gallbladder, obscuring the gallbladder walls. There may be stones along with the tumor, causing posterior shadowing. The differential diagnosis of carcinoma, empyema, and xanthogranulomatous cholecystitis is virtually impossible by ultrasound and surgical intervention may be the only recourse (Fig. 11-47).

Polyp

A polyp appears sonographically as a low-level echo mass adjacent to the wall of the gallbladder. Generally it will not change in position or produce an acoustic shadow as will a gallstone. It is usually attached to the gallbladder wall by a short stalk (Figs. 11-48 and 11-49).

REFERENCES

1. Bartrum, R.J., and Crow, H.C.: Inflammatory diseases of the biliary system, Semin. Ultrasound, Vol. 1, no. 2, 1980.
2. Carter, S.J., Rutledge, J., Hirch, J.H., et al.: Papillary adenoma of the gallbladder; ultrasonic demonstration, J. Clin. Ultrasound 6:433, 1978.
3. Conrad, M.R., James, J.O., and Dietchy, J.: Significance of low level echoes within the gallbladder, A.J.R. 132:967, 1979.
4. Conrad, M.R., Landay, M.J., and James, J.O.: Sonographic parallel channel sign of biliary tree enlargement in mild to moderate obstructive jaundice, A.J.R. 130:279, 1978.
4a. Engel, J.M., Deitch, E.A., and Sikkema, W.: Gallbladder wall thickness: sonographic accuracy and relation to disease, A.J.R. 134:907, 1980.
5. Filly, R.A., Allen, B., Minton, M.J., et al.: In vitro investigation of the origin of echoes within biliary sludge, J. Clin. Ultrasound 8:193, 1980.
6. Filly, R.A., Moss, A.A., and Way, L.W.: In vitro investigation of gallstone shadowing with ultrasound tomography, J. Clin. Ultrasound 7:255, 1979.
7. Finberg, J.J., and Birnholz, J.C.: Ultrasound evaluation of the gallbladder wall, Radiology 133:693, 1979.
8. Fiski, C.E., Laing, F.C., and Brown, T.W.: Ultrasonographic evidence of gallbladder wall thickening in association with hypoalbuminemia, Radiology 135:713, 1980.
9. Gonzalez, L., and MacIntyre, W.J.: Acoustic shadow formation by gallstones, Radiology 135:217, 1980.
10. Graham, M.F., Cooperberg, P.L., Cohen, M.M., et al.: The size of the normal common hepatic duct following cholecystectomy; an ultrasonic study, Radiology 135:137, 1980.
10a. Kane, R.A.: Ultrasonographic diagnosis of gangrenous cholecystitis and empyema of the gallbladder, Radiology 134:191, 1980.
11. Laing, F.C., London, L.A., and Filly, R.A.: Ultrasonographic identification of dilated intrahepatic bile ducts and their differentiation from portal venous structures, J. Clin. Ultrasound 6:73, 1978.
12. Marchal, G.J.F., Casaer, M., Baert, A.L., et al.: Gallbladder wall sonolucency in acute cholecystitis, Radiology 133:429, 1979.
13. Marchal, G., Van de Voorde, P., Van Dooren, W., et al.: Ultrasonic appearance of the filled and contracted normal gallbladder, J. Clin. Ultrasound 8:439, 1980.
14. Parulekar, S.G.: Ultrasound evaluation of common bile duct size, Radiology 133:703, 1979.
15. Sanders, R.C.: The significance of sonographic gallbladder wall thickening, J. Clin. Ultrasound 8:143, 1980.
16. Scheske, G.A., Cooperberg, P.L., Cohen, M.M., et al.: Floating gallstones; the role of contrast material, J. Clin. Ultrasound 8:227, 1980.

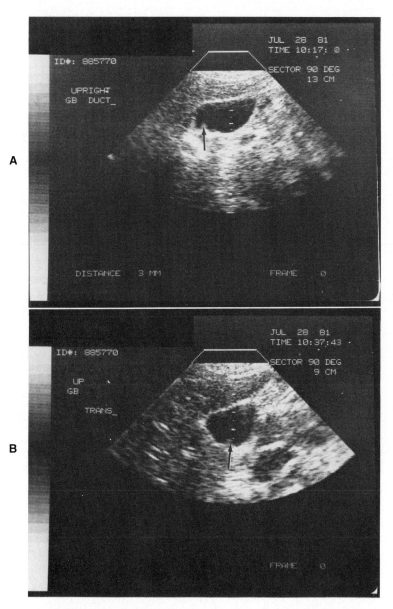

Fig. 11-49. A, This patient presented with burning epigastric pain, nausea, and vomiting for several weeks. Laboratory values were normal. The upright sagittal scan shows the gallbladder with a low-level echo, which represents a polyp. **B,** Upright transverse scan of the gallbladder and polyp *(arrow).*

12 Pancreas

With the advent of each new medical procedure, efforts to visualize the pancreas accurately have met with varying degrees of success. Prior to the relatively recent use of diagnostic ultrasound, other noninvasive procedures were unsuccessful in accurate visualization of the pancreas. The plain film of the abdomen is diagnostic of pancreatitis if calcification is visible in the pancreatic area; however, calcification does not occur in all cases. Localized ileus ("paralyzed gut," gas, and fluid accumulation near the area of inflammation) may be shown on the plain radiograph in patients with pancreatitis. The upper gastrointestinal test series provides indirect information about the pancreas when the widened duodenal loop is visualized. Other diagnostic methods such as hypotonic duodenography, isotope examination, arteriography, fiberoptic gastroscopy, and intravenous cholangiography all provide indirect information about the pancreas or prove limited in their diagnostic ability. Thus investigators have been striving to develop an examination that will be accurate, readily repeatable, and safe. Diagnostic ultrasound appears to be such an examination.

The normal pancreas can be visualized in the majority of patients by using the neighboring organs and vascular landmarks as an aid for locating it. The gland appears echographically as dense as or slightly denser than the hepatic parenchyma. Variations in patient positioning or utilization of contrast media through the stomach aids in visualizing the entire gland.

Difficulties encountered in making the proper diagnosis have been presented to give the sonographer a better understanding of the diagnostic signs of pancreatic disease.

At the present time there are still a few problems in pancreatic visualization with the ultrasonic technique. Familiar impediments are the reflections and absorptions caused by bone, gas, and air. If these occur over the area of interest, it becomes impossible to outline prevertebral vessels and thus visualization of the pancreas is limited. Obesity presents a problem in some cases. The far gain (or the overall gain) of the equipment may need adjustment for properly penetrating these patients. Normal organ movement makes exact repetition difficult in some cases, and several scans may have to be made before a confident analysis is possible. However, real time has overcome this problem, enabling the sonographer to follow the course of the prevertebral vessels accurately and delineate the borders of the pancreas with more precision.

For many reasons the pancreas may be a more difficult organ to visualize than the liver, gallbladder, spleen, or kidneys. Filly and Freimanis[3] have presented evidence that the normal pancreas is difficult to visualize by conventional bistable ultrasonic equipment since the gland produces many echoes at normal sensitivity due to multiple interfaces within it. With gray scale ultrasound a normal pancreas can possess a degree of echogenicity greater than or equal to, but not less than, that of the liver.[4]

ANATOMY

The pancreas lies in the retroperitoneal cavity. It is usually 10 to 15 cm long, anterior to the first and second vertebral bodies. It is located deep in the epigastrium and left hypochondrium behind the lesser omental sac. Thus it is hidden from direct physical examination.

There is some variation in the size of the gland, for it has been described as sausage shaped, dumbbell shaped, or gradually tapering from its head to its tail. The gland is relatively larger (thicker) in children than in adults. It subsequently becomes smaller with advancing age. Several clinical studies have been made in efforts to determine the size of the normal gland (Table 12-1). Our own experience corresponds with the measurements by Arger et al.[1]: head = 2.5 cm; body = 2 cm; and tail = 2 cm.

Table 12-1. Ultrasound correlations of size (cm)

AP	Haber et al. (A.J.R. 1976)	Weill et al. (Radiology, 1977)	Degraaff et al. (Radiology, 1978)	Arger et al. (J. Clin. Ultrasound, 1979)
Head	2.7 ± 0.7	3.0	2.01	2.5
Neck		2.1	1.00	
Body	2.2 ± 0.7	2.8	1.18	2.0
Tail	2.0 ± 0.4	2.8		2.0

173

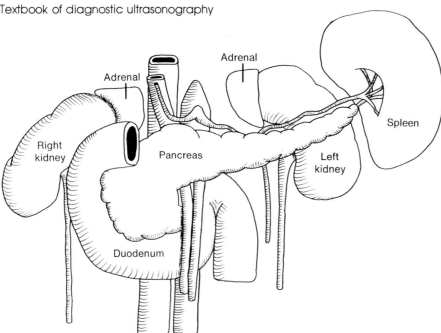

Fig. 12-1. Relationship of the pancreas to other retroperitoneal structures.

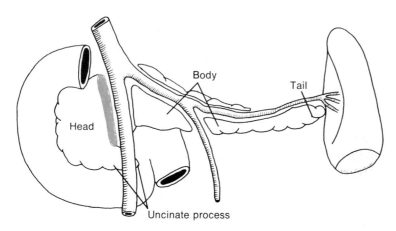

Fig. 12-2. Four parts of the pancreas: head, uncinate process, body, and tail.

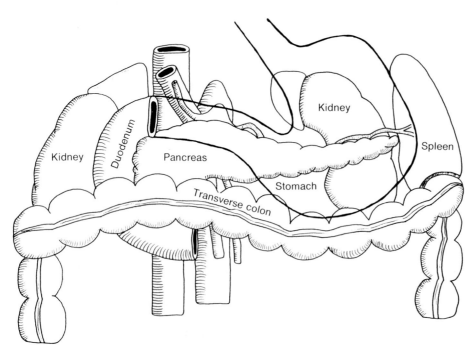

Fig. 12-3. The pancreas is hidden by the stomach, pylorus, and transverse colon.

The pancreas is generally found in a horizontal oblique lie, extending from the concavity of the duodenum to the hilum of the spleen (Fig. 12-1). Other variations of the gland are transverse, horseshoe, sigmoid, L shaped, and inverted V.[11]

The gland is divided into three major areas: head, neck/body, and tail. Each will be discussed as it relates to its surrounding anatomy (Fig. 12-2).

Head

The head of the pancreas is anterior to the inferior vena cava and left renal vein, inferior to the caudate lobe of the liver and the portal vein (Fig. 12-3), and lateral to the second portion of the duodenum. It lies in the "lap" of the duodenum. These structures pass posterior to the superior mesenteric vessels. It is also located posterior to the antrum of the stomach. The uncinate process is posterior to the superior mesenteric vessels. The common bile duct passes through a groove posterior to the pancreatic head (Fig. 12-4), and the gastroduodenal artery serves as the anterolateral border (Fig. 12-5).

Neck/body

The neck/body, the largest part of the gland, lies on an angle from caudal right to cephalic left posterior to the stomach and anterior to the origin of the portal vein (Fig. 12-6). It rests posteriorly against the aorta, the origin of the superior mesenteric artery, the left renal vessels, the left adrenal gland, and the left kidney. The tortuous splenic artery is usually the superior border of the pancreas. The anterior surface is separated by the omental bursa from the posterior wall of the stomach. The inferior surface, below the attachment of the transverse mesocolon, is related to the duodenojejunal junction and the splenic flexure of the colon.

Tail

The tail of the pancreas lies in front of the left kidney close to the spleen and the left colic flexure. The splenic artery forms the anterior border, the splenic vein the posterior border, and the stomach the superoanterior border.

Pancreatic ducts

To aid in the transport of pancreatic fluid, the ducts have smooth muscle surrounding them. The *duct of Wirsung* is a primary duct extending the entire length of the gland. It receives tributaries from lobules at right angles and enters the medial second part of the duodenum with the common bile duct at the *ampulla of Vater* (guarded by the *sphinc-*

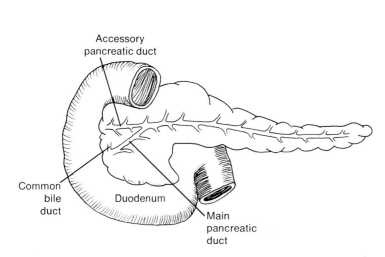

Fig. 12-4. The main pancreatic duct runs along the middle of the gland to join the common bile duct at the lateral margin of the head.

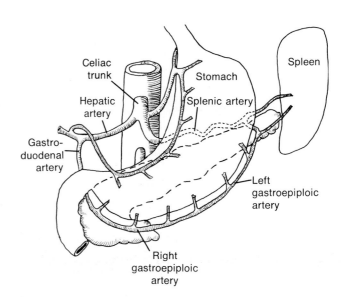

Fig. 12-5. The gastroduodenal artery serves as the anterolateral border of the pancreatic head.

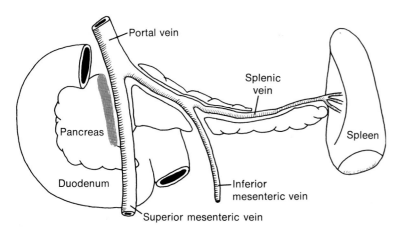

Fig. 12-6. Venous structures serve as the posterior border to most of the pancreatic tissue.

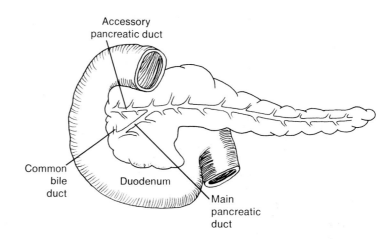

Fig. 12-7. Pancreatic duct.

ter of Oddi) (Fig. 12-7). The *duct of Santorini* is a secondary duct that drains the upper anterior head. It enters the duodenum at the minor papilla about 2 cm proximal to the ampulla of Vater.

Relational anatomy

The important structures related to the posterior surface of the pancreas include the inferior vena cava, the aorta, the superior mesenteric vessels, the splenic and portal veins, and the common bile duct. The splenic artery and stomach lie along the superior border of the pancreas, and the hilus of the spleen lies in contact with the tail of the gland. The anterior pancreatic surface is bounded by the stomach and the lesser peritoneal cavity whereas the inferior surface lies along the greater peritoneal cavity.

Because of the unyielding nature of the posterior abdominal wall, any enlargement of the gland will extend anteriorly.

PHYSIOLOGY

The pancreas is both an exocrine and an endocrine gland. Its exocrine function is to produce *pancreatic juice*, which enters the duodenum together with bile. The exocrine secretions of the pancreas and those of the liver, which are delivered into the duodenum through duct systems, are essential for normal intestinal digestion and absorption of food. Pancreatic secretion is under the control of the vagus nerve and two hormonal agents, secretin and pancreozymin, that are released when food enters the duodenum. The endocrine function is to produce the hormone *insulin*. Failure of the pancreas to furnish sufficient insulin leads to diabetes mellitus.

The enzymes of the pancreatic juice are lipase, amylase, carboxypeptidase, trypsin, and chymotrypsin. The last three are secreted as inactive enzyme precursors to be activated when they have entered the duodenum. The pancreas contains acinar cells, exocrine secretory cells that are arranged in saclike clusters (acini) connected by small intercalated ducts to larger excretory ducts. The excretory ducts converge into one or two main ducts, which deliver the exocrine secretion of the pancreas into the duodenum.

Pancreatic juice is the most versatile and active of the digestive secretions. Its enzymes are capable of nearly completing the digestion of food in the absence of all other digestive secretions. Because the digestive enzymes that are secreted into the lumen of the small intestine require an almost neutral pH for best activity, the acidity of the con-

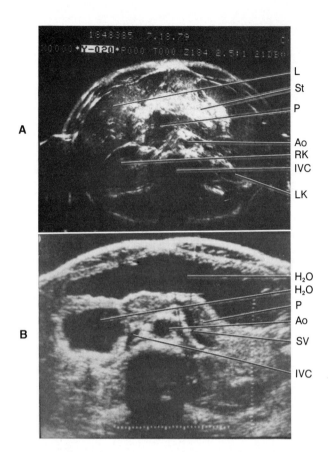

Fig. 12-8. A, The stomach, *St*, can serve as an acoustic impediment or an acoustic enhancement if properly hydrated. This transverse scan shows the collapsed walls of a stomach that has just enough fluid within to permit adequate visualization of the posterior pancreas. **B,** This scan shows an extremely distended stomach, which helps to visualize the pancreas and prevertebral vessels posterior to its border. Water, *H₂O*; pancreas, *P*; aorta, *Ao*; inferior vena cava, *IVC*; splenic vein, *SV*. (Courtesy John Dietz, B.S., Philadelphia.)

tents entering the duodenum must be reduced. Thus the pancreatic juice contains a relatively high concentration of sodium bicarbonate, and this alkaline salt is largely responsible for the neutralization of gastric acid.

The nervous secretion of pancreatic juice is thick and rich in enzymes and proteins. The chemical secretion, resulting from pancreozymin activity, also is thick, watery, and rich in enzymes. Pancreatic juice is alkaline and becomes more so with increasing rates of secretion. This is because of a simultaneous increase in bicarbonates and decrease in chloride concentration.

The proteolytic enzyme trypsin may hydrolyze protein molecules to polypeptides. Chymotrypsinogen is activated by trypsin. Amylase causes hydrolysis of starch with the production of maltose, which is further hydrolyzed to glucose. Lipase is capable of hydrolyzing some fats to monoglycerides and some to glycerol and fatty acids. Although lipases are also secreted by the small intestine, what is secreted by the pancreas ac-

counts for 80% of all fat digestion. Thus impaired fat digestion is an important indicator of pancreatic dysfunction.

LABORATORY TESTS
Amylase

In certain types of pancreatic disease the digestive enzymes of the pancreas escape into the surrounding tissue, producing necrosis with severe pain and inflammation. Under these circumstances there is an increase in serum amylase. A serum amylase level of twice normal usually indicates acute pancreatitis. Other conditions causing increased amylase are intestinal obstruction, mumps, and other disease of the salivary glands or ducts.

Glucose

The glucose tolerance test is performed to discover whether there is a disorder of glucose metabolism. An increased blood glucose level is found in severe diabetes, chronic liver disease, and overactivity of several of the endocrine glands. There may be a de-

creased blood sugar level in tumors of the *islets of Langerhans* in the pancreas.

Lipase

The lipase test is performed to assess damage to the pancreas. Lipase is secreted by the pancreas, and small amounts pass into the blood. The lipase level rises in acute pancreatitis and in carcinoma of the pancreas. (Both amylase and lipase rise at the same rate, but the elevation in lipase concentration persists for a longer period.)

SONOGRAPHIC TECHNIQUES
Patient preparation

If the biliary system is to be evaluated along with the pancreas, the patient should be NPO for 8 hours. If just the pancreas is the main concern, however, I have found it helpful for the patient to be adequately hydrated. Often a full stomach serves as an advantage in outlining the more posterior pancreatic parenchyma. The patient may drink large quantities (16 to 32 ounces) of water or tomato or orange juice prior to or following the initial examination in efforts to distend the stomach and fill the duodenal cap to outline the gland (Fig. 12-8).

Several investigators have used glucagon (1 mg) intravenously followed by 500 ml of water after 2 to 3 minutes.[14] The glucagon reduces the peristaltic action of the stomach and thus maintains a fluid-filled window for almost an hour. Simethicone and other "gas-eliminating" drugs have proved to be of little success. We have often found that they are more gas producing in the difficult "gassy" patients. Generally alterations in patient position and ingestion of fluid are more conducive to obtaining an adequate examination.

Ultrasound should be performed prior to barium studies, for barium inhibits the transmission of sound.

Difficulties in visualization may be due to bowel gas, a transverse stomach obscuring the anatomy, or a small left lobe of the liver (Fig. 12-9). A left lobe measuring 2 to 2.5 cm makes an excellent sonic window for pancreatic visualization (Fig. 12-10). It can be utilized with a caudal tilt of the transducer (15 to 20 degrees) for better visualization of the gland. The distended gallbladder also can be utilized to bypass air in the duodenal cap for better visualizing the pancreatic head.

The patient is initially examined in the supine position. Subsequent RAO or LAO positions may be utilized to avoid bowel interference. A very effective alternative has been the erect position.[9] In this case air moves from the gastric antrum to the fundus.

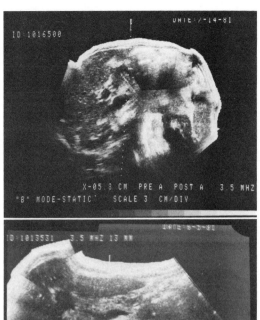

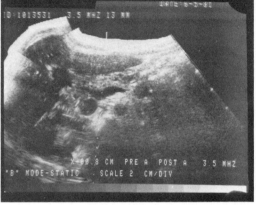

Fig. 12-9. A, Transverse scan of the upper abdomen showing a distended air-filled stomach and colon obscuring the area of the pancreas. **B,** It is more difficult to visualize the body and tail of the pancreas in patients with a small left lobe of the liver.

The upper viscera move downward from under the ribs. The liver moves caudad for an improved hepatic window. The erect position also results in distention of the venous structures, which aids in further localizing the pancreas.

Normal texture pattern

The echogenicity pattern of the pancreas is discussed in terms of how it relates to the liver's homogeneous "soft" echo pattern. Arger et al.[1] have stated that the normal pancreas has an echo pattern which is homogeneous and finer in texture than that of the surrounding retroperitoneum. The echo intensity is usually slightly less than that of the surrounding soft tissues. The echo intensity of the pancreas is moderately greater than that of the liver (Fig. 12-11).

Filly and London[4] have noted that retroperitoneal fat is strongly echogenic. Extensive fatty infiltrations of the pancreas are difficult to visualize by ultrasound. The pancreatic tissue blends with the surrounding retroperitoneal fat.

A lesser degree of fatty infiltration may not

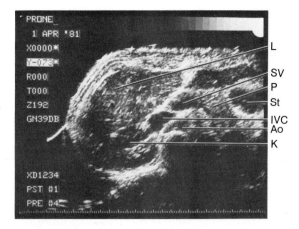

Fig. 12-10. The left lobe of the liver, which measures at least 2 cm, aids in visualization of the body and tail of the pancreas. The liver may further be used as an acoustic window by angling the transducer 10 to 15 degrees caudad in an effort to project even more liver between the transducer and the pancreas.

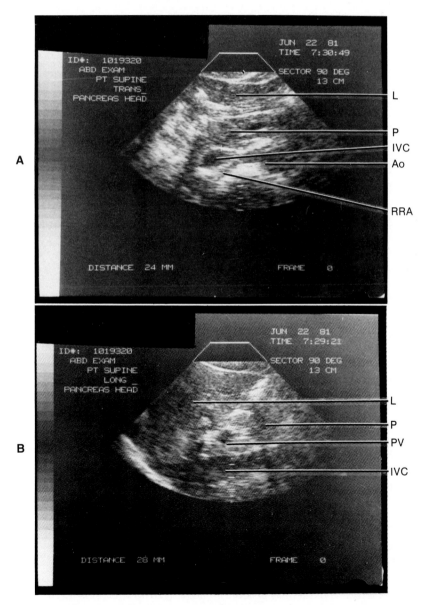

Fig. 12-11. A, Normal transverse pancreas. The head measures 24 mm. **B,** Normal sagittal scan of the pancreatic head anterior to the IVC and inferior to the portal vein. In this patient the texture has the same echogenicity as the liver.

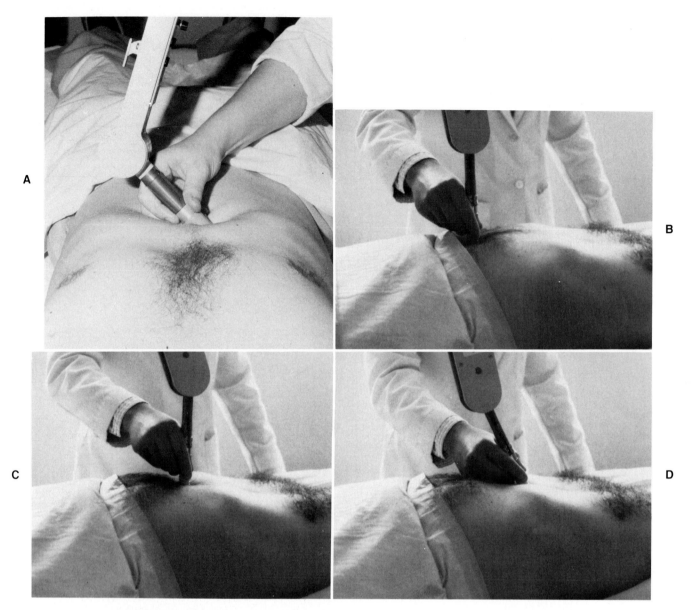

Fig. 12-12. A, Initial scans are made at the level of the xyphoid to search for the prevertebral vessels and pancreatic tissue. **B,** Single pie-sweep technique for better visualizing the midline structures such as the pancreas, superior mesenteric vessels, and great vessels. **C,** The sagittal scan should be performed in full inspiration to outline the vessels for locating the pancreas. A single sweep is used for maximum resolution. **D,** A slight arc motion of the transducer allows the beam to sweep under the xyphoid or costal margin.

render the pancreas invisible but may raise the amplitude of returning *pancreatic* echoes, resulting in the clinical observation that the pancreas returns stronger echoes than the liver.[4]

Marks, Filly, and Callen[10] further investigated the echogenicity of the gland when they observed that a higher-amplitude pancreatic echogenicity is due to more than fat infiltration alone. Fibrous tissue may account for the portion of increased echogenicity not attributable to fat. Increased deposition of fat that has infiltrated along the pancreatic

septa is a major determining factor of pancreatic echogenicity.

Sarti[12] and Sample et al.[11] have described a very effective technique for visualizing this echogenic organ. Pancreatic echoes will be in the highest shade (darkest) of gray when liver echoes register in the higher shades. Thus the pancreatic echoes will be lost in the high-amplitude echoes of the surrounding fatty retroperitoneum. The gain settings should be adjusted so the liver echoes register in the middle to lighter shades. The pancreas will then register one to two shades

darker than the liver but will not be viewed in the darkest shade.

Scanning technique

Transverse scans are used to make the initial visualization of the gland. The patient should be in full inspiration to distend the venous structures that act as landmarks in visualizing the pancreas. The pie-sweep or single-sector scans should be used if real time is not available (Fig. 12-12, *A*). Generally we begin at the level of the xyphoid and proceed at 1-cm intervals until gas

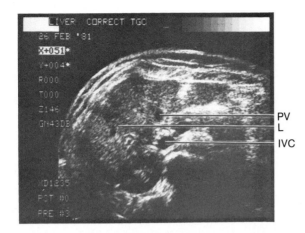

Fig. 12-13. The portal vein can be seen as an ovoid structure anterior to the inferior vena cava.

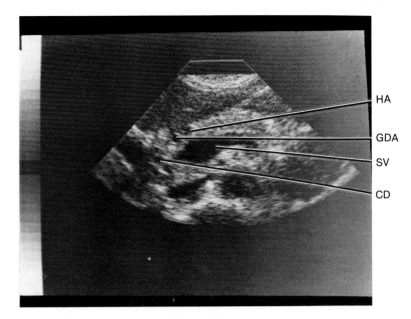

Fig. 12-14. Transverse scan of the pancreas with the common duct, *CD*, hepatic artery, *HA*, and gastroduodenal artery, *GDA*. The splenic vein, *SV*, serves as the posteromedial border of the pancreas.

encumbers the examination. When the pancreas has been imaged, alterations in the angle of the transducer arm are made for more complete visualization. Alterations in patient positioning may be useful for fully visualizing the head or tail of the gland (Fig. 12-12, *B* to *D*).

Sagittal scans are begun at the midline and directed first to the patient's right at 1-cm intervals and then to the left at similar increments.

NORMAL ANATOMIC RELATIONSHIPS
Transverse scan

The left lobe of the liver should be used as an ultrasonic window. The portal vein can be seen as an ovoid-circular structure anterior to the inferior vena cava (Fig. 12-13). Just anterior to the portal vein lie two small circular structures. The common duct is the more lateral, the hepatic artery the more medial (Fig. 12-14). This relationship has been termed by Bartrum and Crow the Mickey Mouse sign—with the portal vein representing Mickey's face, the common duct his right ear, and the hepatic artery his left ear. Pancreatic reflections are usually seen at the junction of the splenic and portal veins. Another useful landmark for the pancreatic head and body is the junction of the superior mesenteric with the splenic/portal veins (Fig. 12-15). The SMV and SMA both are posterior to the head and anterior to the uncinate process (Fig. 12-16). The head is medial to the second and third parts of the duodenum. The fluid-filled duodenum can be a valuable landmark in identifying the pancreas. It is especially useful to evaluate the peristaltic action of the duodenum in efforts to separate it from the lateral margin of the head. The collapsed duodenum appears ultrasonically as a dense central core with an echo-free periphery

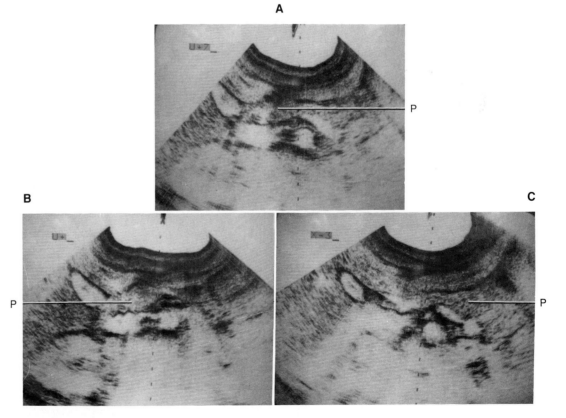

Fig. 12-15. A, Transverse scan of the body and tail of the pancreas draping over the splenic vein and great vessels. **B,** Transverse scan of the pancreatic head just medial to the gallbladder. **C,** Transverse scan of the tail of the pancreas inferior to the left lobe of the liver.

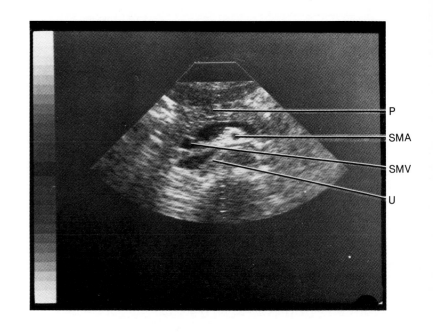

Fig. 12-16. Transverse scan of the superior mesenteric vessels and pancreas. The uncinate process is posterior to the superior mesenteric vein.

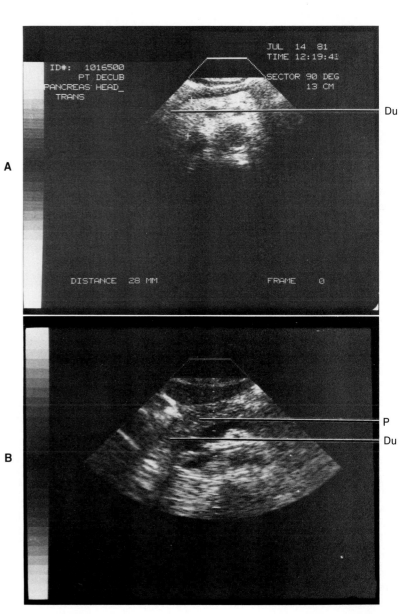

Fig. 12-17. A, Transverse scan of the head of the pancreas as surrounded on the lateral border by the duodenum, *Du.* **B,** The duodenum often casts a shadow. It may be filled with fluid and thus serve as an excellent landmark for outlining the lateral margin of the pancreas.

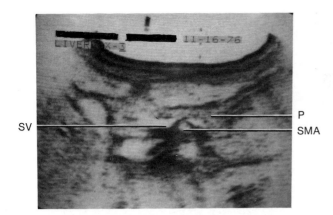

Fig. 12-18. Transverse scan of the body and tail of the pancreas draping over the splenic vein.

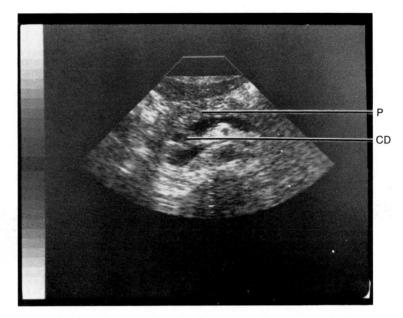

Fig. 12-19. The common bile duct is a circular structure on the lateral margin of the head of the pancreas at its junction with the duodenum.

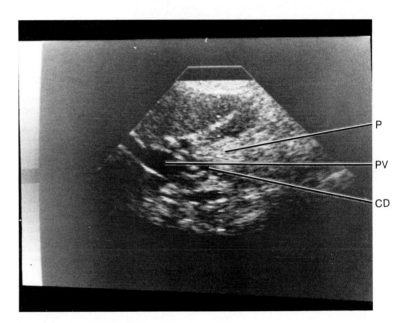

Fig. 12-20. On the sagittal scan the common bile duct can be seen directly anterior to the portal vein as a small tubular structure coursing posterior to the pancreatic head.

(Fig. 12-17). It may be mistaken for part of the pancreas if not carefully evaluated.

The body of the pancreas lies anterior to the SMV and SMA (Fig. 12-18). Shortly after the SMA originates, the curvilinear lucency of the left renal vein courses posterior to it and anterior to the aorta and can serve as a posterior landmark for the body of the gland.

The common bile duct is seen as a circular structure on the lateral margin of the pancreatic head at its junction with the duodenum (Fig. 12-19). Often anterior to the common duct the gastroduodenal artery or one of its branches is seen as a second circular structure.

Sagittal scan

The portal vein is seen as a circular sonolucent structure anterior to the IVC and superior to the head of the pancreas. As one moves slightly toward midline, the common bile duct can be seen directly anterior to the portal vein as a small tubular structure posterior to the pancreatic head (Fig. 12-20). The gastroduodenal artery can sometimes be seen anterior and over the pancreatic head.

As the SMV flows cephalad to join the portal vein, it is seen as a long tubular sonolucency posterior to the neck of the pancreas and anterior to the uncinate process (Fig. 12-21).

The antrum of the stomach appears as a collapsed (Fig. 12-22) bull's-eye and is identified anterior and slightly caudal to the head/body. The splenic vein is a circular sonolucency posterior to the cephalic portion of the gland whereas the aorta, celiac axis, and SMA are posterior to the body of the gland. The left renal vein is a slitlike sonolucency between the aorta and the SMA and serves as a posterior border of the pancreas.

Fig. 12-21. The superior mesenteric vein flows cephalad to join the portal vein. It is seen as a long tubular sonolucency posterior to the neck of the pancreas and anterior to the uncinate process.

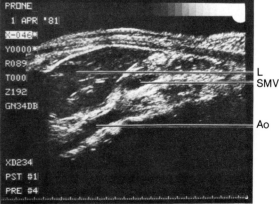

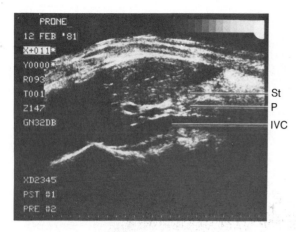

Fig. 12-22. The stomach may be seen as a collapsed bull's-eye anterior to the body of the pancreas on this sagittal scan.

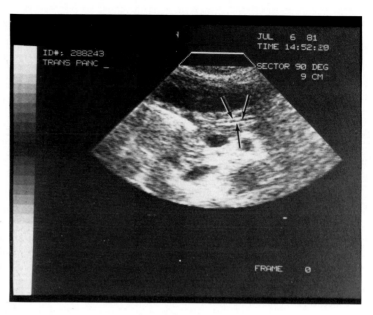

Fig. 12-24. Pancreatic tissue must be identified on each side of the duct *(arrows)* so the duct can be distinguished from a collapsed antrum of the stomach or the splenic vein.

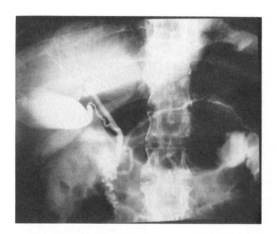

Fig. 12-23. Endoscopic retrograde pancreatogram demonstrating the pancreatic duct, common bile duct, and hepatic ducts.

Pancreatic duct

Because it takes a straighter course in the body of the pancreas, the pancreatic duct can often be visualized on transverse scans as an echo-free tubular structure in this part of the gland (Fig. 12-23). Although the duct is largest in the head, its course is variable. Its smallest diameter is in the tail, and thus it is very difficult to detect by ultrasound.

The normal caliber of the duct is generally considered to be 2 to 3 mm.[15] One should identify pancreatic tissue on both sides of the duct so as not to become confused by vascular structures that may overlie it (Fig. 12-24). However, the splenic vein is actually too posterior and the hepatic artery too anterior to be confused with the duct.

The duct appears as an echo-free area sharply marginated by two parallel echogenic lines (Fig. 12-25). A thin strip of retroperi-

toneal fat may underlie the anterior aspect of the pancreas. This sonolucent linear pattern must not be mistaken for a simple duct structure.[2]

The posterior wall of the antrum can be seen on transverse scans as a relatively echo-free tubular structure overlying the anterior aspect of the pancreas. Again, one must not confuse this with a dilated duct. Confirmation can be made with the sagittal scan.[15]

Generally any degree of duct dilation is indicative of pancreatic disease (Fig. 12-26).

PITFALLS OF PANCREATIC ECHOGRAPHY

Pancreatic echography can be obscured for any of the following reasons:

1. A small echo-free area medial to the liver may be fluid-containing duodenum that could be mistaken for the pancreas. Slight right anterior oblique decubitus scans should enable the sonographer to distinguish the duodenum from the pancreas. The patient may also be instructed to drink fluids to distend the stomach and fill the duodenum.

2. The pancreas may be difficult to visualize because of overlying structures such as stomach fat, muscles, and costal cartilage—in which case the position of the patient should be altered to avoid the interference.

3. Other solid masses in the retroperitoneal region, such as those of lymphadenopathy, may cause some confusion

in the identification of the pancreatic region since the lymph nodes drape across the prevertebral vessels within the region where the pancreas may lie.

PATHOLOGIC CONDITIONS OF THE PANCREAS
Congenital anomalies

Ectopic pancreatic tissue. This is the most common pancreatic anomaly, usually in the form of intramural nodules. The ectopic tissue may be found in various places in the gastrointestinal tract. Frequent sites are the stomach, duodenum, small bowel, and large bowel. On palpation these lesions may seem polypoid, and they characteristically have a central dimple. They are composed of elements of the pancreas, usually the acinar and ductal structures and less frequently the islets of Langerhans. They are generally small (0.5 to 2 cm), and acute pancreatitis or tumor may occur in them.

Annular pancreas. Annular pancreas is a rare anomaly in which the head of the pancreas surrounds the second portion of the duodenum. It is more common in males than in females, and all grades (from an overlapping of the posterior duodenal wall to a complete ring) may be found. It may be associated with complete or partial atresia of the duodenum and is susceptible to any of the diseases of the pancreas.

Fibrocystic disease of the pancreas. This hereditary disorder of the exocrine glands is seen frequently in children and young adults. The pancreas is usually firm

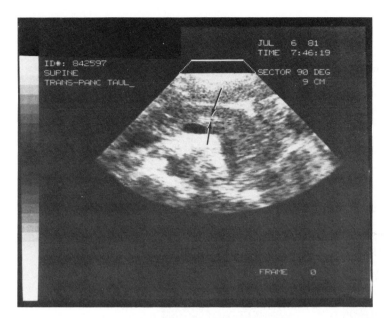

Fig. 12-25. The duct is very small when seen in the normal patient, appearing as a sonolucent area sharply marginated by two parallel echogenic lines *(arrow).*

and of normal size. Cysts are very small but may be present in the advanced stages. The acini and ducts are dilated. The acini are usually atrophic and may be totally replaced by fibrous tissue in many of the lobules. Nausea and vomiting may also occur, thus leading to malnourishment. The pancreatic secretion is gradually lost. With advancing pancreatic fibrosis, jaundice may develop from the common duct obstruction. A late manifestation is diabetes. Grossly the pancreas is found to be somewhat nodular and firm. There may be edema and fat necrosis, but gradually fibrous replacement occurs in much of the parenchyma. Ducts may dilate and contain calculi. Calcification of the gland is seen radiographically in as many as 50% of the patients.

Pancreatitis

Causes. The most common cause of pancreatitis in the United States is biliary tract disease. Gallstone pancreatitis causes a relatively sudden onset of constant biliary pain. As the pancreatic parenchyma is further damaged, the pain becomes more severe and the abdomen becomes rigid and tender.

Alcohol abuse is the second most common cause of pancreatitis; and then comes trauma (surgical or blunt) to the abdomen, which may lead to ascites, the formation of a pancreatic pseudocyst, or pancreatitis (Fig. 12-27).

Acute pancreatitis

Physical findings. The patient presents with moderate to severe tenderness in the

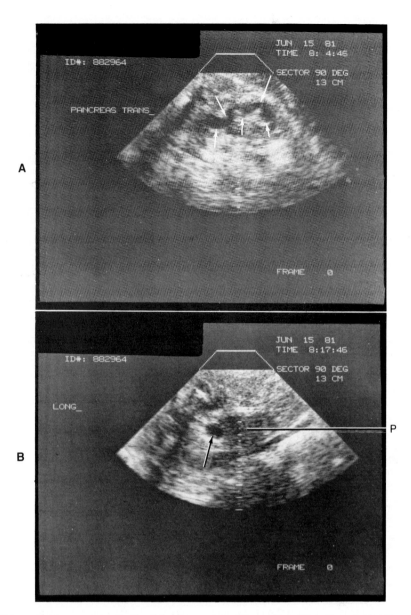

Fig. 12-26. This patient presented with chronic pancreatitis and a dilated pancreatic duct. **A,** Transverse scan showing the dilated and tortuous pancreatic duct. Often such ducts will calcify and shadow. **B,** Sagittal scan of the prominent head of the pancreas and dilated pancreatic duct *(arrow).*

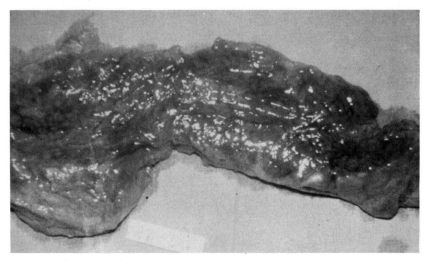

Fig. 12-27. Gross specimen of a pancreas with acute pancreatitis.

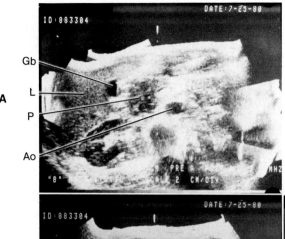

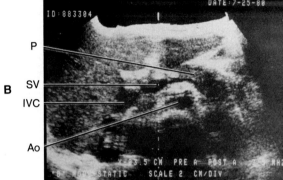

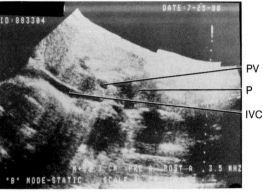

Fig. 12-28. This 51-year-old man was in good health until upper abdominal pain developed and recurred every few months. His amylase level was elevated (962). **A,** Transverse scan showing an irregular margin of the pancreatic head. **B,** Transverse showing the body and tail to be somewhat prominent. **C,** Sagittal scan of the enlarged pancreas. The differential diagnosis would be pancreatitis or tumor.

epigastrium radiating to the back. The abdomen may be distended secondary to an ileus. Generally no jaundice is present. The pancreatitis may be either localized (associated with biliary disease or trauma) or generalized (associated with alcoholism).

Sonographic findings. In the early stages of acute pancreatitis the gland becomes very swollen due to the increased prominence of lobulations and congested vessels. The early stage may clear completely only to recur with more severe symptoms and further damage to the pancreas.

By sonography the pancreas is normally as echogenic as or more echogenic than the liver. With pancreatitis the swollen gland becomes less echogenic than the liver parenchyma (Fig. 12-28). If localized enlargement is present, it may be difficult to separate from neoplastic involvement of the gland. Analysis of patient history and laboratory values should enable the clinician to make the distinction (Fig. 12-29). On longitudinal scans anterior compression of the inferior vena cava by the swollen head of the pancreas may be apparent.

The pancreatic duct may be obstructed in acute pancreatitis due to inflammation, spasm, edema, swelling of the papilla, or pseudocyst formation.[15]

Acute hemorrhagic pancreatitis. This disease is a rapid progression of acute pancreatitis. Patient symptoms may include intense and severe pain radiating to the back,

shock, and ileus. In addition to the typical sonographic signs of pancreatitis, Sarti[12] states that one may find areas of necrosis of the parenchyma. Foci of freshly extravasated blood and fat necrosis are also seen. Necrosis of blood vessels results in the development of hemorrhagic areas referred to as Grey Turner's sign (discoloration of the flanks).

Chronic pancreatitis. Chronic pancreatitis results from recurrent attacks of acute pancreatitis and causes continuing destruction of the pancreatic parenchyma. It generally is associated with chronic alcoholism or biliary disease. Patient symptoms may include epigastric pain progressing with the disease, gastrointestinal problems, and jaundice secondary to common duct obstruction. The duct may dilate and contain calculi. There is calcification of the gland in 20% to 40% of the patients[15] (Fig. 12-30).

Sonographic findings. Chronic pancreatitis may appear as a diffuse or localized involvement of the gland. The irregular borders of the gland are seen with an echogenic parenchyma if fibrosis or calcification is present. Shadowing will occur posterior to the calcification if the calculi are large enough.

The pancreatic duct may show strictures, stenosis, irregularities, and dilation (Fig. 12-31). The most common sites of obstruction are the papilla and the origin of the main pancreatic duct.[15]

Pancreatic abscess

An abscess may arise from a neighboring infection such as a perforated peptic ulcer, acute appendicitis, or acute cholecystitis. The sonographic appearance depends on the amount of debris present. The walls are thick, irregular, and highly echogenic. If air bubbles are present, an echogenic region with a shadow posterior will exist.

Pancreatic cysts

There are two types of pancreatic cysts—true cysts and pseudocysts. They may be either unilocular or multilocular.

True cysts. These microscopic sacs can be congenital or acquired. They arise from within the gland, usually in the head, then in the body, and then the tail. They have a lining epithelium (which may be lost with inflammation), and they contain pancreatic enzymes or are found to be continuous with a pancreatic duct.

Pseudocysts. In contrast, pancreatic pseudocysts are always acquired; they result from trauma to the gland or from acute or chronic pancreatitis. Approximately 11% to 18% of patients with acute pancreatitis develop pseudocysts. Encapsulated collections of pancreatic juice, blood, and debris form the pseudocyst. As Sarti[12] states, "the pancreatic enzymes that escape the ductal system cause enzymatic digestion of the surrounding tissue and pseudocyst development. The walls of the pseudocyst form in

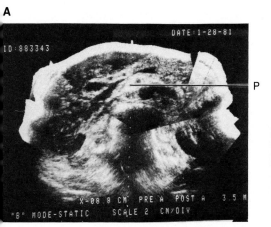

A
P
IVC
Ao

B
P

C
St
SMA
SMV
IVC
Ao

D
P
St
P
Gb

E
L
IVC
P

Fig. 12-29. In this young woman receiving chemotherapy for acute lymphocytic leukemia, epigastric pain developed and radiated to her back. The serum amylase level was 966. The sonogram showed findings of acute pancreatitis. **A,** Transverse scan showing the sonolucent pancreatic tissue anterior to the great vessels. **B,** Sagittal scan of the inflamed pancreas. Subsequent follow-up scans 1 month later showed resolution of the drug induced pancreatitis. **C,** Transverse scan with fluid in the stomach. **D,** Normal pancreas and vessels. **E,** Upright scan of normal pancreas and inferior vena cava.

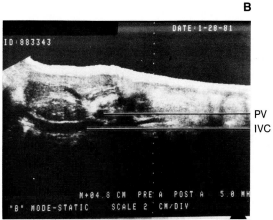

A

B
P
PV
IVC

Fig. 12-30. A, Patient with chronic pancreatitis presents echographically with a very dense pancreas. **B,** Sagittal scan of the pancreas showing bowel interference over the head of the gland. The patient should be scanned in the upright position to penetrate this area and to displace the gas.

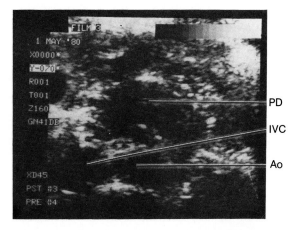

PD
IVC
Ao

Fig. 12-31. Prominent pancreatic duct in a patient with acute pancreatitis.

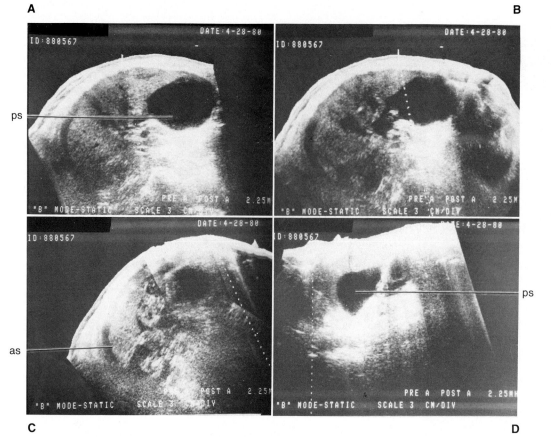

Fig. 12-32. Pancreatic pseudocysts present with a number of sonographic patterns. The most typical is fairly homogeneous with low-level debris, smooth borders, and good through-transmission; the sac assumes the available space in the retroperitoneum. **A,** Transverse scan of a pancreatic pseudocyst, *ps*, in the LUQ. This must be separated from a liver cyst or a fluid-filled stomach. **B,** Transverse scan showing the good transmission of the cyst. **C,** There is also some ascites, *as*, along the lateral and medial walls of the liver. **D,** Sagittal scan showing the pseudocyst to occupy the available space in the retroperitoneum.

the various potential spaces in which the escaped pancreatic enzymes are found."[1] The pseudocyst usually presents few symptoms until it becomes large enough to cause pressure on surrounding organs.

Both pseudocysts and true cysts may protrude anteriorly in any direction, although the true cyst is generally associated directly with the pancreatic area. Pseudocysts usually develop through the lesser omentum, displacing the stomach or widening the duodenal loop.

A pseudocyst develops when pancreatic enzymes escape from the gland and break down tissue to form a sterile abscess somewhere in the abdomen. Its walls are not true cyst walls; hence the name *pseudo-* or false cyst. Pseudocysts may develop anywhere in the abdominal cavity and have been found as low as the groin and as high as the mediastinum. They generally take on the contour of the available space around them and therefore are not always spherical, as are normal cysts (Fig. 12-32). There may be more than

one pseudocyst, so the sonographer should search for daughter collections when performing an echogram.

Sonographically pseudocysts usually appear as well-defined masses with essentially sonolucent echo-free interiors. Because of debris, scattered echoes may be seen at the bottom of the cysts and increased through-transmission is present (Fig. 12-33). The borders are very echogenic, and the cysts usually are thicker than other simple cysts. When a suspected pseudocyst is located near the stomach, the stomach should be drained so the cyst is not mistaken for a fluid-filled stomach. If the patient has been on continual drainage prior to the ultrasonic examination, this problem is eliminated.

Unusual sonographic patterns. Laing et al.[7] have reported a series of pseudocysts found to contain unusual internal echoes. There were three classifications: (1) septated, which presented with multiple internal septations; (2) excessive internal echoes, caused

by an associated inflammatory mass, hemorrhage, or clot formation; and (3) pseudocyst, with absence of posterior enhancement due to the rim of calcification.

Spontaneous rupture. Spontaneous rupture is the most common complication of a pancreatic pseudocyst, occurring in 5% of the patients.[8]

In half of this 5% the drainage is directly into the peritoneal cavity. Clinical symptoms are sudden shock and peritonitis. The mortality rate is 50%. Ascites developing as a consequence of spontaneous rupture may be differentiated from that associated with cirrhosis in patients who have known rupture of a pseudocyst by analysis of the fluid for elevated amylase and protein content.[7]

In the other half of the 5% of patients the rupture is into the gastrointestinal tract. Such patients may present a confusing picture sonographically. The initial scan will show a typical pattern for a pseudocyst formation, but the patient may develop intense pain secondary to the rupture and consequent examination will show the disappearance of the mass.

Benign tumors

Islet cell tumors. These are the most frequent benign tumor of the pancreas. Their size is small, diameter usually 1 to 2 cm, and they are well encapsulated with a good vascular supply. The tumors may be multiple and often are found in the tail of the gland. A large percentage occur in patients with hyperinsulinism and hypoglycemia.

Sonographically islet cell tumors are difficult to image due to their small size. Greatest success is when they are located in the head of the gland.

Duct cell adenoma. This tumor may develop in the main pancreatic duct and cause obstruction. It has been responsible for the appearance of acute pancreatitis.[6]

Papilloma of the duct. These are found in the region of the ampulla and cause duct obstruction.

Cystadenoma. This lesion is a rare benign neoplasm arising from the pancreatic duct, most commonly in the tail of the pancreas. It occurs more commonly in women. Its size may range from 2 to 15 cm. The coarsely lobulated cystic tumors sometimes present sonographically with cyst walls thicker than the membranes between multilocular cysts.

Neoplasms of the pancreas

Adenocarcinoma. The most common primary neoplasm of the pancreas is adeno-

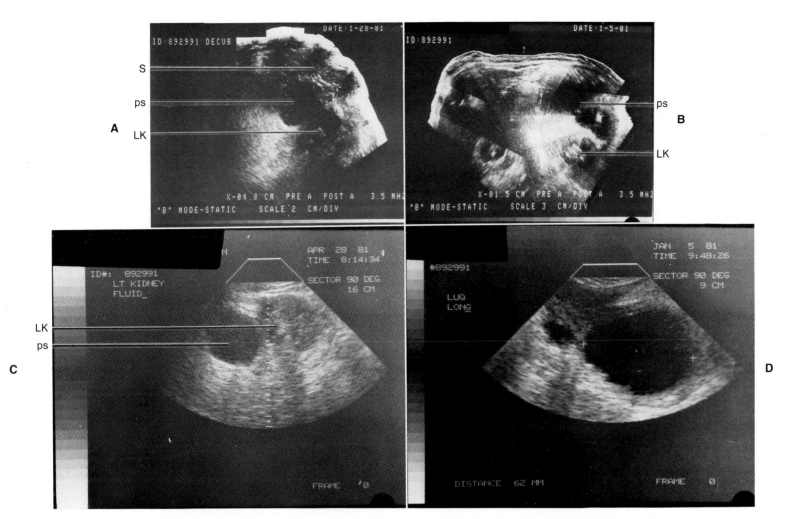

Fig. 12-33. This patient presented 11 days after surgery with LUQ pain. A pseudocyst, *ps*, was found by ultrasound and was demonstrated to be separate from the left kidney and spleen. It was well encapsulated, which ruled out an abscess formation. **A,** Transverse decubitus of the spleen, pseudocyst, and left kidney. **B,** Transverse supine. **C,** Real time showing the mass separate from the kidney. **D,** Longitudinal real time of the pseudocyst.

carcinoma, which usually occurs in the head. It is more commonly found in middle-aged men than in women. Symptoms usually appear late, the most common being pain radiating to the back or a dull steadily aching mid-epigastrium pain. Weight loss, painless jaundice, nausea, vomiting, and changes in stools are also clinical symptoms. The painless jaundice usually appears first, followed by nausea and vomiting. The presence of a dilated gallbladder and a palpable mass is strongly suggestive of carcinoma (Courvoisier's law). A cyst or pancreatitis may occur behind the neoplastic obstruction of the duct. With obstruction of the pancreatic ducts, enzymes will be absent or present only in small amounts (Fig. 12-34).

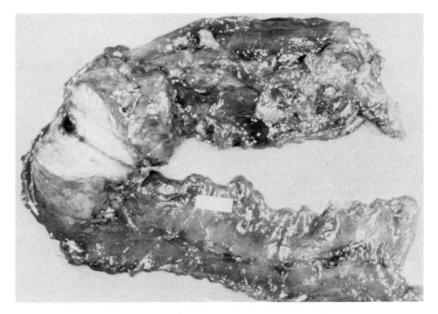

Fig. 12-34. Gross specimen of a pancreatic tumor in the body of the gland.

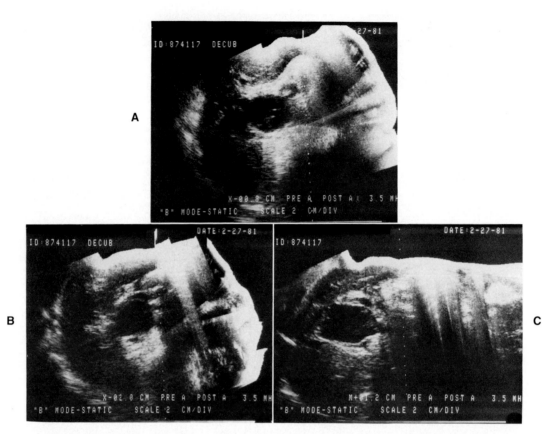

Fig. 12-35. An elderly woman presented with weight loss, gastrointestinal symptoms, and bowel obstruction. Ultrasound demonstrated the presence of a mass between the inferior vena cava and portal vein that was thought to be solid. It lay adjacent to the pancreatic head and most likely represented peripancreatic nodes. **A,** Transverse scan of the solid peripancreatic mass. **B,** The pancreas and vessels were displaced by the mass. **C,** Sagittal scan showing the mass in the area of the porta hepatis. This was found to be adenocarcinoma of the small intestine with invasion.

The sonographic appearance of adenocarcinoma is a general loss of the normal pancreatic parenchymal pattern. The gland becomes enlarged, with an irregular nodular border (Fig. 12-35). There may be secondary enlargement of the common duct due to enlargement of the pancreatic head (Fig. 12-36). A dilated pancreatic duct may be present.

Cystadenocarcinoma. Cystadenocarcinoma may be difficult to separate from carcinoma arising in a true cyst or cystic degeneration of a solid carcinoma. It is an irregular lobulated cystic tumor with thick cellular walls. Metastases arise most commonly in the lymph nodes and liver. The course of this tumor may be slowly progressive with a tendency for the recurrent disease to remain localized.

Sonographic criteria for carcinoma. The detection of tumors less than 2 cm in diameter is difficult for the sonographer. Carcinoma of the pancreas often appears as an irregular mass with ill-defined borders and scattered internal echoes (Fig. 12-37). Arger

et al.[1] state that their series of patients with a pancreatic neoplasm demonstrated these findings: (1) echo production less than in a normal pancreas; (2) unhomogeneous echoes, scattered larger echoes, and more intense echoes within the mass; (3) reduced sound transmission; and (4) areas of dense echogenicity in the large tumors. The detection of carcinoma of the pancreas can be difficult, especially if the tumor is infiltrating; therefore the examiner should be aware of other echographic findings. A large noncontracting gallbladder may be tested with a fatty meal. After waiting 40 minutes from the administration of the fatty meal, rescan the patient to note full contraction of the gallbladder. Sokoloff et al.[13] state that typically large unobstructed gallbladders are seen in fasting normal or vagotomized patients, in the presence of diabetes mellitus, or with contiguous inflammatory process. Weight loss following pancreatitis or with alcohol abuse in association with little pain is highly suggestive of pancreatic carcinoma if there is an ultrasonically detected enlargement of the pan-

creas. Other clinical signs are jaundice with a palpable mass, increased bilirubin, and increased alkaline phosphatase. The liver may be enlarged due to common duct obstruction, tumor, or metastatic disease.

Lymph node enlargement secondary to lymphoma or metastatic carcinoma may be confused with pancreatic carcinoma or pancreatitis. This diagnosis can be made by detecting splenic enlargement or the presence of nodes elsewhere in the abdomen. It is often difficult to differentiate carcinoma from pancreatitis. With pancreatitis the borders tend to be well defined whereas with carcinoma they are often poorly defined. If the pancreas is diffusely involved, this is highly suggestive of inflammatory disease. However, these findings in association with a mass in the region of the head of the pancreas do not exclude carcinoma, since pancreatitis and tumor can coexist. In these cases serial examinations may be very helpful in the evaluation of size changes in the gland.

Other "soft" signs for a pancreatic neo-

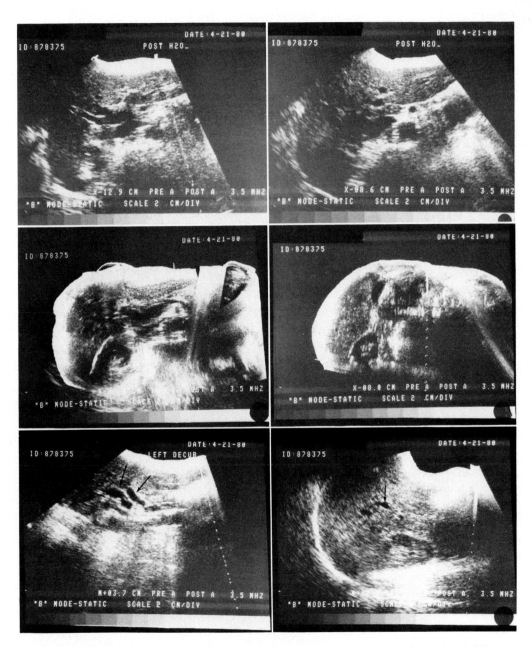

Fig. 12-36. This 68-year-old man presented with severe abdominal pain and weight loss of 3 months' duration. A pancreatic carcinoma was found in the head of the gland. It had caused the biliary ducts to dilate *(arrows)*.

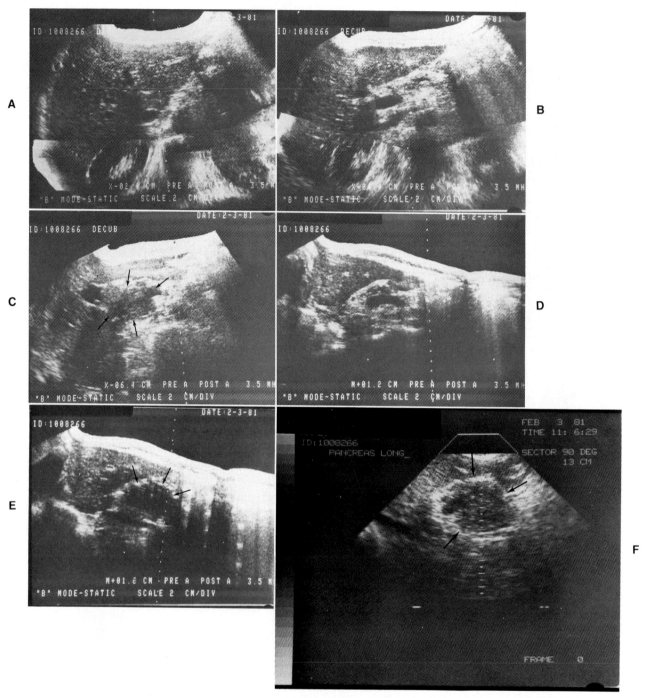

Fig. 12-37. This 49-year-old man had a history of alcohol abuse, weight loss, and abdominal pain. An irregular mass was found in the head of the pancreas. **A,** Supine transverse scan of the upper abdomen. **B,** Area of the pancreas. The body appears to be of normal size and texture. **C,** Enlarged pancreatic head. **D,** Sagittal scan of the superior mesenteric vein as it bisects the body and uncinate process. **E,** Sagittal scan of the prominent pancreatic head. **F,** Real time of the pancreatic head mass.

plasm by ultrasound include anterior indentation of the inferior vena cava due to enlargement of the pancreatic head, anterior displacement of the superior mesenteric vein due to enlargement of the head or uncinate process, and posterior displacement of the superior mesenteric vein due to enlargement of the head or body of the gland.[16]

Pancreatic duct in carcinoma

The majority of pancreatic carcinomas arise from duct epithelium that causes duct dilation secondary to tumor. The pancreas may be poorly visualized if there is marked duct obstruction by tumor.[15]

When the lesion has so progressed that obstructive jaundice is apparent, the identification of a dilated pancreatic duct in conjunction with the dilated biliary tree helps pinpoint the distal site of the lesion. In patients in whom the lesion is small and has not obstructed the CBD, the presence of a periampullary lesion can be suggested by the dilated pancreatic duct.[5]

REFERENCES

1. Arger, P.H., Mulhern, C.B., Bonavita, J.A., et al.: Analysis of pancreatic sonography in suspected pancreatic disease, J. Clin. Ultrasound **7**:91, 1979.
2. Eisenscher, A., and Weill, F.: Ultrasonic visualization of Wirsung's duct: dream or reality? J. Clin. Ultrasound **7**:41, 1979.
3. Filly, R.A., and Freimanis, A.K.: Echographic diagnosis of pancreatic lesions, Radiology **96**:575, 1970.
4. Filly, R.A., and London, S.S.: The normal pancreas: acoustic characteristics and frequency of imaging, J. Clin. Ultrasound **7**:121, 1979.
5. Gosink, B.B., and Leopold, G.R.: The dilated pancreatic duct: ultrasonic evaluation, Radiology **126**: 475, 1978.
6. Hassani, S.N., Smulewicz, J.J., and Bard, R.: Pattern of pancreatic carcinoma by real time and gray scale ultrasonography, Appl. Radiol., September-October 1977.
7. Laing, F.C., Gooding, G.A.W., Brown, T., and Leopold, G.R.: Atypical pseudocysts of the pancreas: an ultrasonographic evaluation, J. Clin. Ultrasound **7**:27, 1979.
8. Leopold, G.R., Berg, R.N., and Reinke, R.T.: Echographic-radiological documentation of spontaneous rupture of a pancreatic pseudocyst into the duodenum, Radiology **120**:699, 1972.
9. Macmahon, H., Bowie, J.D., and Beezhold, C.: Erect scanning of pancreas using a gastric window, A.J.R. **132**:587, 1979.
10. Marks, W.M., Filly, R.A., and Callen, P.W.: Ultrasonic evaluation of normal pancreatic echogenicity and its relationship to fat deposition, Radiology **137**:475, 1980.
11. Sample, W.F., Po, J.B., Gray, R.K., and Cahill, P.J.: Gray scale in ultrasonography techniques in pancreatic scanning, Appl. Radiol., September-October, 1975.
12. Sarti, D.A.: Rapid development and spontaneous regression of pancreatic pseudocysts documented by ultrasound, Radiology **125**:789, 1977.
13. Sokoloff, J., et al.: Pitfalls in the echographic evaluation of pancreatic disease, J. Clin. Ultrasound **2**: 321, 1974.
14. Weighall, S.L., Wolfman, N.T., and Watson, N.: The fluid-filled stomach: a new sonic window, J. Clin. Ultrasound **7**:353, 1979.
15. Weinstein, B.J., Weinstein, D.P., and Brodmerkel, G.J.: Ultrasonography of pancreatic lithiasis, Radiology **134**:185, 1980.
16. Wright, C.H., Maklad, F., and Rosenthal, S.: Grey scale in ultrasonic characteristics of carcinoma of the pancreas, Br. J. Radiol. **52**:281, 1979.

Kidneys

The evaluation of the kidneys with ultrasound is a noninvasive approach to diagnosing renal problems. Generally sonography is utilized after an *intravenous pyelogram* (IVP) has disclosed the need to investigate the acoustic properties of a mass (cystic or solid) or to further delineate an abnormal lie due to an extrarenal mass. In patients who cannot tolerate an IVP because of allergic reaction or other reason, sonography may be selected as the examination of choice to rule out renal disease.

In addition to delineating a renal mass, ultrasound can define perirenal fluid collections (e.g., hematoma or abscess), determine renal size and parenchymal detail, and detect enlarged ureters and hydronephrosis as well as congenital anomalies.

NORMAL ANATOMY

The kidneys lie in the retroperitoneal space under the cover of the costal margin (Fig. 13-1). The right kidney lies slightly lower than the left due to the right lobe of the liver. During inspiration both kidneys move downward by as much as 2.5 cm.

The normal adult kidney varies from 9 to 12 cm in length, 2.5 to 3 cm in thickness, and some 4 to 5 cm in width. Generally both kidneys will attain approximately the same dimensions. A difference of more than 1.5 to 2 cm is significant.

The kidney is surrounded by a fibrous capsule, called the *true capsule,* that is closely applied to the renal cortex. Outside this capsule is a covering of perinephric fat. The perinephric fascia surrounds the perinephric fat and encloses the kidney and adrenal glands. The renal fascia (Gerota's fascia) surrounds the true capsule and perinephric fat (Fig. 13-2).

The ureter is 25 cm long and resembles the esophagus in having three constrictions along its course: (1) where it joins the kidney, (2) where it is kinked as it crosses the pelvic brim, and (3) where it pierces the bladder wall. The pelvis of the ureter is funnel shaped in its expanded upper end. It lies within the hilum of the kidney and receives the major calyces. The ureter emerges from the hilum and runs downward along the psoas, which separates it from the tips of the transverse processes of the lumbar vertebrae. It enters the pelvis by crossing the bifurcation of the common iliac artery in front of the sacroiliac. It then runs along the lateral wall of the pelvis to the region of the ischial spine and turns forward to enter the lateral angle of the bladder.

On the medial border of each kidney is the renal hilum, which contains the renal vein, two branches of the renal artery, the ureter, and the third branch of the renal artery (Fig. 13-3).

The kidney is composed of an internal medullary portion and an external cortical substance (Fig. 13-4). The medullary substance consists of a series of striated conical masses, called the *renal pyramids,* that vary from 8 to 18 in number and their bases are directed toward the outer circumference of the kidney. Their apices converge toward the renal sinus, where their prominent papillae project into the lumina of the minor calyces.

Within the kidney's upper expanded end (or pelvis) the ureter divides into two or three major calyces, each of which divides into two or three minor calyces. The 4 to 13 minor calyces are cup-shaped tubes that usually come into contact with at least one but

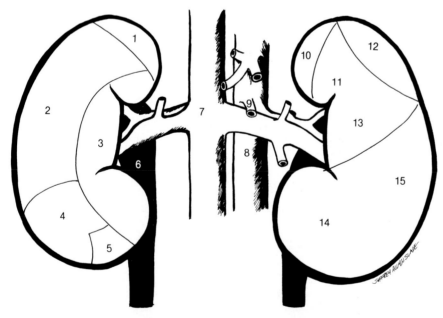

Fig. 13-1. Anatomic structures related to the anterior surfaces of the kidneys. *1,* Right adrenal gland; *2,* liver; *3,* duodenum; *4,* right colic flexure; *5,* small intestine; *6,* ureter; *7,* inferior vena cava; *8,* aorta; *9,* superior mesenteric artery; *10,* left adrenal gland; *11,* stomach; *12,* spleen; *13,* pancreas; *14,* jejunum; *15,* descending colon.

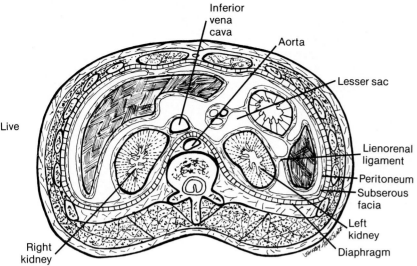

Inferior vena cava
Aorta
Lesser sac
Live
Lienorenal ligament
Peritoneum
Subserous facia
Right kidney
Left kidney
Diaphragm

Fig. 13-2. Transverse section of the abdominal cavity through the epiploic foramen.

Fig. 13-3. Vascular relationship of the great vessels and their tributaries to the kidneys. Aorta, *Ao;* inferior vena cava, *IVC;* right renal vein, *RRV;* right renal artery, *RRA;* left renal vein, *LRV;* left renal artery, *LRA;* superior mesenteric artery, *SMA;* splenic artery, *SA;* hepatic artery, *HA;* left gastric artery, *LGA.*

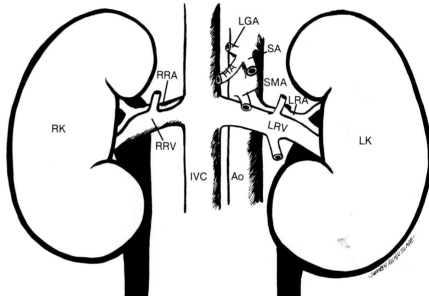

LGA
SA
RRA
SMA
LRA
RK
LRV
LK
RRV
IVC
Ao

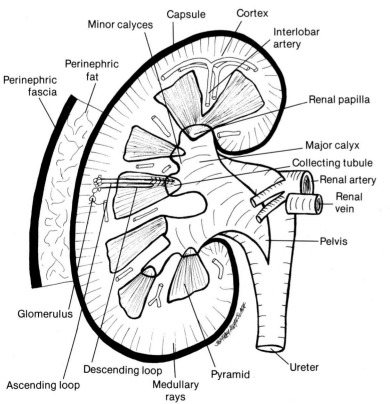

Minor calyces
Capsule
Cortex
Interlobar artery
Perinephric fat
Perinephric fascia
Renal papilla
Major calyx
Collecting tubule
Renal artery
Renal vein
Pelvis
Glomerulus
Descending loop
Ascending loop
Medullary rays
Pyramid
Ureter

Fig. 13-4. Kidney cut longitudinally to show the internal structure.

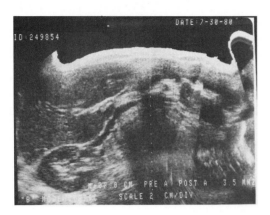

Fig. 13-5. Transverse of the right renal vein as it drains into the inferior vena cava.

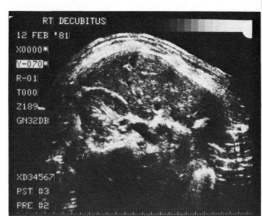

A

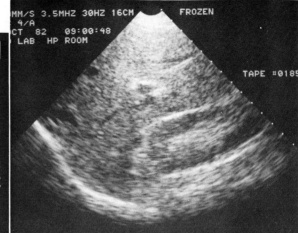

B

Fig. 13-6. A, Transverse of the normal right kidney and liver. The renal parenchyma is less echogenic than the liver. **B,** Sagittal of the liver and right kidney.

occasionally two or more of the renal papillae (forming the blunted apex of the renal pyramid). The minor calyces unite to form two or three short tubes, the major calyces; these, in turn, unite to form a funnel-shaped sac, the renal pelvis. Spirally arranged muscles surround the calyces and may exert a milking action on these tubes, aiding in the flow of urine into the renal pelvis. As the pelvis leaves the renal sinus, it rapidly becomes smaller and ultimately merges with the ureter.

The filtration-reabsorption system relies on a tubular excretory unit called the nephron, which is the structural and functional unit of the kidney. Each nephron contains a *capsula glomeruli* (Bowman's capsule), which consists of two layers of flat epithelial cells with a space between them and within which a cluster of nonanastomosing capillaries (the glomerulus) is enclosed. These two structures, the capsule and the glomerulus, together are named the renal corpuscle or malpighian body. Blood flows into each glomerulus via an afferent arteriole and out via an efferent arteriole. Extending from each Bowman's capsule is a renal tubule that contains several sections: the proximal tubule, descending limb (or loop of Henle), ascending limb, and distal convoluted tubule (which terminates in a straight or collecting tubule). These collecting tubules join larger tubules of one renal pyramid and converge to form a tube that opens at a renal papilla into one of the small calyces. Bowman's capsule and the convoluted tubules lie in the cortex of the kidney whereas the loops of Henle and the collecting tubules lie in the medulla.

The kidney is supplied with blood by the renal artery. Before entering the renal substance, branches of the renal artery vary in number and direction. In most cases the renal artery divides into two primary branches, a larger anterior and a smaller posterior. These arteries break down finally to minute arterioles and are called interlobar arteries. In the portion of the kidney between the cortex and medulla, these arteries are called arcuate arteries.

Likewise, veins of the kidney also break down into these categories. Five or six veins join to form the renal vein, which merges from the hilum anterior to the renal artery. The renal vein drains into the inferior vena cava (Fig. 13-5). Further breakdown of the veins and arteries leads to the afferent and efferent glomerular vessels.

FUNCTION

The function of the kidney is to excrete urine. More than any other organ in the body, the kidneys adjust the amounts of water and electrolytes leaving the body so that these equal the amounts of these substances entering the body.

The major function of the urinary system is to remove urea from the bloodstream so it does not accumulate in the body and become toxic. Urea is formed in the liver from ammonia, which in turn is derived from the simple proteins (amino acids) in body cells. The urea is carried in the bloodstream to the kidneys, where it is passed with water, salts, and acids out of the bloodstream and into the kidney tubules as urine.

The kidneys perform three functions to rid the body of unwanted material, which is excreted in the urine. The first is *filtration* of substances from the blood into Bowman's capsule. This occurs in the glomeruli. The second is *reabsorption* of most of the water and part of the solutes from the tubular filtrate into the blood. Most of the substances in the blood are needed by the body. Re-

absorption is accomplished by the cells that compose the walls of the convoluted tubules, loop of Henle, and collecting tubules. The third process is *tubular secretion*, whereby acids and other substances that the body does not need are secreted into the distal renal tubules from the bloodstream. The distal renal tubules, carrying urine, merge to form the renal pelvis.

CLINICAL SIGNS AND SYMPTOMS

Analysis of the patient's chart and medical history may disclose signs of renal disease such as a palpable flank mass, hematuria, polyuria, oliguria, pain, fever, urgency, or generalized edema. There may already be an acute onset of renal failure present.

Laboratory data that may indicate renal failure are an elevated blood urea nitrogen (BUN) and creatinine and an increased protein in the urine. Since the kidneys possess a significant reserve, loss of up to 60% of functioning renal parenchyma will not lead to elevation of either BUN or creatinine. Renal function is severely impaired when these levels are elevated.

SONOGRAPHIC ANATOMY AND TECHNIQUE

The kidneys are imaged by ultrasound as an organ with a smooth outer contour surrounded by reflected echoes of perirenal fat. The renal parenchyma surrounds the fatty central renal sinus, which contains the calyces, infundibula, pelvis, vessels, and lymphatics (Fig. 13-6). Because of the fat interface, the renal sinus is imaged as an area of intense echoes with variable contour. If two separate collections of renal sinus fat are identified, a double collecting system should be suspected.

Sinus fat and fibrous tissue, known as renal

sinus fibrolipomatosis, may show ill-defined zones of low-level echoes within the renal sinus. It may be distinguished from hydronephrosis by its lack of well-defined borders but may be identical to a tumor within the renal sinus.[5]

Generally patients will be NPO prior to their ultrasound or IVP examination. This state of dehydration causes the infundibula and renal pelvis to be collapsed and thus indistinguishable from the echo-dense renal sinus fat. If, on the other hand, the bladder is distended from rehydration, the intrarenal collecting system will also become distended.[3] An extrarenal pelvis may be seen as a fluid-filled structure medial to the kidney on transverse scans. Differentiation of the normal variant from obstruction is made by noting the absence of a distended intrasinus portion of the renal pelvis and infundibula.[1] Dilation of the collecting system has also been noted in pregnant patients. The right kidney is generally involved with a mild degree of hydronephrosis. This distension returns to normal shortly after delivery.

Renal parenchyma

The parenchyma is the area from the renal sinus to the outer renal surface (Fig. 13-7). The arcuate and interlobar vessels are found within and are best demonstrated as intense specular echoes in cross section or oblique section at the corticomedullary junction.[4]

The cortex generally is echo producing (Fig. 13-8) (though its echoes are less intense than those from normal liver) whereas the medullary pyramids are echo free (Fig. 13-9). The two are separated from each other by bands of cortical tissue, called columns of Bertin, that extend inward to the renal sinus.

Rosenfield et al.[5] divided diseases of the renal parenchyma into those that accentuate cortical echoes but preserve or exaggerate the corticomedullary junction (Type I) and those that distort the normal anatomy, obliterating the corticomedullary differentiation in either a focal or diffuse manner (Type II).

The criteria for Type I changes were that (a) the echo intensity in the cortex be equal to or greater than that in the adjacent liver or spleen and (b) the echo intensity in the cortex equal that in the adjacent renal sinus. Minor signs would include the loss of identifiable arcuate vessels or the accentuation of corticomedullary definition.

Type II changes can be seen in a focal disruption of normal anatomy with any mass lesion, including cysts, tumors, abscesses, and hematomas.

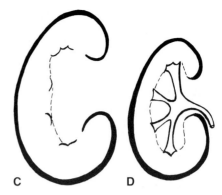
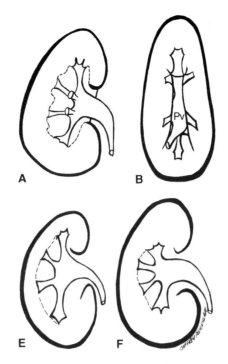

Fig. 13-7. Thickness of the renal substance. **A,** Maximal in the polar regions, medium in the middle zone. **B,** Medial plane showing the pelvis, *Pv,* emerging through the hilum and minimal thickness anteriorly and posteriorly. **C,** Hypertrophy. **D,** Normal adult proportions of the renal substance. **E,** Senile atrophy. **F,** Normal appearance in a 2-year-old child.

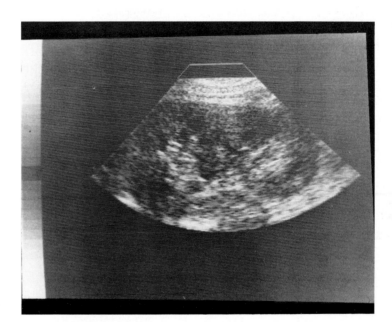

Fig. 13-8. Sagittal scan of a normal renal cortex.

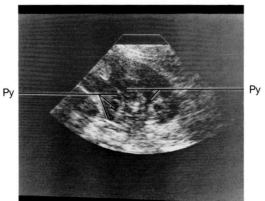

Fig. 13-9. Normal transverse showing sonolucent medullary pyramids, *Py.*

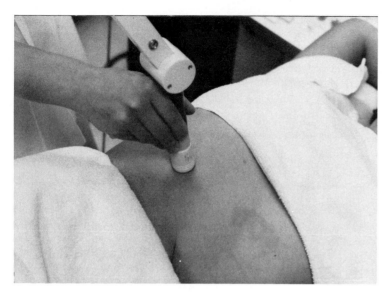

Fig. 13-10. The slight decubitus position is very effective for demonstrating the right kidney when the liver is used as an acoustic window.

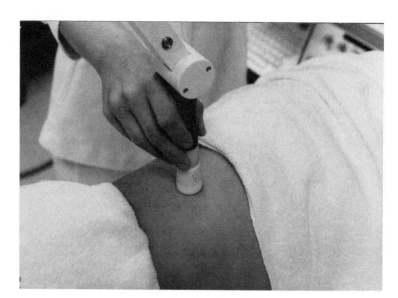

Fig. 13-11. The patient may be rolled into a right decubitus position to image the left kidney in a coronal plane.

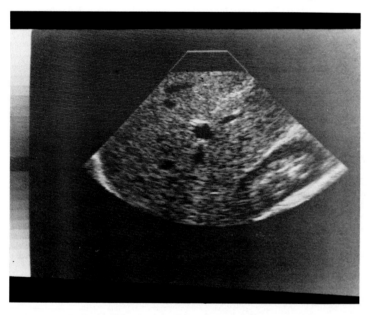

Fig. 13-12. The sagittal scan of the liver and renal parenchyma demonstrates correct TGC and sensitivity settings to permit the liver parenchyma to be more echogenic than the renal.

Technique. The most efficient way to evaluate the kidneys is through the liver for the right kidney (Fig. 13-10) or through the spleen for the left kidney (Fig. 13-11). The patient should be in a supine or decubitus position. The parenchymal echoes of the liver and spleen must be compared to the echo pattern of the renal parenchyma.

A proper adjustment of time gain compensation (TGC) with adequate sensitivity settings will allow a uniform acoustic pattern in the image. The renal cortical echo amplitude should be compared to the liver parenchymal echo amplitude at the same depth so the

effect of an inappropriate TGC setting will be reduced[1] (Fig. 13-12).

If the patient has a significant amount of perirenal fat, a high-frequency transducer may not penetrate the area properly and give the appearance as hypoechoic in the deeper areas of the kidney. Renal detail may also be obscured if the patient has hepatocellular disease, gallstones, or other abnormal mass collections between the liver and kidney.

Transverse, coronal, and longitudinal scans may be made through the intercostal margins to image the renal parenchyma. Relational anatomy should be identified to

rule out possible metastases, abscess formation, or other incidental abnormality.

The upper pole of the left kidney may be difficult to image with the patient supine, and an upright prone or coronal approach through the spleen and left kidney may be more effective.

Real time sector allows the rapid visualization of the lie of the kidney, which may be useful for accurate renal size determination.

Renal vascular structures

The renal vessels are best seen on transverse scans at the level of the hilus. Patency of the renal vein is a very important workup of renal carcinoma. Tumor extension into the renal vein or inferior vena cava may appear as low-level echoes within a dilated vascular structure.

The renal arteries flow posterior to the renal veins. On longitudinal scans the right renal artery is retrocaval and may be seen as a circular structure posterior to the IVC. The left renal vein is preaortic and may be seen as it passes anterior to the aorta and posterior to the SMA before flowing into the inferior vena cava.

Anatomic variations

A common renal variation is the dromedary hump, which is a localized bulge on the lateral border of the kidney. This hump will present the same echographic pattern as the rest of the renal parenchyma and thus will not be mistaken for a mass.

A double collecting system or elongated upper pole infundibulum may show a large column of Bertin in the midportion of the kidney. This has the appearance of a large and occasionally masslike zone of tissue, with echo characteristics much like cortex, insinuated between two separated portions of the echodense renal sinus.[2]

ULTRASONIC IDENTIFICATION OF PATHOLOGIC CONDITIONS
Congenital deformities

Agenesis. Congenital agenesis, absence of one kidney and ureter, may be difficult to assess clinically. Ultrasound can outline the normal kidney and tell with certainty whether one kidney is absent or pathologically afflicted.

Supernumerary kidney. Although rare, supernumerary kidney is a complete duplication of the renal system. It generally is found in the pelvis but occasionally will ascend with the other renal structures. Ultrasound may be able to outline two separate kidneys if they are within the normal renal area but may overlook the extra system if it is in the pelvis.

Horseshoe kidney. Horseshoe kidney occurs during fetal development, with fusion of the upper or lower poles. It does not ascend to its normal position in the retroperitoneal cavity. Generally the isthmus is found near the level of the iliac crest. It has separate ureters from either side of the kidney but is connected by tissue (the isthmus) draping across the midline.

Ultrasonically a horseshoe kidney should be evaluated from the supine position, since the kidneys generally appear lower in the abdomen and may be attenuated by the iliac crest in the prone position. The isthmus is best recorded with single-sweep technique and is seen as a sonolucent band draping over the great vessels. Lymphadenopathy is difficult to diagnose in a patient with a horseshoe kidney, since the isthmus may mimic the lymph nodes. Real time equipment should allow visualization of the renal parenchyma with the isthmus connecting the two capsules and thus may aid in distinguishing other disease from the isthmus (Figs. 13-13 and 13-14, A).

Renal masses

Prior to the ultrasound examination for a renal mass, a complete review of the patient's chart and previous diagnostic examinations should be made. In most patients an IVP will already have been obtained; and these films should be utilized for assessing the size and shape of the kidneys, determining the location of the mass, detecting any distortion of the renal outline or pericalyceal

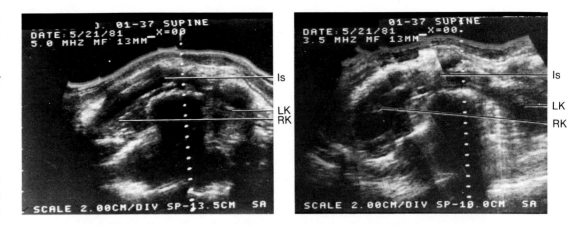

Fig. 13-13. Supine scan of a horseshoe kidney. Isthmus, *Is;* right kidney, *RK;* left kidney, *LK.* (Courtesy VA Hospital, Madison, Wis.)

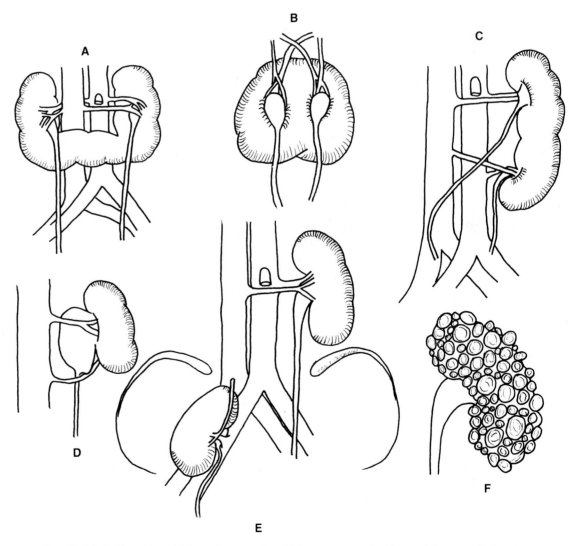

Fig. 13-14. A, Horseshoe kidney shown as two kidneys connected by an isthmus anterior to the great vessels and inferior to the inferior mesenteric artery. **B,** Cake kidney with a double collecting system. **C,** Double collecting system in a single kidney. **D,** Obstruction of the renal pelvis resulting in hydronephrosis. **E,** Pelvic kidneys with one kidney in the normal retroperitoneal position. **F,** Polycystic disease.

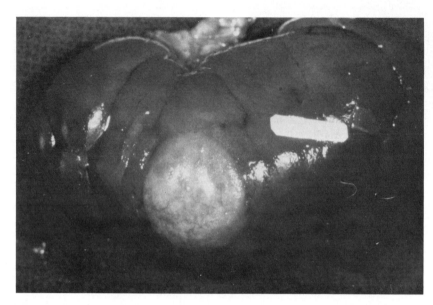

Fig. 13-15. Gross specimen of a renal cyst in the midpole of the right kidney.

system, and establishing the presence or absence of calcium or gas.

Renal masses are categorized as cystic, solid, or complex. A *cystic* mass will present sonographically with several characteristic features: smooth well-defined circular borders, a sharp interface between the cyst and renal parenchyma, no internal echoes (aside from reverberations), and excellent through-transmission. On the other hand, a *solid* lesion will project as a nongeometric shape with irregular borders, a poorly defined interface between the mass and the kidney, low-level internal echoes, a poor posterior border due to the increased attenuation of the tumor, and very poor through-transmission. Areas of necrosis, hemorrhage, or calcification within the tumor may alter the above classification slightly and cause the mass to fall into the *complex* category.

In our experience the real time sector scan allows a more complete evaluation of renal masses than does the articulated arm scan. If the mass is very small, respiration may cause it to move out of the field of view just enough to be missed on the articulated arm scan. The flexibility of the real time sector enables the sonographer to do multiple rotations of the transducer and to view

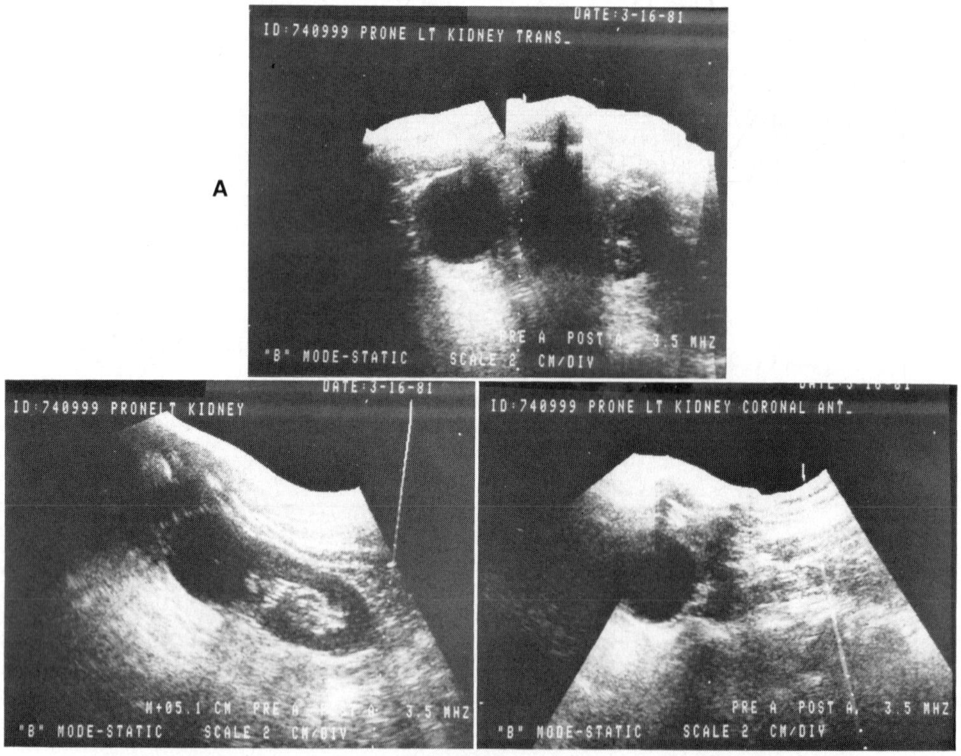

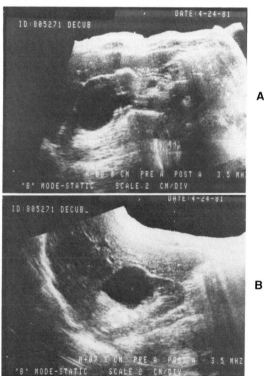

Fig. 13-16. A, Prone transverse scan of a left renal cyst. The borders are well defined and sharply marginated. Good through-transmission is present due to the lack of attenuation by the cystic fluid. **B,** Sagittal scan of the left kidney in the prone position. **C,** Coronal view of the left renal cyst.

Fig. 13-17. A, Supine transverse view of a right renal cyst. **B,** Sagittal supine view of the renal cyst as it compresses the calyceal echo pattern.

the kidney with the patient in normal respiration.

Simple cyst. These cysts may be located anywhere in the kidney and, if benign, are of no clinical significance unless they cause distortion of adjacent calyces to produce hydronephrosis or pain (Fig. 13-15).

Peripelvic cysts are found within the region of the renal pelvis. Parapelvic cysts are outside the renal capsule but in the region of the pelvis.

Sonographic features include a smooth wall, a circular anechoic mass with good through-transmission, and the tadpole sign (Fig. 13-16) (i.e., narrow bands of acoustic shadowing posterior to the margins of the cyst at the borders of enhancement). A septum may occasionally be seen within the cyst as a well-defined linear line (Fig. 13-17). Sometimes small sacculations or infoldings of the cyst wall produce irregularity of the wall, and cyst puncture should be employed to ascertain that the mass is a cyst (Fig. 13-18).

Reverberation echoes may be seen along the anterior margin of the cyst. A change in transducer diameter and frequency may help to "clean up" the reverberation artifacts, especially in smaller cysts. Thus a higher-frequency smaller-diameter transducer would cause a small cyst to appear more sharply defined.

Ultrasonic aspiration techniques. Once a renal mass has met the criteria for a cystic mass, a needle aspiration may be recommended to obtain fluid from the lesion for further evaluation of its internal composition.

The patient should be positioned with sandbags under the abdomen to help push the kidneys toward the posterior abdominal wall and provide a flat scanning surface. The cyst should be located in the transverse and longitudinal planes with scans performed at midinspiration. The depth of the mass should be noted from its anterior to posterior borders so the exact depth can be given to aid in placement of the needle.

A special aspiration transducer with a hole in its central core will allow the sonographer to observe the A-mode trace of the cystic mass. If a metal needle is used, the tip will be shown as a sharp spike between the walls as the needle enters the cyst. This allows close monitoring of the mass as the fluid is withdrawn. Special B-mode aspiration transducers are available to both make the scan *and* visualize the needle insertion; thus the two-dimensional B-scan and A-mode allow for an accurate puncture (Fig. 13-19).

A beveled needle will cause multiple echoes within the walls of the cyst. If the needle is slightly bent, many echoes will appear until the bent needle is completely out of the transducer's path. The larger the needle gauge, the stronger the reflection will be. Needles made of Teflon or other plastics will not produce a strong echo within the cust on A-mode.

Most aspiration transducers are 2.25 MHz, with higher frequencies used for superficial structures. To prevent wobbling or misdirection of the needle, the size of the lumen within the transducer should be close to the needle gauge.

Sterile technique is used for aspiration and biopsy procedures. The transducer must be gas sterilized. (The lumen of the transducer should be cleaned as well with a small brush and alcohol after each procedure.) Sterile lubricant is used to couple the transducer to the patient's skin.

When the area of aspiration is outlined on the patient's back, the distance is measured from the anterior surface to the middle of the cyst. This distance is added to the height of the transducer to give a total depth of the lesion. Special needle-stops act as a guide in preventing the needle from exceeding this precise distance.

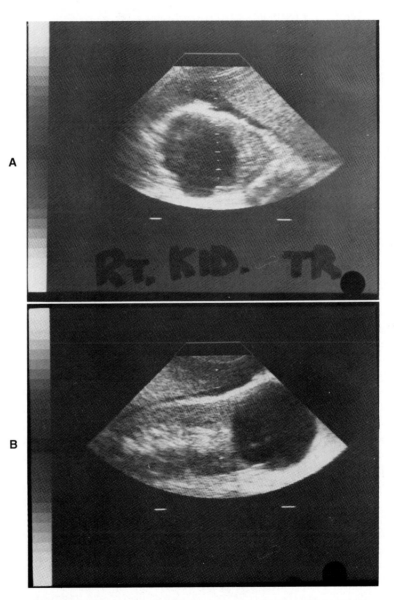

Fig. 13-18. A, Transverse real time of a patient with multiple problems. The primary tumor was adenocarcinoma of the pancreas. The right renal cyst was an incidental finding. Because of this history and the irregularity of the wall, a renal cyst aspiration was recommended. **B,** Sagittal scan. The right renal cyst on the lower pole of the kidney is now well defined and sharply marginated as compared to its appearance on the transverse scan.

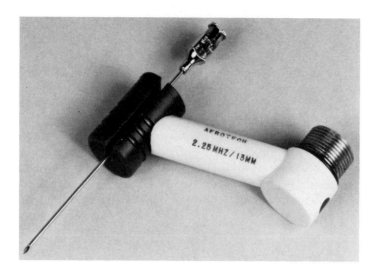

Fig. 13-19. The B-mode aspiration transducer allows placement of the needle, and the slit within the transducer head enables one to move the apparatus away when the needle is placed correctly.

The volume of the cyst may be determined by measuring the radius of the mass and using the following formula:

$$V = \frac{4}{3} \pi r^3$$

The diameter of the mass can be applied to this formula:

$$V = d^3 \div 2$$

The patient's skin is painted with tincture of benzalkonium (Zephiran) and sterile drapes are applied. A local anesthetic is administered over the area of interest, and the sterile transducer is used to relocate the cyst. This may be done with A-mode or B-scan, depending on the type of transducer. The needle is inserted through the lumen of the transducer into the central core of the cyst. The needle stop will help in making sure that the needle does not go through the cyst. The fluid is then withdrawn according to the volume calculations.

Inflammatory cyst. A simple renal cyst that becomes infected may present a complex echo pattern with thick walls, low-level echoes, and ill-defined borders.

Hemorrhagic cyst. This cyst may be difficult to define sonographically. Approximately 6% of simple cysts will hemorrhage, and the pattern may be hard to separate from that of a cystic neoplasm. Patterns range from one belonging to a simple cyst to one having irregular walls with low-level echoes and good through-transmission.

Calcified cyst. A cyst with calcified walls will present decreased through-transmission and echogenic walls. A cyst aspiration should be performed to rule out the presence of malignancy.

Cyst with milk of calcium.[1] These masses are calyceal diverticula that may or may not have lost their communication with the calyceal system. The condition presents no symptoms and generally is found incidentally at radiography. Within the cystic mass there is a layering, a linear band of strong echoes that are associated with an acoustic shadow.

Cystic mass with tumor.[1] The presence of a tumor mass in the cyst may signify a rapidly expanding cyst adjacent to a tumor. The tumor becomes incorporated into the expanding cyst. A cyst puncture should be made to define cellular contents.

Renal sinus lipomatosis. This is generally found by sonography to present as an area of low-level echoes within the cystic area comparable to the pattern from the surrounding parenchyma.

Renal hematoma. Depending on the age of the hematoma, this process has a variety of sonographic findings. A fresh hematoma will present as a cystic structure without a smooth wall. As clot formation occurs, low-level echoes appear. Eventually the hematoma will liquefy or become organized, and its appearance will then become more cystic or complex.

Vascular cystic masses. Saccular aneurysms and arteriovenous malformations may appear as cystic multiloculations and cystic masses respectively.

Hydronephrosis.[4] A cyst found at the upper pole of the kidney should elicit the question of a possible second dilated upper collecting system. If it is hydronephrotic, a tubular echo-free structure may be seen passing medial to the lower collecting system; this represents the dilated ureter. Septa may be seen if more than one calyx is involved.

General hydronephrosis presents as the loss of a pelvicalyceal system with cysts of similiar size. Generally there is an absence of renal parenchyma (Fig. 13-20). This may be associated with a large extrarenal pelvis (one large medial cyst surrounded by and communicating with several laterally placed equal-sized smaller cysts). In another form of hydronephrosis a single cystic mass may be seen replacing the kidney. It may have a slightly lobulated border.

To separate a multicystic kidney from hydronephrosis, one must establish the presence or absence of a pelvicalyceal echo complex.

Multicystic kidney. This is a common cause of a mass in the neonatal abdomen. The kidneys have decreased or absent blood supply and are connected to an atretic ureter. Sonographically multiple cysts may be seen with no evidence of renal parenchyma or pelvicalyceal echo patterns (Fig. 13-21).

Adult multicystic disease. Sonographically these patients will display calcified cysts with a small kidney and absent renal pelvis.

Adult polycystic disease. In this disease a cyst may arise from any portion of a collecting system (Fig. 13-22). Small cysts (under 1 cm) may not be readily detected although renal enlargement will be present. As the cysts grow, they become visible by sonography, with variable shapes and sizes and irregular walls. The pelvicalyceal echoes are seen, although they may be distorted by the cysts (Fig. 13-23).

Associated cysts in the liver (30% to 40%), pancreas (10%), and spleen (5%) have also been reported. Pitfalls in diagnosing them may arise if one becomes infected or hemorrhages. Severe hydronephrosis superimposed on chronic pyelonephritis may be distinguished from polycystic kidney disease by the communication of cysts with a longitudinal configuration. Polycystic cysts have a more circular lobulated appearance (Fig. 13-24).

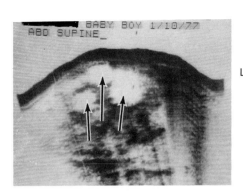

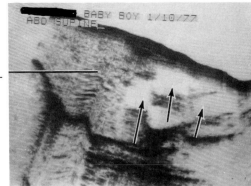

Fig. 13-20. Sagittal of a patient with right hydronephrosis. There is loss of the pelvicalyceal system, with cysts of similar size representing the distended pelvis.

Fig. 13-21. Infant multicystic disease. Multiple small cysts are shown within the right kidney on the supine scans.

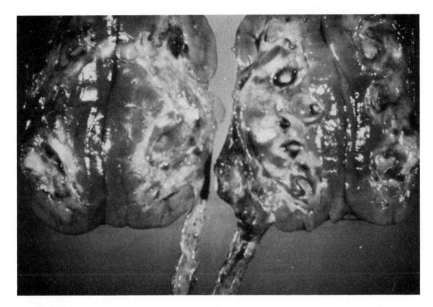

Fig. 13-22. Gross specimen of polycystic disease showing enlarged kidneys with multiple cystic pockets.

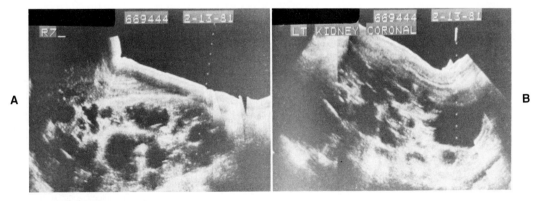

Fig. 13-23. Adult polycystic disease is shown on these sagittal scans of the right, **A,** and left, **B,** kidney. The kidneys are enlarged and filled with multiple cysts of varying sizes throughout the entire parenchyma.

Infantile polycystic disease.[3] This form of tubular ectasia causes the tubules in the distal collecting systems to dilate and form small cystic structures. Sonographically they may appear as hepatic and portal fibrosis with renal enlargement with increased reflections throughout the parenchyma due to defined cystic masses in the cortex and medulla.

Hypernephroma[3] **(renal adenocarcinoma).** In contrast to a smoothly outlined cystic mass, hypernephromas are irregular in shape (Fig. 13-25). The margins are well demarcated from the surrounding tissue, but the mass does not separate itself sonically from the renal parenchyma. Its edges are irregular, and low-level internal echoes are seen (Fig. 13-26). Usually these tumors will produce a "bump" on the IVP. The tumor may grow so large as to replace the renal volume. The smaller tumors, which do not distort the renal outline, are difficult to detect; one must look for subtle renal parenchymal widening or slight calyceal displacement (as seen on the IVP).

The amount of internal echo reflections may depend on the presence or absence of hemorrhage or necrosis within the tumor (Fig. 13-27).

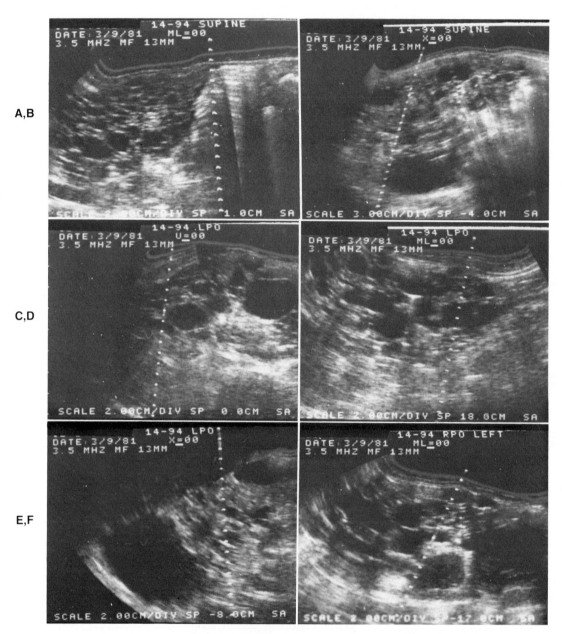

Fig. 13-24. Patient with polycystic kidneys and liver disease. Multiple cysts are seen throughout the parenchyma of both organs. **A,** Supine transverse of the liver and kidney. It is difficult to separate the borders with so many cysts replacing the parenchyma. **B,** Supine transverse scan. **C** and **D,** LPO of the right kidney. **E,** LPO of a large cyst within the right kidney. **F,** RPO of the left polycystic kidney. (Courtesy VA Hospital, Madison, Wis.)

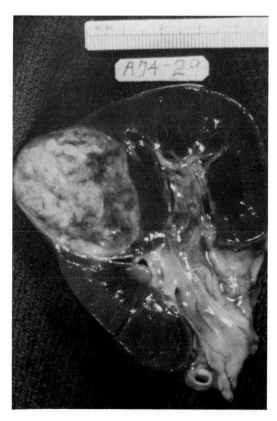

Fig. 13-25. Gross specimen of a renal tumor.

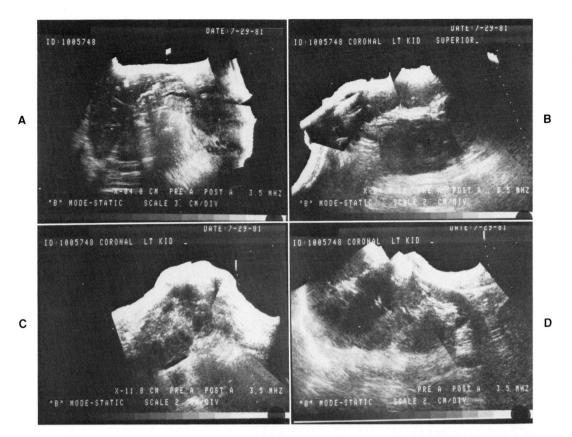

Fig. 13-26. Multiple scans of a large solid renal mass arising from the left kidney in a patient with a previous left renal carcinoma. **A,** Supine transverse showing the mass arising from the anterior border of the kidney. **B,** Coronal showing the left kidney displaced by the mass. **C,** Coronal transverse over the solid mass. **D,** Coronal longitudinal with the solid mass arising from the left upper pole of the kidney.

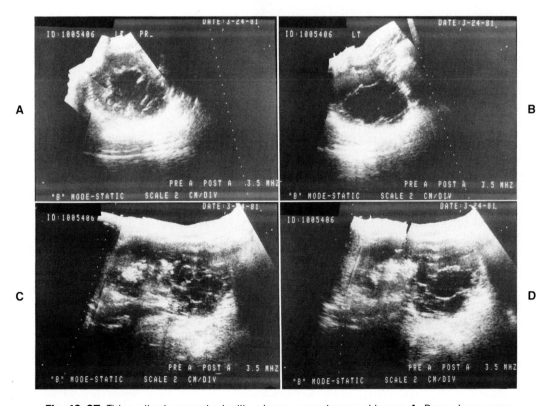

Fig. 13-27. This patient presented with a large complex renal tumor. **A,** Prone transverse scan over the mass. **B,** On this scan the mass appears somewhat homogeneous with good transmission, but the margins are very irregular. **C,** Sagittal prone scan showing the complex nature of the mass as it hangs from the lower pole of the kidney. **D,** Sagittal prone scan.

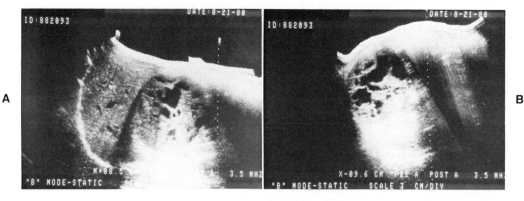

Fig. 13-28. This patient with a renal cell carcinoma presented at ultrasonography with a large solid mass that contained multiple necrotic areas arising from the right kidney. Since a clear margin was seen to separate the mass from the liver, its origin was thought to be renal or retroperitoneal. **A,** Sagittal supine scan. **B,** Transverse supine scan over the complex tumor.

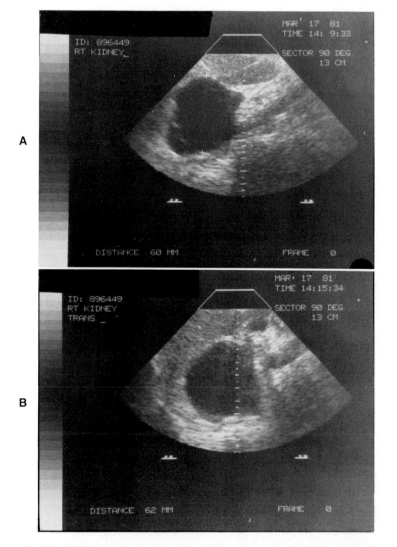

Fig. 13-29. This patient presented with an elevated WBC and spiking fevers. **A,** The supine sagittal scan reveals a homogeneous slightly irregular mass arising from the upper pole of the right kidney. **B,** Transverse scan of the renal abscess. Note the decreased through-transmission posterior to the abscess wall.

If the mass appears to show evidence of a hypernephroma, attention should be directed to other structures and organs (e.g., the renal vein, inferior vena cava, liver) for possible metastases and to the retroperitoneum for the presence of enlarged nodes.

Transitional cell carcinoma. Symptoms generally range from incidental hematuria to grossly bloody urine. Most of these tumors are invasive without the presence of a bulky mass. When a bulky mass is found, it appears to be anechoic or to contain low-level echoes. These tumors become difficult to classify by sonographic findings alone, and thus a differential diagnoses must be given (Fig. 13-28).

Renal lymphoma. Patients with disseminated lymphomatous malignancies may have renal involvement that presents as nonspecific enlargement. If the lymphoma is focal in nature, a defined anechoic or low-level mass will be seen and through-transmission will not be as great as seen with a simple cyst.

Angiomyolipoma (benign renal tumor). This mass presents as a homogeneous strongly echogenic area with significant acoustic impedance. These characteristics are related to its high vascularity and increased fat content.

Inflammatory masses. Symptoms for inflammatory masses include fever, chills, and flank pain. Two acute inflammatory processes in the kidney can produce mass lesions capable of being mistaken for a renal tumor.[3] A *carbuncle or abscess* may present as a sonolucent mass with low-level echoes and shaggy margins. *Inflammatory cells* may be seen in the renal parenchyma and can cause swelling and edema of the kidney with no discrete mass (Fig. 13-29).

A chronic renal abscess may produce a mass in the absence of clinical symptoms and present sonographically as a complex lesion.

Xanthogranulomatous pyelonephritis

Xanthogranulomatous pyelonephritis produces renal enlargement with multiple anechoic areas having central echogenic foci associated with acoustic shadowing.

Perinephric fluid collections

Fluid collections that lie adjacent to the kidney in the intraperitoneal or retroperitoneal space will show sonographically as a somewhat well-defined sonolucent area outside the kidney. To separate this collection from an intrarenal mass requires that the renal outline be well defined. The patient should be scanned in the supine, prone, and decubitus positions so the collection can be visualized outside the kidney (Fig. 13-30).

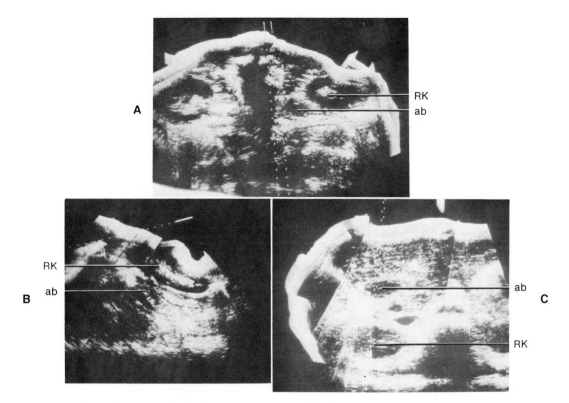

Fig. 13-30. A, Prone transverse scan of an abscess anterior to the right kidney. **B,** Prone sagittal scan of the complex mass. **C,** Supine transverse scan of the abscess anterior to the right kidney.

RENAL FAILURE
Hydronephrosis

Sonographic findings of moderate bilateral hydronephrosis were encountered by Morin and Baker[3] in a dehydrated patient undergoing rehydration. Renal sonography is most reliable in hydronephrosis if performed with the bladder empty and prior to initiation of rehydration.

Increased pressure in the kidney can affect the calyces or pelvis. A common pattern is calyceal distension without a prominent pelvis. By sonography this appears as a group of similiar-sized cystic structures located in the central renal area. It may be distinguished from multicystic disease by the fact that the cysts are of similiar size and there is an absence of echoes from the renal pelvic fat (Fig. 13-31).

Resnick and Sanders[4] state that severe hydronephrosis may take on one of three patterns: a central septation, a blown-out (ovoid) sac, or the dumbbell or hourglass shape (Figs. 13-32 and 13-33).

In patients with ureteropelvic junction obstruction the extrarenal pelvis is larger than the dilated infundibular component of the pelvicalyceal system. This type is the dumbbell pattern.

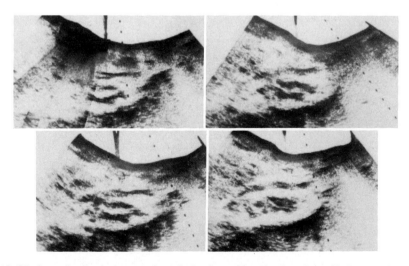

Fig. 13-31. Longitudinal scans of early hydronephrosis showing dilation of the renal pelvis.

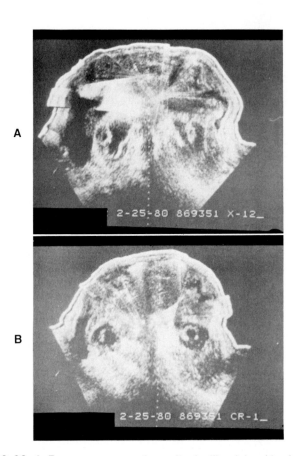

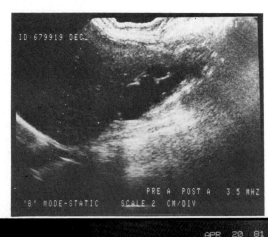

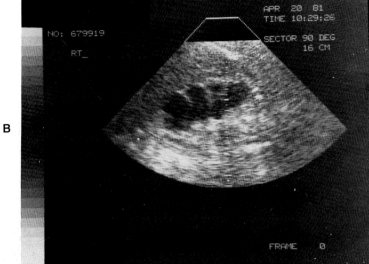

Fig. 13-32. A, Transverse scan of a patient with minimal hydronephrosis. **B,** The bilateral dilation of the central collecting system is well seen in this patient with renal failure.

Fig. 13-33. A, This patient was sent for further evaluation of a nonfunctioning right kidney. Her creatine and BUN values were elevated. Hydronephrosis was seen on the sagittal scan. **B,** Real time helps distinguish between hydronephrosis and multicystic disease by following the contour of the renal pelvis. With hydronephrosis the medial aspect of the renal pelvis will form a triangular shape, whereas with a cyst it will remain spherical.

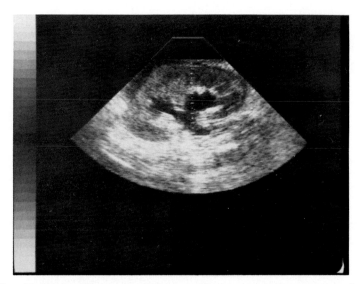

Fig. 13-34. Sagittal scan of the cauliflower appearance of hydronephrosis.

A rim of renal parenchyma surrounding the dilation may or may not be seen. The width of the remaining renal parenchyma may help in determining renal function and the prognosis of the disease.

Another pattern of hydronephrosis shows distended calyces with a medially located larger cystic structure representing the pelvis and upper ureter.[4] This has a sausage shape and may lead into the intrarenal component without a definite segmental narrowing. The cauliflower appearance of calyces flowing to the dilated pelvis may also be seen (Fig. 13-34).

Besides cystic structures mimicking hydronephrosis, or vice versa, the presence of a staghorn calculus within a dilated collecting system may be a source of confusion. To distinguish this finding from another lesion,

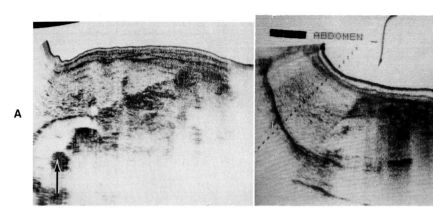

Fig. 13-35. Staghorn calculus is displayed as strong echoes within the renal parenchyma. Complete attenuation of sound may be due to the density of the calculi. **A,** Supine transverse scan demonstrating the anterior border of the kidney and the dense internal echoes with shadowing posterior. **B,** The longitudinal scan demonstrates the shadowing from calculi within the renal parenchyma.

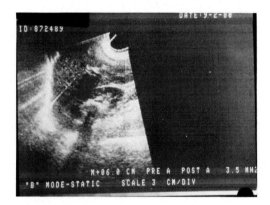

Fig. 13-36. Sagittal scan of a staghorn calculus without obstruction to the renal pelvis.

one should be able to see a prominent acoustic shadow posterior to the dense calculus (Figs. 13-35 and 13-36).

Pyonephrosis may be another variant of hydronephrosis. It will present as a dilated system with low-level echoes from the pus and may be difficult to distinguish from a tumor mass. Careful evaluation of the patient's chart and laboratory values may help make the diagnosis.

Small kidneys

Small kidneys represent end-stage renal disease. In general, when compared to the liver, the renal parenchyma is more echogenic. Renal vascular disease may be another cause of small kidneys. If the infarct is focal, areas of decreased echoes will be seen. Within the infarcted small area, the kidneys will expand and contain fewer parenchymal echoes before shrinking to be echogenic.

REFERENCES

1. Elyaderani, M.K., and Gabriele, O.F.: Ultrasound of renal masses, Semin. Ultrasound 11(1):21, 1981.
2. Finberg, H.: Renal ultrasound: anatomy and technique, Semin. Ultrasound 11(1):7, 1981.
3. Morin, M.E., and Baker, D.A.: The influence of hydration and bladder distention on the sonographic diagnosis of hydronephrosis, J. Clin. Ultrasound 7:192, 1979.
4. Resnick, M.I., and Sanders, R.C.: Ultrasound in urology, Baltimore, 1979, The Williams & Wilkins Co.
5. Rosenfield, A.T., Taylor, K.J.W., Crade, M., and DeGraaf, C.S.: Anatomy and pathology of the kidney by gray scale ultrasound, Radiology 128:737, 1978.

14 Renal transplant

BECKY LEVZOW

SANDRA L. HAGEN-ANSERT

Since 1954 more than 25,000 renal transplants have been performed on patients suffering from renal failure. Renal transplantation and dialysis are currently utilized for the treatment of chronic renal failure or end-stage renal disease. Ultrasound has emerged as an excellent tool in monitoring such transplant patients and may complement nuclear medicine and laboratory values in distinguishing the course of rejection. Since the sonogram does not rely on the function of the kidney, serial studies can be readily incorporated in determining the diagnosis and the treatment to be administered.

A number of complications may arise following transplantation: rejection, acute tubular necrosis (ATN), obstructive nephropathy, extraperitoneal fluid collections, hemorrhage or infarction, recurrent glomerulonephritis, graft rupture, and renal emphysema. Decreased renal function is commonly the main indication for ultrasonic evaluation.

THE PROCEDURE

Most renal transplant patients have had long-standing renal failure without obstructive nephropathy. Before the procedure, patient risk factors to be considered are age, primary diagnosis, secondary medical complications, and transplant source. It is found that recipients between 16 and 45 years of age with primary renal disease have the lowest risk for morbidity and mortality.

The major problem encountered with transplantation is graft rejection. The success of the transplant is directly related to the source of the donated kidney. There are two types of donors: living relatives and cadavers.

The surgical procedure begins with removal of the donor's left kidney, which is then rotated and placed in the recipient's right iliac fossa or groin region. The renal artery is attached by an end-to-end anastomosis with either the common or the external iliac artery (Fig. 14-1).

The ureter is inserted into the bladder above the normal ureteral orifice through a submucosal tunnel in the bladder wall. The tunnel creates a valve in the terminal ureter to prevent reflux of urine into the transplanted kidney.

Although the kidney is more vulnerable to trauma when it is placed in the iliopelvic region, this has rarely been a problem. The advantage of such a location is its observation accessibility. There are complications that may arise following transplantation, however, and thus a variety of examinations may be incorporated to detect and follow the transplant. Useful information may be accumulated through laboratory tests, nuclear medicine, sonography, intravenous pyelography, and renal arteriography.

SONOGRAPHIC EVALUATION

As early as 48 hours after surgery a baseline sonographic examination is performed for the determination of renal size, calyceal pattern, and extrarenal fluid collections. Hydronephrosis can be easily recognized sonographically as the calyceal pattern dilates. Perirenal fluid collections (hematoma, abscess, lymphocele, or urinoma) can be diagnosed reliably and differentiated from acute rejection. Serial scans at 3-to-6-month intervals may be made to detect fluid collections at an early asymptomatic stage. The patient should be examined at the first sign of tenderness in the graft area or mass development.

Technique for sonographic examination

The patient is placed in the supine position. A full urinary bladder is required but should be monitored carefully since overdistension after surgery may result in urinary leakage at the neoureterocystostomy or cause pseudohydronephrosis (Fig. 14-2).

To locate the kidney precisely by ultra-

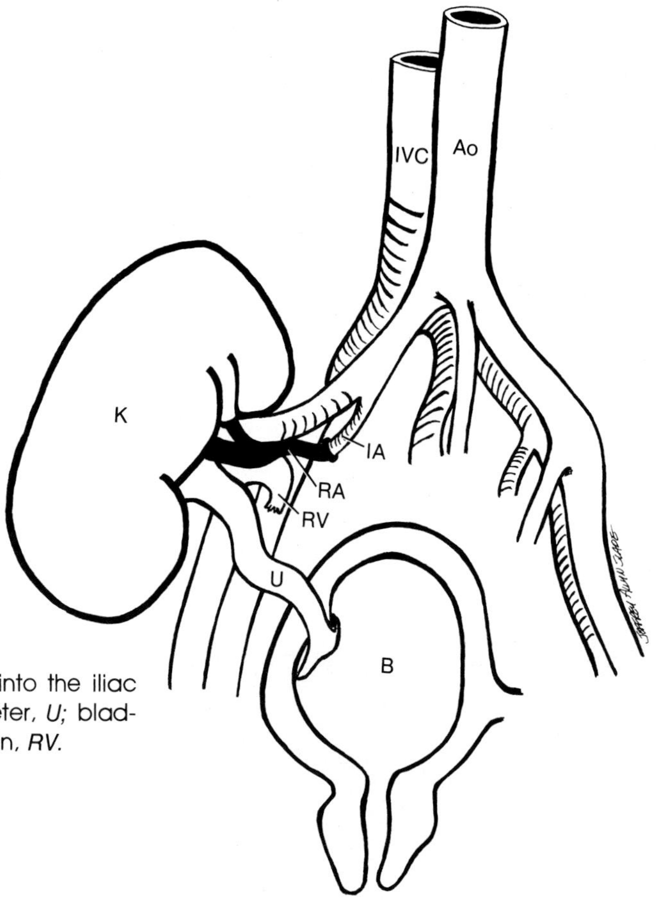

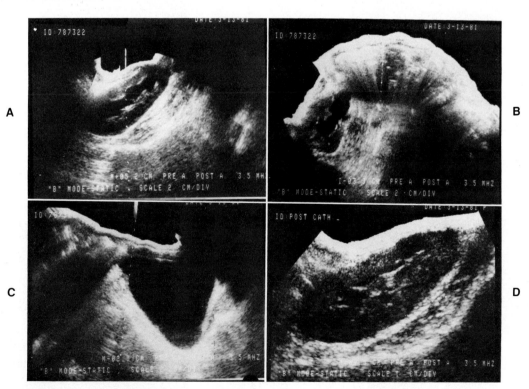

Fig. 14-1. Surgical placement of the renal transplant into the iliac fossa. Aorta, *Ao;* inferior vena cava, *IVC;* kidney, *K;* ureter, *U;* bladder, *B;* internal iliac artery, *IA;* renal artery, *RA;* renal vein, *RV.*

Fig. 14-2. A, Sagittal scan of a renal transplant patient showing distension of the calyceal system. **B,** Transverse scan of the hydronephrosis. **C,** The bladder was extremely overdistended and was the cause of the patient's pseudohydronephrosis. **D,** Scan of the transplant after patient voiding; a normal compact calyceal system.

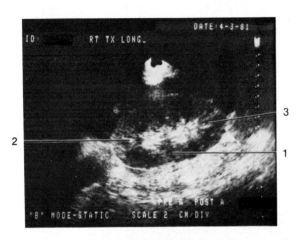

Fig. 14-3. When scanning the transplant, place the transducer over the midportion of the kidney, *1*, and gently arc to the superior pole, *2*. Now begin the scan and sweep the transducer to the inferior pole of the kidney, *3*.

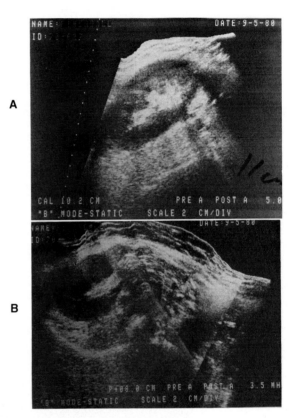

Fig. 14-4. A, Sagittal and, **B,** transverse. Normal appearance of the renal transplant. The homogeneous renal parenchyma surrounds the dense band of echoes from the renal pelvis, calyces, blood vessels, and fibrofatty tissues.

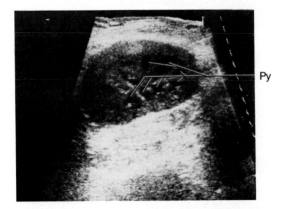

Fig. 14-5. The renal pyramids, *Py*, are discrete sonolucent structures.

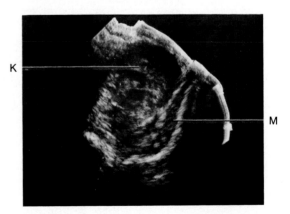

Fig. 14-6. The iliopsoas, *M,* appears as a parallel linear group of echoes posterior to the kidney, *K.*

sound, transverse scans are made from the pubic symphysis to above the level of the graft. A mark is placed on the skin at the location of the superior and inferior poles, with an imaginary line drawn between the two points to determine the long axis of the kidney. If real time is available, rapid determination of the graft orientation may be obtained. Longitudinal and transverse scans at 1-cm intervals are then made parallel with and perpendicular to the long axis of the kidney (Fig. 14-3). From these scans accurate measurements of the renal length, width, and anteroposterior dimensions can be determined.

The normal transplant should appear as a smooth structure surrounding the homogeneous parenchymal pattern. A dense band of echoes in the midportion of the transplant represents the renal pelvis, calcyces, blood vessels, and fatty fibrous tissues (Fig. 14-4). The medullary pyramids are discrete sonolucent structures surrounded by the homogeneous grainy texture of the cortex (Fig. 14-5). The psoas appears as parallel linear echoes posterior to the kidney transplant (Fig. 14-6).

A sonolucent appearance of the anterior portion of the kidney and, at times, an increased echogenic band across the anterior kidney occur on some scans due to inaccurate settings in the near field (Fig. 14-7). Decreased amplification of the near gain in the first few centimeters of the slope will obliterate the decreased echoes of the near field and allow for better fill-in of the anterior portion of the kidney. This difference in anterior structure delineation is probably due to the attenuation of sound by subcutaneous fat, muscle thickness, skin texture, and scarring or to the fact that some patients transmit the sound frequency more readily than others.

The opposite is true for the problem of increased echoes in the near field. By decrease in the near gain, suppression of the echoes in the near field yields an image with uniform texture. Thus it is important to maintain proper penetration and delineation of internal structures with a good outline of adjacent musculature.

To record echoes from the parenchyma and distinguish the cortex from the medulla, the sonographer should scan the patient with low-gain and high-gain settings. The scans will include both kidneys as well as the pararenal area (i.e., iliac wing, iliacus, iliopsoas).

A high-frequency small-diameter transducer is utilized to image the superficial transplant. We have found that a 5.0-MHz 13-mm transducer produces the most acceptable image (Fig. 14-8). The 5.0-MHz 19-mm instrument focuses beyond the kidney and thus produces an image with less definition of the renal parenchyma.

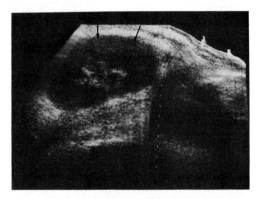

Fig. 14-7. The problem of a band of increased artifactual echoes *(arrows)* across the anterior portion of the kidney was obliterated by suppression of the near gain echoes.

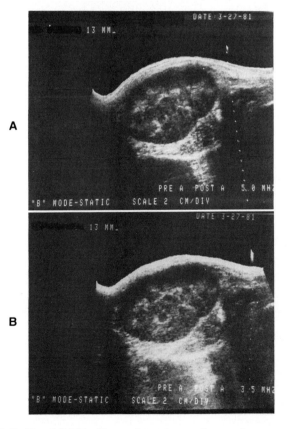

Fig. 14-8. The 5.0-MHz 13-mm transducer, **A,** produces a more acceptable image than does the 3.5-MHz 13-mm transducer, **B.**

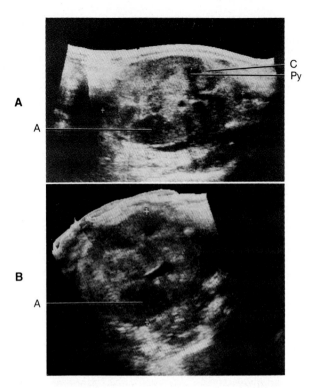

Fig. 14-9. A, Enlargement and decreased echogenicity of the pyramids, *Py,* due to edema and congestion with hemorrhage of the interstitial tissue. Ischemia and cellular infiltration (fibrosis) result in hyperechogenicity of the cortex, *C.* Anechoic, *A,* areas, the product of infarcts, usually occur in the polar regions. **B,** Transverse scan of the same patient demonstrating the extent of the anechoic area.

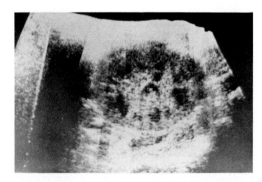

Fig. 14-10. Enlargement and decreased echogenic pyramids with a hyperechoic cortex.

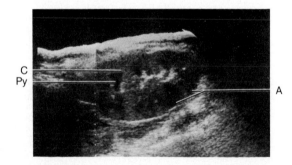

Fig. 14-11. This patient presented with enlargement and decreased echogenic pyramids, *Py,* hyperechogenic cortex, *C,* and a localized anechoic area of renal parenchyma, *A.* This correlated with pathology data of an edematous hemorrhagic cortex and medulla, with fibrin deposited throughout the kidney.

RENAL TRANSPLANT REJECTION

Sonography can be useful in the diagnosis of rejection. Care must be taken to observe the size and shape; the appearance of the pyramids, cortex, and parenchyma; and the presence of any surrounding fluid collections. Maklad et al.[1] summarize the appearance of renal rejection by stating that there are five changes in the renal parenchymal echo pattern that have been observed during the process of rejection:

1. Enlargement and decreased echogenicity of the pyramids. This appearance is not at all uniform, and only a few pyramids may appear as such (Fig. 14-9).
2. Hyperechogenic cortex. The swollen sonolucent pyramids stand out against the background of increased echogenicity of the outer and interpyramidal cortex (Fig. 14-10).
3. A localized area of renal parenchyma, including both the cortex and the medulla presenting an anechoic appearance, is very difficult to fill in even when high sensitivity and TGC settings are used. This is usually seen in polar regions (Fig. 14-11).
4. Distortion of the renal outline due to localized areas of swelling involving both the cortex and the pyramids. The renal sinus echoes may appear compressed and displaced (Fig. 14-12).
5. Patchy sonolucent areas involving both cortex and medulla with coalescence on follow-up studies. These areas can become quite extensive, affecting a large portion of the renal parenchyma.

In long-standing rejection, Maklad et al.[1] state that two patterns have been observed: (1) a normal-sized renal transplant with very little differentiation between the parenchymal and renal sinus echoes and (2) a small kidney with irregular margins and an irregular parenchymal echo pattern.

These sonographic appearances correlate with the pathologic occurrences. When swelling with increased internal echoes within the cortex is present, rejection can be diagnosed. Edema, congestion, and hemorrhage of the interstitium produce swelling of the pyramids, which appears as decreased echogenicity (Fig. 14-13). Ischemia and cellular infiltration produce the increased echogenicity of the cortex. Increased areas of sonolucency may also occur in the cortex due to necrosis and infarction. These areas are usually seen in the polar regions of the transplant. If actual necrosis begins, the affected part appears as an area of decreased echogenicity, which suggests partial liquefaction. Irregular parenchymal echo patterns may result from parenchymal atrophy with fibrosis and shrinkage due to long-standing renal rejection.

Acute tubular necrosis

ATN is a common cause of acute post-transplant failure. Some degree occurs in almost every transplant patient, and it has been stated that as many as 50% of the recipients of cadaver kidneys experience ATN following transplantation. The incidence of ATN is usually higher in cadaver transplants than in donor-relative transplants or in kidneys that undergo warm ischemia or prolonged preservation, kidneys with multiple renal arteries, or kidneys obtained from elderly donors.

ATN usually resolves early in the postoperative period. Uncomplicated ATN is often reversible and can be treated by immediate use of diuretics and satisfactory hydration. It is important to recognize uncomplicated ATN and distinguish it from acute rejection, because the therapy for the two conditions is very different.

Clinically ATN may present a variety of different patterns. Urine volumes may be good initially, followed by oliguria or anuria, or there may be low urine output from the time of transplantation. The serum creatine level is always elevated. If urine output remains low and BUN and creatinine remain elevated, ATN may be difficult to distinguish from rejection. Other indications of rejection (e.g., hematuria, elevated eosinophile counts, or pain over the transplant) are helpful but may be late signs.

Sonographically there are usually no changes seen within the renal parenchyma. In the initial postoperative period the kidney may enlarge slightly due to secondary hypertrophy. This is believed to be a normal physiologic response of the newly transplanted kidney or is caused by swelling that often regresses within a week. However, if the swelling persists, then either ATN or rejection should be considered. With ATN the renal parenchymal pattern remains unchanged, in contrast to the earlier description of the parenchymal changes during rejection. If these changes are lacking and the transplant fails to function, the cause is most likely ATN, provided the radionuclide evaluation has confirmed the patency of the vascular supply to the transplant.

Extraperitoneal fluid collections

There are numerous extraperitoneal fluid collections that may occur following transplantation: lymphoceles and lymph fistulas,

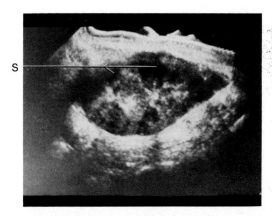

Fig. 14-12. The distortion of the renal outline is seen due to localized areas of swelling in the cortex and pyramids and patchy sonolucent, *S*, areas involving both the cortex and the medulla with coalescence on follow-up studies.

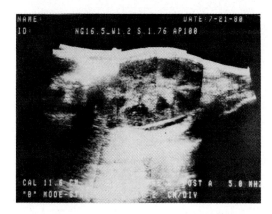

Fig. 14-13. Renal transplant rejection with prominent pyramids and echogenic renal cortex. A small amount of ascites is seen posterior to the transplant.

urinary fistula and urinoma, perinephric abscess, and hematoma. These collections consist of lymph, blood, urine, pus, or a combination of the substances. A sign common to several of the complications is a decrease in renal function manifested by increased creatinine values. Sonographically the fluid collections may appear as round or oval structures with irregular and slightly thickened walls. Usually clinical or laboratory correlation will suggest the etiology of the fluid. Because the transplant is superficial, scans can easily be made and, if necessary, sonographic guidance can be rendered for aspiration of the contents for further analysis.

Lymphocele and lymph fistula. Lymphoceles are a common complication of transplantation, occurring in approximately 12% of all transplant patients. The source of the lymph collection is probably vessels severed during the preparation of recipient vessels,

or it may be the kidney itself in the form of leakage from injured capsular and hilar lymphatics. The lymph drains into the peritoneal cavity, provoking a fibrous reaction and eventually walling itself off. Primary clinical signs are deterioration of renal function (usually within 2 weeks to 6 months of transplantation), development of painless fluctuant swelling over the transplant, ipsilateral leg edema, or wound drainage of lymph cells. If an IVP was performed, a mass indenting the bladder, ureteral deviation, ureteral obstruction, or kidney deviation will be seen.

Sonographically the lymphocele is a well-defined anechoic area, occasionally with numerous septations (Fig. 14-14). Urinomas may appear similar to lymphoceles, although usually they appear early whereas lymphoceles are more common chronically. If the mass is complex with solid components, hematoma or abscess must be considered.

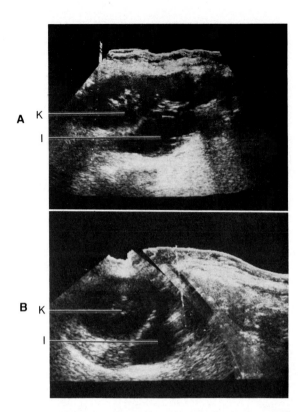

Fig. 14-14. A, Sagittal scan of a renal transplant, *K,* with a lymphocele, *I,* formation along the medial posterior border. **B,** Transverse scan of the transplant and lymphocele.

Urinary fistula and urinoma. Abnormal collections of fluid surrounding the transplant may be readily detected by sonography.

Bladder leaks are derived from the anterior cystostomy or from the ureteroneocystostomy due to faulty surgical technique or bladder overdistension. Clinical signs include local tenderness, fever, sudden decrease in urine output, or urine leakage from the wound. Most fistulas become manifest in the first 2 postoperative weeks, but presentation may be delayed for over a month.

A collection of urine may be present within the pelvis as either a walled-off urinoma or free fluid. These collections are usually echo free. Differentiation of free urine from a loculated urinoma can easily be made by shifting the patient's position and repeating the examination in the same plane to show redistribution of the fluid.

Perinephric abscess. Perinephric infections can be very hazardous to the transplant patient undergoing immunosuppressive therapy. It is an uncommon complication reported as early as 12 days or many months after transplantation. If the patient presents with a fever of unknown origin, care must be taken to rule out an abscess formation. Sonographically an abscess may appear with septa in it. Edema and inflammation may be pres-

ent around the mass, making the borders appear less distinct as compared to those found with lymphoceles and hematomas.

Hematoma. A hematoma may develop shortly after surgery. One of the major indications for an ultrasound scan may be a drop in the hematocrit value. Other clinical findings pertinent to hematomas include signs of bleeding, perinephric hemorrhage, a palpable mass, hypertension, and impaired renal function; or the hematoma may be an incidental finding during scanning. Hematomas appear as walled-off well-defined areas whose sonolucent echo production is dependent on the age or stage of the hematoma. It may appear sonolucent while the blood is fresh and be difficult to distinguish from a lymphocele or urinoma. As the clot becomes organized, the hematoma may tend to fragment and develop low-level internal echoes. The mass will then appear complex and eventually solid. After a time it may revert to a sonolucent mass and form a seroma.

Obstructive nephropathy

Early signs of obstruction are anuria or severe oliguria in a patient with satisfactory renal volumes. Numerous conditions may cause obstruction such as ureteral necrosis, abscess, lymphocele, fungus ball, retroperitoneal fibrosis, stricture at the ureterovesical

junction, ureteral calculus, and hemorrhage into the collecting system with obstruction from clots. Sonographically obstruction appears as a splaying of the normally compact renal sinus echoes by echo-free spaces, which represent dilated calyces and renal pelvis. If a renal calculus is the cause of obstruction, a dense echo with an acoustic shadow may be seen on the sonogram.

Graft rupture

Graft ruptures can occur in the first 2 postoperative weeks, presenting with an abrupt onset of pain and swelling over the graft, oliguria, and shock. Sonographically graft ruptures appear as a gross distortion of the graft contour and a perinephric or paranephric hematoma.

SUMMARY

During the past 10 to 15 years renal transplants have gained wide acceptance in the management of chronic renal failure. Although the functional success rate of the transplant has not significantly improved, patient survival has increased with earlier recognition and management of complications following transplantation.

A baseline sonogram should be obtained as soon as possible following transplantation to document the texture, size, and lie of the kidney. In addition to acute rejection, the most commonly encountered complications are ATN, abscess, lymphocele, hematoma, hydronephrosis, urine leaks, and changes in the vessels supplying the kidneys. The therapeutic approach depends on a prompt and accurate diagnosis. Radionuclide studies provide a quantitative perfusion value, an IVP contributes to the functional value, and sonograms are found more accurate in delineating fluid collections and parenchymal changes.

Sonography is a reliable method for differentiating the previously mentioned lesions from acute rejection. They may appear similar, but with the incorporation of ultrasound-guided aspiration an accurate diagnosis can be obtained. Because of its noninvasive nature, excellent display of anatomic detail, and ability to operate in the absence of renal function, ultrasound has proved to be a reliable examination in the serial evaluation of renal transplant patients.

REFERENCE

1. Maklad, N.F., Wright, C.H., and Rosenthal, S.J.: Gray scale ultrasonic appearances of renal transplant rejection, Radiology **131:**711, 1979.

15   Adrenal glands

The adrenal glands are small structures lying along the superomedial border of both kidneys. Ultrasound visualization of them may be a very tedious task in the normal patient. However, enlarged adrenal glands are imaged quite adequately with proper patient position, transducer selection, and time gain compensation settings.

ANATOMY

The adrenal glands are retroperitoneal organs that lie on the upper pole of each kidney (Fig. 15-1). At birth the ratio of their size to body weight is 20 times what it will be by adulthood, but by 1 year of age they are more proportional to body size. They are surrounded by perinephric fascia and are separated from the kidneys by the perinephric fat. Each gland as a cortex and a medulla.

The right adrenal gland is triangular or pyramidal and caps the upper pole of the right kidney. It lies posterior to the right lobe of the liver and extends medially behind the inferior vena cava. It rests posteriorly on the diaphragm.

The left adrenal gland is semilunar and extends along the medial border of the left kidney from the upper pole to the hilus. It lies posterior to the pancreas, the lesser sac, and the stomach. It also rests posteriorly on the diaphragm.

There are three arteries supplying each gland: (1) the suprarenal branch of the inferior phrenic artery, (2) the suprarenal branch of the aorta, and (3) the suprarenal branch of the renal artery. A single vein arises from the hilus of each gland and drains into the inferior vena cava on the right and into the renal vein on the left.

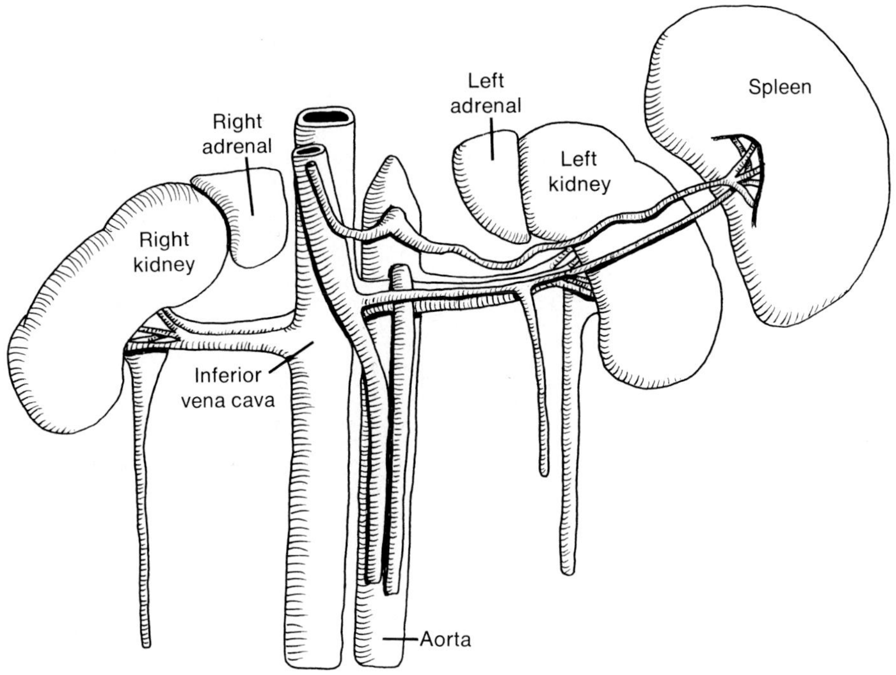

PHYSIOLOGY

Each adrenal gland is comprised of two endocrine glands. The cortex, or outer part, secretes a range of steroid hormones; the medulla, or core, secretes epinephrine and norepinephrine.

Cortex

The steroids secreted by the adrenal cortex fall into three main categories:

1. Mineralocorticoids—regulate electrolyte metabolism. Aldosterone is the principal mineralocorticoid. It has a regulatory effect on the relative concentrations of mineral ions in the body fluids and therefore on the water content of tissues. An insufficiency of this steroid leads to increased excretion of sodium and chloride ions and water into the urine. This is accompanied by a fall in sodium, chloride, and bicarbonate concentrations in the blood, resulting in a lowered pH or acidosis.
2. Glucocorticoids—play a principal role in carbohydrate metabolism. They promote deposition of liver glycogen from proteins and inhibit the utilization of glucose by the cells, thus increasing blood sugar level. Cortisone and hydrocortisone are the primary glucocorticoids. They diminish allergic re-

Fig. 15-1. AP view of the medial location of both adrenal glands.

sponse, especially the more serious inflammatory types (rheumatoid arthritis and rheumatic fever).

3. Sex hormones—androgens (male) and estrogens (female). The adrenal gland secretes both types of hormones regardless of the patient's sex. Normally these are secreted in minute quantities and have almost insignificant effects. With oversecretion, however, a marked effect is seen. Adrenal tumors in women can promote aggressive homosexuality and secondary masculine characteristics. Hypersecretion of the hormone in prepubertal boys accelerates adult masculine development and the growth of pubic hair. The adrenal cortex is controlled by ACTH (adrenocorticotropic hormone) from the pituitary. A diminished glucocorticoid blood concentration stimulates the secretion of ACTH. Consequent increase in adrenal cortex activity inhibits further ACTH secretion.

Hypofunction of the adrenal cortex in humans is called Addison's disease. Symptoms and signs include hypotension, general weakness, loss of appetite and weight, and a characteristic bronzing of the skin.

Oversecretion of the adrenal cortex may be caused by an overproduction of ACTH due to a pituitary tumor or by a tumor in the cortex itself. Cushing's disease is one type of oversecretion disease of the adrenal cortex.

Symptoms include increased sodium retention—which leads to tissue edema, increased plasma volume, and a mild alkalosis. Muscle and bone weakness is common. Secretion of androgens is increased and causes masculinizing effects in women.

Medulla[1]

The adrenal medulla makes up the core of the gland, in which groups of irregular cells are located amidst veins that collect blood from the sinusoids. This gland produces epinephrine and norepinephrine. Both of these hormones are amines, sometimes referred to as catecholamines. They elevate the blood pressure, the former working as an accelerator of the heart rate and the latter as a vasoconstrictor. The two hormones together promote glycogenolysis, the breakdown of liver glycogen to glucose, which causes an increase in blood sugar concentration.

The adrenal medulla is not essential for life and can be removed surgically without causing untreatable damage.

ULTRASOUND ANATOMY AND TECHNIQUE[5]

Although sonography has proved useful in evaluating most soft tissue structures within the abdomen, visualization of the adrenal gland has been very difficult because of its small size, medial location, and surrounding perinephric fat (Fig. 15-2).

If the adrenal gland is enlarged due to disease, it becomes an easy task to separate it from the renal parenchyma and thus determine whether the mass is cystic, solid, or somewhat calcified.

The right adrenal gland is located between the right lobe of the liver and the right crus of the diaphragm. The liver may serve as an acoustic window to visualize the echogenic adrenal gland. The gland is intimately related to the posterior aspect of the inferior vena cava and closely attached to Gerota's fascia.

The right adrenal has a comma or triangular shape in the transaxial plane. Best visualization is obtained by a transverse scan with the patient in a left lateral decubitus posi-

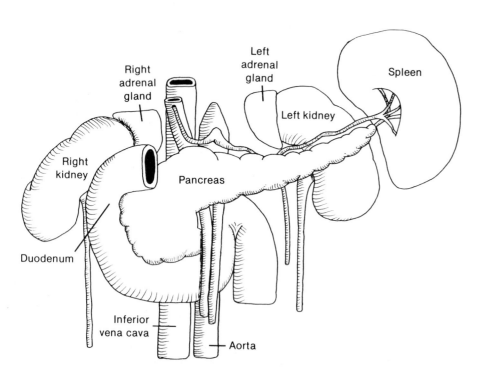

Fig. 15-2. The adrenals are often difficult to visualize because of their small size and the inability of the ultrasound beam to penetrate the duodenum, small bowel, and colon.

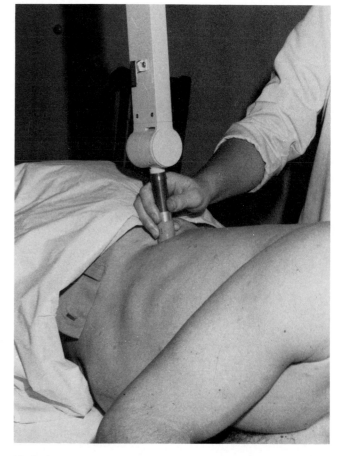

Fig. 15-3. Left decubitus position for visualizing the right adrenal gland.

tion (Fig. 15-3). As the patient assumes this position, the inferior vena cava moves forward and the aorta rolls over the crus of the diaphragm thus offering good visualization of the right kidney and adrenal area (Fig. 15-4). The pie-sweep or single-sweep technique should be utilized with the patient in mid-inspiration (Fig. 15-5). If the patient is obese, it may be difficult to recognize the triangular or crescent-shaped adrenal gland. The adrenal should not appear rounded, for this would most likely represent some sort of abnormality.

On the longitudinal scan one may sector through the right lobe of the liver perpendicular to the right crus of the diaphragm. Care must be taken to separate the retroperitoneal fat reflections from reflections of the liver, crus, and normal adrenal tissue.

The left adrenal gland is closely related to the left crus of the diaphragm and the anterosuperomedial aspect of the left kidney. It may be more difficult to image the left adrenal due to stomach interference. The patient should be placed in a right lateral decubitus position and transverse scans made in an attempt to align the left kidney and the aorta (Fig. 15-6). The longitudinal plane has both a coronal and an oblique orientation.

The left adrenal is more triangular than the right. Variations in patient respiration may help to differentiate it from the superior pole of the left kidney.

Talmont[8] states that the exact coronal or longitudinal scanning plane may be determined by making transverse scans at the level of the lower, middle, and upper poles of the kidney. A mark is placed on the patient's abdominal side to show the relationship between the kidneys and great vessels. From these points the longitudinal oblique scan can be made to image the adrenal. A slightly anterior angulation of the trans-

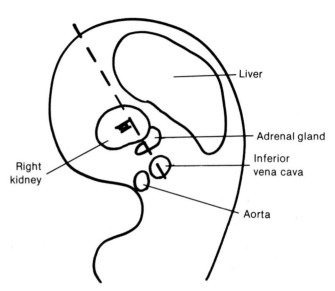

Fig. 15-4. The inferior vena cava moves forward and the aorta rolls over the crus of the diaphragm to provide good visualization of the right kidney and adrenal.

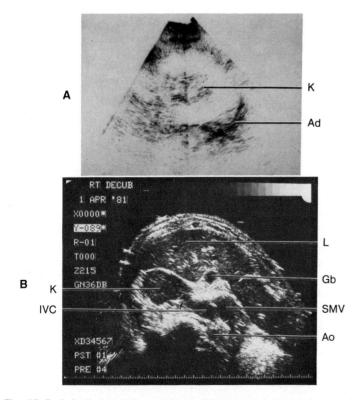

Fig. 15-5. A, Left decubitus position of the normal right adrenal gland, *Ad,* and kidney, *K.* **B,** Arrow indicates the area of the adrenal gland. Liver, *L;* kidney, *K;* gallbladder, *Gb;* inferior vena cava, *IVC;* superior mesenteric vein, *SMV;* aorta, *Ao.*

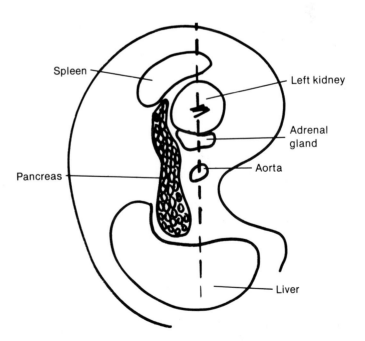

Fig. 15-6. Right decubitus position for visualizing the left adrenal gland.

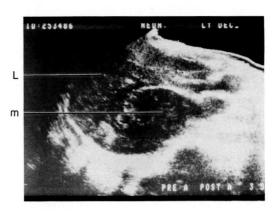

Fig. 15-7. Sagittal scan of a patient with a large pheochromocytoma in the right upper quadrant. *L*, Liver; *m*, mass. (Courtesy Marcia Lavery, R.D.M.S., New England Deaconess Hospital, Boston.)

ducer may be necessary to image the great vessels, diaphragmatic crus, and major organs adequately.

Ultrasound pitfalls[5]

1. Right crus of the diaphragm
2. Second portion of the duodenum
3. Esophagogastric junction (cephalad to the left adrenal gland)[2]
4. Medial lobulations of the spleen[7]
5. Splenic vasculature
6. Body-tail region of the pancreas
7. Fourth portion of the duodenum

Sample[3] states the normal right adrenal gland can be visualized in over 90% of patients whereas the left is seen in 80% of patients.[4]

PATHOLOGY

Sonographically adrenal cysts present a typical cystic pattern, as seen in other organs of the body having a strong back wall, no internal echoes, and good through-transmission. Adrenal cysts have the tendency to become calcified, which gives them the ultrasound appearance of a somewhat solid mass with no internal echoes (a sharp posterior border with poor through-transmission). The cyst may have hemorrhaged, and then it appears as a complex mass with multiple internal echoes and good through-transmission.

Further pathology of the adrenal glands is related to the tumors arising within them and their hyposecretion or hypersecretion of hormones. Endocrine deficiencies may be produced when the glands are destroyed by hemorrhage, infarction, or tumor.[8] Pituitary dysfunction may also play a role in the function of the adrenals and their control of hormones.

There are several cortical syndromes that

the sonographer may encounter while scanning for an adrenal mass.[8]

1. Addison's disease. This may be of adrenal or pituitary origin and is the chronic result of adrenal hypofunction. The deficiency may be due to a primary adrenal tumor or to metastases.
2. Adrenogenital syndrome. This is due to excessive secretion of the sex hormones.
3. Conn's syndrome. This is caused by excessive secretion of aldosterone, usually due to a cortical adenoma.
4. Cushing's syndrome. This is produced by excessive secretion of glucocorticoids due to hyperplasia, a benign tumor, or carcinoma. The syndrome can also be caused by an anterior pituitary tumor.
5. Waterhouse-Friderichsen syndrome. This is commonly due to bilateral hemorrhage into the adrenal glands.

The pheochromocytes of the adrenal medulla may produce a tumor called a pheochromocytoma that secretes epinephrine and norepinephrine in excessive quantities. These patients present with intermittent hypertension. The tumor has a homogeneous pattern that can be differentiated from a cyst by its weak posterior wall and poor through-transmission. Pheochromocytomas may be large bulky tumors with a variety of sonographic patterns including cystic, solid, and calcified components[6] (Fig. 15-7).

Most adrenal carcinomas are not functional, but they may account for Cushing's syndrome or hyperaldosteronemia.[6] The origin of the tumor should be clearly defined. Metastases to the adrenals vary in size and echogenicity (Figs. 15-8 and 15-9). Often central necrosis will cause areas of sonolucency within the tumor.

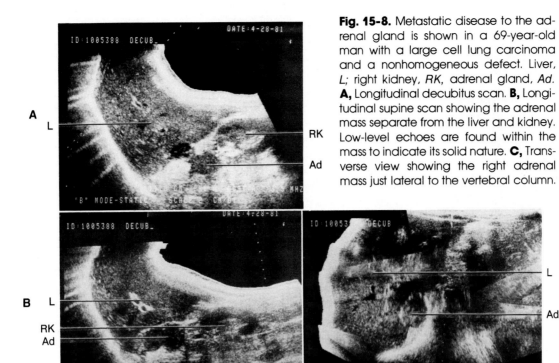

Fig. 15-8. Metastatic disease to the adrenal gland is shown in a 69-year-old man with a large cell lung carcinoma and a nonhomogeneous defect. Liver, *L*; right kidney, *RK*, adrenal gland, *Ad*. **A,** Longitudinal decubitus scan. **B,** Longitudinal supine scan showing the adrenal mass separate from the liver and kidney. Low-level echoes are found within the mass to indicate its solid nature. **C,** Transverse view showing the right adrenal mass just lateral to the vertebral column.

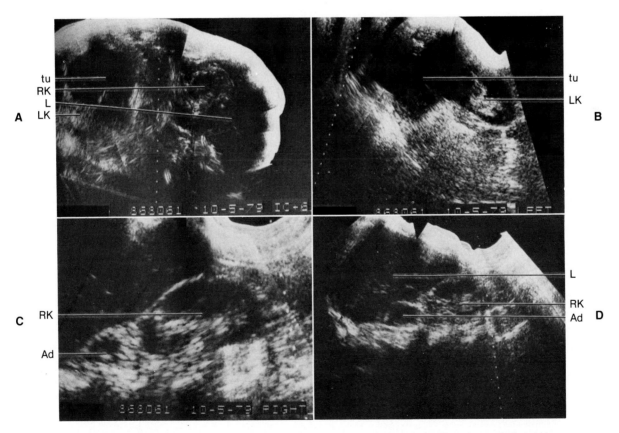

Fig. 15-9. Metastatic disease to the adrenal gland in a patient with a large left renal tumor. **A,** Transverse prone scan. **B,** Sagittal scan. The tumor is growing off the upper pole of the left kidney. **C,** Supine sagittal scan of the right kidney and adrenal metastases. **D,** Supine sagittal scan through the liver, right kidney, and adrenal mass. The liver offers an excellent window to visualize the right kidney and adrenal gland. Left kidney, *LK*; tumor, *tu*; right kidney, *RK*; liver, *L*; adrenal gland, *Ad*.

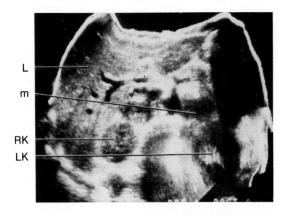

Fig. 15-10. Transverse scan of a patient with bilateral adrenal metastases secondary to oat cell carcinoma. *L,* liver; *RK,* right kidney; *LK,* left kidney; *m,* mass. (Courtesy Marcia Lavery, R.D.M.S., New England Deaconess Hospital, Boston.)

The adrenal neuroblastoma is the commonest malignancy of the adrenal glands in childhood and the most common tumor of infancy. Generally it arises within the adrenal medulla. Although children are usually asymptomatic, some do present with a palpable abdominal mass that must be differentiated from a neonatal hemorrhage and hydronephrosis.[6] Sonographically the tumor appears as an echogenic mass. It may be large, and evaluation of the surrounding retroperitoneum and liver should be made to rule out metastases (Fig. 15-10).

REFERENCES

1. Anderson, P.D.: Clinical anatomy and physiology for allied health sciences, Philadelphia, 1976, W.B. Saunders Co.
2. Rao, A.K.R., and Silver, T.M.: Normal pancreas and splenic variants simulating suprarenal and renal tumors, A.J.R. **126:**530, 1976.
3. Sample, W.F.: A new technique for the evaluation of the adrenal gland with gray scale ultrasonography, Radiology **124:**463, 1977.
4. Sample, W.F.: Adrenal ultrasonography, Radiology **127:**461, 1978.
5. Sample, W.F.: Ultrasonography of the adrenal gland. In Resnick, M.I., and Sanders, R.C., editors: Ultrasound in urology, Baltimore, 1979, The Williams & Wilkins Co.
6. Sample, W.F.: Renal, adrenal, retroperitoneal, and scrotal ultrasonography. In Sarti, D.A., and Sample, W.F., editors: Diagnostic ultrasound; text and cases, Boston, 1980, G.K. Hall & Co.
7. Sample, W.F., and Sarti, D.A.: Computed tomography and gray scale ultrasonography of the adrenal gland; a comparative study, Radiology **128:**377, 1978.
8. Talmont, C.A.: Adrenal glands. In Taylor, K.J.W., et al., editors: Manual of ultrasonography, New York, 1980, Churchill Livingstone, Inc.

16 Spleen

ANATOMY
Normal anatomy

The spleen lies in the left hypochondrium, with its axis along the shaft of the tenth rib. Its lower pole extends forward as far as the midaxillary line. It is of variable size and shape but generally is considered to be ovoid with a convex superior and a concave inferior surface. The vessels that supply it enter at the hilum. The spleen is an intraperitoneal organ, being covered with peritoneum over its entire extent except for a small area at its hilum. Regardless of its shape, the ends of the spleen are called its posterior and anterior extremities; and its borders are superior and inferior. Accessory spleens occasionally are found near the hilum of the spleen.

The spleen is the largest single mass of lymphoid tissue in the body. It is active in blood formation during the initial part of fetal life. This function decreases so that by the fifth or sixth month of gestation the spleen assumes its adult character and discontinues its hematopoietic activity.

Relational anatomy

Anterior to the spleen lie the stomach, tail of the pancreas, and left colic flexure (Fig. 16-1). The left kidney lies along its medial border. Posteriorly the diaphragm, left pleura, left lung, and ninth, tenth, and eleventh ribs are in contact with the spleen (Fig. 16-2).

Blood is supplied by the splenic artery, which travels along the superior border of the pancreas. Upon entering the spleen at the hilum, this artery immediately divides into about six branches.

The splenic vein leaves the hilum and joins the superior mesenteric vein to form the portal vein. This vessel travels along the posterior medial aspect of the pancreas.

The lymph vessels emerging from the hilum pass through a few lymph nodes along the course of the splenic artery and drain into the celiac nodes. The nerves to the spleen accompany the splenic artery and are derived from the celiac plexus.

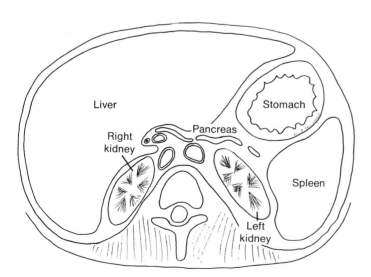

Fig. 16-1. Transverse diagram of the upper abdomen demonstrating the posterior position of the spleen posterior to the stomach and lateral to the left kidney.

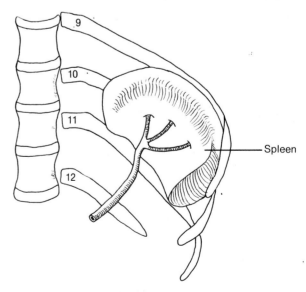

Fig. 16-2. Anteroposterior location of the spleen against the costal margin of the ninth, tenth, and eleventh ribs.

PHYSIOLOGY

The red pulp of the spleen is composed of two principal elements—the splenic *sinuses* alternating with splenic *cords*. The sinuses are long irregular channels lined by endothelial cells or flattened reticular cells. A recent study indicated that there are pores or gaps between the lining cells, implying that the circulation is open and that blood cells can freely leave the sinuses to enter the intervening cords. The membrane shared by a cord and its adjacent sinuses is also perforated. Reticular cells with delicate processes sometimes bridge the cords. Thus these highly phagocytic cells create an open meshwork with the cords. The blood that leaves the splenic sinuses to enter the reticular cords passes through a complex filter.

The venous drainage of the sinuses and cords is not well defined, but it is assumed that tributaries of the splenic vein connect with the sinuses of the red pulp. From here the splenic vein follows the course of the artery, eventually joining the superior mesenteric vein to form the portal vein.

The white pulp of the spleen consists of the malpighian corpuscles, small nodular masses of lymphoid tissue attached to the smaller arterial branches. Extending from the splenic capsule inward are the trabeculae, containing blood vessels and lymphatics. The lymphoid tissue, or malpighian corpuscles, has the same structure as the follicles in the lymph nodes; but it differs in that the splenic follicles surround arteries, so that on cross section each contains a central artery. These follicles are scattered throughout the organ and are not confined to the peripheral layer or cortex, as are lymph nodes.

The spleen as part of the reticuloendothelial system plays an important role in the defense mechanism of the body and is also implicated in pigment and lipid metabolism. It is not essential to life, and it can be removed with no ill effects. The functions of the spleen may be classified under two general headings—those which reflect the functions of the reticuloendothelial system and those which are characteristic of the organ itself.

The functions of the spleen as an organ of the reticuloendothelial system are (1) the production of lymphocytes and plasma cells, (2) the production of antibodies, (3) the storage of iron, and (4) the storage of other metabolites. The functions characteristic of the organ include (1) maturation of the surface of erythrocytes, (2) reservoir function, (3)

culling function, (4) pitting function, and (5) disposal of senescent or abnormal erythrocytes; also included are functions related to platelet life span and leukocyte life span.

The role of the spleen as an immunologic organ concerns the production of cells capable of making antibodies (lymphocytes and plasma cells); however, it should be understood that antibodies are also produced at other sites.

Phagocytosis of erythrocytes and the breakdown of the hemoglobin occur throughout the entire reticuloendothelial system, but roughly half the catabolic activity is localized in the normal spleen. In splenomegaly the major portion of hemoglobin breakdown occurs in the spleen. The iron that is liberated is stored in the splenic phagocytes. In anomalies such as the hemolytic anemias, the splenic phagocytes become engorged with hemosiderin when erythrocyte destruction is accelerated.

In addition to storing iron, the spleen is subject to the storage diseases such as Gaucher's disease and Niemann-Pick disease. Abnormal lipid metabolites accumulate in all phagocytic reticuloendothelial cells but may also involve the phagocytes in the spleen, producing gross splenomegaly.

The functions of the spleen that are characteristic of the organ relate primarily to the circulation of erythrocytes through it. In a normal individual the spleen contains only about 20 to 30 ml of erythrocytes. In splenomegaly the reservoir function is greatly increased, and the abnormally enlarged spleen contains many times this volume of red blood cells. The transit time is lengthened, and the erythrocytes are subject to destructive effects for a long time. In part, ptosis causes consumption of glucose, on which the erythrocyte is dependent for the maintenance of normal metabolism, and the erythrocyte is destroyed. Selective destruction of abnormal erythrocytes is also accelerated by the splenic pooling.

As erythrocytes pass through the spleen, the organ inspects them for imperfections and destroys those it recognizes as abnormal or senescent. This is called the *culling* function. The *pitting* function is a process by which the spleen removes granular inclusions without destroying the erythrocytes. The normal function of the spleen keeps the number of circulating erythrocytes with inclusions at a minimum.

The spleen also pools platelets in large numbers. The entry of platelets into the splenic pool and their return to the circula-

tion are extensive. In splenomegaly the splenic pool may be so large that it produces thrombocytopenia. Sequestration of leukocytes in the enlarged spleen may produce leukopenia.

PATHOLOGIC CONDITIONS

As the largest unit of the reticuloendothelial system the spleen is involved in all systemic inflammations and generalized hematopoietic disorders, and many metabolic disturbances. It is rarely the primary site of disease. Whenever the spleen is involved in systemic disease, splenic enlargement usually develops; and therefore splenomegaly is a major manifestation of disorders of this organ.[7]

Congenital anomalies

Complete absence of the spleen (asplenia or agenesis of the spleen) is rare and, by itself, causes no difficulties. Often, however, asplenia is associated with congenital heart disease (e.g., defects in or absence of the atrial or atrioventricular canal, pulmonary stenosis or atresia, transposition of the great vessels).

Accessory spleen is a more common congenital anomaly. One of every six accessory spleens is located in the tail of the pancreas. Lesions affecting the main spleen usually affect the accessory spleen as well.

Regressive changes

Hyalinization. Hyaline degeneration of the arterial wall may be found in persons of any age and is nonspecific. In young patients it often accompanies hypertension.

Amyloidosis. In systemic diseases leading to amyloidosis the spleen is the organ most frequently involved. It may be of normal size or decidedly enlarged depending on the amount and distribution of amyloid. Two types of involvement are seen—modular and diffuse. In the modular type, amyloid is found in the walls of the sheathed arteries and within the follicles but not in the red pulp. In the diffuse type the follicles are not involved, the red pulp is prominently involved, and the spleen is usually greatly enlarged and firm.

Atrophy. Atrophy of the spleen (50 to 70 g) is not uncommon in normal individuals. It may also occur in wasting diseases. In chronic hemolytic anemias, particularly sickle cell anemia, there is excessive loss of pulp, increasing fibrosis, scarring from multiple infarcts, and incrustation with iron and calcium deposits. In the final stages of atrophy the spleen may be so small that it is hardly recognizable. Advanced atrophy is sometimes referred to as autosplenectomy.

Pigmentation

The pigments found in the spleen are (1) hemosiderin and hematoidin, which are derived from hemoglobin; (2) malarial pigment; and (3) anthracotic pigments. Large amounts of hemosiderin are deposited in all phagocytic cells of the reticuloendothelial system when there is iron excess, as in chronic hemolytic anemia or after many blood transfusions. Deposits of hemosiderin iron in the spleen in abnormally large amounts is called siderosis. In moderate amounts it produces little effect on the tissue. In large amounts it stimulates proliferation of fibrous tissue. The nature of the pigment called hematoidin is largely unknown. It is formed in areas of hemorrhage or infarction.

In malaria the black pigment imparts a dark brown color to the pulp of the spleen. The pigment is of the hematin type and is found within phagocytes.

Anthracotic pigmentation of the spleen is rare.

Rupture

Rupture of the spleen is usually caused by a crushing injury or a severe blow. Much less often it is encountered in the apparent absence of trauma and is described as spontaneous rupture. Spontaneous rupture is encountered most often when the spleen is enlarged and soft in diseases such as infectious mononucleosis, leukemia, malaria, typhoid fever, and other types of acute splenitis.

Nonspecific acute splenitis

In nonspecific acute splenitis the spleen is enlarged by 200 to 400 g and is soft. On section the pulp is often diffluent. The most common disease conditions producing acute splenitis are bacteremia, as in vegetative endocarditis; but any other severe systemic inflammatory disorder such as diphtheria, bacillary dysentery, or pneumonia may effect similar splenic changes. Acute splenitis may be induced by noninfectious disease and is encountered in any extensive tissue destruction of chemical or physical nature, presumably because the spleen is active in resorption of necrotic cell products.

Nonspecific subacute or chronic splenitis

The organ with nonspecific subacute or chronic splenitis is enlarged, but rarely as much as 1000 g, and is firm. This condition is seen most commonly in certain diseases that will be described later. The next most frequent cause is vegetative (bacterial) endocarditis.

Specific forms of splenitis

The specific infections that may affect the spleen are tuberculosis, syphilis, typhoid fever, brucellosis, malaria, sarcoid infectious mononucleosis, kala azar, histoplasmosis, torulosis, schistosomiasis, anthrax, actinomycosis, blastomycosis, echinococcosis, and cysticercosis. The more common infections will be discussed.

Tuberculosis. Although rare in adults, splenic involvement is common in children with pulmonary tuberculosis. The spleen is enlarged but usually does not exceed 500 or 600 g. The tubercles are usually found in the malpighian corpuscles.

Syphilis. The spleen is often enlarged in congenital syphilis, but rarely more than twice its normal size. It is firm and microscopically shows an infiltration of lymphocytes and plasma cells and an increase in connective tissue. In both congenital syphilis and acquired syphilis, gummas occur rarely. Splenomegaly in the tertiary stage usually follows the congestive changes induced by luetic cirrhosis of the liver.

Typhoid fever. The spleen is characteristically enlarged in the range of 250 to 500 g. The outstanding feature is the filling of the pulp with histiocytic cells containing numerous phagocytized red cells, although focal necrosis similar to that seen in other organs is present. The lining cells of the sinuses are hypertrophic and often display active phagocytosis of red cells and other cellular debris.

Malaria. In the acute stage of malaria the spleen is enlarged and soft. In the chronic stage it is greatly swollen, usually in the range of 1000 g but possibly as much as 4000 g, and is firm.

Sarcoid infectious mononucleosis. The spleen is enlarged in at least 50% of cases, usually two or three times its normal size. It is generally soft, fleshy, and hyperemic.

Vascular disease

Acute congestion. Active hyperemia accompanies the reaction in the spleen to acute systemic infections. The spleen is moderately enlarged, rarely over 250 g.

Chronic congestion. Chronic venous congestion may cause enlargement of the spleen, a condition referred to as congestive splenomegaly. The venous congestion may be of systemic origin, caused by intrahepatic obstruction to portal venous drainage or by obstructive venous disorders in the portal or splenic veins. Systemic venous congestion is found in cardiac decompensation involving the right side of the heart. It is particularly severe in tricuspid or pulmonary valvular disease and in chronic cor pulmonale.

The most common causes of striking congestive splenomegaly are the various forms of cirrhosis of the liver. It is also caused by obstruction to the extrahepatic portal or splenic vein (e.g., spontaneous portal vein thrombosis).

Long-standing congestive splenomegaly results in severe swelling of the spleen (1000 g or more).

Hypersplenism. Hypersplenism is a symptom complex characterized by congestive splenomegaly, leukopenia, and anemia (McMichael, 1934). It was referred to as Bonti's disease and was considered a primary hematologic disorder with secondary involvement of the spleen. Currently splenic involvement is believed to be primary.

The hypersplenic syndrome has been divided into primary and secondary types. In primary hypersplenism there is increased splenic activity and size of unknown cause. Secondary hypersplenism may occur in patients whose splenomegaly has a known origin, such as leukemia or lymphoma. In both forms the spleen is almost always enlarged.

Infarcts. Splenic infarcts are comparatively common lesions caused by occlusion of the major splenic artery or any of its branches. They are almost always due to emboli that arise in the heart, produced either from mural thrombi in the left auricle or ventricle or from vegetation on the valves of the left side of the heart.

Hemolytic anemia

Hemolytic anemia is the general term applied to anemia referable to decreased life of the erythrocytes. When the rate of destruction is greater than can be compensated by the bone marrow, then anemia results.

Disorders involving red cells

Hereditary or congenital spherocytosis. In this disorder the spleen may be enlarged and sometimes weighs over 1000 g. An intrinsic abnormality of the red cells gives rise to erythrocytes that are small and spheroid rather than the normal, flattened, biconcave disks. The two results of this disease are the production by the bone marrow

Table 16-1. Pathologic classification of splenic disorders

Hematopoietic	Reticuloendothelial hyperactivity (normal)
Granulocytopoiesis	Still's disease
Reactive hyperplasia to acute and chronic infection (low sonodensity)	Wilson's disease
Noncaseous granulomatous inflammation	Felty's syndrome
	Reticulum cell sarcoma
Myeloproliferative syndromes (normal)	
Chronic myelogenous leukemia	**Congestion (normal or low sonodensity)**
Acute myelogenous leukemia	Hepatocellular disease
Lymphopoiesis (low sonodensity or focal sonolucent)	
Chronic lymphocytic leukemia	**Nonspecific**
Lymphoma	Neoplasm-metastasis (focal sonodense)
Hodgkin's disease	Cyst (focal sonolucent)
Erythropoiesis (normal)	Abscess (focal sonolucent)
Sickle cell disease	Malignant neoplasm (focal sonolucent)
Hereditary spherocytosis	Hodgkin's disease
Hemolytic anemia	Lymphoma
Chronic anemia	Benign neoplasm (focal sonolucent)
Myeloproliferative syndrome	Lymphangiomatosis
Chronic myelogenous leukemia	Hematoma (perisplenic)
Acute myelogenous leukemia	
Other	
Multiple myeloma (low sonodensity)	

From Mittelstaedt, C.A., and Partain, C.L.: Radiology **134:**697, 1980.

of spherocytic erythrocytes and the increased destruction of these cells in the spleen. The spleen destroys spherocytes selectively.

Sickle cell anemia. In the earlier stage of this disease, as seen in infants and children, the spleen is enlarged with marked congestion of the red pulp. Later the spleen undergoes progressive infarction and fibrosis and decreases in size until, in adults, only a small mass of fibrous tissue may be found, weighing less than 1 g (autosplenectomy). It is generally believed that these changes result when sickled cells plug the vasculature of the splenic substance, effectively producing ischemic destruction of the spleen.

Polycythemia vera. The spleen is variably enlarged, rather firm, and blue-red. It usually weighs about 350 g, and infarcts and thrombosis are common.

Thalassemia. The spleen is severely involved. This hemoglobinopathy differs from the others in that an abnormal molecular form of hemoglobin is not present. Instead, there is a suppression of synthesis of beta or alpha polypeptide chains, resulting in deficient synthesis of normal hemoglobin. The erythrocytes are not only deficient in normal hemoglobin but also abnormal in shape; many are target cells whereas others vary considerably in size and shape. Their life span is short because they are destroyed by the spleen in large numbers.

The disease ranges from mild to severe. The changes in the spleen are greatest in the severe form, called thalassemia major. The spleen is very large, often seeming to fill the entire abdominal cavity.

Autoimmune hemolytic anemia. This type of anemia can occur in its primary form without underlying disease, or it may be seen as a secondary disorder in patients already suffering from some disorder of the reticuloendothelial or hematopoietic systems, such as lymphoma, leukemia, or infectious mononucleosis. In the secondary form the splenic changes are dominated by the underlying disease; in the primary form the spleen is variably enlarged.

Disorders involving white cells

Leukemia. Chronic myelogenous leukemia may be responsible for more extreme splenomegaly than is any other disease. Depending on the duration of the disorder, the spleen may weigh anywhere from 1000 to 3000 g. Weights of 6000 to 8000 g are not rare. The organ is symmetrically enlarged and firm, and its capsule may be quite thickened.

Chronic lymphatic leukemia. This disorder produces less severe degrees of splenomegaly. The spleen rarely exceeds 2000 g.

Monocytic leukemia. This kind of leukemia causes mild splenomegaly, rarely producing a spleen over 500 g.

Reticuloendotheliosis

Gaucher's disease. All age groups can be affected by Gaucher's disease. About 50% of patients are under the age of 8 years and 17% under 1 year. Clinical features follow a chronic course, with changes in skin pigmentation and bone pain. Usually the first sign is splenomegaly, enlarging the spleen to as much as 8000 g.

Niemann-Pick disease. This rapidly fatal disease predominantly affects female infants. The clinical features consist of hepatomegaly, digestive disturbances, and lymphadenopathy.

Letterer-Siwe disease. This is sometimes called nonlipid reticuloendotheliosis, and there is proliferation of reticuloendothelial cells in all tissues but particularly in the spleen lymph nodes and bone marrow. Usually the spleen is only moderately enlarged, although the change may be more severe in affected older infants. This disease is generally found in children below the age of 2 years. Clinical features are hepatosplenomegaly, fever, and pulmonary involvement. It is rapidly fatal, as well.

Hand-Schüller-Christian disease. This disorder is benign and chronic in spite of many features similar to those of Letterer-Siwe disease. It usually affects children over 2 years of age. This clinical features are a chronic course, diabetes, and moderate hepatosplenomegaly.

Primary tumors of the spleen

In general, primary tumors of the spleen, either benign or malignant, are rare.

Benign tumors. The cavernous hemangioma is the most common primary tumor of the spleen. Next in frequency is the lymphangioma. These may be very large, consisting of multicystic lesions. Other tumors that may arise in the spleen are fibromas, osteomas, and chondromas.

Malignant tumors. Any of the types of lymphomas or Hodgkin's disease found in the lymph nodes may be primary in the spleen, and they have the same characteristics as in the lymph nodes. Hemangiosarcomas with metastases, especially to the liver, are also known to occur.

The most common secondary tumors are sarcomas, principally the so-called malignant lymphoma group, and Hodgkin's disease.

Metastases of other types of tumors, especially carcinomas, are rare and usually occur only when generalized carcinomatosis has developed. An exception is widely disseminated melanocarcinoma that involves the spleen in about half the cases.

Summary of splenic disorders

Disorders that usually cause massive enlargement of the spleen (over 1000 g) are chronic myelogenous leukemia, chronic lymphatic leukemia (less massive than the myelogenous form), lymphomas, primary or secondary, Gaucher's disease, myeloproliferative syndrome, primary tumors of the spleen (extremely uncommon, but both benign and malignant tumors may cause massive irregular splenomegaly), malaria, kala azar, and other parasitic infestations such as an *Echinococcus* cyst. Congestive splenomegaly due to portal or splenic vein obstruction usually causes moderate enlargement (500 to 1000 g). Disorders brought about by this condition include chronic splenitis (particularly vegetative bacterial endocarditis), tuberculosis, sarcoid tumor, typhoid fever, chronic congestive splenomegaly, sickle cell anemia in early stages, hereditary spherocytosis, metastatic carcinoma or sarcoma, infectious mononucleosis, acute leukemias, Niemann-Pick disease, Hand-Schüller-Christian disease, thalassemia, autoimmune hemolytic anemia, idiopathic thrombocytopenia, and Hodgkin's disease. Conditions causing minimal splenomegaly (usually under 500 g) are acute splenitis, acute splenic congestion, and miscellaneous acute febrile disorders such as bacteremic states, systemic toxemias, systemic lupus erythematosus, and intraabdominal infections (Table 16-1).

ULTRASONIC EVALUATION OF THE SPLEEN
Normal texture and patterns

Sonographically the spleen should stipple in with fine homogeneous low-level echoes as is seen within the liver parenchyma (Fig. 16-3). Cooperberg[1] states that the spleen has two components joined at the hilum. On transverse scans it has a crescentic appearance usually with a large medial component. As one moves inferiorly, only the lateral component is imaged. On longitudinal scans the superior component extends more medially than the inferior component. The irregularity of these components makes it difficult to assess mild splenomegaly accurately.

Patient position and technique

On transverse supine scans the transducer should be moved to the far left posterior side of the patient and angled sharply anteriomedially between the ribs. Generally the stomach and ribs prohibit such visualization of the spleen, and only an outline can be noted from a scan along the left upper abdomen. If adequate visualization cannot be made from the supine position, the patient should be rotated to a prone or right lateral decubitus position in an effort to eliminate interference from the stomach and bowel.

The prone scan is obtained with a slight cephalic angulation of the transducer head. Transverse scans are probably the easiest in which to orient the transducer (Fig. 16-4). When the left kidney is well seen, serial scans are made by moving the transducer gradually cephalad in 1-cm steps. As the scan moves superiorly from the caliceal area of the kidney, the spleen should be identified along the left lateral border (Fig. 16-5). Single scans are probably the best for avoiding rib artifacts. This view may give additional information about the splenic parenchyma, but the best information is probably obtained from the right lateral decubitus position.

The decubitus, or axillary, position enables the sonographer to scan in an oblique fashion between the ribs (Fig. 16-6). The scan arm should be angled slightly medially to allow the spleen to be visualized inferior to the diaphragm and superior and lateral to the left kidney. If the intercostal spaces are narrow, a smaller-diameter transducer may be used to provide more sector capability.

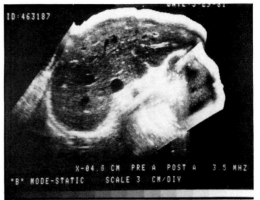
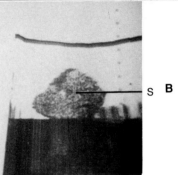

Fig. 16-3. A, The normal texture of the spleen should be stippled with fine homogeneous echoes, as seen in the liver parenchyma. **B,** Normal pattern of splenic parenchyma as shown in a water bath.

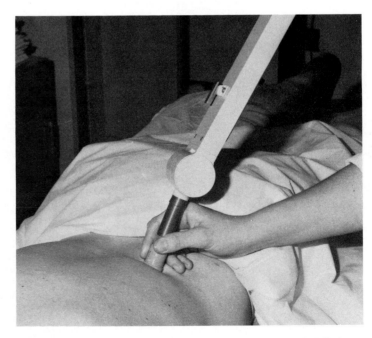

Fig. 16-4. The arm of the transducer should be angled slightly toward the midline of the spine.

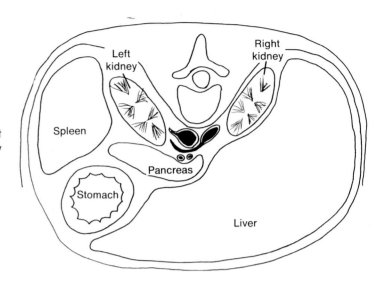

Fig. 16-5. Prone transverse schematic showing the relation of the left kidney to the spleen, pancreas, and stomach and the right kidney to the liver.

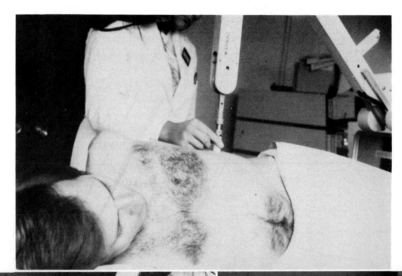

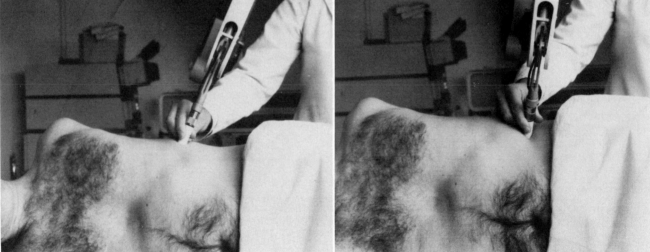

Fig. 16-6. The decubitus position permits scanning between the ribs to record maximal information from the splenic parenchyma.

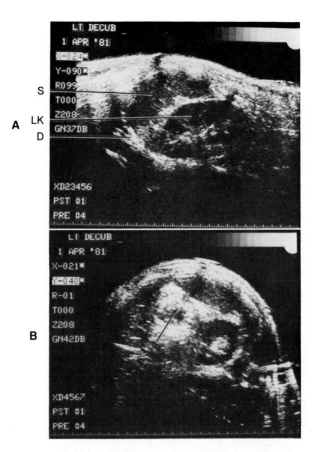

Fig. 16-8. A, Sagittal scan of the left upper quadrant with the patient in a decubitus position demonstrating the left kidney, *LK*, spleen, *S*, and diaphragm, *D*. **B,** Transverse view showing the stomach *(arrow)* anterior to the spleen and left kidney.

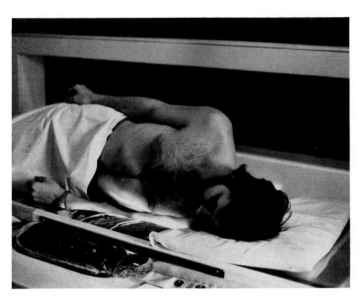

Fig. 16-7. A water path delay scanner, the Octoson, allows visualization of the left upper quadrant without rib interference.

Table 16-2. Ultrasonic-pathologic classification of splenic disorders

Uniform splenic sonodensity		Focal defects		Perisplenic defects
Normal sonodensity	**Low sonodensity**	**Sonodense**	**Sonolucent**	
Erythropoiesis (including myeloproliferative disorders) Reticuloendothelial hyperactivity Congestion	Granulocytopoiesis (excluding myelo-disorders) Lymphopoiesis Other (multiple myeloma) Congestion	Nonspecific (metasta-sis)	Nonspecific (benign primary neoplasm, cyst, abscess, malignant neoplasm [lymphopoietic])	Nonspecific (hematoma)

From Mittelstaedt, C.A., and Partain, C.L.: Radiology **134:**697, 1980.

Various degrees of arcing the transducer through the costal margins may be necessary to demonstrate the fine homogeneous splenic parenchyma. Longitudinal decubitus scans can also be performed for an additional view. One avoids the ribs by merely skipping over them as the scan is being made.

The automated scanners with a water path delay are excellent machines, in which visualization of the splenic parenchyma is made without rib interference (Fig. 16-7).

They enable the sonographer to glide over the splenic area without transducer hangup at the ribs (Fig. 16-8).

Real time sector transducers are also excellent for visualizing the left upper quadrant. They allow more freedom of movement than the articulated arm transducer. Thus the sonographer can successfully manipulate the transducer between costal margins to image the left kidney, spleen, and diaphragm adequately (Table 16-2).

Pathology

Splenomegaly. Although the spleen is sometimes difficult to visualize when the patient is supine, this position often allows a clearer insight into splenic enlargement. One can compare the size of the spleen with that of the liver. Usually the spleen is not well visualized until 9 to 11 cm above the umbilicus. Generally most of the liver is well visualized at the time of splenic visualization. In patients with splenomegaly the spleen may be seen as low as the umbilicus (Fig. 16-9).

Leopold and Asher reported (1975) that one of the echo signs of splenic enlargement in the supine position is visualization of the tip of the spleen exceeding the vertebral column in the transverse lateral projection (Fig. 16-10). However, the examiner must be careful not to use this guide as the sole criterion for a diagnosis of enlargement. Like the liver, the spleen has various shapes and sizes and can be normal even when it exceeds the border of the vertebral column. Generally the spleen lies posterior in the left upper quadrant, but occasionally it will lie

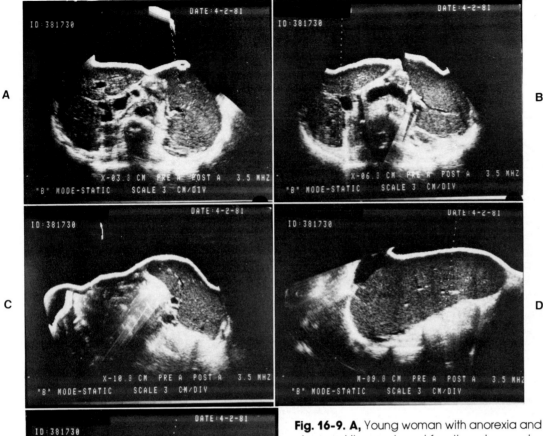

Fig. 16-9. A, Young woman with anorexia and abnormal liver and renal functions shows splenomegaly in this scan taken 3.8 cm below the xyphoid. **B,** Subsequent scan demonstrating a prominent splenic hilum. **C,** The enlarged spleen is still seen at the level of the umbilicus. No liver parenchyma is seen. **D,** Sagittal scan of the splenomegaly with fine uniform parenchymal echoes. **E,** Sagittal scan over the prominent splenic hilum.

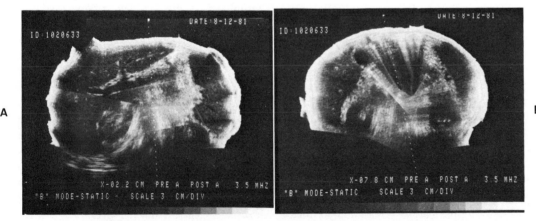

Fig. 16-10. A, A young alcoholic with hepatitis shows hepatosplenomegaly. **B,** The spleen extends along the lateral margin almost to the anterior abdominal wall. Because of the splenomegaly, the left kidney is well seen.

fairly lateral along the left abdominal wall. In this instance visualization of the left kidney and tail of the pancreas may be enhanced.

The determination of splenic enlargement is essential; once that has been established, the pathway to analyzing the cause for enlargement can be evaluated. It may be a general splenomegaly due to a blood disorder, alcoholic cirrhosis, or other reasons; or it may be splenomegaly secondary to a hemorrhage, tumor, or cyst (Figs. 16-11 and 16-12).

Splenic volume. Numerous authors have described a method for calculating splenic volume that correlates well with autopsy results. Koga's method[3] utilizes the decubitus long axis of the spleen. The splenic volume (V) in cubic centimeters is calculated as a function of the sectional area (S) in square centimeters by the following formula:

$$V = 7.53S - 77.56$$

Congenital anomalies. Splenic agenesis may be ruled out by the demonstration of a spleen. The sonographer should be alert not to confuse the bowel, which may lie in the same area, with the spleen. Evaluation of the left upper quadrant with real time should enable one to make the distinction.

An accessory spleen may be difficult to demonstrate by sonography if it is very small. When seen, it may appear as a low-level mass near the splenic hilum.

Splenic trauma. If the patient has left upper quadrant pain secondary to trauma, a splenic hematoma or subcapsular hematoma should be considered (Fig. 16-13). The patient should be scanned in the supine position first; then scans should be made in the prone and decubitus positions to define the hematoma (Fig. 16-14). Increased gain settings can be used to define the extent of the hematoma. If the blood has organized, it may appear as an echo-free area within the spleen. If it has clotted, it may appear as a complex mass. A subcapsular hematoma generally will appear as a complex mass partially surrounding the splenic capsule. If the patient has a slightly enlarged spleen without signs of organized hematoma, serial scans performed 6 hours apart may be helpful in the clinical diagnosis. The serial scans are especially helpful for trauma patients who can afford to wait the 5 or 6 hours necessary between scans for a determination of enlargement to be made. A baseline scan is done as soon as the patient arrives, with follow-up serial scans to a 24-hour period.

Splenic cyst. Echographically a splenic cyst appears as an echo-free area with smooth

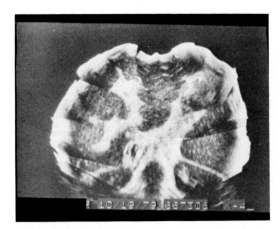

Fig. 16-11. Transverse scan over the upper abdomen in a patient with lymphoma showing a prominent spleen with no focal defects.

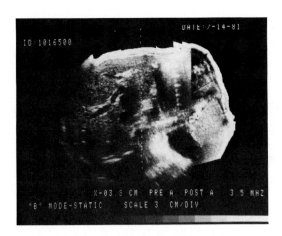

Fig. 16-12. Transverse scan over the upper abdomen in a patient with splenomegaly and a very echogenic parenchyma.

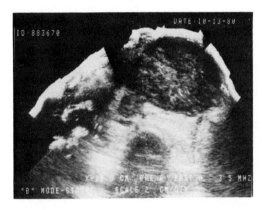

Fig. 16-13. A young soccer player presented 2 days after suffering a severe blow to his left flank. A splenic hematoma was demonstrated.

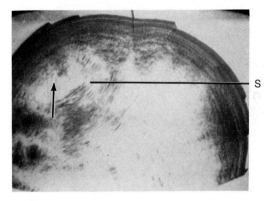

Fig. 16-14. Prone scan of an echo-free area within the periphery of the spleen. This proved to be a splenic hematoma. The patient had a filling defect on the nuclear medicine scan as well.

well-defined borders and good enhancement posterior to its border. Large cysts will be seen to cause splenomegaly and compression of normal splenic tissue whereas smaller cysts may be demonstrated within the outline of the spleen.[1]

It may be difficult to distinguish a splenic cyst from a renal cyst or pseudocyst. Careful evaluation of these other organ systems should define their normal contour and obviate the problem. Compression of normal structures sometimes is helpful in determining the origin of the mass. A splenic cyst may compress the renal parenchyma or even the tail of the pancreas. Of course, clinical evaluation of the patient is important in determining the differential diagnosis.

The sonographic appearance of a hemorrhagic splenic cyst has been described as a cystic mass with a gravity-dependent layering of two fluids each with distinctly different reflectivities. The difference in reflectivity is thought to be related to the amount of particulate matter within each fluid layer.[6]

Neoplasms. Splenic tumors are not seen as commonly as other tumors in the abdomen, and thus experience in their ultrasonic evaluation is limited.

Increased echogenicity of the spleen was reported by Siler et al.,[8] who stated that the spleen is often pathologically involved in patients with leukemia and lymphoma. In leukemia, spleens were grossly enlarged and firm and microscopically showed diffuse and focal infiltrates of leukemic cells. Numerous small infarcts could be seen throughout the parenchyma. Progression of the disease brought further disruption of architecture throughout the spleen. In non-Hodgkin lymphoma, diffuse or nodular masses of cells were demonstrated. This underlying structural similiarity between these diseases may be the reason for the increased echogenicity in infiltrating hematopoietic malignancies of the spleen. The particular stage at which the patient presents for a sonogram may also influence the echogenicity of the spleen.

In another study, by Murphy and Bernar-

dino,[5] a limited number of patients with metastases to the spleen were studied by sonography. Hypoechoic lesions were seen in patients with histiocytic lymphoma, and both echogenic and hypoechoic lesions were seen in patients with melanoma. The dense echoes in patients with melanoma could be related to multiple microscopic metastases and a high tissue density. Although melanoma is one of the most frequent primary tumors to metastasize to the spleen, metastases from the breast, lung, or ovaries also may go to the spleen. Many of these patients are asymptomatic. Occasionally an enlarged spleen secondary to tumor may produce pain in the left upper quadrant or even cause a splenic rupture. A splenic infarction secondary to tumor emboli may also produce acute abdominal pain (Fig. 16-15). Thus splenomegaly may be found only incidentally at physical or sonographic evaluation.

The sonographic findings of lymphoma generally are low-level echoes emanating

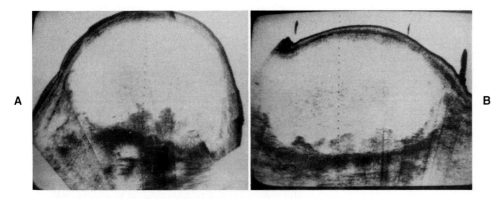

Fig. 16-15. Transverse, **A,** and longitudinal, **B,** scans demonstrating a huge dilated spleen secondary to an infarction.

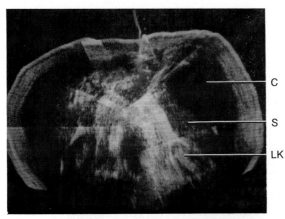

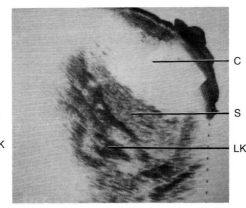

Fig. 16-16. This young patient presented with a large echo-free area within the splenic capsule. There was no history of trauma or other symptoms. A cyst versus tumor was considered.

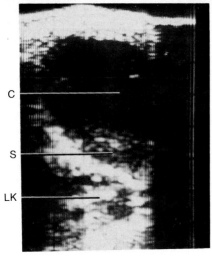

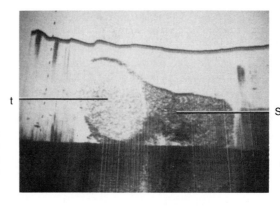

Fig. 16-17. The gross specimen was scanned, and the large sonolucent area within the spleen displayed multiple fine stippled echoes at high sensitivities. This was a benign tumor of the spleen.

from splenomegaly.[9] The spleen may be of normal size and yet contain tumor in 33% of patients with Hodgkin's or non-Hodgkin's disease,[5] and another 33% with Hodgkin's disease may have splenomegaly with a pathologically normal spleen.

Cunningham[2] reports that both isolated lymphoma in the spleen and splenic abscess may give rise to ultrasonic images that show irregular zones of below-normal echo activity with unimpeded acoustic transmission. Since the clinical features of the two diseases are very similar, it may be difficult to separate the entities by sonographic evaluation.

Benign splenic tumors. Benign splenic tumors are occasionally seen by sonography. Generally splenomegaly will be the first indication of an abnormality. As the sensitivity is increased, the normal splenic parenchyma will fill in while the tumor will not (Figs. 16-16 and 16-17).

REFERENCES

1. Cooperberg, P.L.: Ultrasonography of the spleen. In Sarti, D.A., and Sample, W.F., editors: Diagnostic ultrasound; text and cases, Boston, 1980, G.K. Hall & Co.
2. Cunningham, J.: Ultrasonic findings in isolated lymphoma of the spleen simulating splenic abscess, J. Clin. Ultrasound **6:**412, 1978.
3. Koga, T.: Correlation between sectional area of the spleen by ultrasonic tomography and actual volume of the removed spleen, J. Clin. Ultrasound **7:**119, 1979.
4. Mittelstaedt, C.A., and Partain, C.L.: Ultrasonic-pathologic classification of splenic abnormalities: gray scale patterns, Radiology **134:**697, 1980.
5. Murphy, J.F., and Bernardino, M.E.: The sonographic findings of splenic metastases, J. Clin. Ultrasound **7:**195, 1979.
6. Propper, R.A., Weinstein, B.J., Skolnick, L., et al.: Ultrasonography of hemorrhagic splenic cysts, J. Clin. Ultrasound **7:**18, 1979.
7. Robbins, S.L., and Cotran, R.S.: Pathologic basis of disease, Philadelphia, 1979, W.B. Saunders, Co.
8. Siler, J., Hunter, T.B., Weiss, J., and Haber, K.: Increased echogenicity of the spleen in benign and malignant disease, A.J.R. **134:**1011, 1980.
9. Taylor, K.J.W., and Moulton, D.: The spleen. In Taylor, K.J.W., editor: Atlas of gray scale ultrasonography, New York, 1978, Churchill Livingstone, Inc.

17

Retroperitoneum

The retroperitoneal space is the area between the posterior portion of the parietal peritoneum and the posterior abdominal wall muscles. It extends from the diaphragm to the pelvis. Laterally the boundaries extend to the extraperitoneal fat planes within the confines of the transversalis fascia, and medially the space encloses the great vessels[1] (Fig. 17-1). It is subdivided into three categories: perinephric space or fascia of Gerota, anterior paranephric space, and posterior paranephric space. The perinephric space surrounds the kidney and perinephric fat, whereas the anterior paranephric space includes the extraperitoneal surfaces of the gut and pancreas. The iliopsoas, fat, and other soft tissues are within the posterior paranephric space.

Because it is protected by the spine, ribs, pelvis, and musculature, the retroperitoneum has been a difficult area to assess clinically; but ultrasound has become a useful diagnostic tool for detecting tumors and fluid collections (urinoma, abscess, hematoma, or ascites) located there.

LYMPHATIC SYSTEM

There are two major node-bearing areas in the retroperitoneum: the iliac and hypogastric nodes within the pelvis and the para-aortic group in the upper retroperitoneum.

The lymphatic chain follows the course of the thoracic aorta, abdominal aorta, and iliac arteries (Fig. 17-2). Normal lymph nodes are smaller than the tip of a finger (less than 1 cm) and are not visualized by current ultrasound techniques. However, if these nodes enlarge because of infection or tumor, they become easier to visualize.

Since the nodes lie along the lateral and anterior margins of the aorta, the best scanning is done with the patient in the supine position. It is important to examine the patient in two planes, since enlarged nodes seen in the longitudinal plane may mimic an abdominal aneurysm at lower-gain settings. As the transverse scan is completed, the differential of an aneurysm versus lymphadenopathy can be made. The aneurysm will enlarge fairly symmetrically, whereas enlarged lymph nodes drape over the prevertebral vessels.

Longitudinal scans may be obtained first to outline the aorta and to search for enlarged lymph nodes. The aorta provides an excellent background for the somewhat sonolucent nodes. Longitudinal scans should begin at the midline and record both to the left and to the right at 0.5-cm increments. If an abnormality is noted on these sagittal scans, the area should be marked with a grease pencil for proper identification in the

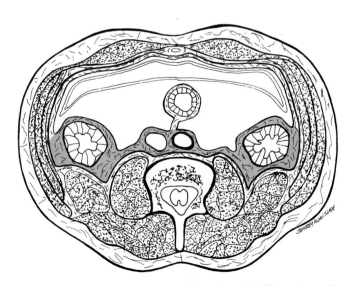

Fig. 17-1. Transverse section of the abdominal cavity at L4. The retroperitoneal space is outlined.

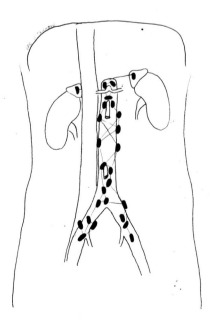

Fig. 17-2. Lymphatic chain along the aorta and iliac artery.

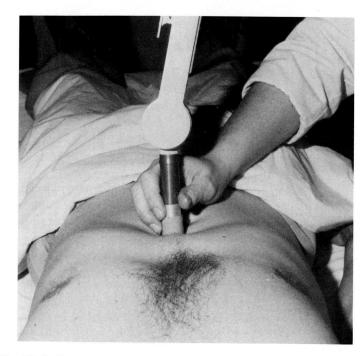

Fig. 17-3. Transverse scans of the lymph node area should be performed in a single-sweep maneuver. Moderate to high gain should be used to evaluate the paraaortic area.

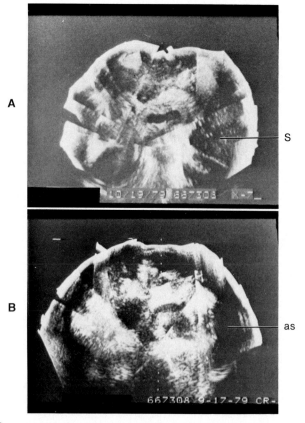

Fig. 17-4. A, Transverse of a patient with lymphadenopathy. Splenomegaly is shown. **B,** The patient also has a large amount of ascitic fluid. Enlarged lymph nodes are seen in the prevertebral area.

transverse plane. Transverse scans are made from the xyphoid to the symphysis at 2-cm intervals (Fig. 17-3). Careful identification of the great vessels, organ structures, and muscle patterns is important. Patterns of a fluid-filled duodenum or bowel may make it difficult to outline the great vessels or may cause confusion in diagnosing lymphadenopathy.

Scans below the umbilicus are more difficult because of interference from the small bowel. Careful attention should be given to the psoas and iliacus within the pelvis, since the iliac arteries run along their medial border. Both muscles serve as a sonolucent marker in the pelvic sidewall. Enlarged lymph nodes can be identified anterior and medial to these margins. A smooth sharp border indicates no nodal involvement. The bladder should be filled to help push the small bowel out of the pelvis.

Splenomegaly should also be evaluated in lymphadenopathy. As the scanner moves caudal from the xyphoid, attention should be on the splenic size and great vessel area (Fig. 17-4).

In our experience lymph nodes remain as consistent patterns whereas bowel and duodenum present changing patterns. As gentle pressure is applied with the transducer in an effort to displace the bowel, the lymph nodes remain constant. The echo pattern posterior to each structure is different. Lymph nodes are homogeneous and thus transmit sound easily; bowel presents a more complex pattern with dense central echoes from its mucosal pattern. Often the duodenum will have some air within its walls, causing a shadow posteriorly. Enlarged lymph nodes should be reproducible on ultrasound. After the abdomen is completely scanned, repeat sections over the enlarged nodes should demonstrate the same pattern as before.

The patient may be asked to return for a serial follow-up visit if there is uncertainty as to whether the pattern indicates enlarged lymph nodes or fluid-filled bowel.

Enlarged lymph nodes are more homogeneous than their surrounding organ structures, such as the pancreas, liver, kidneys, or spleen (Fig. 17-5). With increased sensitivity, diffuse low-level echoes may be seen within the nodes. Proper adjustment of the enhance control on most equipment is necessary for recording these fine echoes on the monitor. Their borders are generally smooth, but as they enlarge they may take on a more irregular appearance (Figs. 17-6 to 17-8).

Asher and Freimanis (1969) stated that periaortic nodes are known to have specific characteristic patterns. They may drape or

Text continued on p. 237.

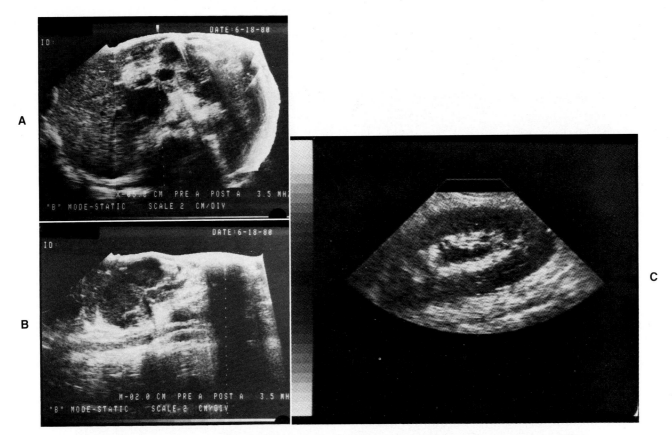

Fig. 17-5. A young man presented with ascites, edema, abdominal pain, and hypoproteinemia. His GI radiograph showed displacement of the duodenum and stomach anteriorly with prominent proximal small bowel folds. Ultrasound showed a large lobulated retroperitoneal mass, ascites, and left hydronephrosis. **A,** Transverse showing splenomegaly and enlarged nodes anterior to the inferior vena cava. **B,** Sagittal of the enlarged nodes in this patient with lymphoma. **C,** Sagittal of the left renal hydronephrosis.

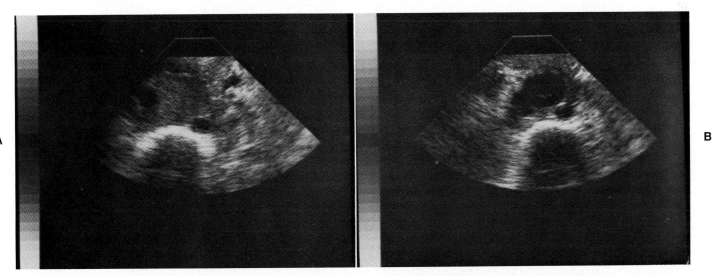

Fig. 17-6. This patient with a lymphoma had been receiving chemotherapy for a number of months. He now presented with fever, and the question of an abscess was raised. Because of his chemotherapy, the enlarged nodes were in various stages of regression, which can make them difficult to distinguish from abscess formation. The area in question was outlined by real time for further needle aspiration and diagnosis. **A,** Transverse of a low-level node anterior to the great vessels. **B,** Transverse of a very homogeneous node anterior to the great vessels.

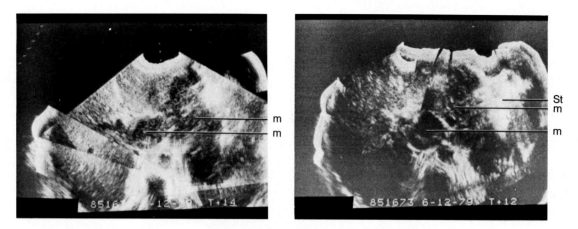

Fig. 17-7. Transverse scans of a 44-year-old man with histocytic lymphoma of the upper abdomen. Ultrasound shows the lymphomatous mass, *m,* surrounding the stomach. The mass extends across the midline into the area of the head of the pancreas.

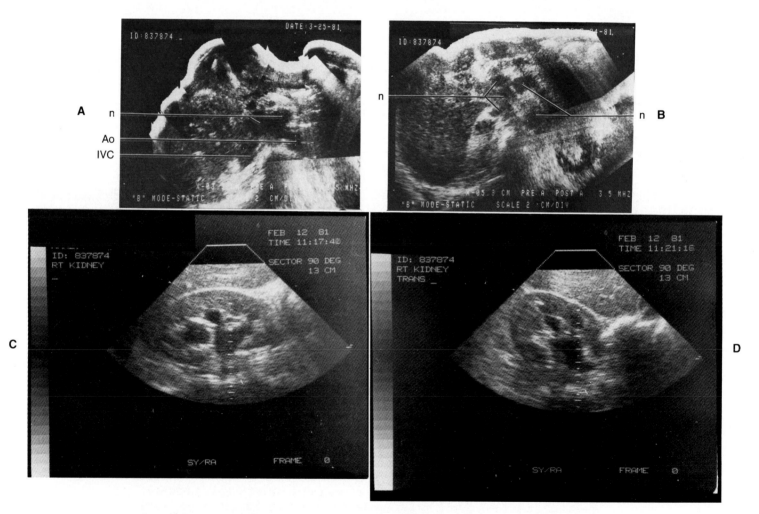

Fig. 17-8. This patient presented with paraaortic node enlargement, an enlarged common bile duct, and right hydronephrosis. **A,** Transverse of the enlarged nodes, *n.* **B,** Several small nodes anterior to the great vessels. **C,** Sagittal of the right hydronephrosis. **D,** Transverse of the hydronephrosis as it narrows to drain into the renal pelvis.

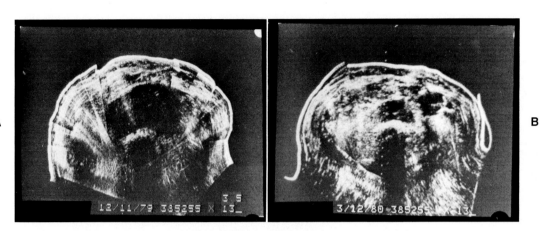

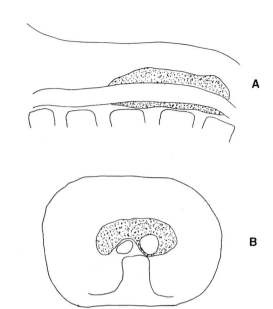

Fig. 17-9. Ultrasound is a very effective tool for monitoring patients with lymphoma. This patient shows a dramatic decrease in the size of the paraaortic mass after treatment. **A,** Initial scan showing the homogeneous lymph mass to encircle the aorta completely. As sensitivity is increased, the aortic border may be seen. **B,** Comparable transverse scan 15 months later. Note the regression in size of the mass surrounding the aorta.

Fig. 17-10. A, Sagittal and, **B,** transverse diagrams of a paraaortic mass that can simulate an abdominal aortic aneurysm if transverse scans are not performed to demonstrate the mantle of the enlarged nodes.

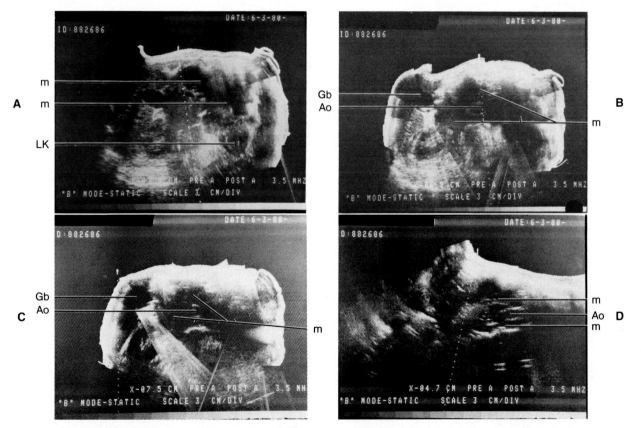

Fig. 17-11. This 56-year-old patient with known laryngeal carcinoma complained of abdominal pain, jaundice, and malaise. Lymphoma was found at biopsy. Ultrasound demonstrated a large solid mass at the level of the porta hepatis obstructing the common bile duct and causing intrahepatic duct dilation and an enlarged gallbladder. Both the inferior vena cava and the aorta were distorted by the mass. **A,** Transverse scan. Mild left hydronephrosis. The mass is seen anterior to the great vessels and kidney. **B,** Transverse scan of the dilated gallbladder, *Gb,* and mass, *m.* **C,** The aorta can just be seen within the mass. **D,** Sagittal scan of the mass encircling the aorta, *Ao.*

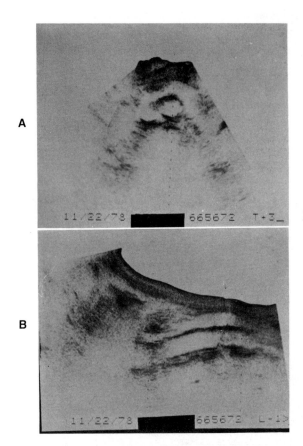

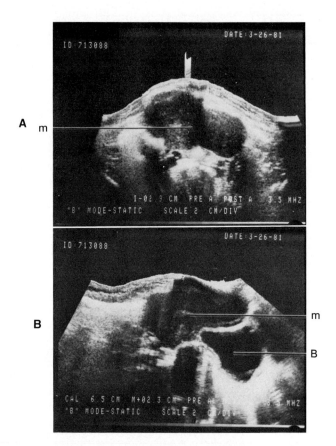

Fig. 17-12. A, Transverse and, **B,** sagittal scans of the patient with retroperitoneal enlarged nodes. Differential diagnosis may include retroperitoneal fibrosis.

Fig. 17-13. A, Transverse and, **B,** sagittal scans of a 12-year-old boy treated 7 years earlier for Burkitt's lymphoma. He now had a scar associated with a fibroma that was enlarging. Bladder, *B;* mass, *m.*

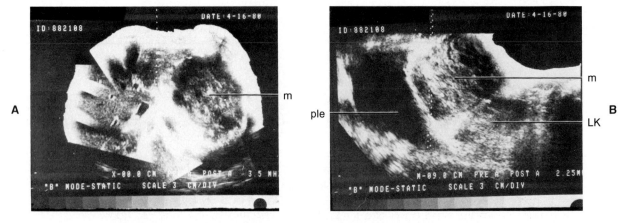

Fig. 17-14. A, Transverse and, **B,** sagittal scans of a patient with a large solid retroperitoneal mass, *m,* separate from the left kidney, *LK.* A large pleural effusion, *ple,* is seen.

mantle the great vessels anteriorly. They may have a lobular, smooth, or scalloped appearance. As mesenteric involvement occurs, the adenopathy may fill most of the abdomen in an irregular complex pattern. (Figs. 17-9 to 17-13).

The diagnosis of lymphadenopathy or a lymphomatous mass can be useful as a baseline study to the clinician. After treatment is administered, follow-up scans may be made to evaluate the shrinkage of the mass. If radiation therapy is used, it is helpful to mark the boundaries of the mass on the patient's skin for therapy planning.

PRIMARY RETROPERITONEAL TUMORS

A primary retroperitoneal tumor is one that originates independently within the retroperitoneal space. The tumor can arise anywhere, and most are malignant. As with other tumors, it may exhibit a variety of sonographic patterns from homogeneous to complex to solid (Fig. 17-14).

Neurogenic tumors are usually encountered in the paravertebral region, where they arise from nerve roots or sympathetic chain ganglia. Sonographically their pattern is quite variable.

Leiomyosarcomas are prone to undergo necrosis and cystic degeneration. Their sonographic pattern is complex. Liposarcomas produce a highly reflective sonographic pattern due to their fat interface.

Fibrosarcomas and rhabdomyosarcomas may be quite invasive and may infiltrate widely into muscles and adjoining soft tissues. They often present with extension across the midline and appear very similar to lymphomas. Sonographically they are highly reflective tumors.

Teratomatous tumors may arise within the upper retroperitoneum and the pelvis. They may contain calcified echoes from bones, cartilage, and teeth as well as soft tissue elements.

Tumors of uniform cell type generally have a homogeneous appearance unless there is hemorrhage or necrosis. Often the presence of necrosis depends on the size and growth of the mass (Fig. 17-15).

SECONDARY RETROPERITONEAL TUMORS

Secondary retroperitoneal tumors are primarily recurrences from previously resected tumors. Recurrent masses from previous renal carcinoma are frequent. Ascitic fluid along with a retroperitoneal tumor usually indicates seeding or invasion of the peritoneal surface. Evaluation of the paraaortic

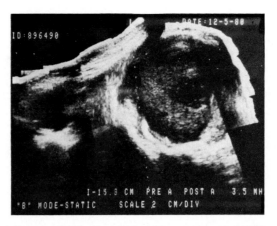

Fig. 17-15. A large retroperitoneal tumor exhibiting central necrosis is surrounded by low-level echoes.

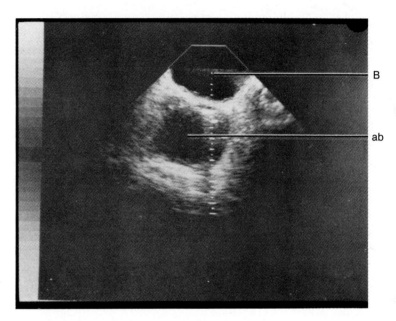

Fig. 17-16. A young man who had been stabbed in the left flank presented with pain, hematuria, urgency, and fever. A large abscess, *ab*, was found anterior to the rectum. Bladder, *B*.

region should be made for extension to the lymph nodes. The liver should also be evaluated for metastatic involvement.

RETROPERITONEAL FLUID COLLECTIONS

Urinoma. A urinoma is a walled-off collection of extravasated urine that develops spontaneously after trauma, surgery, or a subacute or chronic urinary obstruction. Urinomas usually collect about the kidney or upper ureter in the perinephric space. Occasionally urinomas dissect into the pelvis and compress the bladder. Generally their sonographic pattern is sonolucent unless they become infected.

Hemorrhage. A retroperitoneal hemorrhage may occur in a variety of conditions, including trauma, vasculitis, bleeding diathesis, leaking aortic aneurysm, or bleeding neoplasm. Sonographically it may be well localized and produce displacement of other organs, or it may present as a poorly defined infiltrative process.

Fresh hematomas present as sonolucent areas whereas organized thrombus and clot formation show echo densities within the mass. Calcification may be seen in longstanding hematomas.

Abscess. Abscess formation may result from surgery, trauma, or perforations of the bowel or duodenum. Sonographically the abscess usually has a more complex pattern with debris. Gas within the abscess will be reflective and cast an acoustic shadow (Fig. 17-16). One should be careful not to miss a gas-containing abscess for "bowel" patterns.

A

B

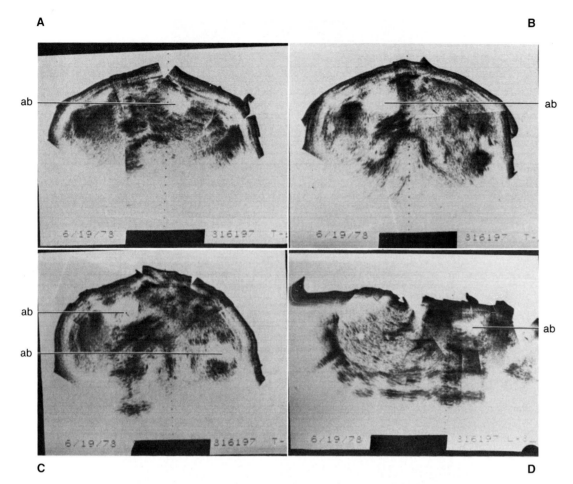

ab

ab

ab

ab

ab

C

D

Fig. 17-17. This young man treated for a ruptured appendix presented with subsequent peritonitis and multiple abscess formations. He continued to spike fevers after drains were placed in the abdomen. Ultrasound found two abscess formations. One was anterior and to the right of midline at the level of the iliac crest. The other collection was far posterior on the left. **A,** Transverse of the abscess, *ab*. **B,** Transverse of the abscess with some ascites along the flanks. **C,** Transverse of both collections of fluid. **D,** Sagittal of the right fluid collection.

The radiograph should be evaluated in this case. The abscess frequently extends along or within the muscle planes, is of an irregular shape, and lies in the most dependent portion of the retroperitoneal space (Fig. 17-17).

RETROPERITONEAL FIBROSIS

Retroperitoneal fibrosis is a disease of unknown etiology characterized by thick sheets of fibrous tissue in the retroperitoneal space. The disease may occur in association with abdominal aortic aneurysms. It may encase and obstruct the ureters and vena cava, with resultant hydronephrosis. A discrete mass of abnormal tissue lying anterior and lateral to the great vessels has been described by Sanders et al.[2] It may mimic lymphoma and thus must be further delineated for benignity or malignancy.

REFERENCES

1. Goldberg, B.B., Pollack, H.M., and Bancks, N.H.: Retroperitoneum. In Resnick, M.I., and Sanders, R.C., editors: Ultrasound in urology, Baltimore, 1979, The Williams & Wilkins Co.
2. Sanders, R.C., Duffy, T., McLaughlin, M.G., et al.: Sonography in the diagnosis of retroperitoneal fibrosis, J. Urol. **118:**944, 1977.

18

High-resolution ultrasonography of superficial structures

LAURA SCHORZMAN

The recent development of high-resolution ultrasound instruments provides a means of effectively evaluating superficial organs and structures. A number of systems have been designed that utilize frequencies in the 7-to-10-MHz range and incorporate water or oil path delays. High-resolution imaging and optimal use of the focal zone are satisfied by such instrumentation. The appellation "small-parts scanning" has been applied to this technology.

The material for this chapter was obtained by a system utilizing a 10-MHz 13-mm diameter transducer. The transducer is focused at a depth of approximately 2.2 cm from the skin surface and provides an axial resolution of 0.4 mm and a lateral resolution of 1 or 2 mm. The transducer is housed in a water bath and mechanically driven back and forth in a linear fashion. This produces a 3 × 4 cm rectangular image format. Update of the information at 30 frames per second provides the real time capability of the system. A thin pliable membrane covering the water bath housing is placed in contact with the skin.

The real time feature of small-parts scanners provides ease and flexibility for rapid and thorough evaluation of structures.

The guidance and support of Dr. William Scheible are gratefully appreciated.

THYROID GLAND
Anatomy

The thyroid gland consists of a right and a left lobe connected in the midline by an isthmus. Each lobe is lateral to the trachea and is bounded posterolaterally by the carotid artery and internal jugular vein (Figs. 18-1 and 18-2). The conical upper pole partly covers the lower portion of the thyroid cartilage, and the rounded lower poles partially cover the third and fourth tracheal rings. The sternocleidomastoid and strap muscles (sternothyroid, sternohyoid, and omohyoid) are situated anterolateral to the thyroid (Fig. 18-2).

The two lobes of the gland are of similar size and shape in most persons, although the right lobe is often slightly larger. The isthmus, which lies anterior to the trachea, is variable in size. A triangular cephalic extension of the isthmus, the pyramidal lobe, is present in 15% to 30% of thyroid glands. When present, it too is of varying size and is more frequently located on the left. A fibrous capsule encloses the gland and gives it a smooth contour.

Blood is supplied to the thyroid via four arteries. Two superior thyroid arteries arise from the external carotids and descend to the upper poles. Two inferior thyroid arteries arise from the thyrocervical trunk of the subclavian artery and ascend to the lower poles. Corresponding veins drain into the internal jugular vein (Fig. 18-1).

239

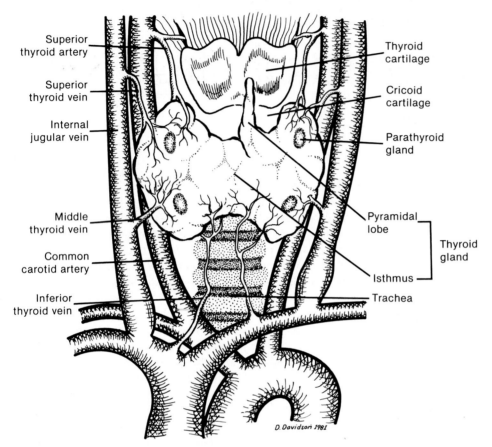

Fig. 18-1. Anterior view of the thyroid and parathyroid regions. (Modified from Forsham, P.H.: Endocrine system and selected metabolic diseases, ed. 3, Summit, N.J., 1974, Ciba Pharmaceutical Co.)

Physiology

The role of the thyroid, an endocrine gland, is to maintain normal body metabolism, growth, and development by the synthesis, storage, and secretion of thyroid hormones.

The mechanism for production of thyroid hormones is iodine metabolism. The thyroid gland traps iodine from the blood and, through a series of chemical reactions, produces the thyroid hormones triiodothyronine (T3) and thyroxine (T4). These are stored in the colloid of the gland. When thyroid hormone is needed, release into the bloodstream is accomplished by the action of thyrotropin or thyroid-stimulating hormone (TSH), produced by the pituitary gland. The secretion of TSH is regulated by thyrotropin-releasing factor, which is produced by the hypothalamus. The level of thyrotropin-releasing factor is controlled by the basal metabolic rate. A decrease in the BMR, which is a result of a low concentration of thyroid hormones, causes an increase in thyrotropin-releasing factor. This causes increased secretion of TSH and a subsequent increase in the release of thyroid hormones. When the blood level of hormones is returned to normal, the BMR returns to normal and TSH secretion stops.

Pathology

Enlargement of the thyroid gland is termed *goiter*. This can be diffuse and symmetric or irregular and nodular (focal). It may be a result of hyperplasia or neoplasia,

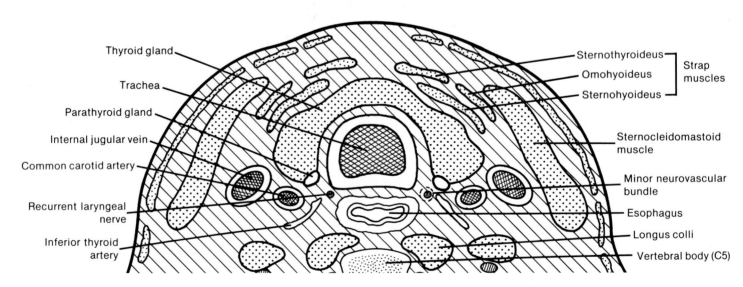

Fig. 18-2. Cross-section of the thyroid region showing organ, vessel, and muscle relationships. (Modified from Forsham, P.H.: Endocrine system and selected metabolic diseases, ed. 3, Summit, N.J., 1974, Ciba Pharmaceutical Co.)

inflammatory processes, or colloid distension of the follicles. A goiter can be associated with normal thyroid function, hyperfunction, or hypofunction.

Hyperthyroidism is a hypermetabolic state in which increased amounts of thyroid hormones are produced as a result of pituitary-thyroid regulatory system failure. The hormonal increase may be caused by an adenoma that independently secretes the thyroid hormone or by an increase in TSH. Manifestations of this condition are weight loss, nervousness, and increased heart rate; exophthalmos may develop when the condition is severe. Hyperthyroidism associated with diffuse goiter is Graves' disease.

Hypothyroidism is a hypometabolic state resulting from inadequate secretion of thyroid hormones. It is usually caused by an abnormality of the gland that restricts production of the hormones. Lethargy, sluggish reactions, and a deep husky voice are manifestations. Congenital hypothyroidism is cretinism.

Benign lesions

Cyst. About 20% of solitary thyroid nodules are cysts. Many are thought to represent cystic degeneration of a follicular adenoma. Blood or debris may be present within them. Cysts are almost uniformly benign.

Adenoma. Adenomas, more common in females, account for approximately 70% of true solitary thyroid nodules. They have a well-developed fibrous capsule encasing distinct internal architecture and are more firm than surrounding thyroid tissue. These solitary discrete lesions, ranging in size from 3 to 10 cm, are typically slow growing but may grow suddenly due to internal hemorrhage.

Diffuse nontoxic goiter (colloid goiter). This compensatory enlargement of the thyroid gland is due to thyroid hormone deficiency. The gland becomes diffusely and uniformly enlarged and is firm but not hard. In the first stage hyperplasia occurs; in the second stage, colloid involution. Progression of this process leads to asymmetric and multinodular glands.

Adenomatous hyperplasia (multinodular goiter). This goiter is one of the most common forms of thyroid disease. Nodularity of the gland can be the end stage of diffuse nontoxic goiter, which can be followed by focal scarring, by focal areas of ischemia and necrosis and cyst formation, or by fibrosis or calcification. Some of the nodules are poorly circumscribed; others appear to be encapsulated. Enlargement can involve one lobe to a greater extent than the other and sometimes causes difficulty in breathing and swallowing.

Thyroiditis. Thyroiditis can be a result of infections or autoimmune causes. The disease may be chronic (lymphocytic and Hashimoto's disease), which presents as mild swelling of the gland, or subacute (De Quervain's), which presents with pain and fever.

Malignant lesions. Thyroid carcinoma is relatively rare and is not a frequent cause of death (approximately 1100 persons die annually versus 100,000 for lung cancer). Evidence suggests an increased risk of thyroid cancer in adults with a childhood history of face, neck, or upper mediastinal radiation. A 7% to 9% prevalence has been cited in these persons.

Any nodule newly discovered or that exhibits a rapid increase in size is suspect for malignancy. In addition, stony hard nodules fixed to surrounding structures and/or palpable cervical lymph nodes are suspect. Primary cancers of the thyroid can be categorized into four types: papillary, follicular, medullary, and anaplastic. Malignant lymphoma and metastatic tumors also occur.

Papillary carcinoma. Papillary carcinoma is the most common thyroid gland malignancy (60% to 70%). The incidence is greatest among young adults (less than 40 years of age), but the lesion also occurs in the older population or in young children. This particular type of thyroid cancer is seen more frequently in females. It is one of the least aggressive and least malignant of human cancers, but in rare instances it can cause death.

The lesions may be tiny or may range up to 10 cm. They grow slowly, tend to infiltrate locally, and spread to cervical lymph nodes.

The clinical presentation is usually the incidental discovery of a nonpainful asymptomatic neck lump. Since metastases to regional cervical and mediastinal nodes are frequent, it is not uncommon for an enlarged lymph node to be detected prior to detection of the primary thyroid nodule.

Papillary carcinomas may be pure or mixed papillary and follicular; however, the long-term behavior is that of pure papillary carcinoma. Whether or not cervical node metastases are present, papillary carcinoma seems to be curable by hemithyroidectomy followed by thyroid hormone therapy.

Follicular carcinoma. This form of thyroid cancer accounts for about 15% to 20% of thyroid cancers. Its frequency increases with advancing age, and again females are more often affected.

An irregular, firm, nodular enlargement or a solitary, seemingly encapsulated, enlarging nodule is characteristic. Enlargement

of the lesion is slow but somewhat more rapid than that of papillary carcinoma.

Metastases travel through the blood to lungs and bone. Lymph node involvement is uncommon. This type of thyroid cancer is more aggressive than papillary cancer; however, the prognosis is good, especially if diagnosed and treated before tissue invasion and before the age of 40 years.

Medullary carcinoma. This form accounts for 5% to 10% of thyroid cancers. It presents as a hard bulky mass that may cause enlargement of a portion of a lobe or involve large areas of the entire gland.

Multiple endocrine neoplasia syndromes (e.g., Sipple's syndrome) have medullary carcinoma associated with pheochromocytoma and parathyroid adenoma. Medullary carcinoma is one type of thyroid carcinoma that may be familial.

Sharply circumscribed but unencapsulated medullary carcinomas frequently invade surrounding structures. They metastasize to cervical lymph nodes and other distant sites. Although their course is rather slow, the 5-year survival rate is 40% to 50%.

Anaplastic (undifferentiated) carcinoma. About 10% to 15% of thyroid cancers are of this form. It usually occurs after 50 years of age, with no predilection for either sex. It is one of the most malignant and deadly of all carcinomas occurring in humans.

The lesion presents as a hard fixed mass with rapid growth and produces pressure symptoms, possibly tenderness. Its growth is locally invasive into surrounding neck structures, and it usually causes death by compression and asphyxiation due to invasion of the trachea. Since there is no effective treatment, most patients die within a year after diagnosis has been established.

Lymphoma. Primary lymphomas of the thyroid arise in the 60-to-70-year-old patient population, with the incidence somewhat greater in females. Although uncommon, they usually occur in a patient with a huge goiter of recent development. The prognosis is generally poor.

Metastatic tumors to the thyroid. Cancers from various organs of the body can metastasize to the thyroid gland. Breast cancer is the most common thyroid metastatic lesion; but metastases also come from the lung, kidney, and colon.

Ultrasound evaluation

Management, whether surgical or medical, of thyroid nodules is handled on the basis of the nodule's being benign or malignant. The date of origin, physical findings, and

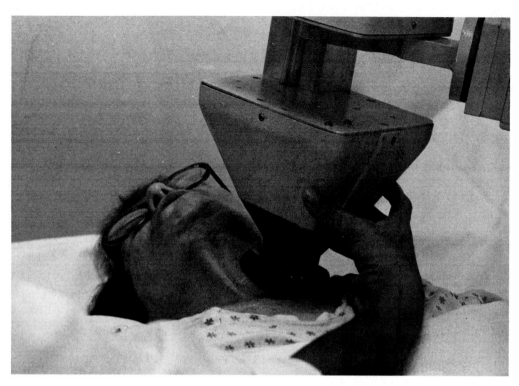

Fig. 18-3. Patient and transducer positions for longitudinal scanning of the thyroid gland.

various laboratory tests are utilized as aids in differentiation. It is frequently impossible to distinguish a single nodule from multiple nodularity by physical examination. A multinodular gland is less likely to be malignant than one with a solitary lesion, excluding patients who have received prior head and neck irradiation; however, benign lesions and carcinomas can coexist.

Although it has resolution limitations (nodules smaller than 1 cm are not demonstrable) and differentiation of cystic from solid lesions is not possible, the radioisotope scan is commonly used in the management of thyroid nodules. After intravenous injection of a radioisotope, ^{131}I or technetium-99^m pertechnetate, a rectilinear scanner or gamma camera is used to detect the concentration of the radioisotope in the nodule and in the remaining gland. The nodules are then classified as cold or hot depending upon how they concentrate the isotope.

Cold nodules concentrate less isotope than the surrounding thyroid tissue. Approximately 20% of cold thyroid nodules are malignant and about 20% are cystic. Most of the remainder are benign adenomas.

Hot nodules represent increased thyroid activity or are nodules that concentrate more radionuclide than the remaining thyroid. They are almost never malignant if hot by ^{131}I scan.

The role of ultrasound is to detect and characterize thyroid nodules. Size and location can be accurately assessed for initial evaluation and for follow-up study. Masses as small as 3 mm can be demonstrated, and differentiation of cystic versus solid nodules easily made, by ultrasound. Sonographic characterization of solid nodules as to benignity or malignancy is a desirable feature that has yet to be clearly established.

Ultrasound is instrumental also in needle aspiration procedures of cystic and solid lesions. Since areas of hemorrhage and necrosis have a poor cytologic yield, they should be avoided. Sonography can provide guidance for accurate needle placement to obtain optimal diagnostic aspirate material.

Scanning technique. When a patient is referred for ultrasound evaluation of a thyroid or neck mass, the isotope examination should be obtained for correlation.

The sonographic examination is begun with the patient lying supine. A sponge or pillow is placed under the neck to hyperextend it. This moves the mandible out of the field of interest and permits better transducer access. The head is turned slightly away from the side being examined, further optimizing transducer access (Fig. 18-3). This position is important for visualization, but one must also consider patient comfort. A comfortable and cooperative patient is instrumental in obtaining a diagnostic examination.

Because of the limited field of view of high-resolution scanners, it is not possible to image the entire thyroid gland in each scan. The lobes must be evaluated independently. In addition, because of the limited view that is ultimately documented, it is prudent for the interpreter of the examination to observe the study being performed.

A methodical routine for thorough investigation of the gland should always be followed. Transverse scanning begins at the lower pole of one lobe and continues up through the entire gland. The transducer is glided over the neck perpendicular to the skin. Because of variations in neck anatomy, experimentation with scanning head angulations may be necessary to achieve maximum transducer-to-skin contact. The carotid artery and jugular vein are utilized as lateral landmarks, and the trachea as a medial reference. If the preliminary survey reveals a normal gland, representative images should be recorded at the lower, middle, and upper poles, care being taken to document the medial and lateral extents of the gland. If an abnormality is encountered, all characteristics of the anomaly (cystic areas, calcifications, halo, etc.) should be demonstrated. It is not uncommon for sonography to demonstrate multiple nodules in a gland previously suspected of having only a solitary lesion.

Longitudinal scans are then performed from the medial aspect of the gland to the lateral surface through the lower, middle, and upper poles. Again, imaging should represent each pole of the thyroid in the normal situation. An abnormality is imaged as in transverse scanning. One lobe is explored in both transverse and longitudinal planes before the opposite lobe is.

After each lobe is evaluated, the isthmus must be scanned. Transverse sections are usually more satisfactory for visualizing this area. The examination is complete when normal and pathologic relationships have been understood and documented.

Ultrasound appearances

Normal. The normal thyroid gland has a smooth homogeneous texture of medium-level echoes. Lateral to the gland the carotid artery and internal jugular vein are identified in the transverse plane (Fig. 18-4, *A*). The vein, which is usually partly collapsed, is lateral and slightly superficial to the artery. A Valsalva maneuver by the patient will cause jugular vein distension. Thyroid vessels are occasionally seen anterior to the gland or coursing within the parenchyma. The strap muscles are anterolateral to the gland and the longus colli can often be identified posteriorly. The trachea is in the midline, posterior to the isthmus.

On longitudinal section the strap muscles and longus colli border the gland anteriorly and posteriorly respectively (Fig. 18-4, *B*). The upper and lower poles appear as conical projections. During swallowing the normal gland glides along the musculature in a cephalocaudad direction.

Cyst. Simple cysts as small as 1 mm can be identified with high-resolution scanners. As in cysts elsewhere, well-demarcated smooth margins and lack of internal echoes are present (Fig. 18-5). Many cysts, however, have internal architecture that may be the result of hemorrhage. Recent hemorrhage can have an echolucent appearance or a fine smooth diffuse echographic pattern. Dense echoes or septations, which represent organization of blood, may be seen within cysts of longer duration. Many clinicians currently postulate that thyroid cysts are simply the result of degeneration of adenomas.

Adenoma. Adenomas, which comprise the majority of "cold" nodules (60%), have a broad spectrum of ultrasound appearances. They range from predominantly echolucent to completely echodense and commonly have a peripheral halo (Fig. 18-6). The echolucent areas are a result of cystic degeneration (probably from hemorrhage) and usually lack a well-rounded margin. This lack of a discrete cystic margin is helpful in differentiation from a simple cyst. Calcification, characteristically rimlike, can also be associated with adenomas. Its acoustic shadow may preclude visualization posteriorly (Fig. 18-6). The halo or thin echolucent rim surrounding the lesion may represent edema of the compressed normal thyroid tissue or the capsule of the adenoma. In a few instances it may be blood around the lesion. Although the halo is a relatively consistent finding in adenomas, additional statistical information is necessary to establish its specificity.

Multinodular goiter. Individual lesions in multinodular goiter have many of the features of true adenomas. The multiple nodules of adenomatous hyperplasia may demonstrate halos and may or may not have discrete margins (Fig. 18-7). The echo texture of the solid portion of the lesion is typically quite similar to that of normal thyroid. Various degrees of cystic degeneration as well as calcification may be present within the nodules.

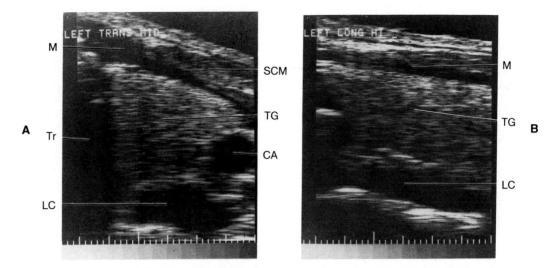

Fig. 18-4. A, Transverse scan of the left lobe of the normal thyroid gland, *TG*, demonstrating the relationships of the carotid artery, *CA*, trachea, *Tr*, and muscles. Note the homogeneous texture of the gland. **B,** Longitudinal scan of the upper pole of the normal thyroid, *TG*. Strap muscles, *M*, border the gland anteriorly and the longus colli, *LC*, borders posteriorly. *SCM,* sternocleidomastoid muscle.

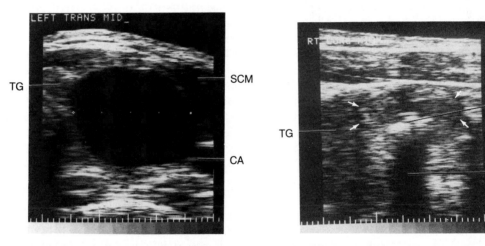

Fig. 18-5. A 2-cm thyroid cyst occupies most of the left lobe on this transverse scan. *TG,* Thyroid gland, isthmus; *CA,* carotid artery; *SCM,* sternocleidomastoid muscle.

Fig. 18-6. Longitudinal scan of a thyroid adenoma demonstrating a halo *(arrows)* and a large central calcification, *c,* with shadow, *sh,* Thyroid gland, *TG.*

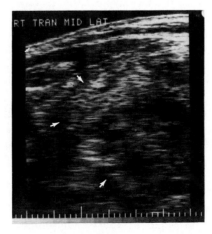

Fig. 18-7. Areas of cystic degeneration and a poorly defined halo *(arrowheads)* can be identified on this transverse scan of a multinodular goiter. Discrete nodule margins are difficult to perceive.

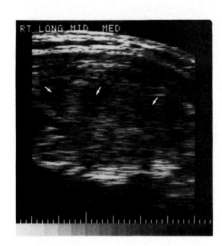

Fig. 18-8. Longitudinal scan of subacute thyroiditis showing diffuse enlargement of the thyroid gland with multiple nodular masses *(arrows).*

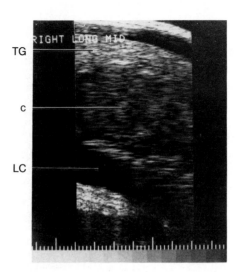

Fig. 18-9. Longitudinal section revealing the 3-cm thyroid carcinoma, *c*, to be less echogenic than the normal thyroid, *TG.* Longus colli, *LC.*

Thyroiditis. Thyroiditis usually appears as an enlarged gland with a generalized lower-amplitude echogenicity than normal thyroid parenchyma. Chronically inflamed glands are inhomogeneous and have disordered parenchymal echoes. Areas of relative sonolucency and/or high reflectivity may be seen as well as discrete solid nodules (Fig. 18-8).

In acute thyroiditis the resultant diffuse edema of the disease produces a homogeneous diminished echo pattern when compared to normal thyroid. The affected lobe or lobes are enlarged.

Carcinoma. Cancers of the thyroid produce areas of lower-amplitude echoes than does normal thyroid parenchyma (Fig. 18-9). The interfaces of the lesion are often poorly defined and a halo is rarely present. Cystic degeneration, if present, is minimal. Specks of calcium, although not common, may also be noted but are seldom peripheral as with adenomas.

PARATHYROID GLANDS
Anatomy

The parathyroid glands are usually closely attached to or embedded in the sheath of the posteromedial surface of the capsule of the thyroid gland (Figs. 18-1 and 18-2). Their numbers and locations are variable. Usually there are two pairs, a superior and an inferior, which lie behind the middle third and lower third of the thyroid. It is the inferior pair that tends to be more variable in position and may be anterior to the thyroid or may be retrosternal in the mediastinum.

The glands are typically somewhat flattened oval structures of approximately 3 × 4 mm in the adult.

Physiology

The parathyroid glands are the calcium-sensing organs in the body. They produce parathormone (PTH) and monitor the serum calcium feedback mechanism.

The stimulus PTH secretion is a decrease in the level of blood calcium. When the serum calcium level decreases, the parathyroid glands are stimulated to release PTH. When the serum calcium level rises, parathyroid activity decreases. PTH acts on bone, kidney, and intestine to enhance calcium absorption.

Pathology

Primary hyperparathyroidism. This is a state of increased function of the parathyroid glands and is characterized by hypercalcemia, hypercalciuria, and low serum levels of phosphate. Kidney damage and bone disease are manifestations of this situation. Primary hyperparathyroidism occurs when increased amounts of PTH are produced by an adenoma, primary hyperplasia, or rarely carcinoma.

Adenoma. By far the most common cause of primary hyperparathyroidism is an adenoma. A single hyperfunctioning lesion is responsible for 80% of cases. This benign tumor is usually very small (rarely larger than 3 cm) and often is not palpable. It is well encapsulated and is most common in the inferior parathyroid glands. Differentiation between adenomas and hyperplasia is difficult on histologic and morphologic grounds.

Primary hyperplasia. Primary hyperplasia is hyperfunction of all parathyroid glands with no apparent cause. Only one gland may significantly enlarge and the remaining glands be only mildly affected, or all glands may be enlarged. In any case, they rarely reach greater than 1 cm in size.

Carcinoma. Histologic differentiation between adenoma and carcinoma is very difficult. Metastases to regional nodes or distant organs, capsular invasion, or local recurrence must be present for the diagnosis of cancer to be made.

Most cancers of the parathyroid glands are small, irregular, and rather firm masses. They sometimes adhere to surrounding structures. If death results, it is more likely to be due to hyperparathyroid complications than to the malignancy itself.

Secondary hyperparathyroidism. A chronic hypocalcemia, caused by renal failure, vitamin D deficiency (rickets), or malabsorption syndromes, induces PTH secretion and leads to secondary hyperparathyroidism. The hyperfunction of the parathyroids is apparently a compensatory reaction; renal insufficiency and intestinal malabsorption cause hypocalcemia, which leads to stimulation of PTH. All four glands are usually affected.

Ultrasound evaluation

Patients with unexplained hypercalcemia detected on routine blood chemistry screening are the most common referrals for parathyroid echography. Symptomatic renal stones, ulcers, and bone pain are other indications.

Scanning technique. The sonographic examination is carried out much like the thyroid examination but with emphasis placed on the anticipated locations of the parathyroid glands (Fig. 18-3).

Transversely the evaluation should begin at the most caudal level possible (sternal notch) and extend as far cephalad as possible (mandible). If no pathology is identified, representative scans should be recorded at the lower, middle, and upper areas of the thyroid gland, which is a major reference organ. Landmarks such as thyroid, trachea, carotid artery, and longus colli should be demonstrated.

Longitudinally the cephalocaudal extent on each side of the neck should be examined from medial to lateral. The trachea represents the medial limit, and the carotid artery the lateral extent. Representative scans of the medial and lateral aspects of the lower, middle, and upper thyroid should be recorded.

Ultrasound appearances

Normal. Theoretically one would expect high-resolution scanners to be capable of resolving the parathyroid glands; however, to date this has not been true. The anatomic relationships (i.e., closely attached to or embedded in the thyroid gland and the apparent lack of acoustic differences between the thyroid and parathyroid glands) are probable explanations.

Since in many cases a prominent longus colli appears as a discrete area posterior to the thyroid, it is important not to confuse this normal anatomy with a mass. Longitudinal sections can usually solve the problem. A linear appearance of the muscle is evident in this plane (Fig. 18-4, *B*). The minor neurovascular bundle, composed of the inferior thyroid artery and recurrent laryngeal nerve, may also be a source of confusion (Fig. 18-2). Again, longitudinal scans can usually eliminate this confusion by identification of its tubular appearance.

Adenoma. Parathyroid adenomas are homogeneous, well-circumscribed, and less echogenic than normal thyroid tissue (Fig. 18-10). A dense sharp outer margin may be present around the lesion and is helpful in determining its extrathyroidal nature.

Hyperplasia. Since hyperplastic parathyroid glands and parathyroid adenomas both appear as relatively sonolucent masses, they cannot be sonographically discriminated. Hyperplasia involves all parathyroid glands to some extent; however, all glands may not be sufficiently enlarged to be seen by sonography.

MISCELLANEOUS NECK MASSES

The role of ultrasound in evaluation of palpable neck masses is to determine site of origin and assess lesion texture.

Developmental cysts

Thyroglossal duct cyst. Thyroglossal duct cysts are congenital anomalies that present in the midline of the neck anterior to the trachea (Fig. 18-11). They are fusiform or spherical masses and are rarely larger than 2 or 3 cm.

A remnant of the tubular development of the thyroid gland may persist between the base of the tongue and the hyoid bone. This narrow hollow tract, which connects the thyroid lobes to the floor of the pharynx, normally atrophies in the adult. Failure to atrophy creates the potential for cystic masses to form anywhere along it.

Branchial cleft cyst. Branchial cleft cysts are cystic formations that are usually located laterally. During embryonic development the branchial cleft is a slender tract extending from the pharyngeal cavity to an opening near the auricle or into the neck. A diverticulum may extend either laterally from the

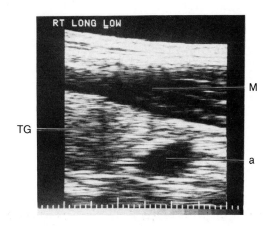

Fig. 18-10. Parathyroid adenoma, *a*, posterior to the lower pole of the thyroid gland, *TG*, on this longitudinal scan. *M*, Strap muscles.

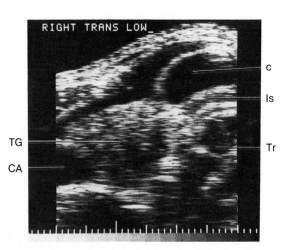

Fig. 18-11. Transverse scan at the level of the thyroid gland, *TG*, demonstrating a thyroglossal duct cyst, *c*, in the midline anterior to the trachea, *Tr*. Carotid artery, *CA*; isthmus of thyroid gland, *Is*.

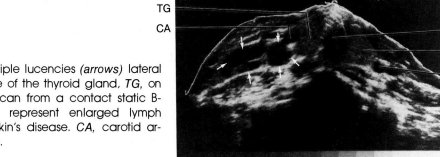

Fig. 18-12. Multiple lucencies *(arrows)* lateral to the right lobe of the thyroid gland, *TG*, on this transverse scan from a contact static B-scanner. These represent enlarged lymph nodes of Hodgkin's disease. *CA*, carotid artery; *Tr*, trachea.

pharynx or medially from the neck.

Although primarily cystic in appearance, these lesions may present with solid components, usually of low-level echogenicity, particularly if they have become infected.

Cystic hygroma. Cystic hygromas of the neck result from congenital modification of the lymphatics. They present from the posterior occiput and are most frequently seen as large cystic masses on the lateral aspect of the neck. They can be multiseptated and multilocular.

Abscesses

Abscesses can arise in any location in the neck. Their sonographic appearance ranges from primarily fluid filled to completely echogenic. Most commonly they are masses of low-level echogenicity with rather irregular walls. Chronic abscesses may be particularly difficult to demonstrate since their indistinct margins blend with surrounding tissue.

The role of ultrasound in evaluation of abscesses is localization for percutaneous needle aspiration and follow-up examination during and after treatment.

Adenopathy

Low-level echogenicity of well-circumscribed masses is the classical sonographic appearance of enlarged lymph nodes. However, in some cases they appear echo free. Inflammatory processes may also exhibit a cystic nature.

Differentiation of inflammatory from neoplastic processes is not always possible by sonographic criteria alone. In some instances, because of the limited field of view of small-parts scanners and the magnitude of the pathologic process, alternative examinations are necessary. A contact static image B-scanner may be required to display the anatomy and pathosis of the questionable area adequately (Fig. 18-12).

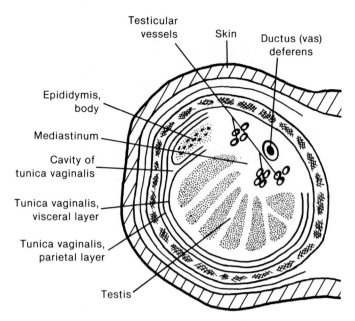

Fig. 18-13. Cross section through the midpoint of the scrotum and right testis. (Redrawn from Anson, B.J.: Morris' human anatomy, ed. 12, New York, 1966, McGraw-Hill Book Co.)

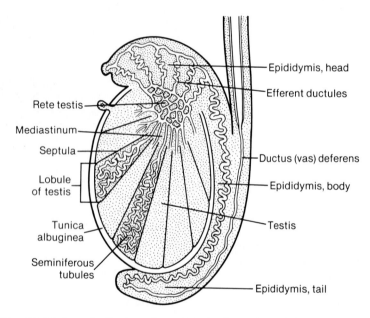

Fig. 18-14. Longitudinal section of the testis and epididymis. (The size of the seminiferous tubules is exaggerated). (Redrawn from Anson, B.J.: Morris' human anatomy, ed. 12, New York, 1966, McGraw-Hill Book Co.)

SCROTUM AND TESTES
Anatomy

Scrotum. The scrotum is a pendant sac that is divided by a septum into two compartments. Each compartment contains a testis, an epididymis, and a portion of spermatic cord and ductus deferens. The left side commonly extends farther caudad than the right.

The innermost investment of the scrotum is formed by the tunica vaginalis. It is a double sac with a parietal or outer layer and a visceral or inner layer (Fig. 18-13). The space between the parietal and visceral layers normally contains a small amount of fluid.

Testes. The two testes, the male organs of reproduction, are ovoid and slightly flattened from side to side. The upper pole is normally a little more anterior than the lower. The average dimensions are 4 to 5 cm long and 2.5 to 3 cm wide. Posteriorly, at the superior and inferior borders of the testes, the head and tail of each epididymis are attached. The spermatic cord is also attached posteriorly. Support of the testes is provided mainly by the spermatic cord and the scrotum.

The visceral layer of the tunica vaginalis covers the testicular surface, except at the epididymis and spermatic cord attachments. Just under the tunica vaginalis is the tunica albuginea, a fibrous capsule encasing the testis (Fig. 18-14). From the fibrous capsule, septa pass into the interior of the testis and form compartments or lobules. These lobules contain the seminiferous tubules, whose lining creates spermatozoa. The union of the septula, ducts, nerves, and vessels is the mediastinum testis. In the mediastinum the tubules join to form the rete testis, from which the efferent ductules open into the epididymis.

Testicular development occurs in the retroperitoneum near the kidneys. Since the testes are attached to the peritoneum, their descent through the future inguinal canal into the scrotum drags the peritoneum with them. The peritoneum then lines each half of the scrotum, covers most of the testes, and is the tunica vaginalis. The passage between the scrotal peritoneum (tunica vaginalis) and the abdominal peritoneum, which was formed during descent of the testicle, is usually obliterated by fusion of the walls. If the connection persists, a congenital hernia results.

Epididymis. The epididymis, which lies along the posterolateral border of the testis, is the first portion of the duct of the testis and is its excretory system. The head (globus major) is at the superior pole of the testis and the tail (globus minor) is attached inferiorly (Fig. 18-14). Laterally and posteriorly the epididymis is covered by the visceral layer of the tunica vaginalis.

The spermatic cord, which ascends from the testis cephalad through the inguinal canal, is formed by the ductus (vas) deferens and testicular vessels and nerves.

Physiology

The testes, which produce spermatozoa, are considered exocrine glands. However, since they also produce male sex hormones, they also can be considered endocrine glands. Testosterone is the hormone responsible for spermatogenesis and the development of male sexual organs and characteristics.

Pathology

Scrotum

Edema. Edema of the scrotum is due to vascular or lymphatic disturbance or stasis. It can be a result of inflammation, allergic states, chronic cardiac insufficiency, enlarged inguinal lymph nodes, or parasitic obstruction of the lymphatics (elephantiasis). Prolonged stasis of the lymphatics causes the scrotal walls to become thickened by connective tissue. Epididymoorchitis frequently has associated scrotal edema.

Hydrocele. A hydrocele is scrotal sac enlargement caused by serous fluid accumulation between the layers of visceral and parietal tunica vaginalis. As much as 300 ml of fluid can be present, but most hydroceles contain 50 to 100 ml. The usual anterior location of a hydrocele causes posterior displacement of the testis within the scrotum.

Acute hydroceles are a result of trauma, infection of the testis or epididymis, or tumor. Chronic hydroceles are frequently idiopathic but can mask an underlying testicular malignancy. Most hydroceles are asymptomatic and are a manifestation of other disease processes.

Hernia. An inguinal hernia occurs when a loop of bowel protrudes into a patent vaginalis-peritoneal communication. When the bowel contains air or fluid, hernia can be confusing since it can have sonographic features similar to those of other scrotal masses.

Testes

Orchitis and epididymitis. Infections limited to the testes are rare. They occur more frequently in the epididymis, with secondary involvement of the testis. Epididymitis is the most common of the intrascrotal inflammations. Organisms from infected urine, the prostate, or the seminal vesicles travel to the epididymis via the vas deferens. Infection can also be lymphatic or blood borne. An acute hydrocele often coexists with intrascrotal infections.

Orchitis and epididymitis can be classified as specific (gonorrhea, syphilis, mumps, tuberculosis), nonspecific, and traumatic. Gonorrhea and tuberculosis affect the epididymis first; syphilis and mumps involve the testis. If the disease is not adequately treated, abscesses can develop.

Nonspecific epididymitis with subsequent orchitis is usually the result of a urinary tract infection.

Traumatic epididymitis can result from strenuous exercise in which infected prostatic secretions or urine are forced into the epididymis.

Testicular abscess is usually a complication of preexisting acute epididymitis. Pain, fever, redness, and edema are the presenting features. It is frequently difficult to assess the epididymal versus testicular nature of this infection because of difficulty on palpation.

Neoplasms. Testicular malignancy is primarily a disease of young men (20 to 40 years of age). It is the second leading cause of cancer death in this age group. There is a higher incidence of malignancy in undescended testes; however, surgical correction before the age of 6 virtually eliminates the risk. Approximately 95% of testicular neoplasms arise from germ (sex) cells of the testes.

Seminoma is the most common type of testicular tumor. For unknown reasons it is more frequent in the right testis than in the left. It is a lobulated homogeneous tumor devoid of hemorrhage or necrosis and is well circumscribed but not encapsulated. Frequently the entire testis is replaced by tumor. Elevated serum titers of follicle-stimulating hormone (FSH) are sometimes present in patients with this tumor.

Being the least malignant of germ cell tumors in its pure form and being highly sensitive to radiation, seminoma has a reasonably good prognosis. With orchiectomy followed by radiation of abdominal and thoracic nodes, the 2-year survival is 92%.

Embryonal carcinoma represents 19% to 25% of malignant testicular tumors. Because of its multiple histology, it is one of the most confusing. Areas of hemorrhage and necrosis are seen within these firm tumors, which typically have poorly demarcated borders. The tumor can partially or completely replace the testis. Elevated serum levels of α-fetoprotein (AFP) and/or human chorionic gonadotropin (hCG) can be found in patients with any nonseminomatous tumor.

The 5-year survival with this aggressive and lethal tumor is only 30% to 35%. It is generally not responsive to radiation and is treated with chemotherapy.

Choriocarcinoma is a highly malignant form of testicular tumor. It is rarely a pure tumor, usually mixed with other cell types. Typically it is small and does not cause testicular enlargement. Elevated serum or urine levels of hCG are usually detected in patients with choriocarcinoma.

Pure testicular choriocarcinoma is fatal. As a result of widespread metastases, almost all patients die within a year of diagnosis.

Teratoma, a tumor consisting of a heterogeneous mixture of tissues, accounts for approximately 7% to 10% of testicular tumors.

Three basic types of testicular teratomas (dermoid, differentiated, and undifferentiated) have been classified and are of varying degrees of malignancy. Because of the possibility of small foci of cancer, many authorities believe that all solid teratomas in adults should be managed as malignant. Abnormal serum levels of hCG and AFP are present in some patients with malignant teratoma.

Orchiectomy with surgical removal of any metastases (usually lymph nodes) is the treatment. The grade of malignancy of teratoma is between those of seminoma and embryonal carcinoma.

Testicular tumors are frequently composed of more than one of the previously discussed cell types (i.e., *mixed tumors*). Approximately 40% are of this nature, with the teratoma–embryonal carcinoma mixture the most common. Teratocarcinomas are those teratomas that have other neoplastic elements.

Ultrasound evaluation

Since it is often difficult to assess the intratesticular versus extratesticular nature of a scrotal mass by physical examination alone, ultrasound evaluation has become an important clinical tool to assist in differentiation.

Scanning technique. For sonographic evaluation the patient is placed in the supine "semifrogleg" position. The scrotum is supported with one hand of the operator while the transducer head is manipulated with the other. Again, because of the limited field of view, each hemiscrotum must be evaluated separately. Examination is made by gentle placement of the water path on the hemiscrotum. The testis and epididymis can be manipulated against the membrane from lateral to medial as scanning is performed.

Longitudinal views are easier to interpret; therefore, it is suggested that they be performed first. A survey through the entire hemiscrotum should be made prior to image recording. The recording sequence begins at the lower pole of the testis with lateral to medial scanning. Static images should document the relationship of the testis to the epididymis, the presence or absence of fluid, and the texture of the testis and epididymis. The midportion and upper pole of the testis are evaluated in a similar fashion. Evaluation of the upper pole should include the epididymis and its texture. The area cephalic to the head of the epididymis is also evaluated and documented. If a pathologic process is identified, characteristics of the abnormality and anatomic relationships should be clearly documented.

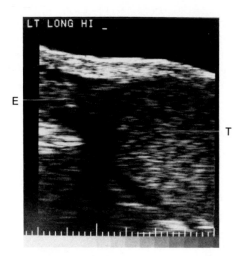

Fig. 18-15. Longitudinal scan showing the homogeneous texture with medium-level echogenicity of the normal testis, T, and the slightly more echogenic epididymis, E. A normal amount of fluid is present around the epididymis and testis.

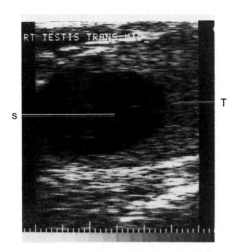

Fig. 18-16. Transverse scan of a testicular seminoma, s, showing less echogenicity than in the normal testicle, T.

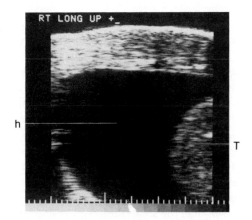

Fig. 18-17. A large hydrocele, h, surrounds the upper pole of the testis, T, on this longitudinal scan.

Transverse scans are performed in a similar manner. Beginning at the lower pole, the testis is manipulated so the lateral to medial examination can be accomplished. The midportion and upper pole and the epididymis are similarly examined, with the same emphasis on pathosis as described for longitudinal scanning. The opposite hemiscrotum is always scanned for comparison.

Ultrasound appearances

Testes. The *normal* testis exhibits a granular homogeneous medium-level echogenicity (Fig. 18-15). A small amount of fluid is present between the layers of the tunica vaginalis and can be identified in most cases.

Inflammation of the testis can be diffuse orchitis or a focal abscess. In orchitis the testicle becomes enlarged and exhibits a lower echogenic pattern than the normal testicle. An abscess appears as a localized area of inhomogeneity within the testis and often has cystic areas.

Testicular *tumors* tend to be of lower echogenicity than normal testicular tissue (Fig. 18-16). They can exhibit rather well-circumscribed borders or may appear to invade the testicular tissue. Although this is the typical pattern for tumor, it is not specific since chronic abscess, hematoma, and granuloma may appear similar. There are no characteristic sonographic patterns for malignant versus benign disease. Reactive hydroceles often coexist with both malignant and benign conditions of the testis.

Epididymis. The epididymis is usually distinguishable because it has a coarser ultrasonic texture than the normal testis (Fig. 18-15). The epididymal head can nearly always be identified and appears to cap the testicular upper pole. The body of the epididymis is more difficult to identify and the tail is not frequently seen.

The most common intrascrotal inflammation is *epididymitis.* It appears sonographically as uniform enlargement of the epididymis and is most evident in the globus major. Compared to normal, the texture is less echodense. In chronic epididymitis the epididymis is very echodense and can contain calcium and shadowing. Focal abscesses may appear as sonolucent areas within the epididymis.

Extratesticular collections. These can be idiopathic or associated with a known disorder.

Hydroceles, as previously mentioned, can be associated with infectious processes or tumors. They appear as a fluid collection surrounding the testis (Fig. 18-17). Depending on their volume, they may surround the testis or be visualized at only the upper or the lower pole.

A *spermatocele* is cystic dilation of the spermatic cord. Since it does not invaginate the tunica vaginalis, it appears cephalad to the testis as a loculated fluid collection often containing low-level echoes.

Hematoceles are uncommon and can be primarily cystic or contain echoes from organization of clotted blood. They also are located cephalic to the testes.

Hydrocele of the cord is the encasement of fluid in a sac of peritoneum within the spermatic cord. It also presents as a cystic mass cephalad to the testis. In contrast to hematoceles and spermatoceles, hydroceles of the cord are almost always entirely echo free.

A *varicocele* is cystic varicose enlargement of the veins of the spermatic cord. The cystic enlargement, cephalic to the testis, is usually of a tortuous nature resembling a bag of worms.

VASCULAR ACCESS FOR HEMODIALYSIS

Approximately 40,000 patients in the United States are undergoing chronic hemodialysis for end-stage renal disease. These are patients whose severely damaged kidneys are not capable of removing toxic products from the blood. Dialysis removes these substances and maintains electrolyte hemostasis by passing the patient's blood through a dialyzing solution.

Anatomy and physiology

Circulatory access for hemodialysis is dependent on creation of an easily accessible high-flow vascular system. This is accomplished by some form of surgical connection between an artery and vein. After anastomosis the veins frequently enlarge due to increased flow of arterialized blood through them. Needles can then be inserted into the arterialized veins to provide adequate flow for dialysis.

Creation of a successful arteriovenous (AV) anastomosis requires a situation in which adequate arteries and veins can be joined without stress and without jeopardy to circulation of the extremity involved. The forearm and thigh are usual locations, with common hookups being radial artery to cephalic vein, brachial artery to antecubital vein, and femoral artery to saphenous vein. The anastomosis can be of the side-to-side, end-to-end, or end-to-side design. This description refers to the respective arterial-venous or graft-venous relationship.

Vascular access systems are of two types. One is a direct AV fistula using the patient's

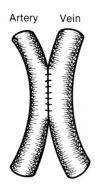

Fig. 18-18. Typical side-to-side arrangement for an arteriovenous fistula. (Redrawn from Massry, S., and Sellers, A.: Clinical aspects of uremia and dialysis, Springfield, Ill., 1976, Charles C Thomas, Publisher.)

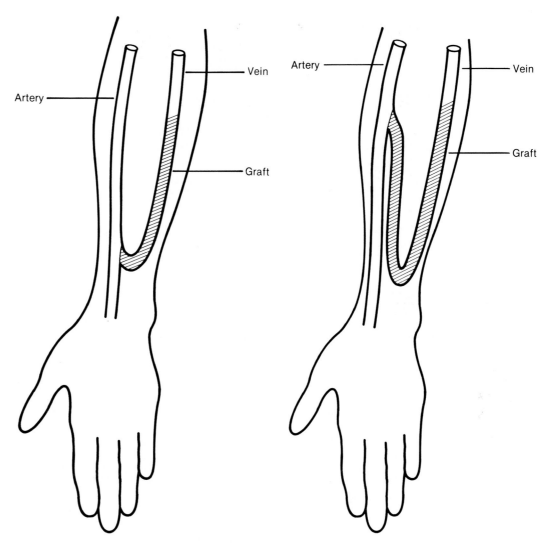

Fig. 18-19. Schematic representation of a bovine heterograft. (Courtesy Christine Skram, R.D.M.S., University of California Medical Center, San Diego.)

Fig. 18-20. Schematic representation of a synthetic graft. (Courtesy Christine Skram, R.D.M.S., University of California Medical Center, San Diego.)

own vessels; the other involves the use of tubes, either heterologous (usually bovine) or synthetic materials.

Arteriovenous fistula. The AV fistula proved to be a major advance over the previously used external Silastic (Scribner) shunts in terms of complications and failures. It is usually the arrangement of choice for initial vascular access.

A side-to-side anastomosis between an artery and the largest available adjacent vein is made (Fig. 18-18). Increased blood flow created by fistula formation causes the subcutaneous veins to become progressively dilated, thereby providing sufficient blood flow for hemodialysis.

Bovine heterograft. Bovine heterografts made from processed carotid arteries of cows are usually reserved for patients whose vessels will not permit establishment of an AV fistula or whose fistula has failed.

The anastomosis is frequently the end-to-side type (Fig. 18-19). A loop fistula between the radial or ulnar artery and the antecubital or a deep vein in the forearm is also common. The thigh is usually reserved as a last resort because of an increased incidence of graft complications in this location.

Synthetic graft. Polytetrafluoroethylene (Gore-Tex) has become a popular material for use in vascular access. Grafts of synthetic material are easier to handle and easier to reoperate on, and they have a better rate of patency than do bovine heterografts.

Straight or U-shaped anastomoses are used with preference for the proximal radial artery and a medial vein at or above the elbow joint (Fig. 18-20).

Pathology

A number of complications can lead to failure of the access. AV fistulas and bovine heterografts have higher complication rates in patients with proved arterial disease. The most likely cause is low blood flow.

Thrombosis. The most common complication to cause access failure is thrombosis. It develops due to low blood flow, which is a result of inadequate arterial inflow or high venous resistance (outflow obstruction). Common sites of thrombosis are anastomotic and puncture sites. Occlusion can develop as a result of thrombus accumulation. Thrombectomy or reconstruction can be performed in an attempt to salvage the access.

Infection. Early detection of infection is crucial in vascular accesses since graft replacement is often required in inadequately treated cases. Infection can result from re- peated venipunctures or after operation. Bovine heterografts are especially susceptible to infection, but it is not a significant problem with radiocephalic AV fistulas. Treatment with systemic and/or topical antibiotics is effective. Localized abscesses can be drained; but if they are grossly infected, the graft must be removed.

Aneurysm. An aneurysm is the result of weakness of the venous wall due to high venous pressure or repeated dialysis trauma. Thrombus can develop within the aneurysm. More ominously, graft degeneration with hemorrhage or infection may occur.

Pseudoaneurysm. A false aneurysm, which probably results from extravasation, may develop as a result of trauma or infection. It is usually found at the site of anastomosis (usually arterial) or at a needle puncture tear.

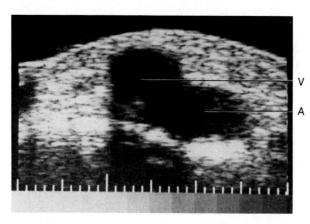

Fig. 18-21. Transverse section through arterial, *A*, to venous, *V*, anastomosis of a normal arteriovenous fistula.

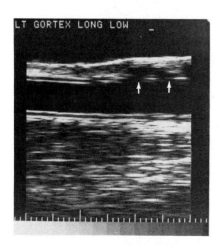

Fig. 18-22. Longitudinal sonogram of a synthetic graft. Note the smooth walls of the graft interrupted at the needle puncture sites (*arrows*).

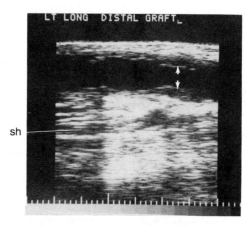

Fig. 18-23. Scan of synthetic graft anastomosis. The junction between the graft and the host vein can be identified by the shadowing, *sh*, deep to the graft. Minimal stenosis (*between arrowheads*) is also present within the vein.

Ultrasound evaluation

Scanning technique. For evaluation of arm fistulas the patient is placed recumbent, primarily for purposes of stability and support of the arm. The arm of interest is closest to the operator and is extended (hand up) and supported on the bed beside the patient. If the arm cannot be positioned as described, a firm flat device for support from shoulder to hand may be utilized. The patient's arm is abducted approximately 45 degrees with the support device positioned under it and the shoulder. If necessary, the examination may be performed with the patient in a wheelchair. Support of the extended arm can be obtained with the device stabilized on the arm of the wheelchair.

For evaluation of leg fistulas the patient is supine on a bed with the leg of interest closest to the operator. A slight frogleg position facilitates transducer access.

A preliminary review of the patient's surgical anatomy (and pathosis if present) should be undertaken prior to image recording.

Since the vein is usually of larger caliber and easier to identify, it is located first and the survey is begun longitudinally near the elbow. With an AV fistula the vein is traced toward the wrist to the anastomosis. After examination of the anastomosis the artery is then traced back to the elbow. A graft is evaluated similarly: scanning is performed toward the wrist through the vein, venous anastomosis, and graft. The arterial anastomosis and artery are then identified, and the sonographer continues to scan back toward the elbow.

After preliminary exploration, scanning is repeated with image documentation of the vein, venous anastomosis, graft, arterial anastomosis, artery, and any pathologic condition that may be present. Transverse scanning is performed utilizing this routine. The flexibility of real time allows the vasculature to be delineated with relative ease.

Ultrasound appearances

Arteriovenous fistula. Since existing vasculature is utilized in creation of an AV fistula, the artery and vein are seen as anechoic tubular channels. With survey through the vessels the anastomosis, usually side-to-side, can be identified where the vein becomes contiguous with the artery (Fig. 18-21). The vascular thrill detected on palpation is helpful in localizing the anastomosis.

Bovine heterograft. The appearance of a normal bovine heterograft is of an anechoic tubular channel whose walls are smooth and regular. It has essentially the same echographic appearance as a patient's normal blood vessels. The anastomoses can be difficult to identify because of the echographic similarity of the heterograft and the native vessel; however, a slight wall irregularity is often evident at the suture site. The end-to-side arterial anastomosis can be identified by tracing the heterograft to its insertion into the side of the artery.

Synthetic graft. The synthetic graft appears as a very discrete anechoic channel (Fig. 18-22). Because of its acoustic properties, synthetic graft material demonstrates a greater beam attenuation than do native vessels. The anastomosis can be clearly identified by the sharp difference in echo attenuation between the graft and the host vessel (Fig. 18-23).

Complications. A number of complications have been reported.

Thrombosis of a vascular access appears as an irregular echo reflection within the otherwise anechoic lumen of the vessel and may create an acoustic shadow. The amount and extent of resultant stenosis can be demonstrated. Special note should be made of wall irregularities from needle puncture, since they may be sites of thrombus deposition.

On rare occasions, soft or early thrombus may not create sufficient acoustic impedance to be sonographically evident. Doppler sonography may be useful in these instances.

Infection can appear as a sonolucent or complex mass around the graft or as vegetations within the graft appearing as echoes projecting from the wall of the lumen. Vegetations may flap with pulsations that can be documented by real time. Special attention should be paid to repeated venipuncture sites since they are potential abscess formation sites.

A palpable mass of vascular grafts is frequently an *aneurysm.* A localized increase in the normal caliber of the vein is characteristic. Thrombus may occur within the aneurysm, which is an area of relative stasis.

A *pseudoaneurysm* occurs most commonly at the anastomotic site or at a needle puncture site. A thrombus may totally fill the pseudoaneurysm (Fig. 18-24).

NEONATAL APPLICATIONS

The newborn infant is especially suited for small-parts scanning since many organ systems in these children are within the depth limits (4 to 5 cm) of the transducer. The real time capability is useful for rapidly surveying areas of interest and diminishing the problem of patient motion.

Technique of neonatal sonography

Examination of the neonate requires a few special considerations. Prior to examination the transducer assembly, especially the water path, must be cleaned with a disinfectant. The operator's hands should be washed and a clean gown should be worn.

Control of the ambient temperature is crucial since premature infants are very sensitive to temperature changes. Overhead heating lamps or an insulated heating pad under the infant can be utilized (Fig. 18-25). The acoustic coupling agent and the water path membrane must also be warmed.

Coordination of the examination between the ultrasound department and the neonatal ward team is especially important. Because of the critical status of many premature infants, unnecessary detainment in the ultrasound department should be avoided. Scheduling must be arranged for equipment availability upon the infant's arrival in the department.

The infant should be recently fed (unless otherwise indicated). A happy child is more likely to be still.

A member of the neonatal ward team should accompany the infant. The sonographer cannot be expected to provide the specialized monitoring sometimes necessary for these infants.

Clinical applications

Abdomen

Urinary tract. A palpable abdominal mass in neonates is usually of renal origin. Ure-

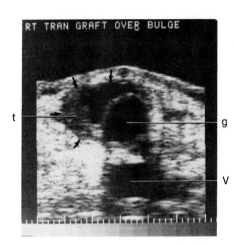

Fig. 18-24. Transverse scan of a synthetic graft, *g,* demonstrating a pseudoaneurysm *(arrows)* partially filled with thrombus, *t.* Native vessel, *V.*

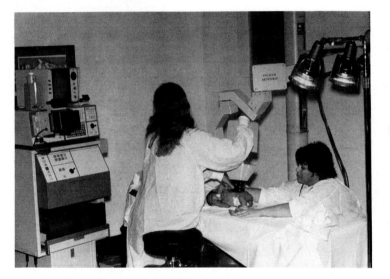

Fig. 18-25. Overhead heating lamps, a clean environment, and a member of the neonatal ward team are necessary for examination of the neonate. (From Canty, T., et al.: Ultrasonography of pediatric surgical disorders, New York, 1981, Grune & Stratton, Inc.)

teropelvic junction obstruction, multicystic dysplastic kidney, and renal vein thrombosis are the most frequent abnormalities.

The ultrasound examination can be performed with the infant in the supine, decubitus, or prone position. If the supine or decubitus position is utilized, examination is performed in the midaxillary line; if prone, examination is from the posterior. Longitudinal scanning of the kidney from medial to lateral is performed followed by transverse scanning cephalad to caudad. Recorded images should be representative of the corticomedullary areas and the renal pelvis.

In the *normal* neonatal kidney the medullary portions (pyramids) are clearly visible as areas of lower echogenicity than the surrounding cortex (Fig. 18-26). An irregular renal outline, called fetal lobulation, can

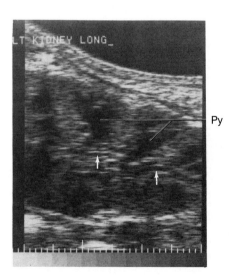

Fig. 18-26. The medullary portions, pyramids, *Py,* of the neonatal kidney, are clearly seen on this prone longitudinal scan. A normal amount of urine within the renal collecting system *(arrows)* is also identified.

often be identified. The normal renal pelvis contains a small amount of urine. Since renal sinus fat is minimal or absent in the neonate, the renal sinus does not appear as dense as in the adult.

In *congenital ureteropelvic junction* (UPJ) *obstruction* the renal pelvis becomes dilated and variable degrees of calyectasis occur (Fig. 18-27). Some normal parenchyma can usually be seen. With other causes of hydronephrosis, especially reflux, the renal pelvis becomes dilated to a lesser degree and more uniformly than with UPJ obstruction.

In *multicystic dysplastic kidney* the contour is quite irregular and the parenchyma disorganized. Multiple cysts of varying size can usually be identified in these nonfunctioning kidneys.

Infants of diabetic mothers and very sick dehydrated babies are at risk for *renal vein thrombosis*. Enlargement of the affected kidney, absence of urine in the renal pelvis, and swollen pyramids are characteristic of this disorder.

Hepatobiliary system. Excellent resolution of the premature infant's liver is possible with small-parts scanners (Fig. 18-28). Depth limitations, however, may preclude complete evaluation of the liver in full-term infants.

In an infant who has not recently been fed, the gallbladder can usually be identified. Sludge, whose significance is unknown at this age, has been seen on occasion; and cholelithiasis, although unusual in newborns, may be demonstrated.

A choledochal cyst, dilation of a segment of the extrahepatic biliary system, may be suspected in an infant who presents with a palpable abdominal mass and jaundice. The sonographic feature is a right upper quadrant cystic mass in the porta hepatis that is separable from the gallbladder. The intrahepatic bile ducts may be dilated or of normal caliber.

Idiopathic hypertrophic pyloric stenosis. Infants who present with vomiting and are suspected of having pyloric stenosis are candidates for sonography. The ultrasonic appearance of pyloric stenosis is a thick (at least 4 mm) circular hypoechoic ring that represents the muscular thickening (Fig. 18-29).

Miscellaneous

Spinal cord. Infants who present with cutaneous defects overlying the sacrum such as a sacral dimple, hairy patch, or hemangioma are at risk for tethering of the cord. A tethered cord is anomalous insertion lower than normal and relatively fixed. Early diagnosis is crucial since it can cause irreversible nerve deficits if not surgically corrected.

Longitudinal imaging is begun in the posterior midline at the midthoracic level. The spinal cord, central canal of the cord, and fluid in the subarachnoid space can be seen (Fig. 18-30). As scanning progresses caudally, the cauda equina and filum terminale can be viewed.

Normally the cord moves freely within the spinal canal. The most striking sonographic features of a tethered cord are the lack of cord motion and thickening of the filum. The cord exhibits a rigid appearance within the spinal canal.

For documentation of dynamic events, the videotape format is necessary. Static photography, however, can be utilized for anatomical representation.

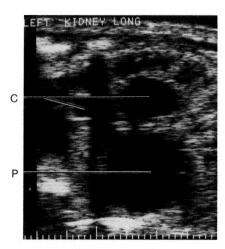

Fig. 18-27. Prone longitudinal scan of a ureteropelvic junction obstruction in a neonate. The renal pelvis, *P,* and calyces, *C,* are grossly dilated.

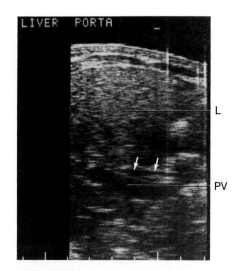

Fig. 18-28. Supine longitudinal scan demonstrating the liver, *L,* and the common bile duct *(arrows)* in this neonate. *PV,* Portal vein.

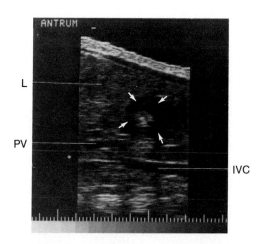

Fig. 18-29. This supine longitudinal scan of the epigastrium shows the thick muscular ring *(arrows)* of pyloric stenosis. *L,* Liver; *PV,* portal vein; *IVC,* inferior vena cava.

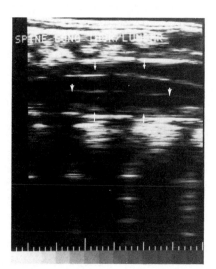

Fig. 18-30. Lumbar spinal cord within the subarachnoid space *(arrows)* on a prone longitudinal scan. The linear echo within the spinal cord is the central canal *(arrowheads).*

19

Breast

MELANIE G. EZO
SANDRA L. HAGEN-ANSERT

One out of eleven American women will develop breast cancer. It is the leading cause of death for the middle-aged woman. Early detection of the tumor is vital since the disease can spread rapidly. Delays in early detection and treatment can be particularly tragic because of the 5-year survival rate for localized breast cancer adequately treated is 98% after 5 years and 95% after 10 years.[7] Metastatic cancer shows survival rates of only 30% to 50% after 10 years.

The clinical diagnosis of breast cancer may fall under several categories depending upon the age of the patient, whether or not the lesion is palpable, the risk factors of the patient, and previous medical history. The practice of self-examination is an important issue in the detection of early lesions, or subtle changes in the breast parenchyma that one may notice only from a regular routine examination.

The purpose of this chapter is to present an overview of breast lesions with particular reference to the aspects with which a sonographer is concerned either directly or indirectly, and its primary emphasis will be on the technique of sonography.

There has been considerable interest in noninvasive methods to image the breast parenchyma (i.e., thermography, diaphanography, and sonography). As early as 1951 the first paper on ultrasound of the breast was published by John Wild using A-mode techniques. The following year Wild utilized the B-mode with a water bag technique to image the breast parenchyma. Several years later, in 1956, the Japanese utilized an overhead water bag method with a 2-MHz transducer and noted that malignancies returned "strong" echoes. In 1967 the Australians developed a similar overhead water bag technique with a 2-MHz transducer and noticed the breast was greatly compressed by this attempt. Contrary to previous work reported, the group at the Ultrasonics Institute discovered that malignancies returned low-level echoes and strong echoes were obtained from the surrounding fibrous connective tissues. The following year Elizabeth

Kelly-Fry developed an overhead water bag method with an open drape allowing the breast to protrude from a hole, held firm by adhesive tape and a plastic drape. In 1969 gray scale instrumentation was developed by the Ultrasonics Institute and had a significant impact on tissue differentiation seen on ultrasound images. In 1974 the Australians modified their instrumentation so the patient would lie in a prone position with her breast immersed in a warm water bath. A single 4-MHz transducer was employed to provide higher resolution. In the succeeding several years three dedicated breast units have become commercially available for clinical use.

ANATOMY

The function of the female breast is to secrete milk during lactation. The breast is a differentiated apocrine sweat gland. Its parenchymal elements are the lobes, ducts, lobules, and acini. Because the mammary gland is a skin derivative, the stromal elements include dense connective tissue, loose connective tissue, and fat. Sonographically fat is the least echogenic tissue within the breast. The interface between fat and loose connective tissue is less echogenic than that between fat and dense connective tissue. The position of these interfaces in relation to the beam determines their reflectivity. The age and functional state of the breast dictate the amount and arrangement of various parenchymal and stromal elements. There may be variation of these elements in women of the same age group, in breasts of similar functioning states, and from region to region in the same breast.

The breast is comprised of 15 to 20 lobes. Each lobe contains the parenchymal elements of the breast. Ducts extend from the lobes through the breast parenchyma to converge in a single papilla, the nipple, which is surrounded by the areola (Fig. 19-1). The ducts are covered with a connective tissue layer that varies in thickness and density from breast to breast. The normal duct usually measures about 2 mm in diameter. The patient who is nursing may have a lac-

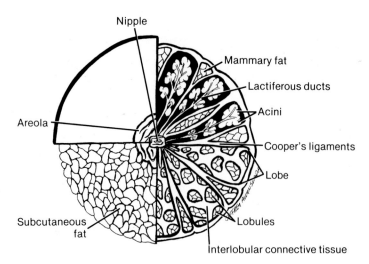

Fig. 19-1. Anatomy of the breast. (Modified from Townsend, C.M.: Clin. Symp. **32**[2]: 1, 1980.)

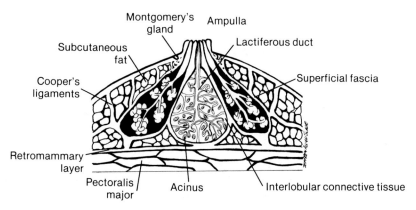

Fig. 19-2. Anatomy of the breast. (Modified from Townsend, C.M.: Clin. Symp. **32**[2]:1, 1980.)

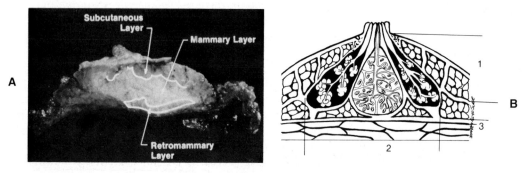

Fig. 19-3. Three layers of breast tissue. **A,** Anatomic section. **B,** Diagram. *1,* Subcutaneous fatty layer; *2,* mammary layer; *3,* retromammary layer. (Modified from Townsend, C.M.: Clin. Symp. **32**[2]:1, 1980.)

There are three well-defined layers in the breast: subcutaneous, mammary, and retromammary (Fig. 19-3). The *subcutaneous* layer is bounded superficially by the dermis and deeply by the superficial connective tissue plane.[1] The principal component of this layer is fat lobules enclosed by connective tissue septa. The *mammary* layer is composed of breast parenchyma and is found between the superficial and deep connective tissue layers. Fat is seen to be interspersed in a lobular fashion throughout the entire breast parenchyma. The sonographic pattern within this layer shows the greatest variation with the patient's age and functional state of the breast.[1] The *retromammary* layer consists of fat lobules that are separated anteriorly from the mammary layer by the deep connective tissue plane and posteriorly by the fascia over the pectoralis major.

During pregnancy the ducts and parenchymal elements of the breast expand to such a degree that the mammary layer takes up the entire breast. The subcutaneous fat layer and the retromammary layer are so squeezed that they appear very narrow on the sonogram. The interfaces in the pregnant breast will be less echogenic.

The major portion of the breast contained within the superficial fascia of the anterior thoracic wall is situated between the second or third rib superiorly, the sixth or seventh costal cartilage inferiorly, the anterior axillary line laterally, and the sternal border medially.[9] The greatest amount of glandular tissue is located in the upper outer quadrant of the breast, which explains why tumors are more frequently found here.

The major pectoral muscle lies posterior to the retromammary layer. The minor pectoral muscle lies superolaterally posterior to it. The pectoralis minor courses from its rib cage origin to the point where it inserts into the coracoid process. The lower border of the pectoralis major forms the anterior border of the axilla. Breast tissue can extend into this region and is referred to as the axillary tail or tail of Spence (Fig. 19-4).

Vascular supply and lymph drainage

The principal blood supply to the breast is from branches of the internal mammary and the lateral thoracic arteries. The intercostal artery plays a subordinant role. Venous drainage is through superficial and deep veins. The superficial veins are usually arranged in a transverse or longitudinal pattern and can be seen on the sonogram. The deep veins are not visible. In the axilla the axillary vein is sonographically visible, with the axil-

tating duct that measures as much as 8 mm.

The entire breast is enveloped in a duplication of superficial pectoral fascia. The posterior part of the fascia is connected to the pectoral musculature; the anterior part to the skin by thin connective septa (Fig. 19-2). The anterior and posterior fascial planes are connected by curvilinear connective tissue septa known as Cooper's ligaments.[3] These ligaments are the supporting structures of the breast and provide the shape and consistency of its parenchyma. The connective tissue septa envelope the lobules and lobes of the breast and become the interlobular and interlobar connective tissues that surround the fat lobules and parenchyma of the breast.

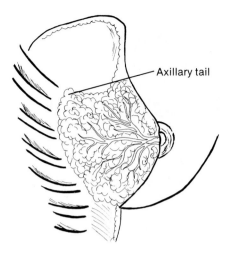

Fig. 19-4. A projection of tissue, called the axillary tail or tail of Spence, usually extends from the upper outer quadrant into the axilla.

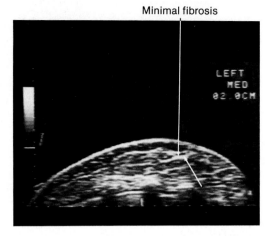

Fig. 19-5. Sagittal scan of the fatty breast. (Courtesy Thomas Jefferson University Hospital, Philadelphia.)

Minimal fibrosis

Fig. 19-6. Sagittal scan of the fatty breast with minimal fibrosis of the connective tissue (compression).

lary artery located superior and a bit posterior to it.

The lymphatics of the breast originate in the lymph capillaries of the mammary connective tissue grid. The lymph capillaries are similar to blood capillaries and are abundant in the breast tissue. They have valves to assure flow in the direction of the venous system (away from the tissues). The lymph vessels empty into lymph nodes; thus when cancer cells invade the lymphatic system, they reach the lymph nodes, which act as a filter and retain the malignant cells. These then grow at the expense of the node and gradually destroy it.

The axillary lymph nodes are closely related to the axillary vein. The majority of the lymph drainage passes to this group of nodes. Other drainage pathways are along the inferior margin of the pectoralis major. Flow may also be directed to groups of lymph nodes around the third, fourth, and fifth prongs of the serratus anterior as well as toward the intercostal and mediastinal node group. Lymph drainage is also routed to the subdiaphragmatic lymph nodes. Medial lymph drainage eventually reaches the peristernal and anterior mediastinal lymph nodes. In addition, there are abundant lymphatic connections to the opposite breast.

Variations in parenchymal patterns

The first pattern, and the one most difficult to image by sonography, is the fatty breast. Fatty replacement of the parenchymal elements of the breast occurs with each pregnancy. With the onset of menopause there is atrophy of the ducts. As a result, all three layers appear fatty. Generally radiogra-

A

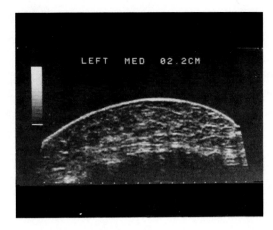

Fig. 19-7. Progressing degress of fibrosis. **A,** Sagittal scan showing dense mammary layer with scalloping of superficial connective tissue plane. **B,** Dense mammary layer with some fatty infiltration (compression). **C,** Fibrosis with extensive fatty infiltration into the mammary layer (compression). (**A** to **C** courtesy Thomas Jefferson University Hospital, Philadelphia.)

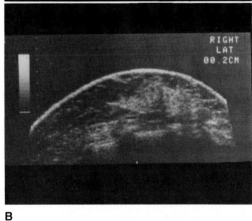

B

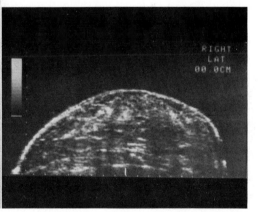

C

phy images this type of breast quite adequately (Fig. 19-5).

The second pattern is still largely fat. Histologically there is some periductal connective tissue, which sonographically presents as bright reflectors. The breast basically appears fatty (Fig. 19-6).

The next pattern is complex. It consists of progressing degrees of fibrosis. Sonographically degrees of coalescence of the dense connective tissue and a scalloped effect of the

superficial connective tissue plane can often be seen (Fig. 19-7). There is still some residual fat present in this pattern.

The last pattern shows no residual fat in the mammary layer. The fat is replaced by dense connective tissue. If this breast is examined with a water path scanner with the patient prone and the breast in a free hanging position, an area of no information occurs in the central portion (Fig. 19-8). The extent of the shadow will depend upon the beam

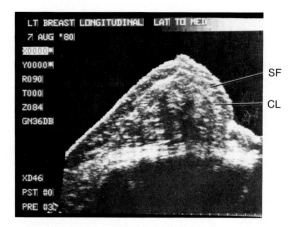

Fig. 19-8. Central shadow in a fatty replaced breast. *SF,* Subcutaneous fat; *CL,* Cooper's ligaments.

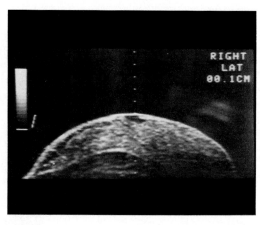

Fig. 19-9. Sagittal scan of a young dense breast in compression.

width, depth of placement of the focus, frequency of the transducer, and tissue structure of the nipple. If multiple transducers are used, a compound scan may help to eliminate this shadow. However, a more effective technique is compression. The use of compression allows the breast tissue to be flattened, thus compressing the dense tissue and allowing the acoustic beam to be perpendicular to more interfaces (Fig. 19-9).

PHYSIOLOGY

The breast is an endocrine gland and is affected in its physical and microscopic state by the changing hormonal levels. The growth of the breast begins before the onset of menstruation. At puberty the combined influences of the hypothalamus and anterior pituitary, and later the ovaries, cause growth of the breast. Although these are the primary endocrine sources responsible for breast growth, complete development also requires normal levels of insulin and thyroid hormone secretions.[4]

During the first year or two of menstruation, ovulation does not occur and there is an increased output of estrogen. This causes the mammary ducts to elongate. Their epithelial lining reduplicates and proliferates as the ends of the mammary tubules form sprouts of future lobules. Estrogen stimulates the vascularity of the breast tissue, increases the volume and elasticity of the connective tissues, and induces fat deposition in the breast.

With the onset of maturity (i.e., when ovulation occurs and the progesterone-secreting corpora lutea are formed) the second stage of mammary development occurs.[8] This is the formation of the lobules and acinar structures and gives the mammary gland the characteristic lobular structure found

during childbearing years. Further acinar development continues in proportion to the intensity of the hormonal stimuli during each menstrual cycle.

During pregnancy, changes occur that make milk production possible. In addition to estrogen and progesterone, hormones such as placental lactogen, prolactin, and chorionic gonadotropin are required for complete gestational development of the breast.[11] At delivery there is a loss of estrogen and progesterone. Prolactin then predominates and the alveolar cells actively synthesize and secrete milk. During the 3 months following cessation of lactation, involution of the breast occurs. The breast remains larger due to the fatty tissue replacement. Postlactation involution is a decrease in the size of the lobular-alveolar components as compared to their enlargement during pregnancy.

EVALUATION OF THE PATIENT WITH A BREAST MASS
Medical history

A complete medical history is very important in assessing the patient with a breast mass. Several pertinent questions may aid the clinician in the final diagnosis:

Age (the greater the age the higher the risk, especially over 35)
Previous cancer of the breast (up to 16% will develop cancer in the other breast)
Family history (40% chance of developing cancer if mother had cancer)
Late first pregnancy (28 or over)
Nulliparous women
Late menopause (54 or older)
Previous biopsy for benign disease
Exposure to radiation at an early age
Mammographic appearance of a prominent duct pattern or marked dysplasia
Obesity
Suppression of emotions (especially anger)

The age of the patient is important since malignancy is rarely found in women under 25 and the incidence steadily increases with age. If the patient or the clinician detects a breast mass, symptoms such as pain, tenderness, or nipple discharge should be noted. The patient is questioned whether these symptoms occur cyclicly, during pregnancy, or in relation to trauma or previous breast disease. Patients with a previous biopsy-proved breast lesion or who have had breast cancer are at an increased risk for cancer. The incidence of cancer is greater in a patient whose mother or sister has had breast cancer. Early menarche and late menopause have also been associated with an increased risk of breast cancer.[8]

The most dramatic decrease in the risk for breast cancer has been found in women who have had a full-term pregnancy before the age of 18.

Diagnostic techniques

A complete physical examination of the patient's breasts should be performed after the medical history has been taken. It is essential that the size, location, consistency, and mobility of the mass be noted, as well as the site of biopsy scars, asymmetry between the breasts, skin changes or discoloration, and the presence of skin dimpling.

One of the most reliable methods for detecting breast masses is palpation, which may be done by either the physician or the patient. The advantages of the physician's performing the examination are threefold: the physician is more skilled in palpation techniques, better prepared to distinguish subtle pathologic changes, and emotionally detached and objective. The disadvantage is that the examination is done only once or twice a year whereas self-examination is done monthly. Premenopausal women should examine their breasts at the same time of the month, preferably 5 to 7 days after cessation of menses, so subtle changes can be detected.

Most breast lumps are benign, with only 20% to 25% of those surgically removed revealing malignancy. More than 90% of the lumps are found by breast self-examination.

Mammography.[8] When a dominant lesion has been found, mammography is used to evaluate the remainder of the breast and the opposite breast for occult lesions that may not be related to the primary mass. Mammography can detect lesions less than 1 cm in diameter, which is smaller than may be clinically palpated. The diagnostic accuracy of mammography is 85% to 90%. Mammography generally is utilized in patients who are at high risk of developing breast cancer, are symptomatic, or are unduly worried about developing breast cancer. It is not used as a routine screening tool for all ages.

Mammography is the most sensitive technique for detecting cancer in the breast whose tissue is predominantly fatty. It also is sensitive in detecting nonpalpable cancers that exhibit malignant calcifications. There is, however, a population for whom mammography may not be the first method of choice in evaluating the breast. This includes young women under 35 and those with dense fibrous glandular breasts. Sonography is far more effective in this population and has been used as a baseline evaluation for following up on these patients.

Diaphanography. This diagnostic technique can distinguish tumors from cysts, detect dilation and twisting of blood vessels that may accompany cancer, and aid in guiding the needle placement for a biopsy.

The principle of diaphanography is that when the breast is illuminated with a light of the appropriate wavelength and photographed with an infrared film malignant tumors appear dark whereas healthy tissue is reddish yellow or translucent. Blood vessels look dark red or black. Cysts with clear fluid show as bright spots within the breast, and benign tumors appear dark red.

The limitation of this technique is that it is not effective in distinguishing cancer from mastitis or from a cyst with hemorrhage. Clinical work is being conducted to further define the benefits of such a noninvasive approach to detecting breast lesions.

Ultrasound. The cautious approach to the use of mammography for the general population in evaluating the breast has caused major commercial companies to push forward with their research and development of dedicated breast water path scanners that can evaluate the entire breast in a systematic manner without the use of ionizing radiation. In 1978 the National Cancer Institute funded a 2-year study to determine the efficacy of ultrasound in detecting breast cancer. At approximately the same time, leading research centers were asked to clinically evaluate dedicated breast ultrasound scanners. From this work, ultrasound was found clinically useful in the following conditions: patients with radiographic dense breasts (any age), younger patients, those with an equivocal mammographic finding, symptomatic patients who were pregnant or lactating, and patients with breast prostheses. It was also of great value in distinguishing a cystic from a solid lesion in a patient with a known breast mass.

Articulated arm technique. Patients who present with a palpable breast lesion may be examined with the articulated arm scanner.

The patient is examined in a supine-oblique position, as she is rolled about 35 degrees toward the side opposite the breast to be examined. A sponge or folded towel is placed under her hips and shoulders to support her position. Her arm (on the side of the breast to be examined) is placed behind her head to help provide a stable scanning surface.

A high-frequency, 5.0- or 7.5-MHz, small-diameter transducer is utilized to image the breast parenchyma. The time gain compensation is adjusted to balance the skin echo, subcutaneous fat, dense breast core or mammary layer, retromammary layer, and pectoral muscles. The sensitivity of the equipment is adjusted to visualize the low-level subcutaneous layer, the echogenic mammary layer, the bright reflection from the retromammary layer, and the medium-level reflection from the pectoral muscles.

The mass is localized and its boundaries noted with a marking pen. The area surrounding the mass in a 3-cm square is then marked off with the marking pen. Scans are made in the transverse direction beginning at the inferior margin and moving cephalad by the smallest intervals possible (most equipment allows 5 mm increments). Subsequent scans are made in the sagittal direction beginning at the medial border of the square and moving laterally by small intervals. Extreme care should be taken to scan very lightly over the breast area so as not to distort the architecture. If the mass is very mobile, you may need to isolate it between two fingers. This will secure the lesion so it will not slip from under the transducer as you are scanning. The characteristics of the mass should be noted: shape, size, definition of borders, amount of transmission or attenuation, presence or absence of internal echoes, and degree of reflection from the anterior or posterior wall. Because the mass must be evaluated so carefully, it is important to assess these characteristics when the beam is directly over the major part of the lesion. Small lesions, under 1 cm, may not be visualized by the articulated arm technique due to the large 5-mm increment system or because the transducer creates a wide beam width, which fails to visualize a mass smaller than the transducer diameter.

The limitations of the articulated arm system are that it deforms the skin and underlying tissues by the direct transducer contact. Generally there is a poor portrayal of skin and subcutaneous detail. In addition, it is very difficult to scan adequately near the nipple area.

Another problem arises in examining the patient with a multicentric process such as fibrocystic disease. Then the entire breast should be evaluated and it becomes very cumbersome to scan the whole breast accurately in small intervals since the breast is such a mobile flaccid structure in the supine position. Thus a dedicated breast water path unit was developed for a complete evaluation of the breast.

Dedicated water path breast instrumentation. The commercially available water path systems allow the patient to lie prone on a special examining bed with the breast suspended in a large water tank (Fig. 19-10).

The transducer or transducers are mounted within the tank (Fig. 19-11). The diameter of the transducer is much larger than found in the conventional hand-held transducer. This allows the beam to be focused more precisely in the breast tissue. The focal length is dependent upon the amount of water present between the breast and the transducer.

The patient lies in the prone swimmer's position with the arm by the breast to be examined placed at her side (Fig. 19-12). This allows the tail of the breast to be coupled with water.

Scans may be performed by small, 1-to-2-mm, intervals in the transverse, sagittal, coronal, or rotational mode (depending upon the particular instrumentation utilized). A mass lesion should be visualized in two axes and its characteristic pattern noted with a single transducer.

There are several approaches to visualizing the breast with the water path system. The multiple transducer approach provides an image with little or no nipple shadow;

however, the multiple transducer *overwrite* may eliminate the attenuation or transmission characteristics of a lesion that might be clearly shown with a single transducer.

Various areas of the breast that cannot be seen on one view may be well shown on another. For example, the blind area on the transverse scan is near the inferomedial margin of the breast whereas on the sagittal scan it is near the inferior margin. Thus a mass may be better shown in one view than another.

Compression techniques. A flexible non-attenuating material may be draped under the breasts or wrapped around the chest to enable the breast tissue to be compressed or flattened.

There are several advantages to the compression technique. Generally if the nipple shadow was present, it will disappear with compression to allow a better view of the subareolar area. Kelly-Fry[5] further states two additional advantages to the compression technique: (1) it decreases the length of the tissue path that the sound field must traverse and allows transducers with higher frequencies to be used; and (2) the problem of the loss of sound at a sharp angle of entrance to the breast is eliminated by the flattening of the tissues and thus delineation of the lesion is improved.

The disadvantages of compression are that it distorts the anatomy and sometimes eliminates the skin line information.

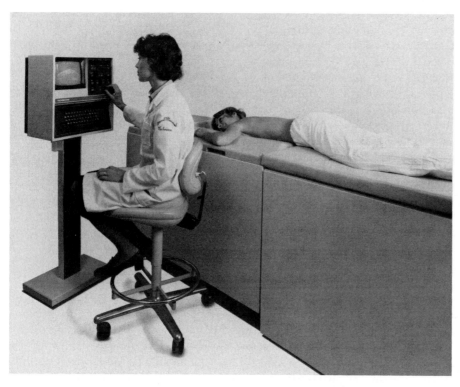

Fig. 19-10. Commercially available real time water path dedicated breast instrument that utilizes a single large-aperture transducer to survey the breast completely.

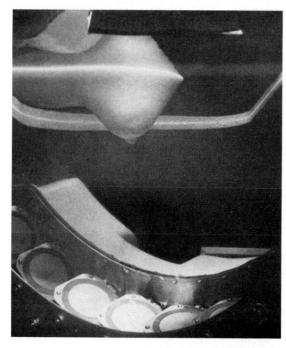

Fig. 19-11. Commercially available water path system that utilizes several large-aperture transducers to examine the breast.

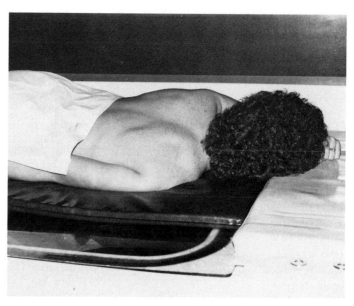

Fig. 19-12. It is necessary that the patient be placed in an oblique position so water contact and perpendicularity of the beam with the breast and the tail of Spence will be maintained.

Ultrasonic description of the normal breast. There are many variations in the normal breast and these must be fully appreciated for interpretation of the sonographic image and differentiation of normal patterns from pathologic processes. The breast of a premenopausal patient will be discussed in detail.

The boundaries of the breast are the skin line, nipple, and retromammary layer. These generally give strong bright echo reflections. The areaolar area may be recognized by the slightly lower echo reflection as compared to the nipple and skin. The internal nipple may show low to bright reflections and is quite variable (Fig. 19-13).

Subcutaneous fat displays areas of generally low reflectivity intermixed with bright reflectors from Cooper's ligaments and other connective tissue (Fig. 19-14). The Cooper ligaments will be seen if the beam strikes them at a perpendicular angle. Often compression of the breast will allow even more ligaments to be visualized.

The mammary layer, often referred to as the breast core or active glandular breast tissue, is generally displayed as a somewhat cone-shaped or triangular area beneath the subcutaneous fat layer and anterior to the retromammary layer. It is shown to converge toward the nipple (Fig. 19-15). The fatty tissue interdispersed throughout the mammary layer will dictate the amount of intensity reflected from the breast parenchyma. If little fat is present, there is a uniform architecture with a strong echogenic pattern (due to collagen and fibrotic tissue) throughout the mammary layer. When fatty tissue is present, areas of low-level echoes become intertwined with areas of strong echoes from the active breast tissue. The analysis of this pattern becomes critical to the final diagnosis, and one must be able to separate lobules of fat from a marginated lesion.

The use of compression may help to determine whether a suspected lesion maintains its shape or loses it, as fatty tissue does when compressed. Some instruments allow one to rotate around a point; thus fatty tissue will be very irregular and merge into the breast parenchyma whereas a lesion will be marginated from the parenchyma. Another technique, the *C-scan,* may be used to record a coronal slice of the area of interest so a lesion can be discerned from fat tissue.

The retromammary layer is similar in texture to the subcutaneous layer, although the boundary echoes resemble skin reflections. The pectoral muscles are shown as low-level

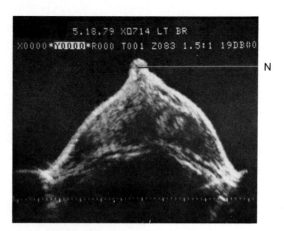

Fig. 19-13. Transverse scan of a noncompressed breast. *N,* Nipple.

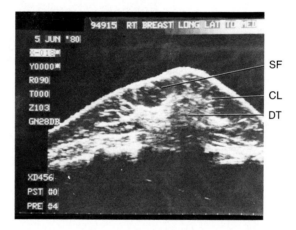

Fig. 19-14. Subcutaneous fat, *SF,* displays areas of low reflectivity interspersed with bright reflectors from Cooper's ligament, *CL.* Dense tissue, *DT.*

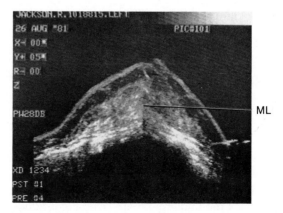

Fig. 19-15. Transverse scan of the mammary layer of the breast, *ML.*

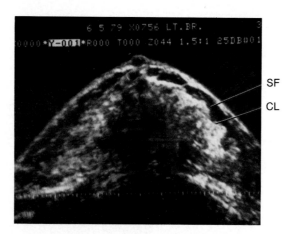

Fig. 19-16. Dense breast. *SF,* Subcutaneous fat; *CL,* Cooper's ligament.

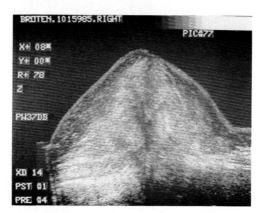

Fig. 19-17. Fatty replaced breast.

echo areas posterior to the retromammary layer. Ribs and intercostal margins are seen as bright and anechoic areas posterior to the pectoral muscles.

The echo appearance of the breast does change with age: the younger the patient, the greater the volume of the mammary layer, the denser the breast, and the more effective sonography is over mammography (Fig. 19-16). The older patient has more fatty tissue, and it is more difficult to distinguish disruptions in architecture than in the younger denser breast (Fig. 19-17).

Many breast lesions occur diffusely within the breast parenchyma (i.e., fibrous infiltration and fibrocystic disease). The recognition of these processes involves assessing the magnitude, texture, and distribution of echoes throughout the breast core.

Changes associated with a diffuse breast lesion may be characterized by
1. Increase in fibrotic tissue (more echogenic)
2. Increase in amplitude of echoes
3. Increase in fatty tissue (less echogenic)
Usually fatty infiltrations are not well circumscribed. Diffuse conditions lack the uniformity and texture seen in normal breast tissue.

Localized lesions may exhibit cystic or solid appearances depending on their particular characteristics. Observation of the lesions should be made using the following criteria:
1. Boundary echoes
2. Attenuation or transmission characteristics
3. Shape and position of the lesion
4. Disruption of normal architecture
5. Nature of surrounding tissues
6. Homogeneity
7. Presence of calcifications
8. Skin changes

Each of these changes will be discussed in the next section as they relate to cystic versus solid lesions and the distinction between benign and malignant breast lesions.

PATHOLOGY OF BREAST MASSES

The most common pathologic lesions of the female breast are, in order of decreasing frequency, fibrocystic disease, carcinoma, fibroadenoma, intraductal papilloma, and duct ectasia.[11] Benign lesions are the most common breast lesions, occurring in 70% of proved lesions biopsied or removed. There are several considerations to utilize when a dominant mass has been palpated: patient's age, physical characteristics of the mass, and previous medical history. Lesions more common to younger women are fibrocystic disease and fibroadenomas. Older or postmenopausal women are more likely to have intraductal papillomas, duct ectasia, and cancer.

The benign and malignant masses will be discussed with their clinical findings and symptoms, mammographic findings,[3] and ultrasound findings.

Characteristic signs of breast masses[9]

Contour or margin
  Smooth
  Irregular
  Spiculated
Shape
  Round
  Oval
  Tubular
  Lobulated
Internal echo pattern
  Anechoic (homogeneous)
    Strong
    Intermediate
    Weak
    Mixed
Boundary echoes
  Anterior and/or posterior
    Strong
    Weak
    Absent
Attenuation effects
  Acoustic enhancement
  Acoustic shadowing
    Central
    Bilateral
    Unilateral
Distal echoes
  Strong
  Intermediate
  Weak
  Absent
Disruption of architecture

Benign disease

Fibrocystic disease. This breast syndrome has histologic changes that occur on the terminal ducts and lobules of the breast in both the epithelial and the connective tissue and is usually accompanied by pain in the breast.

Its etiology is thought to be a disturbance in the estrogen-progesterone balance since it does not occur during puberty. It is a cyclic dysplasia, with signs and symptoms that vary according to the menstrual cycle. (Other diseases such as mammary dysplasia, fibroadenoma, cystosarcoma phylloides, and papillomas do not change with the menstrual cycle.)

The changes in fibrocystic disease occur in the breast parenchyma according to the patient's age. General symptoms are pain, nodularity, a dominant mass, cysts, and occasional nipple discharge.

There are three distinct stages:

1. Mastodynia or mazoplasia
2. Adenosis
3. Cystic disease

Stage 1, *mazoplasia*, is characterized by an increased proliferation of the stroma and by the small number of lobules or acini.[10] Stage 2, *adenosis*, is hyperplasia and proliferation of the epithelial component of the ducts.[10] Stage 3, *cystic disease*, is the involution of the lobules and hyperplasia of the surrounding stroma, leading to the formation of cysts.[10]

Another facet of fibrocystic disease is the dilation of the ducts, known as *comedomastitis*. This is seen in middle-aged women and is characterized by the dilation of ducts filled with a secretion produced by desquamated cells from the duct wall. The secretion will be manifested clinically by a multicolored and sticky nipple discharge. It often is accompanied by a retroareolar or periareolar redness and burning pain and itching. If untreated, the terminal ducts dilate and thicken. If the process is chronic, the ducts become tortuous (varicocele of Bloodgood) and may cause nipple retraction that simulates cancer.

Fibrocystic disease is a benign condition although a patient with duct hyperplasia and atypia is subject to a five-times greater risk of developing breast cancer.[10]

Apocrine metaplasia with atypia carries a similar but slightly decreased risk factor and has been termed *precancerous mastopathy* by Haagensen.[2]

Gross cystic disease and breast cancer occur in the same age group of patients, 40 to 50 years. Thus the method for diagnosis and treatment must be specific, to rule out a benign process versus a malignant one.

In the stage of mastodynia or mazoplasia the breasts are very painful, especially in the premenstrual period. The upper outer quadrants seem to be the most sensitive. This process is commonly seen in young women. Since it is a benign condition, it may subside spontaneously with time, medication, or pregnancy.

Stage 2 or adenosis is commonly seen in women 25 to 40 years of age. The pain is premenstrual and less severe. The patient may also have nipple discharge. (To be clinically significant, the discharge must be spontaneous and unprovoked.) The breast parenchyma is more pronounced and irregular due to nodularity. The nodules are usually of small size; they are considered more dominant as they reach 1 cm.

If the hyperplasia is surrounded by an intense proliferation of fibrous tissue, these areas may form a dominant mass that may be

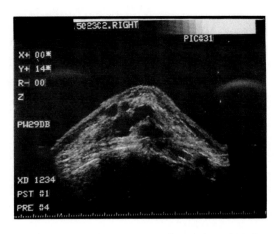

Fig. 19-18. Transverse noncompression scan of a patient with fibrocystic disease showing multiple characteristic cystic structures throughout the breast.

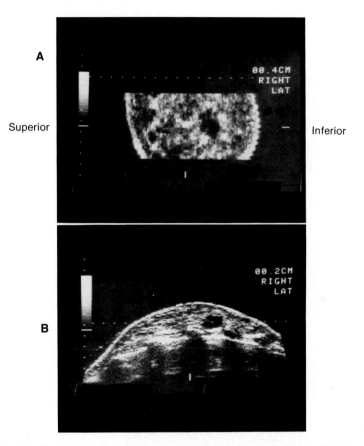

Fig. 19-19. A, The C-scan coronal slice of this cystic mass is taken parallel with the chest wall. It demonstrates the medial to lateral extent of the mass at this particular mass. **B,** Sagittal compression scan of the cystic mass with a septation. (Courtesy University of California, San Francisco.)

mistaken clinically for cancer. It is helpful to distinguish a tumor, which will have three dimensions (height, width and depth) and occupy space, whereas a mass will have only two dimensions (height and width) and represents thickening.

Mammographic findings
1. Scattered fine, coarse, round, or lobulated densities and masses in combination with proliferation of parenchyma and linear strands of fibrous (stromal) tissue

Ultrasound findings (Fig. 19-18)
1. Average amount of subcutaneous fat
2. Areas of fibrous stroma that appear brighter than the parenchyma
3. Small cysts scattered throughout the breast (cystic stage)
4. Large cysts may also be present (Fig. 19-19).

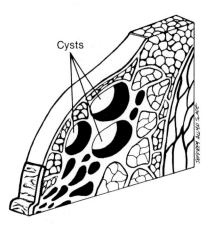

Cysts

Fig. 19-20. Schematic of multiple cysts in a breast. (Modified from Townsend, C.M.: Clin. Symp. **32**[2]:1, 1980.)

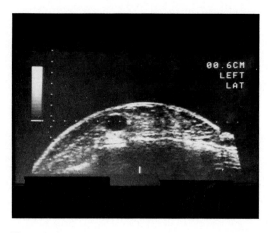

Fig. 19-21. Sagittal scan of a simple cyst with smooth well-defined borders. (Courtesy University of California, San Francisco.)

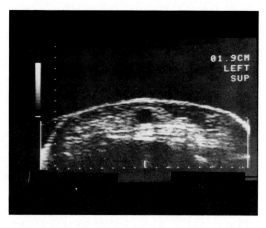

Fig. 19-22. Sagittal scan of a simple cyst with lateral edge shadowing posterior to the mass. (Courtesy University of California, San Francisco.)

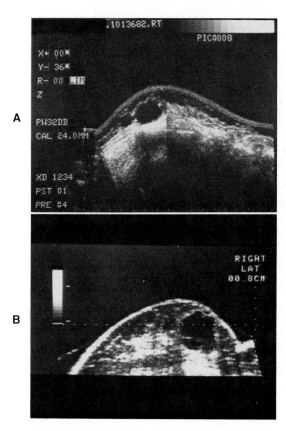

Fig. 19-23. A, Transverse scan of a cystic anechoic mass. **B,** Postoperative sagittal scan of a complex hemorrhagic mass with layering (Courtesy M.D. Anderson Medical Center, Houston.)

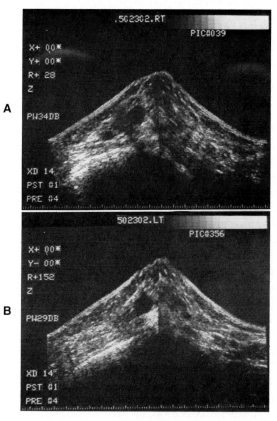

Fig. 19-24. Rotational view of a patient with fibrocystic disease. **A,** The multiple cysts do not appear to exhibit posterior enhancement probably because of transducer positioning in relation to the mass. **B,** The transducer is correctly positioned to record the transmission properties of the cysts.

Cystic disease. This disease is commonly seen in women 35 to 55 years of age. Symptoms include history of a changing menstrual cycle, pain (especially when the cyst is growing rapidly), recent lump, and tenderness. The disease may be microcystic or macrocystic. The small cyst may regress incompletely during the premenstrual phase. In the microcystic form, the cysts are multiple with some pain and tenderness of the breast. The macrocystic form has three-dimensional lesions, well delineated and slightly mobile (Fig. 19-20). These cysts may be aspirated for analysis of the fluid.

Mammographic findings
1. Usually smooth walled with sharp borders
2. Hard to differentiate between a cyst and a noncalcified fibroadenoma
3. Lucent rim of fat around cyst

Ultrasound findings[4]

1. Smooth, sharp, well-defined borders (Fig. 19-21)
2. Lateral edge shadowing (arises from the low energy loss as the beam passes normally through the distal cyst wall, leaving sufficient energy to cause multireflections between the distal cyst wall and the chest wall[6]) (Fig. 19-22)
3. Anechoic (Fig. 19-23)
4. Posterior enhancement (Fig. 19-24)

Fibroadenoma. This is one of the most common benign breast tumors, *the* most common in childhood, and occurs primarily in young adult women. It may be found in one breast only or bilaterally.

The growth of the fibroadenoma is stimulated by the administration of estrogen. Under normal circumstances hormonal influences on the breast (estrogen) result in the proliferation of epithelial cells in lactiferous ducts and in stromal tissue during the first half of the menstrual cycle. During the second half this condition regresses allowing breast tissue to return to its normal resting state. In certain disturbances of this hormonal mechanism the regression fails to occur and results in the development of fibrous and epithelial nodules that become fibroadenomas, fibromas, or adenomas depending on the predominant cell type. They may also be related to pregnancy and lactation.

Clinically the fibroadenoma is firm, rubbery, freely mobile, and clearly delineated from the surrounding breast tissue (Fig. 19-25). It is round or ovoid, smooth or lobulated, and usually does not cause loss of contour of the breast unless it develops to a large size. It rarely causes mastodynia, and it does not change size during the menstrual cycle. It grows very slowly. A sudden increase in size with acute pain may be due to hemorrhage within the tumor. Calcification may follow hemorrhage or infarction, and thus the tumor may mimic a carcinoma.

Mammographic findings

1. Smooth contour
2. Difficult to differentiate from a cyst (except when lobulated)
3. May contain calcium deposits, which make differential diagnosis easier; as degeneration of tumor progresses, size and number of deposits increase

Ultrasound findings[1]

1. Smooth or lobulated borders (Fig. 19-26)
2. Strong anterior wall
3. Intermediate posterior enhancement (Fig. 19-27)
4. Low-level homogeneous internal echoes (sometimes strong) (Fig. 19-28)

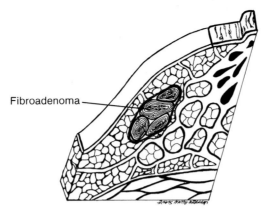

Fig. **19-25.** Schematic of a fibroadenoma. The lesion is palpated as a solitary, smooth, firm, well-demarcated nodule. (Modified from Townsend, C.M.: Clin. Symp. **32**[2]:1, 1980.)

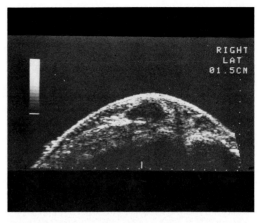

Fig. **19-26.** Sagittal scan of a fibroadenoma in a 33-year-old breast showing a solid mass with lobulated borders. (Courtesy M.D. Anderson Medical Center, Houston.)

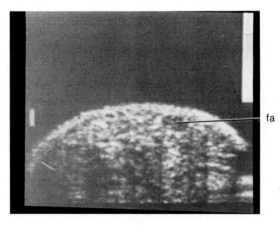

Fig. **19-27.** Sagittal scan of a typical benign-appearing solid mass, *fa*, in a 17-year-old breast. Fibroadenoma with bilateral wall shadowing. (Courtesy Thomas Jefferson University Hospital, Philadelphia.)

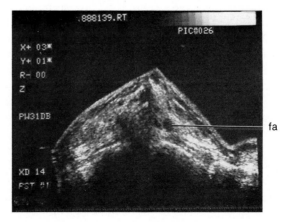

Fig. **19-28.** Transverse scan of a small fibroadenoma, *fa*, displaying low-level internal echoes.

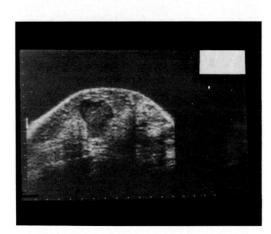

Fig. 19-29. Sagittal scan showing a lobulated complex mass in a 48-year-old breast. Cystosarcoma phyllodes. (Courtesy Thomas Jefferson University Hospital, Philadelphia.)

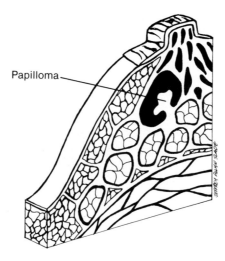

Fig. 19-30. Solitary intraductal papilloma. (Modified from Townsend, C.M.: Clin. Symp. **32**[2]:1, 1980.)

Cystosarcoma phyllodes. This disease is an uncommon breast neoplasia, yet it is the most frequent sarcoma of the breast. It is more commonly found in women in their 50s and usually is unilateral. It may arise from a fibroadenoma as well as de novo. Many patients may notice a small breast mass that has been present for a long time suddenly begin to grow rapidly. At least 27% of these tumors are malignant; 12% will metastasize.

When the tumor is small, it is well delineated, firm, and mobile, much like a fibroadenoma. As it enlarges, the surface may become irregular and lobulated. Skin changes can develop due to increasing pressure. Edema may produce a skin change. As pressure increases, it causes trophic changes and eventual skin ulcerations. Infection and abscess formation may be a secondary complication. The tumor never adheres to the adjacent soft tissue or underlying pectoral muscle, and therefore dimpling of the skin or fixation of the tumor is not observed.[10]

Mammographic findings
1. May be solitary and extremely large or a conglomerate of several masses
2. Borders smooth and sharp
3. Calcifications not usually seen as with fibroadenomas
4. Overlying skin thickened and stretched
5. More difficult to recognize in the young dense breast, where tumor occupies most of the breast

Ultrasound findings (Fig. 19-29)
1. Borders somewhat irregular
2. Anechoic or low level
3. Usually very large
4. Weak posterior margin
5. Architectural disruption

Lipoma. A pure lipoma is entirely composed of fatty tissue. Other forms of lipoma consist of fat with fibrous and glandular elements interspersed (fibroadenolipoma). The lipoma may assume a large size before it is clinically detected. It is usually found in middle-aged or menopausal women.

Clinically on palpation a large, soft, poorly demarcated mass is felt that cannot be clearly separated from the surrounding parenchyma. There is no thinning or fixation of the overlying skin.

Mammographic findings
1. Sharply defined capsule
2. Radiolucent (fat cells)
3. No calcification; appears benign and homogeneous
4. May extend to beneath the skin and displace the subcutaneous fat

Ultrasound findings
1. Difficult or impossible to detect in the fatty breast
2. Internal low-level echo content similar to that of fat
3. Posterior enhancement
4. Smooth walls

Intraductal papilloma. This disease occurs most frequently in women 40 to 50 years of age. The predominant symptom is spontaneous nipple discharge arising from a single duct. When the discharge is copious, it is usually preceded by a sensation of fullness or pain in the areola or nipple area and is relieved as the fluid is expelled.

Papillomas are usually small, multiple, and multicentric. They consist of simple proliferations of duct epithelium projecting outward into a dilated lumen from one or more focal points (Fig. 19-30) each supported by a vascular stalk from which it receives the

blood supply. Trauma may rupture the stalk, filling the duct with blood or serum. Papillomas may also grow to a large size and thus become palpable lesions. They are somewhat linear, resembling the terminal duct, and are usually benign.

Fat necrosis. Fat necrosis may be caused by trauma to the breast or plasma cell mastitis; or it may be related to an involutional process or other disease present in the breast, such as cancer. It is more frequently found in older women.

Clinical palpation reveals a spherical nodule that is generally superficial under a layer of calcified necrosis. A deep-lying focus of necrosis may cause scarring with skin retraction and thus mimic carcinoma.

Mammographic findings
1. Area of nodular fibrosis or typical linear cystlike calcifications

Ultrasound findings
1. Irregular complex mass with low-level echoes
2. May mimic a malignant lesion
3. May appear as fat but is separate and different from the rest of the breast parenchyma

Acute mastitis. This process may be due to infection, trauma, mechanical obstruction in the breast ducts, or other reasons. It often occurs during a lactation, beginning in the lactiferous ducts and spreading via the lymphatics or blood (Fig. 19-31). Acute mastitis is often confined to one area of the breast.

Diffuse mastitis results from the infection's being carried via the blood or breast lymphatics and thus affecting the entire breast.

Mammographic findings
1. Increased density, ill defined
2. Difficult to diagnose in the dense lactating breast unless sufficient fat is interspersed to provide differences in density
3. Skin thickening due to edema

Chronic mastitis. An inflammation of the glandular tissue is considered to be chronic mastitis. It is very difficult to differentiate by ultrasound; the echo pattern will be mixed and diffuse with sound absorption. It usually is found in elderly women. There is a thickening of the connective tissue that results in narrowing of the lumina of the milk ducts. The cause is inspissated intraductal secretions, which are forced into the periductal connective tissue.

Clinically the patient usually has a nipple discharge, and frequently the nipple has retracted over a period of years. Palpation reveals some subareolar thickening but no dominant mass.

Mammographic findings
1. Coarse road-type calcifications
2. Skin thickening
3. Nipple retraction (may or may not be present)

Abscess. This complication may be single or multiple. Acute abscesses have a poorly defined border, whereas mature abscesses are well encapsulated with sharp borders. A definite diagnosis cannot be made from the mammogram alone. Aspiration is needed.

Clinical findings will show pain, swelling, and reddening of the overlying skin. The patient may be febrile, and swollen painful axillary nodes may be present.

Ultrasound findings
1. Diffuse mottled appearance of the breast
2. Dense breast
3. Irregular borders (some may be smooth)
4. Posterior enhancement
5. May have low-level internal echoes

Differential diagnosis of breast masses

The symptoms include pain, a palpable mass, spontaneous or induced nipple discharge, skin dimpling, ulceration, or nipple retraction. The benign process is usually associated with pain, tumor, and nipple discharge. Skin dimpling or ulceration and nipple retraction are nearly always due to cancer. *Solid tumors* are rubbery, mobile, and well delineated (as seen in a fibroadenoma) or stone hard and irregular (as in a carcinoma). Soft tumors usually represent a lipoma (fat tissue). *Cystic masses* are like a balloon of water, well delineated but not as mobile as fibroadenomas because they form part of the breast parenchyma whereas a fibroadenoma has a capsule (Fig. 19-32).

Malignant disease generally develops over a long period. It is not unusual for several years to pass from the first appearance of atypical hyperplasia to the final diagnosis of in situ cancer. This becomes the critical time for detection and treatment.

Malignant cells will grow along a line of least resistance, such as in fatty tissue. In fibrotic tissue most cancer growth occurs along the borders. Lymphatics and blood vessels are frequently used as pathways for new tumor development (Fig. 19-33). If the tumor is encapsulated, it will continue to grow in one area compressing and distorting the surrounding architecture. When the carcinoma is contained and has not invaded the basal membrane structure, it is considered *in situ*. Most cancer will originate in the ducts whereas a smaller percentage will originate in the glandular tissue.

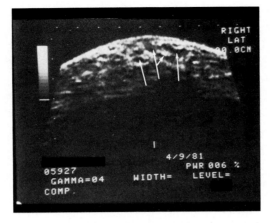

Fig. 19-31. Young breast with dilated milk-filled ducts. (Courtesy M.D. Anderson Medical Center, Houston.)

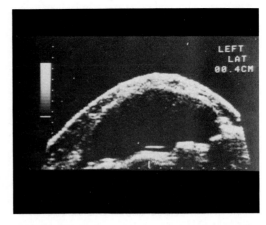

Fig. 19-32. The posterior wall is artifactually displaced posteriorly due to a change in the velocity of sound as it penetrates the silicone bag. (Courtesy University of California, Los Angeles.)

Cancer of the breast is of two types: sarcoma and carcinoma. *Sarcoma* refers to breast tumors that arise from the supportive or connective tissues. Sarcoma is the usual type, growing rapidly and invading fibrous tissue. *Carcinoma* refers to breast tumors that arise from the epithelium, in the ductal and glandular tissue, and usually has tentacles. Other malignant diseases affecting the breast are a result of systemic neoplasms such as leukemia or lymphoma.

Cancer is further classified as infiltrating and noninfiltrating. *Infiltrating* carcinoma has infiltrated the tissue beyond the basement membrane and into adjacent tissue. Chances of metastases are enhanced with the time and type of growth present. Infiltrating carcinomas are histologically designated into several types. Some produce more fibrosis and therefore are categorized as infiltrating ductal carcinoma with productive fibrosis. Others, such as medullary carcinoma, have little associated fibrosis. Colloid carcinoma is a type of cancer in which mucin production occurs and the fibrotic reaction may be variable. Over 80% of carcinomas fall into the category of infiltrating ductal carcinoma with productive fibrosis. *Noninfiltrating* carcinoma is carcinoma of the lactiferous ducts that has not infiltrated the basement membrane but is proliferating within the confines of the ducts and its branches. There is no danger of metastases under these circumstances. This also may be referred to as carcinoma in situ. Most in situ lesions develop from longstanding epithelial hyperplasia of ducts and lobules.

The more favorable cancers, which remain localized to the breast longer and have a 75% survival after 10 years, represent only 10% to 12% of all breast cancer.[12] This group includes medullary, intracystic papillary,

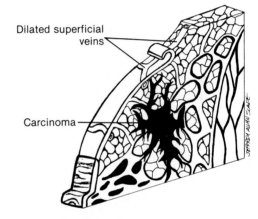

Fig. 19-33. Vascular signs of malignant disease. (Modified from Townsend, C.M.: Clin. Symp. **32**[2]:1, 1980.)

Dilated superficial veins

Carcinoma

papillary, colloid, adenoid cystic, and tubular carcinoma.

Malignant cystosarcoma phyllodes and stromal sarcomas rarely metastasize to regional nodes and have a better than average prognosis after treatment. Occasional spread to distant areas of the body has been reported with these tumors.

The exact type of tumor can be determined only by a histologic diagnosis, not by other noninvasive means. It is the role of mammography and ultrasound to clarify whether a mass is present and whether it has cystic or solid characteristics; then a differential can be made as to its benign or malignant probabilities.

The characteristics most often seen by ultrasound in a malignant mass are as follows:
1. Irregular spiculated contour or margin
2. Round or lobulated
3. Weak nonuniform internal echoes

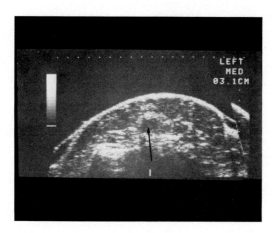

Fig. 19-34. Sagittal scan of a 57-year-old breast with an infiltrating duct carcinoma *(arrow)*. The mass had irregular borders with increased fibrosis surrounding it. (Courtesy Massachusetts General Hospital, Boston.)

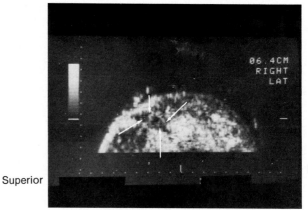

Fig. 19-35. C-scan of an infiltrating duct carcinoma showing the lesion infiltrating from the mammary layer through the subcutaneous fat to the skin, where focal skin thickening is exhibited. (Courtesy University of California, San Francisco.)

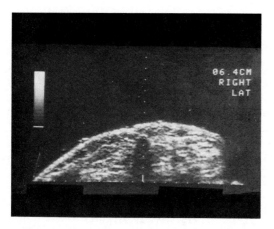

Fig. 19-36. Sagittal scan of the breast in Fig. 19-35 showing the typical appearance of a scirrhous carcinoma attenuating the sound. (Courtesy University of California, San Francisco.)

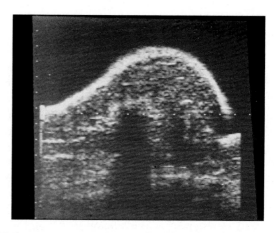

Fig. 19-37. Sagittal scan of an infiltrating duct carcinoma with acute attenuation of the sound. (Courtesy Thomas Jefferson University Hospital, Philadelphia.)

4. Intermediate anterior and absent or weak posterior boundary echoes
5. Great attenuation effects

The exception to this list of criteria is medullary carcinoma. Due to its cellularity and occasional encapsulation, it may present more like a fibroadenoma. Its characteristics are smooth borders and round uniform to absent internal echoes.

Intraductal solid carcinoma (comedocarcinoma). Macroscopically the lactiferous ducts are filled with a yellow pastelike material that looks like small plugs (comedones) when sectioned. Histologically the ducts are filled with plugs of epithelial tumor that have a central necrosis, giving rise to the pastelike material. Both invasive and noninvasive forms exist.

The clinical picture depends upon the stage of the disease. Noninvasive forms may lack any clinical or palpatory findings. If there is a nipple discharge, it is more frequently clear than bloody (unlike papillary carcinoma, in which bloody discharge is typical). The patient may complain of pain or the sensation of insects crawling on the breast. With early invasion, minimal thickening of the surrounding breast tissue may be palpated. In the advanced stage the clinical signs are nipple retraction, dominant mass, and fixation (Fig. 19-33).

Mammographic findings
1. Microcalcifications

Ultrasound findings
1. Irregular border (Fig. 19-34)
2. Diffuse internal echo pattern (Fig. 19-35)
3. Attenuation with shadowing (Figs. 19-36 and 19-37)

Juvenile breast cancer. This disease is similar to the intraductal carcinoma and infiltrating ductal carcinoma found in adults. Generally it occurs in young females, between 8 and 15 years of age, and has a good prognosis when treated.

Papillary carcinoma. This tumor initially arises as an intraductal mass. It may also take the form of an intracystic tumor, but that is rare.

The early stage of papillary carcinoma is noninfiltrating. The tumor occasionally arises from a benign ductal papilloma. It is associated with little fibrotic reaction.

Both intraductal and intracystic forms exist, and these represent 1% to 2% of all breast carcinomas. The earliest clinical sign of *intraductal* papillary carcinoma is bloody nipple discharge. Occasionally a mass can be palpated as a small, firm, well-circumscribed area; this may be mistaken for a fibroadenoma. There may be nodules of blue or red discoloration under the skin with central ulceration. A diffusely nodular appearance overlying the skin is a special variant of multiple intraductal papillary carcinoma. *Intracystic* papillary carcinoma is clinically indistinguishable in its early stages from a cyst or fibroadenoma. When the tumor has invaded through the cyst wall, it is palpable as a poorly circumscribed mass.

Mammographic findings
1. Intraductal—not often diagnosed in early stages
2. Intracystic—recognized when invasion beyond the wall of the cyst occurs; the sharp contours of the cyst are lost because of surrounding edema and infiltration

Ultrasound findings
1. Irregular borders
2. Heterogeneous internal echo pattern
3. Attenuation with acoustic shadowing

Paget's disease. Paget's disease arises in the superficial subareolar or deeper lactiferous ducts and grows in the direction of the nipple, spreading into the intraepidermal region of the nipple and areola. It may be confused with a melanoma.

The disease induces changes of the nipple and areola. Any ulceration, enlargement, or deformity of the nipple and areola should suggest Paget's disease. This is a relatively rare tumor, accounting for 2.5% of all breast cancers. It occurs in older women, over 50 years of age. Differential diagnosis includes benign inflammatory eczematous condition of the nipple, since palpatory findings are frequently not present. The primary duct cancer may be quite deep or embedded in fibrotic tissue.

Mammographic findings
1. Thickened areolar tissue due to eczema or tumor infiltration
2. Solid tumor mass occasionally
3. Microcalcifications (if seen in either a punctate or a linear display, strongly suggestive of duct carcinoma)

Ultrasound findings
1. Irregular borders
2. Heterogeneous internal echoes
3. Attenuation with posterior shadow
4. Subareolar solid mass
5. Skin echo thin and deformed, suggesting infiltration

Scirrhous carcinoma. This tumor is a type of duct carcinoma with extensive fibrous tissue proliferation (productive fibrosis). There may also be focal calcification present. Histologically the cells are found in narrow files or strands, clusters, or columns and may form lumina with varying frequency.

Scirrhous is the most common form of breast cancer. The classical clinical signs are a firm, nodular, frequently nonmovable mass often with fixation as well as flattening of overlying skin and nipple retraction. The retraction is a result of an infiltrative shortening of Cooper's ligaments due to productive fibrosis (Fig. 19-38). Fixation and retraction of the nipple may be the result of a subareolar carcinoma but may also be caused by benign fibrosis of the breast. It is important to note that some patients normally have inverted nipples. The size of the cancer may vary from a few millimeters to involvement of nearly the entire breast. The deep-lying scirrhous carcinoma may grow into and become fixed to the thoracic wall. A sanguineous discharge is rare in this tumor.

Mammographic findings
1. Central mass with lobular and ill-defined contour from which numerous fibrous stands extend into surrounding breast tissue
2. Diagnosis easier in the fatty breast than in the dense breast
3. Microcalcification present in 35%

Ultrasound findings
1. Irregular mass with ill-defined borders
2. Attenuation with posterior shadow
3. Disruption of architecture

Medullary carcinoma. This type of duct carcinoma is a densely cellular tumor containing large, round, or oval tumor cells. It usually is a well-circumscribed mass whose center is frequently necrotic as well as hemorrhagic and cystic.

Medullary carcinoma is relatively rare, comprising less than 5% of breast cancers. The age of occurrence is slightly lower than for the average breast cancer. The skin fixation over the mass is an infrequent finding. It will occasionally reach large proportions and may have a diameter up to 10 cm. Discoloration of the overlying skin is often seen. Bilateral occurrence is more frequent than in other cancers.

Mammographic findings
1. Round, oval, or lobulated mass
2. Margins appear to be smooth, but with nonuniformity and adjacent edema
3. Connective tissue strands occasionally
4. In larger tumors, secondary signs of subcutaneous fatty tissue infiltration, skin thickening, and increased vascularity

Ultrasound findings
1. May resemble fibroadenoma (Fig. 19-39)

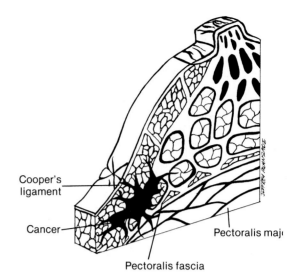

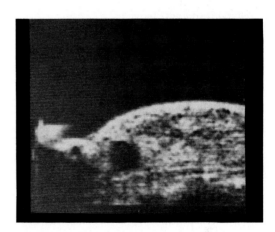

Fig. 19-38. Skin dimpling. (Modified from Townsend, C.M.: Clin. Symp. **32**[2]:1, 1980.)

Fig. 19-39. This benign-appearing solid mass was pathologically proved to be a medullary carcinoma. (Courtesy Thomas Jefferson University Hospital, Philadelphia.)

2. Well-defined border
3. Homogeneous internal echoes
4. Posterior enhancement

Colloid carcinoma (mucinous). This is also a type of duct carcinoma. The cells of the tumor produce secretions that fill lactiferous ducts or the stromal tissues that the tumor cells are invading.

Clinically it presents as a smooth not particularly firm mass at palpation. Due to its smooth nonfibrosing nature, one does not see plateauing or fixation, as with scirrhous carcinoma.

Mammographic findings
1. Smoothly contoured mass resembling a benign tumor

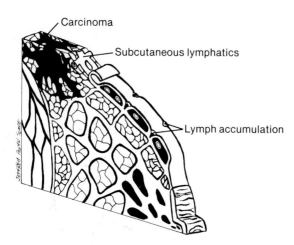

Fig. 19-40. Skin edema. (Modified from Townsend, C.M.: Clin. Symp. **32**[2]:1, 1980.)

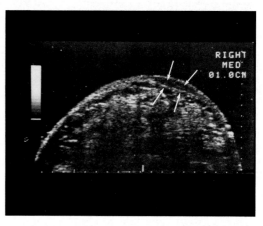

Fig. 19-41. Sagittal scan of a breast with metastatic carcinoma. The area of skin thickening shows decreased echogenicity due to the collection of lymphatic fluid. (Courtesy Massachusetts General Hospital, Boston.)

Ultrasound findings
1. Similar to a fibroadenoma
2. Well defined borders
3. Posterior enhancement

Lobular carcinoma. This disease originates in the ductules of the lobules. When the basement membrane is not invaded and there are no signs of infiltration, the disease is called lobular carcinoma in situ. Secondary involvement of adjacent terminal ductules and neighboring lobules may occur. Multiple foci of lobular carcinoma throughout the breast are not rare.

It most commonly is found in women between the ages of 40 and 50. Frequently it is found in the upper outer quadrants, perhaps because in the involuted breast the residual breast tissue remains in the upper outer quadrants whereas the other areas are replaced by fat. There are no typical clinical symptoms that indicate lobular carcinoma in situ. The indication for biopsy depends on abnormal palpatory findings. It commonly occurs bilaterally; thus prophylactic biopsy and mammography of the opposite breast are recommended.

Mammographic findings
1. Microcalcifications (Some clinicians believe that the tumor is adjacent to the calcifications. However, it is not certain whether the calcifications occur as a result of the lobular carcinoma itself or whether the two processes have an increased tendency to occur together.)

Ultrasound findings
1. Weak internal echo pattern, irregular distribution
2. Intermediate anterior and lateral wall echoes
3. Absent posterior wall

4. Irregular central shadow present
5. Tumor surrounded by bright punctate echoes of breast stroma, especially in the mammary layer

Diffuse carcinoma (inflammatory carcinoma). This tumor presents with all infiltrative types of breast carcinoma (scirrhous, medullary, colloid, etc.). Characteristically there is a diffuse spread of disease throughout the breast due to capillary invasion and involvement of lymphatics of the skin (Fig. 19-40).

It usually is found in middle-aged to older women. The breast is often very large, the progression of inflammatory carcinoma very rapid, and the course very short. The skin shows an erythematous blotchy pattern, and the nipple may be retracted. There is diffuse skin thickening.

Mammographic findings
1. Generalized skin thickening
2. Parenchyma not as cloudy as with inflammatory mastitis, but proliferation of abnormal tissue of increased density
3. Occasionally a dominant mass from which the carcinoma originates
4. Sometimes malignant calcifications in linear or intraductal forms

Ultrasound findings
1. If dominant mass present, borders irregular with high attenuation by shadow (Fig. 19-41)
2. Skin thickening in comparison with the normal breast

BIOPSY TECHNIQUES FOR BREAST TUMORS

Three events have occurred that affect the number and type of invasive procedures on women with breast masses.

First, women are becoming more informed about their diagnostic choices. They are asking their physicians to order an ultrasound examination to determine whether the mass is cystic or solid before subjecting themselves to an excisional biopsy.

Second, as physicians have the availability of ultrasound, they are being more confident in its use and are more willing to perform a needle aspiration of a cystic area rather than the more invasive excisional biopsy. This judgment depends upon the physical characteristics of the breast mass, the age of the patient, and the associated risk factors determined from the patient's history.

Third, needle biopsy is more acceptable to both patients and physicians. Although it is not as accurate as the open biopsy, it has become a useful diagnostic tool in breast lesions suspected of being carcinomatous. The advantages of the technique are that it is an office procedure, it is cost effective, it is simple to perform, and it is relatively atraumatic. Needle biopsy or excisional biopsy is the only reliable method for determining the exact malignancy of a breast mass.

SUMMARY

The death rate from breast cancer has not decreased over the past 40 years. Although most women never get breast cancer, those who do can benefit from advances in detection and treatment of the disease that have occurred. The use of monthly self-examination and palpation techniques combined with mammography and ultrasound will increase the detection of breast tumors. Ultrasound has been found to be effective in younger patients, those with dense breasts, and those for whom subsequent follow-up is needed because of fibrocystic disease. Mammography, on the other hand, has been found effective in patients with fatty breasts, those in the high-risk group, and those over 35 years of age. Many laboratories with dedicated breast ultrasound equipment are doing simultaneous mammography and ultrasonography on patients, and many do subsequent follow-up studies with ultrasound rather than mammography (or take limited follow-up views with mammography). The computer analysis with ultrasound will enable physicians to review the right and left breast simultaneously as well as view the current image with a previous image at the same time. Further histologic classification of attenuation properties of breast masses may make the ultrasound diagnosis more specific as to the particular tumor type found in the breast.

REFERENCES

1. Cole-Beuglet, C.M., Goldberg, B.B., Patchefsky, A.S., et al.: Atlas of breast ultrasound; correlation of anatomy, pathology, mammography, and ultrasonography, Denver, 1980, Technicare Corp.
2. Haagensen, E.D.: Diseases of the breast, ed. 2, Philadelphia, 1971, W.B. Saunders Co.
3. Hoeffken, W., and Lanyi, M.: Mammography, Philadelphia, 1977, W.B. Saunders Co.
4. Jellins, J., Kossoff, G., and Reeve, T.S.: Detection and classification of liquid filled masses in the breast by grey scale echography, Radiology **125:**205, 1977.
5. Kelly-Fry, E.: Breast imaging. In Sabbagha, R.E.: Diagnostic ultrasound applied to obstetrics and gynecology, New York, 1980, Harper & Row, Publishers.
6. Kobayashi, T.: Clinical ultrasound of the breast, New York, 1978, Plenum Publishing Corp.
7. Laing, F.C.: Ultrasonographic evaluation of breast masses, J. Assoc. Can. Radiol. **27:**278, 1976.
8. Netter, F.: Reproductive system. In Ciba collection of medical illustrations, vol. 2, Summit, N.J., 1965, Ciba Pharmaceutical Co.
9. Omni Education: [module] Breast examination, New York, 1974, Ortho Pharmaceutical Corp.
10. Pilnik, S.: Clinical diagnosis of benign breast diseases, J. Reprod. Med. **22**(6):277, 1979.
11. Townsend, C.M.: Breast lumps, Clin. Symp. **32**(2): 1, 1980.
12. Urban, J.: Diseases of the breast, In Danforth, D.N., editor: Obstetrics and gynecology, ed. 3, New York, 1980, Harper & Row, Publishers.

20

Ultrasound evaluation of the neonatal brain

KEVIN E. APPARETI
MICHAEL L. JOHNSON
CAROL RUMACK

Ultrasound evaluation of the brain has advanced by leaps and bounds since its introduction in 1956.[10,25] At that point anatomic structures were being identified by A-mode techniques alone. Because A-mode is a one-dimensional imaging modality, spatial orientation is completely lost. Consequently there is a very real potential of misinterpreting the data, for just the slightest movement of the transducer can alter the display dramatically. It took an extremely skilled person to produce the required information and to read out the diagnosis accurately.

Fortunately technology has continued to move ahead, with many new advances enabling us to see more and more information with higher reliability and accuracy. The first advance was the compound scanner developed in the early 1960s. This gave for the first time a means of visualizing anatomy in cross section and the ability to retain spacial orientation of structures.[3,28] The compound scanner had a dramatic impact on the ultrasound community; however, it lacked adequate penetration of the adult cranium. Not until the advent of gray scale in 1973 did the true potentials of ultrasonic visualization of the neonatal brain become realized. With gray scale came the ability to see much finer detail in the head. This led many investigators (Kossoff et al.[21] Garrett et al.,[9] and Johnson et al.[17]) to describe the various intracranial structures and correlate them with CT and cadaver sections. Much hard work has been done to prove that ultrasound can indeed accurately demonstrate intracranial structures in the neonate.[4,24,30,40]

The next advance came with high-quality

real time technology. With this it was possible to see high-quality gray scale with retained spatial relationships. We can also appreciate movement and continuity of structures. This becomes extremely important when following structures such as the choroid plexus in the lateral ventricles. Real time has added another dimension to the evaluation of the neonatal brain, rounding out our arsenal of state-of-the-art technology. What will come in the future to add to our diagnostic arsenal? Time will have to answer that question. Looking at the significant leaps we have made already, I can only get excited about the strides we will be making in the next few years. The aim of this chapter is to present an approach to visualizing the normal and abnormal neonatal brain. To do so completely, we must first cover fetal brain anatomy. The importance of thoroughly understanding this anatomy cannot be overemphasized. Then a discussion of techniques of evaluation will lead us into the ultrasonic visualization of both normal and abnormal brain. Finally we will look at the many different parameters we can use to help us interpret the results.

BRAIN DEVELOPMENT

Brain development in the human begins early and continues to be active through birth. At approximately 18 days of embryonic life the neural plate starts to develop. From this neural plate the neural tube will form, eventually differentiating into the central nervous system (brain and spinal cord). The cranial end of the neural tube, which will form the brain, differentiates and grows the fastest.[29] At approximately the fourth week of development the expanding neural folds fuse to form three primary brain vesicles: the forebrain or prosencephalon, the midbrain

We would like to thank Ms. Judith Caplan for her excellent secretarial assistance.

or mesencephalon, and the hindbrain or rhombencephalon. From these three primary vesicles will arise all the anatomic landmarks necessary for neonatal brain evaluation. An understanding of this development may help in appreciating the normal anatomy and abnormal anatomy you might encounter. The following is not by any means an exhaustive discussion of embryology but rather is a short summary to help put into perspective the amazing development that goes on within the fetal brain.

As the neural tube folds, forming the primary brain vesicles, there is also some associated flexing ventrally. The rapid growth of the brain causes this bending; and two flexures result, the midbrain flexure and the cervical flexure. Later another flexure, caused by uneven growth, will form; this is the pontine flexure. The pontine flexure, midbrain flexure, and cervical flexure all shape the evolving brain for the final stages of development.

The pontine flexure divides the hindbrain into caudal (myelencephalon) and rostral (metencephalon) parts. The myelencephalon becomes the medulla oblongata, and the metencephalon gives rise to the pons and cerebellum. The fourth ventricle arises from the cavity of the hindbrain.

The midbrain (mesencephalon) undergoes relatively few changes. The third and fourth ventricles are joined by the cerebral aqueduct as the neural canal narrows. Just rostral to the developing cerebellum the cerebral peduncles are formed of fibers growing down from the cerebrum. The cerebral peduncles get more prominent as more descending fibers pass through the developing midbrain on their way to the brain stem.

The forebrain or prosencephalon has a central part called the diencephalon and lateral expansions called the telencephalon. The walls of the diencephalon become the thalami, and the cavity forms the third ventricle. The thalamus on each side develops rapidly and bulges into the cavity of the third ventricle. This pressure on the third ventricle reduces it to a narrow slit, which explains why the third ventricle is so difficult to see in the normal state by ultrasound. In approximately 70% of brains the thalami meet and fuse in the midline.[29] This forms a bridge of gray matter across the third ventricle, called the massa intermedia, which can be seen by ultrasound only in the abnormal state.

The cavity of the telencephalon forms the lateral ventricles and the extreme anterior part of the third ventricle. At first the lateral ventricles (at this early stage called cerebral vesicles) are in wide communication with the third ventricle through the interventricular foramina. As the cerebral hemispheres expand, they cover the diencephalon, midbrain, and hindbrain. Eventually the hemispheres meet at the midline, flattening their medial surfaces. This decreases the size of the interventricular foramina and forms the longitudinal fissure between them, called the falx cerebri. As the hemispheres grow, they assume a C shape. This differential growth and curvature also affect the shape of the developing lateral ventricles. The ventricles likewise assume a C shape, with frontal, posterior, and temporal horns forming. As the cerebral cortex differentiates, fibers passing to and from it divide into the caudate and lentiform nuclei. The caudate nucleus, which we are more interested in, becomes elongated and C shaped, conforming to the outline of the lateral ventricle. Its head and body lie in the floor of the anterior horn and body of the lateral ventricle. Its tail makes a U-shaped turn winding up on the roof of the temporal horn of the lateral ventricle.

As the ventricles and cerebrum are developing and taking shape, changes are occurring that will produce the choroid plexus. All four ventricles are lined by an ependymal membrane. This ependymal lining, covered externally by vascular pia mater, forms the tela choroidea. The very active proliferation of the vascular pia mater causes the tela choroidea to invaginate into the ventricular cavity. There is further differentiation until the tufted choroid plexuses form. This process takes place at four sites to form the choroid plexus: roof of the fourth ventricle, roof of the third ventricle, and posteromedial walls of the lateral ventricles. The choroid plexuses when formed are responsible for the secretion and absorption of cerebrospinal fluid.

The rate of growth differs tremendously between the different parts of the brain. The ventricles grow much more slowly than the cerebral hemispheres. This explains the high ventricular-to-hemispheric ratio at 15 weeks (40% to 70%) versus the low ventricular/hemispheric ratio at term (23% to 33%).[16] The growth and development of the different parts of the brain are also very complicated in the early stages. Fortunately most of the complicated differential growth occurs before we evaluate the intracranial structures in the neonate by ultrasound. After 20 to 35 weeks the brain is essentially developed and is just increasing in size and maturing.[29]

BRAIN ANATOMY

At this point we need to take a good look at the cross-sectional relationship of structures in the brain so correlation can be made with ultrasound. There are many ways to divide the brain cross-sectionally. We will deal only with the three sections that are commonly used in ultrasound—axial, coronal, and sagittal.

An axial section of the brain is one in which we slice the brain from one lateral side to the other parallel with the canthomeatal line (Fig. 20-1). By looking at the upper surface of the cut we can see a cross-sectional plane that displays both hemispheres and midline structures. Making this slice at approximately 15 to 20 degrees above the canthomeatal line gives us a section used by CT and ultrasound. Starting just above the external auditory meatus, we can see many anatomic landmarks that are important for ultrasound evaluation[27] (Fig. 20-2). Posteriorly the cerebellum can be seen with the tentorium separating it from the cerebrum. As we move anteriorly on this section, we can see the cerebral peduncles with the fourth ventricle just behind. In front of the peduncles we find the suprasellar cistern, containing the cerebrovascular circle of Willis. Taking a slice approximately 5 mm above the external auditory meatus reveals the ambient cisterns between the hippocampal gyrus and the cerebral peduncles and inferior colliculi (Fig. 20-3). More anteriorly and laterally we see the sylvian fissures bilaterally, which contain the middle cerebral arteries. Another slice 5 mm higher displays the thalami as two symmetric areas on each side of the midline (Fig. 20-4). The third ventricle lies right between the thalami. Anterior to the thalami are the frontal horns of the lateral ventricles. Posterolateral to each frontal horn is the region of the caudate nucleus. In premature infants the germinal matrix lies in the subependymal layer along the caudate nuclei. This is of critical anatomic importance since it is the most common site of intracranial hemorrhage in premature infants. Posterior to the thalami are the occipital horns of the lateral ventricles. Between the occipital horns and frontal horns is the area of the interhemispheric fissure.

In the next 5-mm slice higher we can see the bodies of the lateral ventricles (Fig. 20-5). The course of the lateral ventricles is from anteromedial to posterolateral, an important relationship in trying to visualize by ultrasound. The corpus callosum is seen between the lateral ventricles. At this level the caudate nuclei lie in the lateral walls of

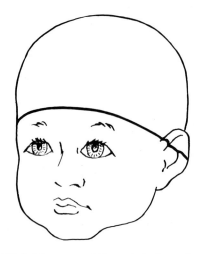

Fig. 20-1. Diagram of the axial plane through the skull.

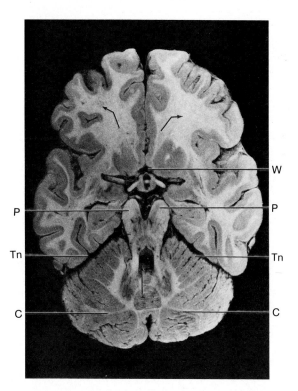

Fig. 20-2. Axial anatomic section showing the, *C*, cerebellum and, *Tn*, tentorium. *curved arrows*, Cerebrum; *arrow*, fourth ventricle; *P*, cerebral peduncles; *W*, circle of Willis. (From Matsui, T., and Hirano, A.: An atlas of the human brain for computerized tomography, New York, 1978, Igaku-Shoin Medical Publishers, Inc. With permission.)

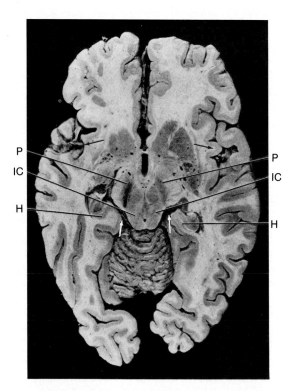

Fig. 20-3. Axial anatomic section 5 mm above the external auditory meatus. White arrows show the ambient cisterns. *H*, Hippocampal gyrus; *P*, cerebral peduncles; *IC*, inferior colliculi. Anterolaterally on each side can be seen the sylvian fissures *(black arrows)*, containing the middle cerebral arteries. (From Matsui, T., and Hirano, A.: An atlas of the human brain for computerized tomography, New York, 1978, Igaku-Shoin Medical Publishers, Inc. With permission.)

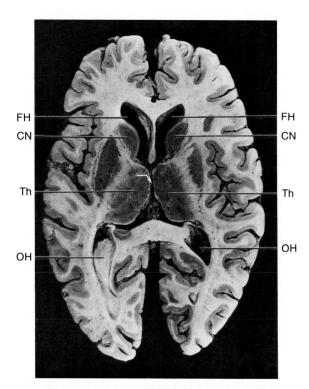

Fig. 20-4. Axial anatomic section approximately 10 mm above the external auditory meatus. Shown are the, *Th*, thalami, *(curved arrow)* third ventricle, *FH*, frontal horns, *CN*, caudate nucleus, and, *OH*, occipital horns. (From Matsui, T., and Hirano, A.: An atlas of the human brain for computerized tomography, New York, 1978, Igaku-Shoin Medical Publishers, Inc. With permission.)

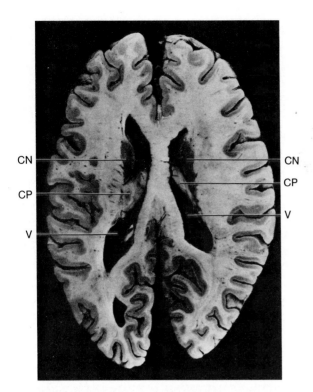

Fig. 20-5. Axial anatomic section 15 to 20 mm above the external auditory meatus. This level shows the lateral ventricle, *V*, and choroid plexus within, *CP*. The caudate nucleus, *CN*, is lateral to the ventricles. The corpus callosum is the tissue between the ventricles. (From Matsui, T., and Hirano, A.: An atlas of the human brain for computerized tomography, New York, 1978, Igaku-Shoin Medical Publishers, Inc. With permission.)

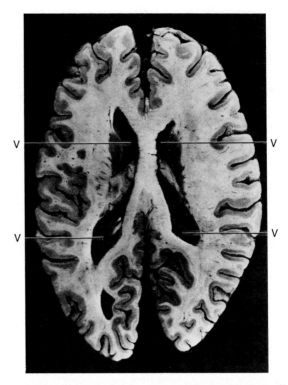

Fig. 20-6. Axial anatomic section 20 to 25 mm above the cantho-meatal line. The lateral ventricles, *V*, can be seen. (From Matsui, T., and Hirano, A.: An atlas of the human brain for computerized tomography, New York, 1978, Igaku-Shoin Medical Publishers, Inc. With permission.)

the lateral ventricles. The choroid plexus can also be seen within the lateral ventricles. At the next higher level only the lateral ventricles can be seen (Fig. 20-6). This level, where there is no choroid plexus showing, is the correct level for measuring ventricular size.

Coronal sections are obtained by making slices approximately 90 degrees from the axial sections (Fig. 20-7). Technically a coronal view is 90 degrees to Reid's baseline. However, a number of different angles to Reid's baseline are used in performing the examination. When we look at the sections, the vertex of the skull is at the top and the left side of the brain is to the right of the image.

Starting anteriorly in the brain, we can see the relationship of the frontal horns of the lateral ventricles to the heads of the caudate nuclei (Fig. 20-8). Each caudate nucleus lies posterolateral to the frontal horn. The interhemispheric fissure can also be seen. As we move posteriorly, the cavum septi pellucidi between the frontal horns becomes visible

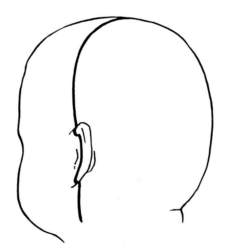

Fig. 20-7. Diagram of a coronal plane through the skull.

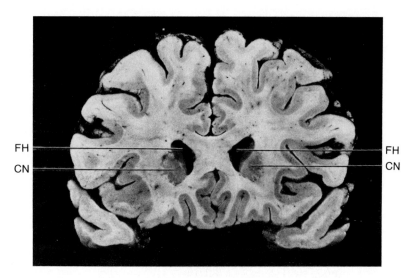

Fig. 20-8. Coronal anatomic section demonstrating frontal horns, *FH*, and caudate nucleus, *CN*. The caudate nucleus lies posterolateral to the frontal horns. (From Matsui, T., and Hirano, A.: An atlas of the human brain for computerized tomography, New York, 1978, Igaku-Shoin Medical Publishers, Inc. With permission.)

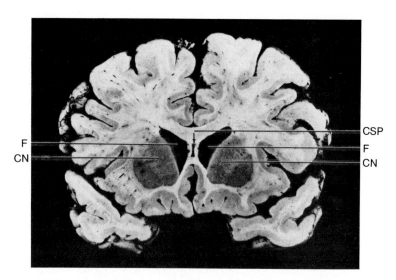

Fig. 20-9. Coronal anatomic section through the area of the cavum septi pellucidi, *CSP.* (From Matsui, T., and Hirano, A.: An atlas of the human brain for computerized tomography, New York, 1978, Igaku-Shoin Medical Publishers, Inc. With permission.)

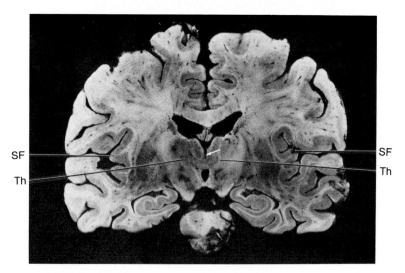

Fig. 20-10. Coronal anatomic section through the thalami, *Th,* third ventricle *(arrow),* and sylvian fissures, *SF.* (From Matsui, T., and Hirano, A.: An atlas of the human brain for computerized tomography, New York, 1978, Igaku-Shoin Medical Publishers, Inc. With permission.)

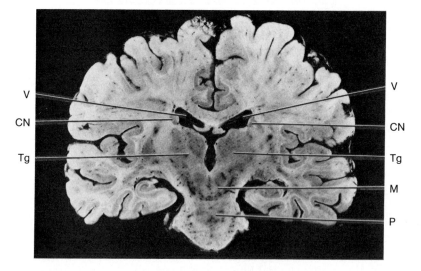

Fig. 20-11. Coronal anatomic section demonstrating the proximity of the caudate nucleus, *CN,* to the body of the lateral ventricle, *V.* The pons, *P,* and midbrain, *M,* can also be seen. *Tg* is the trigonum. (From Matsui, T., and Hirano, A.: An atlas of the human brain for computerized tomography, New York, 1978, Igaku-Shoin Medical Publishers, Inc. With permission.)

(Fig. 20-9). This is a normal developmental structure.[38] The cavum septi pellucidi has been mistaken for the third ventricle. Remember, the third ventricle is more inferior and between the thalami.

The next slice more posteriorly shows the thalami and third ventricle (Fig. 20-10). Also the region of the foramen of Monro, connecting the lateral ventricles, and the third ventricle appears. The sylvian fissures, containing the middle cerebral arteries, become visible; and as we continue posteriorly, we can now see the pons and hippocampal gyrus (Fig. 20-11). The bodies of the lateral ventricles can also be seen with the adjacent caudate nuclei. Finally, as we move back, we see the trigonum of the lateral ventricle and the choroid plexus within (Fig. 20-12). The lie of the lateral ventricles at this level is more superomedial to inferolateral. The cerebellum and tentorium can also be seen.

Sagittal sections are done by rotating the coronal plane approximately 90 degrees (Fig. 20-13). Sagittal sections are viewed with the anterior brain to the left and occipital portion of the brain to the right. Three sagittal sections of the brain are usually used—one of each lateral ventricle and one of the midline structures. The sections of the lateral ventricles demonstrate the lie of the caudate nuclei and choroid plexus. The caudate nuclei are just posterior and lateral to the lateral ventricles. The choroid plexus is on the floor of the body and occipital horn of each lateral ventricle and on the roof of the temporal horn. In the midline starting superiorly are the corpus callosum and cavum septi pellucidi. The posterior extension of the cavum septi pellucidi is called the cavum vergi, which regresses after birth. Below the corpus callosum lies the third ventricle with the massa intermedia. The aqueduct joins the third ventricle with the fourth ventricle, which is posterior to the pons and other midbrain structures.

METHODS OF EVALUATION
Axial scans (static scanner)

There are many approaches to examining the neonatal brain, each having specific advantages and disadvantages. An attempt will be made to cover the major approaches, explain their utility, and point out trouble spots. Ultrasound examples will be shown to demonstrate the anatomy just covered.

Axial scanning was the first approach to neonatal brain evaluation. This technique offers important information about the relative sizes of the ventricles but is hindered by the boney calvarium, which limits resolution of important structures. Since the articulated arm scanner is not portable, axial scans are done when the neonate is healthy enough to come to the department.

In preparing the ultrasound room for axial scans, a number of considerations must be heeded. First, even though the neonate may be well enough to come to your laboratory, he is still very fragile and susceptible to any environmental changes. Consequently blankets, radiant heaters, oxygen hookups, and heating pads are all essential to making the environment in the laboratory suitable. Second, if there are any problems with the child, a crash cart and life support systems must be immediately available. Very often a nurse will accompany the child for monitoring purposes.

When the laboratory is set up, the child is brought in and placed on the examining table with the head in a true lateral position. A pair of extra hands is essential to stabilize the baby's head during the examination. Mineral oil is spread on the head and the canthomeatal line is noted. The transducer is aligned 15 to 20 degrees above this line to obtain sections that correspond to the normal CT sections. The highest-frequency transducer should be used that will permit adequate penetration. This is usually a 3.5-MHz medium-focused transducer. The TGC should be set so the knee of the slope is positioned at the echo arising from the far side of the calvarium. The initial gain is then set to produce an even gray level of echoes from brain parenchyma in the near field to

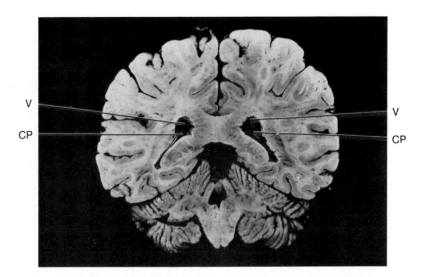

Fig. 20-12. Coronal anatomic section in the region of the trigonum of the lateral ventricles, *V.* The choroid plexus, *CP,* is seen within the ventricles. (From Matsui, T., and Hirano, A.: An atlas of the human brain for computerized tomography, New York, 1978, Igaku-Shoin Medical Publishers, Inc. With permission.)

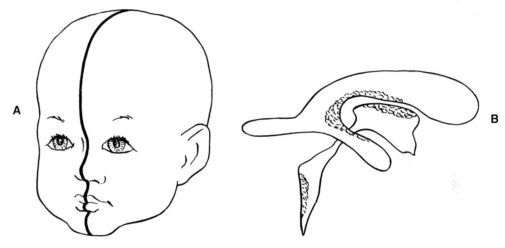

Fig. 20-13. Diagrams of, **A,** a sagittal section through the head and, **B,** the ventricular system with the choroid plexuses.

the far field. Gain settings must be set high to produce low-to-medium-level echoes arising from the brain parenchyma while leaving fluid-filled structures anechoic.

Axial sections are taken at 5-mm intervals starting approximately 5 mm above the external auditory meatus and going rostrally. The transducer is moved back and forth in linear and sector sweeps to get the needed information. The flatter the baby's head, the more linear your technique is and the less overwriting you have to do. When overwriting cannot be avoided, it will be important for the holder to maintain the baby's head position. Care must be taken to get as much

information anteriorly and posteriorly as possible. These areas contain important anatomic landmarks.

The inner table of the skull and the first centimeter of brain near the face of the transducer are not well visualized as a result of the main bang artifact. Therefore information on the up-side hemisphere cannot be adequately obtained. Consequently the infant's head is turned 180 degrees and the procedure is repeated. If there are intraventricular catheters or other tubing connected to the baby, care must be taken when moving the infant not to disturb them. Sections low in the brain demonstrate the

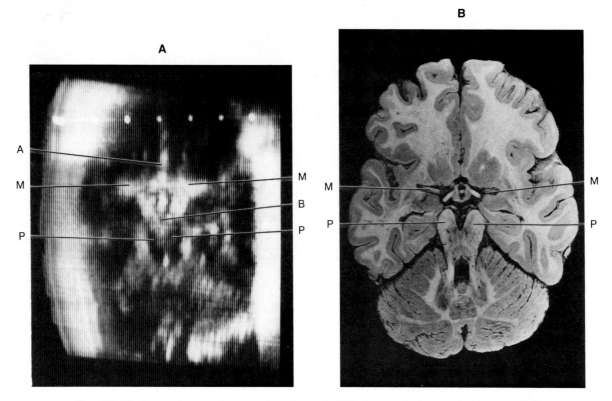

Fig. 20-14. A, Axial scan showing the circle of Willis. The anterior cerebral, *A*, middle cerebral, *M*, and basilar, *B*, arteries can be seen. The echolucent peduncles, *P*, are also visible posterior to the circle of Willis. **B,** Anatomic section demonstrating the same anatomy.

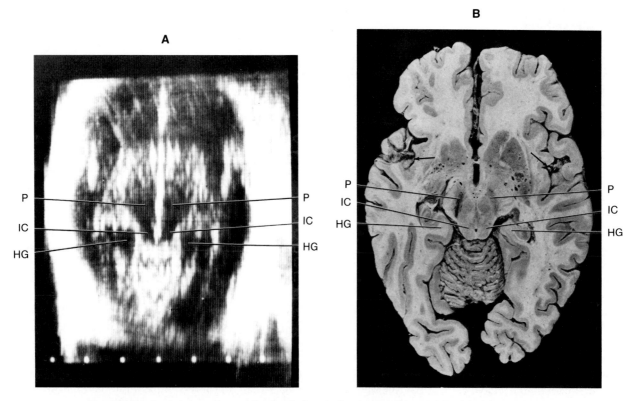

Fig. 20-15. A, Axial section of the brain low in the head. The ambient cisterns appear as dense echoes between the hippocampal gyri, *HG*, and the peduncles, *P*. The inferior colliculi, *IC*, can also be seen. **B,** Anatomic section demonstrating the same anatomy. The sylvian fissures appear as dark echoes *(arrows).*

A

B

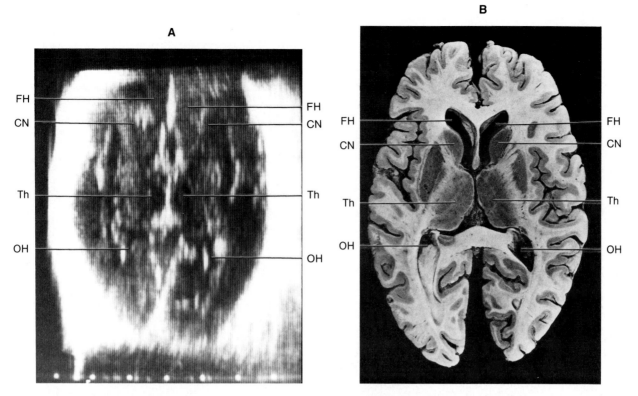

Fig. 20-16. A, Axial section demonstrating the mildly echogenic thalami, *Th.* The frontal, *FH,* and occipital, *OH,* horns can also be seen. The caudate nucleus, *CN,* is lateral to the frontal horns. **B,** Anatomic section demonstrating the same anatomy.

circle of Willis (Fig. 20-14). Since there are many arteries in this area that produce high-level echoes, the circle of Willis is seen as an echogenic area just in front of the cerebral peduncles. These vascular structures are confirmed by real time evaluation. The peduncles show up as less echogenic structures. The area of the fourth ventricle is found just behind the peduncles. The fourth ventricle is not commonly seen unless there is a related pathologic process.

Five millimeters above the external auditory meatus we can see the tentorial incisura (Fig. 20-15). This V-shaped densely echogenic structure surrounds the vermis of the cerebellum. Anterior to the vermis is the quadrigeminal cistern, with the ambient wings extending laterally. The less echogenic hippocampal gyrus is situated posterior to the ambient wings and lateral to the tentorium. Medial and anterior to the ambient wings is the sonolucent midbrain. The inferior colliculi project posteriorly, and the cerebral peduncles anteriorly. The long echogenic structure anterior to the midbrain is the interhemispheric fissure. A little anterior and lateral are the sylvian fissures. These are represented by a very dense echogenic line.

The thalami are seen at the next 5-mm level rostrally (Fig. 20-16). They appear as mildly echogenic symmetric structures on each side of the midline. The third ventricle lies between the thalami and is not usually seen unless abnormal. The sonolucent structures just anterior to the thalami are the frontal horns of the lateral ventricles. Just lateral and posterior to the frontal horns lie the caudate nuclei. The echogenicity of the caudate nucleus is just a little greater than that of the thalamus. Depending on the projection, the occipital horns can sometimes be seen posterior to the thalami.

The lateral ventricles are at the next higher level (Fig. 20-17). They lie on each side of the dense midline echo arising from the corpus callosum. The choroid plexus can be seen as a very dense structure running anteromedial to posterolateral in the ventricles. The next level will give the correct area for lateral ventricle measurements (Fig. 20-18). At this level we are just above the choroid plexus.

Axial scans can also be done using a water path system.[2] Water is warmed to body temperature and allowed to stand to eliminate bubbles. Ordinary liquid soap can be used as a surfactant to help eliminate bubbles. Only

a small amount is needed to obtain the required results. It is important to have the depth of the water slightly greater than the BPD so there will be no artifacts within the brain image. With the increased depth of the brain a longer focal length is required. Mineral oil is applied to the infant's head and to the plastic membrane. The water path assembly is positioned over the head, care being taken not to put too much pressure on the skull. One advantage of using a water path system is that it enables better visualization of the frontal and occipital areas and may result in better image quality. However, the setup is more cumbersome and can sometimes be tricky when trying to eliminate artifacts.

Sedation is usually not necessary. When examined after a feeding and with a nipple or pacifier in place, most infants tolerate the examination with little restraint. The entire axial scan exam should take approximately twenty minutes.

Coronal scans (static scanner)

Initially coronal scans were done through the calvarium with the patient in the axial position. This obviously limited the resolution and produced less than adequate im-

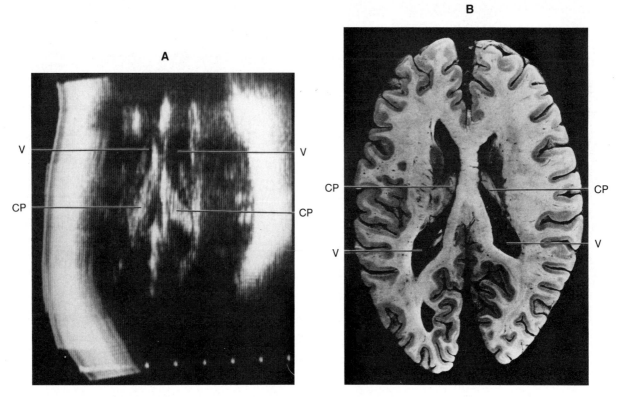

Fig. 20-17. A, Axial section showing the lateral ventricles, *V,* and the choroid plexus, *CP,* within. **B,** Anatomic section demonstrating the same anatomy.

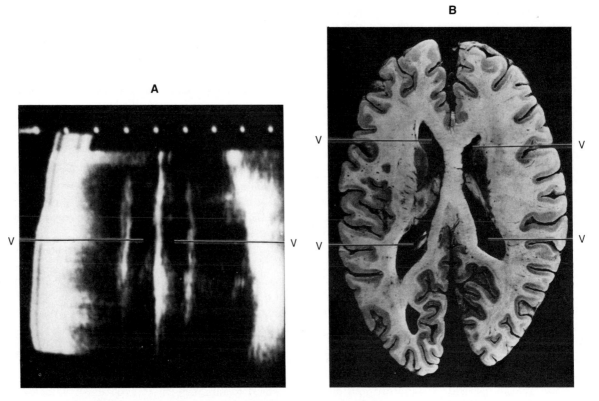

Fig. 20-18. A, Axial section showing the ventricles just above the level of the choroid plexus. **B,** Anatomic section demonstrating the same anatomy.

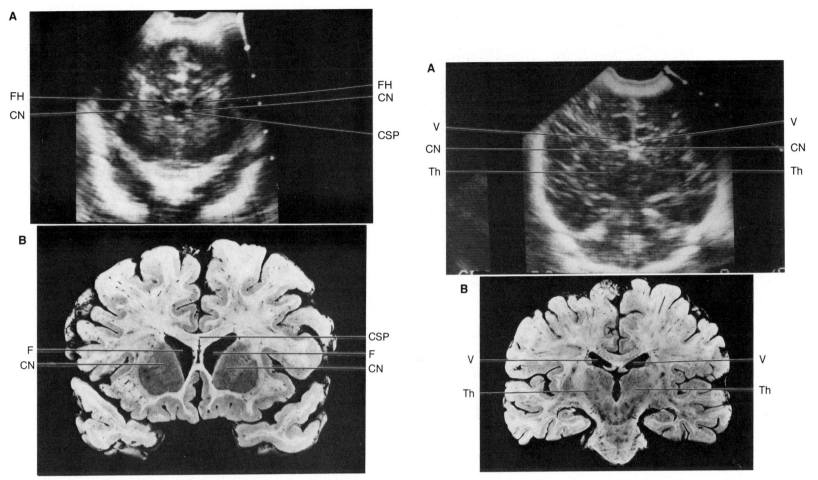

Fig. 20-19. A, Coronal section demonstrating the frontal horns, *FH*, and position of the caudate nucleus, *CN*. Also seen is the cavum septi pellucidi, *CSP*. **B,** Anatomic section demonstrating the same anatomy.

Fig. 20-20. A, Coronal section demonstrating the bodies of the lateral ventricles, *V*. The choroid plexus, *CP*, and thalami, *Th*, can also be seen. **B,** Anatomic section demonstrating the same anatomy.

ages. By repositioning the transducer or moving the infant, scans through the anterior fontanelle can be obtained.[1,7,11,15] These scans, approximately 90 degrees to the axial plane, provide much better resolution and have added tremendously to our ability to visualize the neonatal brain.

Patients can be held in a sitting position or placed on a very thick sponge for the coronal scans. Depending on the particular machine and the laboratory setup, either method will work. Because the anterior fontanelle can be very small or very large, one position of the scanning arm is not possible for the whole study. Depending on where and how big the fontanelle is, a number of modified coronal angles must be used. Starting anteriorly, the transducer is angled and moved posteriorly while always staying in the fontanelle. Single sector sweeps are employed. Because of the number of sources of unwanted movement, overwriting and compounding should be avoided. A higher-frequency transducer can be used because no

bony surfaces will be encountered. A 5-MHz medium-focus transducer is a good one to start with. Acoustic gel is used instead of mineral oil to provide a thicker medium that will stay in place.

Sections very anterior will demonstrate the sonolucent frontal horns of the lateral ventricles (Fig. 20-19). Posterolateral are the heads of the caudate nuclei, appearing as low-level echogenic structures. Often there is a sonolucent structure between the frontal horns, the cavum septi pellucidi. This is a normal developmental structure that should not be confused with the third ventricle. The gain settings should be set high enough to give the brain parenchyma mild echogenicity. As the transducer is moved posteriorly, the bodies of the lateral ventricles can be seen (Fig. 20-20). These appear as sonolucent slits with echodensities on their posterior surface representing the normal appearance of the choroid plexus. Just beneath the ventricles are the mildly echogenic thalami. Posterior to the thalami are

the mildly echogenic midbrain structures. The very dense echoes from the sylvian fissures can also be seen lateral to the thalami. Finally, as the transducer sweeps posteriorly the occipital horns come in view (Fig. 20-21). They are sonolucent and contain the echodense choroid plexus. Posterior to the occipital horns is the cerebellum, separated from the cerebrum by the echodense tentorium.

Sagittal views (static scanner)

By moving the transducer 90 degrees to the coronal plane, a sagittal section can be obtained. With the anterior fontanelle as a window the lateral ventricles and midline structures can be visualized. The lateral ventricles lie in an anteromedial to posterolateral plane. Therefore when setting the scanning arm follow this same plane for each of the ventricles. Best results are obtained when angling the transducer from the opposite side of the midline from the ventricle you are trying to visualize.

When imaged properly, the lateral ven-

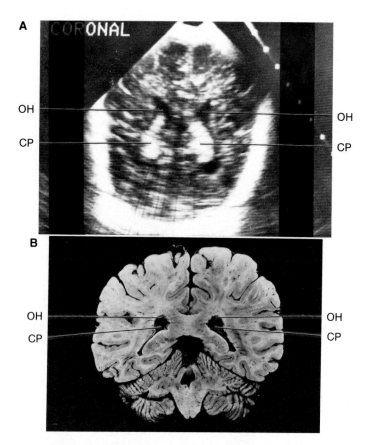

Fig. 20-21. A, Coronal section demonstrating the occipital horns, *OH*, and choroid plexus, *CP*, within. **B,** Anatomic section demonstrating the same anatomy.

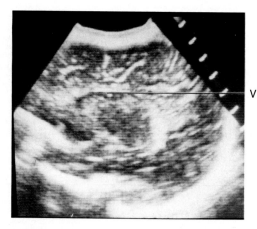

Fig. 20-22. Sagittal section of the lateral ventricle.

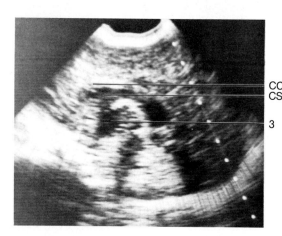

Fig. 20-23. Sagittal section of midline structures. The corpus callosum, *CC*, cavum septi pellucidi, *CSP*, and third ventricle, *3*, can be seen.

tricle shows up as a thin sonolucent C-shaped structure with a small tail (Fig. 20-22). The C-shaped ventricle drapes around the mildly echogenic thalamus, with the frontal horn anterior and the temporal horn inferior. The tail extends posteriorly and represents the occipital horn of the lateral ventricle. The densely echogenic choroid plexus lies on the floor of the body of the ventricle and extends posteriorly to the occipital horn, ending up on the roof of the temporal horn.

Midline sections display the echogenic corpus callosum with the echolucent cavum septi pellucidi (Fig. 20-23). The sonolucent third ventricle can be seen joining the fourth ventricle via the aqueduct. Anterior to the sonolucent fourth ventricle are the mildly echodense midbrain structures.

The sagittal sections of the lateral ventricles give a tremendous amount of information about pathology. The normal tapering of the choroid plexus is altered in caudate nucleus hemorrhage.[11] The occipital horns are best seen and measured here for monitoring for early signs of hydrocephalus, since they tend to be the first to dilate.

Real time examination

Static scans in all three projections give high-resolution images of the various areas of the brain. However, a certain degree of continuity is lost between the images. With the advent of high-resolution real time, the needed continuity of structures is gained. The ability to follow structures rapidly and get immediate feedback has added to the efficacy of the examination. Real time mobility and maneuverability on the patient have added another dimension to our role as sonographers. Very unstable infants can now be examined at bedside without risking their life support needs. Many infants are examined entirely by real time; and, as will be discussed later, the results are more than adequate.[6,19,39]

The real time examination takes only 5 to 10 minutes and can be done at bedside or in the laboratory with static scanning. Acoustic gel is used and applied to the anterior fontanelle. The transducer is placed in the fontanelle, and gain settings are adjusted for adequate penetration of the brain. A 5-MHz transducer with fairly high gain settings will usually produce ample parenchymal texture.

The orientation of the coronal image is set so the baby's left side is to the right side of the scope.

The occipital horns are visualized first, and the transducer is swept slowly anteriorly. As it sweeps, look at two things: first, make sure the image remains symmetric (to assure that you are in the correct plane); second, follow the continuity of the structures. Of most importance are the choroid plexuses. As the transducer sweeps anteriorly, they taper down until fading out. Any disruption of this pattern should be cause for concern. Slow sweeping from occipital to frontal horns is essential for proper interpretation. If a videotape player is available, two or three sweeps should be recorded with narration for the interpreter. Freeze frame images of frontal, midbody, and occipital horns should be photographed for permanent records.

Next, sagittal views should be done, sweeping from one ventricle through midline to the other ventricle. The sagittal views are very important, and enough time should be spent to get adequate images. Remembering the oblique lie of each ventricle, position the transducer to get the entire ventricular system. Again videotaping the sweeps and photographing the freeze frame images are essential. A photograph should be taken of the midline structures as well as of both lateral ventricles.

Finally, axial planes should be done with real time. Angle the transducer 15 to 20 degrees above the canthomeatal line and sweep the transducer rostrally. When the lateral ventricles are in view just above the choroid plexus, take a photograph of the freeze frame for measurement purposes.

All three views using the real time scanner give the exact anatomy seen on static scans (Fig. 20-24); but, in addition, there is the added benefit of portability, maneuverability, detection of motion, and continuity. Real time has become the modality of choice in evaluating the neonatal head.

PATHOLOGY
Hydrocephalus

Hydrocephalus has been detected by ultrasound on a routine basis for many years.[9,18,24,30,41] The axial anatomy just described in the lateral ventricular region can be seen quite easily by ultrasound. Both static scans and real time imaging will demonstrate the ventricular system.

Hydrocephalus can be caused by a number of abnormalities that interfere with the normal circulation or absorption of cerebral spinal fluid.[14] The accumulation of fluid in many cases is quite subtle, and significant loss of brain parenchyma may result before it is clinically suspected.[20,22] Therefore an inexpensive, noninvasive, and nonionizing modality such as ultrasound is ideal for screening early on patients who are at risk for hydrocephalus—neonates with meningomyelocele, intraventricular hemorrhage or meningitis and infants with congenital malformations that have associated brain abnormalities.

The best method of recognizing hydrocephalus and following its course is via the lateral ventricular-to-hemispheric ratio.[18] An axial scan is obtained of the lateral ventricles just rostral to the choroid plexus. Measurements of hemispheric dimension are taken from the midline echo to the first echo arising from the downside skull. Then the dimension from the midline echo to the echo

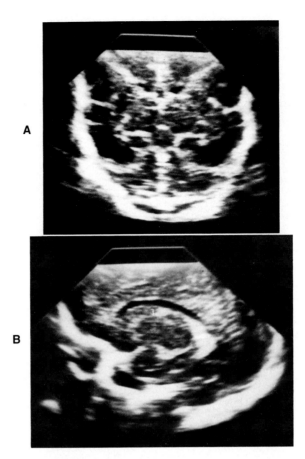

Fig. 20-24. Real time freeze frame images of the coronal, **A,** and sagittal, **B,** planes.

arising from the lateral wall of the lateral ventricle is taken (Fig. 20-25). This dimension divided by the hemispheric dimension is the ventricular/hemispheric ratio, which for neonates ranges from 24% to 30%.[17] The ratio for premature infants weighing less than 1500 g and gestational age less than 32 weeks is 24% to 34%.[17,21] The correlation between ultrasound and the gold standard CT scan has been reported to be excellent.[17,30]

Because multiple scans can be performed safely and without great expense, serial evaluations of ventricular size following shunting procedures or repeated lumbar punctures can be easily done.[31]

It should be pointed out that the measurement from the midline to the lateral ventricle is not the true dimension of the lateral ventricle. The medial border of the lateral ventricle is not perpendicular to the transducer, so an echo does not arise. Therefore the true measurement of the lateral ventricle is less than our measurements.

Cystic lesions other than hydrocephalus

Other cystic lesions may be seen by ultrasound with both the static and real time machines. Porencephaly, a communication be-

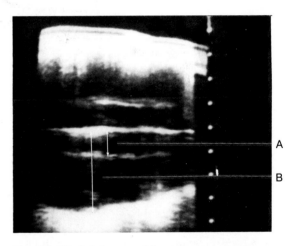

Fig. 20-25. Axial scan of the lateral ventricles. The width of the lateral ventricle, *A,* divided by the hemispheric dimension, *B,* is the ventricular/hemispheric ratio.

tween the ventricular system and the subarachnoid space, can be nicely demonstrated by ultrasound.[5,35] Areas of porencephaly can be associated with intracranial hemorrhage.[12] Other cystic lesions seen by ultrasound include Dandy-Walker cysts, hydranencephaly, and subdural hematomas.[1,5]

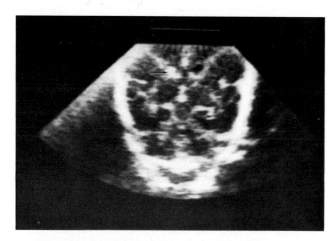

Fig. 20-26. Coronal section demonstrating a small caudate nucleus hemorrhage *(arrow)*.

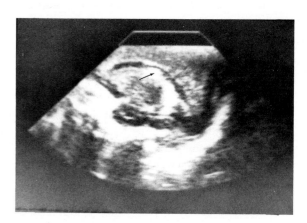

Fig. 20-27. Sagittal section of the lateral ventricle demonstrating a small caudate nucleus hemorrhage. Note the tapering of the choroid plexus anteriorly and the bulging density of the hemorrhage.

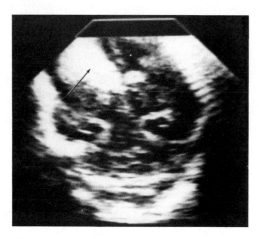

Fig. 20-28. Coronal section demonstrating intraparenchymal hemorrhage in its initial stage. Note the high level of echogenicity.

Intracranial hemorrhage

Recently much work has been done in the detection of intracranial hemorrhage. This has come about for two reasons. *First,* premature nurseries have developed rapidly in their ability to sustain life. The technology is available now to keep alive premature infants born well before 32 weeks. With this life-sustaining technology has come new problems that must be dealt with. One of these has been the high incidence of intracranial hemorrhage and its sequelae.[23,37] *Second,* ultrasound has advanced technologically as well. With high-resolution scanners we can now readily see brain structures and evaluate them for pathosis. Ultrasound has become very active in the management of neonates.

Premature infants of less than 32 weeks gestational age have intracranial hemorrhage 40% to 60% of the time.[4,33,34,37] The hemorrhage usually occurs in the subependymal layer of the germinal matrix, which is located in the caudate nucleus.[13] As the fetus develops, the germinal matrix matures; and by term there is only a 5% incidence of hemorrhage in this area. Ultrasonically a subependymal hemorrhage (SEH) looks very echodense in the region of the caudate nucleus.[11,32] In the coronal sections this will be lateral and inferior to the frontal horns of the lateral ventricles (Fig. 20-26). The most common site of a hemorrhage is the head of the caudate nucleus.[13] Often this echodense bleed will bulge into the ventricle, which can make it difficult to tell whether there is also intraventricular hemorrhage (IVH).

Real time is the most accurate way of confidently detecting a SEH.[11,39] Sweeps from occipital to frontal horns in a coronal plane demonstrate the tapering of the choroid plexus, which is thick posteriorly and thins out anteriorly. If there is another large echodense area after the choroid has tapered, this is characteristic of a SEH. As in other ultrasound examinations, if pathosis is seen in one plane you must search for it in another plane. Sagittal sections show nicely the tapering of the choroid and formation of a SEH (Fig. 20-27).

If there is a large amount of bulging into the ventricle, you should try to confirm intraventricular extension of the hemorrhage. This can be done by noting dense echoes arising from clot that occupies the most dependent part of the ventricular system. Moving the neonate, if possible, will demonstrate the mobility of this clot from an IVH.

A subependymal hemorrhage can extend into the brain parenchyma. This is called an intraparenchymal hemorrhage (IPH). Both IPH and SEH will appear as very echodense masses (Fig. 20-28), probably because of the large number of interfaces created by blood and vessels and brain parenchyma. As the area of IPH matures, some centralized changes begin to appear and sonolucent areas develop (Fig. 20-29). This usually occurs within 10 to 14 days. With the passage of more time, 3 or 4 weeks, a sonolucent rim appears as the clot retracts and separates from the brain (Fig. 20-30). Finally, this now cystic area of clot communicates with the ventricle; and the condition then is termed porencephaly (Fig. 20-31).

The echo intensity of SEH, IVH, and IPH looks exactly like the echo intensity arising from the choroid plexus. Therefore it is vitally important to demonstrate an abnormal area on two planes. Also the correct symmetry and sweeps help prevent misinterpretation. Remember, both static and real time

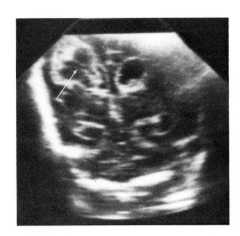

Fig. 20-29. Same patient as in Fig. 20-28 showing centralized sonolucency occurring after 10 to 14 days.

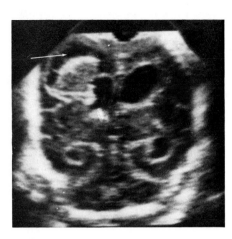

Fig. 20-30. Same patient as in Fig. 20-28 showing a sonolucent rim appearing at 4 weeks.

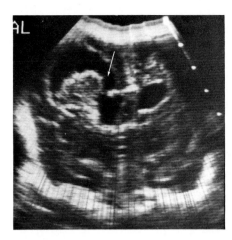

Fig. 20-31. Coronal section on same patient as in Fig. 20-28 demonstrating an area of porencephaly.

scanners achieve the same results when viewing the brain from the three views (coronal, axial, sagittal). Static scanners produce extremely high-resolution images but require movement of the patient to the laboratory and a longer examination time. Real time scanners provide flexibility and mobility and adequate resolution if the correct transducer is used.

The sensitivity of ultrasound in the detection of ICH is very encouraging. Detection of ICH by axial static ultrasound examinations is 91%. The sensitivity and specificity of ICH detection by real time are 100% compared to those by CT.[11] Although CT is used as a standard,[8] remember that hemorrhages can be seen ultrasonically for a much longer time than they can by CT because after 5 to 10 days they become isodense on the CT scan.

In approximately 60% to 70% of premature infants who have ICH the hemorrhage appears in the first 48 hours.[36] Hemorrhages have been seen to develop as late as 8 days. This creates a problem in detection because a single examination may not give the answer. Therefore a single screening examination should be done between 5 and 7 days.[36] If ICH is found, weekly examinations should be done for approximately a month to watch for hydrocephalus.

CONCLUSION

Ultrasound has proved to be an ideal imaging modality for the neonatal brain. Thorough understanding of anatomy will enable us to evaluate the normal and abnormal brain. High-resolution images can be generated by static scanners. Real time offers rapid, inexpensive, portable means of brain evaluation with little sacrifice of resolution. Cystic and solid lesions as well as hydrocephalus and ICH can be detected by ultrasound. With further investigation and technologic advancements will come greater accuracy, thus providing invaluable information for the neonatologists.

REFERENCES

1. Babcock, D.S., Han, B.K., LeQuesne, G.W., et al.: B-mode gray scale ultrasound of the head in the newborn and young infant, A.J.R. **134**:457, 1980.
2. Ben-Ora, A., Eddy, L., Hatch, G., et al.: The anterior fontanelle as an acoustic window to the neonatal ventricular system, J. Clin. Ultrasound **8**:65, 1980.
3. Brinker, R.A., and Taveras, J.M.: Ultrasound cross sectional pictures of the head, Acta Radiol. [Diagn.] **5**:745, 1966.
4. Burstein, J., Papile, L., and Burstein, R.: Intraventricular hemorrhage and hydrocephalus in premature newborns: a prospective study with CT, A.J.R. **132**:631, 1979.
5. Cantu, R.C., and LeMay, M.: Porencephaly caused by intracerebral hemorrhage, Radiology **88**:526, 1967.
6. Donat, J.F., Okazaki, H., Kleinberg, F., and Regan, T.J.: Intraventricular hemorrhages in full term and premature infants, Mayo Clin. Proc. **53**:437, 1978.
7. Edwards, M.K., Brown, D.L., Muller, J., et al.: Cribside neurosonography: real time sonography for intracranial investigation of the neonate, A.J.R. **136**:271, 1981.
8. Fitz, C.R., and Harwood-Nash, D.C.: Computed tomography in hydrocephalus, C.T. **2**:91, 1978.
9. Garrett, W.J., Kossoff, G., and Jones, R.F.C.: Ultrasonic cross sectional visualization of hydrocephalus in infants, Neuroradiology **8**:279, 1975.
10. Gordon, D.: Echoencephalography, Br. Med. J. **3**:1500, 1959.
11. Grant, E.J., Schellinger, D., Borts, F.T., et al.: Real time sonography of the neonatal and infant head, A.J.R. **136**:265, 1981.
12. Haber, K., et al.: Ultrasonic evaluation of intracranial pathology in infants: a new technique, Radiology **134**:173, 1980.
13. Hambleton, G., and Wigglesworth, J.S.: Origin of intraventricular hemorrhage in the preterm infant, Arch. Dis. Child. **51**:651, 1976.
14. Harwood-Nash, D.C., and Fitz, C.R.: Neuroradiology in infants and children, St. Louis, 1976, The C.V. Mosby Co.
15. Horbar, J.O., Walters, C.L., and Phillips, A.G., et al.: Ultrasound detection of changing ventricular size in posthemorrhagic hydrocephalus, Pediatrics **66**:674, 1980.
16. Johnson, M.L., Dunne, M.G., Mack, L.A., et al.: Evaluation of fetal intracranial anatomy by static and real-time ultrasound, J. Clin. Ultrasound **8**:311, 1980.
17. Johnson, M.L., Mack, L.A., Rumack, C.M., et al.: B-mode echoencephalography in the normal and high risk infant, A.J.R. **133**:375, 1979.
18. Johnson, M.L., and Rumack, C.M.: Ultrasonic evaluation of the neonatal brain, Radiol. Clin. North Am. **18**(1):117, 1980.
19. Johnson, M.L., Rumack, C.M., Mannes, E.J., et al.: Detection of neonatal intracranial hemorrhage utilizing real time and static ultrasound, J. Clin. Ultrasound, 1981.
20. Korobkin, R.: The relationship between head circumference and the development of communicating hydrocephalus in infants following interventricular hemorrhage, Pediatrics **56**:74, 1975.
21. Kossoff, G., Garrett, W.J., and Radavanovich, G.: Ultrasonic atlas of normal brain of infant, Ultrasound Med. Biol. **1**:259, 1974.
22. Larroche, J.C.: Post-hemorrhagic hydrocephalus in infancy. Anatomical study, Biol. Neonate **20**:287, 1972.
23. Lee, B.C.P., Grassi, A.E., Schechner, S., et al.: Neonatal intraventricular hemorrhage. A serial computed tomography study. J. Comput. Assist. Tomogr. **3**(4):483, 1979.
24. Lees, R.F., Harrison, R.B., and Sims, T.L.: Gray-scale ultrasonography in the evaluation of hydrocephalus and associated abnormalities in infants, Am. J. Dis. Child. **132**:376, 1978.

25. Leksell, L.: Echoencephalography in detection of intracranial complications following head injury, Acta Chir. Scand. **110**:301, 1956.

26. Mack, L.A., Rumack, C.M., and Johnson, M.L.: Ultrasound evaluation of cystic intracranial lesions in the neonate, Radiology **137**:451, 1980.

27. Matsui, T., and Hirano, A.: An atlas of the human brain for computerized tomography, New York, 1978, Igukn-Shoin Medical Publishers, Inc.

28. McRae, D.L., and Makow, M.: Horizontal laminography of the head with ultrasound. J. Can. Assoc. Radiol. **17**:75, 1966.

29. Moore, K.L.: The developing human, Philadelphia, 1977, W.B. Saunders Co.

30. Morgan, C.L., Trought, W.S., Rothman, S.J., and Jiminez, J.P.: Comparison of gray-scale ultrasonography and computed tomography in the evaluation of macrocrania in infants, Radiology **132**:119, 1979.

31. Murtaugh, F.R., Quencer, R.M., and Poole, C.A.: Cerebrospinal fluid shunt function and hydrocephalus in the pediatric age group, Radiology **132**:385, 1979.

32. Pape, K.E., Blackwell, R.J., Cusick, G., et al.: Ultrasound detection of brain damage in preterm infants, Lancet **1**:1261, 1979.

33. Papile, L., Burstein, J., Burstein, R., et al.: Incidence and evolution of subependymal and intraventricular hemorrhage: a study of infants with birth weights less than 1500 grams, J. Pediatr. **92**:529, 1978.

34. Persner, P.H., Garcia-Bunuel, R., Leeds, N., et al.: Subependymal and intraventricular hemorrhage in neonates, Radiology **119**:111, 1976.

35. Ramsey, R.G., and Hackman, H.S.: Computed tomography of porencephaly and other cerebrospinal fluid-containing lesions, Radiology **123**:73, 1977.

36. Rumack, C.M., McDonald, M.M., O'Meara, O.P., et al.: CT detection and course of intracranial hemorrhage in premature infants, A.J.R. **131**:493, 1978.

37. Rumack, C.M., Rumack, B.H., Peterson, R.G., et al.: Intracranial hemorrhage and aspirin: maternal use as a factor in neonatal intracranial hemorrhage, Obstet. Gynecol. **58**(suppl. 5):525, 1981.

38. Shaw, C.M., and Alvord, E.C., Jr.: Cava septi pellucidi et vergae: their normal and pathological states, Brain **92**:213, 1979.

39. Skelly, A.C., Appareti, K.E., Johnson, M.L.: Real time evaluation of normal intracranial anatomy in the premature infant, Med. Ultrasound **5**:11, 1981.

40. Skolnick, M.L., Rosenbaum, E., Matzuk, T., et al.: Detection of dilated cerebral ventricles in infants: a correlative study between ultrasound and computed tomography, Radiology **131**:447, 1979.

41. Slovis, T.I., Kuhns, L.R.: Real-time sonography of the brain through the anterior fontanelle, A.J.R. **136**:277, 1981.

21

Gynecologic ultrasound

LINDA LONDON

The ultrasound examination of the pelvis has been used for years as a tool in evaluating gynecologic pathology. It is a painless and noninvasive examination in the assessment of pelvic masses. In most cases a clinician refers a patient when there is a question as to location, origin, size, and consistency of a mass or masses. In some cases a patient will be referred for pain with no palpable mass. The use of B-scanning and real time ultrasonography together allows for rapid anatomic identification and correlation of structures.

Selection of equipment

In imaging the adult pelvis a 3.5- or 5.0-MHz with a long internal focus has been the transducer of choice. In a child or infant a 5.0-MHz transducer with a short or medium internal focus is generally used. The articulated arm B-scanner should have a late generation analog or digital scan converter with maximum use of the gray scale low-level echo pattern. If possible, a table that tilts should be used to help visualize the more superior structures in the pelvis when using the Trendelenburg position (head tilted approximately 30 degrees lower than the feet).

The optimal type of real time instrument would be a sector scanner with a small scan head that is easily maneuvered to visualize the anatomic structures in the somewhat U-shaped pelvis. The head is easily positioned at various angles to maximize visualization of the entire pelvic region so long as the urinary bladder is full (Fig. 21-1).

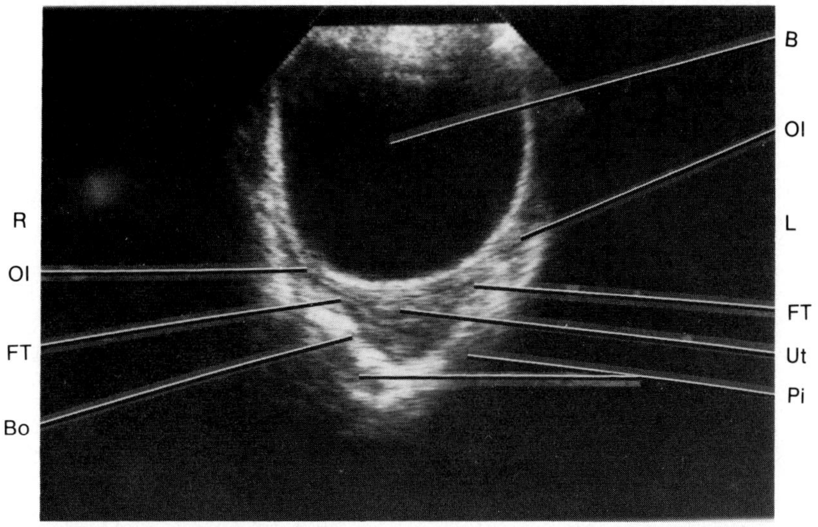

PREPARATION OF THE PATIENT

The proper preparation for a pelvic ultrasonogram begins with the patient having a full urinary bladder. This usually requires that she drink four to six 8-ounce glasses of clear fluids 1 hour prior to the examination and not void. If the patient is unable to drink, an intravenous fluid may be started or a Foley catheter inserted with retrograde filling of a sterile fluid or whatever is feasible for the particular situation.

The full urinary bladder has a low attenuation factor that acts as a window for visualization of deep posterior pelvic structures. It also displaces loops of small bowel out of the pelvis in a cephalic direction so a comparison can be made in assessing the fluid versus soft tissue consistency of other pelvic structures.

When the bladder is used as a tool in evaluating masses, care must be taken not to overfill it and thereby compress or displace a mass or the uterus and ovaries. One must also use caution not to confuse the bladder with other fluid-filled structures. A useful aid in distinguishing the bladder from a pelvic mass is to have the patient partially or completely void. Partial voiding may be accomplished by giving the patient a large cup or small basin and having her void into the container once or twice leaving some urine in the bladder.

The patient is placed in the supine position and the area between the symphysis

Fig. 21-1. Real time sector transverse scan showing the bladder, *B*, uterus, *Ut*, obturator internus, *OI*, bowel, *Bo*, piriformis, *Pi*, and fallopian tubes, *FT*. **R,** Right. **L,** Left.

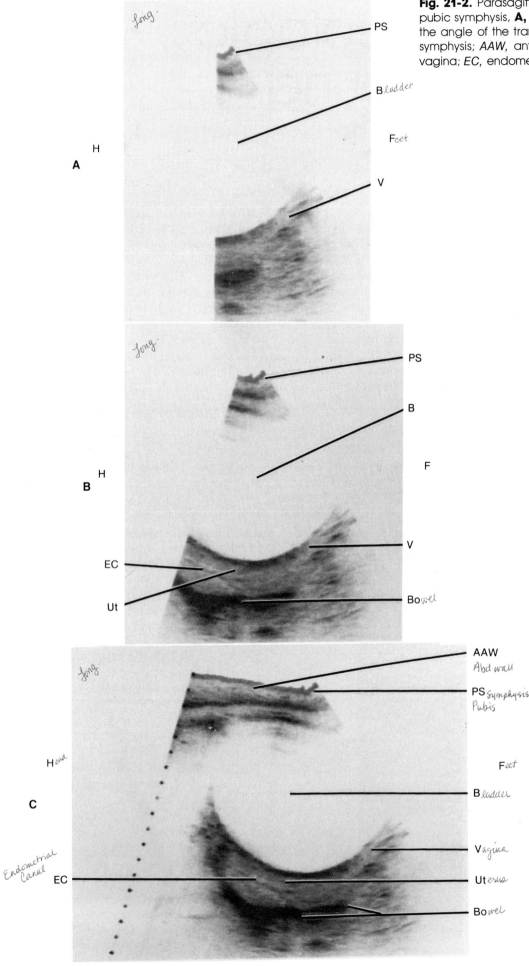

Fig. 21-2. Parasagittal single sweep of the midline starting from the pubic symphysis, **A,** and sliding toward the umbilicus, **B** and **C.** Note the angle of the transducer as indicated by dotted lines. *PS,* Pubic symphysis; *AAW,* anterior abdominal wall; *B,* bladder; *Ut,* uterus; *V,* vagina; *EC,* endometrial canal; *Bo,* bowel. **H,** Head. **F,** Foot.

pubis and umbilicus exposed. A coupling agent of mineral oil or water-soluble gel is applied to the skin or the transducer head. Lack of the appropriate amount of coupling agent may result in loss of echoes received by the transducer and improper setting of the time-gain compensation (TGC) curve on the equipment.

Technique

A B-scan of the pelvis usually begins with a single-sector pass of the transducer at the midline in a longitudinal plane of section. The transducer is placed at the symphysis pubis and angled caudally. The transducer begins by sweeping in a cephalic direction and slides toward the patient's umbilicus, approaching a perpendicular orientation to the floor. It then remains perpendicular and slides toward the umbilicus (Fig. 21-2).

At this point one must stop to assess the TGC curve. A good pelvic technique shows the body wall clearly with a minimal line of dark echoes at the transducer interface. The bladder is clear of noise artifacts, and a minimal low-level echo pattern is seen in the near field at its anterior surface. This is due to the inherent structure of the receiving mechanism in the transducer. By angling the transducer in a caudal or cephalic direction, one can differentiate these echoes from real structures.

In a normal study the area between the bladder and the uterus is undetectable because the uterus abuts on the posterior bladder wall when the bladder is filled to the desired level. A normal uterus should be a homogeneous echogenic structure with a dark linear echo representing the endometrial cavity. The area posterior to the uterus is sometimes visualized or may be blocked totally by bowel gas. This area will vary in appearance with each individual.

A good TGC curve will produce all the above structures with the highest-frequency transducer available (Fig. 21-3). If available, one should use a far field suppressant to clean up the noise posterior to the pelvis for a more desirable image.

When the TGC curve is set up, serial scans beginning at the iliopsoas and proceeding from the right side to the left side every centimeter should be recorded. The arm is

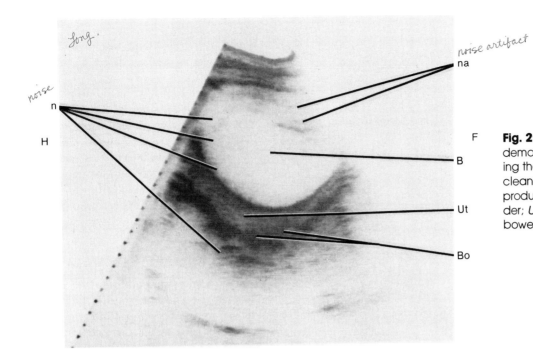

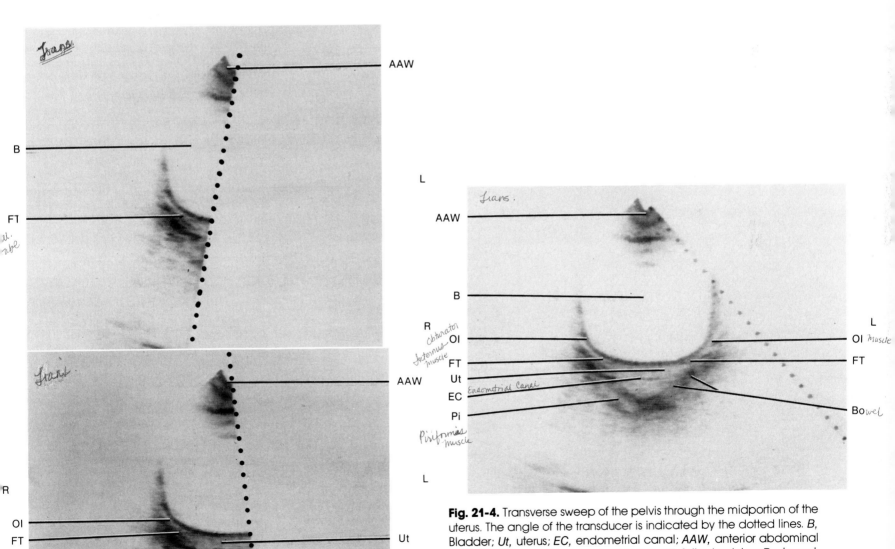

Fig. 21-3. Parasagittal scan through the uterus demonstrating too steep a TGC curve. Adjusting the slope to a more horizontal position will clean up the noise throughout the image and produce a scan similar to Fig. 21-2, *C. B*, Bladder; *Ut*, uterus; *n*, noise; *na*, noise artifact; *Bo*, bowel. **H,** Head. **F,** Foot.

Fig. 21-4. Transverse sweep of the pelvis through the midportion of the uterus. The angle of the transducer is indicated by the dotted lines. *B*, Bladder; *Ut*, uterus; *EC*, endometrial canal; *AAW*, anterior abdominal wall; *Pi*, piriformis; *OI*, obturator internus; *FT*, fallopian tube; *Bo*, bowel. **R,** Right. **L,** Left.

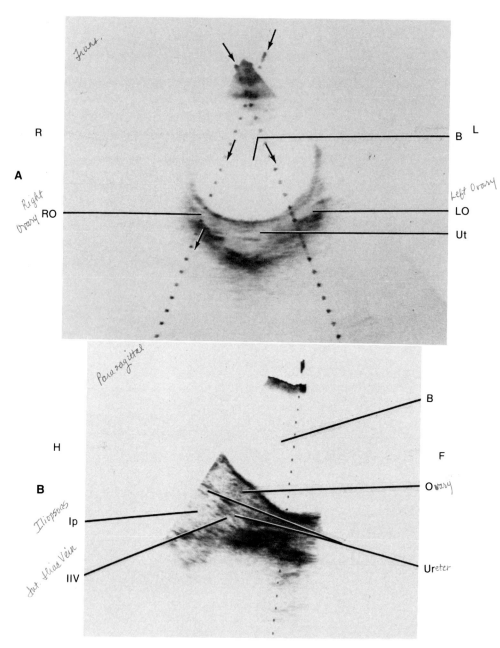

Fig. 21-5. A, Transverse scan of the pelvis indicating the angle necessary to produce a longitudinal scan of the ovary (dotted lines and arrows). **B,** Parasagittal scan of the ovary obtained by angling the transducer perpendicular to the ovarian plane indicated in **A.** Ut, Uterus; LO, left ovary; RO, right ovary; AAW, anterior abdominal wall; B, bladder; O, ovary; IIV, internal iliac vein; Ur, ureter; Ip, iliopsoas. **R,** Right. **L,** Left. **H,** Head. **F,** Foot.

duce the best anatomic images of the uterus and ovaries as well as delineate any pelvic disorder.

When a full B-scan has been completed, a real time examination of the pelvis may be done. The same routine is employed to scan with a real time unit as with a B-scanner. By real time a loop of bowel is easily differentiated from another soft tissue structure. Because a large amount of bowel lies adjacent to the pelvic structures, real time scanning should be employed whenever possible.

NORMAL ANATOMIC CONSIDERATIONS

In a normal longitudinal plane of section the vagina, cervix, and uterine body and fundus are routinely demonstrated. The vaginal canal is imaged as a strong echogenic reflective interface directly posterior to the bladder wall in the most caudal direction. On longitudinal section the imaged length is variable due to individual bladder configuration but the width is usually around 5 mm (Fig. 21-2, B). In a transverse plane of section the canal appears flat and wide. One should be aware of the possibility of fluid in the vagina, either urine from the bladder or blood during menstruation. When the vagina is full of fluid, a sonolucent region will be imaged. A tampon in the vaginal vault will be imaged as multiple linear lines paralleling the vaginal wall. In patients who have had a hysterectomy, the vaginal cuff appears quite prominent, often giving a masslike appearance. Caution must be exercised not to misinterpret appearances.

The uterus is best identified in the longitudinal plane of section. A scan of the endometrial canal in its entirety best identifies the uterus and its position in the pelvis. The endometrial cavity produces a strong reflective echo. Sometimes in the fundal portion the endometrial canal appears thick and may even have a sonolucent region within the central cavity. To distinguish endometrial pathosis from early gestation or a variation in the canal during the menstrual cycle may require serial scans.

The uterus may be identified in various forms of anteversion or retroversion (Fig. 21-6). In cases of retroversion one must overfill the bladder to distinguish the normal retroverted uterus from a myomatous uterus. In some cases the normal uterine texture will vary, and loss of echoes may result from the increased angle of the uterine-bladder interface. The uterus may also take a leftward or rightward course in the transverse plane of section (Fig. 21-7). To distinguish the uterus from an adnexal mass, one must carefully

then moved 90 degrees to a transverse plane of section and is angled 15 degrees caudad. One begins a sweep angling the arm from right to left while sliding the transducer from right to left (Fig. 21-4). Three to four scans should be recorded of the vaginal vault with a caudal angle. The arm is then angled perpendicular to the floor and a few scans of the cervix are recorded. Next, the arm is angled cephalad so the transducer is perpendicular to the bladder wall and body of the uterus. One then proceeds to record images every

centimeter until the bladder is no longer imaged and the transducer approaches the umbilicus.

At this point random scans of the uterus and ovaries in the longitudinal and transverse planes of section are recorded. The ovary is best visualized in the longitudinal section with the transducer angled perpendicular to the ovary at the angle established in the transverse plane. One should use a short linear or sector motion to obtain random scans (Fig. 21-5). These scans often pro-

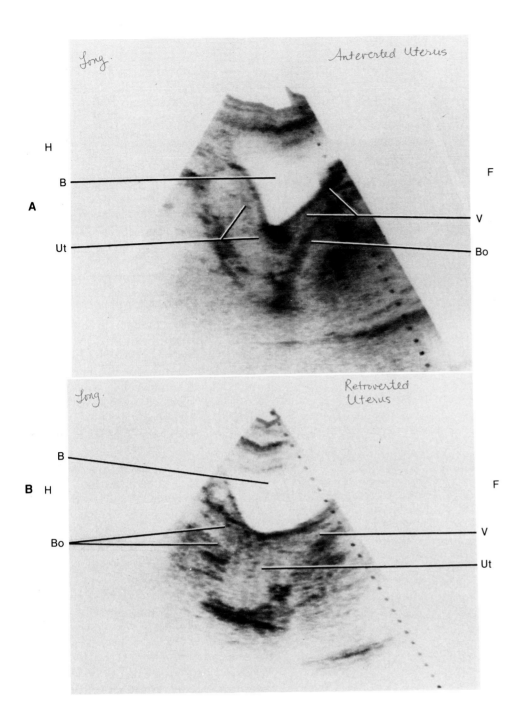

Long.   Anteverted Uterus

H

B

A

Ut   V

                                                                 Bo

Fig. 21-6. Parasagittal scan of an anteverted, **A,** and a retroverted, **B,** uterus demonstrating normal variations of size and shape. *B,* Bladder; *Ut,* uterus; *V,* vagina; *Bo,* bowel. **H,** Head. **F,** Foot.

Long.   Retroverted Uterus

B

B H   F

Bo   V

                                                                 Ut

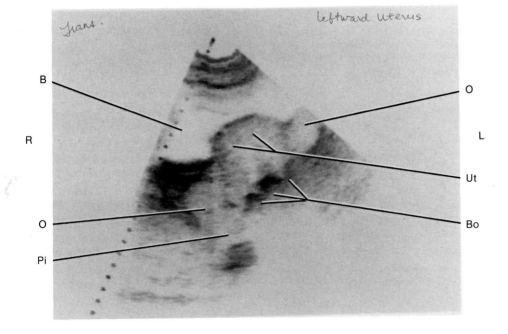

Trans.   Leftward Uterus

B   O

R   L

                                                                 Ut

O   Bo

Pi

Fig. 21-7. Transverse scan of the pelvis demonstrating a leftward uterus and the upper limits of normal sized ovaries. *B,* Bladder; *Ut,* uterus; *O,* ovary; *Pi,* piriformis; *Bo,* bowel. **R,** Right. **L,** Left.

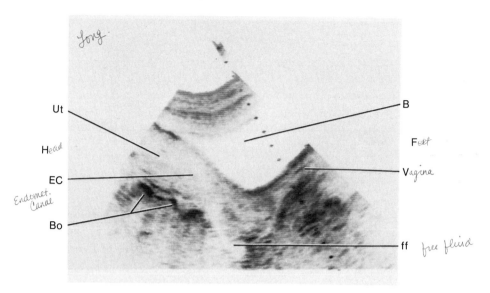

Fig. 21-8. Parasagittal scan of the uterus demonstrating free fluid in the cul-de-sac in a normal patient. *B*, Bladder; *Ut*, uterus; *EC*, endometrial canal; *ff*, free fluid; *Bo*, bowel; *V*, vagina. **H,** Head. **F,** Foot.

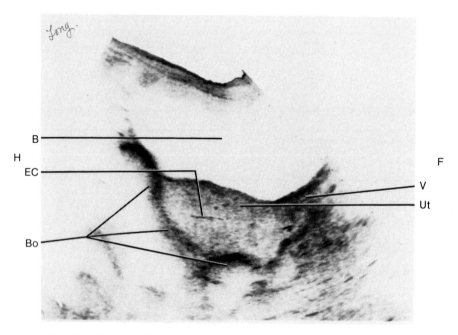

Fig. 21-9. Parasagittal scan of the uterus demonstrating a strongly reflective endometrial canal. Note the strong curvilinear echo produced by bowel and sometimes mistaken for a mass. *B*, Bladder; *Ut*, uterus; *V*, vagina; *EC*, endometrial canal; *Bo*, bowel. **H,** Head. **F,** Foot.

identify the endometrial canal and follow its course.

The normal uterus at birth is small. In an unstimulated uterus with an adult shape but no discernible endometrial canal, the size and shape usually remain the same until menarche. At puberty the normal uterus varies in length from 5 to 8 cm and in thickness from 1.5 to 3 cm. The postmenopausal uterus is usually atrophic.

The ovary is an intraperitoneal structure attached to the uterus by the fallopian tube and to the pelvic sidewall by the lateral pelvic segment. The normal ovary varies slightly in size from birth until puberty. After 2 years of age it can be visualized sonographically with tedious scanning techniques.

In the postpubertal patient the ovaries usually lie in the ovarian fossa, which is posterior to the psoas and the exterior iliac ves-

sels and anterior to the piriformis. The ovary may vary in position as the ovarian ligament changes size in accordance with phases of the menstrual cycle. The normal postpubertal ovary averages $1 \times 3 \times 2$ cm, thus giving a normal range for ovarian volumes of 1.8 to 5.7 cm according to Sample (½ × width × thickness × length).

Location of the normal ovary on a sonogram can be aided by using the major adnexal structures. The major pelvic sidewall muscles are the obturator internus, pubococcygeus, and iliopsoas. The obturator internus is best seen in the transverse plane at an angle perpendicular to the floor or slightly caudal, depending on the fullness of the bladder. Medial and anterior to this muscle in the transverse plane of section lies the ovary, which can be identified lying caudal and medial to the ovarian blood vessels within the infundibulopelvic ligament. These vessels are stable in relation to the ovary and are a most reliable reference in identifying the ovary in the longitudinal plane of section (Fig. 21-5, *B*). To identify these vessels and the ovary requires a longitudinal scan at an angle determined on the transverse plane of section. A single sweep of the right ovary is obtained by angling the transducer at a predetermined angle to the right while scanning to the left of the midline. These vessels usually lie directly medial and caudal to the iliopsoas.

The appearance of normal ovarian tissue is homogeneous with low-level gray scale echoes. During changes of the menstrual cycle, in response to hormonal flux, the ovary may contain cystic elements. At ovulation follicular cysts may be abundant, measuring approximately 1 cm in diameter. After ovulation the corpus luteum develops and cysts averaging 2 cm may develop, regressing with the onset of menses. Such physiologic phenomena should not be confused with pathologic processes. Reexamination at a later date may help differentiate such conditions. Similarly, free peritoneal fluid mimicking ascites, some inflammatory process, or a possible ectopic pregnancy is frequently seen; and if clinically permitted, reexamination at a later date may be necessary (Fig. 21-8).

The sonographic appearance of the rectosigmoid portion of the gastrointestinal tract varies; but usually some bowel gas is present, producing a strong curvilinear echo with posterior shadowing (Fig. 21-9). Fecal material or fluid in the bowel may mimic a pelvic mass. Real time may distinguish the movement of bowel from a mass, or reexamination after a water enema may be helpful. If all these attempts do not clarify the issue, additional studies such as computed tomography with contrast media may be done.

INTRAUTERINE CONTRACEPTIVE DEVICE

At the present time the IUCD is one of the most common methods of birth control. Accompanying the improvements in the second generation of devices is a corresponding increase in complications. These may include unknown expulsion of the device, pregnancy while using the device, pelvic inflammatory disease, and uterine rupture. Along with any of these complications one may experience discomfort and irregular bleeding.

Ultrasonography has been useful in imaging a lost IUCD along with verification of any of the above complications. Since the consequences of a false-positive or false-negative sonogram are clinically significant in the management of the patient, a precise diagnosis is imperative. When a sonogram is inconclusive, a single radiograph of the pelvis may be made as a supplemental examination.

Most IUCDs are sufficiently different in acoustic impedance from the normal uterus and can easily be detected. The most common pitfall in the evaluation of the uterus for an IUCD is attributed to the high-amplitude specular reflection generated from the endometrial canal (Fig. 21-9).

Knowledge of the specific type of device used and its position relative to the position of the transducer will aid in correct identification of an IUCD. The Lippes loop is still commonly used and is easiest to recognize by the two to five distinct echoes in the longitudinal plane of section (Fig. 21-10). The transverse plane of section produces a series of linear horizontal echoes within the uterus.

Although the Dalkon shield has been discontinued at the present time, many are still in use. This is the smallest and most difficult device to image. It is frequently displayed as a small line of linear echoes within the uterus on all planes of section.

The Saf-T-Coil is a double coil with a central arm. It can have several sonographic appearances. If the coils are scanned, they may produce separate echoes similar to those of a Lippes loop. If the arm of the device is scanned, a long linear echo similar to that from the endometrial cavity may be viewed in the longitudinal plane of section.

The Copper-7 and Copper-T are similar in appearance. They both have a long base limb and a short cross limb (Fig. 21-11).

When the anatomy of an IUCD is identified, one must obtain an acoustic shadow caused by the difference in velocity from

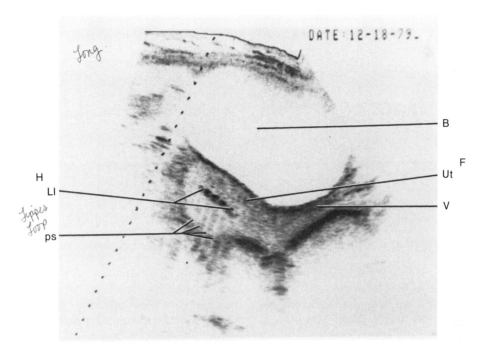

Fig. 21-10. Parasagittal scan of the uterus demonstrating posterior shadowing, *ps*, and parallel echoes of a Lippes loop, *LI*, intrauterine contraceptive device. *B*, Bladder; *Ut*, uterus; *V*, vagina. **H**, Head. **F**, Foot.

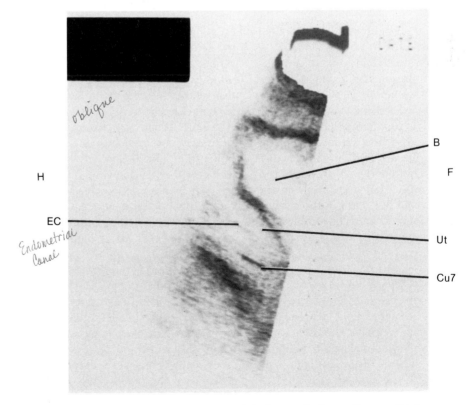

Fig. 21-11. Oblique scan of the pelvis demonstrating a Copper-7 intrauterine contraceptive device, *Cu7*, outside the uterus. *B*, Bladder; *Ut*, uterus; *EC*, endometrial canal. **H**, Head. **F**, Foot.

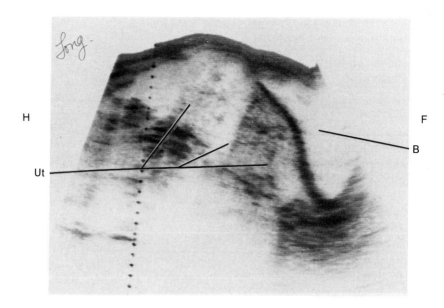

Fig. 21-12. Parasagittal scan of the pelvis demonstrating a large, nonhomogeneous, irregular myomatous uterus. *B,* Bladder; *Ut,* uterus. **H,** Head. **F,** Foot.

surrounding tissues. When a shadow is not seen, the scan is inconclusive. Another feature of an IUCD in utero is parallel echoes generated by the device. Though unproved, these may represent entrance-exit reflections from the anterior and posterior interfaces of the IUCD. To demonstrate this requires high-frequency transducers with appropriate focal zones for good axial resolution (Fig. 21-10).

PATHOLOGIC PROCESSES
Uterine neoplasms

Leiomyoma. Benign leiomyoma is the most commonly encountered uterine tumor and is easily detected by ultrasonography. It is composed of smooth and connective tissue and commonly presents as a palpable mass in middle-aged women.

The consistency of a leiomyoma varies in relation to the distribution of the elements of the tumor. Its growth is stimulated by the hormone estrogen, and it often enlarges during pregnancy. Myomas may develop anywhere in the uterus but are usually in the fundus or body and less often in the cervical region. The tumors may be intramural, subserosal, or submucosal and may extend into the broad ligament or may even detach from the uterus.

Leiomyomas of the uterus are usually multiple and of varying sizes. As they increase in size, they may become degenerative as they outgrow their blood supply. Their degeneration may be benign or malignant, although malignancy is seldom diagnosed preoperatively because of the lack of characteristic symptoms.

The most common symptom of myomas is uterine bleeding. Pain is unusual except in degenerative changes or torsion of a submucosal myoma on a pedicle. Discomfort may be caused by larger tumors pressing on other pelvic structures. Infection may occur from pelvic inflammatory disease by direct extension, through the lymphatics, or by extrusion of a myoma into the cervical canal.

The sonographic appearance of a leiomyoma is that of an enlarged or irregularly shaped uterus (Fig. 21-12). There may be distortion of the endometrial canal or indentation of the bladder wall at the anterior surface of the uterus. These masses are often inseparable from the uterus, except in the case of a pedunculated mass. The echogenicity depends upon the organization or degeneration of the elements of the tumor. In some cases myomas are more homogeneous than normal uterine tissue and have a poor far-wall delineation due to attenuation of the ultrasonic beam. A characteristic circular pattern is observed in some cases. Calcifications may appear as highly echogenic areas with or without shadowing. Cystic degeneration may be observed as areas of sonolucency within highly echogenic areas of the uterus.

The most common pitfall in the ultrasonographic diagnosis of a leiomyoma of the uterus is the inappropriate use of the TCG curve. One must carefully set the slope of the curve according to the size of the patient and the size and consistency of the tumor (Fig. 21-13). Insufficient amplification of the far field (too shallow a slope) may result in an incorrect diagnosis of the size, shape, consistency, or even existence of a tumor. Careful scanning of the pelvis must be done with a full and half-full bladder so all areas under suspicion for pedunculated tumors or highly attenuating fundal masses will be visualized.

Other uterine masses. Included among these are leiomyosarcomas, carcinosarcomas, and mixed mesodermal tumors. They all appear similar to the leiomyoma although they are less common. Malignant ascites as well as distinct areas of metastases may accompany such tumors.

Cervical or endometrial carcinoma is rarely distinguishable by ultrasound. Often it is diagnosed by clinical laboratory tests such as the Pap smear. When detectable on the ultrasonogram, the tumor may be followed with treatment. Patients should be observed after hysterectomy for recurrence of tumor.

Congenital anomalies. Congenital anomalies of the uterus detectable ultrasonographically include various formations of the bicornuate uterus. The uterus and vagina, formed as paired structures, eventually fuse in the midline. Incomplete fusion results in a septated or bicornuate uterus. Discovery of such an anomaly usually occurs during pregnancy with palpation of a nodular mass. The ultrasonographic appearance of a nongravid uterus is the image of a binodular mass in the transverse plane (Fig. 21-14). A bicornuate uterus is rarely distinguished after the first trimester of pregnancy. Scans of the kidneys should be obtained in such cases since renal anomalies may accompany the disorder.

Hydrometrocolpos. This condition results from accumulation of secretions within the uterus and vagina due to obstruction at the level of the uterine horn. Hydrocolpos implies accumulation of fluid in the vagina alone. Patients may present with symptoms including delayed menstruation, pain, or dysuria from compression of the mass. On the ultrasonogram the uterus and vagina ap-

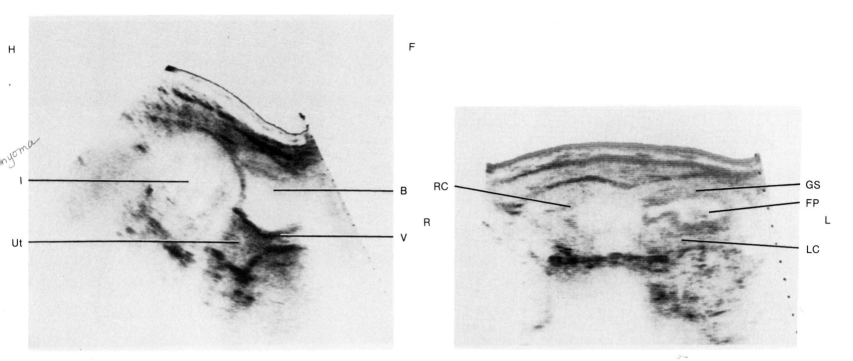

Fig. 21-13. Parasagittal scan of the pelvis demonstrating a large fundal leiomyoma attenuating the sound beam. Note the difference in texture of the normal uterus compared to the myomatous fundus. *B,* Bladder; *Ut,* uterus; *I,* leiomyoma. **H,** Head. **F,** Foot.

Fig. 21-14. Transverse scan of a bicornuate uterus with a 6-week gestational sac in the left cornu. *RC,* Right cornu; *LC,* left cornu; *GS,* gestational sac; *FP,* fetal pole. **R,** Right. **L,** Left.

pear markedly distended and some clot may be distinguished.

Ovarian masses

The most common extrauterine masses seen by ultrasonography are often cystic and usually clinically insignificant.

Cysts. The types of ovarian cysts that may present include follicular, corpus luteal, and paraovarian. Normal follicles are sometimes as large as 3 cm before being considered a true mass.

Follicular cysts generally are smaller than 5 to 6 cm but can be as large as 10 cm (Fig. 21-15). They may be multiple and usually are thin walled, have smooth borders, and are unilocular.

Corpus luteal cysts are indistinguishable from follicular cysts by sonography. They are common during pregnancy and regress during the second trimester. They are luteinized follicles that have accumulated fluid or blood, sometimes appearing to have soft internal echoes and good through-transmission. They are small, unilateral, and thin-walled. Theca-lutein cysts are luteinized and usually large, multiple, and bilateral when associated with hydatidiform mole, multiple pregnancy, erythroblastosis fetalis, and gonadotrophin administration (Fig. 21-16).

Fimbrial or *paraovarian* cysts are thin-walled and may grow up to 18 cm. They

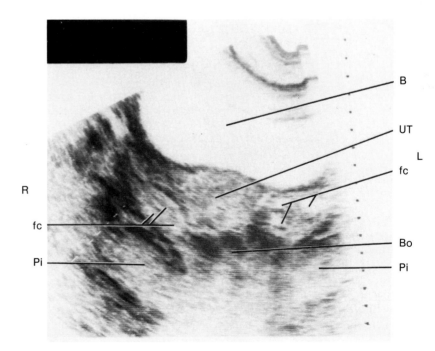

Fig. 21-15. Transverse scan of the pelvis demonstrating bilateral follicular cysts of the ovaries. *B,* Bladder; *Ut,* uterus; *fc,* follicular cysts; *Pi,* piriformis; *Bo,* bowel. **R,** Right. **L,** Left.

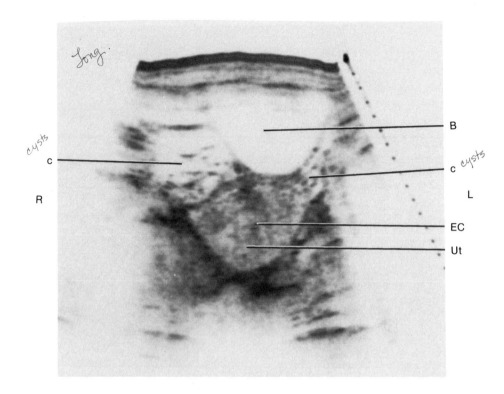

A

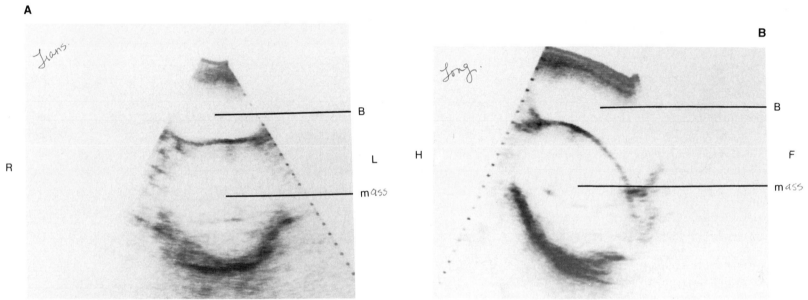

Fig. 21-16. Transverse scan of a hydatidiform mole with theca-lutein cysts. Note the abnormal pattern of the uterus. *B*, Bladder; *Ut*, uterus; *EC*, endometrial canal; *c*, cysts. **R**, Right. **L**, Left.

Fig. 21-17. Transverse, **A**, and parasagittal, **B**, sections of the pelvis demonstrating a serous cystadenoma of the ovary. *B*, Bladder; *m*, mass. **R**, Right. **L**, Left. **H**, Head. **F**, Foot.

may be unilocular or may have thin septa. Their ultrasound characteristics resemble those of follicular cysts or cystadenomas though with growth they may assume a position very anterior in the pelvis. Ovarian and paraovarian cysts may be followed by serial sonograms for determination of their status of growth or regression.

Polycystic ovaries. Polycystic ovaries may be seen in the Stein-Leventhal syndrome. Occurring in women during their late teens and upward, this syndrome consists of menstrual irregularity, reduced fertility,

obesity, excessive growth of hair (hirsutism), and bilateral cystic ovaries. Other types of polycystic ovaries are unilateral and are follicular or luteal in origin. Common symptoms include dysmenorrhea, menstrual irregularity, and pelvic discomfort associated with pelvic inflammatory disease, endometriosis, uterine leiomyomas, or pituitary hormonal stimulation.

Primary tumors of the ovary. These are highly fatal tumors. Their histologic classification varies with pathologic appearance, but most are serous or mucinous cystadeno-

mas or cystadenocarcinomas. Clinically the ovarian tumor may produce no symptoms until it is large enough to be palpated or cause distension of the abdomen. Then the symptoms include abdominal discomfort, vomiting, shortness of breath, and irregularity of bowel or urinary habits.

Rapid growth or menstrual irregularity may be seen in both benign and malignant ovarian tumors. The development of ascites, pain in one leg or the sacrum, palpation of hard nodules, and immobility are the clinical symptoms most likely caused by a malignant tumor. The typical ultrasonographic appearance of an ovarian neoplasm may include a spherical mass or bilateral masses with well-defined borders.

Serous cystadenoma is usually thin walled with occasional septa. It may vary in size and may be bilateral. Some solid components are sometimes seen within the cyst (Fig. 21-17). Most tumors are histologically malignant.

Serous cystadenocarcinoma is complex, solid, and cystic. It can be capsular or may infiltrate into the pelvis. Ascites and nodal metastases may be associated with this tumor (Fig. 21-18).

Mucinous cystadenoma can become very large and multilocular with thin opaque septa. It may contain solid components and is rarely bilateral.

Mucinous cystadenocarcinoma is difficult to assess for malignancy by ultrasound since it tends to have the same features as a benign mass of the same type. It is a complex solid and cystic mass that presents bilaterally with loss of definition, capsular infiltration, and fixation. Often these masses are accompanied by ascites, but they do not metastasize to the lymph nodes.

Metastatic neoplasms. Metastatic neoplasms to the ovary are common and can originate from the gastrointestinal tract, breast, or genital organs and are classified as Krukenberg tumors. They usually present bilaterally and are accompanied by ascites. They vary in size and appear to have a homogeneous echo pattern with cystic to solid components and good through-transmission of the sound beam.

Clear cell tumor. This lesion is predominantly solid or cystic, can be borderline benign or malignant, and is occasionally bilateral. It is commonly referred to as chocolate cyst from the hemorrhagic chocolate-covered material it contains.

Brenner tumor. This uncommon solid tumor varies in size from small (nodules) to 20 cm in diameter. It is associated with mucinous cystadenoma.

Germ cell tumor. In the germ cell tumor category cystic teratoma or dermoid cyst is frequently seen. This tumor may be bilateral and is benign, varying in size but rarely larger than 10 cm. It is usually a spherical well-defined fluid mass with a localized solid portion of hair, teeth, or bone. There may be a layer of fat and other materials (Fig. 21-19). Ultrasonographically the dermoid in adults is characterized by a fluid-filled level and a highly echo-producing solid internal component casting acoustic shadows. When there is a strong reflective shadow bordering the

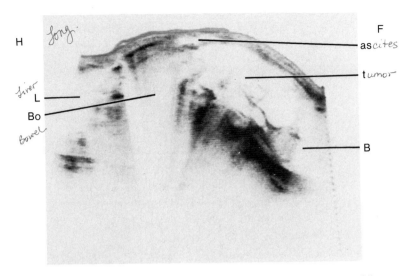

Fig. 21-18. Parasagittal scan of a serous cystadenocarcinoma of the ovary. Note the thin line of ascites anterior to the tumor. *B,* Bladder; *t,* tumor; *as,* ascites; *Bo,* bowel; *L,* liver. **H,** Head. **F,** Foot.

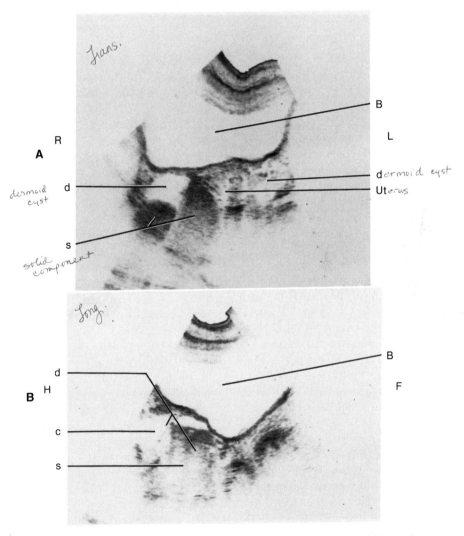

Fig. 21-19. A, Transverse scan of the pelvis demonstrating bilateral dermoid cysts. **B,** Parasagittal scan of the right dermoid cyst demonstrating the cystic and solid components of the tumor. *B,* Bladder; *Ut,* uterus; *d,* dermoid; *c,* cystic component; *s,* solid component. **R,** Right. **L,** Left. **H,** Head. **F,** Foot.

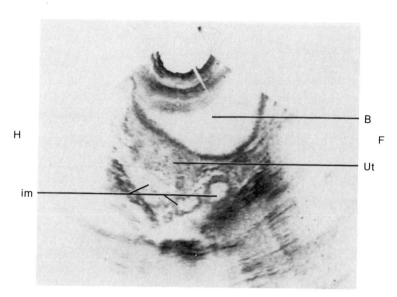

Fig. 21-20. Parasagittal section of the pelvis demonstrating pelvic inflammatory disease making definition of the uterus and other tissue planes difficult. *B,* Bladder; *Ut,* uterus; *im,* inflammatory masses. **H,** Head. **F,** Foot.

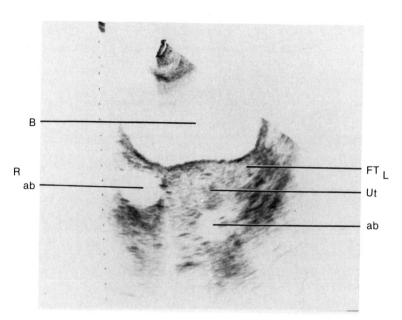

Fig. 21-21. Transverse scan of the pelvis demonstrating a pyosalpinx on the right and an abscess in the cul-de-sac in a patient with pelvic inflammatory disease. *B,* Bladder; *Ut,* uterus; *ab,* abscess; *FT,* fallopian tube. **R,** Right. **L,** Left.

bowel, one must be careful not to confuse it with bowel gas. Pelvic x-ray examination may be helpful in differentiating bowel from dermoid. In children, dermoids appear as solid masses.

Other ovarian tumors. Included with this group are fibroma, fibroadenoma, mesenchymal tumor, dysgerminoma, granulosa cell tumor, and choriocarcinoma. All these tend not to have any specific ultrasonographic feature characterizing them, and they are difficult to differentiate from other ovarian tumors.

Pelvic inflammatory disease

PID is classified as a gonococcal, pyogenic, and tuberculous infection of the genital system. It may be categorized anatomically as endometritis, salpingitis, or oophoritis. In the acute phase of the disease the initial sonographic findings include a slight increase in the visibility of the fallopian tubes, ovaries, and ligaments with a decrease in the intensity of internal echoes. The uterus may become less echogenic, and definition of the various tissue planes is more difficult and at times impossible (Fig. 21-20). Similarly the borders of the uterus cannot be identified; and in the transverse plane an inflammatory mass may take the shape of the pelvis whereas on longitudinal scans the cephalic extent of the mass may be difficult to distinguish from bowel. The use of careful scanning and a focused high-frequency transducer is necessary for visualizing the endometrial canal and possibly the outline of the

uterus. The adnexal regions appear thickened and blend into the pelvic sidewall musculature, again making it difficult to distinguish fallopian tubes and ovaries.

The usual treatment for PID is antibiotic therapy. A series of scans may be obtained during and after treatment for assessment of the pelvic organs. Often the disease will clear with therapy and the uterus and adnexa will again appear as normal structures.

In the chronic stage of the disease the uterus appears normal with possibly some thickening around the uterine wall and often dilation of the fallopian tubes. The tubes may appear as a single sausage-shaped structure, or there may be multiple small fluid-filled areas surrounding them (Fig. 21-21). There may be adhesions, giving a thickened sonographic appearance to adnexal structures, although the pelvic sidewall can usually be distinguished. This appearance can be unilateral but often appears bilaterally.

Not uncommonly a tubo-ovarian abscess or pyosalpinx will present with gonococcal forms of the disease. Single or multiple fluid-filled masses may appear as cystic structures with or without internal components. The ovary usually cannot be distinguished as a separate structure (Fig. 21-21). Often there will be fluid in the pouch of Douglas or cul-de-sac region. In cases of hydrosalpinx the ovary may be distinguished and a thick-walled cystic mass with or without septa will be visualized.

PID may take on an atypical ultrasono-

graphic appearance; and if present with other forms of pelvic pathology such as ovarian cysts, ectopic pregnancies, or a dermoid, the possibility of distinction may be difficult or even overlooked.

Endometriosis

Endometriosis is a common disease in menstruating women and is defined as the ectopic location of the functioning endometrial glands and stroma outside the uterus. Most commonly it is located in the ovaries, uterine ligaments, and pelvic peritoneum; less commonly it occurs at other locations in the pelvis, lymph nodes, scars, and rarely the extremities. Symptoms include pelvic pain, dysmenorrhea, and infertility. Often changes occur with the menstrual cycle, and bleeding may occur during menstruation. Ovarian involvement alone may not produce pain but may be discovered as an adnexal mass at routine pelvic examination.

Adenomyosis is a special form of endometriosis defined as a benign invasion of the endometrium into myometrium. In most cases there is no specific ultrasonographic appearance other than some uterine enlargement.

The ultrasonographic appearance of endometriosis is variable, depending on cystic changes and location. An endometrioma may appear cystic, solid, or mixed. A *cystic* mass tends to have thick irregular walls and may have septations, making it difficult to distinguish from other pelvic cystic structures. A *solid* lesion without other sonographic appearances may be confused with an ovarian tumor. If a pelvic mass is a *mixed* lesion, it can be confused with PID or a dermoid tumor.

Two common ultrasonographic appearances include a solid thickening of the adnexal region and a unilocular thick-walled cystic mass with or without internal components from clot, fibrosis, and liquefaction (Fig. 21-22).

Postpartum uterus

The normal uterus remains enlarged for 6 to 8 weeks after delivery. Enlargement is due to atrophied muscle wall and a slight amount of residual debris within the uterine cavity. The ultrasonographic appearance of the uterus is normal in texture with a prominent and sometimes lucent endometrial cavity.

Indications for ultrasonography in the postpartum patient include retained products of conception such as placenta or fetal parts or a uterine or parauterine hematoma. Symptoms may include bleeding, pain, and sometimes elevated temperature.

Pelvic lymphadenopathy

Normal masses in the pelvis appear by ultrasonography to be lobular along the distribution of the iliac vessels anterior to the iliopsoas and in the presacral area. On transverse sections asymmetry is noted along the pelvic sidewalls. Large nodal masses can impinge upon the posterior or lateral borders of the bladder.

Nodal masses may vary in their sonographic appearance. Lymphomatous masses appear as sonolucent and well-defined concentric accumulations located laterally. Although the documentation of enlarged nodes by ultrasonography is not specific for tumor, this finding usually does indicate metastatic disease.

Nongynecologic solid masses

A malignant tumor of abdominal origin can present as an extrauterine mass. Carcinoma of the colon is the most common disease entity. It may have an echogenic center resembling bowel. A barium enema will show the origin of this mass to be different from that of other masses (e.g., embryonal tumor, neural element tumor, soft tissue sarcoma). Aside from assisting in location of such masses, ultrasonography is nonspecific for origin. CT is the modality most often used for follow-up of tumors of the bony pelvis.

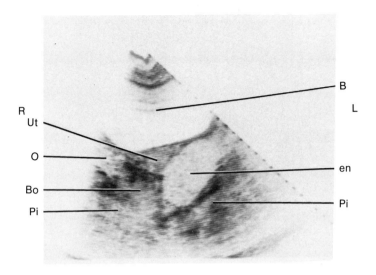

Fig. 21-22. Transverse scan of the pelvis demonstrating a blood-filled endometrioma on the left. *B*, Bladder; *Ut*, uterus; *O*, ovary; *en*, endometrioma; *Bo*, bowel; *Pi*, piriformis. **R,** Right. **L,** Left.

Hematoma or abscess

Because of the vascularity of the uterus, hematoma after cesarean section or other pelvic surgery is no uncommon. Symptoms include pain, fever, drop in hematocrit, and tenderness. A hematoma usually develops in the abdominal wall, uterine wall, cul-de-sac, or adnexa.

Hematoma and abscess are similar in appearance. They are usually well defined and may be either echogenic or cystic in appearance. Some abscesses, however, may not be well defined because they contain gas or are overshadowed by loops of bowel.

An abscess may result from operative procedures, hematogenous spread, or penetrating trauma. It tends to displace adjacent structures. A diaphragmatic abscess is easily imaged by using the liver as a window on the right and scanning the left side posteriorly in the erect position. Ultrasonography easily detects an intraperitoneal abscess but is nonspecific for blood, pus, or fluid types. An appendicial abscess is similar to other abscesses, and the clinical picture is helpful for diagnosis in cases of a questionable mass. A pelvic abscess is seen with the help of a full bladder and tends to occur in the cul-de-sac and adnexal regions.

Lymphocele and urinoma

A lymphocele or urinoma will appear as a fluid-filled mass within the cul-de-sac or anterior to the psoas. It is cystic and may be multiloculated with septa. Its ultrasonographic image is similar to that of an abscess or hematoma.

A lymphocele is usually secondary to renal transplant surgery or a nodal dissection in which there has been trauma to the lymphatic system. A urinoma is secondary to trauma. Both masses can mimic the urinary bladder. It is necessary to do the initial ultrasonogram with a full bladder and then postvoid scans. This procedure will clear up such an error in diagnosis and is discussed in depth in Chapter 14.

Bladder*

Ultrasonography of the urinary bladder is easily done for recognition of bladder masses, calculi, and foreign bodies. The normal bladder must be full for evaluation of the smooth surfaces of its walls. A tumor will be an echogenic protrusion off the wall into the lumen. Overdistension of the bladder can mean a functional abnormality, and underdistension may suggest invasion by a tumor. Calculi are echogenic and demonstrate acoustic shadowing.

Pelvic pseudomasses

Ascites and fluid-filled loops of bowel are most commonly mistaken for masses in the lower abdomen and pelvis.

Loculated ascites may be distinguished by the loops of bowel floating within it and by its

*The prostate may be studied by means of transverse and longitudinal scans angled caudally through the bladder. The use of a small scan head is necessary for real time imaging. An abnormal prostate will appear inhomogeneous with irregular walls. Hypertrophy will appear more homogeneous.

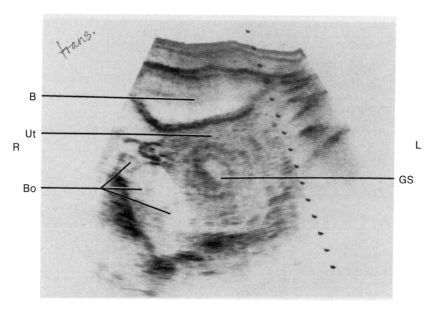

Fig. 21-23. Transverse scan of the pelvis in a patient with an early intrauterine pregnancy presenting with pain. B-scan of the pelvis demonstrated multiple fluid-filled masses consistent with bowel loops that showed peristalsis by real time. *B,* Bladder; *Ut,* uterus; *Bo,* bowel; *GS,* gestational sac. **R,** Right. **L,** Left.

irregular margins. As previously mentioned, true pelvic masses will move adjacent structures.

Loops of fluid-filled bowel are easily mistaken on static images, especially after recent ingestion of fluids. They usually change shape and position with time. Peristalsis will be apparent by real time imaging (Fig. 21-23).

Feces in the rectum and sigmoid area can mimic a cul-de-sac mass. A cleansing enema may be helpful or a repeat scan at another time after a special cleansing preparation. Feces in the bowel cannot be distinguished as readily as bowel in the adnexal regions.

SUMMARY

Pelvic ultrasonography tends to be a sensitive area for diagnosis of size, shape, and consistency of pelvic processes. The appropriate technical goal of the sonographer should be to produce images that will locate and describe the characteristics of masses, thereby helping in the clinical management of the patient.

22 Obstetric ultrasound

LINDA LONDON

Obstetric ultrasonography is probably the area most widely affected by the technical advances in the field of ultrasound. Pulsed diagnostic ultrasound, because it appears to be safe and noninvasive, has become a principal method for obtaining information about the intrauterine contents and surrounding structures. An ultrasonogram can aid in evaluating the size, shape, and variations in structure of the uterus, placenta, and fetal anatomy and in following the growth and development of the fetus. With the advent of dynamic high-resolution real time scanning, it has become possible to evaluate three-dimensional intrauterine structures swiftly and accurately.

Obstetricians are now more dependent upon information obtained from an ultrasonogram pertaining to the condition of the fetus and related structures than ever before and are using ultrasonography as guidance for such procedures as amniocentesis, fetoscopy, intrauterine transfusion, and fetal surgery. This chapter is devoted to the applications of ultrasonography in the area of obstetrics.

Selection of equipment

In evaluating the geometry of intrauterine structures, the sonographer can use the ultrasonogram to make a carefully organized assessment of the two-dimensional images obtained; but to do this properly requires choosing an instrument by the size and location of the structure to be studied. Both static B-scan equipment and dynamic high-resolution real time equipment have advantages in achieving this objective.[29]

A total static B-scan of the pregnant uterus achieves maximum information of the uterine contents. It enables projections from large and deep structures in a series of scans to be built up to form a three-dimensional image of the uterus. In the hands of an ex-perienced sonographer, a total static B-scan can be completed within 20 minutes. One should choose the highest-frequency transducer available to allow through-transmission of the sound beam and follow a set routine of imaging.

When a total B-scan has been completed, the use of real time scanning is then necessary to detect changes ni size and shape of structures, especially in a moving fetus. The main advantages of using a real time scanner are *detection* and evaluation of fetal movement and rapid accurate *measurements* of fetal anatomy. A real time unit is less dependent on operational expertise and in most cases is easily moved from one area to another.[29]

At the present time a linear-array scanner is the most common real time equipment used in the area of obstetrics. The cost of the instrument is low compared to the cost of other types of real time equipment, and the size and shape of the transducer allow significant image width to achieve head and body measurements with minimal distortion.[29] Because of the increased detail of the image and the ease of handling the transducer, sector real time scanners are becoming more widely used. The main disadvantages are the limited field of view and the somewhat higher cost of the equipment.

Technique

An examination of the pregnant uterus begins by preparing the patient as for a gynecologic ultrasonogram. A full bladder is especially necessary in early pregnancy to act as a window for viewing pelvic structures and to move the loops of bowel out of the pelvis. In later pregnancy a full bladder (1) allows evaluation of the lower uterine segment for placental location and fluid in the cervical os and (2) moves the fetus in a direction more perpendicular to the transducer for better imaging of fetal structures in the caudal portion of the uterus.

After a full explanation of the procedure

I wish to thank Barbara Robnett for her assistance in obtaining images for this chapter.

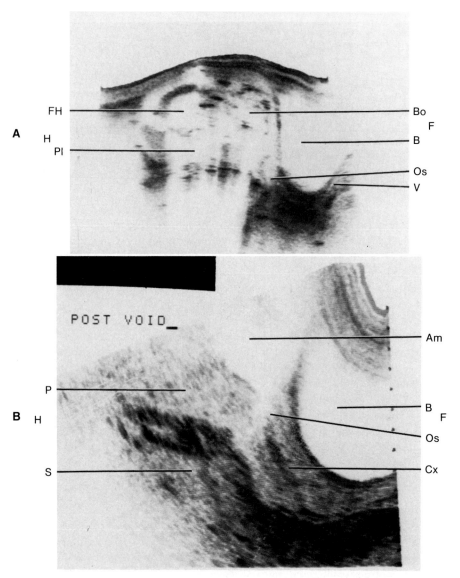

Fig. 22-1. A, Parasagittal scan of a 32-week fetus for placental location. The bladder appears to be overfilled, suggesting a complete placenta previa. **B,** Postvoid parasagittal scan of the cervical os demonstrating a low-lying placenta instead of complete previa. *B,* Bladder; *Cx,* cervix; *Os,* cervical os; *Pl,* placenta; *Am,* amniotic fluid; *S,* sacrum; *FH,* fetal head; *Bo,* fetal body; *V,* vagina. **H,** Head. **F,** Foot.

position and the apparent extent of the placenta (Fig. 22-1, *A*). At this point the operator may want to have the patient partially void to achieve a better view of such structures.

A set of transverse scans is then obtained for verification of findings seen on the sagittal scans as well as to obtain measurements of the fetal head and body in cases of cephalic presentation. Scans are begun at the pubic bone by carefully placing the transducer at an angle perpendicular to the uterine surface with each successive scan. Because of the rounded shape of the maternal abdomen, some sectoring may be necessary to obtain scans at the midportion of the uterus. Scans are obtained in small increments from the symphysis pubis to the fundus, care being taken to visualize the adnexal regions for any abnormalities. At this point random scans of the fetal head and body are obtained for measurement of the diameter or circumference, and pertinent small-sector scans are made of any anatomy of interest. In view of the differing clinical data, gestational ages, and abilities to visualize certain structures, random images will vary from patient to patient.

If available, a real time scanner is then employed for quick assessment of fetal movement, breathing, or heart rate if necessary and to confirm the biparietal diameter and obtain certain random images of the fetus and surrounding structures. When real time imaging is the only modality used, the protocol should be similar to that for static scans whether or not one is recording the images being viewed.

Fertilization

Fertilization takes place when the ovum, with the mass of surrounding granulosa cells that formed the cumulus oophorus, is shed into the fimbriated end of the fallopian tube. The ovum is moved by muscular and ciliary activity into the ampulla. There it encounters the spermatozoa that have ascended through the uterus.[20]

When the spermatozoa and ovum meet in the tube, syngamy takes place. A spermatozoon must penetrate the outer layer of the ovum, the zona pellucida, which may consist of one or two layers. When it has entered the zona, a reaction occurs making the zona impervious to other sperm. A diploid chromosome number is thereby reestablished and mitotic cell division of a new individual can begin[20] (Fig. 22-2).

has been given the patient, she is put in a supine position on the examination table and the lower abdominal skin is coated with mineral oil for the static scan. Mineral oil is used for the static B-scan because it is relatively inexpensive, spreads easily, and tends not to dry out as water-soluble couplants have a tendency to do. However, some real time equipment manufacturers suggest using water-soluble couplants to protect the outer transducer casing. In such cases water-soluble gel may be purchased less expensively in liter form.

The examination begins with a series of longitudinal scans obtained with the patient supine. The transducer is placed at the pubic bone and carefully moved cephalad while

angling to remain perpendicular to the structures being visualized. After a midline sagittal scan has been achieved, the sonographer carefully adjusts the TGC curve to balance out the image. In obstetric imaging this may be time consuming since there are so many different levels of attenuation in one section from fetal structures. When a satisfactory image is obtained, a series of sagittal scans moving from the right side of the uterus to the left in small intervals is recorded. Centimeter markers must be placed on every scan. At the completion of this set of scans, the sonographer has an idea of placental location, fetal position, number of fetuses, and extent of the urinary bladder. Often a too full bladder will change fetal

Timing of pregnancy

Clinically pregnancy is dated from the first day of the last menstrual period (LMP), when this is known. From that date an expected date of labor or confinement (EDL or EDC) is calculated by assuming a duration of 280 days. Since in an idealized cycle ovulation occurs on the fourteenth day, the actual duration of pregnancy is 266 days. When cycles are irregular or artificially induced, timing must be based on a presumed date of ovulation or fertilization and 266 days added.[20]

PHYSIOLOGY AND DEVELOPMENT OF THE FETUS AND PLACENTA

After fertilization mitotic division begins—slowly at first but with increasing speed—so that during its time in the fallopian tube the ovum undergoes considerable growth, in terms more of number of cells than of actual size. During most of the period of its existence in the tube, the fertilized ovum is a solid mass of cells. Blastocyst formation begins at about the fifth day (Fig. 22-2). On the fifth or sixth day the blastocyst arrives in the uterine lumen, where it continues a free-floating existence for at least 24 hours.[17,20]

The formation of the corpus luteum in the ovary and the consequent secretion of progesterone in large quantities begin to alter the endometrium in preparation for implantation. Implantation ordinarily takes place on the surface epithelium of the uterine wall among a series of openings of endometrial glands, directly over endometrial stroma[20] (Fig. 22-2).

Within 24 hours the blastocyst apparently is able to bury itself deeply into the endometrium, and the surface epithelium of the endometrium begins to proliferate over it. By 7 to 8 days after ovulation this implantation, which is referred to as *interstitial* since the blastocyst burrows into the endometrium, is complete; and shortly thereafter the surface epithelium is healed over the blastocyst.[20]

The advancing trophoblast, being provided with ready gas exchange and in the glycogen-rich endometrium, a ready source of energy, begins to develop rapidly into the primitive placenta. This consists of large masses of syncytiotrophoblast among which spaces begin to form. These are the primitive lacunae, which are destined to form the intervillous space. Columns of trophoblast, the primary villi, then form; and some attach themselves to the decidua as anchoring villi. On about the eleventh day the advanc-

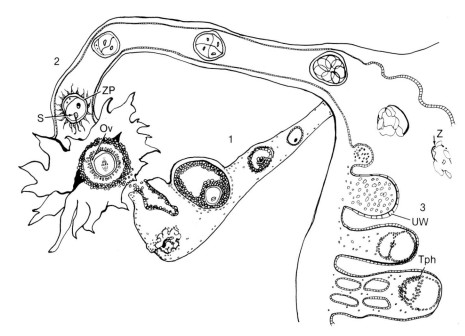

Fig. 22-2. Schematic representation of ovulation, fertilization, and implantation. *1*, If fertilization takes place, the egg undergoes a series of mitotic divisions resulting in a ball of cells (morula). *2*, A cavity then appears within the morula, converting it into the blastocyst. The outer wall of the blastocyst consists of ectodermal cells (trophoblast) that are directly involved in the implantation process and later in the formation of the placenta. *3*, Implantation takes place about the seventh day after ovulation. *Ov*, Ovum; *S*, sperm; *ZP*, zona pellucida; *Z*, zona; *Tph*, trophoblast; *UW*, uterine wall. (Modified from Danforth, D.N.: Obstetrics and gynecology, ed. 3, New York, 1977. Harper & Row, Publishers.)

ing cytotrophoblast penetrates a maternal capillary and initiates a flow of blood into the lacunae of the primitive placenta. The perforation of maternal blood vessels by the syncytiotrophoblast also makes possible the direct injection into the maternal circulation of human chorionic gonadotropin (hCG), which within the next few days is able to convert the corpus luteum on the ovary into a corpus luteum of pregnancy, thereby preventing the withdrawal of hormonal support from the endometrium and allowing the continuation of pregnancy.[20] The greatest growth is toward the endometrium, close to the maternal circulation. This sets the stage for the development of the definitive placenta at the site of implantation. The healing of surface epithelium over the ovum (blastocyst) effectively keeps the trophoblast from contact with the opposite uterine wall in the course of its further growth and development; and therefore the placenta forms on only one side.[17,20]

The margin of the amniotic sac is attached to the periphery of the embryonic disc. As the disc grows, its lateral margins fold ventrally. Ultimately only a thin strand of mesoderm, the body stalk, connects the placenta to the embryo. This is known later as the umbilical cord.[17]

The amniotic sac grows rapidly. On its ventral portion a layer of endoderm (destined to become fetal gut) forms the roof of the yolk sac. The amniotic sac appears on the dorsal portion of the cavity. During the second month the amniotic cavity enlarges at the expense of the yolk sac and former cavity of the blastocyst.[17] The yolk sac is visualized in early first trimester pregnancies as a small circle.

With advancing pregnancy the endometrium is virtually entirely changed into decidua. Although *decidua* means that which is shed, remnants are retained within the uterus and are later the source of relining the uterine cavity by endometrium at the conclusion of the pregnancy.[17,20]

FIRST TRIMESTER PREGNANCY

The most common complication of early pregnancy is death of the embryo. The first objective of the ultrasonographer in early pregnancy is to establish whether there is an intrauterine pregnancy with a live embryo. By means of modern ultrasound equipment and the use of high-frequency transducers, the gestational sac can be imaged as early as 4 to 5 weeks past the LMP and a fetal pole can be imaged by 5 to 6 weeks.[17] Fetal activity can be assessed shortly thereafter.

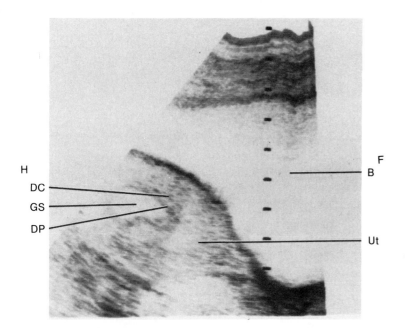

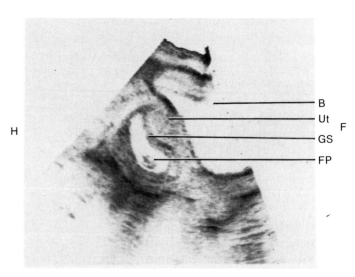

Fig. 22-3. Parasagittal scan of the uterus demonstrating a double ring of echoes representing the space between the decidua parietalis, *DP*, on the inside and the decidua capsularis, *DC*, on the outside. *B*, Bladder; *Ut*, uterus; *GS*, gestational sac. **H**, Head. **F**, Foot.

Fig. 22-4. Parasagittal scan of the uterus repeated after 10 days demonstrating a well-defined gestational sac with a fetal pole. *B*, Bladder; *GS*, gestational sac; *FP*, fetal pole; *U*, uterus. **H**, Head. **F**, Foot.

Bleeding is the most common indicator for an ultrasonogram in the first trimester.[38] The patient may also present with cramping or a history of spontaneous abortion or ectopic pregnancy. In some cases an embryonic pregnancy or fetal demise may be the cause for such symptoms. The patient usually has taken a pregnancy blood test (more reliable than a urine test) and pregnancy may be detected within 10 days of conception. The ultrasonogram is then obtained as a second means for making an assessment of embryonic status.

The visualization of a gestational sac on the ultrasonogram has been described as a reliable indicator of early pregnancy.[17,38,40] The gestational sac first appears 3 weeks past conception as a complete circle of echoes in the fundus or midportion of the uterus. Initially it is circular to ovoid, representing the blastocyst embedded in the uterine wall with decidua fairly evenly distributed over the entire blastocyst and the developing villous system. A double ring of echoes is visualized as the sac grows further into the uterus (Fig. 22-3). This is thought to represent the space between the decidua parietalis and the outer portion of the sac, the decidua capsularis.[17] The decidua basalis is the area that remains in contact with the chorion frondosum, which develops into the placenta. Because of its complex blood supply, this area is thought to produce higher-level echoes than the surrounding tissue.[40]

The gestational sac increases rapidly in mean gestational diameter from 1 to 6 cm, allowing accuracy in dating a pregnancy.[38] A repeat examination in 10 days to 2 weeks gives an accurate and reliable means of dating a living fetus when there is question of a viable pregnancy (Fig. 22-4). With advancing gestation the blastocyst enlarges and the decidua capsularis fuses with the decidua parietalis.[17] At approximately 11 menstrual weeks the sac disappears due to the lesser amount of blood leaving the amniotic cavity.[17] During the first 10 weeks the gestational sac may take on various shapes due to compression by the bladder, uterine wall, or bowel (Fig. 22-5). This variation should not be misinterpreted as abnormal. With the advent of high-resolution real time equipment the fetal pole can now easily be imaged as early as 5 to 6 menstrual weeks. More accurate measurement of the fetal complex of echoes at around 8 weeks gives rise to the fetal crown-rump measurement (Fig. 22-6). The fetus measures approximately 5 to 8 mm at 5 weeks postconception and 20 to 30 mm at 8 weeks.[28,31]

Single as well as multiple gestational sacs can be detected in utero. A cause of first trimester bleeding may be the abortion of one twin when there are two fetuses. Recent reports[12] have confirmed a higher incidence of twins conceived than delivered. The image of an empty amniotic cavity can confirm this diagnosis (Fig. 22-7). A follow-up scan may be indicated to confirm the growth of both fetuses when multiple gestations in early pregnancy are diagnosed.

Early gestations can be accompanied by a variety of complications—the most common being variations of clinical abortion, ectopic pregnancies, corpus luteum cysts, associated pelvic masses, pseudocyesis, and bicornuate uterus. Abortions may be classified according to gestational age, fetal weight, etiology, or clinical picture. Clinically they are divided into four categories: (1) *inevitable* or threatened, when the cervical os is dilated to the point that a finger can be introduced and the patient has uterine contractions and vaginal bleeding; (2) *incomplete*, when fragments of the products of conception protrude from the external os, are found in the vagina, or have been passed; (3) *complete*, following curettage for reduction of infection; and (4) *missed*, when the conceptus is retained within the uterine cavity 4 weeks after death of the embryo.[17] In cases of first trimester bleeding the ultrasonogram will be used as a tool for evaluating incomplete abortion or retained products of conception.[38] If an empty or normal uterus is imaged, the patient may not need a dilation and curettage. However, recently curettage has been thought to speed up recovery time.[17] If there are retained products of conception or blood clots within the uterus, a surgical procedure is usually required.[17,40]

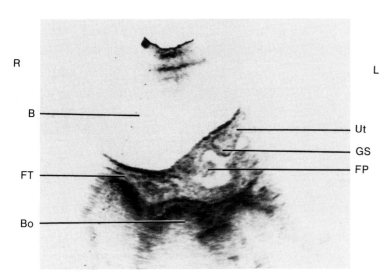

Fig. 22-5. Transverse oblique scan of the uterus demonstrating an unusual configuration of the uterus in a normal 7-week pregnancy. *B,* Bladder; *Ut,* uterus; *GS,* gestational sac; *FP,* fetal pole; *FT,* fallopian tube; *Bo,* bowel. **R,** Right. **L,** Left.

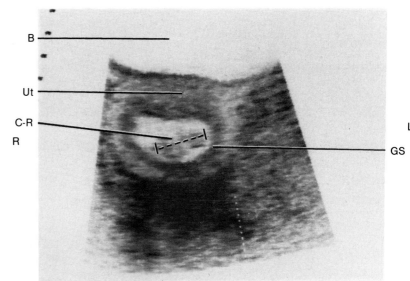

Fig. 22-6. Transverse scan of a 7-week pregnancy showing the fetal crown-rump length *(dotted lines). B,* Bladder; *Ut,* uterus; *C-R,* crown-rump length; *GS,* gestational sac. **R,** Right. **L,** Left.

Several signs have been described indicating an abnormal gestational sac:

1. Single break or fragmentation
2. Lack of growth
3. Weak surrounding echoes
4. Lack of fetal echoes by the seventh to eighth week
5. Low implantation of the sac within the uterus
6. Double gestational sac with a single fetus[38,40]

Of these, the most reliable is the lack of adequate growth. If the gestational sac has not grown at least 1 cm in diameter in 10 days or 2 weeks, a nonviable pregnancy is strongly suggested. The second most reliable sign is lack of fetal echoes within the gestational sac (Fig. 22-8). By 8 to 10 weeks an embryo as well as some fetal activity should be noted.[38,40] The other signs are suggestive and help if visualized together with either of the first two.

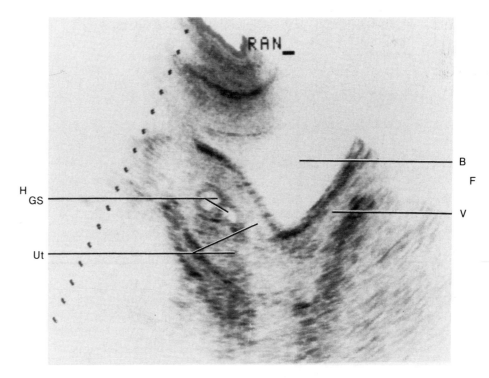

Fig. 22-7. Parasagittal scan of an early intrauterine pregnancy with two gestational sacs. The patient subsequently had an episode of bleeding, and a later sonogram revealed one live fetus in the second trimester. *B,* Bladder; *Ut,* uterus; *V,* vagina; *GS,* gestational sac. **H,** Head. **F,** Foot.

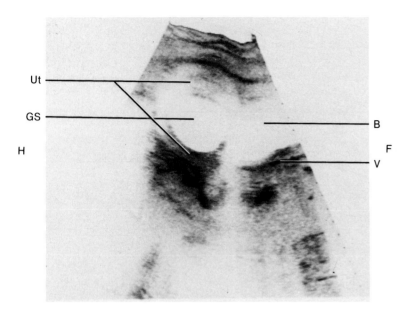

Fig. 22-8. Parasagittal scan of an 8-week gestational sac with no evidence of a fetal pole by B-scan or real time examination. *B,* Bladder; *Ut,* uterus; *V,* vagina; *GS,* gestational sac. **H,** Head. **F,** Foot.

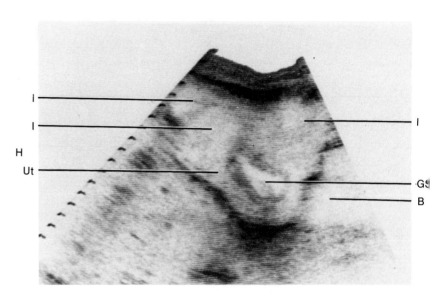

Fig. 22-9. Parasagittal scan of a 6-week gestation within a myomatous uterus. *B,* Bladder; *Ut,* uterus; *GS,* gestational sac; *I,* leiomyoma. **H,** Head. **F,** Foot.

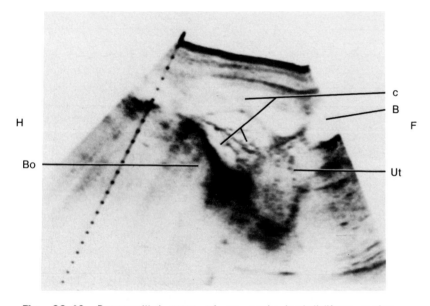

Fig. 22-10. Parasagittal scan of an early hydatidiform molar pregnancy with multiple theca lutein cysts. *B,* Bladder; *Ut,* uterus; *c,* cysts; *Bo,* bowel. **H,** Head. **F,** Foot.

MASSES ASSOCIATED WITH PREGNANCY

A variety of masses associated with early pregnancy are imaged ultrasonographically. Leiomyomas are commonly seen and followed for complications of edema, growth, and degeneration (Fig. 22-9). They may cause pain and abnormal fetal growth, and in the case of a large cervical myoma a cesarean section will be performed. Other masses include ovarian cysts, or theca lutein cysts.

Sonography is helpful in differentiating the above masses and following them by serial examination for growth or spontaneous resolution.[13,40]

Leiomyomas may appear in any portion of the uterus and have been described in Chapter 21. Multiple theca lutein cysts are usually asymptomatic and are commonly seen in association with an abnormal pregnancy such as hydatidiform mole[13] (Fig. 22-10). Ovarian cysts appear as sonolucent pelvic masses in-

distinguishable from corpus luteum cysts, which are common in early pregnancy and are sometimes confused with an ectopic gestation.[13]

Pseudocyesis can be easily diagnosed by lack of a gestational sac and a normal-sized uterus.[40] Bicornuate uterus is usually a known entity by clinical examination but can be demonstrated ultrasonographically in the early first trimester. A double-horned uterus can be visualized with the development of a gestational sac in one horn. Later in pregnancy the nongravid section of the uterus becomes difficult to identify.[40]

ECTOPIC PREGNANCY

The clinical diagnosis of ectopic gestation is often difficult. The patient can present with pain, bleeding, and a positive pregnancy test or any one of the these.[8] Hormonal stimulation can cause uterine atrophy and the development of decidua, as in a normal pregnancy except for the absence of chorionic villi.[3,8,27] A hematoma may develop after rupture of the sac into adjacent tissue, and fluid may collect in the cul-de-sac. With an acute ectopic pregnancy symptoms include pain, sycope, and shock from blood loss. In a chronic ectopic pregnancy there may be irregular vaginal bleeding, fever, and a palpable mass.[8]

The problem is less difficult when a reliable beta subunit of hCG pregnancy test is available. Other pregnancy tests yield less accurate results.[3,8] If the pregnancy test is

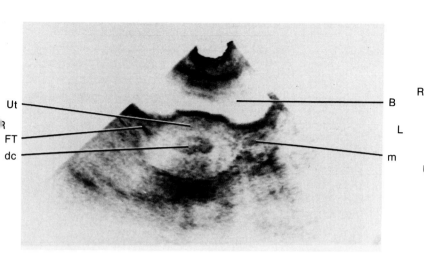

Fig. 22-11. Transverse scan of the pelvis demonstrating a decidual cast within the uterus and an adnexal mass in a patient with a positive hCG pregnancy test. *B,* Bladder; *Ut,* uterus; *dc,* decidual cast; *FT,* fallopian tube; *m,* mass. **R,** Right. **L,** Left.

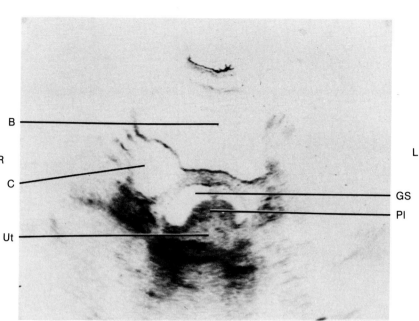

Fig. 22-12. Transverse scan demonstrating a 7-week intrauterine pregnancy and a corpus luteum cyst in a patient presenting with RLQ pain. *B,* Bladder; *Ut,* uterus; *GS,* gestational sac; *c,* cyst; *Pl,* placenta. **R,** Right. **L,** Left.

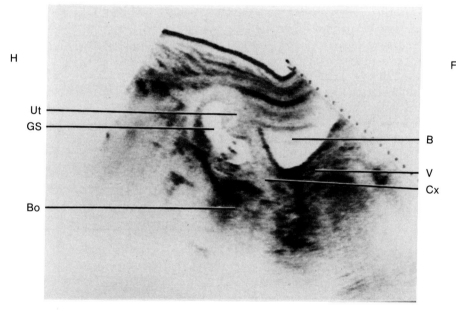

Fig. 22-13. Random parasagittal scan of a uterus demonstrating a 7-week intrauterine gestation. *B,* Bladder; *GS,* gestational sac; *Ut,* uterus; *V,* vagina; *Cx,* cervix; *Bo,* bowel. **H,** Head. **F,** Foot.

positive and the ultrasonogram demonstrates an intrauterine gestational sac, the diagnosis of ectopic can be excluded. However, one must not confuse this with the decidual cast that accompanies an ectopic gestation, leading to a false-negative diagnosis.[27] A decidual cast within the uterus may be a less echogenic rind of echoes or, in some cases, may have a double rim of high-amplitude echoes mimicking a normal gestational sac (Fig. 22-11). A definite diagnosis of normal intrauterine pregnancy cannot be made until a fetal pole is demonstrated. Then one can be fairly confident that there is no ectopic gestation, keeping in mind that there could be an intrauterine and extrauterine gestation (extremely rare).[27]

In the case of a positive pregnancy test with absence of an intrauterine pregnancy, one must carefully evaluate the adnexal regions. If no abnormalities exist, such as adnexal masses or fluid in the cul-de-sac, ectopic pregnancy may be excluded since the majority of cases have abnormal findings.[3] In patients with adnexal masses laparoscopy is indicated to rule out ectopic pregnancy.[3]

With a negative pregnancy test the intrauterine findings become less helpful and the adnexal findings more relevant. If the ultrasonogram reveals no abnormal adnexal or cul-de-sac findings, the diagnosis of ectopic is unlikely. If, however, an adnexal mass or fluid in the cul-de-sac is demonstrated, an

ectopic pregnancy may or may not be present (therefore yielding an indefinite diagnosis).[3] Laparoscopy will be performed in cases of high clinical suspicion. With findings of an adnexal mass (with or without a positive pregnancy test), one must consider extrauterine pregnancy or a variety of other situations including pelvic inflammatory disease and ovarian masses[3,8] (Fig. 22-12).

To eliminate the presence of false masses, all patients should have a full bladder when the examination is performed. A total B-scan is obtained with a high-frequency transducer. Random scans of the adnexal region are then done to visualize the ovaries. Random scans of the uterine cavity may be performed for imaging of a decidual cast and a fetal pole as well as fluid in the cul-de-sac (Fig. 22-13).

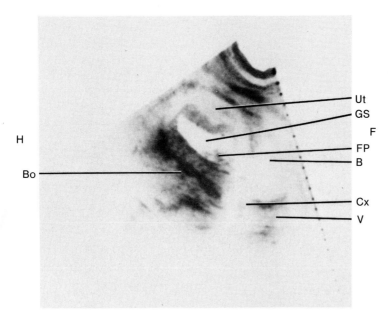

Fig. 22-14. Parasagittal scan of a 7-week intrauterine pregnancy scanned with a half-full bladder. Note the anteroposterior position of the uterus. *B*, Bladder; *V*, vagina; *Cx*, cervix; *Ut*, uterus; *GS*, gestational sac; *FP*, fetal pole; *Bo*, bowel. **H,** Head. **F,** Foot.

ULTRASONIC MEASUREMENT IN PREGNANCY

In the area of obstetrics an ultrasonogram is most commonly requested to determine fetal age, for up to 40% of women have unknown or inaccurate dates of their last menstrual cycle.[34,35,40] Because of its relative simplicity, safety, and accuracy within the first two trimesters of pregnancy, ultrasound has gained wide acceptance as the preferred method for assessing gestational age.

Correlation between sonar crown-rump length, biparietal diameter, and gestational age has been well established.[21,31] The CRL is a technique that can be accurately used up to the thirteenth week of gestation. From then on the BPD is the preferred technique. From 13 until 32 weeks after the last menstrual period the BPD can be considered accurate to within 10 days. After 32 weeks its accuracy decreases because of the variability of fetal head growth.[34,35]

Early studies by Robinson,[31] Jouppila,[19] and other workers presented the first useful data on the growth of the uterus and the *gestational sac*. The information, however, was accurate to within only ±2 weeks of gestational age. The methods used included the mean diameter of various planes of the uterus and gestational sac. Other workers followed with published data still well beyond +1 week of accuracy. The potential source of error with all these measurements is the variation of the sac and uterine size with different stages of bladder filling.[31]

In 1975 Robinson[31a] published a method for obtaining gestational sac volumes by taking multiple scans of the sac and measuring the area of each using a planimeter and applying a simple formula to obtain volume. Results were within 10%, giving a chance of error within ±9 days.

In 1973 Robinson[31] introduced the method of measuring the fetal *crown-rump length* (CRL) to estimate gestational age. This method involves measuring the longest demonstrable length of the fetus excluding the limbs. Attempts at obtaining a static B-scan image of the fetus may be made at two different stages, one with the bladder full and one with the bladder almost empty (Fig. 22-14). With an almost empty bladder, the uterus stands erect and the fetal pole is easily viewed in the transverse plane since the uterus acts as a window. The most accurate CRL is obtained by use of high-resolution real time scanning. Then the small scan head is helpful in chasing and maneuvering around a moving fetus. The accuracy of fetal CRL is within ±5 days, thus making it the most reliable method of assessing early gestational age apart from fertilization or implantation studies.[31]

Numerous methods for obtaining a *biparietal diameter* (BPD) have been reported in the past.[4,22,35-37] This may be due partly to rapid changes in diagnostic equipment that have permitted visualization of fetal cranial anatomy in greater detail. With the advent of high-resolution real time images and static

digital scan converters, it is now possible to assess the neuroanatomy of a fetal skull and obtain the same planes of section in every fetus studied.

A BPD can be obtained with either real time or a static B-scanner. Real time is almost always the faster method. The fetal lie is observed during the initial examination, making it easy to assess the longitudinal axis of the fetus. If the fetus is in a cephalic lie, the transducer is rotated to the transverse plan, approximately 90 degrees to the longitudinal axis of the fetus (Fig. 22-15). It is then angled cephalad to accommodate the posterior inclination of the fetal head. The amount of this angulation will vary with inclination, and one must use anatomic structures to vary the angle of the transducer. Scanning begins at the base of the skull. Recognizable landmarks include the bony petrous ridges and the greater sphenoid wing, which form an X-shaped structure at the base of the skull. One then moves higher in the head, visualizing the peduncles and midbrain and then the thalami and third ventricle. At this point several scans may be obtained if the following are true (Fig. 22-16):

1. Measurements from midline to inner skull tables are equal.
2. The head is ovoid instead of round or distorted.
3. Each image is taken after moving the transducer to the top of the skull and back to achieve more accurate results with the reproduction of equal measurements.

The use of a full bladder and the Trendelenburg position may be necessary in the case of a low-lying fetal skull. If the BPD is unobtainable with a full bladder, the patient may empty her bladder causing the fetus to rotate. In cases of a prone or supine fetus, having the patient walk, roll over, or rock her pelvis on hands and knees may aid in rotating a stubborn fetus.

A great deal of controversy surrounds the methodology of recording the fetal BPD as well as the actual description of anatomic detail.[22,40] I believe that an accurate BPD can be obtained in most cases if exact criteria on fetal neuroanatomy are used to identify the same plane of section in each patient examined. Also the sonographers measuring the BPDs must use the same criteria for points of measurement on the fetal skull borders.

In the breech or transverse lie the BPD is obtained in a similar manner excluding the angle of the transducer since the fetal skull tends to lie in a more horizontal plane. The

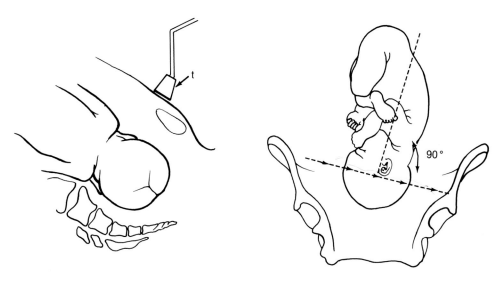

Fig. 22-15. Diagram of a fetus in cephalic presentation. The trans-ducer, *t*, is placed perpendicular to the posterior inclination of the fetal skull and rotated approximately 90 degrees to the longitudinal axis of the fetus to obtain the correct transverse plane of section for measuring the BPD.

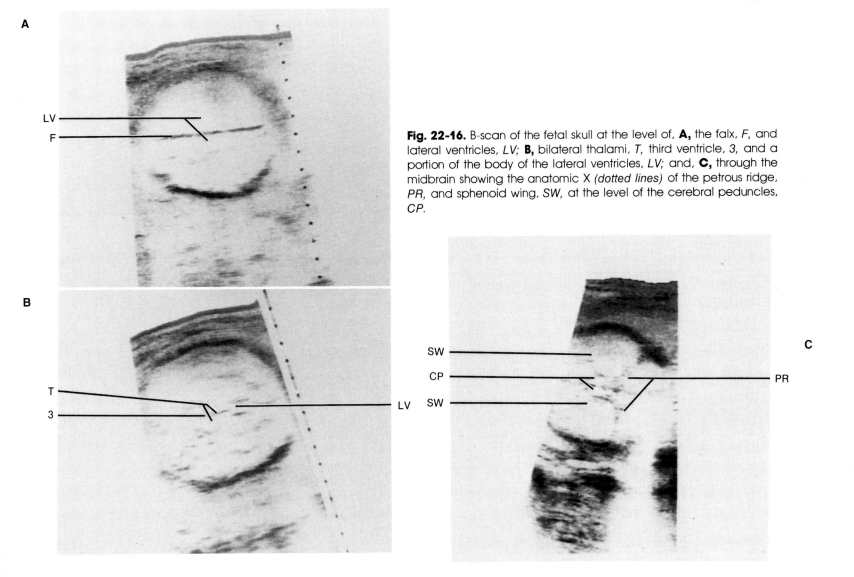

Fig. 22-16. B-scan of the fetal skull at the level of, **A,** the falx, *F*, and lateral ventricles, *LV*; **B,** bilateral thalami, *T*, third ventricle, *3*, and a portion of the body of the lateral ventricles, *LV*; and, **C,** through the midbrain showing the anatomic X *(dotted lines)* of the petrous ridge, *PR*, and sphenoid wing, *SW*, at the level of the cerebral peduncles, *CP*.

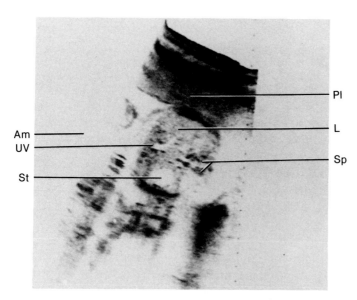

Fig. 22-17. Transverse section of the fetal body at the level of the umbilical vein, *UV.* Liver, *L;* stomach, *St;* spine, *Sp;* amniotic fluid, *Am;* placenta, *Pl.*

same steps are taken to achieve the appropriate shape of the skull and pertinent anatomic structures.

From the sixteenth to the thirtieth week the BPD increases approximately 3 mm per week. After 30 weeks it increases approximately 1.8 mm per week and becomes a less reliable indicator in the last trimester.[34,35,40] In the beginning of the last trimester the fetal abdomen should equal the BPD. One can then use the head-body symmetry as an indicator of a small or growth-retarded fetus.[33,39] The fetal abdomen grows rapidly in the third trimester and by term can be well over 1 cm larger than the skull.[39] The fetal body diameter is obtained at the level where the umbilical vein enters the liver (Fig. 22-17). Using other images, including the fetal liver and stomach and a portion of the umbilical vein, will assure a more transverse plane of section than will using one identifiable structure.

As with every method of measuring human growth, the many biologic variables of the individual examined can offset the charts that one may be using. It therefore is necessary to do serial gestational age measurements of any fetus at risk for slow or rapid growth. Serial scans performed every 2 or 3 weeks of the first and second trimesters will allow the clinician the evaluate the individual fetus based on its own growth.

Sabbagha et al.[36,37] have shown that by employing serial cephalometry it is possible to place fetuses in large, average, or small cephalic categories. This is known as *growth-adjusted sonar age* (GASA). Even though in an individual pregnancy it is not possible to predict birth weight precisely on the basis of the BPD rank, it is helpful to know the growth bracket for each BPD category. By using GASA, estimates of gestational age based on second trimester BPDs are enhanced, yielding smaller 95% confidence limits of approximately 1 to 3 days.[35]

According to Sabbaga[35] the best intervals for serial BPD measurements are (1) 20 to 24 weeks, (2) 30 to 33 weeks, and (3) 35 to 38 weeks. The first two readings are used to assign fetuses a GASA and a specific BPD percentile growth rank. The third is used to evaluate growth attained in relation to each fetus' growth potential, defining any risk for intrauterine growth retardation.

Another method for determining gestational age is *limb length* (femur or humerus). It has been shown that femur length correlated with BPD is helpful in detecting fetal limb malformation. Data are now available for use in measurement.[11,16]

There are other reported methods of ultrasonographic measurement in pregnancy, but it is beyond the scope of this chapter to review them in detail. The methods discussed are widely accepted as appropriate for defining gestational age. Whichever one chooses, care must be taken to define the data reported as being either the gestational age (menstrual dating) or the fetal age (date of conception or approximately 14 days past the first day of the LMP).

INTRAUTERINE GROWTH RETARDATION

The diagnosis of IUGR is generally made at birth by pediatricians who relate the infant's weight to gestational age. This condition accounts for a large percentage of prenatal morbidity.[9] Growth-retarded babies are subject to numerous problems during the immediate postpartum period—intrapartum asphyxia, neonatal hypoglycemia, acidosis, hypoglycemia, polyglycemia.[9] The majority of growth-retarded neonates belong to a heterogeneous group called small for gestational age (SGA), which is defined as a baby at or below the tenth percentile of weight for gestation. This group is heterogeneous because in it are both normal small infants and infants who are small because severe or chronic insult has produced IUGR. In turn, IUGR infants are also a heterogeneous group composed of symmetric and asymmetric categories.[2] Symmetric growth retardation occurs before the twenty-eighth week of gestation and is associated with body and head growth lag, accounting for approximately 25% of IUGR infants.[9] Asymmetric IUGR occurs during the second and third trimester with body growth lag and relatively little cephalic growth lag, resulting in both cell reduction and diminished cell size of all organs—an abnormality that may lead to CNS deficits.[9]

Factors that adversely influence fetal growth are as follows[33]:

Genetic defects
Chromosomal aberrations
Antigen relationships
Chronic fetal infections
Maternal ingestion of cytotoxic agents
Maternal smoking
Maternal diseases (cardiovascular, metabolic)
Poor maternal nutrition
High altitude
Multiple pregnancy
Irradiation

Because hyperplasia normally ceases at some time during fetal life, the early onset of growth retardation is likely to affect cell division adversely and lead to diminution in organ size and possibly organ function.[33] By contrast, delayed onset of growth retardation (after organ cell number is completed) is known to decrease only cell size—an insult that is reversible.

The application of ultrasound in the prenatal detection of IUGR is related to three diagnostic goals[2]: First, the fetus' gestational age must be defined as precisely as possible. Second, fetal size must be estimated well enough to distinguish SGA fetuses from average or above average fetuses. Third, an effort must be made specifically to diagnose growth retardation within the SGA group and sometimes in larger babies.

An SGA fetus usually is discerned on the basis of one or more of the following clinical criteria[12]:

1. Patient history
2. Maternal weight gain
3. Fundal height
4. Estimation of fetal weight[12]

Ultrasonographically the fetus will demonstrate initially discordant head and body measurements with slow body growth. Exceptions include fetuses with congenital anomalies resulting in symmetric growth retardation. In other cases the BPD rarely lags in growth prior to 30 weeks.[9] It is therefore necessary to assess the BPD, the head-body correlation, and if possible the total intrauterine volume (although the TIUV has been reported as inaccurate for detecting growth-retarded fetuses).[6]

For head-body correlation the head (circumference or diameter) is normally larger than the body until 30 weeks, and from 30 to 36 weeks they appear approximately the same; after 36 weeks the body (diameter and circumference) is larger. In the growth-retarded fetus this does not occur. The findings most suggestive of IUGR are (1) asymmetry between head size and abdomen size, (2) decreased amniotic fluid, (3) small or advanced-grade placenta, (4) decreased intrauterine volume, (5) poor growth of BPD, and (6) slow BPD for gestational age.[2]

To obtain a body circumference or diameter, one takes a cross-sectional scan of the fetus at the level of the umbilical vein showing a section of the liver and usually the stomach. The correctly obtained section should be round. At this level a diameter or circumference may be measured. A BPD is then obtained at the level of the thalami and third ventricle. Again a diameter or circumference is measured and compared for concordance. Actual measurement of the abdominal circumference can be done with a map measurer or electronic plotting device. The standard measurement is a line around the outside of the abdomen, and the maximum measured circumference is used. Abdominal circumference appears to be the best single estimator of fetal size in combination with the BPD.[2,43]

The ratio of head circumference to body circumference is a good estimator of symmetry. The head circumference is taken at the level of the thalamus, using the largest circumference obtained. Standard plots of

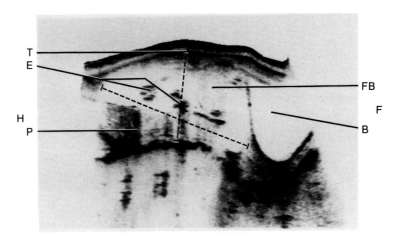

Fig. 22-18. Parasagittal scan of the uterus demonstrating the level for measurement of the TIUV. Dotted lines indicate levels of measurement. At level *T* a transverse scan is obtained for measuring the width of the uterus. *B,* Bladder; *FB,* fetal body; *P,* placenta; *E,* fetal extremities. **H,** Head. **F,** Foot.

head circumference to abdominal circumference versus gestational age are available. There is evidence that asymmetry is detected by the the head circumference to abdominal circumference and is a good predictor of IUGR.[4]

Oligohydramnios is often associated with the appearance of IUGR in the third trimester but can be seen normally late in pregnancy. It is possible to estimate amniotic fluid by measuring the fluid areas on sequential scans with an area measurer or by measuring intrauterine volume. If there is crowding of limbs and little or no space is seen between the fetus and surrounding uterus or placenta, oligohydramnios is usually present. When oligohydramnios is suspected the two other common causes, congenital abnormalities and ruptured membranes, should be excluded.[2,30]

To obtain a total intrauterine volume (TIUV), one takes a sagittal scan through the cervical os at the longest section of the uterus (usually midline). This will demonstrate the largest anteroposterior dimension and the longest sagittal section (Fig. 22-18). Centimeter markers are made on the scan in both the horizontal and the vertical plane, for there may be variation in the x-y characteristics on the photograph obtained. The transverse scan is then made at the level of the largest anteroposterior dimension (Fig. 22-16). Again, horizontal markers are placed on the image and the largest diameter between the walls of the myometrium is taken. The TIUV is calculated by the following formula:

$$Volume = 0.5233 \times Length \times Height \times Width \text{ of uterus}$$

derived from the formula for an ellipse. In the literature there are several monograms for TIUV to compare the volume with the mean.[2,14] Three problems exist with this measurement.[2,6] First, it is difficult to reproduce. Second, there are both false-positives (when a normal SGA is scanned for example) and false-negatives (most notable with polyhydramnios). Third, if the gestational age is not known, there can be errors in determining whether the TIUV is normal or not.

Other observations are helpful in diagnosing IUGR.[24] First is the identification of a fetal anomaly, since over one third of affected babies may have fetal anomalies.[2] Second is depressed fetal activity. This may be noted by observing cardiac activity, limb movement, and fetal breathing. Third is observation of a grade III or mature placenta. If this occurs before 34 weeks, it is suggestive of IUGR.

THE PLACENTA

Formation of the placenta begins at the time of implantation. The placenta rapidly develops into a relatively complex structure. The function of the placenta is to interchange gases, water and nutritive materials.[8,20] The placenta develops from mesodermal cells that later develop into chorionic villi. Ultimately, on a relatively thin strand of mesoderm, the body stalk connects the lateral placenta to the caudal end of the embryo. This eventually is known as the umbilical cord.[17] During the first trimester the fetal and maternal portions of the placenta develop the structures necessary for their function. The villous tree is formed by structures of the chorion whereas the maternal

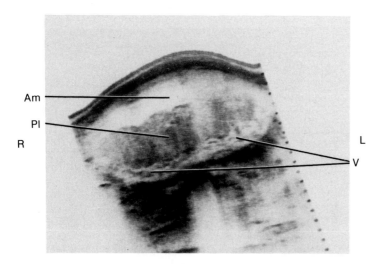

Fig. 22-19. Transverse scan of a fundal placenta demonstrating the maternal vascular structures in the basal area of the uterus. *Am,* Amniotic fluid; *Pl,* placenta; *V,* vessels. **R,** Right. **L,** Left.

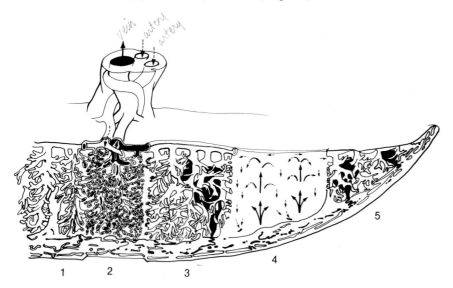

Fig. 22-20. Schematic representation showing circulation of the human placental blood flow. Direction of the placental blood flow is indicated by arrows. Section *1* demonstrates the villous tree structure; section *2,* the fetal circulation; section *3* the maternal circulation within the intervillous spaces; section *4,* the intervillous space flow; section *5,* a marginal pattern. (Modified from Danforth, D.N.: Obstetrics and gynecology, ed. 3, New York, 1977, Harper & Row, Publishers.)

side of the placenta is derived from the decidua basalis.

On the fetal side of the placenta a layer of amnion is fused to chorion, forming a thick layer of vascular structures and trophoblastic tissue that disappears at term. Below the chorionic tissue, sometimes referred to as the chorionic *plate*, lies the villous tree, or cotyledons, made up of the major villi and multiple branches. The major villi are separated by septa and can be recognized ultrasonographically as thick dense echoes. The fetal circulation of the placenta begins in the umbilical arteries and is passed through the placenta via the villous tree, returning via the umbilical vein.[17,20,42]

The maternal circulation begins in the uterine arteries, which pass through the basal plate and send blood into the intervillous space to return to the maternal circulation via the uterine veins. By means of high-frequency transducers these vessels are sometimes seen ultrasonographically as vascular tubular structures within the myometrial wall[20,42] (Figs. 22-19 and 22-20).

High-resolution equipment shows the placenta early in the first trimester. With a high-frequency transducer the placenta appears as a thickened echodense section of a large portion of the wall along the gestational sac. At approximately 9 to 10 menstrual weeks the decidua capsularis and decidua parietalis

begin to fuse and the placenta is more easily recognized as a separate structure from the myometrial echoes (Fig. 22-11). At around 12 fetal weeks the placental implantation site is recognizable as the gestational sac disappears and only the amnion is visible. The placenta is more echogenic than the rest of the uterine wall and occupies approximately 50% of the volume of the uterus. The uterus continues to grow more rapidly than the placenta so that by term the placenta occupies only 25% of it. As the uterus grows, the placenta appears to change position. Actually this movement is the growth and rotation of the uterus on its axis, and with the uterine wall moves the placenta. In most cases the placenta moves toward the fundus since the lower uterine segment is the last to grow.[17,20,42]

Early in pregnancy the placenta can appear to be on two separate surfaces of the uterus. This may be due to a myometrial contraction of the wall, giving an echogenic thickened appearance, or to an unsoftened portion of the uterine wall with the same ultrasonographic characteristic.[40]

The most common indication for placental evaluation is painless vaginal bleeding or transverse fetal lie caused by placenta previa or abruptio placentae. The question of placenta previa can be easily evaluated in over 95% of all referred cases.[15,40] Abruption is a more difficult diagnosis by ultrasound, especially in very late pregnancy, when the amniotic fluid diminishes.

An examination of the placenta should begin with a full bladder and the routine longitudinal and transverse scans of the uterus to assess size, margins, internal structure, and surfaces. After the routine scans have been performed, a high-frequency transducer may be used (especially with an anterior placenta) for assessment of internal structure. Magnified longitudinal and transverse scans of the cervical os are recorded to help identify the placental margin. By having the patient partially void, one can assess whether there is a change in position of a low-lying placenta. This technique often will clear up the question of a marginal placenta previa (Fig. 22-1).

The placenta has a speckled appearance during the second trimester and is more echogenic than the surrounding myometrium.[42] At times small cystic areas are seen within the placenta. These may represent macroscopic lesions and are of no clinical significance. As the placenta matures, it may develop a variety of inhomogeneities such as small dense areas thought to be calcifications, more echogenic interfaces in the villous tree, and a denser basal plate along the maternal surface[15,42] (Fig. 22-21). An anterior placenta is easier to examine ultrasonographically than a posterior placenta because there may be areas in a posterior placenta shadowed by various parts of the fetus. With different patient positions and a lower-frequency transducer a posterior placenta can usually be well outlined. With a low-lying head in the cephalic position the patient may be put in the Trendelenburg position and the fetal head may move up by itself or with gentle maneuvering. If all fails and the lower margin of the posterior placenta is not visualized, the margin between the maternal sacrum and posterior cranial wall may be measured for thickness. If the distance is less than 15 mm, a low-lying placenta is usually excluded.[15] This technique must be carefully undertaken, with particular identification of the cervical os and appropriate anatomy. A small scan head on a real time sector scanner proves to be most helpful in borderline posterior placentas.

As the placenta matures, echogenic densities appear on the ultrasonogram that are randomly dispersed within the substance of the placenta.[42] These are 1 to 4 mm in size and have their long axis parallel with the long axis of the placenta. The basal layer remains devoid of such densities according to Grannum et al.[15] This is known as a Grade I placenta.[15] In a Grade II placenta, echogenic densities appear in the bassal area and their long axis parallels the base of the placenta. They appear numerous and are randomly dispersed. The chorionic plate becomes more markedly indented (Fig. 22-21). In a Grade III placenta, the most mature, the densities contiguous with the chorionic plate extend to the basal area, dividing the placenta into compartments. Often areas devoid of echoes leave holes to be imaged along with large irregular densities that cast acoustic shadows.[15]

In early pregnancy all placentas appear as Grade 0. In each pregnancy the placenta matures at various rates. Many placentas will appear as Grade I or II at term, suggesting that the placenta does not go through the entire maturation process with each pregnancy. The value of grading placental maturation lies in detecting a Grade III placenta in a patient prior to 34 weeks (premature aging), especially when there is suspected IUGR or hypertension.[15]

The most common ultrasonographic finding with abruptio placentae is separation of a portion of the placenta from the uterine wall. Sometimes an abrupted placenta will appear thickened as clots form between the myometrium and placenta. Small abruptions may not be visible on the scan, and therefore a negative ultrasonogram does not exclude the possibility of an abrupted placenta. The scan should be approached with caution so a false diagnosis is not produced.[41]

Another area of importance in imaging is assessment of placental size. As already mentioned, the placenta occupies less volume later in pregnancy than in the beginning stages. In the last two trimesters of pregnancy one can begin to assess the placenta for thickness. A normal placenta is 2 to 4 cm thick.[15,42] A placenta of 5 cm or more is considered abnormal. When assessing placental size, one must take a scan at the midpoint of a true transverse and sagittal section of the placental location (Fig. 22-22) avoiding an oblique or tangential view that can cause a measurement to be falsely thick.

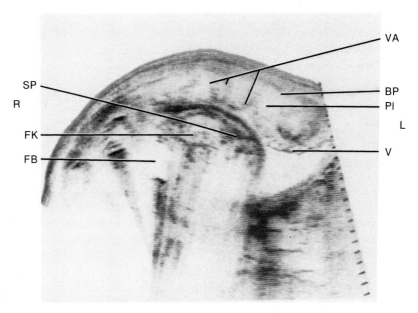

Fig. 22-21. Transverse scan of a third trimester pregnancy demonstrating the structural areas in the placenta. *FB,* Fetal bladder; *FS,* fetal spine; *FK,* fetal kidney; *Pl,* placenta; *VA,* villous areas; *BP,* basal plate; *V,* vessels. **R,** Right. **L,** Left.

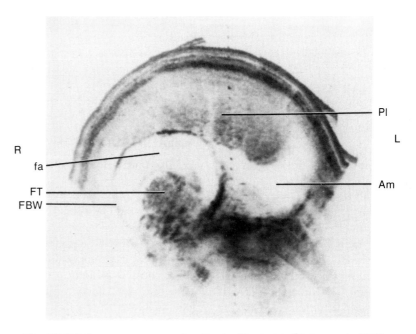

Fig. 22-22. Transverse scan of patient with severe Rh incompatibility. Note the enlarged placenta and severe ascites. *Pl,* Placenta; *Am,* amniotic fluid; *FBW,* fetal body wall; *fa,* fetal ascites; *FT,* fetal trunk.

In diabetes mellitus everything intrauterine can be enlarged, including the fetus and placenta. In Rh incompatibility the placenta may also be enlarged accompanied by fetal ascites or edema.[15,39,42] In Rh incompatibility the pregnancy is carefully monitored for fetal ascites or edema, since fetal blood transfusions may be performed and are more successful prior to the severe onset of such conditions. Careful scanning of the entire fetus with multiple cross sections of the head and body is necessary for assessment of fluid or edema. Both real time and static images should be obtained for serial follow-up comparison examinations during the pregnancy. Other less frequent causes of a thickened placenta include transplacental syphilis and a hydatidiform molar pregnancy with a fetus.[8]

SPECIAL PROCEDURES

Another use of ultrasound in placental location is for invasive procedures such as amniocentesis, fetal blood transfusions, fetoscopy, and fetal surgery. The use of ultrasonographic guidance in such procedures has proved invaluable to the specialist, and the chance of fatality has been decreased significantly.

Amniocentesis is a procedure done in early pregnancy to provide information for karyotyping and neural tube defects (levels of α-fetoprotein) and facilitates screening for many hereditary metabolic disorders. In later pregnancy amniotic fluid samples are used to assess fetal pulmonic maturity, gestational age, and the presence or absence of isoimmunization syndromes.[1,30] A linear-array real time scanner may be used to identify the placenta, fetus, and amniotic fluid. Locating a large area of fluid away from the placenta and umbilical cord is invaluable for needle insertion. The procedure is performed with sterile technique. After the amniotic fluid has been obtained, the fetal heart should always be monitored for rate and irregularity.

In prior years *intrauterine blood transfusion* (IUT) was accomplished by x-ray fluoroscopy. More recently IUT has been done as a therapeutic procedure for Rh isoimmunization pregnancy under the guidance of real time ultrasonography.[12] The patient is carefully scanned prior to the procedure for fetal position and evaluation, placental location, and amniotic fluid volume. Complete sterile procedure is used, including masks, gowns, and gloves. A sterile biopsy transducer is used to direct the needle into the fetal abdomen. Needle placement is confirmed by

the injection of a few centimeters of air, the bubbles imaged by real time sonography. Blood is then introduced into the peritoneal cavity. The fetal heart is monitored after the procedure for rate and irregularity.

Fetoscopy is performed in a manner similar to amniocentesis. The uterus is scanned prior to the procedure for assessment of fetal position and well-being and for placental location and amniotic fluid volume. Sterile procedure is then used in preparing the site for insertion of the fetoscope. The scope will be inserted near the area of interest but not too close to the umbilical cord on the fetal side of the placenta. A sterile transducer is used to guide the scope to the area of interest. The fetoscope is used to identify areas of the placenta for fetal blood sampling to detect a variety of genetic blood disorders. Fetoscopy is also used to do various intrauterine biopsies of the fetus, for identification of abnormalities that may not be seen by ultrasonography, and to guide the placement of shunt tubes, catheters, and various drainage tubes in fetuses with hydrocephaly, posterior urethral valves, or other abnormalities.

Fetal surgery is a new procedure currently being tried after successful attempts on animals. Ultrasonography will play a huge role in this procedure as the method of guidance and assessment of fetal well-being.

NORMAL FETAL ANATOMY

A routine obstetric ultrasonographic procedure usually includes a set of scans with transverse and sagittal sections of the uterus plus some random fetal head and body sections for measurement. In most cases this is considered to be adequate; but if there is any clinical question of abnormality or if an abnormality is picked up on a routine ultrasonogram, one must carefully evaluate the fetal anatomy. To do this requires assessing the fetal position and lie on routine scans for the appropriate section of the fetal anatomy. In each plane of section the TGC curve must be adjusted as well as the transducer angle and arm position for the optimal image. Real time imaging is invaluable for rapid surveying with good fetal anatomic detail and for locating static scan planes.

When the fetal position has been ascertained, the spine is located. The position of the fetal spine allows the examiner to determine which is the left and which the right side of the fetus. For example, if there is a breech fetus and the spine is on the maternal left, the fetus is lying on its right side; conversely, if the fetus is cephalic and the spine

is on the maternal left, the fetus is lying on its left side.[10] This position may be easily demonstrated in transverse section by viewing a cross section of the fetal body, identifying the spine and stomach.

One carefully begins a survey with either real time or a static B-scanner at the top of the skull, taking multiple scans in cross section approximately 15 degrees cephalad from the canthomeatal line of the fetus (Fig. 22-16). One should first visualize the well-established anatomic structures known as the falx cerebri and the interhemispheric fissure. This strong echo complex should be equidistant from the right and left lateral borders of the fetal skull. If so, the side-to-side rotation of the transducer is correct. The anatomy of the lateral ventricles of a normal fetal skull is hard to visualize in this plane at the present time. A linear echo reflection from the lateral ventricular walls will usually be visualized near the top of the fetal skull. The precise nature of this anatomy is still in question.[10] More caudad the falx cerebri echo complex breaks up to form the midline structures of the brain. At this level one will visualize a portion of the falx cerebri–interhemispheric fissure complex, the thalami on each side of the anterior third ventricle, the third ventricle, and the trilinear structure thought to represent a portion of the bodies of the lateral ventricles. Slightly more caudad the brain stem–cerebral peduncle complex of echoes is seen. The next strongly reflected group of echoes comes from the base of the skull. The petrous ridges and greater wing of the sphenoid meet to form an X-shaped structure considered to be the base of the skull.[10] At this level another sweep of the skull should be made in the cranial direction (Fig. 22-16).

The BPD measurement should be taken at a level that is constantly in a plane of section at the largest diameter of the fetal skull. The thalami are paired structures situated at the largest diameter of most fetal skulls. They are sonolucent, adjacent to the third ventricle at the midline, and centrally located (Fig. 22-16, *B*). These consistent landmarks suggest that the BPD measurement be taken at this section of the cranial anatomy.

At the base of the skull the transducer is rotated to the level of the canthomeatal line to image the orbits and bony structures of the facial area. Such details as the lens of the eye, soft tissue of the outer ear, mouth, tongue, and fetal hair have been imaged, especially by real time.

When the skull has been surveyed, the transducer is rotated approximately 90 degrees to a sagittal view of the fetal spine. The spine appears as two high-amplitude parallel bands of echoes representing the posterior ossification centers (Fig. 22-23). Just anterior to the spine the abdominal aorta can be imaged and followed into the thorax, where it forms the aortic arch after its origin from the heart (Fig. 22-24). On each side of the spine the kidneys are imaged as two reniform objects with echogenic centers representing the calyceal structures[10] (Fig. 22-25).

After viewing the spine in the sagittal plane, the operator rotates the transducer 90 degrees and views transverse sections of the fetal thorax starting from the cervical spine at the base of the skull. The transverse image of the spine has a somewhat triangular shape (Fig. 22-26). The base represents the posterior ossification center, and the apex the vertebral body.[10] The transducer moves caudally from the neck region into the thorax, where the fetal heart is easily imaged. Surrounding the chest cavity, the ribs are de-

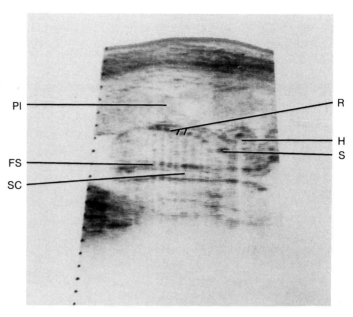

Fig. 22-23. Parasagittal scan of the fetal spine demonstrating the spinal canal. *Pl*, Placenta; *R*, fetal ribs; *H*, fetal humerus; *S*, fetal scapula; *FS*, fetal spine and, *SC*, spinal canal.

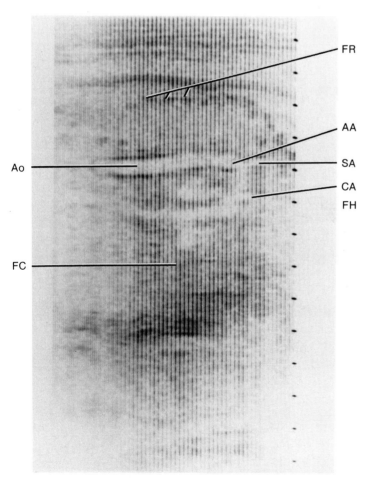

Fig. 22-24. Real time scan of the fetal aorta, *Ao*, and aortic arch, *AA*. Note the subclavian, *SA*, and carotid, *CA*, arteries. *FC*, Fetal chest; *FR*, fetal ribs. **FH**, Fetal head.

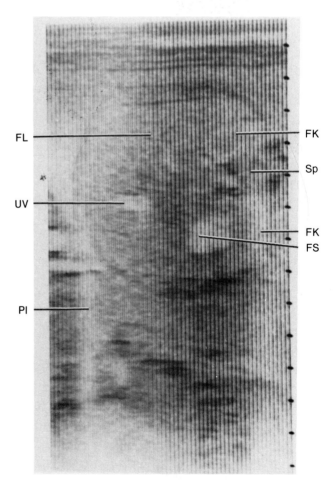

Fig. 22-25. Transverse scan of the fetal abdomen demonstrating fetal kidneys, *FK*, fetal stomach, *FS*, fetal spine, *Sp*, umbilical vein, *UV*, fetal liver, *FL*, and a posterior placenta, *Pl*.

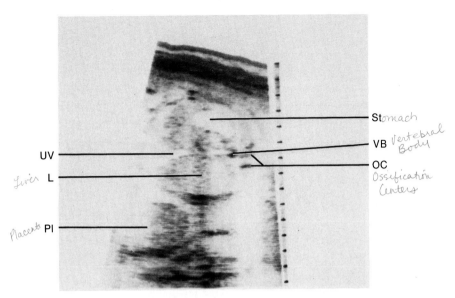

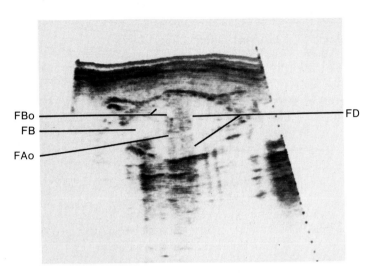

Fig. 22-26. Transverse scan of the fetal abdomen demonstrating the triangular shape of the fetal spine. *VB,* Vertebral body; *OC,* posterior ossification centers; *UV,* umbilical vein; *St,* stomach; *L,* liver; *Pl,* placenta.

Fig. 22-27. Parasagittal scan of a 30-week pregnancy demonstrating the fetal diaphragm, *FD,* fetal bowel, *FBo,* fetal abdominal aorta, *FAo,* and fetal bladder, *FB.*

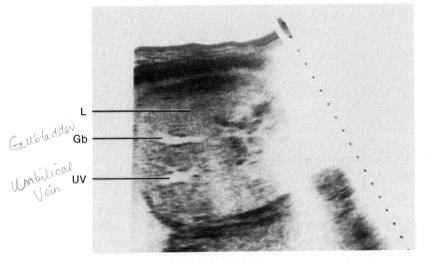

Fig. 22-28. Transverse scan of the fetal abdomen demonstrating the fetal gallbladder, *Gb,* surrounded by liver tissue, *L,* and situated to the right of the umbilical vein, *UV.*

tected as equally spaced echogenic structures producing barlike shadows in the sagittal plane (Fig. 22-23). At the beginning of the second trimester the heart can be imaged as a fluid-filled pulsatile organ. Real time imaging of the heart shows its pulsatile structure and function. Detailed fetal echocardiograms are now being made to evaluate the heart for abnormalities.

As the transducer moves caudally, the fetal diaphragm is viewed in part and may be seen in detail on sagittal scans (Fig. 22-27). The first abdominal structure to be recognized is usually the fetal stomach, which appears as a fluid-filled prominent ovoid structure in the left side of the fetal abdomen when distended. At the same plane of section the umbilical vein can be imaged as a vascular structure entering the area of umbilicus, coursing cranially and posterior at the midline of the abdomen. To the right of the umbilical vein a similar-appearing structure is recognizable, the gallbladder. This organ lies slightly toward the right anterior abdominal wall. The surrounding homogeneous echogenic tissue is the liver parenchyma[10] (Fig. 22-28).

As the transducer moves caudally, the fetal kidneys appear. These round discrete structures are less echogenic than the liver. They are more easily identified in the third trimester and sometimes seen earlier depending on the equipment used and the tissue character of surrounding structures. The fetal bowel is imaged anterior to the kidneys. It is a nondiscrete echogenic tissue unless fluid filled, in which case loops of bowel are visualized as small sonolucent structures.[10] Real time scanning can differentiate fluid-filled loops of bowel from other sonolucent structures by demonstrating peristalsis of the bowel. (As a fetus reaches term gestation, the bowel loops have been seen as nonhomogeneous echogenic tissue.) When the transducer moves into the pelvis, the fetal bladder is recognized as a round and prominent fluid-filled structure when full (Fig. 22-28). It should change size with time as the fetus voids, a fact to remember when looking for the bladder. The iliac wings are commonly identified as strongly reflective structures on each side of the bladder that produce shadows. By the third trimester the scrotum should be visualized in many male fetuses. The scrotum and penis can be viewed by angling the transducer in a slightly caudal and anterior direction from the fetal bladder (Fig. 22-29).

When the fetal abdomen has been imaged, the fetal extremities are visualized. Fetal skeletal structures are among the first to be consistently identified in the first trimester. The fetal extremities most accessible to ul-

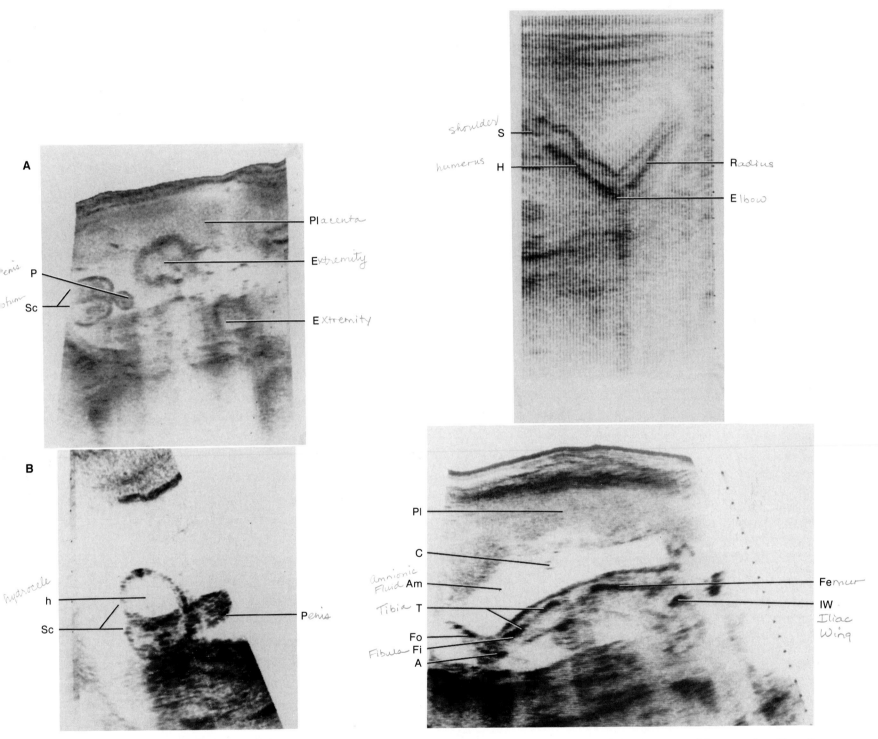

Fig. 22-29. Random B-scans of two male fetuses demonstrating a normal scrotum, **A,** and a fetus with a hydrocele, **B.** *Sc,* Scrotum; *P,* penis; *E,* extremity; *Pl,* placenta; *h,* hydrocele.

Fig. 22-30. Random scans of the upper and lower extremities. *S,* Shoulder; *H,* humerus; *E,* elbow; *R,* radius; *Pl,* placenta; *C,* cord; *Am,* amniotic fluid; *IW,* iliac wing; *Fe,* femur; *T,* tibia; *Fi,* fibula; *A,* ankle; *Fo,* foot.

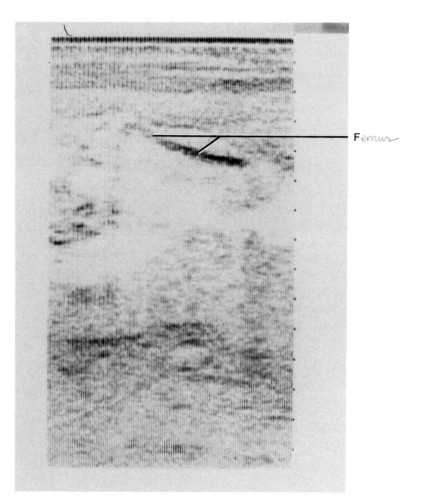

Fig. 22-31. Real time scan of a fetal femur, *F.*

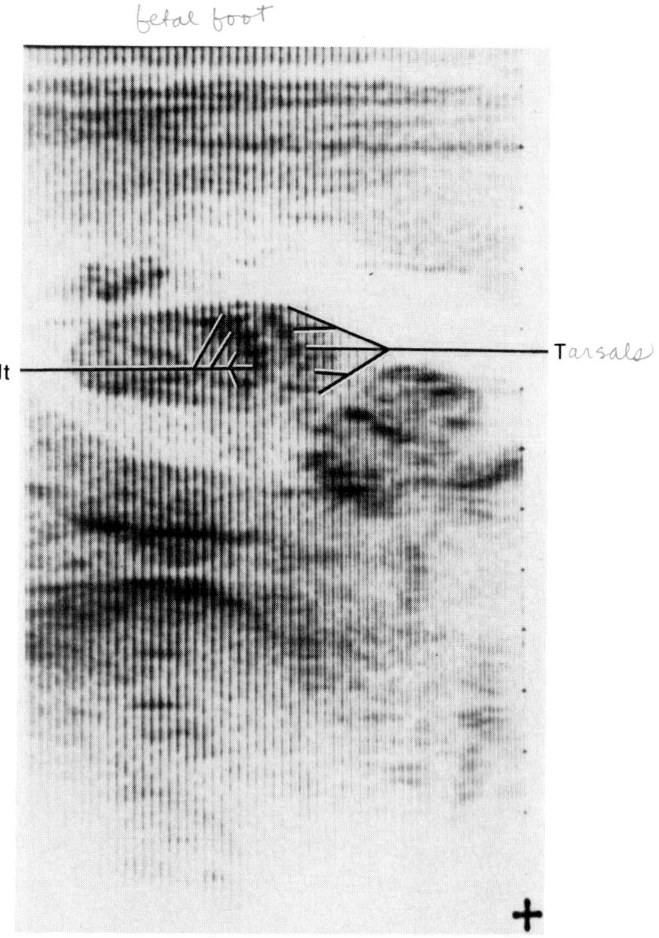

Fig. 22-32. Real time image of a fetal foot demonstrating the tarsals, *T*, and metatarsals, *Mt.*

trasonography are the long bones (Fig. 22-30). By real time the femur is easily accessible, for in most cases it comes off the body at a right angle to the long axis of the fetus[10] (Fig. 22-31). It is best seen with a linear-array transducer. The entire femur must be visualized for measurement of its length. Multiple images should be stored for use later in estimating fetal age and diagnosing conditions like short-limbed dwarfism. This is usually done in the second and third trimester as data become available to refer to.[11] The hands and feet are easily recognized, though distinguishing each toe and finger is a time-consuming process (Fig. 22-32). Other conditions involving anomalous metacarpals and fingers are now being demonstrated by ultrasonography. Careful screening of fetal limbs can diagnose skeletal dysplasias as well as pathologic fractures of the long bones. The scapulas may also easily be identified by the third trimester as linear high-amplitude echoes in the posterior upper thorax.

The umbilical cord is the final structure to be noted. It is seen floating in the am-niotic fluid with its arteries and vein in transverse sections through the cord (Fig. 22-33). The vein is then seen entering the fetal abdomen. At this level in the abdomen one also can see a small sonolucent band known as *pseudoascites*. Care must be taken not to confuse this with a minute amount of ascites.[10]

SMALL-FOR-GESTATIONAL-AGE UTERINE GROWTH

Categorized with the question of fetal age, uterine growth is the next most commonly posed diagnostic question to be addressed by ultrasound. A uterus too small for dates will usually be a growth-retarded fetus or oligohydramnios from some abnormality. Oligohydramnios can also be seen in a patient who is overdue (post-EDC dates), in a patient with twin transfusion syndrome (in which one fetus has polyhydramnios causing the other to have oligohydramnios), or in a patient with leaking premature rupture of the membranes.[16]

The urinary tract contributes to amniotic volume; and when a patient presents with oligohydramnios, one should look for a renal cause of the abnormality.[16] The fetal kidneys should be approximately the same size and lie on each side of the spine. They should not occupy more than one third of the intra-abdominal area (Fig. 22-25). In renal agenesis one expects to find the following: TIUV several standard deviations below the mean for gestational age, absent fetal kidneys, and no fetal urinary bladder.[16] In a lower urinary tract obstruction one expects to find hydronephrotic kidneys and oligohydramnios.[16] Other causes of oligohydramnios include polycystic kidney disease and atresia of the ureter.[7]

GREATER THAN ANTICIPATED UTERINE GROWTH

A greater than anticipated uterus for menstrual dates can be accounted for by disclosing a fetus more mature than the patient's last menstrual period, when she is unsure of dates, or has had functional bleeding after her last period, thereby solving the discrepancy problem. A multiple gestation is another frequent cause for a large uterus. Twins

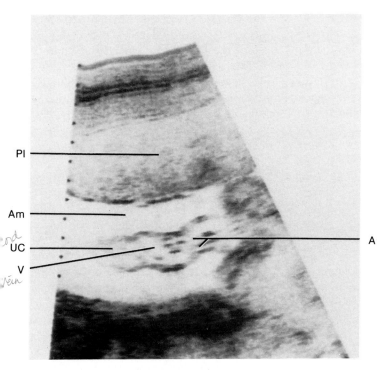

PI

Am

rd
UC

V
ein

A rteries

Fig. 22-33. Random B-scan through the umbilical cord demonstrating the umbilical vein, *UV,* and arteries, *A.* Placenta, *PI;* amniotic fluid, *Am;* umbilical cord, *UC.*

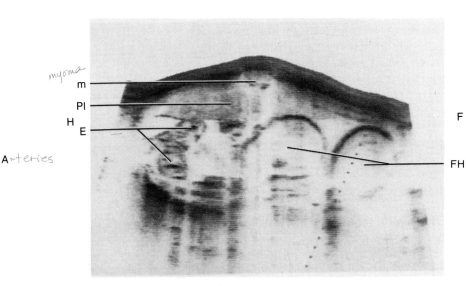

myoma
m

PI

H
E

F

FH

Fig. 22-34. Parasagittal scan of a patient presenting too large for menstrual dates. B-scan demonstrates two fetuses and a myoma, *m,* in the anterior uterine wall. *PI,* Placenta; *E,* fetal extremity; *FH,* fetal heads. **H,** Head. **F,** Foot.

can be visualized in the first trimester as two gestational sacs (Fig. 22-34). The BPD of one twin may be difficult to assess because of fetal lie, especially in the third trimester, when there is less amniotic fluid and larger fetal parts are attenuating the sound beam. In the case of difficult BPDs, bodies may be used as another indication of growth. The reported growth of twins should be similar to that of a singleton.[2]

A routine ultrasonography for twins or other multiple gestation should include transverse and sagittal scans of the uterus, an oblique scan showing more than one fetal head and body, and a sagittal scan of each fetus showing the entire fetus on one scan as well as BPDs and body measurements of all fetuses. A real time examination should then be done to confirm all of the above and any cardiac activity.

Another reason for a large uterus can be polyhydramnios. The true incidence of polyhydramnios is difficult to calculate but has been estimated to be 1:1000 deliveries. In approximately 25% of patients with polyhydramnios, major anomalies of the fetus are present.[8] Polyhydramnios appears as a large fluid-filled area surrounding the fetus. In many cases the fetus is located along the posterior uterine wall (Fig. 22-35). The diagnosis is easily recognized on an ultrasonogram, but confirmation of a TIUV over 2

standard deviations of the mean for gestational age will confirm suspicion. Because a percentage of cases are associated with fetal anomalies, the ultrasonogram can detect these antenatally[7,25,26,28] (Table 22-1). A patient will usually be observed for resolving fluid in the case of no abnormalities visualized.

A hydatidiform mole may also present with a large uterus. The incidence of molar pregnancy in North America is 1:2000 pregnancies.[15] Other symptoms include vaginal bleeding, elevated hCG levels, and high blood pressure. The ultrasound image of a molar pregnancy will show an enlarged uterus filled with echogenic tissue and small

sonolucent structures representing placental tissue but no fetus (except in the case of a fetus and a mole)[15] (Fig. 22-18). Theca lutein cysts frequently accompany molar pregnancies and appear as somewhat large adnexal structures. (See Chapter 21.) When scanning, the examiner must be careful to search the adnexal regions for these cysts since they aid in the diagnosis. Ultrasonography can follow the staging of a choriocarcinoma, which develops from the malignant form of hydatidiform mole.

Another explanation of a larger than anticipated uterus is pregnancy associated with a mass. A patient who is pregnant with a pelvic mass can present a special problem.

Table 22-1. Causes for polyhydramnios* (University of Wisconsin, 1981)

Miscellaneous causes	Fetal malformations	Failure to swallow	Obstruction of venous circulation	Multiple pregnancies	Maternal disorders
Fetal polyuria Enlarged placenta	Nonclosure of cavities Anencephaly Spina bifida Umbilical hernia Ectopic vesica Meningocele Achondroplasia Hypoplastic lungs	Esophageal atresia Duodenal atresia Cerebral malformations Hyperextended neck Tumors Goiterous enlargement of thyroid	Vascular (fetal heart disease, cord stenosis, cirrhosis)	Conjoined twins Twin transfusion (one twin with polyhydramnios, one with oligohydramnios)	Diabetes mellitus Chronic heart, liver, kidney disease Chorioangioma of placenta Preeclampsia Hydrops fetalis

*Defined as more than 2000 ml of fluid.

Any invasive diagnostic procedure may cause premature labor. On physical examination it is difficult to establish the size and shape of a mass with a pregnancy. If a mass appears to be more than 5 cm in diameter or to be enlarging during pregnancy, surgical intervention is usually indicated.[13] The ultrasonogram will provide the obstetrician with the consistency, size, and mobility of a mass and whether it is intrauterine or extrauterine.

One of the most common masses encountered during pregnancy is the uterine leiomyoma. Ultrasonographically its appearance varies from homogeneous to complex with areas of cystic degeneration or diffuse echogenicity. It may be located within the uterine wall or be subserosal and pedunculated.[13] In cases of a pedunculated leiomyoma careful scanning of the patient in the Trendelenburg position may indicate whether a mass is extrauterine or, in fact, a myoma. If a leiomyoma consists primarily of smooth muscle, it may appear sonolucent. The differentiation of a leiomyoma from a cystic mass would depend on the lack of acoustic enhancement in the area of the posterior wall. An intramural leiomyoma may cause nodular enlargement in the uterine wall[13] (Fig. 22-9). Myomas are stimulated by hormonal increases during pregnancy and show increased growth. Follow-up examinations for position and size should be done because some may cause difficulty in delivery if they are located near the cervical os.

Adnexal masses associated with pregnancy include simple cysts of the ovary. Ovarian cysts can be large and show some septations in an otherwise purely cystic mass. These are followed ultrasonographically for size and are not to be confused with corpus luteum cysts that disappear after the first trimester. Other less frequent masses include dermoid tumors, tubo-ovarian abscesses, and hematomas.

INCOMPETENT CERVIX

The ultrasonographic picture of an incompetent cervix will show a fluid-filled section of the endocervical canal[40] (Fig. 22-36). The technique of scanning the cervix must be done carefully, for the endocervical canal rarely lies in a straight sagittal section. Transverse scans must be done with the transducer perpendicular to the long axis of the cervix. When the course of the cervix has been mapped out in transverse scans, sagittal scans of the entire cervix from right to left are taken. The endocervical canal will show up as a highly reflective linear echo within the cervix. The entire canal must be visualized for evaluation; therefore the bladder must be adequately filled. If the bladder is overfilled, the cervix may collapse from the pressure.

Incompetent cervix usually presents in the second trimester as a painless bloodless abortion with minimal warning. Etiologies include a weak cervix from a previous delivery or surgery, emotional factors, or a weak cervical ring.[40] Most patients present with a history of previous abortions. Follow-up examinations are usually done through the end of the second trimester.

FETAL DEATH IN LATER PREGNANCY

The diagnosis of fetal death in the second and third trimester is usually made clinically and through use of a Doppler monitor. At this point a patient will be referred to ultrasound for confirmation of fetal death, especially in cases of questionable dates, obesity, or an inexperienced clinical examiner. In some cases the position of the fetus is unknown, making the detection of a fetal heartbeat difficult without the use of ultrasound imaging.

A routine B-scan for fetal position and any nonspecific signs of fetal death will usually be done first. In some cases the fetus may appear normal; however, depending on the time of death, a macerated fetus may be imaged. A macerated fetus will exhibit collapse of the fetal head, abdomen, and extremities.[38] The uterus may be decreased in size.

In late pregnancy a dead fetus may appear to have a coarse outline and later become edematous as fluid penetrates the tissues. Edema, especially scalp edema, must not be taken as a sign of fetal death, however, since scalp edema is visualized in live fetuses with other conditions (e.g., diabetes). In some cases of fetal death the skull bones overlap and there may be loss of visualization of the anatomy of the midline structures in the fetal skull. In some cases of polyhydramnios, a dead fetus will appear extended along the posterior wall of the uterus.[38]

When real time is not available, a B-scan over the fetal heart will locate the area where an M-mode or A-mode scan may be done. A real time scan is preferred for diagnosing fetal death (the signs of fetal death are more reliable with this technique). Two 3-minute examinations should be performed by separate examiners before fetal death is confirmed. The transducer is placed over the fetal thorax in the region of the heart to look for cardiac motion. In cases of oligohydramnios or unrecognizable anatomic structures the head is localized first and the transducer is rotated 90 degrees to find the long axis of the spine. It is then moved anterior into the region of the thorax. The diagnosis of fetal death can be made only after the entire fetal thorax has been examined using all available techniques. If no head, body, limb, or heart motions are seen, fetal death can then accurately be diagnosed.

ABNORMAL FETAL ANATOMY

With the advancement of technology, the delineation of intrafetal structures by ultrasound is becoming extremely intricate; and this diagnostic modality has definitely become the preferred method of examining fetuses at high risk for anomalies. Generally patients with a history of a previous anomaly or abnormal condition are referred to a center with experienced ultrasonographers and obstetricians in the field of genetics. However, many unsuspected cases of anomalies are picked up in general ultrasound centers; and it is therefore necessary for the sonographer to recognize the signs of these abnormalities.

Because of its highly reflective borders,[10] the fetal skull is perhaps the easiest structure to locate on an ultrasonogram. The cranium can be seen as early as 7 fetal weeks. The diagnosis of hydrocephaly has been made early in the second trimester on the basis of a large head-body discrepancy. In hydrocephaly abnormal dilation of the lateral ventricles precedes distension of the calvarium[16,26] (Fig. 22-37). Therefore in normal fetuses the border of the lateral ventricle should not extend halfway between the falx and the outer skull outline. In the second trimester the structure of the midbrain appears echogenic and the lateral ventricles undelineated. In hydrocephaly the lateral ventricles become apparent. In the third trimester growth of the head will accelerate over that of the body. Serial BPDs will confirm excessive growth. In severe cases the lateral ventricular dilation will be obvious and there may be a shift of the midline structures. In diabetic patients care must be taken not to confuse a large head with hydrocephaly. Most macrocephalic fetuses have a large body diameter as well.

Anencephaly is diagnosed by ultrasonography on the basis of an absent fetal skull. The occurrence is 1:1000 pregnancies (1:25 after one, and 1:10 after two affected fetuses).[16,26] Polyhydramnios can accompany anencephaly. Any patient who is large for dates or who has an elevated serum α-fetoprotein level or a previous fetus with a neural

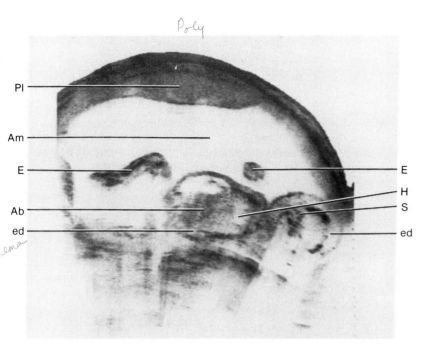

Poly

Fig. 22-35. Parasagittal scan of a twin pregnancy demonstrating polyhydramnios, fetal skull, and body edema in a fetus with twin transfusion syndrome. *Pl*, Placenta; *Am*, amniotic fluid; *E*, fetal extremities; *Ab*, fetal abdomen; *H*, fetal heart; *S*, fetal skull; *ed*, edema.

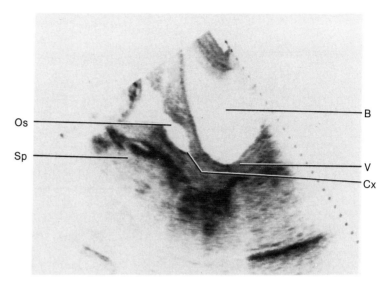

Fig. 22-36. Parasagittal scan of a second trimester pregnancy patient with a history of multiple spontaneous abortions demonstrating fluid in the region of the cervical canal. *B*, Bladder; *Cx*, cervix; *Os*, cervical os; *Sp*, spine; *V*, vagina.

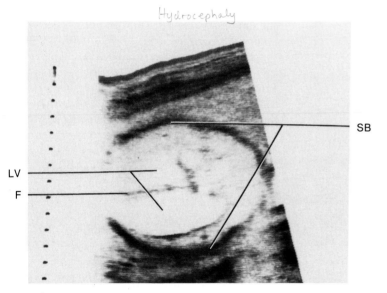

Hydrocephaly

Fig. 22-37. Random scan of a third trimester fetus with severe hydrocephaly. *LV*, Lateral ventricles; *SB*, skull borders; *F*, falx.

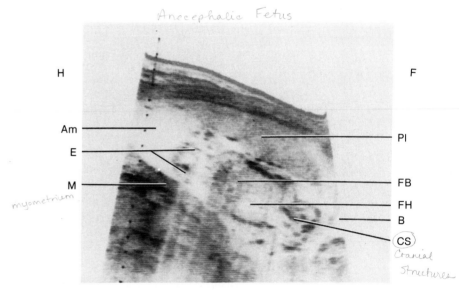

Anencephalic Fetus

myometrium

Cranial Structures

Fig. 22-38. Parasagittal scan of a second trimester pregnancy demonstrating an anencephalic fetus in a patient with an elevated AFP. *Pl*, Placenta; *Am*, amniotic fluid; *B*, bladder; *M*, myometrium; *FH*, fetal heart; *FB*, fetal body; *E*, fetal extremities and, *CS*, cranial structures. **H,** Head. **F,** Foot.

tube defect will be screened in the second trimester for abnormalities. The fetal body will appear normal, with cardiac activity in many cases. The region of the skull may project a variation of dense echoes depending on the development of the cranial structures (Fig. 22-38).

Microcephaly will appear as a small fetal skull in proportion to the fetal body. The fetal body must be diagnosed as normal in size prior to diagnosis of microcephaly by ultrasonography.[16] Normal growth of the fetal abdomen is similar to normal growth of the fetal head except after 35 to 36 weeks, when the fetal abdomen may grow up to 10 mm larger than the fetal head by term.

A variety of extracranial structures may be identified contiguous with the fetal skull. Cystic hygromas and lymphangiectasia are two such reported conditions.[26] A cystic hygroma will appear as a multicystic mass in the region of the fetal neck area contiguous with the skull and upper thorax region (Fig. 22-39).

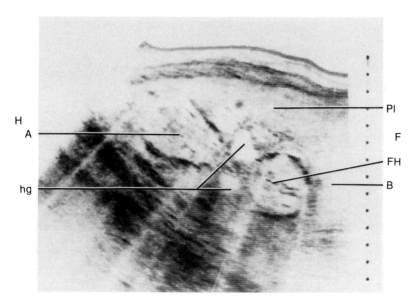

Fig. 22-39. Parasagittal scan demonstrating a fetus with a cystic hygroma. Note the lack of definition due to oligohydramnios. *B*, Bladder, *FH*, fetal head; *hg*, hygromas; *A*, fetal abdomen; *Pl*, placenta. **H,** Head. **F,** Foot.

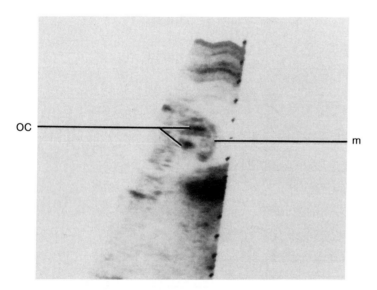

Fig. 22-40. Parasagittal scan of a fetal spine demonstrating a meningomyelocele, *m*, protruding through a defect between the ossification centers, *OC*.

Spinal defects result from incomplete closure of the neural tube. Leakage of α-fetoprotein (AFP) may occur resulting in elevated AFP levels.[16] Ultrasonography will be performed in cases of previous neural tube defects or elevated AFP levels. Although spinal defects may be detected on sagittal views of the spine by seeing a defect or widening of the parallel structure of the posterior ossification centers of the spine, transverse scans are more reliable in detecting the entire spine.[10,16] A series of carefully spaced transverse scans should be made by an experienced ultrasonographer. A meningomyelocele is a saclike protrusion of a spinal defect that may or may not contain neural tissue.[16] On transverse scans the sac can be seen contiguous with the defect (Fig. 22-40). Other more rare spinal abnormalities such as tumors of the spine may be visualized.

The fetal thorax can be affected by multiple anomalies. The size and configuration of the chest cavity may aid in the diagnosis of such conditions. These include skeletal dys-plasias, masses of the chest, and abnormal diaphragm.[16,26] Ultrasonographic images of the fetal thorax will vary in appearance with each abnormality, although in the third trimester abnormalities are more easily recognized than earlier in pregnancy.

In the fetal abdomen careful evaluation must be made of any unrecognizable fluid-filled structures for any gastrointestinal or renal anomalies. Obstruction of the GI tract proximal to the ileum is associated with polyhydramnios. Obstruction may occur in the esophagus, duodenum, or small bowel. Obstructions distal to the stomach will markedly distend the stomach. A duodenal atresia may present with a double fluid-filled area in the upper abdomen.[25] Various lower GI obstructions may present with large dilated loops of bowel.[16,23,24]

Renal anomalies affect the uterine volume. Oligohydramnios is a finding associated with nonfunctioning or obstructed kidneys.[16] Examination of the fetus may be difficult with oligohydramnios; therefore the best way to exclude this possibility is to visualize a fetal bladder by ultrasonography. If a fetal bladder is not demonstrated on the initial scan, the patient should return in an hour because a normal fetal bladder will fill out with time.

Cystic abnormalities of the fetal kidneys involve bilateral or unilateral enlargement. Infantile polycystic disease produces bilateral kidney enlargement with disordered architecture. Multiple small cysts are present, causing an increased echo pattern in the parenchyma. A multicystic kidney and hydronephrosis from a ureteropelvic junction obstruction are usually unilateral with normal function of the opposite kidney.[7,16]

Obstructions of the urinary tract seen by ultrasound include ureteral stricture, which causes gross dilation of the fetal bladder. This may be accompanied by oligohydramnios (Fig. 22-41). Bilateral hydronephrosis and hydroureter occur in severe cases. At the present time attempts are being made to relieve the obstruction in utero with the aid of ultrasound-guided techniques.

Renal agenesis may be diagnosed by nonvisualized kidneys, an empty bladder, or severe oligohydramnios. This is referred to as Potter's syndrome and is accompanied by the typical Potter's facies and some form of pulmonary hypoplasia. Other conditions (e.g., renal hamartoma, Wilms' tumor, neuroblastoma) are seen as enlarged solid renal structures. Ascites usually accompanies a hamartoma.

Conditions of the genitalia such as hydroceles are easily detected on an ultrasonogram as cystic areas in the male scrotum (Fig. 22-26, *B*). Female abnormalities are less easily detected but may include hydrometrocolpos and ovarian cystic masses arising out of the fetal pelvis.[7]

Some anomalous conditions are associated with fetal ascites. The most common are urinary tract obstruction, prune-belly syndrome, and multiple-anomaly syndromes.[16] When ascites is noted on an ultrasonogram, a fluid interface is readily noted between the bowel and abdominal wall of the fetus. In the case of nonimmunologic disease, ascites is usually associated with multisystem anomalies and the prognosis is usually hopeless.

Defects in the abdominal wall leading to abnormal position of the fetal bowel, as in gastroschisis and omphalocele, can be made with careful scanning of the fetal abdomen (Fig. 22-42). In gastroschisis dilated loops of bowel are seen floating outside the fetal abdomen.[28] In an omphalocele the bowel is confined to a membrane. Careful examination is necessary to differentiate the organs outside the confines of the abdomen by ultrasonography. A rare diagnosis of conjoined twins in utero can be made by ultrasound,[16] but care must be taken to differentiate the organs and their separation.

FETAL ECHOCARDIOGRAPHY

Fetal echocardiography is a method dependent upon technical expertise. Time-motion (T-M) mode echocardiography of the fetal mitral or tricuspid valve provides an excellent method for measuring beat-to-beat variability because it is more distinct than the fetal phonocardiogram and it is not plagued with the artifacts seen on the fetal electrocardiograms. It can therefore be combined with the stress test for more accurate evaluation of change in heart rate.[32]

The potential of T-M mode and two-dimensional real time echocardiology in detection of congenital fetal heart defects in utero will most likely govern the future applications of this modality. Any anatomic abnormality that does not depend on physiologic changes in the heart chamber size after birth should be detectable. These abnormalities include atrioventricular canal, valvular atresia, truncus arteriosis, tetrology of Fallot, and hypoplasia of the heart chamber.[32] When standard fetal heart dimensions have been established for each gestational age, they can be used to diagnose chamber dilation.

In performance of fetal echocardiography a B-scan or real time section of the fetal

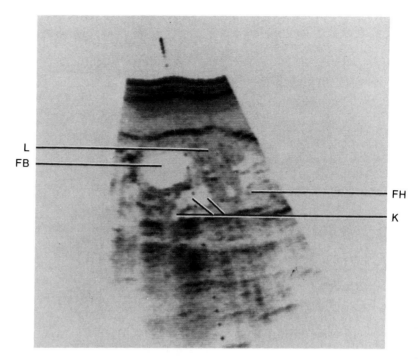

Fig. 22-41. Parasagittal scan of a fetal abdomen demonstrating a posterior urethral valve obstruction. Note the thick-walled fetal bladder, *FB*, and severely hydronephrotic fetal kidney, *K*. Fetal heart, *FH*; fetal liver, *L*.

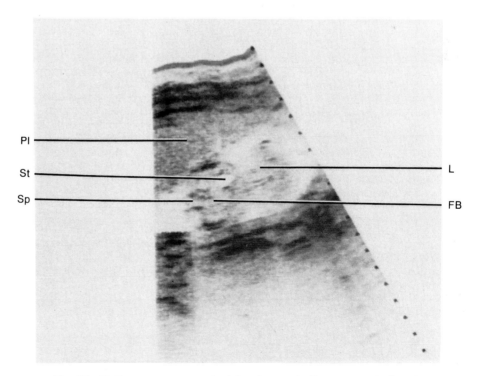

Fig. 22-42. Transverse scan of a fetus demonstrating an omphalocele with the liver protruding through the defect in the abdominal wall. *Pl*, Placenta; *Sp*, fetal spine; *FB*, fetal body; *St*, fetal stomach; *L*, fetal liver.

thorax will reveal the location of the heart and spine to establish the fetal lie. The plane of the long axis of the heart is marked, and careful sectioning of the heart is done until the greatest cardiac dimensions are obtained. A hand-held transducer is used for versatility of movement. The TGC curve is manipulated to remove extraneous echoes and enhance dynamic structures. The transducer is then manipulated to image the structures of the fetal heart.[32]

SUMMARY

Since the field of ultrasonography has progressed so rapidly, it is difficult to find the current concepts of all aspects of ultrasound in one text. With this in mind, I organized this chapter on obstetrics to include all the basic aspects of technique and a synopsis of the many areas of diagnosis. These areas are covered in greater detail in the literature and specialty texts as listed in the references. I hope the information in this chapter will be used as a technical guide to produce the most diagnostic examination possible.

REFERENCES

1. Arger, P.H., et al.: Ultrasound assisted amniocentesis in prenatal genetic counseling, Radiology **120:** 155, 1976.
2. Bowie, J.D.: Syllabus for the categorical course in ultrasonography. American Roentgen Ray Society, March, 1981.
3. Brown, T.W., Filly, R.A., Laing, F.C., and Barton, J.: Analysis of ultrasonic criteria in the evaluation for ectopic pregnancy, A.J.R. **131:**967, 1978.
4. Campbell, S.: An improved method of fetal cephalometry by ultrasound, J. Obstet. Gynaecol. Br. Commonw. **75:**568, 1968.
5. Campbell, S.: Ultrasound measurement of the fetal head to abdomen circumference ratio in assessment of growth retardation, Br. J. Gynaecol. **84:**165, 1977.
6. Chinn, D.H., Filly, R.A., and Callen, P.W.: Prediction of intrauterine growth retardation by sonographic estimation of total intrauterine volume, J. Clin. Ultrasound **9:**175, 1981.
7. Cooperberg, P.L.: Abnormalities of the fetal genitourinary tract. In Sanders, R.C., and James, A.E., Jr., editors: Ultrasonography in obstetrics and gynecology, ed. 2, New York, 1980, Appleton-Century-Crofts.
8. Danforth, D.N., editor: Obstetrics and gynecology, ed. 3, New York, 1977, Harper & Row, Publishers.
9. DeVore, G.R., and Hobbins, J.C.: Fetal growth and development: the diagnosis of intrauterine growth retardation. In Clinics in diagnostic ultrasound. Vol. 3. Diagnostic ultrasound in obstetircs (J.C. Hobbins, editor), New York, 1979, Churchill Livingstone, Inc.
10. Filly, R.A., and Callen, P.C.: Normal fetal anatomy as visualized with gray-scale ultrasonography. In Sanders, R.C., and James, A.E., Jr., editors: Ultrasonography in obstetrics and gynecology, ed. 2, New York, 1980, Appleton-Century-Crofts.
11. Filly, R.A., Golbus, M.S., Carey, J.C., et al.: Short-limbed dwarfism: ultrasonographic diagnosis by menstruation of fetal femoral length, Radiology **138:**653, 1981.
12. Finberg, H.J., and Birnholz, J.C.: Ultrasound observations in multiple gestation with first trimester bleeding: the blighted twin, Radiology **132:**137, 1979.
13. Fleisher, A.C., Bolehm, F.H., and James, A.E.: Sonographic evaluation of pelvic masses occurring during pregnancy. In Sanders, R.C., and James, A.E., Jr., editors: Ultrasonography in obstetrics and gynecology, ed. 2, New York, 1980, Appleton-Century-Crofts.
14. Gohari, P., and Berkowitz, R., and Hobbins, J.C.: Prediction of intrauterine growth retardation by determination of total intrauterine volume, Am. J. Obstet. Gynecol. **113:**823, 1972.
15. Grannum, P., Berkowitz, R., and Hobbins, J.C.: The ultrasonic changes in the maturing placenta and their relation to fetal pulmonic maturity, Am. J. Obstet. Gynecol. **133:**915, 1979.
16. Hobbins, J.C., and Venus, I.: Congenital anomalies. In Clinics in diagnostic ultrasound. Vol. 3. Diagnostic ultrasound in obstetrics (J.C. Hobbins, ed.), New York, 1979, Churchill Livingstone, Inc.
17. James, A.E., Howerton, H.C., Weinstein, M.L., et al.: Embryologic foundation of obstetrical sonography. In Sanders, R.C., and James, A.E., Jr. editors: Ultrasonography in obstetrics and gynecology, ed. 2, New York, 1980, Appleton-Century-Crofts.
18. Jeanty, P., Kirkpatrick, C., Dramaix-Wilmet, M., and Struyven, J.: Ultrasonic evaluation of fetal limb growth, Radiology **140:**165, 1981.
19. Jouppila, P.: Ultrasound in the diagnosis of early pregnancy and its complications, Acta Obstet. Gynecol. Scand., suppl. 15, 1971.
20. Kaiser, I.H.: Fertilization and the physiology and development of fetus and placenta. In Danforth, D.N., editor: Obstetrics and gynecology, ed. 3, New York, 1977, Harper & Row, Publishers.
21. Kurjak, A., Cecuk, S., and Breyer, B.: Prediction of maturity in first trimester of pregnancy by ultrasonic measurement of fetal crown-rump length, J. Clin. Ultrasound **4:**83, 1976.
22. Kurtz, A.B., et al.: Analysis of biparietal diameter as an accurate indicator of gestational age, J. Clin. Ultrasound **8:**319, 1980.
23. Lee, T.G., and Blake, S.: Prenatal fetal abdominal ultrasonography and diagnosis, Radiology **124:**475, 1977.
24. Lee, T.G., and Warren, B.H.: Antenatal demonstration of fetal bowel, Radiology **124:**471, 1977.
25. Lees, R., Alford, B., Benbridge, N., et al.: Sonographic appearance of duodenal atresia in utero, A.J.R. **131:**701, 1978.
26. Little, D.J., and Campbell, S.: The diagnosis of spina bifida and intracranial abnormalities. In Sanders, R.C., and James, A.E., Jr., editors: Ultrasonography in obstetrics and gynecology, ed. 2, New York, 1980, Appleton-Century-Crofts.
27. Marks, W.M., Filly, R.A., Callen, P.W., and Laing, F.C.: The decidual cast of ectopic pregnancy: a confusing ultrasonic appearance, Radiology **133:**451, 1979.
28. Morgan, C.L., Haney, A., Christakos, A., and Phillips, J.: Antenatal detection of fetal structural defects with ultrasound, J. Clin. Ultrasound **3:**287, 1978.
29. Morgan, C.L., Trought, W.S., Haney, A., and Clark, W.M.: Application of real-time ultrasound in obstetrics: the linear and dynamically focused phased arrays, J. Clin. Ultrasound **7:**108, 1979.
30. Platt, L.D., and Manning, F.A.: Special procedures. In Clinics in diagnostic ultrasound. Vol. 3. Diagnostic ultrasound in obstetrics (J.C. Hobbins), New York, 1979, Churchill Livingstone, Inc.
31. Robinson, H.P.: Sonar measurement of fetal crown-rump length as a means of assessing maturity in the first trimester of pregnancy, Br. Med. J. **4:**28, 1973.
31a. Robinson, H.P.: Gestational sac volumes as determined by sonar in the first trimester of pregnancy, Br. J. Obstet. Gynaecol. **82:**100, 1975.
32. Rocaen, R.S.: Fetal echocardiography: present and future applications, J. Clin. Ultrasound **9:**223, 1981.
33. Sabbagha, R.E.: Intrauterine growth retardation: antenatal diagnosis by ultrasound, Surg. Obstet. Gynecol. **52:**252, 1978.
34. Sabbagha, R.E.: The use of ultrasound in defining gestational age. In Clinics in diagnostic ultrasound. Vol. 3. Diagnostic ultrasound in obstetrics (J.C. Hobbins, editor), New York, 1979, Churchill Livingstone, Inc.
35. Sabbagha, R.E.: Biparietal diameter and gestational age. In Sabbagha, R.E., editor: Diagnostic ultrasound applied to obstetrics and gynecology, New York, 1980, Harper & Row, Publishers.
36. Sabbagha, R.E., Barton, F.B., and Barton, B.A.: Sonar biparietal diameter: analysis of percentile growth differences in two normal populations using same methodology, Am. J. Obstet. Gynecol. **126:** 479, 1976.
37. Sabbagha, R.E., Barton, F.B., Barton, B.A., and Kingas, E.: Sonar biparietal diameter. II. Predictive of three fetal growth patterns leading to a closer assessment of gestational age and neonatal weight, Am. J. Obstet. Gynecol. **126:**485, 1976.
38. Sanders, R.C.: Ultrasound in the diagnosis of fetal death. In Sanders, R.C., and James, A.E., Jr., editors: Ultrasonography in obstetrics and gynecology, ed. 2, New York, 1980, Appleton-Century-Crofts.
39. Sarti, D.A., Crandall, B.F., Winter, J., et al.: Correlation of biparietal and fetal body diameters: 12-26 weeks gestation, A.J.R. **137:**87, 1981.
40. Shaug, M.S.: Obstetrical ultrasonography. In Sarti, D.A., and Sample, W.F., editors: Ultrasound: text and cases, Boston, 1980, D.K. Hall & Co.
41. Spirit, B.A., Kagan, E.H., and Rozanski, R.M.: Abruptio placentae: sonographic and pathologic correlation, A.J.R. **133:**877, 1979.
42. Spirit, B.A., Kagan, E.H., and Rozanski, R.M.: Sonographic anatomy of the normal placenta, J. Clin. Ultrasound **7:**204, 1979.
43. Tamura, R.K., and Sabbagha, R.E.: Percentile ranks of sonar fetal abdominal circumference measurements, Am. J. Obstet. Gynecol. **138:**475, 1980.

23

Peripheral vascular Doppler examinations

RICHARD E. RAE II

Throughout medical history the circulatory system has been a source of great mystery and puzzlement. Many diseases and conditions in the human body have led investigators to discover a vascular etiology where a completely different diagnosis was expected. Unfortunately the source often has not been found in time to save a diseased organ or limb or has been discovered only after the patient's death.

The introduction of radiographic imaging of the arterial system in 1923 made possible accurate vascular diagnosis and greatly enhanced the potential for surgical repair of vascular lesions. The first carotid arteriogram was performed in 1927,[21] and the first translumbar aortogram in 1929.[7] Many years were required for perfection of angiographic equipment and techniques, but angiography has become the standard method for the assessment of vascular anatomy.

The drawbacks of angiography are numerous. There are risks from reactions to the iodine-based contrast media. Furthermore, the examination is performed with the patient in an immobile position; needle punctures or cutdowns and rapid injections of contrast are required,[3,12] all of which contribute to patient anxiety and occasionally result in the patient's refusing the examination. Even the recent introduction of digital subtraction angiography has not eliminated certain risks and discomforts.

There are several noninvasive or non-arteriographic methods for assessing the circulatory system in the body that involve various methods and techniques depending on the vessels and location of the area of interest. Unfortunately they often rely on complex or time-consuming equipment setups, may be uncomfortable or actually invasive, and are open to any number of variables that can adversely affect their results. Their accuracy can vary from poor to excellent when correlated with angiographic studies and depending on the disease condition being ruled out.[3,8,12]

The varying specificity and accuracy level of certain of these nonradiographic alternatives has caused many physicians to search for a vascular diagnostic method that is truly noninvasive, has a high level of accuracy, is atraumatic and comfortable to the patient, can be performed quickly, and does not require bulky equipment or long setup procedures. Doppler ultrasonic methods fulfill these requirements. The use of Doppler techniques has become increasingly widespread since their inception 24 years ago and as initial physician wariness has given way in response to documented accuracy. Many clinical and laboratory studies have been performed comparing Doppler methods to angiography, with 95% to 98% accuracy for some types of examination.[3,6,8,12]

This chapter describes Doppler ultrasound techniques for arterial and venous examination, including the extremity vessels and the cerebrovascular system. Descriptions of spectral analysis of Doppler signals, Doppler vascular scanning, and real time B-mode duplex sonography of the carotid system are also given. Each vascular system is considered independently, including pertinent anatomy, pathology, and equipment needs; and a complete explanation of commonly used examination procedures based on the techniques described by Barnes et al.[2-4] Data on examination variations, normal results, and interpretation of abnormal findings are presented as well as illustrative cases.

Doppler principles and instrumentation

It is essential to understand the principles of a diagnostic procedure before becoming involved with it. This section considers the Doppler effect and how it applies to the

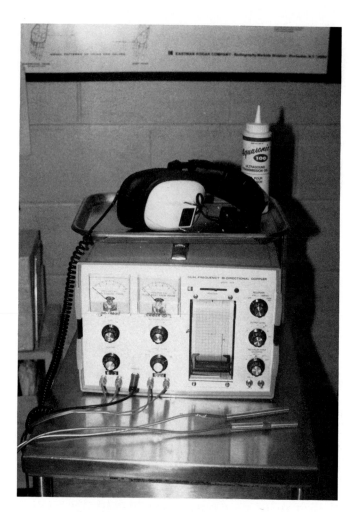

Fig. 23-1. Directional Doppler device.

vascular examination, along with the equipment and its use.

The Doppler ultrasound apparatus makes use of the Doppler effect, which was described by the mathematician Christian Doppler in 1842. He observed that the frequency of sound waves varied depending on the speed of the sound transmitter relative to the listener. Having developed an equation to express this phenomenon, he devised an experiment to test its validity.

Doppler assembled a small group of musicians with perfect pitch near a railroad track. He then had some trumpet players on a flatcar pulled past these musical observers while the trumpeters played a series of notes at previously established pitches. The observers wrote down what pitches they heard as the train pulled the trumpeters back and forth at different speeds. The variations in tone heard by the observers versus what was actually being played proved Doppler's equation.[14]

In the continuous-wave Doppler blood-flow device (Fig. 23-1) the sound source is a small probe housing one transmitting and one receiving crystal. Red blood cells reflect ultrasound impulses, and the frequency of the reflected sound wave is shifted to either a higher or a lower pitch depending on the flow velocity. In all devices a change or shift in frequency is detected only if the flow velocity is greater than 6 cm/sec; therefore an absent signal at a vascular site may imply anything from totally absent flow to flow moving at a velocity slower than 6 cm/sec.[3]

In the directional Doppler device the probe is held so the sound beam intersects the vessel at an angle of approximately 45 degrees *against* the flow. Flow is then interpreted by the circuitry as being *toward* the probe and is considered *antegrade flow*. That away from the probe is considered *retrograde flow*. A directional Doppler therefore is capable of showing the *direction* as well as the *relative velocity* of flow. Most equipment features two gauges, one for *flow toward* and one for *flow away* from the probe, and these gauges are calibrated to show relative velocity of the blood flow in the direction specified. It is important that the transducer be correctly directed relative to the direction of

flow in the vessel being examined so that false diagnoses of flows seeming to go in the wrong direction will be avoided.

In practice the probe is placed against the skin and is coupled by means of a water-soluble acoustic gel, which serves to eliminate air pockets and ensure optimal acoustic transmission and reception. The transmitted sound waves strike the red corpuscles and bounce back. The reflected signals are shifted in pitch, either higher or lower, depending on the relative velocity. The direction of flow also affects the reflected sound. As the reflected waveforms strike the receiving crystal, they are converted into electric signals via the piezoelectric principle. The circuitry of the Doppler device then separates the signals of increased frequency from those of decreased frequency and distinguishes between signals reflected by flow toward or away from the probe face. The signals are then fed to outputs that convert them to audible sound (heard by speakers or headphones) and/or are fed to a strip-chart or tape recording device.[3]

Probes are available in frequencies manufactured in ranges from 2.25 to 10 MHz. The lower frequencies are usually found in fetal monitoring devices or Doppler stethoscopes intended for intraabdominal vessels, wherein sound penetration and large beam widths are desirable. The higher frequencies, from 5 to 10 MHz, are the ones most frequently used in extremity and cerebrovascular Doppler examinations. The probes also vary in size and shape, from flat transducers with a fixed beam angle used often in surgery for brachial pulse monitoring to large pocket-sized devices that incorporate the transducer and signal processors into one unit.

The most versatile probe, and the one that will be referred to exclusively in the discussion to follow, is the pencil-style probe. This probe is also available in many configurations, depending on the manufacturer. It can vary from a simple aluminum tube with the crystals epoxied into the end to a completely enclosed plastic probe with complex circuitry incorporated into the probe housing. The simpler the probe, however, the better, when maintenance and cost are prime concerns. The simple probes are light as well as practical and are easier to repair than a complex probe. Their lower cost usually means that several can be placed in reserve for the same price as one more sophisticated probe. Usually the complex probes require attached modules to allow frequency-circuit matching. The simple probes are calibrated to one set frequency and are matched to calibrated input and output jacks. The latter system has advantages in that faulty frequency-matching modules may ruin both probe and Doppler device whereas calibrated jacks and transducers require no modules between probe and Doppler system. Although the complex probe-module systems allow easier interchanging of different frequency probes, the devices utilizing simpler probes are optionally equipped with two sets of calibrated outlets and a selection knob so higher and lower frequencies can be used alternatively.

The audible Doppler flow information requires a method of permanent recording if later interpretation and diagnosis are required. The most commonly used system is the *strip-chart recorder*. This device has a *zero-crossing circuit*, which discriminates between antegrade and retrograde flow, much as the directional gauges in the main device do. In the standard recording format antegrade flow is placed on the positive (upward) side of a zero baseline and retrograde flow on the negative (downward) side. The examiner is thus able to determine the flow direction and flow patterns visually.

Some Doppler devices are equipped with a signal-select switch, which can be set to show retrograde flow on the positive side of the graph to facilitate determination of the amount of flow reversal. Other devices have a separate knob that allows only positive, only negative, inverted net flow, or normal net flow to be recorded.

Strip charts are usually single graph, but some recorders have provisions for two readouts simultaneously. One readout is usually set for net flow and the other for antegrade flow, retrograde flow, ECG, or any other tracing that may be useful while the Doppler examination is being recorded. For most purposes one graph is sufficient, and all examples in Appendix I are shown with net flow on a single-graph chart.

The directional Doppler audible signal is stereophonic, which allows easy distinguishing between antegrade and retrograde flow. Antegrade flow is usually heard in the left ear and retrograde flow in the right ear (although occasionally the opposite is true). A nondirectional Doppler is monophonic since both antegrade and retrograde signals are processed together and no directional distinction is made. Regardless of whether the audible signals are stereophonic or monophonic, the sounds can be recorded on a stereophonic tape recorder to preserve interesting flow patterns for reference or if spectral analysis is to be performed at a later time. (See "Spectral Analysis of Doppler Signals," p. 353.)

ARTERIAL DOPPLER EXAMINATIONS

The Doppler examinations pertaining to the arterial system are probably the simplest to learn and interpret. The techniques still require a high degree of examiner familiarity and a thorough knowledge of the arterial anatomy to enable confident and accurate diagnoses to be made. This section will discuss basic arterial occlusive syndromes and disease processes, Doppler signal characteristics, flow physiology, anatomy, examination of the lower and upper extremities, and related studies. Interpretations with illustrative examples appear in Appendix I.

Types of arterial occlusive conditions

Occlusive diseases and other pathologic conditions are common to arteries anywhere in the body and present clinically in various manners. Extensive coverage of these is beyond the scope of this work, but several of the more common diseases and pathoses that the examiner is likely to encounter will be discussed.

Atherosclerosis accounts for the greatest percentage of occlusive diseases in which the arteries are constricted or narrowed, preventing adequate flow to the distal portion of the arterial tributaries. Atherosclerosis is distinguished from arteriosclerosis by the fact that the former is usually a focal accumulation of lipids, calcium, fibrous tissue, and blood products in the intima of an artery whereas the latter is a generalized aging process in the entire system, shown by intimal thickening, calcification, and loss of vascular wall elasticity.

Focal atherosclerotic areas are also known as *plaques*. Plaques are usually elevated lesions of the intima that can be fatty or fibrous and that project into the lumen of an artery, narrowing the flow path and reducing flow. They have amorphous, or atheromatous, cores and may calcify or become ulcerated and thromboembolic. Cast-off emboli from plaques may occlude distal capillaries and tributaries, causing ischemia (deficiency of blood) to the areas they supply. These thrombi are composed of platelet material, and it is thought that platelet secretions may interact with vessel walls and actually initiate atherosclerosis. The causes of arterial thrombosis are often related to plaque formations but may also be due to embolization from cardiac diseases, such as occurs in subacute bacterial endocarditis with vegetation formation or myocardial infarctions with an accompanying thrombus. Atherosclerosis may also be referred to in severe cases as *atherosclerosis obliterans* (ASO).[2,5,21]

Congenital arterial anomalies, such as congenital arteriovenous fistulas that cause abnormal communication between arteries and veins, can occur. Coarctation, or kinking, of an artery is also possible. Some other anomalies include variations in the anatomic course of an artery, absence of a normal vessel, and separate branches appearing in different locations or at unusual origins. The use of real time B-scanning may help in questionable cases.[3,12]

Raynaud's phenomenon is related to cold and abrupt temperature changes, which cause vascular spasm in the digits and resulting obstruction. Purplish fingers and toes are often seen in this disorder. Vasospasm occurring by itself is termed Raynaud's disease, whereas vasospasm resulting from another condition is Raynaud's phenomenon. The latter is often seen in lupus erythematosus, arthritis, and other diseases.[21,26]

Buerger's disease is a form of presenile spontaneous gangrene that affects the distal arteries in the digits and toes. It is caused by heavy cigarette smoking and can be distinguished from atherosclerotic disease on an arteriogram by a smooth well-defined artery proximal to a distinct occlusion point. The fingers and toes are usually involved simultaneously, and Raynaud's phenomenon may also occur with this syndrome. The onset is much more acute than that of atherosclerotic occlusion and usually presents as a sudden total arterial occlusion. Intense rest pain may occur independently in Buerger's disease, rather than as a progressive process following claudication. (See "Symptoms of arterial disease.") This disease is also termed thromboangiitis obliterans (TAO). It is treated by selective amputation and/or sympathectomy in extreme cases.[8]

Frostbite involves the actual freezing of tissue. The cause of arterial occlusion has been attributed to permanent vasoconstriction in response to the cold with or without freezing of blood or fluids. The exact cause of tissue injury is not fully understood. The emergency treatment of warming the affected part is an attempt to restore circulation by relaxing the vasospasm. If flow is not restored in time to save viable tissue, necrosis of the ischemic parts will occur and amputation may be necessary.[21]

Arteritis is usually caused by collagen-related diseases. In cases such as Takayasu's syndrome the media of the artery becomes thickened and swollen, occluding the arterial lumen without changing the external configuration of the vessel itself. This process is usually detected by a diminishing pulse

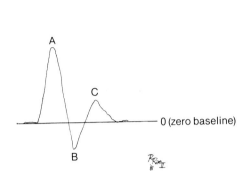

Fig. 23-2. Normal arterial waveform in the extremities. *A* is the first diastolic component, *B* the brief period of reversal, and *C* the diastolic component.

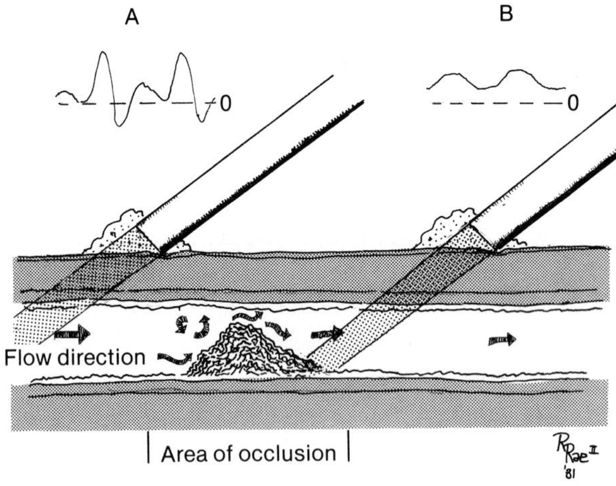

Fig. 23-3. Diagram of flow patterns proximal and distal to an occlusion. *A* shows the waveform obtained proximally, with all normal components present. *B* shows the characteristic loss of components and flow diminishing found in the segment distal to the block.

noted over a time. Takayasu's does not localize but usually occurs in the entire arterial system from the aortic root outward. Other types may occur in isolated vessels.[21]

Mechanical compression of an artery involves obstruction by compression of the vessel between or against another part of the body. Examples are thoracic outlet syndrome, in which the arteries, veins, and nerve plexuses are compressed against the first rib or muscle groups by arm flexion and abduction, and loculated infections, which may cause purulent lesions or masses that compromise nearby vasculature and compress the vessels against other areas of the body.

Symptoms of arterial disease*

Claudication. This term comes from the Latin verb "to limp."[14] Patients with claudication notice tiring and pain in the limb distal to the occlusion with exertion. A walking patient may feel pain in the calf first, often within a measurable distance. The pain and tiring will progress to muscle cramping if the patient persists (e.g., for a city block). If the patient rests, the cramping and pain will resolve completely. The symptoms will resume with the onset of activity. In the arms a patient may feel pain, tiring, and cramping if extensive lifting or elevation of the affected arm is performed. In either legs or arms the affected limb may give way if too much demand is placed upon it.

Dependent rubor and elevation pallor. Erythema is often seen in patients with advancing arterial disease, along with drying

*References 2, 3, 5, 8, 13, 21.

and flaking of skin and thickening of the nails. If the extremity is hung dependent, it will usually present puffy and red digits and even the entire forefoot or hand in advanced disease. If the limb is elevated, the redness will disappear and the limb will become increasingly pale.

Rest pain. This symptom of very severe arterial insufficiency is usually found in cases of lower-than-normal resting blood flow. The pain will be localized in specific areas of inadequate perfusion (e.g., toes, heel, calf). It is often described as a burning pain that will keep the patient awake at night. The skin is red and thin, often shiny. This symptom is a definite sign that arterial reconstruction or some other means must be undertaken to prevent loss of the limb.

Coldness of the limb. This is due to inadequate arterial flow and is readily noticed by the examiner.

Gangrene. When the disease advances to near cessation of flow, circulation to the distal portion of the digits (with the most easily occluded vessels) will often be blocked completely. The tissue will necrose and gangrene will set in, appearing as a black shriveling spot or region that progresses and from which fluids exude. Amputation is often the only course, although recent advances in hyperbaric pressure chamber medicine have enabled many largely necrosed limbs to be saved in whole or in part.

Regardless of the symptoms and signs, arterial disease is a dangerous entity. It depletes the blood flow to vital organs, impairs normal activity, and often acts as a precursor to more serious conditions.

Flow dynamics in the arterial system

The normal arterial Doppler flow signal is evaluated by the chart tracing as well as by the audio signals. Both positive and negative chart deflections exist in the arterial signal, again with antegrade flow being positive and retrograde flow being negative. Probe position is critical in the arterial examination. If the sound beam is perpendicular to the direction of flow, no Doppler shift will occur and a flat tracing will result. The examiner should utilize the flow direction gauges and the signal strength as heard through the speakers to determine the precise angle for optimal blood flow sampling.

The normal arterial Doppler flow signal in the extremities consists of three components: a large *positive deflection* with *systole*, a period of *net flow reversal* to the *negative side* of the zero line, and a lesser *diastolic positive* deflection (Fig. 23-2). The period of reversal is due to the high resistance of the vascular bed in the extremities. In vasodilated conditions the flow will be seen primarily on the positive side, but the three deflections will still be present. The normal arterial flow signal, because of the three components, is said to be *triphasic*.[3]

In cases of arterial obstruction the flow signal begins to lose one or more components, becoming *biphasic* or *monophasic*. The flow pattern will tend to remain triphasic proximal to the obstruction but will begin to show diminished systolic components and lose the diastolic component distally, secondary to narrowing across the occlusion site and in some cases to ischemia-induced vasodilation in the distal vascular bed (Fig. 23-3).

Physiology of flow pressures[3]

Segmental blood pressure measurement in the limb is the basis of the Doppler examination in the extremities. To understand what happens, the examiner must understand some basic physiology of blood flow dynamics.

Poiseuille's law pertains to pressure gradients of fluids through arterial segments in the body. Two factors determine the flow: (1) the pressure difference across the segment and (2) the resistance of the segment. Poiseuille's law is stated as the following equation:

$$\Delta P = Q8Lv/\pi r^4$$

where the flow, Q, as determined by the length of the segment, L, viscosity of the blood, v, and radius of the segment, r, varies directly with the pressure gradient, ΔP, across the segment and indirectly with the resistance (interaction of L, v, and r) across it. ($8/\pi$ is a mathematical constant.) This can best be applied physiologically to arteries in which the pressure gradient across the segment can be increased by increasing the flow through the segment or decreasing the radius of the lumen.

When obstructions are present, blood is forced through collateral channels, where the resistance is higher than in the normal vessel (Fig. 23-4). Thus, as flow is forced around the obstruction and into collaterals, the pressure drop along that segment is increased. This information is important for the arterial Doppler examination since the examiner must be aware of pressure drops that can occur and must understand the mechanism of the pressure drop distal to an occlusive site.

Doppler lower extremity arterial examination

Arterial anatomy of the lower extremities.[16]
To understand the Doppler lower extremity examination, one needs to have a thorough knowledge of the vascular anatomy as it pertains to the Doppler examination. Only the arteries that are directly accessible and that figure into the examination will be discussed.

Flow to the extremities comes from the *abdominal aorta*. The aorta bifurcates about the level of the umbilicus to form the *common iliac* arteries. The common iliac vessels then bifurcate into the *internal* and *external iliac* arteries. The internal iliac (hypogastric) supplies the buttock and genital area. The external iliac supplies the leg and becomes the *common femoral* artery at approximately the level of the inguinal ligament. Several branches are given off, of which the *profunda*

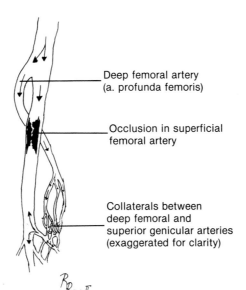

Deep femoral artery (a. profunda femoris)

Occlusion in superficial femoral artery

Collaterals between deep femoral and superior genicular arteries (exaggerated for clarity)

Fig. 23-4. Diagram of recovery in a segment distal to a superficial femoral occlusion due to collateralization from the profunda femoris.

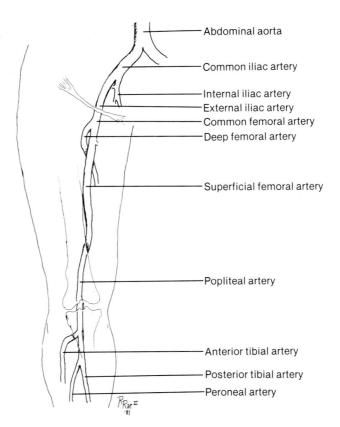

Abdominal aorta
Common iliac artery
Internal iliac artery
External iliac artery
Common femoral artery
Deep femoral artery
Superficial femoral artery
Popliteal artery
Anterior tibial artery
Posterior tibial artery
Peroneal artery

Fig. 23-5. Arterial blood supply to the lower extremity.

femoris is the most important. It comes off about 2 to 5 cm below the inguinal ligament and supplies the bone and muscles of the thigh.

At this point the common femoral becomes the *superficial femoral* artery. It runs along the medial surface of the thigh and curves posteriorly behind the knee to become the *popliteal* artery.

The popliteal artery continues behind the knee joint and gives off the *anterior tibial*

artery 3 to 6 cm below the popliteal fossa. The popliteal then terminates as the *posterior tibial* and *peroneal* arteries (Fig. 23-5).

The anterior tibial descends through muscles along the tibia and becomes the *dorsalis pedis* at the level of the ankle. The dorsalis pedis then runs superficially and dorsally on the medial side of the foot to terminate in the deep plantar arch between the first and second metatarsals.

The posterior tibial artery descends along

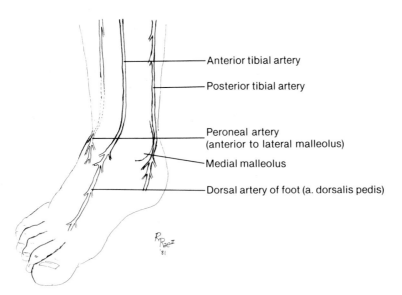

Fig. 23-6. Arteries at the ankle that are accessible to the Doppler probe.

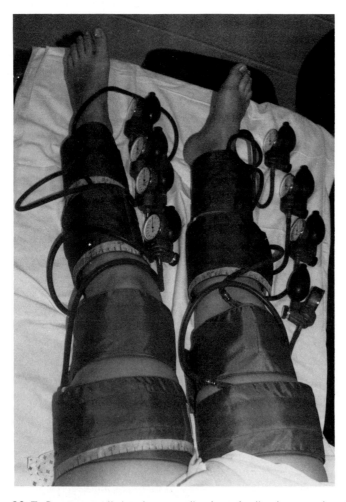

Fig. 23-7. Pressure cuffs in place on the legs for the lower extremity arterial study.

the posterior surface of the tibia to run posterior to the medial malleolus.

The peroneal artery descends deeply on the fibular side of the leg and becomes accessible anterior to the lateral malleolus (Fig. 23-6).

Routine lower extremity arterial examination. There are several points that should be emphasized in connection with this examination.

The first step is to obtain as complete a history as possible from the patient, the patient's chart, or both. The emphasis should be placed on the following information:

1. If the patient is *claudicating*, note whether one or both legs are affected, where the pain is felt (calf, thigh, hip, etc.), and if it is a tiring or a cramp in the muscle. The distance the patient can ambulate prior to stopping because of the pain should be noted and whether the symptoms are relieved by rest.
2. Palpate the *pulses* at the femoral, popliteal, posterior tibial, and dorsalis pedis arteries. Weak or absent pulses should be noted.
3. Check for *night cramping* or *rest pain*.
4. Note the *skin color and condition*. Check for dry skin, erythema of the toes, thickened nails, gangrenous spots, and unhealed ulcers.
5. Check for *known vascular diseases, past bypass surgeries, diabetes, cardiac disease, smoking, hypertension*, and *family history*.

Blood pressure cuffs are then applied to the legs for measuring the pressure gradients. The cuffs are placed in four locations on each leg: one on the *ankle*, one just below the knee on the *calf*, one just above the knee on the *lower thigh*, and one just below the groin on the *upper thigh* (Fig. 23-7).

The main requirement is that the cuffs be long enough to wrap around the patient's legs. Narrow cuffs should be used for the thigh pressures despite the higher-than-normal pressure readings that can be expected there. An aneroid manometer should be attached to each cuff or a friction or Luer-Lok type of fitting installed to permit easy transfer of the manometer from cuff to cuff.

When the four cuffs have been placed on the legs, another one is placed on the arm to take a brachial blood pressure.

The brachial artery is examined at its site on the medial side of the antecubital fossa, and the probe is angled cephalad until the most satisfactory signal is obtained. A tracing is made of the Doppler signal. With the probe still in place, the cuff is inflated above the point at which the signal disappears. It is then deflated about 2 to 4 mm/sec until the systolic pulse is heard. This breakthrough point is the systolic pressure. Deflation continues until the fourth returning sound corresponding to the diastolic antegrade component on the waveform is heard and the flow resumes its normal pattern. The point where the "slurred" sound of the third and fourth component is heard marks the diastolic pressure. Recording the pulse tracing is not necessary but can help the examiner locate the point where the flow resumes its normal pattern until proficiency or "ear training" is attained. For purposes of the Doppler examination, recording the diastolic pressure is not necessary since the systolic pressure is the only component needed for calculation of the ankle/brachial index.

The foregoing steps are repeated for the other arm. The examiner then should move to the patient's feet to commence examination of the ankle arteries and pressures.

The posterior tibial artery is monitored and recorded at its site posterior to the medial malleolus. The probe is angled until the strongest signal is obtained. It is then kept in place, and the ankle cuff is inflated past the point where the signal disappears. Deflation begins until the systolic signal is heard, and the pressure at that point is recorded (Fig. 23-8).

The examiner then moves the probe to examine the dorsalis pedis at its sites on the dorsum of the foot. Once again, the best signal is obtained and an ankle pressure is recorded in the same manner as for the posterior tibial artery (Fig. 23-9).

Before continuing, the examiner should compare waveforms and pressures of the two arteries. The artery with the higher pressure should be used to take the remaining pressures in the leg.

If flow in either the dorsalis pedis or the posterior tibial artery is unsatisfactory or absent, the peroneal artery should be examined at its site anterior to the lateral malleolus. It is examined in the same manner as were the other ankle vessels.

The artery that is selected is then monitored. Each cuff from calf to upper thigh is inflated and deflated in turn, and the systolic blood pressure taken at each level. It is not necessary to record a tracing from the artery while the pressures are being taken. It *is* a must, however, to keep the probe stationary and motionless to prevent the systolic signal from being lost as the cuff is deflated.

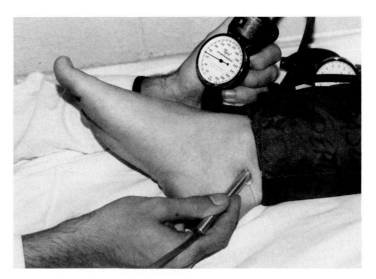

Fig. 23-8. Examining the posterior tibial artery.

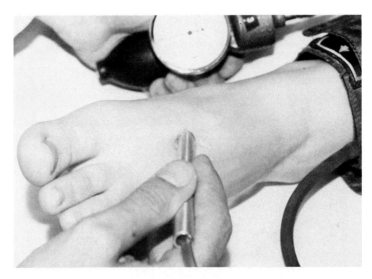

Fig. 23-9. Examining the dorsalis pedis.

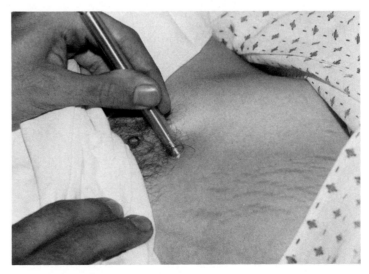

Fig. 23-10. Examining the common femoral artery.

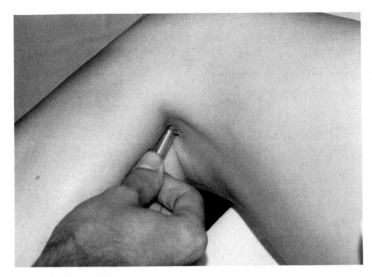

Fig. 23-11. Supine examination of the popliteal artery.

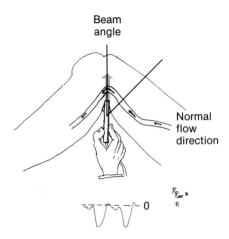

Fig. 23-12. Diagram showing how improper probe placement can cause a false reading of retrograde or diminished flow if the beam is not angled against the flow of the vessel.

When the tracings and pressures from one extremity have been taken, the procedure is repeated for the other.

After pressures have been taken at all cuff sites in both legs, the cuffs are removed. The examiner then palpates the superior border of the inguinal ligament and places the probe in position just above the ligament to determine the site for monitoring of the femoral artery (Fig. 23-10). The external iliac is actually being monitored at this level rather than the common femoral. It is better to obtain the signal here, however, than to listen below the ligament, where the bifurcation of the profunda femoris can cause confusion. The common femoral arteries are then monitored and recorded bilaterally. Some pressure on the probe may be needed to obtain a clear signal. The signals will be found lateral to the common femoral venous signals (heard as a "windstorm" sound). An arterial signal found *medial* to the vein is probably the hypogastric artery and must not be mistaken for the femoral. If in doubt, move the probe laterally and medially to locate the vein and determine the vessel's relationship. The hypogastric also may appear as a retrograde signal when the probe is angled cephalad.

The popliteal arteries are next to be examined and are found at their sites behind the knees. There are two methods of examining the popliteal arteries: *supine* and *prone.*

In the supine position the patient's knees are bent to a 90-degree angle and the probe is placed in the popliteal fossa and angled cephalad (Fig. 23-11). An ample quantity of gel is required to ensure good probe-skin contact. Firm pressure may be needed to displace fat and tissue. Be careful not to occlude

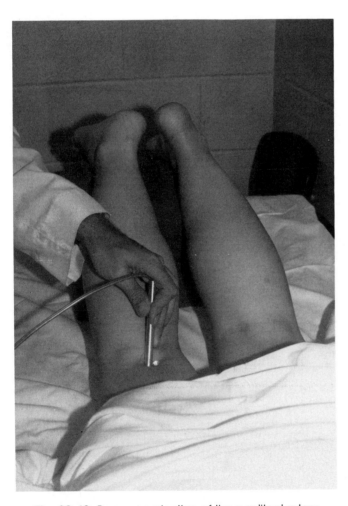

Fig. 23-13. Prone examination of the popliteal artery.

the artery. The probe should be angled to obtain the clearest signal with distinct waveform patterns. This segment of the study requires an accurate tracing, for the popliteal signal may be the determining factor in decisions as to whether an occlusion exists above the knee or in the trifurcation vessels below the knee. The best signal is obtained with the probe more toward the calf than toward the knee, to avoid catching the flow at an angle that could suggest occluded flow or even retrograde flow in the artery (Fig. 23-12).

In the prone position the patient's legs are elevated 30 to 45 degrees and are supported with a bolster or pillow (Fig. 23-13). The same basic examination technique is used as in the supine position, and the probe is angled cephalad. The advantage of this position is the ability actually to see the relationship of the popliteal fossa and the probe. It is a good position to use for the examiner-in-training.

I have found that both positions give excellent results. A major advantage of the supine position is that the patient does not need to move after the initial portion of the examination has been completed. This is especially beneficial to the postoperative or invalid patient who cannot turn over. The choice of examination positions is best left to the examiner's preference.

In summary, these are the steps in the lower extremity arterial examination:

1. Take the patient's history, with emphasis on symptoms and past vascular disease and surgery.
2. With the patient supine, place blood pressure cuffs over the ankles, calves, lower thighs, and upper thighs bilaterally.
3. Apply cuffs to the upper arms and take bilateral brachial tracings and blood pressures.
4. Take tracings and systolic pressures from the dorsalis pedis and posterior tibial arteries at the ankle. Use the artery with the higher ankle pressure to take segmental pressures from the rest of the leg.
5. Obtain systolic pressures sequentially from the calf, lower thigh, and upper thigh cuffs in the artery selected.
6. Examine the other leg, repeating steps 4 and 5, and remove the cuffs.
7. Check the common femoral arteries and make tracings bilaterally.
8. With the patient either supine or prone, check and record the popliteal artery pressures.

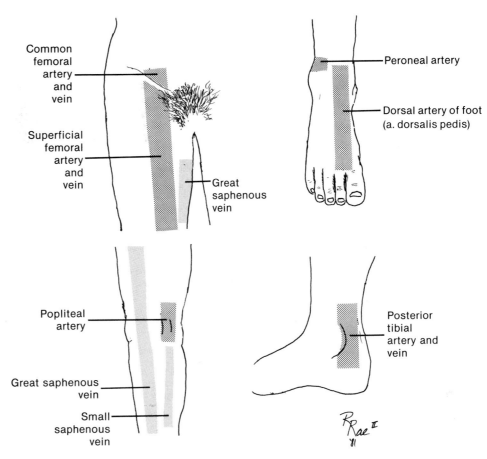

Fig. 23-14. Sites where both arterial and venous signals can be obtained in the lower extremity.

9. (Optional) If there is a loss of triphasicity between the femoral and popliteal sites, examination of the superficial femoral artery may be made at its sites in the midportion of the thigh.
10. Mount the tracings and calculate the ankle/brachial indices.

Fig. 23-14 shows the probe sites for both arterial and venous Doppler examinations. Examples of normal and abnormal examinations can be seen in the illustrative case section.

Interpretation of the lower extremity arterial examination. To determine the flow status of the extremities, one must calculate ratios of the ankle systolic pressures divided by the brachial systolic pressures. The *ankle/brachial index* is thus obtained. The higher systolic pressure of the two arteries examined at the ankle is divided by the higher systolic pressure of the two arms. This is done for each leg. The higher brachial pressure should be used for both legs to ensure uniformity.

In normal individuals the ankle/brachial index should be greater than 1.00. Patients who are asymptomatic or with slight symptoms will have indices from 0.90 to 1.00. Patients with claudication show indices of 0.50 to 0.90. Anything less than 0.50 implies rest pain or gangrene.[3,6]

My own experience with follow-up studies has shown that in normal individuals the ankle/brachial index can vary from 0.85 to as much as 1.10. This factor seems to depend on the relative blood pressure that a patient may have on the day of examination and whether it may change between the time the arm is checked and when the ankle pressures are taken. Therefore the examiner and interpreting physician should not expect the same index in a normal patient to be completely reproducible from examination to examination and should be aware that a lower index may not imply disease if a strong triphasic signal is found.

It should also be noted that patients with calcific arteries will often have abnormally or unusually high ankle/brachial indices, such as 1.20 to 3.00. In these individuals the quality of the waveform is the best indicator of occlusion since the vessels are incompressible. Patients with extremely obese legs or diabetes also may have abnormally high indices.[8]

Further information about the circulation may be obtained by comparison of the segmental pressures. In a normal patient there will usually be no greater than 40 mm Hg of difference between any two cuffs. The pressure reading will increase as the circumference of the extremity increases. An accurate pressure at the thigh could be obtained only with an extremely wide cuff but it is unnecessary for Doppler readings since the difference *between* cuffs is used as an indicator of a pressure drop. The upper thigh pressure should not exceed 50 mm Hg above the brachial pressure.

As mentioned, extremely high pressures (as in noncompressible arteries or other situations with pressures >300 mm Hg) in the ankle or calf imply a calcified segment. This should be noted on the report form so there will be no confusion during interpretation.

If an upper thigh pressure is significantly *less* than the brachial pressure, this implies iliac artery occlusion.

If there is a significant pressure drop between the lower and upper thigh cuffs, this implies a superficial femoral artery obstruction.

If there is a significant pressure drop between the lower thigh and calf cuffs, a popliteal artery occlusion is implied.

If there is a significant pressure drop between the ankle and calf cuffs, this implies occlusion of the anterior tibial, posterior tibial, or peroneal arteries.

A normal arterial signal will be triphasic. Diminution or loss of any of the components implies obstruction proximal to the probe site. If flow is triphasic at the ankle, it must be triphasic at all sites above the ankle. The absence of a triphasic pattern in the popliteal artery in the presence of a normal triphasic pattern in the femoral and ankle areas implies technical error, and the artery should be rechecked.

Following is a guide to interpretation of the waveforms in cases of disease:

1. If the waveforms are triphasic in the femoral, popliteal, dorsalis pedis, and posterior tibial arteries, the flow in the leg is within normal limits.
2. If the waveforms are triphasic in the femoral and popliteal but biphasic or monophasic in either of the ankle vessels where the other is triphasic, the abnormal artery is likely the only one diseased.
3. If flow is triphasic in the femoral and popliteal but biphasic or monophasic in both ankle arteries, there is likely disease below the popliteal involving the trifurcation vessels.
4. If flow is triphasic in the femoral but biphasic or monophasic at the popliteal and ankle vessels, this implies superficial femoral artery stenoses or occlusions. Examination of the proximal and distal superficial femoral artery can help locate the level of obstruction.
5. Finally, biphasic or monophasic flow at the femoral and all sites below implies an iliac artery occlusion.

The use of segmental pressures compared to the waveform readout and audible information is quite accurate in helping to determine the relative flow status of the extremity. However, errors in interpretation can occur and are often the result of poor examination technique. The next section will discuss these problems.

False-positive conditions and their rectification

Absent signal. The Doppler signal may be absent in cases of extreme atherosclerosis obliterans. The examiner must be aware, however, that absence of flow should not be observed in patients with strong pulses. The probe site should be rechecked and a careful search made for the artery by slowly moving the probe laterally and medially. Care must also be taken that an even but not extreme amount of pressure is being applied; otherwise, the vessel may be occluded by the force on the probe. Careful examination is often required to register flow when there is not enough pressure in the segment to create a palpable pulse. One suggestion is to apply a generous amount of acoustic couplant to the skin at the various probe sites along the arterial segment and place the probe within the mound of gel without actually touching the skin. The gel acts as an acoustic path, thereby allowing minimal flow information to be obtained without inadvertent pressure on the artery being examined, which might occlude it.

False diagnosis of biphasic or monophasic flow at the popliteal site. This is most often due to poor technique and is usually noticed because the femoral and ankle arteries exhibit normal triphasic flow. Precise positioning of the probe, careful pressure judgment, moving the probe more toward the calf than toward the thigh, and angling cephalad with respect to the course of the artery should resolve this problem. If in doubt, another attempt should be made.

False diagnosis of biphasic or monophasic flow at the femoral site. This occurs when triphasic signals are found in the distal vessels in the postsurgical or obese patient. It is due to fatty tissue or scarring in the groin. The probe should be moved lateral to the vein and placed on either side of the scar, or with the fat held back out of the way. Angling medially or laterally into the desired area should give good results. Remember also that the beam should be 45 degrees to the *flow*, not to the skin surface. If it is impossible to obtain an accurate signal above the ligament, the report form should be noted to that effect and the proximal segment of the superficial femoral artery away from the profunda bifurcation should be obtained.

False diagnosis of retrograde flow in a major limb artery. This occurs when the beam is angled through a segment at a point where flow is perceived as receding from the probe. In the femoral region the hypogastric artery can be wrongly monitored medial to the common femoral vein. The probe should be moved lateral to the vein for the correct signal. This can also occur if the probe is angled incorrectly. In the popliteal area the probe should be moved toward the calf to allow the beam to intersect flow at the correct angle (see Fig. 23-12).

False reversal in the posterior tibial artery and the dorsalis pedis occurs most often when flow below the knee is so reduced that pulsatility nearly vanishes and the accompanying vein sounds are mistaken for those from the artery. Careful listening is necessary to detect any trace of a pulse. The vein can be ruled out by squeezing the fleshy part of the foot and listening for a rush of flow, which will not occur in the artery.

There are several other factors that must be constantly checked to maintain accuracy. The probes must be monitored periodically for wire and electric damage, epoxy decay, or crystal damage. Manometers and cuffs should be calibrated and checked for leakage every 2 or 3 weeks.

For the examiner, concentration is required as well as practice at keeping the probe in place with one hand while inflating and releasing the cuff with the other. Cultivation of ambidextrous independence is useful to provide flexibility. Maintaining constant probe position also should be practiced to avoid losing the signal during cuff inflation and release. Experience and practice are the best ways to develop the examination technique.

Doppler examination of the postoperative patient. This section will deal with the variations in the examination needed to provide adequate results in the patient who has recently undergone vascular surgery.

The basic format of the routine examination is adhered to. The brachial arteries are examined as in the routine examination unless an arterial monitor line or IV prevents it.

One of the two arms is required for the ankle/brachial index determination, especially since the success or failure of the surgery often depends on the results obtained by the examiner. Again, either the higher of the two arm pressures or the single arm pressure is utilized.

The history is taken, and the type of surgery and graft material (either the patient's own vein or a synthetic) is noted. If possible, a drawing of the surgical connections should be made for future reference if included in the chart, showing the vessels that were resected and/or ligated, the levels where the graft is attached to the artery, and the course of the graft in the extremity.

There are many different types of grafts and graft materials.* Their purpose is to shunt the main blood flow around the obstructed area to the patent sections of the artery at a lower level. Fig. 23-15 illustrates several of the most common bypasses in the lower limb.

Types of grafts and the surgical conditions for which they are used include the following:

1. *Aortoiliac.* Commonly a synthetic bifurcated graft, employed in cases of abdominal aortal aneurysm at the bifurcation of the common iliac arteries
2. *Aortofemoral.* Also synthetic, either unilateral or bilateral, used to bypass iliac obstructions or aneurysms extending past the common iliac regions
3. *Femorofemoral.* Synthetic, placed subcutaneously across the lower abdomen to shunt flow from a patent femoral to a point distal to the obstruction in the opposite femoral artery
4. *Femoropopliteal.* Synthetic or autogenous saphenous vein; in the latter case the patient's own great or small saphenous vein is removed and sutured into place around superficial femoral obstructions
5. *Femorotibial.* Same materials as in the femoropopliteal graft, but insertion is in either the anterior or the posterior tibial arteries; it is passed subcutaneously on the medial surface of the leg and may be palpated easily at the knee area; used to bypass obstructions extending through the popliteal artery and/or involving the trifurcation vessels
6. *Femoroperoneal.* Used in the same circumstances as the femorotibial graft but may be passed through the popliteal fossa rather than the medial side of the knee

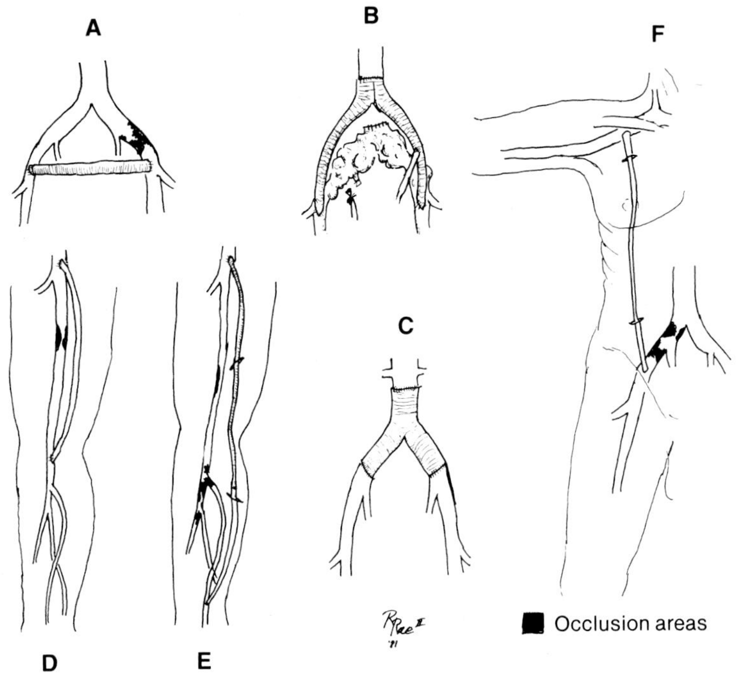

Fig. 23-15. Various types of bypass graft operations. **A,** Femorofemoral. **B,** Aortofemoral. **C,** Aortoiliac. **D,** Femoropopliteal. **E,** Femorotibial. **F,** Axillofemoral.

7. *Axillofemoral.* Rarely performed although occasionally encountered; usually synthetic, passed from the axillary artery subcutaneously across the chest and lower abdomen to the ipsilateral femoral artery; can also be palpated along its length

There are many variations on these methods.[7] To avoid confusion, the examiner should be aware of the extent and exact type of surgery performed.

There is a definite rule to follow in postoperative examination: *Never put a pressure cuff over a graft, whether new or old, because you might occlude the graft.* It is far safer to use just the ankle and calf cuffs or just the ankle cuff if the graft extends that far down (as in femorotibial bypasses). Only the ankle pressure is required for the ankle/brachial index. The use of segmental cuffs is not actually necessary since in most patients a prior examination or arteriogram will have been given to confirm the occlusion preoperatively. If the patient has undergone an endarterectomy or embolectomy rather than a bypass, the same guidelines should be observed.

The procedure is as follows:

1. Monitor and record the brachial artery pressures. If one arm has an arterial line or IV in it, use the other arm for taking blood pressures.
2. Place pressure cuffs on the ankles and calves (ankles only if the patient has received a femorotibial graft).

3. Routinely take tracings and pressures from the ankle arteries.
4. Remove the cuffs and take tracings from the femoral or superficial femoral arteries. If a dressing prevents a site from being examined, note this on the report form.
5. Take popliteal tracings if dressings and conditions permit. In case of a femorotibial bypass, record the signal at the medial side of the knee since the graft is superficial and subcutaneous.

The tracings are mounted. Any pertinent comments noted are included with the examination.

Examination of the patient after percutaneous transluminal angioplasty. Many obstructive cases have been found to be of a nature that does not necessarily indicate bypass surgery as the only method of relief. When the plaque is soft and atheromatous, a recent technique known as percutaneous transluminal angioplasty may be utilized. This involves methods similar to those used for arteriography; special catheters, fluoroscopic guidance, and contrast injections are needed. A catheter designed by Dr. A. Gruntzig (formerly in Switzerland, now at Emory University in Atlanta) is used that has a balloon in its tip with the boundaries marked radiopaquely. This balloon catheter is threaded through the artery along a guide wire to the point of obstruction or stenosis. It is then threaded through the obstructed section until the balloon lies along the area

---

*References 4, 7, 11, 18, 22.

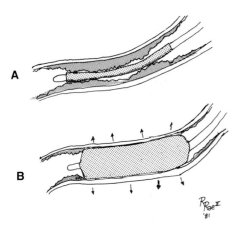

Fig. 23-16. Percutaneous transluminal angioplasty. **A,** Positioning the balloon along the diseased segment. **B,** Inflation of the balloon and dispersion of the plaque.

marked for dilation. The balloon is inflated to a pressure of 5 atm. This compresses and disperses the plaque against the arterial walls, where it is absorbed (Fig. 23-16). The method does not work well with calcific, severe, or multiple obstructions; bypassing is indicated in these cases.

The Doppler examination after angioplasty does not differ from the normal examination, except that thigh cuffs and tracings in the region of the catheterization site may be omitted if the patient is feeling tenderness in that area.

Examination of the patient with a false-negative diagnosis. Occasionally the examiner will encounter a patient who presents with the typical symptoms of lower extremity claudication (often severely) but has normal tracings and indices. This type of symptomatic patient is difficult to evaluate, for the pain and claudication present only with exercise. The symptoms often are due to a neuropathic rather than a vascular disorder.

In these patients frequently the exercise or hyperemic test will determine whether or not obstruction is present. The main aim is to increase demand for blood flow in the extremity either with exercising the patient on a treadmill or by inducing hyperemia through transient application of a tourniquet (inflated blood pressure cuff). The intention in both cases is to recreate or simulate the conditions that bring on the claudication and then measure the amount of time required for normal flow patterns to resume.

Although there are many current attitudes concerning the treadmill versus the hyperemic test,[14,20,31] I will discuss both without attempting to prove one over the other. The final decision will be left to individual opinion, and further reading is encouraged on these subjects.

Physiologic responses to exercise.[3,21] The normal response to exercise in the leg is a demand for increased blood flow in the muscular vascular bed, causing a decreased vascular resistance. Flow is increased in the main arteries of the leg, and an adequate oxygen supply is thus provided. The normal muscular metabolism is maintained, as is the flow pattern.

In cases of obstruction, however, exercise results in the same demand for blood in the vascular bed and decreased resistance but the obstructed vessels and collaterals cannot supply enough blood to meet the demand. The pressure in the major arteries (including the ankle arteries) drops, and the waveform diminishes. Metabolic waste products accumulate, causing the pain, cramping, and muscle tiring of claudication.

Doppler treadmill examination. The criteria and examination techniques quoted here are based on information given by Barnes et al.[3]

The Doppler treadmill examination requires a stopwatch, three pressure cuffs, and a treadmill set for a constant load of 2 mph at a 12% grade.

Brachial and ankle systolic pressures are taken, as in the routine examination, and recorded. The patient keeps the ankle cuffs in place and walks on the treadmill for 5 minutes or until claudication forces him to stop. He should tell the examiner where and when pain is noticed and then walk until he would normally stop because of the pain.

At the end of 5 minutes, or when the patients reaches his tolerance limit, the treadmill is stopped and the patient resumes the supine position. The arm with the higher pressure and both ankle pressures are taken and recorded at 1, 2, 4, 6, 10, 15, and 20 minutes following the exercise. Ankle pressures are usually taken until either the preexercise pressure or the time limit is reached.

It should be noted that experience with patients with neuropathic etiologies has shown a return to normal pressures and waveforms within the first minute following exercise, making the first time measurement on the scale of Barnes et al.[3] almost unusable. The severely obstructed or neuropathic patient may take longer than 2 minutes to recover, but the preexercise level is reached usually in less time. Shorter intervals may be required for determining the recovery rate within the first minute after exercise.

If an ECG treadmill examination is also performed, it is often advantageous to do the Doppler treadmill simultaneously; but cardiac and respiratory factors may not allow the patient to lie quickly supine, especially if the heart rate is being evaluated.[3]

Doppler hyperemic postocclusion examination. This method requires the thigh and ankle cuffs and is often performed after the routine Doppler resting examination.

Instead of ambulation, the patient rests supine and the femoral artery is occluded at the upper thigh to simulate exercise and induce metabolic changes. This examination is advantageous when the patient is unable to walk.

Pressure cuffs are placed bilaterally on the ankles and high thighs, and the brachial pressure is taken and recorded. The higher of the two systolic arm pressures is again used for the ankle/brachial indices. One leg is examined at a time.

Before the thigh cuff is inflated, a preocclusive resting waveform and ankle pressure should be taken in the ankle vessels and recorded. The artery with the higher pressure is used for the examination. The probe is held in place, and the thigh cuff is inflated well above the point at which the signal disappears. The pump is then locked off, and the stopwatch is started. It is important to monitor the artery and maintain the occlusive pressure for 3 minutes. After that time, the thigh pressure is released all at once and an immediate waveform and ankle pressure are taken and recorded. Waveforms and pressures are continually taken every 15 seconds until the artery reaches its preocclusion pressure and waveform pattern. The technique is repeated for the other extremity.

Most patients will resume normal pressures and waveforms within 15 to 30 seconds. The individual pressures at each interval are divided by the brachial pressure to give sequential ankle/brachial indices up to the preocclusion level. Normal ratios taken immediately after occlusion should be above 0.80. Lower indices or longer recovery times imply neurologic or obstructive disease.

The disadvantages to this method include possible probe slippage during the occlusive period, intolerance of high thigh cuff pressure by some individuals, and varying results depending on the examiner's ability to take tracings and cuff pressures one after the other every 15 seconds. This examination also fails to work on patients with obese thighs or noncompressible arteries.

There are other methods of hyperemic and treadmill testing as well as studies that have used treadles pumped by the patient in a supine position. However, the results are similar to those reported; reports are available in current journals.[8,12,20,31]

Doppler penile blood flow test. Recently studies have been undertaken to show that impotence is not always psychologic but is often physical in nature. Tests have shown that many patients with arteriosclerotic vascular disease present with reduced or non-existant sexual function. Doppler has been a great aid in the noninvasive diagnosis of physical impotence due to impaired blood flow.

Blood to the penis comes from the right and left cavernosal (profunda) arteries, the right and left dorsal arteries, and the right and left spongiosal arteries. These branches of the internal pudendal arteries arise from their respective internal iliac arteries[16,24] (Fig. 23-17).

The dorsal arteries have no part in the erectile function and lie superficially on the dorsum of the penis.[24] The cavernosal arteries run through the center of their respective corpora cavernosa. During sexual arousal, if either or both arteries are occluded, a reduced amount of blood will pool in the corpus and erection of the occluded sides will not occur. "Lopsided" erections result.

The penile Doppler examination begins with a history obtained as in the lower extremity examination, with attention paid to claudication and arterial insufficiency symptoms. Buttock cramping is often a sign of internal iliac occlusion.

Next, a specific set of questions is asked pertaining to the patient's impotence[24]:

1. Is he able to obtain and maintain erections, and are they full or partial?
2. Do positional changes or activity cause a loss of function?
3. How long has the dysfunction been occurring, especially if it coincides with the onset of claudication?
4. Does erection occur upon waking up, and does it disappear with urination?
5. Does he have spontaneous nocturnal erections?
6. How is his libido?
7. Is he able to ejaculate?
8. Is there a history of diabetes? What about alcohol intake? What medications is he presently taking?

The patient first should receive a routine lower extremity examination to determine the state of his limb circulation.

When the lower extremity examination is completed, a small digit cuff is placed around the base of the penis. It should be strong enough to withstand pressures greater than 250 mm Hg and have extra-strong Velcro fastenings to prevent its coming undone. A regular manometer is used with the cuff.

For purposes of hygiene the examiner should wear rubber gloves during the examination. Gel is applied to the probe sites and the vessels are monitored.

The cavernosal vessels are examined close to the glans of the penis bilaterally (Fig. 23-18). When an adequate tracing is obtained, the cuff is slowly inflated to the point at which the signal is obliterated. The examiner should note the ponit where the flow *disappears* rather than the point where it returns when the cuff is let down. This is done three times, and the pressure is obtained by averaging the three readings.

The dorsal arteries may next be examined by checking their sites carefully on the dorsum of the penis. Pressures are taken as with the cavernosal arteries. It should be mentioned that the dorsal arteries are not involved in the erection mechanism and are not diagnostic in determining vasculogenic impotence.[24] Flow decrease in these arteries should not be considered significant if the arteries are patent and show good pressure indices.

Interpretation of the penile examination. A penile/brachial index is obtained by dividing the systolic brachial pressure into the averaged pressure for each artery. On the basis of studies performed by various vascular laboratories, an index of less than 0.86 is significant of vascular impotence.[24] Current studies also show that a variety of normal waveforms exist in the penile arteries and that monophasic and biphasic waveforms should not be automatically interpreted as diseased.[16]

Arteriovenous fistulas. An arteriovenous (A-V) fistula is an abnormal direct communication between an artery and an adjacent vein. A-V fistulas can be either congenital or acquired.[3] *Congenital* A-V fistulas involve multiple communications with arteries and veins in a specific area of the body and are present at birth. *Acquired* A-V fistulas are localized communications that may have been caused by trauma, aneurysmal erosion, or infection.[10,23]

A-V fistulas are also classified by size. *Microfistulas* are too small to be seen with the naked eye. *Macrofistulas* are readily seen.[3]

The flow dynamics of the A-V fistulas are extremely complicated, involving turbulence and cross channeling of oxygenated and non-oxygenated blood between the two systems (Fig. 23-19). Physical symptoms in the extremities usually consist of swelling, purplish discoloration, pallor, palpable thrills and bruits, and pain. The limb may or may not become incapacitated and may possibly de-

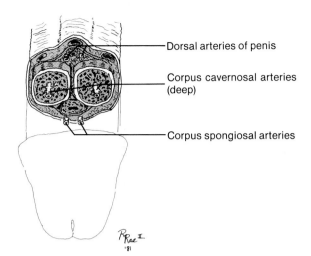

Fig. 23-17. Arterial blood supply to the penis.

Dorsal arteries of penis

Corpus cavernosal arteries (deep)

Corpus spongiosal arteries

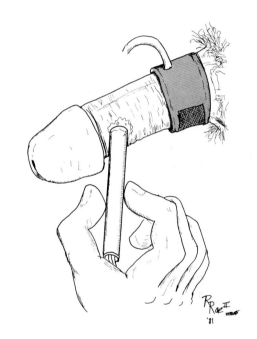

Fig. 23-18. Examination of the cavernosal arteries.

velop ischemia depending on the extent of the fistula.

By using the Doppler, one can map out the major arterial and venous pathways to show areas of increased turbulence and changes in flow dynamics. A characteristic Doppler examination may show signs of turbulence, monophasic and biphasic flow in arteries, retrograde flow in arteries due to collaterals and venous connections, absence of flow in a major vessel, pulsatile flow in a vein, etc. These may occur individually or in combination.

Surgical intervention is almost always required,[10,23] with amputation often being necessary in severely affected limbs. Because of the extensive network found in patients with congenital A-V fistulas, individual liga-

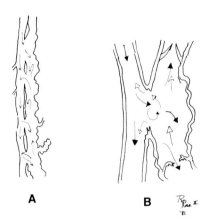

A   **B**

Fig. 23-19. Arteriovenous fistulas. **A,** Multiple connections in a congenital malformation. **B,** Flow dynamics occurring in an A-V fistula. Arterial flow *(black arrows)* progresses partly through the arterial segment and partly through the fistula to move either antegrade or retrograde in the vein. The pressure can destroy the valves in the distal venous segment and create insufficiency in the veins. Venous flow *(white arrows)* can also enter the arterial segment and disrupt the flow of oxygenated blood to the distal arterial branches.

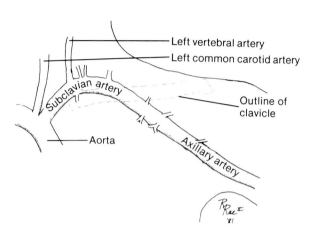

Fig. 23-20. Arteries of the upper extremity from the aorta to the axilla.

tion of the site is usually impractical and nearly impossible. Microfistulas pose the biggest problem in this regard. A recent technique that has had varying success is therapeutic embolization, which involves injecting a saline solution of tiny sponge balls (Ivalon or other materials) into the main connecting arteries. The suspension travels to the various fistula points and occludes them, sealing many of the more threatening connections and allowing easier ligation or revascularization.

The general technique for Doppler examination of a patient with suspected or known A-V fistulas will vary with the individual. The best approach is to bear the following criteria in mind:

1. Collateral channels may exist that shunt flow around a fistula and cause retrograde flow in a given segment immediately distal to the fistula.
2. Venous valves will become incompetent. Thus flow will be reversed in the venous segment *distal* to the fistula and may mimic arterial flow, whereas it will be continuous in the *proximal* venous segment.
3. Manual occlusion of the fistula will cause flow in the distal arterial segment to resume normal characteristics.
4. If the standard Doppler extremity examination is performed, there will be a pressure drop distal to the fistula.

Knowledge of these characteristics will facilitate discrimination among A-V fistulas.

An example of a congenital A-V fistula in the upper extremity can be found in Appendix I.

Doppler upper extremity arterial examination

The Doppler examination of the upper extremities is performed in a manner similar to the examination of the lower extremities. It is not done as frequently as the lower extremity examination, but it is important that the examiner be familiar with these techniques since many of them are used in cooperation with the Doppler cerebrovascular examination.

Arterial anatomy of the upper extremities.[16] This section will cover Doppler-related anatomy in the upper extremity and upper thorax.

The *subclavian artery* is the first major artery to arise from the *aortic arch.* It has a different origin on each side. On the *right* it arises from the *brachiocephalic (innominate) artery,* and on the *left* directly from the aortic arch.

The first branch of the subclavian artery is the *vertebral artery.* Its anatomy will be discussed in more detail in the cerebrovascular anatomy section.

Many other arteries are given off between the arch and the shoulder. At the level of the first rib, the subclavian becomes the *axillary* artery. The axillary artery tends to run superficially through the axilla and then slightly more deeply at the tendon of the teres major. Here it becomes the *brachial* artery (Fig. 23-20).

The brachial artery runs medially along the arm to the elbow. Approximately 1 cm distal to the elbow, it bifurcates into the *radial* and *ulnar* arteries.

These continue on to the wrist on the anterior surface of the arm, the radial on the radial side and the ulnar on the ulnar side. The ulnar artery gives off a *medial interosseus branch,* which may occasionally be heard between the radial and ulnar. Each artery passes into the hand and terminates at respective *radial and ulnar palmar arches,* which are connected by collaterals (Fig. 23-21).

Routine upper extremity arterial examination. The equipment needed for the upper extremity examination is the same as for examination of the lower extremities: a directional Doppler device and pressure cuffs.

A thorough history is obtained once again, with emphasis on upper extremity occlusive disease. The classic symptoms consist of claudication of the arm that occurs with lifting objects or holding the arms raised over the head for short periods.[17] The afflicted arm will also feel colder to the touch than the unobstructed arm, and occasionally numbness and discoloration of the fingers will occur. Systolic blood pressures will usually show a discrepancy between the two sides. Microembolic activity can be assumed in cases of digital discoloration when the rest of the arm is normal. Note should be made also of whether the patient notices discoloration with exposure to cold or temperature changes.[7,21]

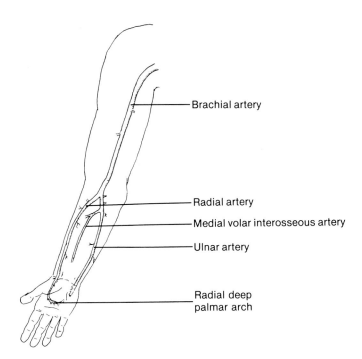

Fig. 23-21. Arteries of the upper extremity from the axilla to the hand.

Brachial artery

Radial artery

Medial volar interosseous artery

Ulnar artery

Radial deep palmar arch

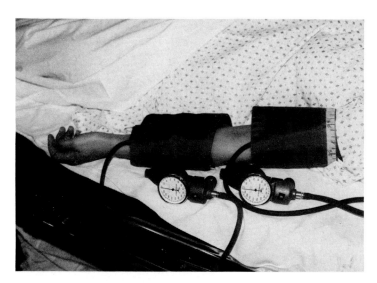

Fig. 23-22. Pressure cuffs in place for the upper extremity arterial study.

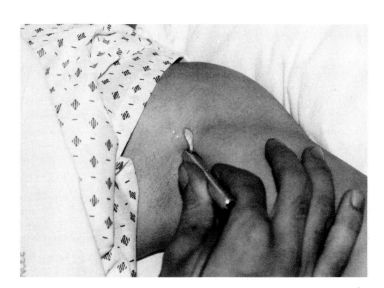

Fig. 23-23. Examination of the axillary artery.

A patient with dizziness accompanying the extremity problems can be suspected of having a subclavian steal syndrome. This is always a possibility when there is a pressure difference of greater than 20 to 40 mm Hg between the two arms.[27,28]

After the history is taken, the patient lies supine. Two pressure cuffs are placed on each arm, one on the *forearm* and one on the *upper arm* (Fig. 23-22).

The brachial artery is the first vessel to be checked. A waveform is recorded and the systolic pressure taken. The examiner then moves down to the wrist and monitors the radial artery and takes a tracing. The probe is kept in place and the arm cuff is inflated past the point at which the signal disappears and is then deflated to obtain the systolic pressure at the point where the signal returns. The examiner then follows the same procedure with the forearm cuff and obtains a forearm pressure.

The probe is then moved to the ulnar artery and the same sequence of tracings with arm and forearm pressures is followed.

Then the examiner monitors the radial artery and compresses the ulnar artery to determine the patency of the palmar arch. Compression is held for four beats and a tracing is made at a slow chart speed to record any changes.

The procedure is repeated, this time monitoring the ulnar artery and compressing the radial artery. The ulnar artery should be recorded for four beats and the radial artery compressed for four beats and then released

for four more. Any audible changes should show up on the tracing as an increase in flow.

The other arm is examined the same way, with the brachial signal recorded and the brachial systolic pressure taken. The radial and ulnar arteries are then examined, with pressures taken, and the palmar arch flow is checked.

The cuffs are removed, and the patient's arms are raised. The examiner locates the axillary artery signal in the axilla (Fig. 23-23) and records the signal with the probe angled cephalad. Both axillary arteries are examined.

The examiner then moves to the head of

the patient, for ease of examination, and monitors the subclavian and vertebral arteries in the supraclavicular fossa. The subclavian artery is located by angling the probe medially and downward in the fossa until a distinct triphasic signal is heard. The clearest signal is then recorded (Fig. 23-24).

The vertebral artery can be heard in a triangle formed by the inferior border of the sternocleidomastoid muscle, the clavicle, and the lateral side of the neck. The probe should be angled downward and medially slightly to just lateral of the sternocleidomastoid until a distinct triphasic signal with a rapid stop at the baseline and a limited pe-

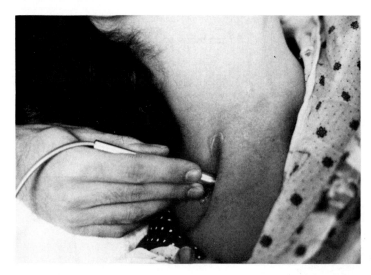

Fig. 23-24. Examination of the subclavian and vertebral arteries.

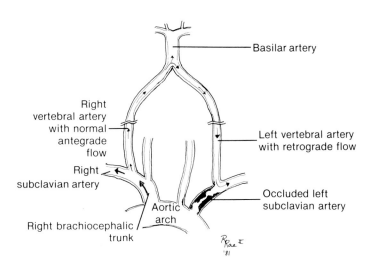

Fig. 23-25. Diagram of the pathway in subclavian steal syndrome.

riod of reversal is heard. (See Appendix I for a normal vertebral tracing.) The subclavian and vertebral arteries should be recorded bilaterally.

When a pressure difference of greater than 20 to 40 mm Hg exists between arms, the examiner must pay careful attention to the direction of the vertebral signal on the side that shows evidence of occlusion. This is a definite indication of subclavian steal syndrome.[27,28]

A subclavian steal occurs when an occlusion develops in one of the subclavian arteries proximal to the vertebral artery. If flow is compromised severely enough, flow from the contralateral patent vertebral will be "stolen" around the vertebrobasilar junction *down* the vertebral on the affected side to the patent portion of the subclavian to supply the arm. Flow is therefore *retrograde* in the vertebral artery on the affected side in this condition (Fig. 23-25). (See the cerebrovascular section, p. 346, for further discussion of vertebrobasilar hemodynamics.)

In vertebral reversal, flow may sound similar to the normal vertebral signal but will be retrograde to the expected direction. The examiner should assume that reversal is real if it is heard on the side with an obstructed subclavian artery rather than suspect an incorrectly placed probe.

Examination for suspected subclavian steal syndrome.[1,28] In a patient presenting with questionably reversed or weak but antegrade vertebral flow, verification should be made as to whether a steal is present. To check for steal syndrome, the examiner has the patient lie supine and places a pressure cuff on the *arm with the occlusion.* The vertebral artery is monitored, with the cuff inflated to at least 50 mm Hg above the systolic

pressure to occlude flow to the arm and induce hyperemia. The monitoring continues with the cuff inflated for 3 minutes. At the end of that time, the cuff pressure is released. The chart recorder should be running prior to release of the cuff to show any changes that occur.

In a patient with vertebral steal a *reversed signal* will *augment* for a short period. An antegrade signal will *momentarily reverse* below the zero line for several beats within the first 5 seconds.

Following is a summary of the steps in the upper extremity arterial examination:

1. Take the patient's history, with emphasis on claudication and numbness of the arm, and note any discoloration or positional problems.
2. Place cuffs bilaterally on the arms and forearms and take a brachial tracing and blood pressure from one arm.
3. Record the radial and ulnar arteries and take pressures at the arm and forearm in each artery.
4. Evaluate the palmar arch by monitoring the radial artery and ulnar artery and compressing the unmonitored vessel while recording to check for flow changes.
5. Examine the other arm using steps 2, 3, and 4.
6. Record both axillary arteries.
7. Examine and record both subclavian arteries in the supraclavicular fossa.
8. Record both vertebral arteries and check the flow direction.
9. If there is evidence of occlusion and a pressure difference of greater than 20 to 40 mm Hg between the two arms, do a subclavian steal examination to rule out vertebral steal.

10. Calculate forearm/brachial indices. Fig. 23-26 shows the probe sites for arterial and venous Doppler examinations. Examples of normal and abnormal upper extremity examinations will be found in Appendix I.

Interpretation of the upper extremity arterial examination. As in the lower extremity examination, the upper extremity flow status is determined with an index of pressures. In the arms the systolic brachial pressure is divided into the higher systolic forearm pressure of the two arteries examined at the wrist for calculation of the *forearm/brachial* index.

The normal patient should have a forearm/brachial index of 1.00 or greater. Indices of less than 1.00 are measured according to the criteria used in the lower extremity ankle/brachial index.[3] (See "Interpretation of the lower extremity arterial examination," p. 331.

A normal upper extremity examination will have triphasic waveforms in the subclavian, axillary, brachial, radial, and ulnar arteries. The vertebral artery may be triphasic or biphasic. Patency of the palmar arch is shown by an augmentation of flow with compression of the ulnar artery when monitoring the radial and with compression of the radial when monitoring the ulnar.

A patient with distal disease will show decreased waveforms in the radial and ulnar arteries as well as a decreased forearm/brachial index. All signals from the brachial to the subclavian artery will be triphasic and normal.

A patient with brachial or low axillary occlusion between the elbow and shoulder will have decreased waveforms at the radial, ulnar, and brachial arteries and a decreased brachial systolic pressure in the affected arm.

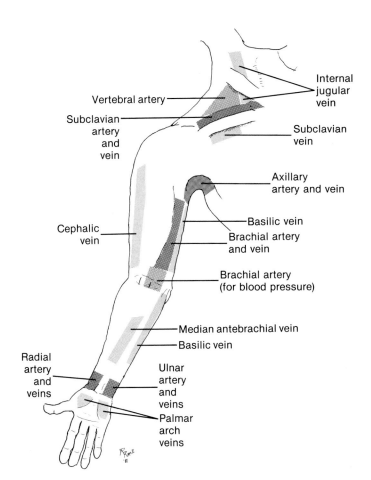

Fig. 23-26. Sites for both arterial and venous examinations of the upper extremity.

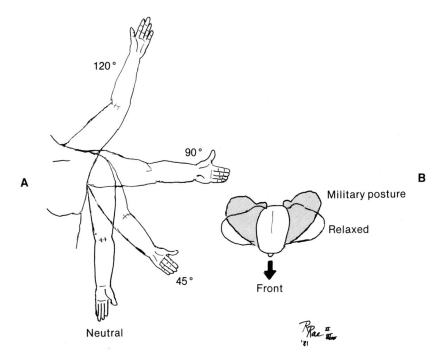

Fig. 23-27. Positions for examination of the patient with thoracic outlet syndrome. **A,** Arm and angles. **B,** Shoulders in relaxed and military postures.

The axillary, subclavian, and vertebral signals will be normal.

A patient with high axillary occlusion will have reduced waveforms at all sites below the shoulder and a corresponding pressure drop. The subclavian and vertebral arteries will be normal.

A patient with subclavian occlusion will show reduced waveforms at all sites, except for the proximal subclavian if the occlusion does not extend as far as the vertebral. Otherwise, decreased waveforms and possibly reversed vertebral waveforms can be expected.

It is important to remember that the forearm/brachial index should be calculated to show the degree of occlusion. If *both* arms show evidence of obstruction, note should be made on the report form that waveforms indicate occlusion and that the forearm/brachial index is ineffective.

Thoracic outlet syndrome examination. Many patients will often show completely normal resting upper extremity pressures even though they have difficulty only when their arms are raised or placed at an unusual angle. These patients usually complain of numbness, tingling, and discoloration if the arm is abducted, lain upon, pulled back behind the shoulder, or held over the head. Changing the position of the arm to a more forward or neutral position resolves the symptoms completely.[21] In these patients a routine upper extremity examination should be performed and then a more specialized examination of the thoracic outlet.

Thoracic outlet syndrome occurs when the arteries, veins, and/or nerves supplying the arm are obstructed by compression between the clavicle and first rib, a cervical rib and the scalene muscles, or the pectoralis minor with hyperabduction of the arm. The vessels usually involved are the subclavian artery and vein and the brachial nerve plexus where it leaves the chest and goes to the arm.[21]

In the thoracic outlet examination the patient should sit either in a chair or on the edge of the examination table with the arms completely relaxed. The examiner takes a tracing from the brachial artery with the arm in a neutral position. Then, with the help of an assistant, the patient's arm is raised to a 45-degree angle. The patient is instructed to let the arm go limp and offer no assistance at all. A tracing is taken from the arm in this position and is marked accordingly. With the arm in this position the patient then is instructed to pull the shoulders back into a military posture and perform a Valsalva maneuver. The examiner keeps the probe in place during the Valsalva and records any changes that occur.

The arm is raised to a 90-degree angle, and the procedure is repeated. A tracing is made both neutrally and with the patient in military posture performing a Valsalva maneuver.

The arm is finally raised to a 120-degree angle, and the same steps are repeated.

Additional maneuvers can include hyperabduction, hyperadduction, and Adson's test. In Adson's test, the patient hyperabducts the arm over the head and turns the head *toward* the side being examined. This position can help reveal the presence of a cervical rib.[21]

Positive findings in thoracic outlet syndrome will be a reduction or cessation of brachial artery flow with the onset of the military posture and Valsalva maneuver or the application of Adson's test. Any comments the patient makes concerning the onset of symptoms with the assumption of a particular position should be noted on the report form.

The positions for the thoracic outlet examination are shown in Fig. 23-27.

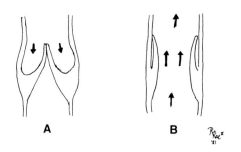

Fig. 23-28. Venous valves. **A,** Closed with inspiration. **B,** Open with expiration.

VENOUS DOPPLER EXAMINATIONS

The incidence of venous disease has been estimated to surpass that of cardiac disease and stroke.[32] Venous thrombosis, varicose veins, and pulmonary embolism are among the most common problems encountered in both outpatients and inpatients.

Pulmonary embolism is among the most dangerous of venous diseases. It occurs as a result of venous thrombosis and can especially affect bedridden, paraplegic or quadriplegic, and/or comatose patients, in whom clots develop because of a lack of muscular activity leading to venous stagnation.[34,42]

Varicose veins are frequently encountered in patients suffering from venous valve insufficiency in the superficial system as an aftereffect of a previous thrombosis or destructive condition. A similar occurrence in the deep system may occur shortly after treatment of thrombosis or phlebitis and is known as *postphlebitic syndrome.*[34]

The diagnosis of venous disease has proved to be one of the most difficult areas for the physician, exceeding a 50% error margin.[32-34] Fortunately many of the classic methods of diagnosis have now been supplemented with newer techniques designed to rule out venous thrombosis or insufficiency.

Contrast phlebography (venography) is the standard method of diagnosing venous thrombosis or embolism.[32,33,35] This is, again, an invasive technique, with many of the same risks found in arteriography (e.g., contrast media reactions, radiation risks). A further complication is that the patient must support his own weight and attempt to remain immobile while tourniquets are applied and irritating contrast medium is injected. The position may, understandably, be difficult to maintain. The examination may also, in rare cases, cause a thrombus to form. Venography remains the "gold standard," however, since small thrombi can be readily detected throughout the superficial and deep venous systems even with no flow obstruction.[32]

Nuclear medicine techniques are also used

to diagnose sources of venous emboli (thrombi).[32,33,35] These involve injecting radionuclides, which are either followed through the deep venous system by a gamma camera or absorbed by the thrombus and shown on a static scan. The former method uses technetium-99[m] pertechnetate and is more efficient for veins above the knee since discrimination of calf veins is impossible due to the diminished resolution. The latter method, using I-125 fibrinogen, allows discrimination of isolated calf thrombi but is not successful in veins above the knee because of the higher background activity from the radionuclide absorption. Both methods eliminate the irritation of the venographic contrast media and are accurate but are not feasible for routine screening of symptomatic patients. Other methods are indicated in these patients.[43]

Another diagnostic technique is impedance phleboplethysmography. The varying methods under this classification involve the measurement of blood flow in the limb based on volume and circumferential changes in response to respiratory variations or automatic inflation of a pressure cuff on the thigh. These methods are prone to error caused by collateral flow, improper respiratory responses, and poor cooperation by the patient.[33,35,43,44]

The Doppler examination of the venous system requires only the use of the Doppler device. Small pocket-sized instruments can be carried for bedside examination, to avoid the need for patient transportation. Strip-chart recording is optional if a record of flow is desired. The use of stethoscope or low-frequency sensitive headphones is imperative, because venous velocity signals tend to be very slow and low pitched and could be missed if external speakers alone are used.

Characteristics of the normal Doppler venous velocity signal[32]

Physiologically, flow dynamics of the venous and arterial systems differs because of the methods by which the blood is moved through them. In the arterial system, blood is pumped directly by the heart and a pulsatile pattern of flow corresponding to the cardiac cycle is heard. In the venous system, however, there is no pump to force the blood back toward the heart so there should be no pulsatility.

Unlike the arteries, the veins possess valves along their courses that prevent blood from backing up into the more distal segments and ensure a steady flow of blood. The blood is moved through the veins by respiratory variations in intraabdominal and intra-

thoracic pressure. During inspiration the pressure is increased, the valves close, and flow stops. During expiration the pressure eases, the valves reopen, and blood flows forward once again (Fig. 23-28).

Familiarity with the normal arterial signal can help the examiner locate the venous signals at their various sites. The venous signal has been described as wind-like; it is of a lower velocity than the arterial signal and rises and falls in pitch with expiration and inspiration respectively. This quality of variation with respiration is called *phasicity*.

There are six normal qualities in the veins that are checked by an examiner at all probe sites.[1]

The first quality is *patency*. This means that a vein allows blood to flow through it without obstruction of the lumen. Flow heard through a venous segment implies patency of that portion of the vein. Complete absence of a flow signal at any given site implies occlusion of that segment.

The second quality is *spontaneity*. This means that a signal is heard through the vein without manipulation of the limb to force flow through the segment being examined. Spontaneity will not occur in vasoconstricted veins (e.g., those in a cold leg). It will also not occur in veins that are drained of blood, as in an elevated leg. Only the posterior tibial vein may not be normally spontaneous and may require compression of the foot to augment flow.

The third normal quality is *phasicity*. As mentioned earlier, this means that normal variations with respiration should occur in a normal vein. Loss of phasicity will result in a steadily rushing, unchanging, *continuous* flow pattern. This always implies disease.

The fourth normal quality is called *augmentation*. This is the technique of compressing the venous pools in the distal portion of the limb to increase, or augment, the flow. Augmentation can also be created by compressing the segment of the vein proximal to the probe site, holding it for several seconds, and then releasing. This creates a backup of flow, which rushes forward upon release. Lack of augmentation implies occlusion between the probe and the compression site.

The fifth quality concerns *competence* of the valves in the limb, or their normal ability to prevent retrograde flow in the venous system. If the valves are destroyed by thrombus or disease, leakage will occur and flow will back up into the distal segment of the vein. Incompetence is often found after treatment of deep vein thrombosis and in varicose veins. Competency is checked by listening for reflux, which may occur with *release* of *distal* compression or the act of *proximal* compression. Any reflux implies lack of valvular competence between the probe and the compression site. The Valsalva maneuver is also a good test for the valves since it should also stop flow and shut the venous valves.

The sixth and final quality is *nonpulsatility*. It is usually abnormal for the venous system to vary with the cardiac cycle *in the lower extremities*. A patient with congestive or right heart failure may have pulsatility due to increased pressure within the venous system. A patient with an extremely irregular breathing pattern may also show a similar pattern to pulsatility. The veins in the upper extremity thoracic area do not show this quality.

In summary, the six qualities of the normal venous velocity signal are:

1. Patency. Flow can be heard through the venous segment spontaneously or with augmenting.
2. Spontaneity. Flow is heard without manipulation of the limb, except in the posterior tibial vein occasionally.
3. Phasicity. Flow varies with the respiratory cycle.
4. Augmentation. Flow increases normally with distal compression and also with release of proximal compression.
5. Competence. The valves prevent retrograde flow in the vein.
6. Nonpulsatility. The venous flow is not affected by the cardiac cycle.

Doppler lower extremity venous examination

The examination of the venous system of the lower extremities requires no equipment other than a Doppler blood flow device and a strip-chart recorder if the waveforms are intended to be recorded. Most patients presenting with venous disease will require the examination of the lower limbs. One of the best ways to determine the presence of venous disease is to check for arterial symptoms first and determine whether a pulse is felt.[34] Purplish discoloration and dark areas on the skin usually characterize venous disease, as do swelling and edema of the ankles and legs. The leg will be warm rather than cool as in arterial disease. Pain will occur with dependence of the limb, and relief is obtained by elevation. Swelling will also diminish with elevation of the extremity. Pain will also appear regardless of whether the patient is walking or resting, and walking may actual-

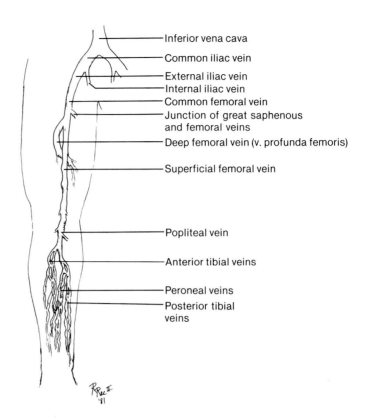

Fig. 23-29. Deep venous system of the lower extremity.

ly alleviate the symptoms. Varicosities and red streaks on the limbs also characterize venous disease. Pulling the toes of the foot back toward the leg (dorsiflexion) may cause sharp pain in the calf if calf vein thrombosis is present (Homan's sign).[34] These symptoms should aid the examiner in making a differential determination.

Venous anatomy of the lower extremities.[38] There is usually a corresponding vein for every artery in the Doppler lower extremity examination. The venous system is divided into deep and superficial systems, however.

In the *deep system* various plantar veins anastomose into larger tributaries that unite with the deep venous plantar arch. These veins come together to form the *posterior tibial* vein.

The posterior tibial vein runs on the medial surface of the leg superiorly and is superficially accessible directly posterior to the medial malleolus. Although there are anterior tibial and peroneal veins, they are not examined in the Doppler lower extremity examination.

The posterior tibial vein ascends through the calf and generally forms two venous plexuses. The anterior tibial and peroneal veins also each form two plexuses. These veins join to form the *popliteal* vein.

The popliteal vein runs alongside the pop-

liteal artery behind the knee and continues upward into the thigh, where it becomes the *superficial femoral* vein. The superficial femoral vein continues cephalad and becomes the *common femoral* vein at the point of anastomosis of the *deep femoral (profunda femoris)* vein, which drains the muscles and bone.

The common femoral vein continues cephalad and becomes the *external iliac* vein, which anastomoses with the *internal iliac* vein to form the *common iliac* vein. The common iliacs from each side come together to join with the *inferior vena cava* (Fig. 23-29).

The *superficial system*, for Doppler purposes, consists mainly of the *great* and *small saphenous* veins.

The great saphenous vein arises from the dorsum of the foot and ascends anterior to the medial malleolus. It runs along the medial surface of the leg superficially, outside the knee to the thigh, and anastomoses with the common femoral vein at the saphenofemoral junction. Accessory saphenous veins can occur randomly along the thigh or calf and empty into the great saphenous vein.

The small saphenous vein arises posterior to the lateral malleolus. It progresses superficially up the back of the calf to the knee, where it penetrates the deep fascia and empties into the popliteal vein (Fig. 23-30).

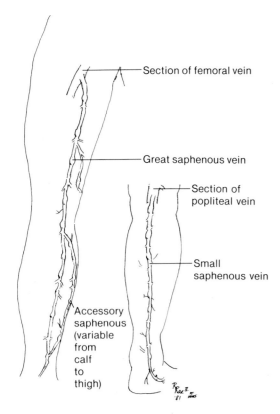

Fig. 23-30. Superficial venous system of the lower extremity.

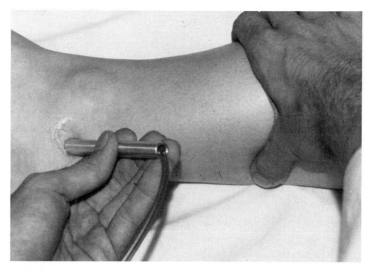

Fig. 23-31. Examination of the posterior tibial vein, with proximial calf compression. Note angling of the transducer against the flow.

Routine lower extremity venous examination. As in all examinations, the first step is to obtain a thorough history from the patient or the chart. Special attention must be paid to the location of the pain, whether it occurs with walking or rest, and whether elevation relieves the discomfort. Areas of swelling are checked. If unilateral disease is present, one leg will appear larger than the other. Areas of dark almost greenish color are signs of venous insufficiency, as are purple patches and prominent varicose veins. Red streaks imply superficial disease. The patient should also be questioned about past surgeries, especially if arterial or coronary artery bypasses have been performed. In these cases the saphenous vein is removed in whole or in part and is used for the bypass. A high percentage of post–coronary bypass patients develop venous disease 6 months to 1 year after surgery.[45]

Finally, it is helpful to document any past history of phlebitis or deep vein thrombosis and determine whether the patient is currently taking anticoagulants such as heparin or warfarin (Coumadin).

The patient should remove all clothing from the lower extremities, including stockings and underwear, and lie supine with the head raised 20 to 30 degrees to ensure venous pooling in the legs.[32,33] The legs should not be elevated and should be relaxed and slightly flexed at the knees to allow good flow dynamics and prevent compression of the popliteal vein against the condyles of the knee joint. The room should be warm to prevent vasoconstriction.

The first vein to be examined is the posterior tibial vein at its site posterior to the medial malleolus. Gel is applied to the site, and the probe is angled caudally. The posterior tibial artery can be used as a landmark for locating the area. The patient is instructed to take in exaggerated breaths to accentuate the phasicity in the veins. A patient with cold feet may have vasoconstriction, and a spontaneous signal may not be heard.

When the site has been determined, the foot may be squeezed to augment flow if spontaneity is not present. The examiner listens for phasicity and nonpulsatility. The amount of augmentation with distal (foot) compression is evaluated; then the leg is grasped at the calf proximally to the probe, compressed for several seconds, and released to elicit augmentation (Fig. 23-31). The flow signal should stop with proximal compression, then resume in a rush, and return to normal with release. Lack of response with either distal or proximal compression implies disease.

The popliteal vein is the next vein to be examined. As with the popliteal artery, there are two ways to position the patient—supine or prone. If the prone method is preferred, examination of the popliteal can be performed as the last step in the examination.

In the supine position the patient's knee should be flexed a bit more, and the probe is placed in the popliteal fossa and angled caudally. (See Fig. 23-11 for relative positioning.) The arterial signal is located, and the probe is angled medially and laterally until a distinct venous signal is heard. The amount of pressure required can vary, for venous collaterals in the fossa should be stopped but the popliteal vein should not be occluded. Gentle pressure usually will not occlude the vein.

When the signal has been found, the examiner checks for patency, spontaneity, phasicity, and nonpulsatility. Augmentation is evaluated by distal compression of the foot and calf (Fig. 23-32) and by proximal compression of the thigh. A Valsalva maneuver may be performed at this point to demonstrate the competence of the proximal venous valves.

In the prone position the patient's feet are elevated approximately 30 degrees by pillows. With this exception, the examination is performed in the exact sequence as described above for the supine position. (See Fig. 23-12 for positioning.)

The common femoral vein is examined next. The best site to examine the vein is superior to the inguinal ligament. The common femoral artery is first located, and the probe is moved medially and angled caudally to obtain the venous signal. Pressure may be applied to the probe gently to occlude the superficial venous collaterals since the femoral vein will not be as easily compressed. Once again, the signal is evaluated for patency, spontaneity, phasicity, and nonpulsatility. Augmentation is elicited by distal compression (calf, thigh) and proximal compression of the vein superior to the probe

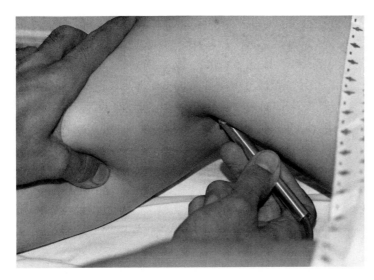

Fig. 23-32. Supine examination of the popliteal vein, with distal calf compression. Note that the transducer is angled against the flow.

site and/or by Valsalva maneuver. Competence is assessed by listening for reflux with compression and by the response to the Valsalva.

If a discrepancy between the groin and knee is noted, the superficial femoral vein may be examined in the groove superior to the vastus medialis and the sartorius on the thigh. The examination should follow the same procedure of signal evaluation, distal and proximal compression, and the Valsalva as used at the other sites. This completes the examination of the deep veins.

The superficial system examination is less involved but requires a finer degree of awareness on the part of the examiner.

The great saphenous vein can be examined anywhere along its course from ankle to the saphenofemoral junction. A light probe pressure is required to avoid compression of the vessel. Flow *may* or *may not* be *spontaneous* and/or *phasic* through the saphenous systems. It is helpful to position the probe at the site on the inside medial thigh and percuss or milk the distal vein to augment its flow.

Whether the responses obtained by augmentation and the relative flow dynamics signify disease will depend on whether a predisposing factor is suspected. Femoral thrombosis extending into the saphenofemoral junction, varicose veins, and evidence of superficial venous thrombic symptoms are all predisposing factors that will affect the flow and/or occlude the vein. Following the saphenous along its length will often help localize small thrombi.

The small saphenous follows the same criteria and can be examined along its course

at the back of the calf from the lateral malleolus to the knee.

The above deep and superficial vein examination is repeated for the other leg.

In summary, these are the steps in the routine lower extremity venous examination:

1. Obtain a history, with emphasis on past phlebitis, graft surgery, pain location, swelling, and discoloration.
2. The patient lies supine with the knees flexed and the head elevated 30 degrees.
3. Examine the posterior tibial vein for flow pattern abnormalities, with distal compression of the foot and proximal compression of the calf to augment flow.
4. Examine the popliteal vein in the supine position. Check the signal for abnormalities and perform distal and proximal compression.
5. Examine the common femoral vein. Check the signal for abnormalities and perform distal compression. Proximal compression and/or Valsalva can also be used for augmentation.
6. Examine the superficial femoral vein if there is evidence of thrombosis between the knee and groin.
7. Check the superficial veins to determine whether thrombosis exists either within or at the points where they anastomose with the deep veins.
8. Repeat steps 1 through 7 for the other leg.
9. If popliteal examination was not performed in the supine position, have the patient turn over, elevate the feet, and examine the vein in the prone position.

See Fig. 23-14 for examination sites in the lower extremity venous study.

Interpretation of the lower extremity venous examination. It may be helpful to reiterate the normal responses obtained in the examination at each site:

1. All deep veins should be patent and phasic, respond well to augmentation, be nonpulsatile, have competent valves, and, with the exception of the posterior tibial vein, be spontaneous.
2. If no spontaneous flow is heard, the vein should be augmented to determine whether flow is present and the vessel patent.
3. Normal distal augmentation will result in an abrupt increase in flow that will then return to normal. Normal proximal augmentation will result in stopping of flow with the act of compression, and a sharp increase in flow with a return to normal will follow release of compression.
4. The normal superficial venous system may or may not be spontaneous and/or phasic but should augment well and allow patency to be determined.

In *calf vein thrombosis* the posterior tibial signal is less phasic or continuous if it is spontaneous. Distal compression will be normal unless the ankle veins are occluded. There will be decreased augmentation upon release of calf compression.

The popliteal signal will usually be continuous or less phasic depending on whether the thrombus extends into the distal popliteal. The signal may not be spontaneous, and there will be decreased augmentation with foot compression. Foot compression will not result in any augmentation of flow through the calf veins.

Both the superficial and the common femoral signals will be normal, with normal responses to augmentation except by calf compression. It may help to compare the affected leg with the unaffected leg if the disease is unilateral.

In *femoropopliteal vein thrombosis* the posterior tibial vein signal is continuous, with normal distal and decreased proximal augmentation.

The popliteal vein will have either no signal or markedly reduced flow. Usually high-pitched collaterals will be heard in the popliteal fossa. Distal and proximal augmentation maneuvers will result in either extremely reduced or absent augmentation.

The common femoral vein will be continuous or less phasic, again depending on whether the thrombus extends into the prox-

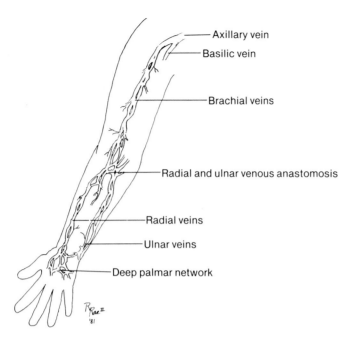

Fig. 23-33. Deep venous system of the upper extremity to the axilla.

Axillary vein

Basilic vein

Brachial veins

Radial and ulnar venous anastomosis

Radial veins

Ulnar veins

Deep palmar network

imal femoral segment. The superficial femoral will be absent, or reduced and continuous. Abnormal augmentation responses can be anticipated. An increased flow signal at the femoral may be due to saphenous shunting around the thrombus.

In *iliofemoral thrombosis* the posterior tibial, popliteal, and superficial femoral veins will be continuous, with reduced augmentation at all sites. The common femoral will have absent or reduced continuous flow with poor or absent responses to augmentation maneuvers. Prominent collaterals may exist in the groin.

The diagnosis of superficial vein thrombosis is often difficult, for there may or may not be spontaneous and/or phasic flow present. The determination of disease should be based on the predisposing factors mentioned earlier and on reduced or absent augmentation.[33,34]

Occasionally patients will present with diminished-sounding flow or flow that seems continuous where normal responses to compression are noted. The examiner should recheck results for the presence of collaterals, by applying gentle pressure to the probe at the site, and should check the patient's breathing pattern and have him inspire more deeply and exhale more forcibly to be certain that a phasic pattern does not exist in the veins.

Findings in postphlebitic patients and examination additions. Postphlebitic syndrome occurs in patients who have had deep vein thrombosis at one time but have undergone anticoagulation treatments. These pa-

tients may have a recurrence of symptoms due to insufficiency resulting from the destruction of the valves by the earlier thrombus. When assessing these patients, the examiner must check their history to help determine whether the insufficiency may be due to a new thrombus or to the destruction of the old valves from the previous phlebitis.

The normal Doppler examination is done with attention given to reflux heard after *proximal* compression or the *release* of *distal* compression. The area of reflux enables one to pinpoint the site of the old thrombus. Valsalva maneuvers will not stop the flow if there are no competent valves proximal to the thrombus site.

In the superficial system, reflux through the saphenous implies destruction of the valves at the saphenofemoral junction.

In evaluations of the perforating venous system between the superficial and deep systems for incompetence, the legs should be elevated and emptied of blood and a tourniquet applied to the calf to prevent superficial reflux. The probe is then moved lightly over the leg, which is covered with couplant, and the thigh is squeezed *above* the tourniquet to determine whether any reflux between the superficial and deep systems is detected. The tourniquet should *not* be tied tightly enough to occlude the calf veins.[32]

Doppler upper extremity venous examination

Though the major incidence of venous disease occurs in the lower extremities, the upper extremities are also the site of venous

occlusions that can be just as serious as those found in the legs. Since the introduction of intravenous solution administration, monitoring catheters, and dialysis operations for the patient in renal failure, the incidence of upper extremity phlebitis has increased.[33,34] As in the legs, the upper extremity veins may also thrombose and give off pulmonary emboli.[34,42] The contrast method of venography may not be suitable, especially in the dialysis patient with a surgically produced A-V fistula. Determining the patency of veins often becomes a factor in decisions on whether to proceed with venography, to intervene surgically, or to attempt anticoagulant therapy to resolve the problem. The Doppler device again provides an easily available method of evaluation.

Venous anatomy of the upper extremities. Both deep and superficial systems exist in the complex upper extremities.

The *deep* venous system is of somewhat small caliber and difficult to examine in the forearm. A decent signal can occasionally be obtained from the *radial* and *ulnar* veins, which arise from venous plexuses in the venous palmar arches. These veins run superiorly along with their respective radial and ulnar arteries and anastomose at the antecubital fossa to form the *brachial* vein.

The brachial vein runs superiorly along either side of the brachial artery and anastomoses with the *axillary* vein at the junction of the basilic (superficial) vein at the shoulder (Fig. 23-33).

The axillary vein continues superiorly into the thorax, where it becomes the *subclavian* vein at approximately the lateral border of the first rib. The subclavian vein then anastomoses with the *internal jugular* vein to form the *brachiocephalic* vein. The right and left brachiocephalic veins join the *superior vena cava*, which then empties into the right atrium of the heart (Fig. 23-34).

The *superficial* venous system of the upper extremity consists of two major veins, the *basilic* and *cephalic* veins.

The basilic vein begins on the ulnar side of the arm. It runs proximally on the posterior surface of the ulnar side of the arm and continues superiorly along the medial aspect of the arm to the axilla, where it joins the axillary vein. The *median antebrachial* vein lies between the radial and ulnar arteries and anastomoses with the basilic vein approximately 2 cm below the antecubital fossa.

The cephalic vein begins in the radial part of the dorsal venous network of the hand. It extends proximally around the radial border of the forearm to the antecubital fossa, where

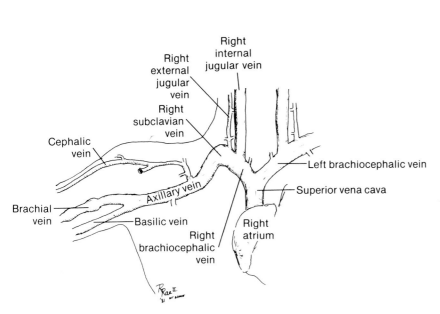

Fig. 23-34. Deep venous system in the thorax to the right atrium.

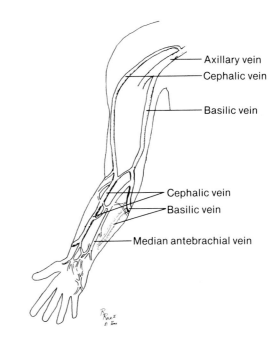

Fig. 23-35. Superficial venous system in the upper extremity.

it anastomoses with the median cubital vein. It then continues up the lateral side of the arm superiorly and enters the shoulder to anastomose with the subclavian vein (Fig. 23-35).

Routine upper extremity venous examination. The patient's history is once again obtained, with emphasis on pain, discoloration, swelling, and history of recent intravenous infusions; and differentiation is made between arterial and venous disease as in the lower extremity examination.

The patient lies supine in a room with the same environmental conditions as for the lower extremity examination.

First, the deep veins are examined. The radial and ulnar veins are located at the wrist by locating their companion arteries. The probe is then angled caudally, and the venous signal is distinguished and evaluated by the standard characteristic qualities of the normal venous signal. Note that expansion of the superior vena cava due to negative intrathoracic pressure may increase venous flow in the upper extremity with *inspiration* rather than expiration.

When the flow signal is evaluated, the forearm is compressed and is released after several seconds for proximal augmentation. Distal augmentation may be performed by compression of the fleshy part of the hand. Both the radial and the ulnar veins are evaluated in this manner.

Next, the brachial vein is examined. It is monitored at its site on the medial side of the arm at the intramuscular septum. Locating the artery first may, once again, aid the

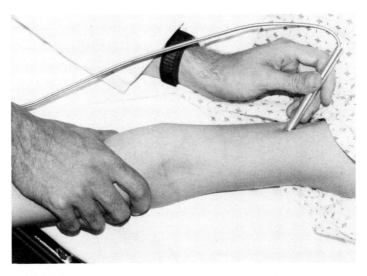

Fig. 23-36. Examination of the brachial vein with distal forearm compression. The transducer is angled against the flow.

examiner. The standard signal qualities are used to evaluate the venous flow signal. Distal compression is performed by compression of the forearm (Fig. 23-36), and the Valsalva maneuver is used for proximal compression. Responses should be the same as in the lower extremity venous examination.

The axillary vein is then located by angling caudally in the axilla, medial to the axillary artery. The axillary signal may be *pulsatile* and is one of the few exceptions to the rule of nonpulsatility. (All pulsatile signals from this site proximally should be interpreted as normal.) Distal compression of the upper arm and forearm should be performed. Proxi-

mal compression consists of the Valsalva maneuver.

The subclavian vein is located by placing the probe either beneath the clavicle and angling superiorly and laterally or in the supraclavicular fossa and angling laterally and inferiorly. This signal is also pulsatile and must be carefully distinguished from the subclavian artery signal. Examination is performed as for the axillary vein.

If axillary or subclavian thrombosis is indicated, the internal jugular vein should be evaluated for determination of the extent of the thrombus.

The internal jugular is located by angling

the probe inferiorly and laterally to either the inferior or the superior border of the sternocleidomastoid muscle. The internal jugular signal can be phasic, continuous, or pulsatile and usually is heard as a high-velocity variable hissing sound. The only maneuver performed is a Valsalva. Diminished augmentation on release implies a proximal brachiocephalic venous thrombus.[32]

The superficial veins are examined in a manner similar to that for the veins of the lower extremity. They can, again, be monitored anywhere along their course; and they also require light probe pressure. Usually a slightly phasic or continuous signal is heard, and augmentation is performed by percussion or light compression. Reduced or absent flow may imply a thrombus near the axillobrachial junction in the cephalic vein and in the subclavian vein with diminished basilic vein flow.

In summary, these are the steps in the venous examination of the upper extremity:

1. Obtain the history.
2. Examine the radial and ulnar veins. Distal compression of the hand and proximal compression of the forearm may be performed for augmentation.
3. Examine the brachial vein. Distal compression of the forearm may be performed, and a Valsalva maneuver for proximal compression.
4. Examine the axillary vein, with distal compression of the forearm and Valsalva maneuver.
5. Examine the subclavian vein in the supraclavicular fossa, or underneath the clavicle the same way as the axillary vein.
6. Examine the internal jugular vein if there is a question of thrombus extending into the brachiocephalic vein. A Valsalva maneuver also may be performed.
7. Evaluate the basilic and cephalic veins. See Fig. 23-36 for upper extremity venous probe site locations.

Interpretation of the upper extremity venous examination. It may be helpful again to reiterate the findings in the upper extremity venous examination.

In *brachial vein thrombosis* there will usually be a continuous signal in the radial and ulnar veins. One or both may be continuous depending on the level of the thrombus. There will be poor augmentation responses with release of upper arm compression or Valsalva.

The brachial venous signal will be either absent or continuous, with a markedly reduced flow rate.

The axillary and subclavian signals will be normal with normal responses to Valsalva but poor distal augmentation responses with arm compression.

The superficial veins will show changes reflecting the extent of the thrombus, especially if it extends into the axillary.

In both *axillary* and *subclavian venous thrombosis* the radial and ulnar vein signals will be continuous. Poor proximal augmentation can be expected.[62]

The axillary signal may be absent or continuous depending on the location of the thrombus and collateral circulation. Both distal compression and Valsalva maneuver responses will be poor.

The subclavian vein will reflect the same conditions as in the axillary; but if thrombosis is suspected in the proximal brachiocephalic vein, the jugular signal should be evaluated.

In the internal jugular vein, a reduced Valsalva response will imply a brachiocephalic venous occlusion. Flow may be reduced depending on the extent of the thrombus.

The use of IV infusions tends to be the greatest cause of superficial phlebitis in the upper extremities.[32] In cases of superficial thrombus in the basilic and cephalic veins, flow will usually be completely absent with poor or limited response to augmentation maneuvers. Evaluation must be based on augmentation and patency, as in the lower extremity veins.

Summary

The Doppler venous study is a technically demanding yet accurate and convenient method of evaluating the peripheral venous system noninvasively. Although the venous examination is probably the most difficult-to-learn and examiner-dependent study of all the Doppler techniques, expertise can be gained with practice on normal subjects to determine the correct differentiation of normal and abnormal signals. Careful examination is required for distinguishing collaterals from deep veins and for determining the correct amount of probe pressure to avoid occluding the veins. False results are almost always due to technical error, so it is important to recheck the results in cases of uncertainty.

In conclusion, here are several guidelines to remember:

1. Arteries and veins are almost always paired, making location of either simple.
2. Exaggerated breathing will accentuate phasicity.
3. Continuous flow in a vein is usually significant of a thrombosis. If a patient is receiving anticoagulant therapy, the flow pattern may be of higher velocity; and this should be noted on the report form. Flow will almost always be phasic distal to an occlusion.
4. Reflux accompanying release of distal compression in a vein or occurring with proximal compression always implies incompetent valves between the compression site and the probe. In stereophonic headphones this will be heard in the ear opposite the side with antegrade flow.
5. Absence of flow in a distal ankle vein implies occlusion only if collaterals are prominent and vasoconstriction is not occurring. Lack of response with foot compression may also imply distal occlusion.

Careful examination and thorough knowledge of characteristic responses will ensure accurate examinations. If performed correctly and with confidence, these examinations can be a valuable adjunct to contrast studies or other diagnostic efforts.[37,44]

Illustrations of lower extremity and upper extremity venous examinations and tracings appear in Appendix J.

DOPPLER EXAMINATION OF THE CEREBROVASCULAR SYSTEM

Cerebral ischemia secondary to arterial occlusion to the brain, known as stroke, is one of the leading causes of death in the world. These occlusions result primarily from atherosclerotic plaques in the carotids.[56,58] A variety of other conditions, including Takayasu's arteritis, fibromuscular disease, arterial dissections, aneurysms, and trauma, may result in stroke.[48,58] Despite the overall decreased stroke incidence over the last few years, occlusion from both calcific and soft plaque (which may embolize) still remains a definite concern. The neurologic symptoms from these processes may manifest themselves as *transient ischemic attacks* (TIAs) until the patient suffers an episode that does *not* resolve as previous episodes may have, which may result in either death or debilitation of the patient for the rest of his life.

Many techniques have been developed over the years to diagnose carotid and cerebral arterial conditions, but cerebral angiography has remained the standard for determining the location of occlusions or the extent of plaque in the arteries. The risks that have been discussed earlier regarding angiography need not be reiterated here. Interestingly the alternative techniques of noninvasive Doppler, carotid real time sonography, Doppler spectral analysis, and Doppler carotid scanning are currently being used by more and more physicians in the screening of patients who present with TIAs, neurologic problems, or asymptomatic bruits.

Anatomy of the cerebrovascular circulation[56,61]

The first major vessels involved in the Doppler examination are the *common carotid* arteries. The right common carotid arises from the *brachiocephalic (innominate)* artery, and the left common carotid arises directly from the aortic arch. Both travel superiorly in the neck to just above the thyroid cartilage. Here the carotids widen into the *carotid bulbs* and bifurcate into the *internal* and *external* carotid arteries.

The internal carotid artery has no branches within the neck. It continues upward to enter the skull through the *carotid canal.* It makes several twists and turns anteriorly and posteriorly and then gives off its first branch intracranially, the *ophthalmic* artery (Fig. 23-37).

The ophthalmic artery continues anteriorly into the orbit, where several branches arise and pass superiorly over the globe and exit the orbit onto the face near the orbital margin. The peripheral branches are the *supraorbital, frontal (supratrochlear),* and *nasal (dorsal nasal)* arteries. These three arteries are the most easily accessible vessels that reflect the hemodynamics of the distal internal carotid.

The supraorbital artery passes through the supraorbital notch or foramen, and branches onto the forehead. The frontal artery exits the orbit at the upper medial angle and also branches onto the forehead. The nasal artery passes out of the orbit at the inferomedial angle and runs alongside the nose to anastomose with the angular artery from the external carotid (Fig. 23-38).

The external carotid supplies extracranial structures mostly. It gives off several branches in the neck, beginning with the superior thyroid artery at the bulb and progressing up to the *occipital* artery, which passes posterosuperiorly toward the ear.

The next branch given off is the *facial* artery, at about the same level. It passes anteriorly around the inferior border of the mandible and continues superiorly to the medial corner of the orbit. It becomes the *angular* artery at about the corner of the mouth.

The external carotid then continues superiorly and bifurcates into the *superficial temporal* and the *internal maxillary* arteries just below the ear.

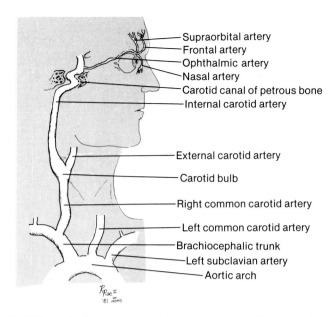

Fig. 23-37. Aortic branches and the internal carotid arterial system.

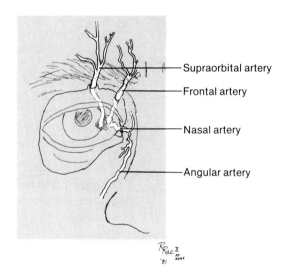

Fig. 23-38. Terminal branches of the ophthalmic artery.

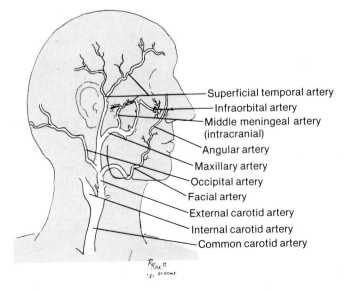

Fig. 23-39. Branches of the external carotid artery.

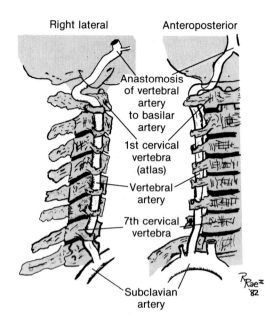

Fig. 23-40. Two views of the vertebral artery.

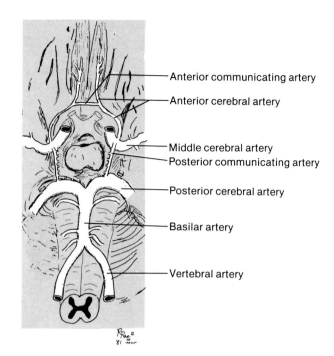

Fig. 23-41. Circle of Willis.

The superficial temporal artery continues upward just in front of the ear and gives off several branches, the anterior of which branches onto the forehead.

The internal maxillary artery gives off the *middle meningeal* artery, which supplies the dura and floor of the cranium and then gives off deep intramaxillary branches before terminating as the *infraorbital* artery, which exits the skull to the superficial facial muscles through the infraorbital foramen (Fig. 23-39).

The next major arteries are the *vertebral* arteries. Each vertebral artery arises from its respective subclavian artery, and travels superiorly and posteriorly to enter the transverse foramen of the sixth cervical vertebra. The vertebral arteries travel through the transverse foramina of the next five vertebrae until they exit the first cervical vertebra, curve anteriorly and posteriorly, and enter the skull through the foramen magnum.

Upon entering the skull the two vertebral arteries anastomose to form the *basilar* artery (Fig. 23-40).

The vertebral, basilar, and internal carotids service or are serviced by the *circle of Willis*, an arterial circle at the base of the brain. It is formed by the following vessels (Fig. 23-41):

1. The *right and left anterior* and *middle cerebral* arteries (which are the terminal branches of the internal carotids)
2. The *posterior cerebral* arteries (terminal branches of the basilar artery)
3. The *anterior* and *posterior communicating* arteries

The cerebral arterial circle of Willis pro-

vides a common collateral pathway in cases of single or multiple arterial obstruction. For example, if one internal carotid artery is diseased or occluded, the other internal carotid artery can supply its needs by shunting flow via the circle of Willis. The basilar artery can also supply either or both carotids in severe obstruction.

Hemodynamics and possible anastomoses in cerebral arterial obstructions[48,49,56]

In the circle of Willis the following routes of shunting occur with obstructive disease of the internal carotid:

1. *One obstructed internal carotid* can be supplied by either the *opposite internal carotid* via the *anterior cerebral and anterior communicating* arteries or by the *vertebrobasilar* arteries via the *posterior cerebral and posterior communicating* arteries.
2. If *both internal carotids are obstructed*, they are supplied by the *vertebrobasilar* arteries via *both posterior cerebral and both posterior communicating* arteries.

Obstruction in the vertebral or carotid arteries is often masked if excellent flow is maintained in the circle of Willis. I have seen cases in which the patient with bilateral total carotid occlusion was asymptomatic and the condition was discovered during examination for a completely unrelated problem.

Obstructions can also cause anastomoses between the internal and external carotid systems. Potential anastomoses include

1. *Superficial temporal artery* (external carotid)–*supraorbital and/or frontal arteries* (internal carotid)—usually on or across the forehead
2. *Facial-angular artery* (external carotid)–*nasal artery* (internal carotid)
3. *Infraorbital artery* (external carotid)–*nasal artery* (internal carotid) via the *angular artery*
4. *Middle meningeal* (external carotid)–*ophthalmic artery* (internal carotid) with a direct intracranial connection

When one subclavian artery is obstructed proximal to the vertebral orifice, the *vertebrovertebral* anastomosis results in a subclavian steal. (See p. 338, for explanation of the hemodynamics involved, and Fig. 23-25 for illustration.)

On rare occasion, *vertebral artery* anastomoses with the *occipital artery* high in the neck may draw flow from the external carotid to counteract vertebral insufficiencies.

Characteristics of the Doppler arterial signal in the cerebral examination

Unlike the signal in the extremities, the normal Doppler signal in the carotid and cerebral circulation is of high velocity, and due to the low resistance of the intracranial vascular bed it does *not* go below the zero line. The same basic components as in the extremity artery signal exist here, but there is a much shorter secondary component and a larger diastolic component. The secondary component may be absent depending on disease or vascular resistance.

In disease blunting of the systolic and

diminishing of the diastolic component will occur as the severity increases. Turbulence due to flow obstruction may cause the zero-crossing circuit to average flow as flat on the chart tracing, depending on the strength of the antegrade and retrograde directional flow patterns. Reversal of flow below the baseline may occur in cases of internal carotid obstruction and should always be considered abnormal.

Routine Doppler cerebrovascular examination

Equipment for the arterial cerebrovascular examination consists of the directional Doppler, one or two blood pressure cuffs, a stethoscope, and a strip-chart recorder.

The first step is to obtain a history from the patient or the chart. Emphasis should be placed on the following details:

1. *Prior history or recent occurrence of cerebrovascular accident (CVA)* and what areas of the body are affected or have resolved since the onset
2. *Transient ischemic attacks (TIAs),* which can result in short duration episodes of dizziness, paralysis, hemiparesis, blurred vision or amaurosis fugax, lost or slurred speech, expressive aphasia or paraphasia, syncope, unusual or irritational behavior, confusion, headache, and nausea with or without vomiting[56] (Recording the number of episodes that have occurred, their duration, and whether one or more of the above symptoms were noted at once is of benefit; any residual symptoms that have not resolved should also be mentioned.)

The carotids should be auscultated with a stethoscope or carotid phonoangiograph for the presence of *bruits.* A bruit will be heard as a low-to-high–pitched squirting noise occurring with systole and may range from soft to loud. It results from intraarterial flow turbulence and is usually heard directly over area of stenosis although it may be detected in the distal portion of the artery as well. Bruits should be considered significant of disease, especially when they occur in the asymptomatic patient, for they may indicate the presence of severe stenosis and atherosclerotic plaque.

Bruitlike sounds can be heard in patients with systolic blowing murmurs of cardiac origin that radiate through the arch to the carotids. The heart should therefore also be checked to determine whether murmurs that could be radiating are present. Simulated bruits occur in patients with low bifurcations, and in young people due to turbulence in

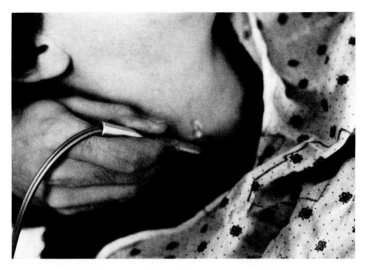

Fig. 23-42. Examination of the common carotid artery.

normal vessels; hence the need to determine objectively whether arterial disease is present.

Next, the patient lies supine with a pillow or bolster placed slightly under the shoulders to extend the head back and expose more of the neck. A pressure cuff is applied to each arm, and the brachial artery signal is monitored and recorded bilaterally. The systolic (and optional diastolic) pressures are then taken from each arm. If there is a greater than 20-to-40-mm Hg difference between arms, with a corresponding reduction of the waveform, a subclavian steal examination should be done during the course of the procedure on the affected side. (See p. 338.) A blood pressure reading also may be taken with the patient sitting if there is dizziness with positional changes, to help determine whether there is an orthostatic blood pressure drop.

The common carotids are examined next, one at a time. The examiner locates the probe site by having the patient turn his head slightly opposite the side being examined, then palpating the superior or inferior border of the sternocleidomastoid muscle. Gel is applied to the neck, and the probe is placed on the intended site and angled caudally. A gentle amount of pressure may be required to displace tissue (Fig. 23-42).

Two obstacles may interfere with obtaining a clear tracing: the sternocleidomastoid muscle and the internal jugular vein. Ideally the probe position should be on either side of the muscle. Retraction of the muscle by the probe may be necessary when examining the middle section of the common carotid. The vein will usually be heard as a loud, phasic or continuous, irregular hissing signal—frequently directly over the low com-

mon carotid—and will mask the pulsatile signal or dominate the negative side of the zero-crossing circuit so as to make recording difficult. If moving the probe medially or laterally and angling around the vein does not work, the vein may be stopped momentarily by having the patient do a Valsalva. The vein may also be manually compressed above the probe site.

When an adequate low or mid–common carotid signal is obtained, the probe is moved to the area directly above and lateral to the superior border of the thyroid cartilage and a tracing of the area of the bifurcation/bulb is made.

The bifurcation level varies in most individuals. It can be found anywhere from the base of the carotid to above the lower angle of the mandible but in the general population is usually found from the thyroid cartilage up. The signals are occasionally obscured if calcified plaque or turbulence is present.

Many times individual examination of the internal and external carotids will help diagnose stenoses or turbulence, especially if the bifurcation/bulb area signal is obscured by plaque.

The external carotid is usually found anteriorly in the neck. It has a distinct signal different from that of the internal carotid. The external signal is much more distinct in the accentuation of the second component and may sound almost like an extremity artery in a patient with a particularly dynamic vascular bed. If the bifurcation area is established, the examiner should move the probe anteriorly while angling caudally to pick up the signal.

Moving posteriorly from the bulb will usually bring in the internal carotid. The internal carotid signal usually is of a higher

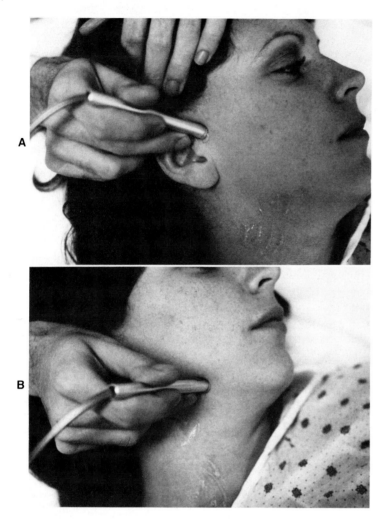

Fig. 23-43. Examination of, **A,** the temporal artery and, **B,** the facial artery.

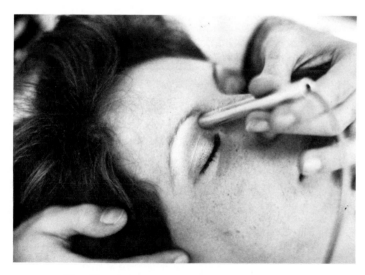

Fig. 23-44. Positioning for the frontal artery.

velocity than that of the external carotid, with no second component and diastolic flow well above the zero line. If the takeoff of the internal carotid is severely stenosed, the signal may be almost of a pulsatile high-pitched hissing nature. This suggests a severe stenosis and is caused by a *jet effect,* similar to holding one's finger over the end of a water hose to make the flow increase.

As can be suspected from previously mentioned cases in the extremities, a pressure drop will occur on the distal side of a stenosis. In the internal carotid, lack of sufficient pressure will cause the collaterals to send blood through the most available collateral channel to compensate for the deficiency of cerebral flow. This fact is the basis for the next portion of the examination, *the Doppler ophthalmic test.*

After the carotids have been evaluated bilaterally, the examiner may wish to take tracings from the *superficial temporal artery* in front of the ear and the *facial artery* at the mandibular notch. These may be of value in determining whether increased flow in either is present, implying possible collateralization, or if there is decreased flow, indicative of external carotid occlusion[53] (Fig. 23-43).

The examiner moves to the head of the examining table, asks the patient to relaxedly close his eyes, and places the probe gently just superior to the inner canthus of the eye within the orbital rim. The probe should be angled medially and cranially until the *frontal artery*[48,54] signal is obtained (Fig. 23-44).

When the signal is located, the chart recorder should be run at slow speed to show the direction of flow. The flow signal is normally antegrade. Retrograde flow implies a greater than 70% internal carotid obstruction.[48,49]

Various compression maneuvers are next performed to determine whether compression of the external carotid branches from the ipsilateral and contralateral sides will cause any increase, decrease, or reversal of the frontal artery signal. The examiner steadies the position of the probe by resting one hand on the patient's chin or by steadying the examining arm in some fashion prior to beginning the compressions. This is to ensure that the probe will not slip off the artery during the time the compression is being attempted.

The first vessel to be compressed is the superficial temporal artery on the side being examined. Normally this either will cause an increase in flow or will not affect the signal. It should be held for at least three beats and then be released.

The facial artery on the same side is then compressed and held for three beats. A normal response to this compression is either an increased or an unchanged signal.

The infraorbital artery on the same side is compressed next. The normal response is an unchanged signal (Fig. 23-45).

With the probe still in place the examiner switches hands and compresses the superficial temporal, facial, and infraorbital arteries of the opposite side of the face in turn. Compression of the contralateral arteries should not affect the frontal artery flow signal.

When the contralateral compressions are completed, the examination procedure is repeated for the remaining frontal artery.

The supraorbital artery should be examined bilaterally by palpating the supraorbital notch and monitoring the artery at that site. This vessel should be included to confirm or add to directional and collateral determination. Compression of the ipsilateral temporal artery usually augments flow.

Carotid compression has been argued as both valid and necessary or worthless and dangerous by many schools of physicians. There is no right answer, for carotid compression may aid in determining cross-channel collaterals from the contralateral side in intracranial collateralization,[49] but there may be severe risk in cases of extreme stenosis.[56] If performed, a physician should always be present, and the artery should be compressed only long enough to determine that it affects the flow pattern. NEVER EXCEED TWO BEATS.

To summarize, these are the steps in the routine cerebrovascular examination:

1. Take a history with emphasis on cerebral insufficiency and symptoms.
2. Examine the neck with a stethoscope for bruits.
3. Take brachial arterial signals and blood pressures and determine the need for subclavian steal examination.
4. Examine and record both common carotids.
5. Check the bifurcation/bulb areas and make internal and external carotid tracings if desired.
6. Check the frontal artery and record the signal through the following compression maneuvers to show changes:
7. Compress the superficial temporal on the side being examined. Either an augmented or an unchanged signal results.
8. Compress the facial artery on the same side. It also will either augment or not change the frontal signal.

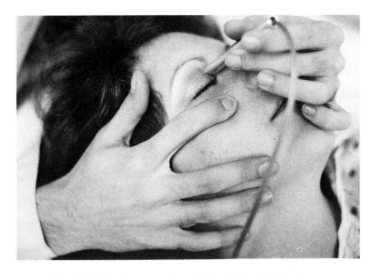

Fig. 23-45. Compression of the infraorbital artery.

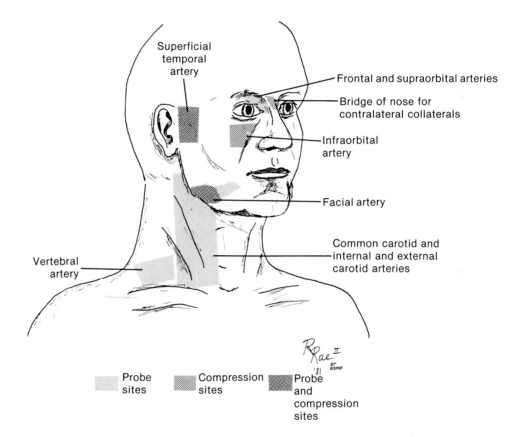

Superficial temporal artery

Frontal and supraorbital arteries

Bridge of nose for contralateral collaterals

Infraorbital artery

Facial artery

Common carotid and internal and external carotid arteries

Vertebral artery

Probe sites   Compression sites   Probe and compression sites

Fig. 23-46. Sites for examination and compression in the cerebrovascular Doppler examination.

9. Compress the infraorbital artery on the same side. It should result in an unchanged signal.
10. Compress the contralateral temporal, facial, and infraorbital arteries. This should not change their signals.
11. Check the supraorbital artery for flow direction and possible collateral flow connections.
12. Repeat steps 7 through 11 for the frontal and supraorbital arteries on the other side.

An optional tracing may be made of the vertebral arteries at their bases to reaffirm patent or occluded cerebral flow from all sources. (See "Routine upper extremity arterial examination," p. 336, for the technique of obtaining this tracing.)

The sites for monitoring and compression in the cerebrovascular examination are shown in Fig. 23-46. Normal and abnormal cerebrovascular examinations are shown in Appendix I.

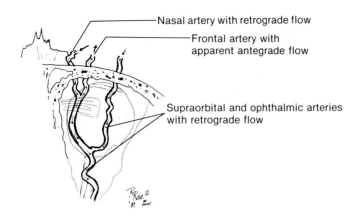

Nasal artery with retrograde flow

Frontal artery with apparent antegrade flow

Supraorbital and ophthalmic arteries with retrograde flow

Fig. 23-47. Diagram of nasal artery flow stolen by the frontal artery.

Interpretations and findings in cerebrovascular obstruction

The normal responses mentioned in the preceding section should be memorized so diagnosis during the examination will be facilitated. Discussion of likely collateralization will be discussed in specific occlusion disorders.

In internal carotid obstruction with an *ipsilateral superficial temporal artery collateral:*

1. Frontal flow will be retrograde, since flow travels *into* instead of *out from* the orbit.
2. Compression of the ipsilateral temporal artery will either *stop* or *reverse the flow pattern to antegrade,* provided there is sufficient internal carotid pressure or another intracranial collateral supply to compensate.
3. Same-sided facial and infraorbital compression will not change the signal.
4. Contralateral compressions will have no effect.

When the internal carotid is obstructed with a *contralateral temporal* collateral, compression of the contralateral temporal will have the same effect as in no. 2 above. Other results will be as stated.

In obstruction with a *facial collateral:*

1. Frontal flow may be either antegrade *or* retrograde.
2. Flow will be unchanged with temporal compression.
3. In retrograde flow, ipsilateral facial compression will stop or reverse the signal. If a *contralateral* facial collateral is present, compression of the contralateral facial rather than the ipsilateral facial will cause the change. Since this latter collateral can come across the *bridge of the nose* due to contralateral angular collateral connections, compression at the bridge should have the same effect as direct facial compression.

4. Other compressions will have no effect.

When flow is antegrade, the signal will still change. The apparent antegrade signal may result from retrograde flow in the angular artery entering the nasal artery and making a "U-turn" to come back out the frontal artery (Fig. 23-47). The examiner should check flow in the supraorbital artery to be certain that retrograde flow in the ophthalmic artery is present.

In internal carotid obstruction with *infra-orbital artery collaterals:*

1. Frontal artery flow will be retrograde, usually.
2. Temporal and facial compressions bilaterally will have no effect on the signal.
3. Either ipsilateral or contralateral infraorbital compression will affect the signal. The contralateral collateral network may also cross the bridge of the nose, as with the facial artery.

Intracranial or *circle of Willis collaterals* may also occur.[47,49,63,64] When the *contralateral internal carotid* is supplying the obstructed artery, the following occurrences will be seen:

1. The frontal artery signal will be *antegrade.*
2. Peripheral external carotid artery branch compressions will cause augmentation or no changes, as in a normal examination.

In this situation it may be necessary to compress the common carotids one at a time, for this is the only definite way to distinguish the abnormality by Doppler.

With a physician, preferably, performing the compression the carotid is located, straddled by the tips of two fingers, and compressed low in the neck for *no more than two beats* while the frontal signal is monitored.

The result of contralateral carotid compression should be *obliteration* or *diminish-*

ing of the signal. Ipsilateral compression will augment flow.

When a *vertebrobasilar collateral* situation exists, contralateral carotid compression will have *no effect.* Having the patient hyperextend the neck may result in successful compression of the vertebrals at their entrance to the foramen, but this is not usually feasible.

Intracranial collaterals are among the hardest to diagnose with Doppler, but proper examination can limit the possibilitites of their being missed.

Discussion of false-positive and false-negative conditions[49]

The Doppler cerebrovascular examination is open to any number of occurrences that can cause errors to take place. Some of these are technical; some are due to the nature of Doppler ultrasound.

A few of the false-negative conditions will be discussed first:

1. Doppler is a fairly reliable indicator of occlusion when the vessel lumen is obstructed by 70% to 80% of its transverse diameter, but the 70-80 figure must be attained before a significant pressure drop occurs in the cerebrovascular system. Diagnosis of a false-normal condition may occur when the artery is not occluded enough to reduce flow. This factor can be reduced if the Doppler examination is performed with a carotid high-resolution real time study as part of the routine examination. (See "Carotid Real Time Sonography," p. 357.)
2. Many deep and nonaccessible arteries and collaterals exist that cannot be compressed or heard with the probe. These may also give a false impression of normal flow.
3. There are some nonstenotic soft tissue plaques that do not obstruct flow and therefore cause no audible change in the signal. With carotid real time sonography these can be seen.
4. Sometimes both the internal and the external carotids can be obstructed when only tracings of the facial and temporal arteries will show the subsequent flow reduction.
5. Inaccurate measurement of the frontal and supraorbital arteries can occur if the examiner places the probe outside the orbital rim and catches the flow signal at an incorrect angle or tries to make a reversed signal "antegrade" if unsure of the probe technique.
6. Using a nondirectional Doppler will not show flow direction and may lead an inexperienced examiner to believe a pa-

tient has normal flow, especially in postoperative patients.

Now some of the false-positive diagnoses:

1. Excessive probe pressure may occlude the frontal or supraorbital, making flow seem reduced or absent. The probe can also slip off the artery without the examiner's noticing it during compression maneuvers, occasionally giving one the idea that compression has affected the flow.

2. Flow caught leaving the forehead by an incorrectly angled probe may lead to false diagnosis of flow reversal.

3. Monitoring the palpebral artery in the eyelid instead of the supraorbital may cause confusion, for the palpebral usually stops with temporal compression and this leads to a false diagnosis.

4. Monitoring the nasal artery can cause problems, especially if the patient fits in the category of retrograde flow (45% of normal individuals).[49] This is rarely encountered with good probe technique.

5. If the ophthalmic artery is occluded, flow will be reversed.[11] The patient will usually show signs of blindness without cerebral symptoms, however. Arteriography is indicated to specify this condition.

Common sense, care, and steady probe positioning will usually produce an accurate examination. Research should be done by the examiner if an unusual situation occurs.

Cerebrovascular examination in the postoperative patient

The most common procedure to alleviate a stenosed internal, external, or common carotid artery is *endarterectomy*. This procedure involves opening the artery at the area of occlusion and resecting and removing the atheromatous deposits and/or diseased intima. Although the carotid is clamped and flushed prior to closing and clamp release, emboli or bits of plaque still can break off and reocclude the artery higher up after surgery. The Doppler examination is of vital importance to normal postoperative hemodynamics.

Various grafts may be used in severe flow problems for shunting. They are usually synthetic and have a variety of applications. Some typical situations are mentioned below and shown in Fig. 23-48.

1. *Common carotid–subclavian.* This is used to correct a subclavian steal by shunting flow distal to the subclavian occlusion and restoring vertebral flow.

2. *Carotocarotid.* This is palpable and can

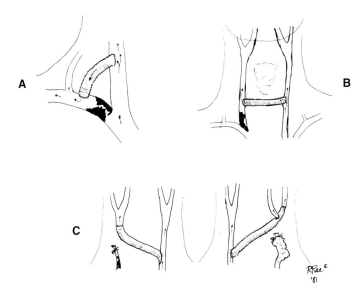

Fig. 23-48. Types of bypass grafts. **A,** Carotosubclavian. **B,** Caroto-carotid. **C,** Two examples of cross-carotid reconstruction.

be found usually extending subcutaneously across the lower thyroid cartilage. It supplements a carotid that is kinked or stenosed in the low portion near the base.

3. *Various cross-carotid.* Connections between the contralateral common carotid and ipsilateral bulb and/or internal carotid may be established depending on the disease and its severity.

Percutaneous transluminal angioplasty has been performed also for stenotic bulb lesions. The risk of embolization, as can be imagined, is much more significant than in the extremities and the procedure is rarely performed.

The examination procedure in the postop patient is the same as in the routine patient, with the possible exception of direct carotid studies on the operative side. Careful documentation of flow direction and flow changes is extremely important. Preoperative examinations should be compared, and an optional carotid real time study performed several days after surgery may assist in follow-up evaluation.

Summary

To conclude, the Doppler cerebrovascular examination is one of the most important and valuable in the specialty. Knowledge of the techniques and results will enable the examiner to screen patients with minimal symptoms or asymptomatic buits accurately and determine whether further investigation is required; it will also assist the vascular surgeon and the neurologist in diagnosing cerebral ischemia. Utilizing the Doppler with carotid real time examination can provide a thorough and noninvasive look at the carotid and cerebral circulation.

SPECTRAL ANALYSIS OF DOPPLER SIGNALS

The most common method of making a permanent record of Doppler flow signals has been through the strip-chart recorder. An organized set of flow tracings by this device also allows delayed interpretation and diagnosis of vascular flow abnormalities. The strip-chart tracing, however, shows only a mean flow velocity analog and does not reveal the complete range of frequencies present in the audible Doppler signal. The clinician interpreting the examination from tracings alone therefore is unable to take into account the various sounds and frequency changes in the Doppler signal that may indicate flow obstructions and stenoses. This may lead to an incorrect diagnosis, especially in the cerebrovascular system, in which normal flow is of high velocity and always above the zero baseline. Unless a lesion occludes a vessel, the high-velocity and high-frequency jet effect distal to the obstruction may often have the parameters of a normal internal carotid signal. A well-trained examiner should be able to hear these changes; unfortunately, many times the examiner and the interpreting clinician are not the same person. The examiner may note, for the benefit of the interpreting clinician, where signals that are suggestive of disease occur; but any inexperience or uncertainty can confuse the diagnosis and cause erroneous interpretation.

Sound spectral analysis of Doppler signals has recently emerged as a technique that

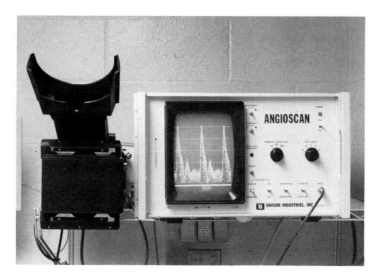

Fig. 23-49. Typical spectral analyzer (unidirectional, gray scale).

allows the information lost in strip-chart recording to be permanently recorded in a visual format. This method involves analyzing the frequencies present in a Doppler-shifted signal by Fourier transformation, with subsequent *sorting* of the frequencies by a series of filters.[65,69] The relative strengths of the sorted frequencies are assigned respective brightness levels or color codes and then displayed as a function of time. Note that the gradients of gray or color levels do *not* signify the relative velocity; this is shown as a deflection above (and below, on bidirectional devices) a zero baseline, as in the strip-chart recorder. Time is represented along the horizontal axis of the screen (Fig. 23-49).

Instrumentation

The spectral analysis device has been available in many forms for a number of years. Early devices required recording several seconds of the signal intended for analysis on a built-in tape. The "sonagram" was traced on a paper-covered rotating drum as the tape played over and over, and the process usually took a minute or longer before the sonagram was complete. This method is still used by some laboratories, but it has many disadvantages. The signals are not analyzed as they are being obtained (real time), and the process is not practical in a heavy case load. This means tape recording the examination for later analysis processing. Another disadvantage is that many of the higher and lower frequencies are lost in the transfer of the sound from tape to tape.

Modern devices intended for Doppler flow analysis present the data in real time and can be directly connected either to the audio or tape-output jacks of the Doppler device or to the audio tape recorder outputs if analysis of prerecorded signals is intended. This display several seconds of signal data and have freeze frame capability for photographic hard copy recording. Some devices have gray scale energy displays, some color-coded displays, and some both. They can be either unidirectional or bidirectional. The unidirectional devices do not show reversal components, making their use limited when extremity flow is being analyzed.

The standard spectral analyzer also has adjustable vertical frequency scales and can range from -6 to 20 kHz (from 0 to 20 kHz on unidirectional devices). The scale setting is changed if the vertical frequency exceeds the limits of the display. A cursor is also provided for numeric readout of the peak vertical frequency at a particular point of a waveform. Different input levels are also selected to ensure the clearest signal and filter out artifacts.

An example of a spectral analysis system is shown in Fig. 23-50.

Examination technique

Although spectral analysis can be performed on the flow in any peripheral artery or vein, the widest current use is in the analysis of carotid system flow signals.[65,66] The technique of examining the carotids is exclusively covered here, but many of the principles and waveform interpretations can be easily adapted to examination of extremity vessels.

Before beginning this section, it may be helpful to review the carotid anatomy given on p. 347.

The procedure for carotid spectral analysis is best performed after the routine cerebro-

vascular Doppler study is completed. The Doppler device is attached to the spectral analyzer, the the appropriate input level is selected to prevent signal overload and artifact production (artifacts will appear as noise interference). The probe is placed against the skin and coupled with gel, as in the standard Doppler examination. Depending on the area of the artery being examined, it may help to angle the probe *cephalad* rather than caudad; personal experience has shown the standard caudad angle to be just as effective, with the cephalad angle useful only on high internal and external carotid branches. Regardless of the angle, the Doppler device and analyzer should be adjusted to show the direction of flow correctly on the screen. In unidirectional analyzers, angle will make no difference since the analyzer has no zero-crossing capability; high-velocity flow will appear properly on the screen regardless of the flow direction.

The following positions are used for routine flow analysis and correspond to direct carotid examination positions in the routine cerebrovascular Doppler examination:

1. *Low to middle common carotid* (see Fig. 23-42)
2. *Carotid bifurcation—bulb area*
3. *Internal carotid*, found by moving slightly posterior and superior to the bifurcation
4. *External carotid*, found by moving anterior and superior to the bifurcation and/or internal carotid signal

The characteristics of the normal common, internal, and external carotid signals have been explained in the cerebrocascular section; to reiterate briefly, flow will be above the baseline in all cerebrovascular vessels normally. The internal carotid flow will generally be of a higher velocity than the external, with no visible second component and with a higher diastolic flow. The external carotid signal has a distinctly heard second component and may almost have flow characteristics similar to those of an extremity artery.

At the selected probe site the examiner angles the probe to obtain the clearest signal and must observe the monitor screen of the analyzer to be certain that the flow pattern seen corresponds with what is being heard. An appropriate vertical frequency scale should be selected to show the waveform to best advantage. If the waveform peaks near the top of the chosen scale, the analyzer should be set to the next highest scale. When a satisfactory waveform has been obtained, the examiner or an assistant freezes

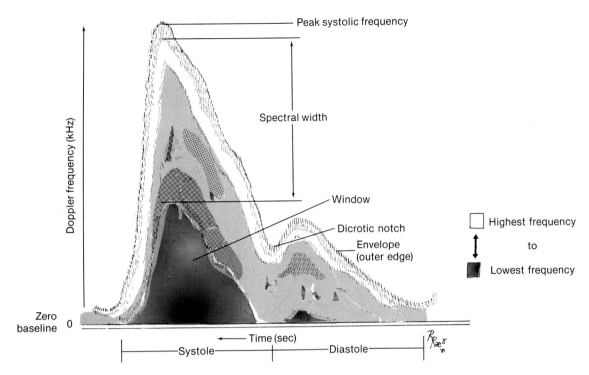

Fig. 23-50. Diagram of spectrally analyzed Doppler waveform, showing diagnostic characteristics.

the image on the monitor so that two or more clear waveforms are distinctly seen. A photographic hard copy can be made at this point, and peak vertical frequency measurements using the cursor may also be made and recorded. The examiner should be certain to note the monitor frequency scale (e.g., 5 kHz, 20 kHz) on the hard copy to ensure accurate interpretation. If the analyzer has the capability, videotape recordings can be made of the real time spectral waveforms and Doppler sounds simultaneously.

Interpretation of the Doppler spectral waveform[65,66,69]

The normal waveform has several characteristics: a high systolic peak frequency, usually at 4 kHz, with a high diastolic flow, about one third that of peak systole. The systolic flow is shown as a concentration of brighter shades of gray or color levels near the upper frequencies, moving at a high velocity, and a darker area within the systolic envelope, caused by a lack of low-velocity blood flow. This dark area is referred to as the *window*. Diastolic flow has a more uniform distribution of intensity levels due to deceleration of flow velocity (Fig. 23-50). The internal carotid will show the same flow characteristics, with a possibly higher velocity. The external carotid signal will have a shorter peak frequency duration, with distinct waves seen in the diastolic components.

In the determination of flow disturbance, certain characteristics of the waveform should be evaluated[69]:

1. The *peak systolic frequency* should be measured. This will determine flow velocity.
2. The shape of the *waveform envelope* should be checked. A well-defined envelope is characteristic of normal or smooth flow; ragged and poorly defined envelopes signify turbulence.
3. The *presence of the window* is an indicator of relatively normal flow. If turbulent or disturbed flow causes a variation in flow distribution, the window may fill in and disappear.
4. The *spectral width* should be measured. This comprises the distribution of the strongest flow intensity levels from the upper border of the window to the peak of the systolic component. Flow intensities in normal flow will usually be along the envelope outline. If the intensities are spread throughout the waveform and cause the disappearance of the window, the spectral width may comprise the entire waveform. Flow intensities centering around the baseline may indicate eddies and turbulence in the flow sample area.

In situations of arterial occlusion, the following characteristics may be seen:

1. Proximal to the stenosis a normal or slightly blunted waveform may be seen. The peak frequency should be normal, and there may or may not be a rounding of the peak. The separation between the first and second components (dicrotic notch) may disappear due to vascular elastic changes along the stenosed area. The window may show some flow scattering throughout.
2. Across the stenosis an increased-frequency (higher-velocity) waveform will usually be seen. The same characteristics as in the proximal waveform may be noted, and the envelope may begin to break up. The velocity will usually increase directly with the degree of stenosis. The window may also begin to disappear. A corresponding increase in pitch will be heard with the Doppler. It may help to remember that cerebrovascular flow remains nearly constant until a severe stenosis (at 60% to 70% luminal reduction) occurs.[1]
3. Immediately distal to the stenotic area, disturbed or turbulent flow may be found ranging from a strained burbling to a high-pitched hissing Doppler signal. The flow stream increases by the jet effect (p. 350), originating at the stenosis; and an area of flow stagnation immediately distal to the plaque or lesion near the artery wall may cause turbulence during systole. The spectral waveform will have a ragged-appearing indistinct envelope, with widely distributed frequencies, and a com-

pletely absent window. The severity of the stenosis may be judged from the level of envelope disruption and frequency distribution. Turbulence and eddy formation will cause an increase in the higher-energy intensities at the baseline[69] and in severe cases may cause a completely disrupted waveform with apparent velocity reductions *at systole* in bidirectional analyzers. Pulsatility may be absent, and the pitch may either increase or decrease with the sound becoming rough and harsh.

4. A signal obtained more distally from the stenosis, away from the turbulent region, may assume the appearance of a reduced waveform with even intensity throughout and no visible components. The peak frequency may be markedly rounded. Severely diminished flow may become almost flat in appearance.

5. In total occlusion a sharp thudding or thumping sound may be heard in the patent portion of the vessel immediately proximal to the block. Flow may actually drop to or below the baseline, and a very irregular-appearing spectral waveform with no distinguishing characteristics may be seen. This is caused from flow eddies within the stump.[65]

The characteristics of flow increase across a stenosis apply to extremity arteries as well. Distal to the stenosis a rounded blunt waveform will be noted, with disappearance of the window and evidence of low flow velocities. As flow decreases, a flattened signal close to the baseline will usually be found. Remember that in the extremity arteries, loss of the second retrograde component signifies occlusion proximally and the flow envelope may remain well defined regardless of the level of flow reduction.

Examples of normal and abnormal spectrally analyzed Doppler signals will be found in Appendix I.

Summary

Using spectral analyzers as an adjunct to the cerebrovascular Doppler study and carotid real time sonography can help increase the accuracy of diagnosis. Spectral analysis will often eliminate the confusion sometimes created when examiner notation of the flow sounds fails to correlate with the results on a strip-chart recording. Spectral analysis adds only a few minutes to an examination, and the results may supply the information needed to confirm or reject a diagnosis of flow obstruction. As with other Doppler techniques, adequate training and thorough

familiarity with the procedures are imperative for accurate examination and interpretation of results. Many articles and papers have been published on the use of spectral analysis,[66,68] and refinements in the technique are occurring constantly with the increase in technology. There are other methods and variations on the above-mentioned techniques, and the reader is encouraged to conduct further research into this subject.

DOPPLER ULTRASONIC ANGIOGRAPHY (DOPPLER SCANNING)

One of the more common uses of Doppler other than for flow measurement has been the noninvasive imaging of arteries and veins based on the creation of an image from Doppler signals on a storage cathode ray tube (CRT). This technique uses a Doppler device connected to a signal-processing unit and an X-Y axis scanning arm, similar to that used in conventional B-scan imaging. A directional Doppler probe is used, and current devices either create the image in bistable on a CRT or use a more sophisticated color image system.[73,75] Directions of flow or flow intensities are assigned color levels, as in spectral analysis, and the image of the artery or vein is a composite of colors showing some flow and morphologic information. The Doppler angiograph can also be connected to spectral analyzers or microcomputers for additional information. Some Doppler arteriographs have integral analyzers and computers[71-75] and show several types of information simultaneously on the monitor.

Examination techniques

The Doppler angiograph can be used for both arteries and veins,[72] but it is most frequently used in scanning the carotid bifurcation. The basic technique involves positioning the patient, immobilizing the area intended for study, and positioning the scanning arm.[73] The examiner coats the area with gel and creates the image by moving the probe back and forth transversely across the artery and/or vein being examined. A Doppler signal received by the probe is heard and shown as a trace on the screen. The examiner steps the arm to another position, thereby building up a series of traces until an image of the vessel is shown on the screen (Fig. 23-51). Lines are also placed on the image to denote the inferior border of the mandible on carotid scans and the skin line on transverse scans. When the image has been created, a hard copy is made photographically.

Further processing is possible at this point. Some devices have a cursor that shows the position of the probe anywhere along the arterial or venous image, which enables simultaneous spectral flow patterns and/or Doppler signals to be recorded showing the point in the artery or vein where the signal is heard. Some devices, such as the MAVIS (Mobile Arterial and Venous Imaging System) (GEC/Picker, Middlesex, England), are equipped with computers to allow beam/vessel angle measurement, measure velocity profiles, and compute blood flow volumes. Flow tracings are also provided.

Either pulsed mode or continuous-wave Doppler is used, with some devices incorporating both. The pulsed Doppler systems tend to provide better resolution of the image (1 mm or more). The probe is often detachable to allow hand-held Doppler studies to be performed in addition to imaging.

Interpretation and discussion

Doppler angiographic images appear as a series of dots or lines making up the profile of a vessel being examined. Areas where no Doppler signal is received appear as gaps or indentations in the profile (Fig. 23-52). In color-coded devices brighter color intensities correspond to higher-frequency flow. Some devices have as few as 3 or as many as 15 color gradients. Others use only red, blue, and yellow, for either frequency categorization or flow direction.

Areas where signals are not received usually correspond to plaques, lesions, or occluded vessels; but calcium deposits may cause false diagnoses of occlusion. Devices coupled with spectral analysis or flow profiling can help in determining the status of flow distal to such areas.

Although these devices have definite benefits, moving plaques (e.g., pseudovalves) may not be detected since unobstructed flow will be received as a normal signal; or if detected on one sweep, they may be obscured on the return sweep of the probe. Some areas (e.g., the carotid bifurcation) may be inaccessible to the probe and prevent accurate flow detection. Prominent branches of the external carotid in internal carotid occlusion may simulate the bifurcation, causing an incorrect image.[73] Vessels lying in the same plane may not be distinguished on longitudinal scans, and external and internal carotids that approximate each other may blend together on transverse images.

Another disadvantage is the length of time required to perform the study. Contrary to some manufacturers' claims, the examination can take from 30 minutes to 1½ hours to perform, even in skilled hands. This, of course, depends on the type of processing to be done on the signal or image, the difficulty of the patient, and the examiner's ability. These devices are extremely operator dependent, and untrained personnel may measurably affect the examination results and performance time. Routine screening can sometimes be impractical.

Summary

Doppler ultrasonic angiography may be beneficial in determining the flow status of arteries and veins and may allow location of some obstructive lesions. Correlating the results with cerebrovascular Doppler studies, carotid real time sonography, and Doppler spectral analysis will give more thorough coverage of the cerebrovascular circulation; but some redundancy may occur when both carotid real time scanners and Doppler angiographs exist in the same department since somewhat more specific information concerning plaque obstruction can be obtained by combined usage of the cerebrovascular Doppler examination, spectral analysis, and a carotid B-mode real time device. The best deployment of the current Doppler angiographic instrumentation seems to be in determining flow volume measurements and profiles and showing respective flow directions and intensities in arteries and veins. As with most Doppler-related examinations, the best overall results are obtained by correlation with the basic Doppler examination and/or another imaging modality.

CAROTID REAL TIME SONOGRAPHY

The introduction of high-resolution small-parts scanners has proved to be a definite breakthrough in the noninvasive examination of small or difficult-to-evaluate structures in the body. Of the many uses of these newer real time devices, examination of the common carotid system has had the most publicity and investigation so far.[77-80] The results of real time sonography are more specific than those of carotid arteriography in visualizing bulb plaques, although the final reports on many of these devices are yet to be published and verified.[77,80] However, real time carotid sonography does not eliminate the need for carotid arteriography to image plaques and occlusions above the carotid bifurcation and the cranial segments, since these are too deep or are inaccessible to the transducer. At the present time carotid sonography is best employed as a correlative screening method alongside Doppler cerebrovascular examination and carotid arteriography.

This subject is mentioned within the Doppler area because most of the scanners available incorporate a provision for Doppler to be done intermittently with imaging of the vessel. The methods of Doppler sampling and technique will be discussed in further detail in the appropriate sections below.

Description of the small-parts scanner

Several companies manufacture small-parts scanners, and improvements in operator-oriented design and resolution are occurring constantly. Most of these scanners utilize one of three methods to obtain a real time image of the area being examined (Fig. 23-53):

1. One system (Advanced Technology Laboratories, Bellevue, Wash.) uses three or more 5-MHz transducers installed in a rotor that rotates rapidly, sweeping the ultrasonic beam through a fluid-filled coupling head and producing a relatively flicker-free image rate.

The Doppler signals are obtained by activating a 5-to-8-MHz pulsed range-gated

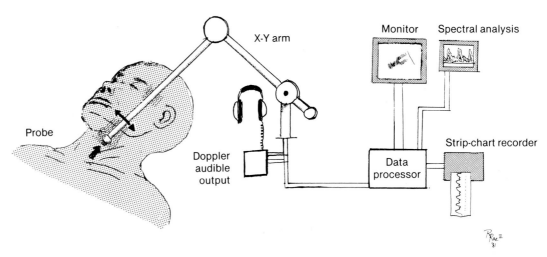

Fig. 23-51. Technique of Doppler angiography.

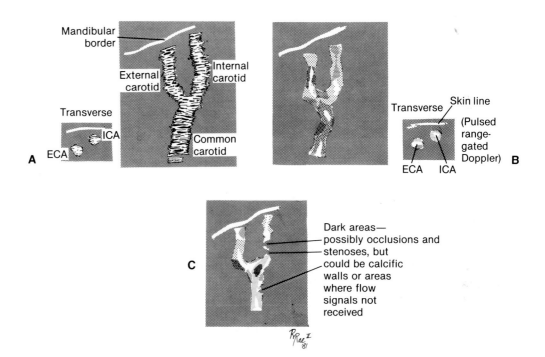

Fig. 23-52. Typical appearances of Doppler angiographic scans of the carotid bifurcation. **A,** Normal image on a CRT. **B,** Normal image on a gray scale or color-coded system. **C,** Abnormal image showing the appearance of nonvisualized areas indicative of vascular stenosis, occlusion, or calcific vessel walls.

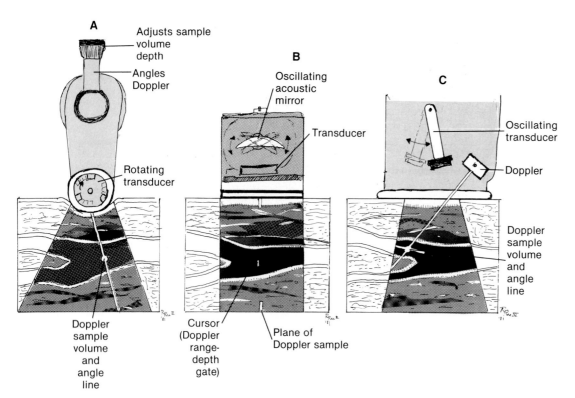

Fig. 23-53. Types of small-parts scanner transducers. **A,** Rotor. **B,** Acoustic mirror. **C,** Oscillating transducer.

Doppler (utilizing one of the scan transducers in the scan rotor) that can be angled relative to the scan plane of the vessel, with the sampling depth of the signal adjusted separately. The main drawback to this system has been the necessity of freezing the image and stopping the rotor while a Doppler signal is being taken. The image on the screen serves as a guide to the placement of the M-line and the sample volume; but to obtain an accurate evaluation of flow at a precise site, the transducer must remain in the same place as when the image was frozen. Looking at a simultaneous A-mode signal helps to locate the sample level, when provided.

2. A second system (Bio-Dynamics, Indianapolis, Ind.) utilizes a fixed 8-MHz transducer with an oscillating acoustic mirror to sweep the beam through a fluid path.

Doppler in this system is obtained through the same 8-MHz transducer as is used for imaging. Activating the Doppler stops the mirror at the midline position and cuts in a simultaneous extended A-mode for reference when range-gating of the Doppler sample depth is being done. The examiner can thus see changes in position and move the transducer to compensate. The angle of the Doppler is fixed, however, and the entire probe head must be angled to obtain the best signal. The company is adding (at the time of

this writing) a feature that allows a choice of A-mode or freeze frame image and the ability to move the mirror to angle the Doppler in long axis views.

3. A third system (Diasonics, Sunnyvale, Calif.) uses an oscillating transducer (5-MHz) for imaging and a separate Doppler transducer (3 MHz).

An advantage of this system is that when the Doppler is activated the device continues to image at a reduced and staggered frame rate with the Doppler pulsing in the intervals when the imaging transducer is off. The image is updated four times per second to allow more exact technique.

It should be mentioned that at the time of this writing no available system has been able to obtain true simultaneous imaging and Doppler since the oscillation or rotor mechanism usually interferes with the Doppler signals, forcing one modality to be disengaged while the other is operating.

Most of these scanners have axial and lateral resolution capabilities of no less than 0.3 mm and enlarge the image to show the detail of the arterial walls or other area being examined. Their sizes vary from large to fairly compact, but a few of them are portable enough for use in bedside examinations. Some companies have introduced miniature versions, enabling the device to be more easily transported and providing an equiva-

lent or better image at roughly half the cost of the larger units.

As can be seen, the differing characteristics of the various machines available demand differing examination techniques. Discussion of the examination methods and idiosyncrasies present with each type is not practicable here. A general explanation of the interpretation of a typical examination will be given, however, along with fairly flexible examination techniques that can be used with most of the systems currently available.

Description of the carotid real time image

Before performing or interpreting an examination, the sonographer must have a thorough knowledge of the appearance and anatomy of the carotid system. This can be reviewed on p. 347 and seen in Figs. 23-37 and 23-39.

The *common, internal, and external carotids* appear to have sonolucent fluid-filled lumina bordered by two bright reflections, the arterial walls. The walls are lined with a low-level gray layer bordered by a fine slightly brigher echo, thought to represent the *intima* of the arteries.

Usually an irregular vessel without the thicker-walled characteristics of an artery is seen either anterior to or on one side of the common carotid. This is the *internal jugular vein.* It can be distinguished by its lack of pulsatility, its phasic dilation and collapse with respiration, its tendency to be irregularly shaped and to widen out at the base, and the ease with which it is collapsed by light pressure from the transducer. This is much more apparent when compared with the even diameter, thicker walls, regular pulsatility, and much more stable appearance of the common carotid.

As the transducer moves up the neck, the carotid will be seen to widen out into the area of the *carotid bulb.* The bulb is the most common site of plaque and intimal thickening, which is usually seen to extend into the internal and/or external carotids directly above the bulb.

Contrary to some beliefs, a perfect Y appearance of the *carotid bifurcation* is infrequently seen. The bifurcation tends to be rotated differently in certain individuals, and the appearance will depend on the ability to obtain both vessels in the same view. For evaluation the internal and external carotids are best examined individually.

1. The *internal carotid* can be seen by moving the transducer in a posterior direction from the area of the bulb. It is

a vessel generally of slightly larger diameter than the external carotid, tapering into regularly spaced walls that come off the bulb.

2. The *external carotid* is seen by moving anteriorly. It is usually of smaller diameter without the prominent widening frequently seen at the takeoff of the internal carotid.

3. The transverse appearance of the *common carotid* is a round lumen posterior or lateral to the irregularly shaped jugular vein. The normal carotid maintains its round appearance up to the bulb, where the diameter of the vessel becomes larger and begins to elongate as the bifurcation approaches.

The internal and external carotids will be seen as two separate round lumina forming from the bulb as the transducer moves superiorly. The internal will be larger than the external and positioned slightly posterior to the smaller round lumen of the external.

Disease in the carotid appears as low-to-moderate gray, soft, and smooth to irregularly edged deformations of the intima extending into the lumen. Calcific plaque is a bright echo with sonic dropout extending past the lesion. Calcific plaque can be incorporated into a "soft" (medium to low echogenic) plaque and is troublesome when the area of dropout obscures the deep wall and a superficial wall plaque is present. Ulcerated plaque can be seen as indentations or erosions in either soft-tissue plaque or the intima.

Examples of normal and abnormal scans with labeling are in Appendix I.

Examination technique in carotid real time sonography

A basic technique and transducer positioning guide are given here, and the respective views should be altered to conform with the capabilities of each examiner's scanner. The examination can be recorded by videotape or hard-copy camera methods.

The patient should either lie supine or sit in a chair. The techniques are applicable to both positions.

The first position used is the *anterior position*. The transducer is held so the patient's head is to the top or left of the screen, depending on the machine being used. (Some institutions will have the head to the bottom of the screen when the left side is being examined, due to inversion by the transducer. This is optional and depends on preference or protocol.) The neck is coated with gel, and the patient's head turned

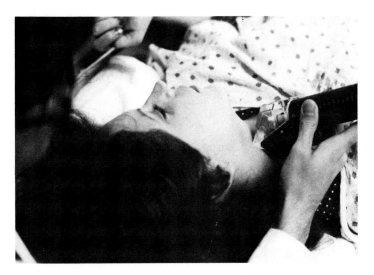

Fig. 23-54. Examination of the carotid artery in the anterior position.

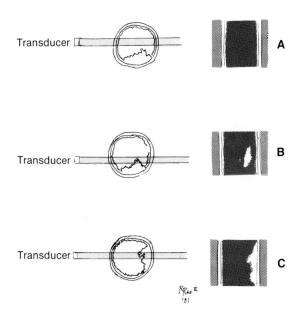

Fig. 23-55. Rocking the transducer. **A,** Plaque on the lateral walls may be missed by the parallel beam. **B,** Slight lateral motion of the transducer enables one to image the peaks of the plaque. **C,** When the transducer is moved to a different examination angle, the plaque is shown in cross section.

slightly away from the side being examined. To obtain as true an anterior view as possible, the examiner should come in directly parallel with the sagittal plane of the neck (Fig. 23-54).

The examiner then examines the common carotid from the base to the bifurcation in long axis, being careful to show the artery continuously. Slight side-to-side motion of the transducer is used to pick up plaque, which may project from a lateral wall parallel with the plane of the examination. It is noted, recorded on the videotape, or photographed for later reference (Fig. 23-55).

Upon reaching the bifurcation, the examiner moves the transducer anteriorly and posteriorly to determine the takeoffs of the external and internal carotids at the bifurcation.

When the position and identification of each artery are determined, the examiner checks to see if any disease is present in the common carotid, bulb, and bifurcation areas. The transducer is moved accordingly to show the extent and degree of occlusion of the disease. Areas of disease are documented and the positioning described.

The examiner then determines the lie of

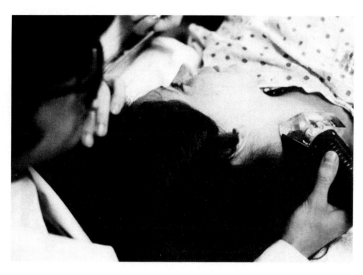

Fig. 23-56. Examination of the carotid artery in lateral position.

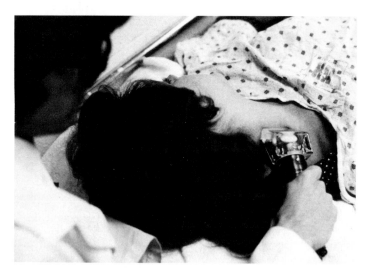

Fig. 23-57. Posterior position.

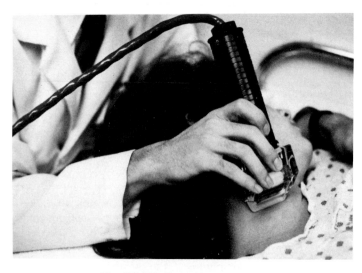

Fig. 23-58. Transverse position.

the internal carotid and moves the transducer posteriorly toward the ear while rotating it slightly along the plane of the long axis of the artery. It is followed up as high as practicable.

The transducer next is moved anteriorly and rotated or angled to demonstrate the external carotid. As much of the artery as possible should be seen.

The anterior view is not the best, for the probe will come against the mandible within the area of the bifurcation. It can, however, show disease that is not well seen in the other long axis views.

The patient should turn his head a little more to facilitate the *lateral* position. The transducer is brought around so the beam intersects the artery perpendicular to the sagittal plane of the *head*. The vessels are examined in the fashion described above (Fig. 23-56).

The patient should then turn his head as far as possible. In the *posterior* position the transducer is brought in from behind the sternocleidomastoid muscle and angled toward the anterior side of the patient. The arteries are located and examined as above. The common and bifurcation vessels may be deep in this view and not readily visualized. The Y appearance of the bifurcation tends to be seen in this position more often than in any other (Fig. 23-57).

When the long axis views of the artery have been obtained, the transducer is turned *transversely*. The medial side of the neck will be at the top or left of the screen in viewing the right carotid and the lateral side to the top or left in viewing the left carotid.

For an accurate determination of the location of the obstruction and the percentage of stenosis, the transducer is moved slowly up the common carotid to the bifurcation. Special attention must be given to documenting any areas that were shown in the anterior, lateral, or posterior views (Fig. 23-58).

The bifurcation should also be examined for circumferential plaques, shown previously, and the transducer then moves superiorly to image the figure 8 of the external and internal carotids.

The internal carotid will be seen posterior to the external. On the right, in machines with the skin surface ot the left side of the screen and medial to the top, this means that the uppermost vessel will usually be the external carotid. On the left this position will be reversed. Positioning is less confusing in equipment with the skin surface to the top of the screen.

If the scanner is equipped with a Doppler,

there are several ways to use it. In longitudinal examination of the vessel, flow sampling should be performed below, across, and above any areas of stenosis encountered. (For a review of signal characteristics and waveforms, see "Doppler Examination of the Cerebrovascular System," p. 346.) This procedure works well with probes utilizing a movable angle and sample line. With probes utilizing the acoustic mirror the entire transducer should be physically angled to best pick up flow. No matter which type of transducer is used, flow should always be checked in the *common*, at the *bifurcation/bulb*, and in the *internal* and *external* carotids.

Special mention should be made here that the Doppler devices in the scanners are not as sensitive as the hand-held probes. Many times an angle may be off just enough to record flow inaccurately, possibly misleading an inexperienced examiner or interpreting physician into making a false diagnosis of flow absence or reduction. If the scanner-mounted Doppler is used, it is best utilized to make a *confirmation* of flow presence or absence and not a definitive diagnostic statement unless a correlative hand-held Doppler examination is also performed, preferably by the same examiner. In short, *the scanner-mounted Doppler should not be used as a substitute for a more sensitive hand-held Doppler probe.* When there is a discrepancy between the hand-held Doppler results at a given arterial site and the signal obtained at an identical location by the scanner's Doppler, the general preference is to trust the former rather than the latter.

In scanners that use the probe with the acoustic mirror Doppler signals may best be obtained in the transverse position, in which there is much more flexibility of transducer movement. Since no separate control exists for angling of the Doppler sample line, the entire transducer must be free to move and find the best angle to intersect the flow. Flow should be checked below, across, and above the stenoses as is done with longitudinal sampling.

Interpretation and appearance of disease

When the examination is complete, it should be interpreted by the physician. Videotape of the studies has been found to cause the least loss of low-level gray areas and to provide the most exact representation of the "live" examination. In hard-copy photography usually there will be a loss of detail and image sharpness, which may cause many diagnostic results to be overlooked.

With careful adjustment of the camera settings this can be reduced.

The normal arteries should have clear lumina with their walls regular and uniform and the intima barely seen. The diseased vessel, however, will take on many different appearances depending on the extent and type of disease.

Soft tissue plaque tends to be the most frequently seen anomaly. It can vary from a soft low-level gray-appearing lesion that may be mistaken for artifact to a brighter homogeneous mass that completely occludes the lumina of the common, internal, and external carotids. It can be a smooth slightly thickened area of the intima or a large irregular-bordered mass jutting into the lumen. Irregular plaques are the more dangerous, for they throw off emboli that travel into the circulation of the brain, block the flow to a small tributary, and cause a TIA or a CVA. Quite often areas of soft tissue plaque may be missed on arterio grams unless they severely compromise the lumen, since they sometimes do not obstruct the flow of contrast. (See Bernstein et al.,[8] p. 239.) This is often to the detriment of the patient, who returns later with a CVA that might have been avoided with an endarterectomy performed in time. Some sonographers may not be aware of soft tissue plaque's importance; one instance was seen at our clinic in which the physician was noting only reflective calcific plaques and not the "soft" areas. These lesions must not be overlooked.

Ulcerated plaque, which is usually found as an erosion of the intima and arterial wall, is seen as depressions or notches in a thickened or fairly irregular intimal lining. The ability of the carotid scan to reveal areas of ulceration has been shown to be excellent compared with pathologic surgery specimens in studies in progress at St. Vincent Hospital, Indianapolis.

Calcific plaque is both significant and troublesome. It appears as a bright reflection on the superficial or deep wall of the artery being examined. Many times smaller patches of calcium can be seen within a larger soft plaque. Calcific plaque will cast a shadow of sonic dropout through the area directly behind it that may obscure the rest of the lumen or other wall if it is superficially located. The difficulty lies in determining whether the plaque or the wall is calcified and whether the portion not seen in the lumen is large. There is also the likelihood that plaque exists on the deep wall but is hidden by the shadowing. The examiner should rock the transducer from side to side

in an attempt to find a window in the plaque or should go to an alternate position that may permit looking around the area of calcification.

Aneurysms will be seen as large dilated areas of the common carotid, bulb, or branches. Plaque will frequently be seen, as may ulcerations or dissection of the walls. The examiner must remember that the internal carotid is normally wide at the point where it comes off the bulb and then tapers into a narrower vessel. An aneurysm will be much more obvious, bulbous, and prominent with irregular-appearing walls.

Total occlusion of the internal, external, and/or common carotids will be seen as a completely filled-in area or a complete segment with none of the totally clear characteristics associated with a blood-filled lumen. The homogeneity of the blocked artery(ies) may blend in with surrounding adipose, connective, and muscle tissue. This situation requires distinction only by visualizing the brighter arterial walls, which should be followed from the base to ascertain that they are continuous with the obstructed vessel. Depending on the nature of the occlusion, some clear areas of flow may be seen above or below the obstructed areas. Occasionally a small lumen will be found at the center or side of an occlusion. Doppler use can aid in verifying the presence of minimal or the absence of flow. A comparative cerebrovascular Doppler study should be done, if it has not been previously, to determine collateral flow and check for carotid flow.

All these diseases can appear in combinations, and careful attention must be given to distinguishing the separate arteries and the parameters of the disease within the vessels.

Obstacles to the performance of the carotid real time scan

There are many variations in anatomy and pathology that can hinder the examination and prevent a complete or accurate study. The following paragraphs will discuss some of these obstacles:

1. The *location of the bifurcation* varies in every individual, even from side to side in some people. Occasionally the bifurcation will be above the lower border of the mandible and will be unreachable by the transducer. Sometimes the proximal areas of the internal and external are visualized, but disease above that level can be missed.

2. *Fat and musculature*, especially in the short-necked patient, will cause the artery to lie deep and be difficult to visualize. The fat and tissue also may attenuate the sound

beam, which cannot always penetrate because of the higher frequency at which the transducer operates.

3. *Calcific plaque*, as mentioned earlier, will cause an area of dropout to occur past the lesion that may obscure part or all of the bifurcation if it appears on the superficial wall of the artery. Once again, either rocking the beam through the artery or repositioning may afford better visualization of areas on the wall opposite the plaque.

4. *Congenital anomalies and variations* can cause the most confusion if their presence has not previously been mentioned. *Tortuousity* (usually of the internal or common carotid artery) is a frequently seen condition, in which the artery's complex twists and turns make long axis and transverse visualization extremely difficult. Patience and perseverance are required for a thorough examination. *Coarctation* or *kinking* is not so much an anomaly as a disease state, due to its flow obstruction. *Anomalous vessels* are occasionally seen. Some examples that I have detected by carotid sonography include a separate origin of the external carotid from the subclavian, absence of the bifurcation with separate internal and external carotids, and bilateral low bifurcations at the clavicle level.

5. The *internal jugular vein* has been confused with the common carotid occasionally but can be easily distinguished by the previously mentioned characteristics.

6. *Inversion of the positions of the internal and external carotids* has caused many inaccurate diagnoses. This often happens when a transposed external is diseased and the internal is not. Since disease tends to be found more in the internal carotid, careless interpretation without checking vessel takeoff and internal diameters could lead to a false-positive report. If a Doppler is installed, the flow characteristics of the separate arteries should be readily distinguishable and assist in verifying the individual vessels.

7. *Machine artifacts* will sometimes simulate the appearance or leading edges of plaques. Careful adjustment of gain, periodic transducer maintenance, and regular flushing and replacement of the fluid path medium will resolve most artifacts. If the examiner is in doubt as to whether an area is artifact or disease, the transducer should be moved. Any lines or gray areas that remain in the same location on the screen will be artifactual.

If there is a case in which distal branches or segments of the carotid cannot be visualized, the Doppler cerebrovascular test will help to determine whether a flow obstruction occurs further up the neck. Conversely, the carotid real time examination can be used to confirm areas of turbulence or implications of internal carotid stenosis found with the Doppler examination. One technique therefore can cover the other and make difficult evaluations more simple.

Postoperative uses

In most patients with carotid obstruction an endarterectomy will be performed to eliminate the blockage. Unfortunately the surgeon can remove only what can be felt or directly seen when the artery is opened. Sometimes residual plaque may remain, acting as a base where plaque can reform above or below the surgery site. An intraoperative probe with a resolution capability of 0.0005 will be available soon and will enable the surgeon to examine the artery above and below the intended surgical site to determine where the disease is and where the vessel should be opened for removal of the plaque.

Postoperatively the artery can be examined after the scar has healed for several days. Sequential follow-up studies can be arranged to evaluate the condition in the months following surgery.

The appearance of the endarterectomized carotid is similar to that of the normal vessel. A bright area on the wall may be seen where the sutures were placed, and the intimal reflections will be missing in the area of the surgery because the intima was resected with the plaques.

Preoperative and postoperative examination will enable much better correlations to be made with subsequent pathology reports and future follow-up care.

Summary

The uses of carotid sonography are only beginning to be realized. The modality provides a simple and quick way of screening the carotid arteries for plaques and may allow a better determination of whether a patient is a candidate for operative management.

Coupled with a Doppler cerebrovascular examination, the carotid real time study can show areas of obstruction and flow disturbance and can enable a more thorough evaluation of the carotid and cerebral circulation to be performed.

As advances in technology continue to be made, the capabilities of small-parts scanners can only improve and should provide a useful adjunct to arteriographic and noninvasive diagnosis of the cerebrovascular system.

FINAL SUMMARY OF PERIPHERAL VASCULAR DOPPLER TECHNIQUES

In this discussion of Doppler vascular methods the complexity and difficulty of many of the techniques have been suggested. The Doppler examinations are probably more difficult than any of the other ultrasound methods, and they require independent decisions and specific knowledge of the techniques and diagnoses to ensure an accurate and thorough study. Among many sonographers there is a general misunderstanding of what Doppler methods are and what they can do. Noninvasive vascular diagnosis is a definite part of ultrasound; but it is too often placed in the background, behind B-scanning and echocardiography. There is a demand for more technicians and sonographers trained in Doppler methods. Any attempt by a sonographer to learn Doppler can be rewarded by the knowledge that the acquired understanding of arterial and vascular hemodynamics will aid in diagnosing and interpreting great vessel B-scans and carotid scanning. The echocardiographer can also apply pulsed Doppler techniques to the M-mode examination. Even a basic understanding of Doppler techniques will open new doors to the sonographer and enable new examinations and abilities to be added to the repertoire of a flexible and valuable diagnostic ultrasound department.

REFERENCES

Arterial Doppler examinations

1. Baker, J.D.: Poststress Doppler ankle pressures: a comparison of treadmill exercise with two other methods of induced hyperemia, Arch. Surg. **113**:1171, 1978.
2. Barnes, R.W.: Axioms on acute arterial occlusion of an extremity, Hosp. Med. **14**(6):34, 1978.
3. Barnes, R.W., et al.: Doppler ultrasonic evaluation of peripheral arterial disease, Iowa City, 1975, University of Iowa Press.
4. Barnes, R.W., and Garrett, W.V.: Intraoperative assessment of arterial reconstruction by Doppler ultrasound, Surg. Obstet. Gynecol. **146**:896, 1978.
5. Baron, H.C.: Chronic arterial insufficiency of the lower limbs, Hosp. Med. **14**(9):33, 1978.
6. Baron, H.C., and Hiesiger, E.: Significance of ankle blood pressure in the diagnosis of peripheral vascular disease, Am. Surg. **45**:289, 1979.
7. Bergan, J.J., and Yao, J.S.T.: Gangrene and severe ischemia of the lower extremities, New York, 1978, Grune & Stratton, Inc.
8. Bernstein, E.F., et al.: Noninvasive diagnostic techniques in vascular disease, St. Louis, 1978, The C.V. Mosby Co.
9. Blackshear, W.M. Jr., et al.: Pulsed Doppler assessment of normal human femoral artery velocity patterns, J. Surg. Res. **27**:73, 1979.
10. Cooperman, M., et al.: Use of Doppler ultrasound in intraoperative localization of intestinal arteriovenous malformation, Ann. Surg. **190**:24, 1979.
11. Corson, J.D., et al.: Doppler ankle systolic blood pressure. Prognostic value in vein bypass grafts of the lower extremity, Arch. Surg. **113**:932, 1978.
12. Diethrich, E.B., editor: Noninvasive cardiovascular diagnosis, Baltimore, 1978, University Park Press.
13. Friedman, S.A.: Guide to diagnosis of peripheral arterial disease, Hosp. Med. **15**(1):87, 1979.
14. Gardner, A.L., et al.: Arterial occlusions and stenosis: when should you order a Doppler study? Diagnosis **1**(5):87, 1979.
15. Gaylis, H.: Penile pressure in the evaluation of impotence in aorto-iliac disease, Surgery **89**(2):277, 1981.
16. Goss, C.M., editor: Gray's anatomy, ed. 29, Philadelphia, 1974, Lea & Febiger.
17. Gross, W.S., Louis, D.S.: Doppler hemodynamic assessment of obscure symptomatology in the upper extremity, J. Hand Surg. **3**(5):467, 1978.
18. Hill, D.A., et al.: Haemodynamic validity of lower limb arterial crossover grafts, J. R. Coll. Surg. Edinb. **24**:170, 1979.
19. Hitchon, P.W., et al.: The Doppler ultrasonic flowmeter as an adjunct to operative management of cerebral arteriovenous malformations, Surg. Neurol. **11**:345, 1979.
20. Hummel, B.W., et al.: Reactive hyperemia versus treadmill testing in arterial disease, Arch. Surg. **113**:95, 1978.
21. Juergens, J.L., Spittell, J.A., and Fairbairn, J.F.: Peripheral vascular diseases, Philadelphia, 1980, W.B. Saunders, Co.
22. Lee, B.Y., et al.: Noninvasive hemodynamic evaluation in selection of amputation level, Surg. Obstet. Gynecol. **149**:241, 1979.
23. Najem, Z., et al.: Arteriovenous malformations of the cecum: operative localization by Doppler ultrasound, Am. Surg. **45**:538, 1979.
24. Nath, R.L., et al.: The multidisciplinary approach to vasculogenic impotence, Surgery **89**(1):124, 1978.

25. Oliver, M.A., et al.: Use of Doppler ultrasound in dissecting aortic aneurysm, Crit. Care Med. **61**(1):45, 1978.
26. O'Reilly, M.J., et al.: Plasma exchange and Raynaud's phenomenon: its assessment by Doppler ultrasonic velocimetry, Br. J. Surg. **66**:712, 1979.
27. Platz, M.: Doppler ultrasound studies of subclavian steal hemodynamics in subclavian stenosis, J. Thorac. Cardiovasc. Surg. **27**(6):404, 1979.
28. von Reutern, G.M., et al.: Dopplersonographische diagnostik von Stenosen und Verschlussen der Vertebralarterien und des Subclavian-Steal-Syndroms, Arch. Psychiatr. Nervenkr. **222**(2-3):209, 1976.
29. White, D.N., et al.: Noninvasive techniques for the recording of vertebral artery flow and their limitations, Ultrasound Med. Biol. **6**:315, 1980.
30. Yeh, H.C., et al.: Ultrasonography of the brachiocephalic arteries, Radiology **132**(2):403, 1979.
31. Zicot, M.J.: Combined study of hyperemia after arterial occlusion and exercise by an isotopic test and a Doppler-ultrasonic method, Angiology **29**:534, 1978.

Venous Doppler examinations

32. Barnes, R.W., et al.: Doppler ultrasonic evaluation of venous disease, Iowa City, 1975, University of Iowa Press.
33. Bernstein, E.F., et al.: Noninvasive diagnostic techniques in vascular disease, St. Louis, 1978, The C.V. Mosby Co.
34. Couch, N.P.: Axioms on venous thrombosis, Hosp. Med. **13**(6):68, 1977.
35. Diethrich, E.B., editor: Noninvasive cardiovascular diagnosis, Baltimore, 1978, University Park Press.
36. Dosick, S.M., and Blakemore, W.S.: The role of Doppler ultrasound in acute deep vein thrombosis, Am. Surg. **13**:265, 1978.
37. Flanigan, D.P., et al.: Vascular laboratory diagnosis of clinically suspected deep vein thrombosis, Lancet **2**:331, 1978.
38. Goss, C.M., editor: Gray's anatomy, ed. 29, Philadelphia, 1974, Lea & Febiger.
39. Greenberg, S.H., et al.: Use of the Doppler stethoscope in the evaluation of varicoceles, J. Urol. **117**:296, 1977.
40. Kiil, J., et al.: Ultrasound and clinical diagnosis of deep vein thrombosis of the leg, Acta Radiol. [Diagn.] **20**:292, 1979.
41. Maryniak, O., and Nicholson, C.G.: Doppler ultrasonography for detection of deep vein thrombosis in lower extremities, Arch. Phys. Med. Rehabil. **60**:277, 1979.
42. Netter, F.H., and Divertie, M.B., editors: Ciba collection of medical illustrations. Vol. 7. Respiratory system, Summit, N.J., 1979, Medical Education Division, Ciba Pharmaceutical Co.
43. Pollak, E.W.: The choice of test for diagnosis of venous thrombosis, Vasc. Surg. **11**:219, 1977.
44. Salles-Cunha, S.X., et al.: Reliability of Doppler and impedance techniques for the diagnosis of thrombophlebitis, Med. Instrum. **12**(2):117, 1978.
45. Strandness, D.E., and Sumner, D.S.: Hemodynamics for surgeons, New York, 1975, Grune & Stratton, Inc.
46. Sumner, D.S., and Lambeth, A.: Reliability of Doppler ultrasound in the diagnosis of venous thrombosis both above and below the knee, Am. J. Surg. **138**:205, 1979.

Doppler examination of cerebrovascular system

47. Baker, W., et al.: The cerebrovascular Doppler examination in patients with nonhemispheric symptoms, Ann. Surg. **186**:190, 1977.
48. Barnes, R.W., et al.: Doppler cerebrovascular examination: improved results with refinements in technique, Stroke **8**:468, 1977.
49. Barnes, R.W., et al.: Doppler ultrasonic evaluation of cerebrovascular disease, Iowa City, 1975, University of Iowa Press.
50. Beach, K.W.: Noninvasive carotid diagnosis—entering the second decade, Bruit **4**(3):9, 1980.
51. Bone, G.E., et al.: Implications of the Doppler cerebrovascular examination: a correlation with angiography, Stroke **7**:271, 1976.
52. Brunner, H.H., et al.: Bestimmung des Schweregrades von Aorteninsuffizienzen mit gepulstem Doppler-Ultraschall an der A. carotis communis, Schweiz. Med. Wochenschr. **105**:1449, 1975.
53. Budingen, H.J., et al.: Die Differenzierung der Halsgefässe mit der direktionellen Doppler-Sonographie, Arch. Psychiatr. Nervenkr. **222**:177, 1976.
54. Burger, R., et al.: Choice of ophthalmic artery branch for Doppler cerebrovascular examination: advantages of the frontal artery, Angiology **28**:421, 1977.
55. Diethrich, E.B., editor: Noninvasive cardiovascular diagnosis, Baltimore, 1978, University Park Press.
56. Fields, W.S.: Aortocranial occlusive vascular disease (stroke), Clin. Sympos. **26**(4):3, 1974.
57. Hodek-Demarin, V., and Muller, H.R.: Reversed ophthalmic artery flow in internal carotid occlusion. A reappraisal based on ultrasonic Doppler investigations, Stroke **10**:461, 1979.
58. Juergens, J.L., Spittell, J.A., and Fairbairn, J.F.: Peripheral vascular diseases, Philadelphia, 1980, W.B. Saunders Co.
59. Keller, H., et al.: Noninvasive angiography for the diagnosis of carotid artery disease using Doppler ultrasound, Stroke **7**:354, 1976.
60. Keller, H., et al.: Noninvasive angiography for the diagnosis of vertebral artery disease using Doppler ultrasound, Stroke **7**:364, 1976.
61. Netter, F.H., Kaplan, A., et al.: Ciba collection of medical illustrations. Vol. 1. Nervous system, Summit, N.J., 1953 (1979 printing), Medical Education Division, Ciba Pharmaceutical Co.
62. Schlagenhauff, R.E., et al.: The value of Doppler ultrasonography in internal carotid disease, Neurology **27**:356, 1976.
63. Towne, J.B., et al.: Periorbital ultrasound findings: hemodynamics in patients with cerebrovascular disease, Arch. Surg. **114**:158, 1979.
64. von Reutern, G.M., et al.: Diagnose und Differenzierung von Stenosen und Verschlussen der Arteria carotis mit der Doppler-Sonographie, Arch. Psychiatr. Nervenkr. **222**(2-3):191, 1976.

Spectral analysis of Doppler signals

65. Barnes, R.W., et al.: Doppler ultrasonic spectrum analysis of carotid velocity signals, Richmond, 1980, Medical College of Virginia.
66. Baskett, J.J., Beasley, M.G., et al.: Screening for carotid junction disease by spectral analysis of Doppler signals, Cardiovasc. Res. **11**:147, 1977.
67. Blackshear, W., et al.: Detection of carotid occlusive disease by ultrasound imaging and pulsed Doppler spectral analysis, Surgery **86**:698, 1979.

68. Johnston, K.W., deMorais, D., et al.: Cerebrovascular assessment using a Doppler carotid scanner and real-time frequency analysis, J. Clin. Ultrasound **9:**443, 1981.

69. Myers, L., Avecilla, L.S., et al.: Correlative studies of color-coded real-time spectral analysis of flow in model arterial systems and selected cerebrovascular pathology. Illustrative display, Bowman Gray School of Medicine. (Personal communication.)

Doppler ultrasonic angiography

70. Blackshear, W., et al.: Detection of carotid occlusive disease by ultrasound imaging and pulsed Doppler spectral analysis, Surgery **86:**698, 1979.

71. Blackwell, E., Merory, J., et al.: Doppler ultrasound scanning of the carotid bifurcation, Arch. Neurol. **34:**145, 1977.

72. Day, T.K., Fish, P.J., et al.: Detection of deep vein thrombosis by Doppler angiography, Br. Med. J. **1:**618, 1976.

73. Johnston, K.W., deMorais, D., et al.: Cerebrovascular assessment using a Doppler carotid scanner and real-time frequency analysis, J. Clin. Ultrasound **9:**443, 1981.

74. Widder, B.: Ein vereinfachtes Doppler-Angiographie-Gerat zur unblutingen Diagnostik von Karotis-Stenosen, Nervenarzt **48:**397, 1979.

75. Wood, C.P.L., and Meire, H.D.: A technique for imaging the vertebral artery using pulsed Doppler ultrasound, Ultrasound Med. Biol. **6:**329, 1980.

Carotid real time sonography

76. Baker, D.W., Barber, F.E., et al.: Ultrasonic duplex echo-Doppler scanner, IEEE Trans. Biomed. Eng. **BME-21:**109, 1974.

77. Cooperberg, P.L., et al.: High-resolution real-time ultrasound of the carotid bifurcation, J. Clin. Ultrasound **7:**13, 1979.

78. Dunnick, N.R., et al.: Ultrasonic demonstration of thrombus in the common carotid artery, A.J.R. **133:**544, 1979.

79. Gompels, B.M.: High-definition imaging of carotid arteries using a standard commercial ultrasound B-scanner. A preliminary report, Br. J. Radiol. **52:**608, 1979.

80. Green, P.S., et al.: A real-time ultrasonic imaging system for carotid arteriography, Ultrasound Med. Biol. **3:**129, 1977.

81. Janowitz, W.R.: Small parts scanning, Radiol. Nucl. Med. **11:**25, 1981.

82. Philips, D.J., et al.: Ultrasonic duplex scanning in peripheral vascular disease, Radiol. Nucl. Med. **8:**6, 1978.

24 Cardiac anatomic and physiologic relationships

The heart is a muscular organ that consists of two separate pumps operating in parallel. The right side of the heart receives blood via the superior and inferior venae cavae and pumps it through the pulmonary arteries to the lungs. In the lungs it is oxygenated, and carbon dioxide is removed. The blood is returned to the heart through the pulmonary veins and is pumped out through the aorta to the body (Fig. 24-1).

THORAX

The thorax constitutes the upper part of the trunk. Within the thorax lies the thoracic cavity. This is separated from the abdominal cavity by the dome-shaped diaphragm, which reaches upward as high as the mid-axillary level of the seventh rib. Superiorly the upper thoracic cavity gives access to the root of the neck. It is bounded by the upper part of the sternum, the first ribs, and the body of the first thoracic vertebra. Anteriorly the sternum consists of three parts: the manubrium, the corpus sterni (body), and the xyphoid. The junction between the manubrium and the body of the sternum is a prominent ridge. Together they form the angle of Louis. This palpable landmark is important in locating the superior mediastinum or the second rib cartilages, which articulate with the sternum at this point.

The greater part of the thoracic cavity is occupied by the two lungs, which are enclosed by the pleura. To understand the pleural sac, imagine a deflated plastic bag covering your fist. Both sides of the bag should be reflected onto your fist to simulate the pleural sac. The internal layer (visceral pleura) is adherent to each lobe of the lung. The external layer (parietal pleura) is adherent to the inner surface of the chest wall (costal pleura), diaphragm (diaphragmatic pleura), and mediastinum (mediastinal pleura). The costophrenic sinus is the pleural reflection between the costal and diaphragmatic portions of the parietal pleura. This space lies lower than the edge of the lung and in most cases is never occupied by the lung. When pleural fluid accumulates, its most common location is in the costophrenic sinus. On radiographic examination the costophrenic angle is blunted by pleural effusion.

The space between the visceral and parietal pleuras is the mediastinum. It extends superiorly to the root of the neck and inferiorly to the diaphragm. Anteriorly it extends to the sternum and posteriorly to the twelfth thoracic vertebra, the thymus, the heart and great blood vessels, the trachea and esophagus, the thoracic duct and lymph nodes, the vagus and phrenic nerves, and the sympathetic trunks.

An imaginary plane from the sternal angle to the lower body of the fourth thoracic vertebra divides the mediastinum into superior and inferior mediastina. The inferior mediastinum is subdivided into three parts: (1) middle, which contains the pericardium and heart; (2) anterior, which is a space between the pericardium and sternum; and (3) posterior, which lies between the pericardium and vertebral column.

It is helpful to remember the anteroposterior locations of the following major mediastinal structures:

1. Superior mediastinum
   a. Thymus
   b. Large veins
   c. Large arteries
   d. Trachea
   e. Esophagus and thoracic duct
   f. Sympathetic trunks
2. Inferior mediastinum
   a. Thymus
   b. Heart within the pericardium, with the phrenic nerves on each side
   c. Esophagus and thoracic duct
   d. Descending aorta
   e. Sympathetic trunks

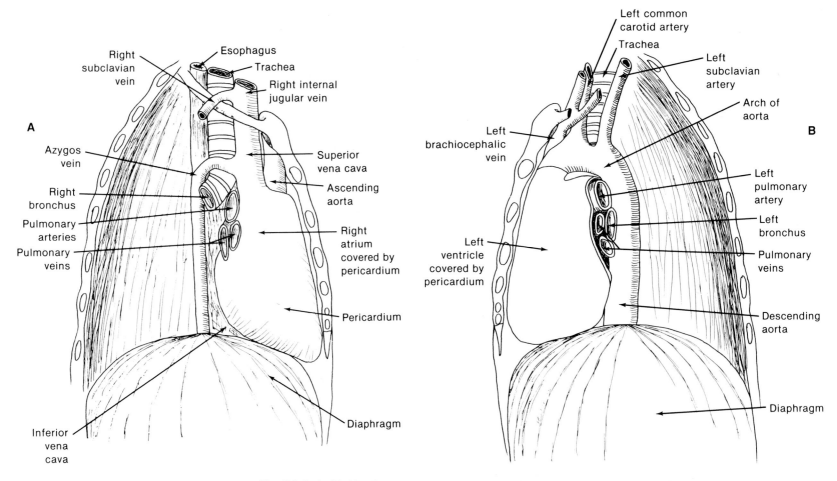

Fig. 24-1. A, Right side and, **B,** left side of the mediastinum.

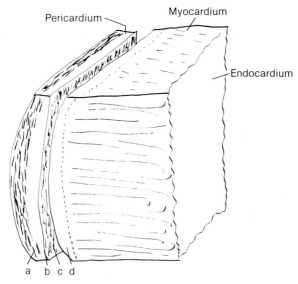

Fig. 24-2. Schematic of the pericardial space, *c,* surrounded by the serous pericardium, *d,* or epicardium and the serous pericardium (parietal layer), *b.* The fibrous pericardium, *a,* surrounds the serous pericardium.

THE HEART

Contrary to the usually illustrated anatomic position, the heart is not situated with its right chambers lying to the right and its left chambers to the left. It may be better considered as an anteroposterior structure with its right chambers more anterior than its left chambers. During embryologic development the heart forms as a right-to-left structure. However, with further development the right side becomes more ventral and the left side remains dorsal. In addition, another change in axis causes the apex (or inferior surface of the heart) to tilt anteriorly. The final development of the heart presents the right atrium anterior to and to the right of the sternum, and the right ventricle anterior and beneath the sternum or slightly to the left. The left atrium becomes the most posterior chamber to the left of the sternum, and the left ventricle swings its posterior apex slightly toward the anterior chest wall.

The heart and roots of the great vessels lie within the pericardial sac. Like the pleura the pericardium is a double sac. The *fibrous* pericardium limits the movement of the heart by attaching to the central tendon of the diaphragm below and the outer coats of the great vessels above. The sternopericardial ligaments attach it in the front. The *serous* pericardium is divided into parietal and visceral layers. The parietal layer lines the fibrous pericardium and is reflected around the roots of the great vessels to become continuous with the visceral layer of serous pericardium. The visceral layer is very closely applied to the heart and is often called the EPICARDIUM (Fig. 24-2). The slit between the parietal and visceral layers is the *pericardial cavity*. This cavity normally contains a small amount of fluid that lubricates the heart as it moves.

The pericardial sac provides the heart protection against friction. If the serous pericardium becomes inflamed (pericarditis) and too much pericardial fluid, fibrin, or pus develops in the pericardial space, the visceral and parietal layers may adhere to one another.

The pericardium does not totally encompass the heart. On the posterior left atrial surface of the heart the reflection of serous pericardium around the pulmonary veins form the recess of the oblique sinus. This is an important landmark in the separation of pericardial effusion from pleural effusion in echocardiography. The transverse sinus lies between the reflection of serous pericardium around the aorta and pulmonary arteries and the reflection around the large veins.

The heart has three surfaces: sternocostal (anterior), diaphragmatic (inferior or apex), and base (posterior) (Fig. 24-3). The right atrium and right ventricle form the sternocostal surface. The right atrium forms the right border of the heart to the right of the sternum. The left border is formed to the left of the sternum by the left ventricle and left atrium. The right and left ventricles are separated by the anterior interventricular groove.

The diaphragmatic surface of the heart is formed principally by the right and left ventricles separated by the posterior interventricular groove. A small part of the inferior surface of the right atrium also forms this surface.

The base of the heart is formed by the left atrium, into which open the four pulmonary veins. The right atrium contributes a small part to this posterior surface. The left ventricle forms the apex of the heart, which can be palpated at the level of the fifth intercostal space, about 9 cm from the midline.

The chambers of the heart are lined by an endothelial layer, the *endocardium*. The *myocardium* is part of the middle layer of the

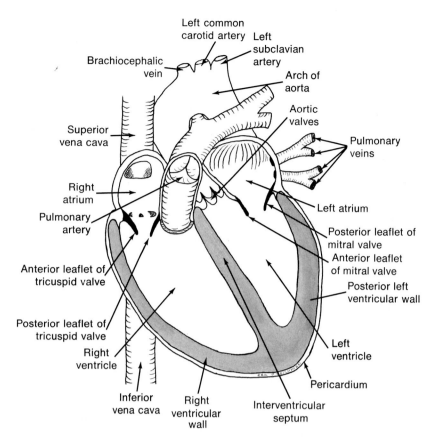

Fig. 24-3. Anatomy of the cardiac structures.

posterior heart wall. The *epicardium* is referred to as the outer or third layer of the heart wall but actually is part of the visceral layer of the pericardium.

Right atrium

The right atrium forms the right border of the heart. The superior vena cava enters the upper posterior border, and the inferior vena cava enters the lower posterior border (Fig. 24-4). The posterior wall of the right atrium is directly related to the pulmonary veins, which flow from the lung to empty into the left atrium. The medial wall is formed by the interatrial septum. The septum angles slightly posterior and to the patient's right, so the atrium lies in front and to the right of the left atrium (Fig. 24-5). The upper part of the medial wall of the right atrium is in direct relationship with the root of the aorta. The two parts of the atrium are separated by a ridge of muscle, the *crista terminalis*.

The anterior and lateral walls of the right atrium are ridged by the *pectinate muscles*. The superior portion of the right atrium, the right atrial appendage, contains the most prominent pectinate muscles. The posterior and medial walls are smooth, probably due to the continual flow of blood from the inferior and superior venae cavae.

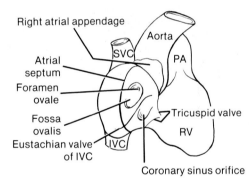

Fig. 24-4. Schematic of the right atrium, atrial septum, foramen ovale, and fossa ovalis. *SVC*, Superior vena cava; *PA*, pulmonary artery; *RV*, right ventricle; *IVC*, inferior vena cava.

The medial wall of the right atrium is formed mainly by the interatrial septum. The central oval portion of this septum is thin and fibrous. Just superior and in front of the opening of the inferior vena cava lies a shallow depression, the *fossa ovalis*. Its borders are the *limbus fossae ovalis* and the *primitive septum primum*. The *foramen ovale* lies under the most superior part of the limbus fossae. The limbus fossae ovalis is the remainder of the atrial septum and forms a ridge around the fossa ovalis.

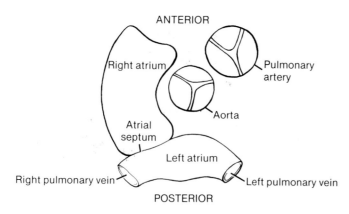

Fig. 24-5. Transverse schematic to show the atrial cavities and relationship of the semilunar valves to one another.

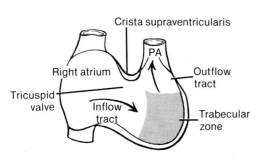

Fig. 24-6. Schematic of the right ventricle's inflow and outflow tracts. *PA,* Pulmonary artery.

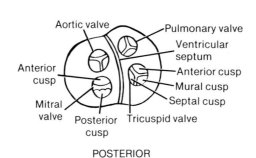

Fig. 24-7. Schematic of the relationship of the atrioventricular to the semilunar valves. There is continuity between the aorta and mitral valve.

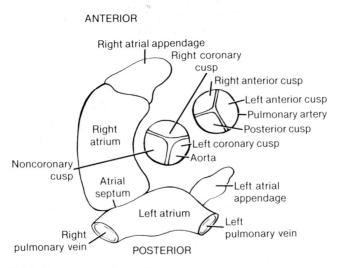

Fig. 24-8. Transverse schematic view of the relationship of the aortic to the pulmonary valve.

The atrioventricular part of the membranous septum separates the right atrium and left ventricle. Atrial septal defects can occur in this area, causing blood to flow from the high-pressured left ventricle into the right atrial cavity. The bundle of *His* arises from the atrioventricular (AV) node and serves as an important structure in the conduction pathway of the heart.

The *coronary sinus* drains the blood supply from the heart wall. It is bordered by the fossa ovalis and the tricuspid valve.

Right ventricle

The base of the right ventricle lies on the diaphragm whereas the roof is occupied by the *crista supraventricularis*, which lies between the tricuspid and pulmonary orifices. The right ventricle is essentially divided into two parts: the posteroinferior inflow portion (containing the tricuspid valve) and the anterosuperior outflow portion (which contains the origin of the pulmonary trunk). The demarcation between these two parts is by a number of prominent bands—*parietal band, supraventricular crest, septal band,* and *moderator band.* Together these form an almost circular orifice that normally is wide and forms no impediment to flow.

The inflow tract of the right ventricle is short and heavily trabeculated. It extends from the tricuspid valve and merges into the trabecular zone (Fig. 24-6). This trabecular zone is known as the body of the right ventricle. The trabeculae carneae enclose an elongated ovoid opening. The inflow tract unites with the outflow tract, which extends to the pulmonary valve. The outflow portion of the right ventricle or *infundibulum* is smooth walled and contains few trabeculae.

The right ventricle has two walls, an anterior (corresponding to the sternocostal surface) and a posterior (formed by the ventricular septum).

Tricuspid valve. The tricuspid valve separates the right atrium from the right ventricle. It has three leaflets—anterior, septal, and inferior (or mural). The septal leaflet may be maldeveloped in association with such conditions as ostium primum defect or ventricular septal defect. The leaflets are attached by their bases to the fibrous atrioventricular ring (Fig. 24-7). The chordae tendineae attach the leaflets to the papillary muscles. As these muscles contract with ventricular contraction, the leaflets are pulled together to prevent their being pulled into the atrial cavity. The septal and anterior leaflets are connected to the same papillary muscle, which helps in this process.

Pulmonary valve and trunk. The pulmonary valve lies at the upper anterior aspect of the right ventricle (Fig. 24-8). It has three cusps—anterior, right, and left. The wall of the pulmonary artery bulges out adjacent to each cusp to form pockets known as the pulmonary sinuses of *Valsalva.*

The pulmonary trunk passes posterior and slightly upward from the right ventricle. It bifurcates into the right and left pulmonary arteries just after leaving the pericardial cavity. The *ligamentum arteriosum* connects the upper aspect of the bifurcation to the anterior surface of the aortic arch. (It is a remnant of the fetal ductus arteriosus.)

Left atrium

The left atrium is a smooth-walled circular sac that lies posterior in the heart. Two pulmonary veins enter posteriorly on each side of the cavity. Occasionally these veins unite prior to entering the atrium, and sometimes there are more than two on each side. The veins may also be congenitally defective and enter the right atrium or other areas in the thoracic cavity. This absence of pulmonary veins entering the left atrial cavity is known as *total anomalous pulmonary venous return* (TAPVR).

The septal surface of the atrium is fairly smooth. A somewhat irregular area indicates the position of the fetal valve of the foramen ovale. The left auricle (left atrial appendage) is a continuation of the left upper anterior part of the left atrium. Small pectinate muscles are located within its lumen.

Left ventricle

The left ventricle is conical or egg shaped. The smaller end represents the apex whereas the larger end lies at the base of the heart. The left ventricle has a short inflow tract from the mitral valve to the trabecular zone that merges with the outflow tract extending to the aortic valve (Fig. 24-9). Unlike the right side of the heart (where there is no continuity between the tricuspid and pulmonary valves), the anterior leaflet of the mitral valve is continuous with the posterior aortic wall and the interventricular septum is continuous with the anterior aortic wall (Fig. 24-10).

The left ventricle has two walls, a lateral and a medial. The medial wall is formed by the ventricular septum. The left ventricular wall is two to three times the thickness of the right ventricular wall. The lateral wall is covered with trabeculae, which are finer and more numerous than those found in the right ventricle.

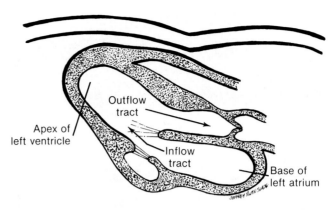

Fig. 24-9. Long axis view of the ventricular cavity. Note the outflow and inflow tracts of the ventricle.

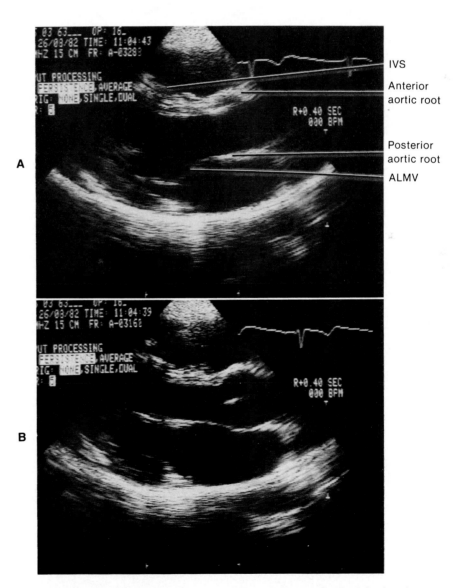

Fig. 24-10. Parasternal long axis in, **A,** systole and, **B,** diastole showing the interventricular septum, *IVS*, continuous with the anterior aortic root and the anterior leaflet of the mitral valve, *ALMV,* continuous with the posterior aortic root.

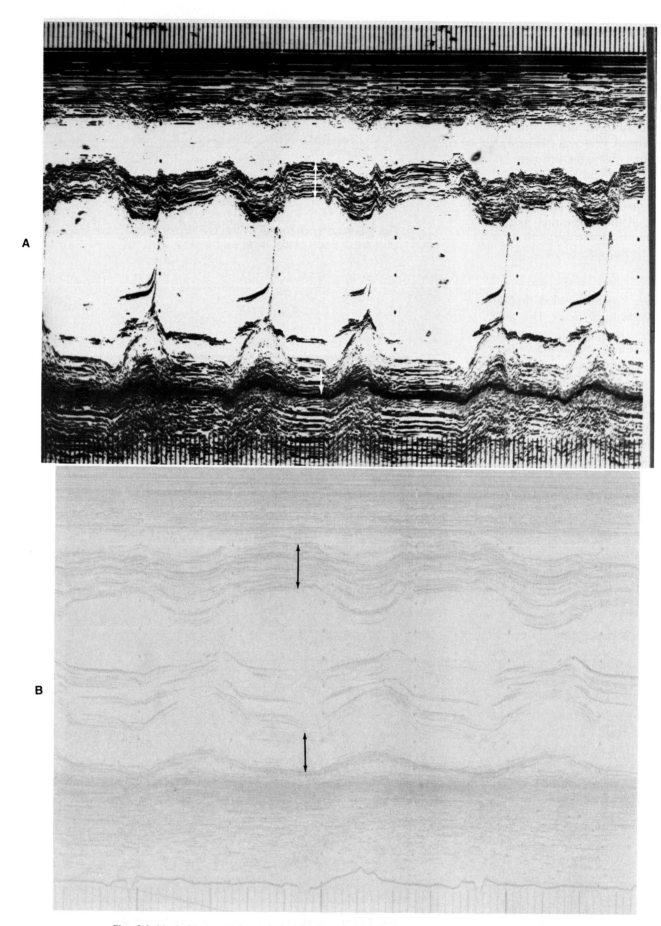

Fig. 24-11. A, Normal M-mode tracing of the interventricular septum, left ventricle, and posterior heart wall. **B,** Scan of a patient with concentric hypertrophy of the septum and posterior wall. A small pericardial effusion is posterior to the epicardium. **C,** Scan of a patient with hypertrophic asymmetric septal hypertrophy of the left ventricle.

Interventricular septum. The septum is triangular in shape, its apex corresponding to the apex of the heart and its base fusing posteriorly and superiorly with the atrial septum. The ventricular septum is formed of four parts—membranous, inflow, trabecular, and infundibular. These parts arise from the endocardial cushions, the primitive ventricle, and the bulbus cordis. The membranous septum varies in size and shape. It merges into the tissue at the aortic root and infundibular septum but is sharply demarcated from the muscular portion of the septum.

Most of the interventricular septum is muscular. It consists of two layers, a thin layer on the right and a thicker layer on the left. The major septal arteries run between these layers. The muscular portion of the septum has approximately the same thickness as the left ventricular wall. (In patients with concentric hypertrophy the septal wall and posterior wall thicken symmetrically whereas in patients with hypertrophic cardiomyopathy there is asymmetric septal thickening, Fig. 24-11.)

Mitral valve. The mitral valve separates the left atrium from the left ventricle. It consists of two large principal leaflets (anterior and posterior) and two small commissural cusps (which usually merge with the posterior leaflet). The anterior leaflet is much longer and larger than the posterior leaflet. It projects downward into the left ventricular cavity. The leaflets are thick membranes that are trapezoidal with fine irregular edges. They originate from the *anulus fibrosus* and are attached to the papillary muscles by *chordae tendineae*. The functions of the chordae tendineae are to prevent the opposing borders of the leaflets from inverting to the atrial cavity, act as mainstays of the valves, and form bands or foldlike structures that may contain muscle.

Aortic valve. The aortic valve lies at the root of the aorta and has three cusps—right, left, and posterior (or noncoronary). The wall of the aorta bulges out adjacent to each cusp to form the sinus of Valsalva (Fig. 24-12). The coronary arteries arise from the right and left aortic cusp. At the center of each cusp is a small fibrous nodule, *Arantius' nodule*, which aids in preventing leakage of blood from the left ventricle when the aortic cusps are closed. Often it becomes the site of calcification in patients in whom arteriosclerosis develops.

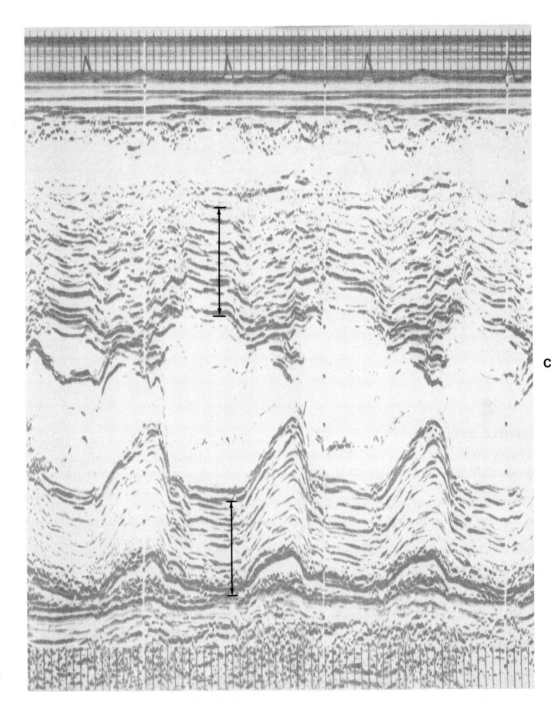

C

Fig. 24-11, cont'd. For legend see opposite page.

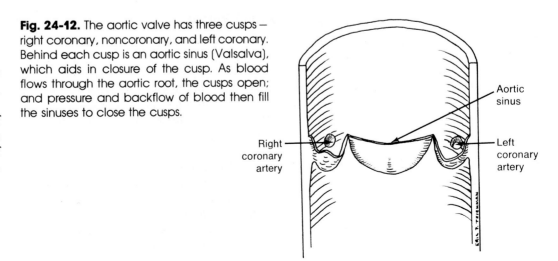

Fig. 24-12. The aortic valve has three cusps — right coronary, noncoronary, and left coronary. Behind each cusp is an aortic sinus (Valsalva), which aids in closure of the cusp. As blood flows through the aortic root, the cusps open; and pressure and backflow of blood then fill the sinuses to close the cusps.

Right coronary artery

Aortic sinus

Left coronary artery

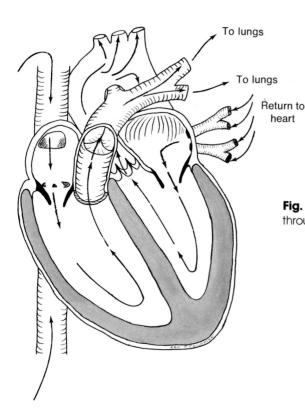

To lungs

To lungs

Return to heart

Fig. 24-13. Arrows indicate blood circulation throughout the cardiac cavity.

CARDIAC CYCLE

The heart is a muscular pump that propels blood to all parts of the body. It is able to act in definite strokes or beats and in the normal adult beats 70 times per minute on the average. The cardiac cycle is the series of changes that the heart undergoes as it fills with blood and empties. Rhythmic contraction of the heart causes blood to be pumped through the chambers of the heart and out through the great vessels (Fig. 24-13). The forceful contraction of the cardiac chambers is *systole*, and the relaxed phase of the cycle is *diastole*.

We shall consider the systematic events of the heartbeat starting from the diastolic phase, when the muscle is relaxed. During this phase venous blood enters the right atrium from the superior and inferior venae cavae. At the same time the oxygenated blood returns from the lungs through the pulmonary veins to enter the left atrium. At this point the atrioventricular valves (tricuspid and mitral) between the atria and ventricles are open so the blood may flow from the atria into the ventricles. The next phase allows atrial contraction to squeeze the remaining blood from the atria into the ventricles. The combination of atrial contraction and increased pressure of the full atrial cavities ultimately drains the atrial blood into the ventricles.

Shortly after this phase the ventricles contract (*ventricular systole*). The rising pressure in the ventricular cavity closes the atrio-ventricular valves. As the pressure increases in the ventricles, the semilunar valves (pulmonary and aortic) open so that blood can be forced into the lungs and body respectively.

The ventricles relax when contraction is completed (*ventricular diastole*). The blood in the aorta is under very high pressure, and the decreased pressure in the ventricles would cause it to flow backward into the ventricle. However, the semilunar valves prevent this reverse flow. The blood fills the sinuses of Valsalva and forces the valves to close. During ventricular contraction the atria relax and the venous blood starts to fill them again. When the ventricles are completely relaxed, the atrioventricular valves open and blood flows into the ventricles to begin the next cardiac cycle.

HEART VALVES

Surface anatomy (Fig. 24-14). The tricuspid valve lies behind the right half of the sternum, opposite the fourth intercostal space. The mitral valve lies behind the left half of the sternum, opposite the fourth costal cartilage. The pulmonary valve lies behind the medial end of the third left costal cartilage and the adjoining part of the sternum. The aortic valve lies behind the left half of the sternum, opposite the third intercostal space.

Auscultation. Heart sounds are associated with the initiation of ventricular systole, closing of the atrioventricular valves, and opening of the semilunar valves (Fig. 24-15).

The first sound is lower in pitch and longer in duration than the second. Both sounds can be heard over the entire area of the heart; but the first sound, "lubb," is heard most clearly in the region of the apex of the heart.

The second sound, "dupp," is sharper and shorter and has a higher pitch. It is heard best over the second right rib, for the aorta approaches nearest the surface at this point. The second sound is caused mainly by the closing of the semilunar valves during ventricular diastole. Following the second sound there is a period of silence. Thus the sequence sounds like this—lubb, dupp, silence, lubb, dupp, silence, etc.

Defects in the valves can cause excessive turbulence or regurgitation of the blood. These are extra abnormal sounds and are called *murmurs* or clicks. If the valves fail to close tightly and blood leaks back, a hissing murmur is heard. The hissing sound is heard in the area of the affected valve; thus if the mitral valve is affected, it will be heard in the first sound. Another condition giving rise to an abnormal sound is stenosis or stiffening of a valve orifice. In this case a rumble is heard in the area of the affected valve.

It is beyond the scope of this text to present an in-depth approach to auscultation, and the reader is referred to the *Bibliography* for additional reading on this subject. An understanding of auscultation will help in understanding the cardiac physiology and echocardiographic differential diagnosis.

ELECTROCARDIOGRAM

On stimulation of a muscle or nerve the cell membranes are depolarized, and on recovery they are repolarized. These electrical events are spread throughout the body and can be detected with suitable instruments applied to the skin surface at considerable distances from the sites of origin. The study of the heart's electrical activity is termed *electrocardiography*.

The electrodes (or leads) are made of metal and are slightly concave so as to make good contact with the skin in the regions of the wrists and ankles. A gel containing an electrolyte is rubbed over the surface of the skin to facilitate conduction of the impulse from the skin through the electrode attached at this area to the machine.

In echocardiography we use lead I. An ECG lead is attached to the patient's right and left wrists, with a ground on the ankle. The ECG has three components: P, QRS, and T waves (Fig. 24-16).

Text continued on p. 377.

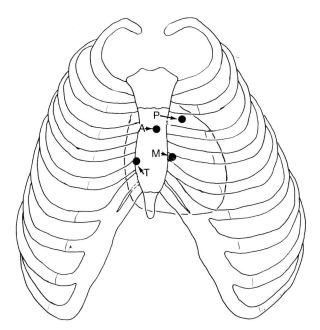

Fig. 24-14. Position of the heart valves. *P*, Pulmonary; *A*, aortic; *M*, mitral; *T*, tricuspid.

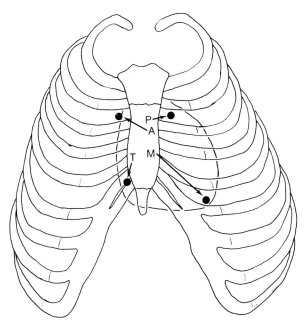

Fig. 24-15. Position of the heart valves. The valve sounds may be heard best with the least interference at the location of the arrows. *P*, Pulmonary; *A*, aortic; *M*, mitral; *T*, tricuspid.

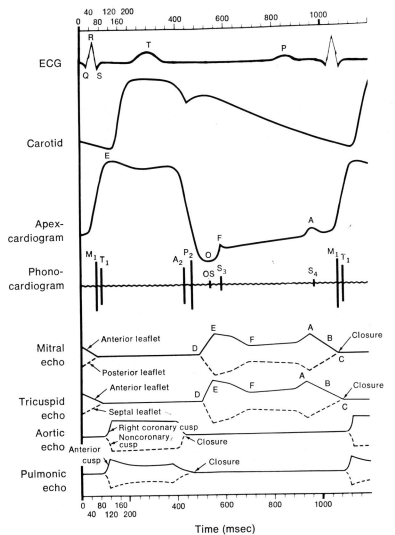

Fig. 24-16. Correlation of heart sounds, pulse tracings, and electric timing with the cardiac valves.

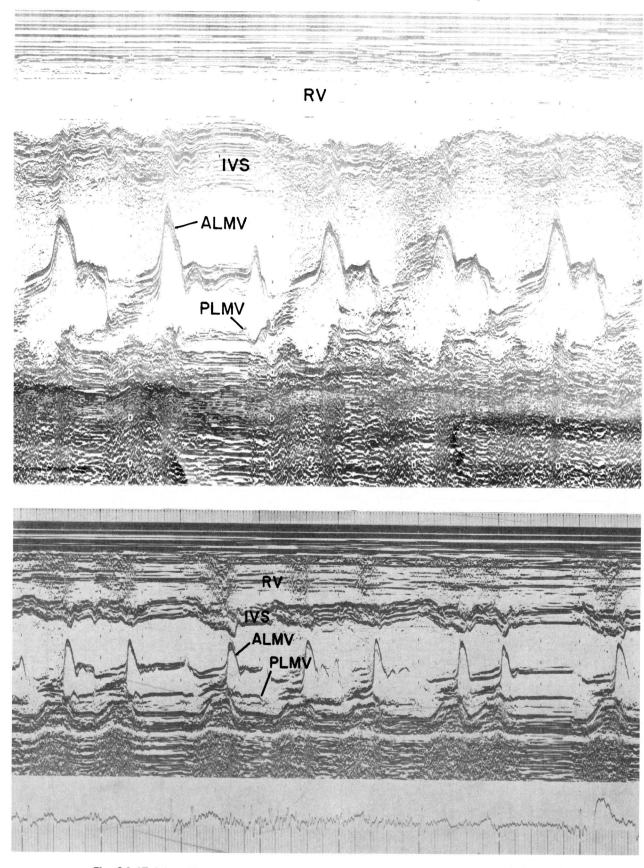

Fig. 24-17. Intermittent prolonged diastolic intervals may be noted occasionally during an echocardiography. The extradiastolic kick should be disregarded when routine cardiac measurements are being taken.

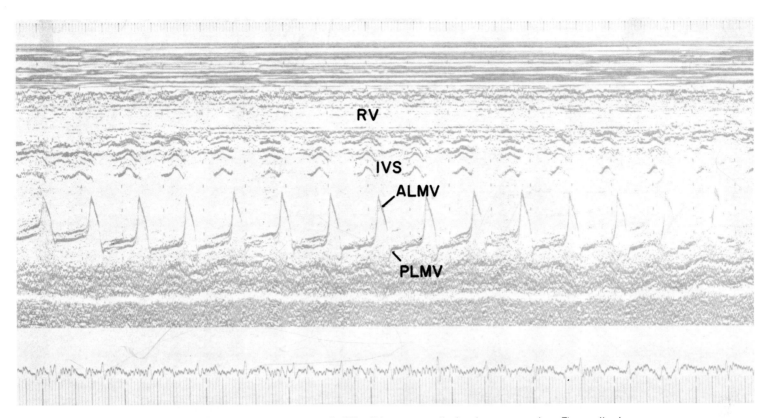

Fig. 24-18. Tachycardia makes it difficult to assess mitral valve parameters. The patient should be reexamined when in normal sinus rhythm.

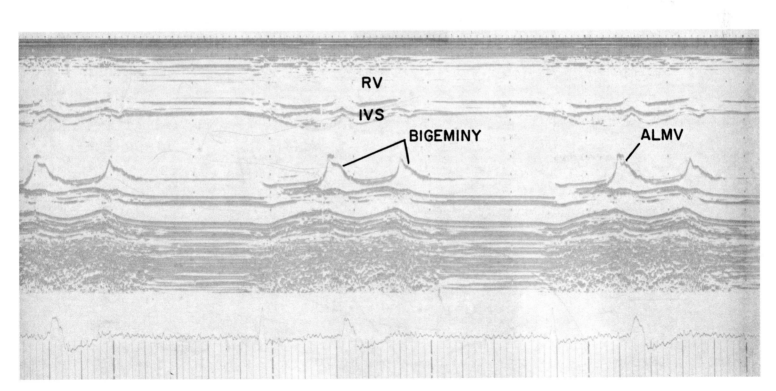

Fig. 24-19. Patient with bigeminy arrhythmia.

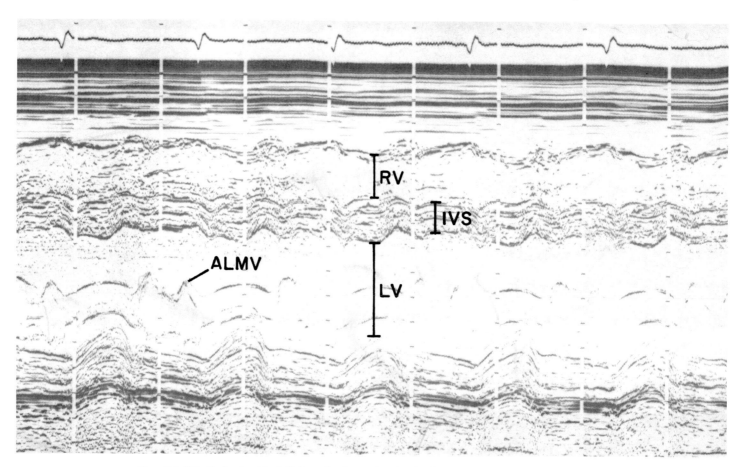

Fig. 24-20. Patient with left bundle branch block demonstrating abnormal septal movement.

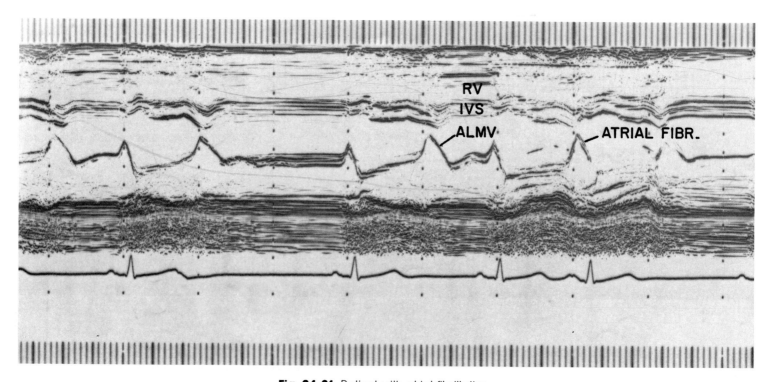

Fig. 24-21. Patient with atrial fibrillation.

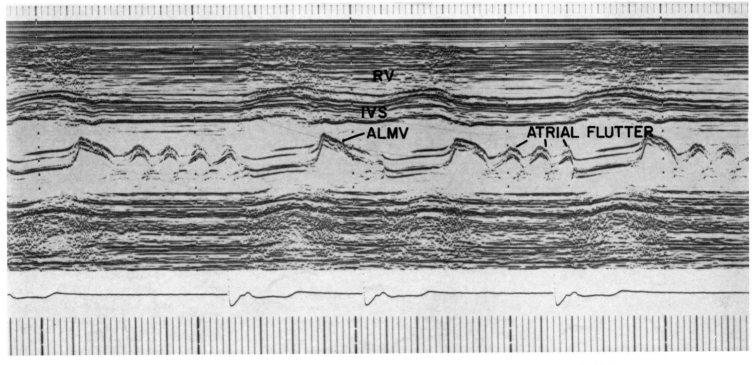

Fig. 24-22. Patient with atrial flutter. Coarse oscillations are evident at the point of atrial contraction (which is fluttering).

P wave. The impulse is initiated by the sinoatrial (SA) node and spreads over the atria. The P wave represents the electrical activity associated with the spread of the impulse over the atria (i.e., the wave of depolarization or activity of the atria).

QRS complex. The wave of depolarization spreads from the SA node over the bundle branches (His) and Purkinje system to activate both ventricles simultaneously. The QRS complex is the result of all electrical activity occurring in the ventricles.

PR interval. This is measured from the beginning of the P wave to the beginning of the QRS complex. It indicates the time that elapses between activation of the SA node and activation of the AV node.

T wave. This represents ventricular repolarization.

• • •

Only a few of the more obvious abnormalities that may be detected by the electrocardiogram and recognized by the cardiac sonographer will be outlined here:

1. Abnormal rates and rhythms. The normal rate is about 70 beats per minute (Fig. 24-17). A very slow rate, bradycardia, is not considered pathologic. An increased rate, tachycardia, is more frequently associated with disease and is demonstrated by rapid beats (175 to 200 per minute) (Figs. 24-18 and 24-19).
2. Heart block. A PR interval in excess of 0.2 second is indicative of this condition, together with an occasional missing QRS complex (Fig. 24-20).
3. Atrial fibrillation. An atrial rate in excess of 180 to 200 is termed atrial fibrillation or flutter (Figs. 24-21 and 24-22).

25 Echocardiographic techniques and evaluation

The evaluation of cardiac structures by echocardiography has many important parameters that must be fully understood and utilized in a daily practice. During the past decade M-mode echocardiography has gained increasing popularity, and this technique is currently regarded as an essential diagnostic tool for the practice of cardiology. The reason for its widespread use is that it is a noninvasive, reproducible, and accurate assessment of cardiac structures in the evaluation of cardiac disease. The M-mode technique is limited, however, in that it provides only a one-dimensional or "icepick" view of the heart. The advent of two-dimensional echocardiology has allowed cardiac structures to be visualized in a real time fashion. Thus observation of contractility, assessment of intracardiac lesions, and the estimation of valvular function can all now be accomplished by the echocardiographer. The combination of real time and M-mode studies provides an extremely accurate means of evaluating wall thickness, valvular orifice and chamber size, and contractility of the left ventricle.

To perform a diagnostic echocardiogram examination, the sonographer must be aware of anatomic and pathophysiologic parameters of the heart as well as understand the physical principles of sonography. These parameters will be discussed relative to M-mode and two-dimensional techniques. The standard M-mode examination will be presented first and followed by the evaluation of the heart by combined two-dimensional and M-mode techniques.

TRANSDUCERS

Several types of transducers are available for echocardiography. Ideally one should use as high a frequency as possible to improve the resolution of returning echoes. However, the higher the frequency, the less the penetration; therefore compromises will have to be made.

Many echocardiographers use a 3.5-MHz transducer with a medium focus. (Fig. 25-1). A larger patient may require a 2.25-MHz transducer, and a barrel-chested, emphysematous patient a 1.6-MHz transducer. The pediatric patient generally requires a 5.0- or a 7.5-MHz transducer for good resolution and near-field definition.

Although many transducers are internally focused to improve resolution by shaping the beam and reducing distortion, most cardiac transducers are of medium focus to concentrate the maximum resolution in the area of the mitral valve.

A smaller crystal or diameter of the transducer allows better skin contact between rib interspaces and also gives more freedom to sweep the beam. Thus the transducer remains in one interspace, but the beam angle is changed to record cardiac structures in an oblique path.

Special transducers may be advantageous depending on the specific patient population and the type of examination offered. An aspiration transducer may be useful in the location of pericardial effusion for pericardiocentesis. The small suprasternal transducer may be employed for measuring the left atrium, ascending aorta, or left brachial cephalic vein and for detection of a dissecting aortic aneurysm, right atrial myxomas, or left atrial thrombi.

DISPLAY OF NORMAL HEART PATTERNS

The conventional M-mode display of echocardiographic techniques reveals the cardiac structures from anterior to posterior, just to the left of the sternal border. The patient is generally examined in the supine or left lateral semidecubitus position. (Fig. 25-2). The cardiac window is usually the fourth intercostal space to the left of the sternal border and may be considered the area on the anterior chest where the heart is just beneath the skin surface free of lung interference (Fig. 25-3). With high gain we have

Text continued on p. 383.

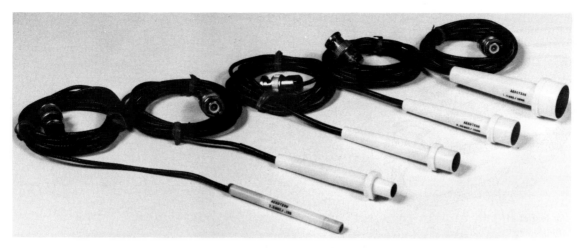

Fig. 25-1. To improve resolution of the cardiac structures, transducers with the highest frequency and smallest diameter should be used. Pediatric transducers may vary in diameter from 3 to 6 mm with varying frequencies of 3.5, 5.0, and 7.5 MHz. Adult transducers also vary in diameter, including those of 6, 13, and 19 mm and frequencies of 3.5, 2.25, and 1.6 MHz. (Courtesy KB-Aerotech, Lewistown, Pa.)

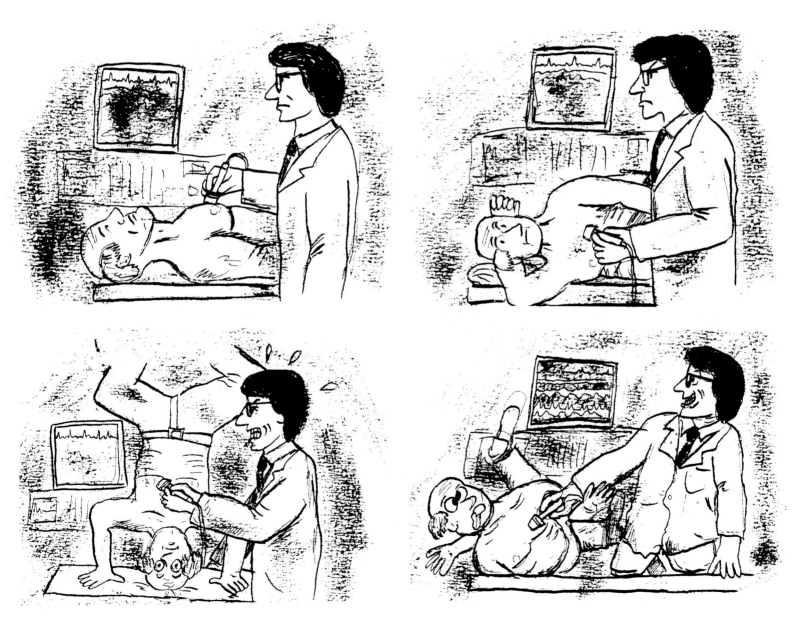

Fig. 25-2. Sometimes the cardiac sonographer thinks it is impossible to find the correct cardiac window in the standard patient position; however, with moderate manipulations success will be obtained. (Illustrated by Richard E. Rae)

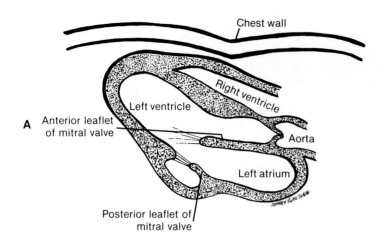

A

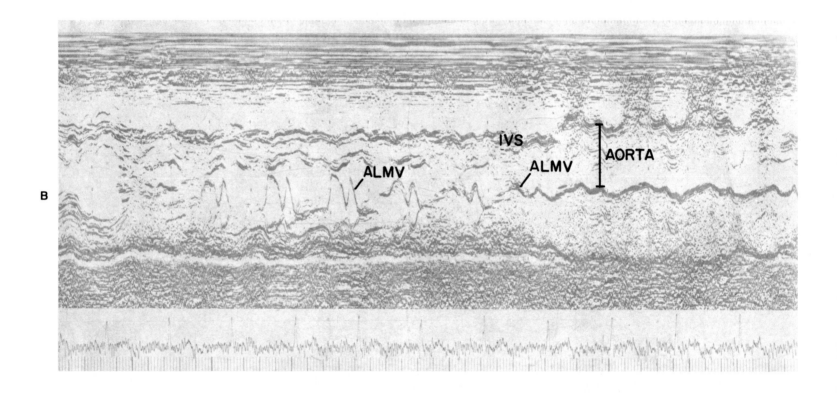

B

Fig. 25-3. A, Schematic of the correct cardiac window to visualize the left heart. **B,** Generally it is best to locate the maximum excursion of the mitral leaflet, *ALMV*, by the cardiac sweep from the left ventricle to the aortic leaflet area. The tip of the mitral valve is seen just before the minor axis of the left ventricle is seen.

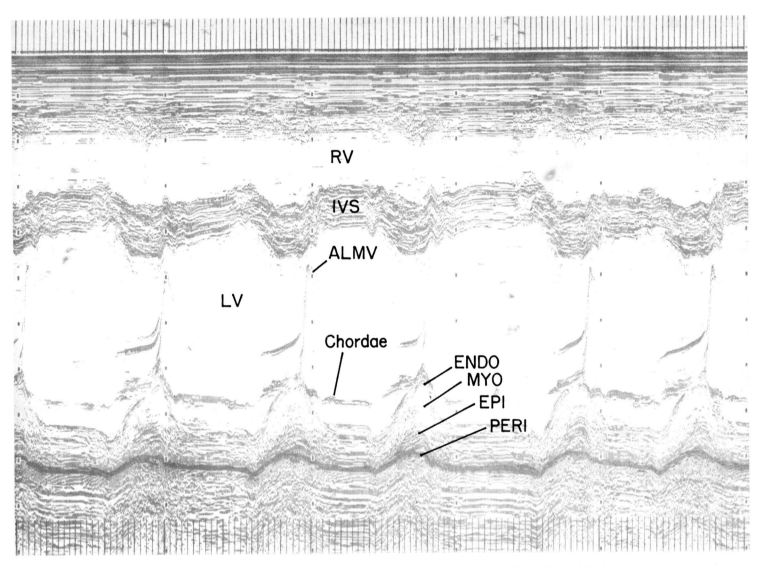

Fig. 25-4. Correct angulation of the transducer should demonstrate the right ventricular cavity, both sides of the septum, the left ventricular cavity containing pieces of the mitral apparatus, and the posterior wall with pericardium.

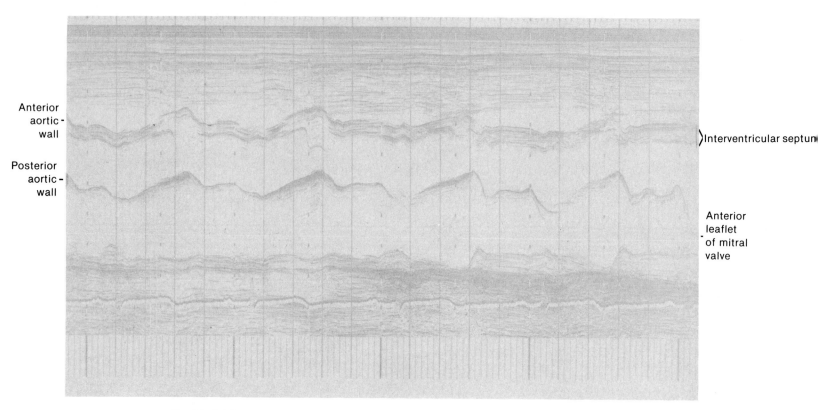

Anterior
aortic-
wall

Posterior
aortic-
wall

Interventricular septum

Anterior
leaflet
of mitral
valve

Fig. 25-5. M-mode sweep of the aortic root to mitral valve area. The anterior wall of the aortic root is continuous with the interventricular septum, and the posterior wall is continuous with the anterior leaflet of the mitral valve, *ALMV*.

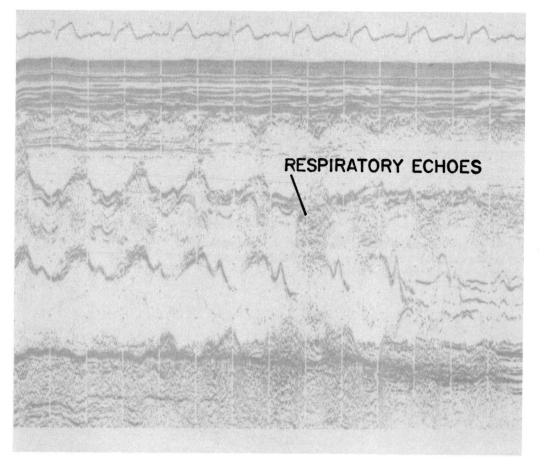

RESPIRATORY ECHOES

Fig. 25-6. Respiratory echoes may interfere with a clean tracing and usually can be avoided by watching the pattern of the patient's respiration and recording when the patient is exhaling.

found it more advantageous to cover a larger area along the sternal border in the initial search for typical echocardiographic patterns to determine which interspace is best. When the transducer is placed along the left sternal border, the examiner should run the transducer up and down the chest wall to define the pericardial echo with the strongest or loudest echo reflection (Fig. 25-4). After the pericardium is defined, one can search for the mitral and aortic valve patterns and determine which interspace is best for demonstrating the continuity of cardiac structures (Fig. 25-5).

The echocardiographer must keep in mind that different body shapes will require variations in transducer position. The following positions are guidelines for the average patient: An obese patient may have a transverse heart, and thus a slight lateral movement from the sternal border may be needed to record cardiac structures. A thin patient may have a long and slender heart, requiring a lower more medial transducer position. Barrel-chested patients may present echographic difficulties because of the lung absorption interference. It may be necessary to turn these patients completely on their left side or even prone to eliminate this lung interference. Sometimes the upright or slightly bent-forward position is useful in forcing the heart close to the anterior chest wall.

In the initial echocardiographic study moving the transducer freely along the left sternal border until all the cardiac structures are easily identified is a better practice than restricting it to one interspace. This saves time and gives the examiner a better understanding of cardiac relationships. If there is difficulty examining the patient in the supine position, a semidecubitus position should be used. Sometimes, if the heart is actually medial, the best study is performed with the patient completely on the left side. If too much lung interference clouds the study, the patient should exhale for as long as possible (Figs. 25-6 and 25-7). This will usually give the examiner enough time to record a valid study.

The gain is usually increased for the initial searching period and decreased to obtain a clear tracing. The highest gain will be in the left ventricle and mitral valve area, but the aorta and tricuspid and pulmonary valves require less gain. Table 25-1 contains locations and characteristics of intracardiac structures as seen by M-mode.

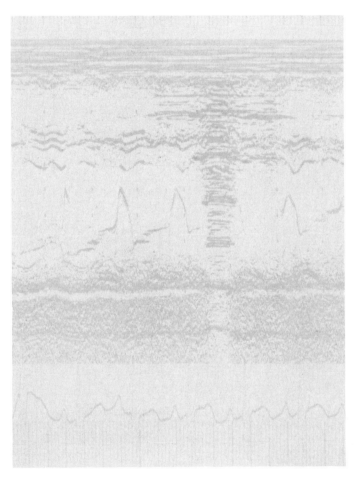

Fig. 25-7. The respiratory echoes are shown to arise from the anterior chest wall and continue throughout the cardiac structures in a vertical line.

Table 25-1. Approximate locations of intracardiac structures

Structure	Distance from transducer (cm)	Transducer position	Characteristics
Posterior heart wall (PW)	9 to 12	Usually found in third, fourth, or fifth interspace with transducer directed perpendicular to chest wall	Strong pulsating echo complex Pericardium strongest reflection in cardiac cavity Three layers of posterior heart wall, endocardium, myocardium, epicardium, are seen anterior to pericardium
Anterior leaflet of mitral valve (ALMV)	6 to 9	Transducer perpendicular to chest wall; may need slight medial or lateral angulation	Biphasic kick (M pattern seen on M-mode) Moves at least 2 to 3 cm in A- or M-mode Strong reflector
Posterior leaflet of mitral valve (PLMV)	9 to 10	From ALMV, angle *slightly* inferiorly and laterally (must maintain part of ALMV and watch for "clapping hands" movement of ALMV and PLMV moving opposite one another)	W pattern on M-mode Weak echo (be careful reject is not turned up to wipe out this echo)
Aortic root	4 to 6	From MV, angle transducer superiorly and medially toward right shoulder	Parallel echo movement on A-mode Anterior part of aorta comes off IVS Posterior part of aorta comes off ALMV Normal aortic valve size: 1.2 to 1.9 cm
Cusps		Slight angulations to record cusp movement (may be medial, lateral inferior, or superior); if there is trouble recording noncoronary cusp, move slightly down and laterally or have patient stop breathing; may have to move up an interspace or roll patient to left side to see cusps	Internal echo seen within parallel echo complex on A-mode When both noncoronary and right coronary cusps recorded, box pattern is seen on M-mode Third cusp (left coronary) moves throughout center of box
Tricuspid valve (TV)	2 to 4	From aortic root, angle inferiorly and slightly medially or from MV, angle medially	Similar in appearance to MV (biphasic kick, wide excursion) Because of location under sternal border, difficult to record completely; usually initial opening recorded
Right ventricle (RV)	1 to 3	Right ventricle seen anterior to IVS and MV, aortic root with transducer on left sternal border	Anterior side of RV can be identified as first moving structure beyond crystal artifact and chest wall Posterior surface anterior side of IVS Normal size less than 2 to 3 cm

Table 25-1. Approximate locations of intracardiac structures—cont'd

Structure	Distance from transducer (cm)	Transducer position	Characteristics
Interventricular septum (IVS)	2 to 4	Usually seen with transducer perpendicular to chest wall or angled inferiorly and lateral to MV	Should be able to identify both sides of septum well by using near gain (suppression) and delay; if too many echoes in RV, turn gear gain up; If not enough, turn near gain down (counterclockwise) (delay should be increased until it breaks off at anterior edge of septum) Should equal posterior wall thickness (ratio 1.3:1)
Left ventricular wall (LVW) (endocardium, myocardium, epicardium, pericardium)	9 to 12	Inferior and lateral to ALMV	Extremely important to sweep from ALMV to left ventricle Chordae tendineae may be demonstrated anterior to LVW (appear as denser echoes than endocardium and have less excursion); endocardium has characteristic notch ⟵ Chordae tendineae ⟵ Endocardium By decreasing gain, three layers of LVW may be demonstrated, with pericardial echo remaining as strongest moving reflection (demonstration of pericardial effusion is done by this method if fluid layer would dampen movement of pericardium)
LV and IVS		Transducer inferior and lateral to ALMV, but may angle slightly superiorly to this position to record IVS (use care to record IVS movement in correct position; when transducer is angled toward aorta, paradoxical motion may be seen)	For LV dimensions important to record IVS and LVW together (in systole they contract, in diastole they relax, and normal movement requires IVS and LVW to move toward one another); conversely, paradoxical septal motion means IVS moving opposite LV in systole
Pulmonary valve (PV)	1 to 3	From aortic root, angle superiorly and laterally toward left shoulder; may have to move up on interspace	Parallel movement on A-mode Cusp echo may be seen within echo complex Usually only posterior cusp seen, which moves posteriorly with systole

NORMAL MITRAL VALVE

The bicuspid atrioventricular valve located between the left atrium and left ventricle is the mitral valve (Fig. 25-8). It consists of the extension of the endocardial layer of the left atrial wall and the lateral posterior wall of the aortic root. The mitral ring or anulus is the superior border of the valve structure, and the multiple sail-like chordae tendineae serve to attach the anterior and posterior leaflets to the papillary muscle of the left ventricular heart wall (Fig. 25-9).

Echographically the mitral valve is one of the easiest cardiac structures to recognize. The transducer should be directed perpendicular to the patient's chest wall, slightly toward the left sternal border, in approximately the fourth intercostal space (Fig. 25-10). With proper gain settings the A-mode and M-mode tracings are often the most sensitive recorder of initial mitral valve motion. The sonographer may recognize the initial echo of the right ventricular wall, the echo-free cavity of the right ventricular cavity, the anterior and posterior walls of the interventricular septum, and, finally, the mitral valve area as shown in the left atrial or left ventricular cavity (depending on transducer angulation) (Fig. 25-11). The mitral valve pattern is usually seen 6 to 9 cm from the patient's skin surface. It has the greatest amplitude and excursion and can be unquestionably recognized by its *double* or biphasic kick. This is caused by the initial opening of the valve in ventricular diastole and the atrial contraction at end diastole. Thus the valve opens with its maximum excursion in early diastole, the ventricle relaxes, and the valve starts to close. The atrium then contracts, forcing the valve open with reduced amplitude. The ventricle is then fully relaxed, the mitral valve closes, and the onset of ventricular systole occurs (Fig. 25-12).

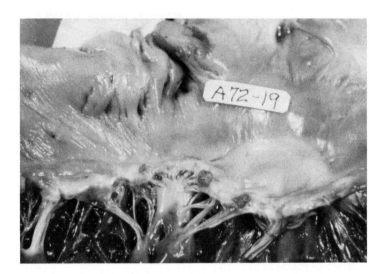

Fig. 25-8. Gross specimen of the mitral leaflet, mitral anulus, and chordae tendineae of the anterior and posterior leaflets.

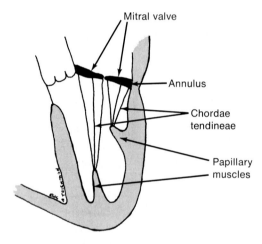

Fig. 25-9. Attachment of the mitral leaflets to the anulus, chordae tendineae, and papillary muscles.

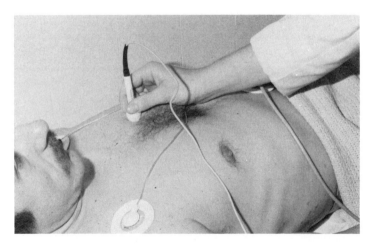

Fig. 25-10. Perpendicular angulation of the transducer to record the mitral valve apparatus by M-mode.

It is critical to find the maximum excursion of the leaflet for recording purposes. The sonographer should glide along the left sternal border to observe the maximum amplitude of the valve. The transducer should be perpendicular to the mitral valve for an adequate scan.

When diastole begins, the anterior mitral leaflet executes a rapid anterior motion, coming to a peak at point e* (Fig. 25-13). As the ventricle fills rapidly with blood from the left atrium, the valve drifts closed—point f. The rate at which this movement takes place represents the rate of left atrial emptying and serves as an important indicator of altered mitral function. As the left atrium contracts, the mitral valve opens in a shorter anterior excursion and terminates at a, which occurs just after the P wave of the ECG. This is followed by a rapid posterior movement from point b to point c, which coincides with the QRS systolic component on the ECG produced by left ventricular contraction's closing the valve.

On the phonocardiogram point c for the mitral valve coincides with the first heart sound, representing the position of maximum closure of the mitral valve (Fig. 25-14). During systole the closed valves move slightly anterior in a smooth continuous manner. This is most likely caused by the emptying of the left ventricular cavity and the drawing of the whole valve and its ring toward the base of the heart. The second heart sound can then be heard, because it indicates the closure of the aortic valve.

*Throughout Chapters 25 to 35, the references to these letter points along the cardiac cycle will be by both lower case and capital letters since both designations are used in the field and the authors have employed the one more familiar to them.

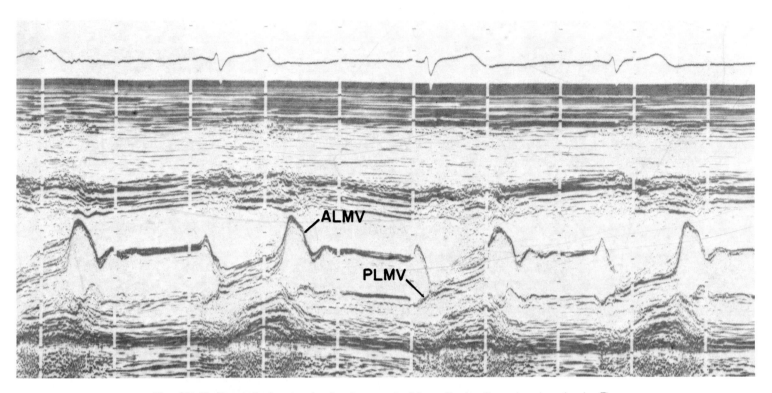

Fig. 25-11. The mitral valve is clearly seen in this patient with a slow heart rate. The systolic segment moves slightly anteriorly until diastole begins, which causes the anterior leaflet to sweep anteriorly while the posterior leaflet dips posteriorly. Atrial contraction gives rise to the smaller *a* kick until the valve closes at end diastole.

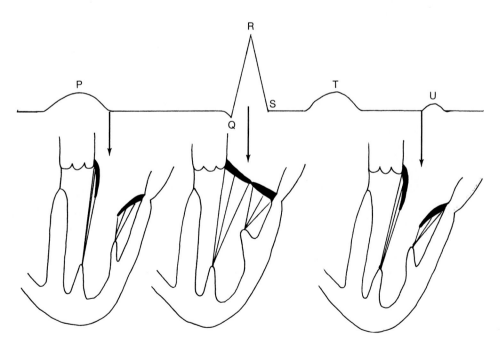

Fig. 25-12. Correlation of the electrocardiogram with the mitral apparatus. The P wave triggers the onset of atrial contraction, which gently forces the mitral leaflet open (*a* wave). The QRS complex is the onset of systole, at which point the mitral valve closes completely to allow blood to flow through the aortic root. The T wave on the ECG signifies the end of systole; and at that point the mitral valve opens to its full extent in early diastole.

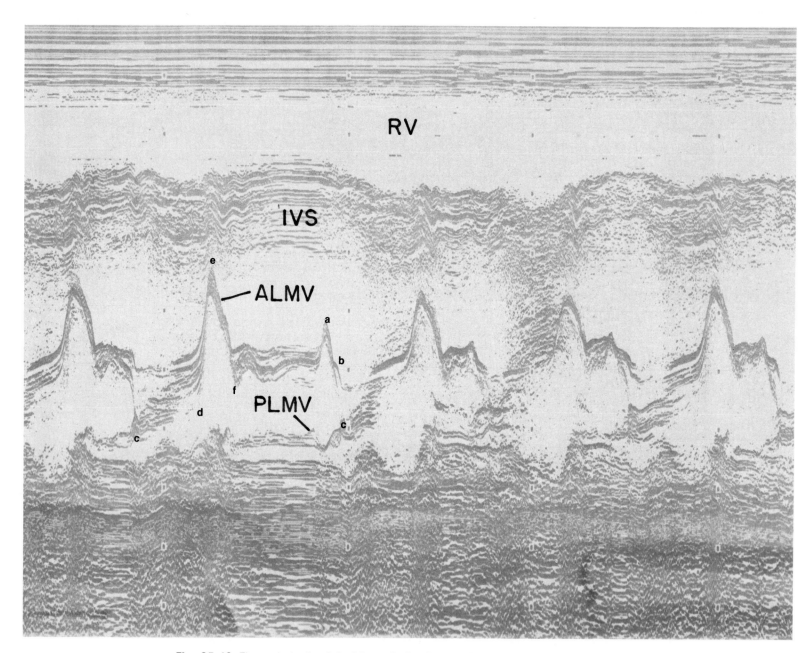

Fig. 25-13. The anterior leaflet of the mitral valve has been assigned standard letters to signify certain systolic and diastolic components. The *c* to *d* points represent systole; *e, f, a,* and *b* points represent diastole.

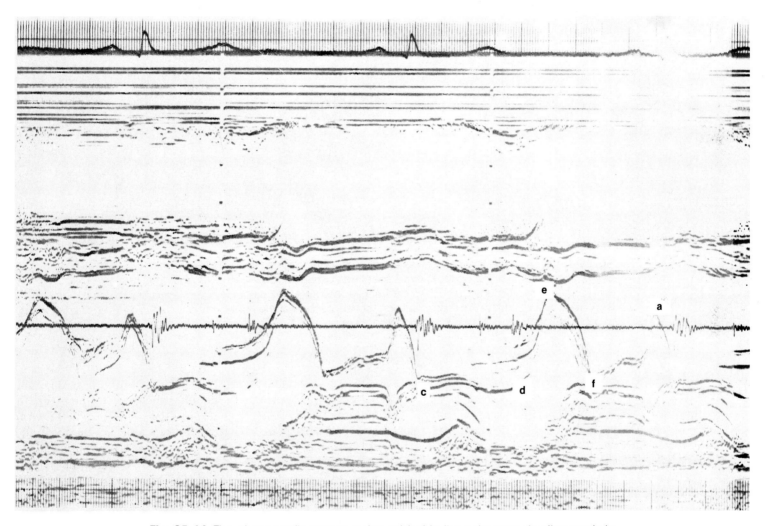

Fig. 25-14. The phonocardiogram may be added to the echogram simultaneously to record the first and second heart sounds in relation to the valve motion (note the mid-systolic click on the phonocardiogram corresponding to the mitral valve prolapse). (Echo courtesy Paul Walinsky, M.D., Philadelphia.)

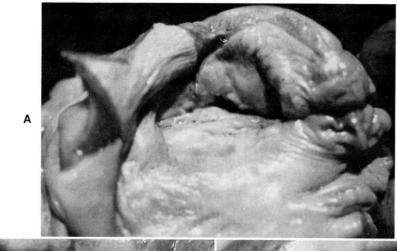

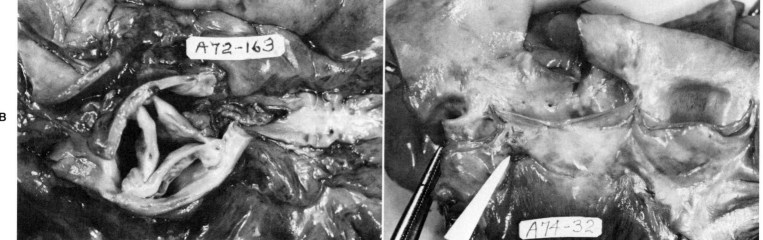

Fig. 25-15. A, Gross specimen of the aortic valve as seen from the inferior to the superior angle, up the barrel of the aorta. **B,** Gross specimen of the aorta viewed down into the ventricular cavity. The aortic sinus lies between each cusp and the wall of the aorta. **C,** A direct view of the aortic root split open for visualization of the right coronary cusp and artery, left coronary cusp, and noncoronary cusp.

NORMAL AORTIC VALVE AND LEFT ATRIUM

The aorta has many subdivisions as it leaves the left ventricle. The base of this vessel is the aortic root, which has three cusps to prohibit a free flow of blood to the body (Fig. 25-15). The ascending aorta rises from the aortic root and begins its posterior descent at the arch of the aorta. The descending aorta then proceeds posteriorly to pierce the diaphragm and enter the abdominal cavity (Fig. 25-16).

In examinations of the aortic root, semilunar cusps, and left atrial cavity, the transducer should be directed from the area of the mitral valve cephalad medial to the patient's right shoulder (Fig. 25-17). The sonographer should be able to identify the anterior leaflet of the mitral valve blending with the posterior aortic wall at the same time the interventricular septum blends into the anterior aortic wall (Fig. 25-18). Often there is a double parallel echo appearance along the anterior and posterior aortic walls denoting wall thickness (Fig. 25-19). Care should be taken to record both wall echoes to ensure proper measurement of the aortic root dimension. Adjustment of the near-gain control allows excellent visualization of the anterior wall. The echoes recorded from the aortic root should be parallel, moving anteriorly in systole and posteriorly in diastole. The chamber posterior to the aortic root is the left atrium, which can be recognized by its immobile wall. As one sweeps from the mitral apparatus medially and superiorly, the left ventricular wall blends into the atrioventricular groove and finally into the left atrial wall (Fig. 25-20). Thus the sweep demonstrates good contractility in the left ventricle, with anterior wall motion in systole to the AV area, where the posterior wall starts to move posteriorly in systole, and then to the left atrium, where there is no movement. Sometimes it is possible to record the left pulmonary vein within the left atrial cavity. This appears as a thin double-walled vessel and can be a problem in determining left atrial measurements. Care should be taken to sweep from the mitral valve to the aortic root and back to the mitral apparatus several times to note the continuity of the posterior ventricular wall to the left atrial wall and to avoid confusion. The pulmonary vein will never appear continuous.

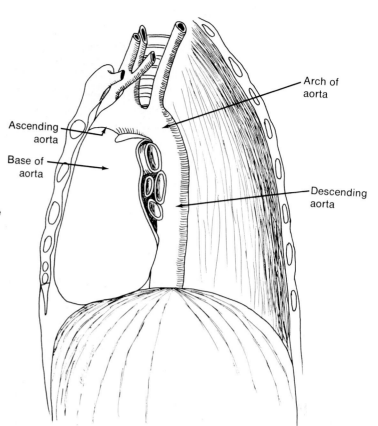

Fig. 25-16. Left side of the mediastinum demonstrating the parts of the aorta.

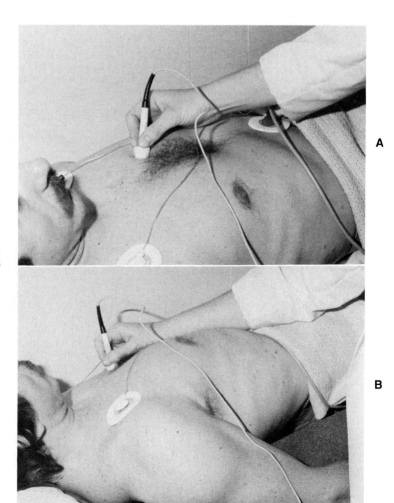

Fig. 25-17. A, Transducer position for locating the aortic valve. **B,** Medical transducer angulation with the patient in a semidecubitus position to record the aortic root and cusps.

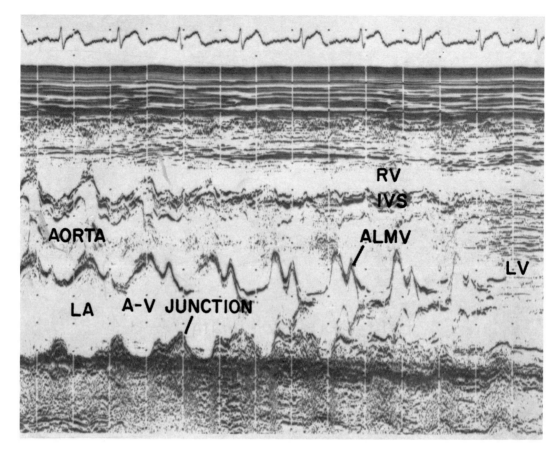

Fig. 25-18. M-mode sweep from the aorta and left atrium to the mitral valve area. The left atrial wall can be seen to blend into the atrioventricular junction behind the mitral valve area.

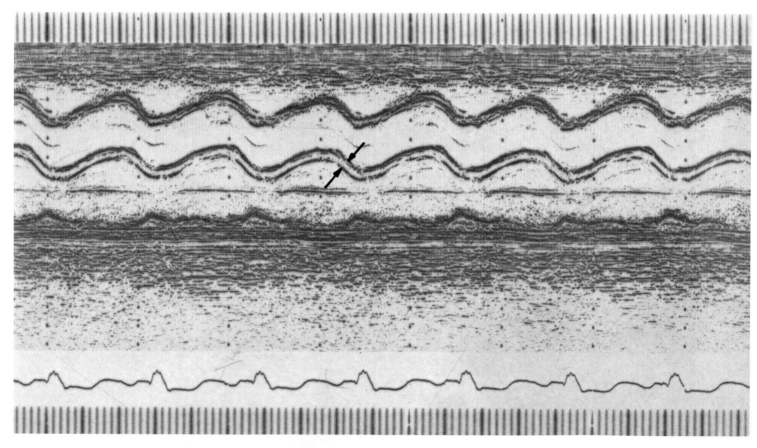

Fig. 25-19. Parallel double lines on the posterior aortic wall demonstrate that the transducer was not exactly perpendicular to the aortic wall. Sometimes it is possible to record the inner and outer dimensions of both anterior and posterior walls of the aorta with good resolution. A dissecting aneurysm would display a widened distance in the aortic wall (more than 1 to 1.6 cm) if the dissection occurred at the root of the aorta.

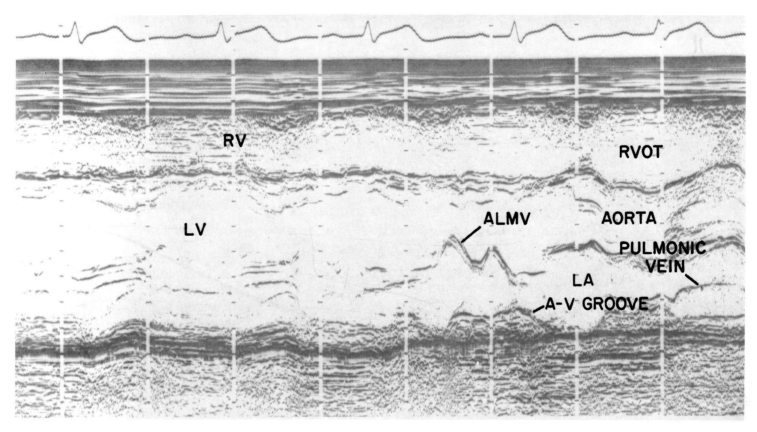

Fig. 25-20. Sweep from the left ventricle to the mitral area to the aortic root demonstrating good posterior wall motion in the left ventricle, a box-type motion in the AV groove, and no motion in the left atrial cavity.

As the transducer is angled slightly medial, two of the three semilunar cusps can be visualized (Fig. 25-21). The right coronary cusp is shown anterior and the noncoronary cusp posterior (Fig. 25-22). When seen, the left coronary cusp is in the midline between these two cusps (Fig. 25-23). The onset of systole causes the cusps to open to the full extent of the aortic root. The extreme force of blood through this opening causes fine flutter to occur during systole. As the pressure relents in the ventricle, the cusps begin to drift to a closed position until they are fully closed in diastole.

Chang (1977) states that the anterior "humping" of the aortic valve following its closure is a common occurrence in patients with efficient cardiac outputs. It may be a total displacement of the aortic root anteriorly following systolic completion and does not seem to denote abnormality (Fig. 25-24).

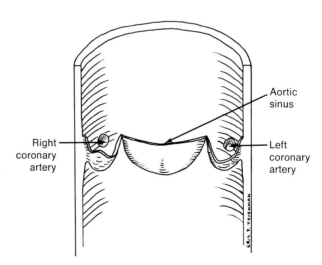

Fig. 25-21. Semilunar cusps with their respective coronary arteries.

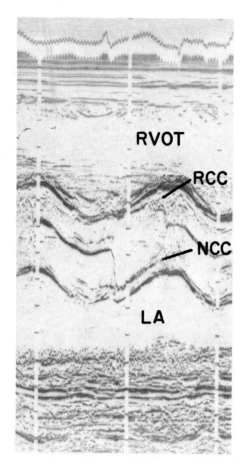

Fig. 25-22. The right coronary cusp is the most anterior cusp seen in the aortic sweep, and the noncoronary cusp is the most posterior.

LEFT ATRIAL CAVITY

The left atrium is located posterior to the aortic root. Normally a 1-to-1 ratio exists between the left atrial cavity and the aortic root. The left atrial dimension should be calculated at the end-systolic dimension from the leading edge of the posterior aortic wall to the leading edge of the left atrial wall (Fig. 25-25). Enlargement of the left atrium most likely reflects mitral valve disease, cardiomyopathy, or congestive heart failure.

INTERVENTRICULAR SEPTUM

The interventricular septum divides the right ventricle from the left ventricle. Its right side is contiguous with the anterior aortic root (Fig. 25-26). At this junction the movement of the septum is influenced by the movement of the aorta, and thus it may appear to move abnormally or paradoxically in relation to the posterior heart wall. As the transducer is angled slightly inferior and lateral to the mitral valve, the septum moves somewhat anteriorly in early systole and posteriorly at the end of systole and early diastole (Fig. 25-27). Both sides of the septum should move symmetrically. If they do not, the transducer should be placed more medial on the chest wall or the patient should be rolled into a slightly steeper decubitus position.

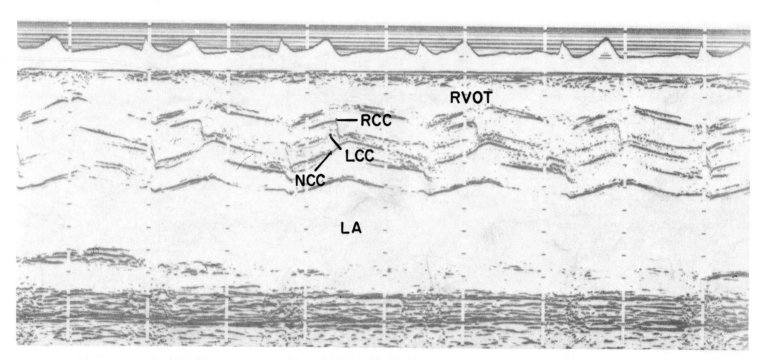

Fig. 25-23. M-mode demonstration of the aortic root with three cusps. *RVOT,* Right ventricular outflow tract; *RCC,* right coronary cusp, *LCC,* left coronary cusp; *NCC,* noncoronary cusp; *LA,* left atrium.

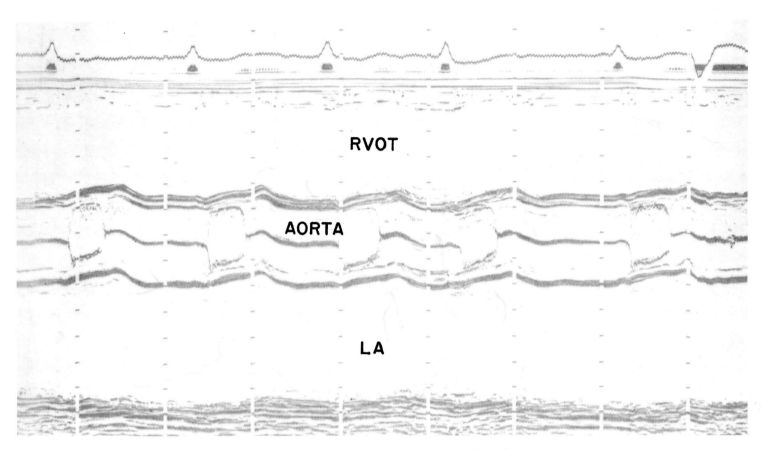

Fig. 25-24. The humping of the aortic valve following its closure is a common occurrence in patients with efficient cardiac outputs.

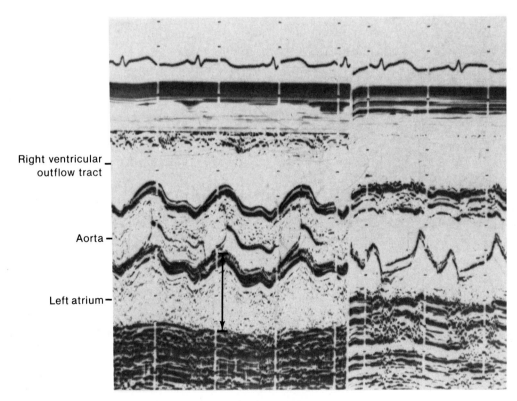

Fig. 25-25. M-mode of the left atrial cavity. Arrows indicate the points at which the chamber should be measured, from leading edge to leading edge.

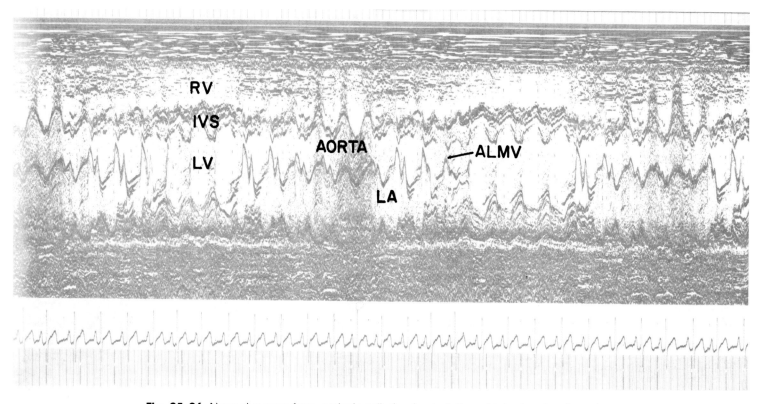

Fig. 25-26. Normal sweep from aorta to mitral valve to left ventricle showing the relationship of the interventricular septum to other cardiac structures.

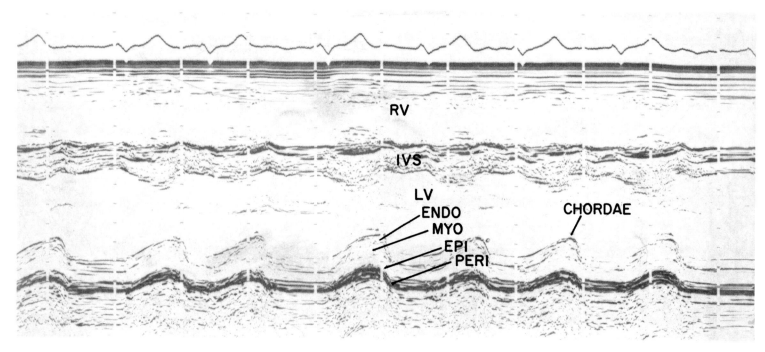

Fig. 25-27. Normal septum moving posteriorly at end systole to contract with the posterior left ventricular wall.

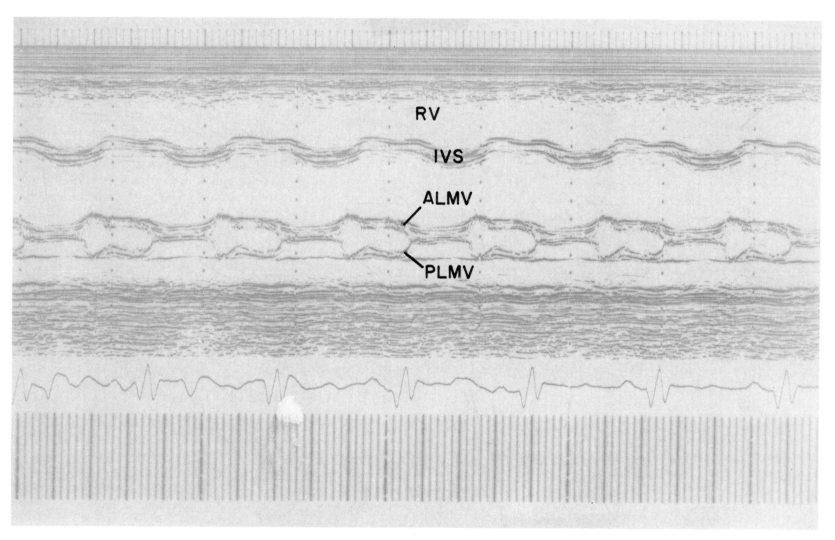

Fig. 25-28. M-mode sweep of the patient with concentric cardiomyopathy. The thin septum is shown, with the double diamond appearance of the mitral anterior and posterior leaflets.

The septum thickens in the midportion of the ventricular cavity. The measurement and evaluation of septal thickness and motion should be made at this point. Normal septal thickness should match that of the posterior left ventricular wall and not exceed 1.2 cm.

Congestive cardiomyopathy usually produces concentric thinning of the septum and posterior wall and reduced septal motion (Fig. 25-28). Coronary artery disease or anterior myocardial infarction can reduce or flatten septal motion or cause paradoxical movement of the septum (Fig. 25-29). Right ventricular volume overload results in paradoxical septal motion when scanned in the left ventricular plane. Thickening of the septum may be produced by asymmetrical septal hypertrophy or poor technique in defining the right ventricular wall (Fig. 25-30). Concentric hypertrophy from hypertension or aortic stenosis results in symmetrical thickening of the septum and posterior wall.

Left bundle branch block reveals an abrupt posterior movement of the septum in early systole followed by a ragged motion in diastole (Fig. 25-31). Post–cardiac surgery patients may reveal abnormal septal motion, but the septum may return to normal in time.

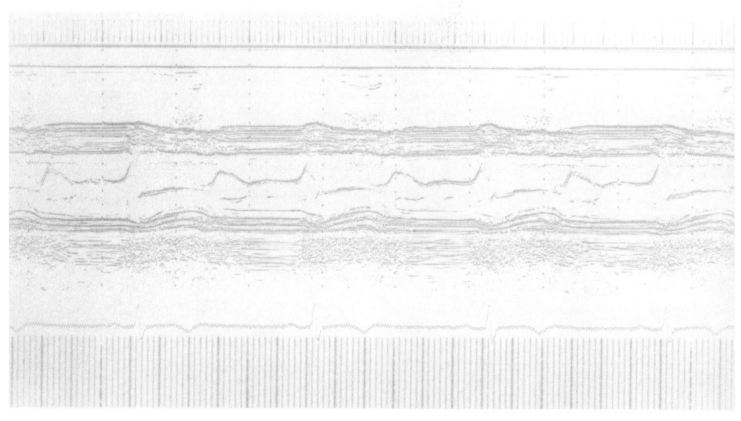

Fig. 25-29. M-mode sweep of a patient with coronary artery disease showing an immobile septum.

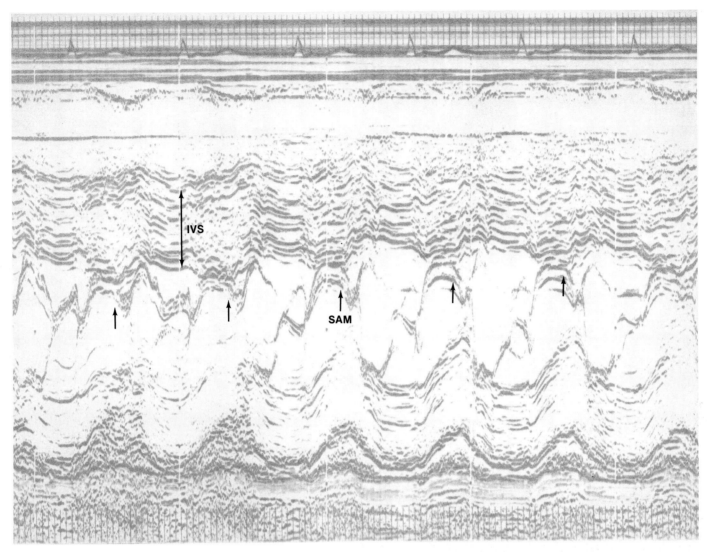

Fig. 25-30. M-mode sweep of a patient with obstructive hypertrophic cardiomyopathy demonstrating a thickened septum, *IVS*, and systolic anterior motion, *SAM*, of the mitral apparatus.

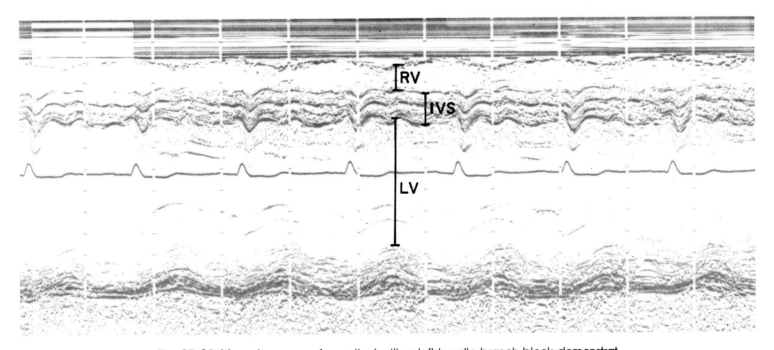

Fig. 25-31. M-mode sweep of a patient with a left bundle branch block demonstrating abnormal septal motion.

LEFT VENTRICLE

Determination of left ventricular volume and function may be made with the routine M-mode sweep. The patient is generally examined in the supine position. If inadequate studies are shown in this position, the left semidecubitus position is used for defining septal motion and posterior wall contraction. The anterior leaflet of the mitral valve should be located and then the beam angled inferior and slightly lateral to record the left ventricular chamber. Correct identification of this chamber may be made when both sides of the septum are seen to contract with the posterior heart wall (Fig. 25-32). If the septum is not well defined or does not appear to move, medial placement of the transducer along the sternal border with a lateral angulation may permit better visualization. The three layers—endocardium (inside layer), myocardium (middle layer), and epicardium (outer layer)—should be identified separately from the pericardium. Some-

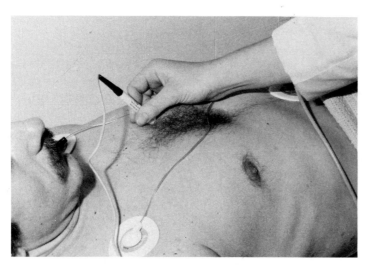

Fig. 25-32. Inferior angulation from the anterior leaflet of the mitral valve to record the left ventricular dimensions.

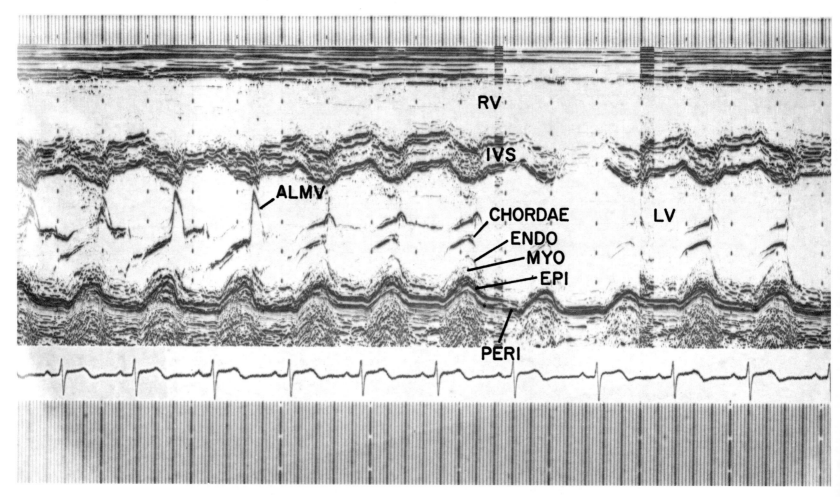

Fig. 25-33. M-mode sweep from the mitral valve area into the left ventricle to differentiate the chordae from the posterior wall. Decrease in gain further defines the pericardial echo.

times it is difficult to separate epicardium from pericardium until the gain is reduced (unless the equipment has a special enhance control built into it). The myocardium may appear echo free or echo producing, and care must be exercised to avoid mistaking it for pericardial fluid (the three layers of the posterior wall must be separated from the pericardium for diagnosis of pericardial effusion). The endocardium is one of the most difficult structures to record since it reflects a very weak echo pattern above the myocardium (Fig. 25-33). Sometimes the multiple chordae tendineae are difficult to separate from the endocardium, and careful evaluation of the posterior wall must be used. The chordae are much denser structures than the endocardium. They generally are shown in the systolic segment along the anterior surface of the endocardium (Fig. 25-34). As the ventricle contracts, the endocardial velocity is greater than the chorda tendineal velocity (Figs. 25-35 and 25-36).

Small pieces of the mitral apparatus seen in the left ventricle ensure that the correct dimension is being evaluated (Fig. 25-37). Posterior papillary muscles are shown near the apex of the ventricle. These appear as a dense fuzzy echo bands and make it difficult to evaluate the posterior wall. If ventricular volume is to be determined, these muscles are a clue that the transducer is directed too far inferior to the desired point of measurement.

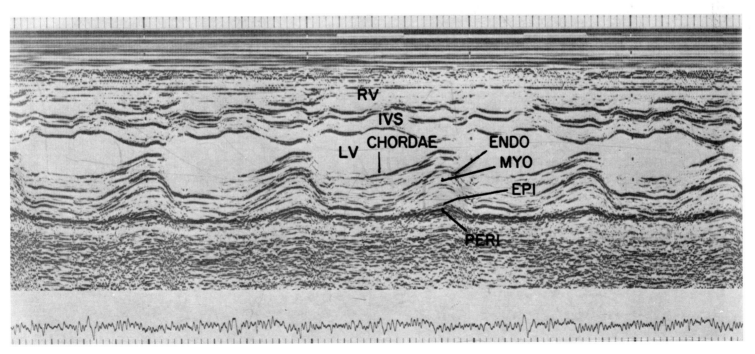

Fig. 25-34. M-mode recording in the left ventricular cavity.

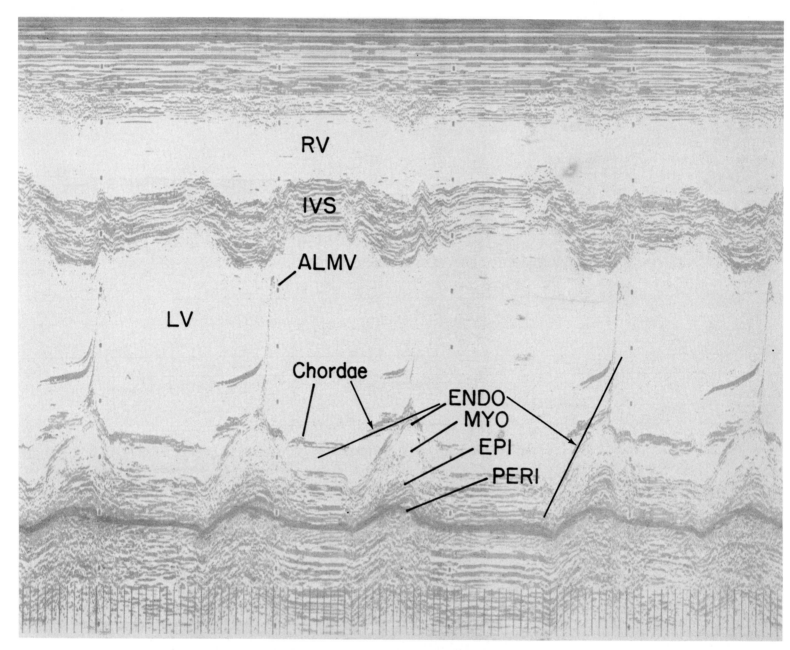

Fig. 25-35. Distinction between the endocardium and chordal structures may be made by assessing the velocity of the two. The normal endocardial velocity is always much greater than the chordal velocity.

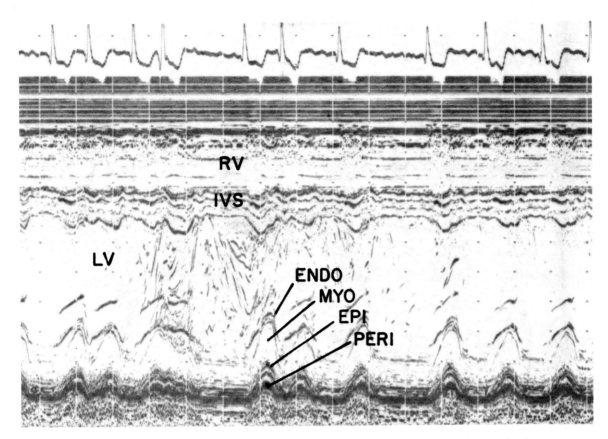

RV

IVS

LV

ENDO
MYO
EPI
PERI

Fig. 25-36. Indocyanine green dye can be injected into the left ventricular cavity during cardiac catheterization. The dye causes the ventricular cavity to fill with echoes and thus differentiates the left side of the septum from the endocardial surface.

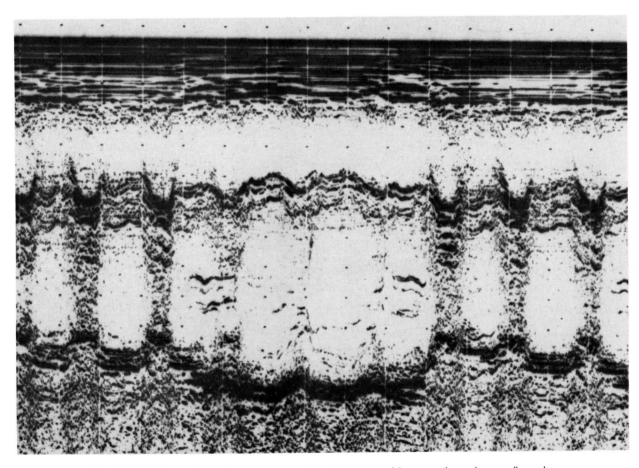

Fig. 25-37. The major-minor sweep, or T sweep, is used to record maximum diameter of the left ventricle. When the ventricle is recorded in the normal position, a horizontal arc is made with the transducer across the minor axis of the ventricle.

RIGHT VENTRICLE

The right ventricle is the most anterior chamber of the heart. Its anterior wall may be demonstrated with proper near-gain settings adjusted so the first moving echo shown after the immobile main bang and chest wall echoes represents the right ventricular wall (Figs. 25-38 and 25-39). If this echo is not clearly defined, Popp has suggested an arbitrary measurement of 0.5 cm from the last nonmoving echo to serve as the right ventricular wall for right ventricular size determination. Most ventricular measurements are made in the supine position and must be adjusted if the patient is examined in an upright or decubitus position.

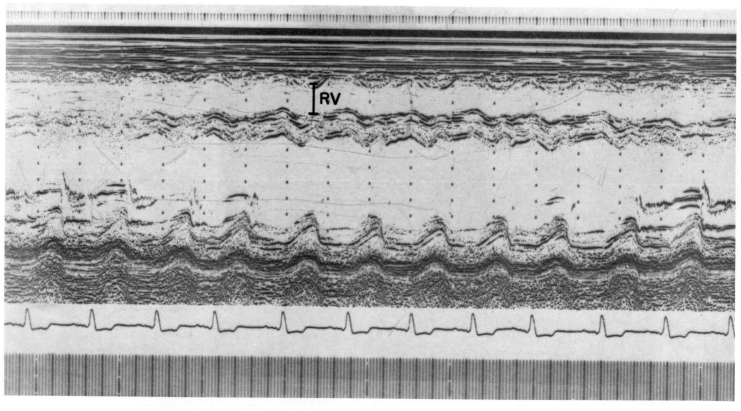

Fig. 25-38. In echocardiography the right ventricular cavity is the first echo-free space seen. The anterior wall of the right ventricle is identified as the first moving echo.

Right ventricular enlargement may result from overload of the right ventricle caused by tricuspid insufficiency, pulmonary insufficiency, or septal defect (Fig. 25-40). Right ventricular pressure overload may result from pulmonary stenosis obstructing the blood flow from the right ventricle. Congestive cardiomyopathy or congestive heart failure will cause right ventricular enlargement along with other chamber enlargement (Fig. 25-41).

The right atrium is best seen on the longitudinal real time or B-mode display as the inferior vena cava empties into it. Suprasternal approach directed toward the right hip also allows visualization of this chamber.

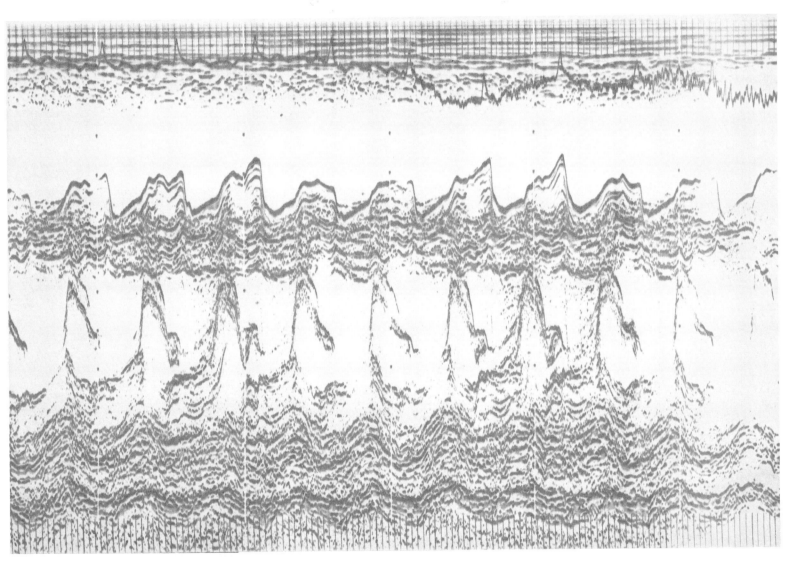

Fig. 25-39. Caution must be used in measuring the right ventricular cavity. Here a catheter in the right ventricle is obscuring the posterior ventricular margin. Other structures (e.g., tricuspid apparatus and chordal pieces) may also interfere in cavity measurements.

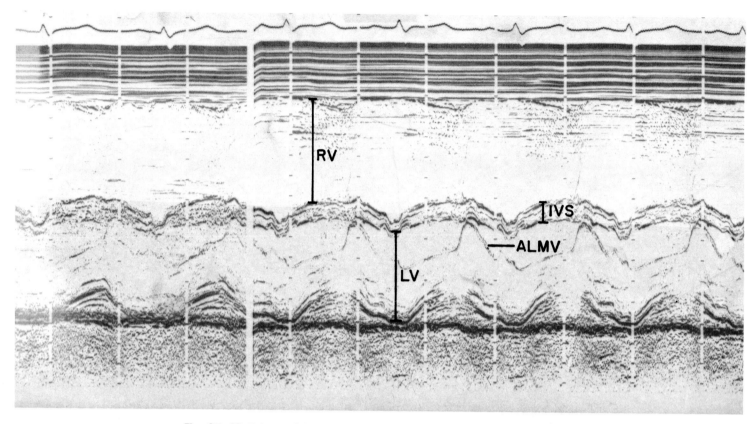

Fig. 25-40. Enlarged right ventricle secondary to an atrial septal defect.

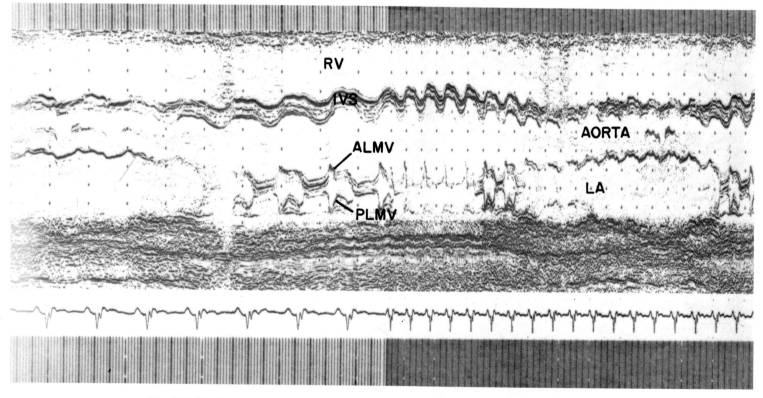

Fig. 25-41. Alcoholic cardiomyopathy shown by dilated cardiac chambers, with reduced amplitude of the mitral valve and multiple echoes in systole from the chordae tendineae.

NORMAL TRICUSPID VALVE

The tricuspid valve is not as easily identified as the mitral valve because of its sub-
sternal location in most patients (Fig. 25-42).
Recordings are easily made if the right ventricle is slightly enlarged or if the heart is
rotated to the left of the sternum. When the
transducer has recorded the mitral apparatus, the beam should be directed slightly
medial to record the tricuspid valve (Fig.
25-43). It is fairly easy to identify the whip-
ping motion of the anterior valve in systole
and early diastole (Fig. 25-44). However,
the diastolic period reveals the pathologic
changes of stenosis and regurgitation; and
careful angulation may allow this phase to be
recorded. An alternate method of recording
is to locate the aortic root. The transducer
beam should sweep inferiorly and medially
toward the patient's right foot to record the
tricuspid valve (Fig. 25-45).

Sometimes it is confusing to differentiate
the tricuspid from the pulmonary valve. In
the normal person the tricuspid valve is always inferior and medial to the aortic root
whereas the pulmonary is superior and lateral. The other difference is that the tricuspid valve moves anteriorly with atrial contraction while the pulmonary *a* valve dips
posteriorly (Fig. 25-46).

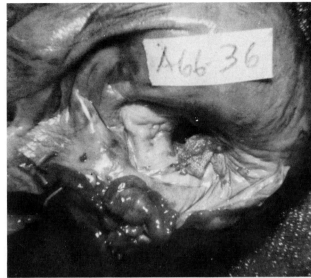

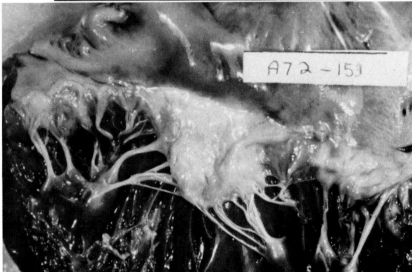

Fig. 25-42. A, Gross specimen of the tricuspid valve as viewed from the superior right
atrium into the barrel of the valve leaflets. **B,** The specimen demonstrates the large anterior leaflet attached by chordae tendineae to both walls of the heart. The posterior
leaflet *(right)* is much smaller and can be seen on the echo posterior to the anterior
leaflet. The septal leaflet *(left)* is not seen by echo, since it parallels the transducer
beam.

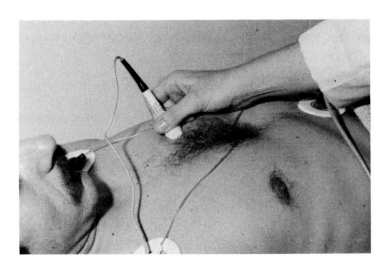

Fig. 25-43. Medial and slightly caudal angulation of the transducer
to demonstrate the tricuspid valve.

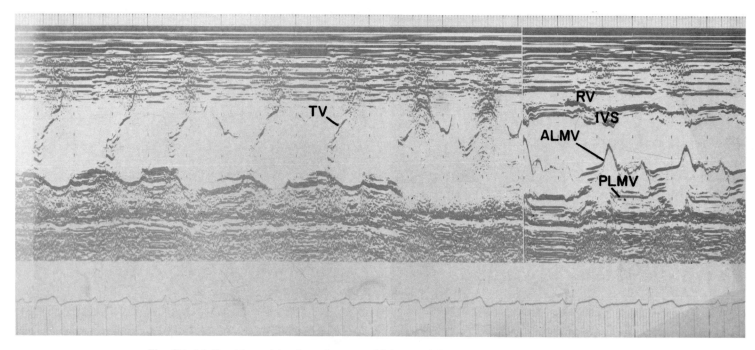

Fig. 25-44. The tricuspid valve of young children, adolescents, and slim adults is easy to record. In most cases the transducer may be held directly over the sternum, or the patient may be rolled into a left decubitus or lateral position to allow the right side of the heart to be viewed.

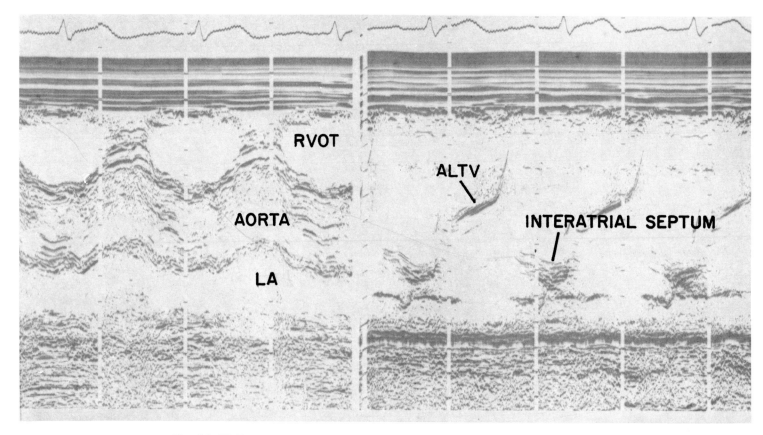

Fig. 25-45. The tricuspid valve is well seen with the interatrial septum posterior.

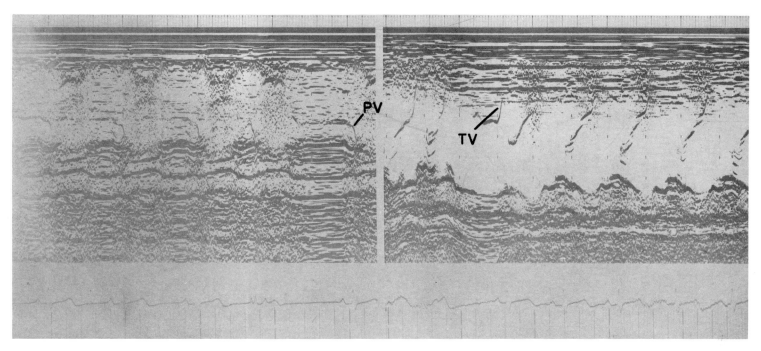

Fig. 25-46. Distinction of the tricuspid valve from the pulmonary valve is one of position and movement. The tricuspid valve moves anteriorly after atrial contraction whereas the pulmonary valve dips posteriorly.

NORMAL PULMONARY VALVE

The normal pulmonary valve was the last of the four valves to be adequately visualized by ultrasound. Gramiak and Nanda (1972) were the first to document its echographic pattern through the aid of contrast studies. Although it is a semilunar three-cusp valve, only the left or posterior cusp can be adequately demonstrated echocardiographically.

A slow sweep from the aortic valve area laterally and superiorly toward the left shoulder should allow visualization of the pulmonary valve area (Fig. 25-47). The parallel aortic echoes serve as a landmark in the sweep to the pulmonary valve. The anterior aortic root forms the posterior boundary of the pulmonary valve area. There should be a 2-to-4-cm space beneath the anterior chest wall and in front of this posterior border in which to visualize the pulmonary valve. Gramiak (1972) identified these posterior structures as the junction of the right ventricular outflow tract with the pulmonary artery and the atriopulmonary sulcus with the left atrium posterior.

When this structure complex is identified, small adjustments in beam position and di-

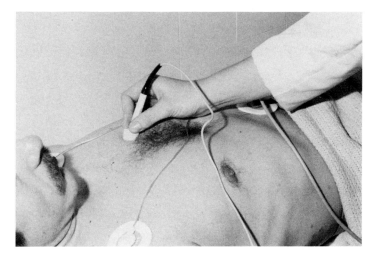

Fig. 25-47. Lateral cephalic angulation from the aortic position to record echoes from the pulmonary valve.

rection will usually pass the beam through the left pulmonary valve cusp, which lies in a posterior position in the right ventricular outflow space (Fig. 25-48). We have found the A-mode trace very helpful in recognizing the fleeting posterior cusp motion of the pulmonary valve. Its appearance is similar to that of the aortic cusp and requires very slight angulation of the beam to demonstrate

fully. We have not found it easier to locate this valve in one particular position. We usually look for the cusp with the patient in a slight left lateral decubitus position; and if unsuccessful, we have the patient lie in a supine position. In patients with increased right heart dimensions the pulmonary valve is easier to visualize.

The other method for locating the pul-

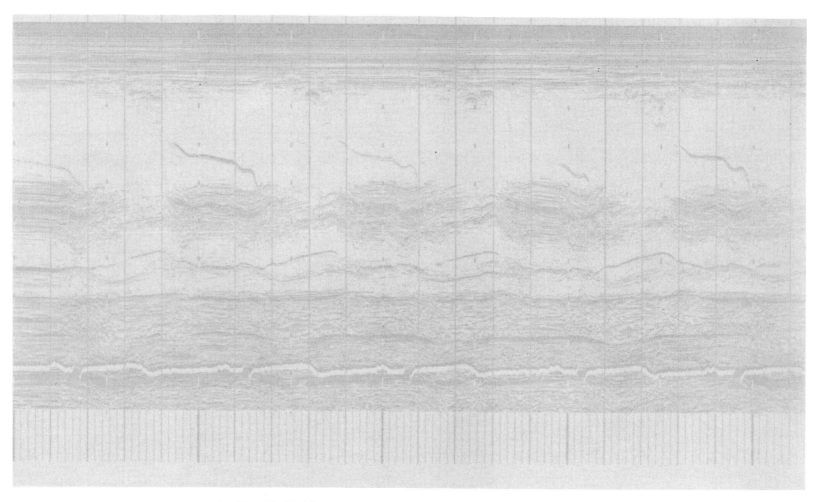

Fig. 25-48. M-mode recording of the normal pulmonary valve.

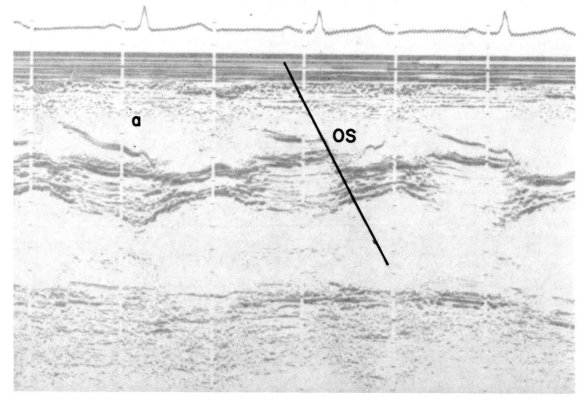

Fig. 25-49. *OS* refers to the opening of the pulmonary valve. The *a* dip corresponds to atrial contraction.

monary valve is to direct the transducer beam from the area of the mitral valve superiorly, without changing the lateral angle. We have found this to be more difficult because of lung interference, but in some cases it succeeds when the aortic sweep fails.

Gramiak (1972) described the physiologic parameters as shown on the echocardiogram. At the beginning of diastole the pulmonary valve is displaced downward and is represented anteriorly on the ultrasound record. The low transducer position with upward beam angulation, together with the vertical inclination of the pulmonary ring, results in examination of the valve from below. All elevations of the pulmonary valve in the stream of flow are represented as posterior movements on the echo. Likewise, downward movements are represented by anterior cusp positions on the trace.

The valve begins to move posteriorly in a gradual manner as the right ventricle fills in diastole. Atrial systole elevates the valve and produces a 3-to-7-mm posterior movement–"a dip" (Fig. 25-49). The valve moves upward with ventricular systole and thus shows a rapid posterior motion on the echo.

OTHER METHODS OF ULTRASOUND EXAMINATION

In a small percentage of the patients scanned, the examiner will not be able to record adequate information from the conventional left sternal approach. This may be a function of lung interference, an unusual angulation of the cardiac structures, or pathosis. Therefore other useful approaches should be employed to obtain the echographic information.

Suprasternal approach. The suprasternal technique was first described by Goldberg (1972). A special flattened transducer is placed in the suprasternal notch with the beam directed caudad. The transducer beam passes through the left brachiocephalic artery, aortic arch, right pulmonary artery, and left atrium. This technique has proved useful in the further detection of aneurysmal growth, tumor invasion, and arterial size in the pediatric and neonatal groups (Fig. 25-50).

Subxyphoid approach. Chang first described the subxyphoid approach as an alternative method in the evaluation of cardiac structures obscured by lung tissue. The transducer is directed in a cephalic angulation from the subxyphoid approach. Recordings can then be made of the left ventricular wall, mitral valve, and aortic valve. Although accurate measurements cannot be obtained

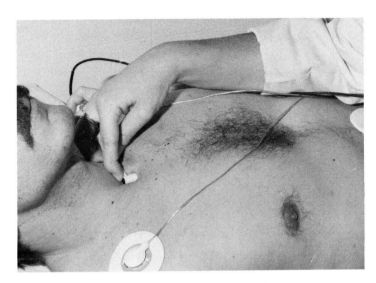

Fig. 25-50. Suprasternal approach demonstrating the aortic arch, right pulmonary artery, and left atrium.

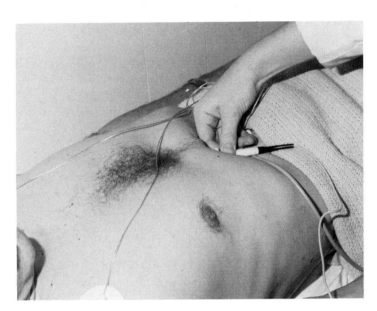

Fig. 25-51. Subxyphoid technique for patients with too much lung interference in the conventional ultrasonic approach.

from this tangential approach, it has proved a useful technique in ruling out certain cardiac problems such as valvular disease, pericardial effusion, and tumor formation (Fig. 25-51).

Pulsed Doppler approach. The pulsed Doppler apparatus has been especially useful in the detection of regurgitation flows, septal defects, and certain kinds of arrhythmias. The transducer is directed over the area of interest while audible and direct printouts are recorded to demonstrate forward and reverse flow.

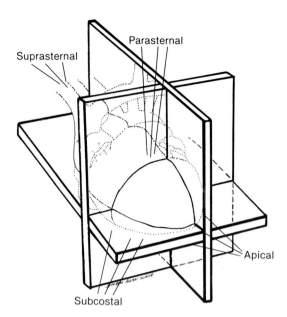

Fig. 25-52. Schematic of the four transducer positions for the two-dimensional echocardiogram. *Suprasternal.* Transducer placed in the suprasternal notch. *Subcostal.* Transducer located near the midline and beneath the costal margin. *Apical.* Transducer located over cardiac apex. *Parasternal.* Area bounded superiorly by the left clavicle, medially by the sternum, and inferiorly by the apical region.

EVALUATION OF THE HEART WITH TWO-DIMENSIONAL ECHO

The Committee on Nomenclature and Standards in Two-Dimensional Echocardiography of the American Society of Echocardiography recommends the following nomenclature and image orientation standards:

Transducer locations (Fig. 25-52)

Suprasternal—transducer placed in suprasternal notch

Subcostal—transducer located near body midline and beneath costal margin

Apical—transducer located over cardiac apex (at *point of maximal impulse,* PMI)

Parasternal—area bounded superiorly by left clavicle, medially by sternum, and inferiorly by apical region

Imaging planes (Fig. 25-53)

Described by manner in which two-dimensional transducer beam transects heart:

Long axis—transects heart perpendicular to dorsal and ventral surfaces of body and parallel with long axis of heart

Short axis—transects heart perpendicular to dorsal and ventral surfaces of body and perpendicular to long axis of heart

Four chamber—transects heart approximately parallel with dorsal and ventral surfaces of body.

A routine two-dimensional examination for the adult and pediatric patient may begin with the patient supine or in a semi–left lateral decubitus position (Fig. 25-54). The decubitus position allows the heart to move away from the sternum and closer to the chest wall, thus allowing a better cardiac window.

Parasternal long axis view. The PLA should be utilized first in the echocardiographic examination. An attempt should be made to record as many of the cardiac structures as possible (from the base to the apex of the heart).

Generally this is accomplished by placing the transducer slightly to the left of the sternum in about the fourth intercostal space (Fig. 25-55). When the bright echo reflection of the pericardium is noted, the transducer is gradually rotated until a long axis view of the heart is obtained (Fig. 25-56).

If it is not possible to record the entire long axis on a single scan, the transducer should be gently rocked cephalad to caudad (icepick fashion) to record information from the base of the heart to the apex (Fig. 25-57).

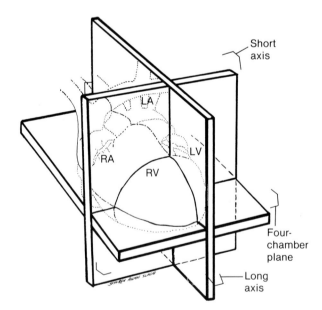

Fig. 25-53. Imaging planes for the two-dimensional study include the short axis, long axis, and four chamber plane.

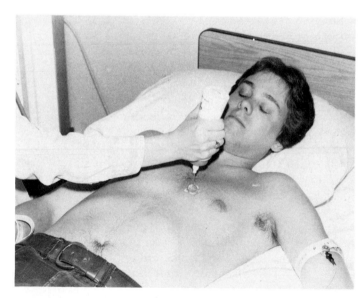

Fig. 25-54. The cardiac sonographer places the coupling material on the patient's chest wall to maintain adequate contact between the transducer and the chest.

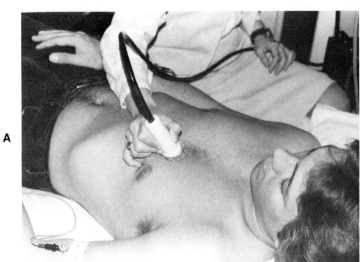

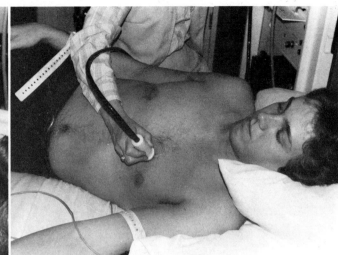

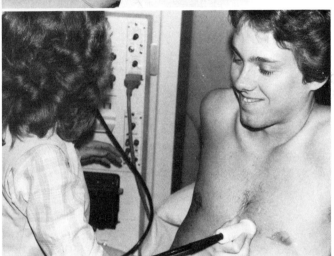

Fig. 25-55. A, The patient is examined in the supine position with the transducer along the parasternal axis. **B,** The patient is rolled into a semi–left decubitus position for better visualization of the cardiac structures along the parasternal axis. **C,** An alternate view is the upright position. In some patients this view permits the cardiac structures to fall against the chest wall and thus avoid lung-air interference.

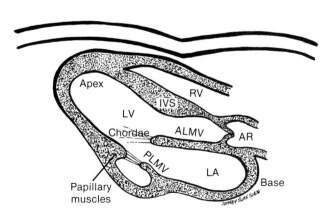

Fig. 25-56. Schematic of the long axis of the heart. *RV,* Right ventricle; *IVS,* interventricular septum; *LV,* left ventricle; *Apex,* apex of left ventricle; *AR,* aortic root; *LA,* left atrium, *ALMV,* anterior leaflet of mitral valve; *PLMV,* posterior leaflet of mitral valve.

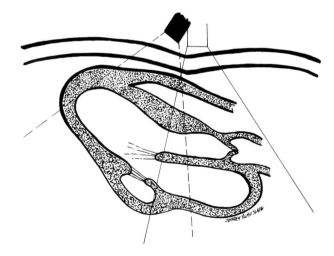

Fig. 25-57. If it is not possible to record all the structures on a long axis scan, the transducer should be gently rocked cephalad to caudad icepick fashion to record the apex to the base of the heart.

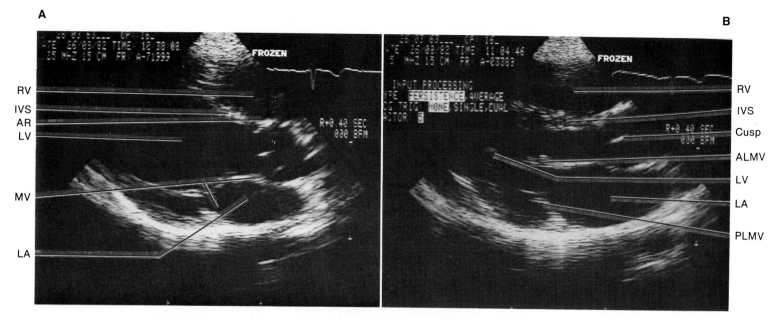

Fig. 25-58. Two-dimensional long axis parasternal views of the heart in, **A,** systole and, **B,** diastole. *RV,* Right ventricle; *IVS,* interventricular septum; *LV,* left ventricle; *MV,* mitral valve; *LA,* left atrium; *Cusp,* aortic cusp; *AR,* aortic root.

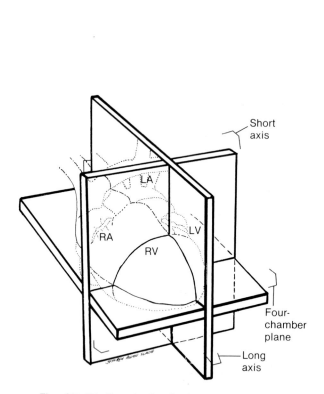

Fig. 25-59. The short axis view of the heart is 90 degrees to the long axis plane.

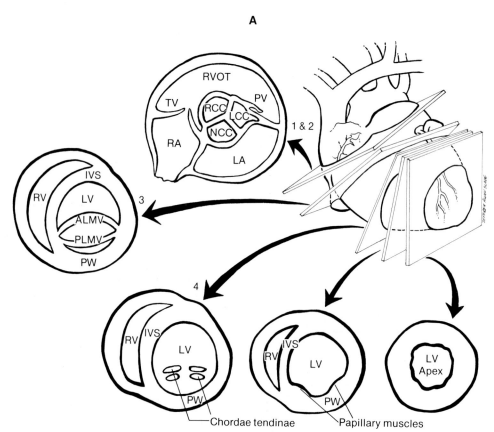

Fig. 25-60. A, The short axis plane may be used to evaluate cardiac structures at the level of, *1,* pulmonary valve, *PV,* right ventricular outflow tract, *RVOT,* tricuspid valve, *TV,* right atrium, *RA,* left atrium, *LA,* right coronary cusp, *RCC,* left coronary cusp, *LCC,* and noncoronary cusp, *NCC; 2,* as above, only better visualization of the aortic cusps; *3,* right ventricle, *RV,* interventricular septum, *IVS,* left ventricle, *LV,* anterior leaflet of mitral valve, *ALMV,* posterior leaflet of mitral valve, *PLMV,* and posterior wall, *PW; 4,* right ventricle, interventricular septum, left ventricle, chordae tendineae, papillary muscles, and posterior wall. •

The sonographer observes the following structures and functions in the long axis view (Fig. 25-58):

1. Composite size of the cardiac chambers
2. Contractility of the RV and LV
3. Thickness of the RV wall
4. Continuity of the IVS with the anterior wall of the aorta
5. Pliability of the atrioventricular and semilunar valves
6. Coaptation of the atrioventricular valves
7. Presence of increased echoes on the atrioventricular and semilunar valves
8. Systolic clearance of the aortic cusps
9. Presence of abnormal echo collections in the chambers or attached to the valve orifices
10. Presence and movement of chordal–papillary muscle structures
11. Thickness of the septum and PWLV
12. Uniform texture of the endocardium-myocardium
13. Size of the aortic root (dilation)

Respective M-mode tracings should then be made in these areas:

1. Record the aortic root, cusps, and left atrium.

2. Sweep from the aortic to the mitral valve:
   a. Demonstrate IVS–anterior aortic wall continuity and posterior aortic wall–MV continuity.
   b. Show transition from LA wall to atrioventricular groove to PWLV.
3. Record the ALMV at the *tip* of the leaflet.
4. Record the ALMV and PLMV.
5. Record the LV at an area inferior to the tip of the mitral apparatus and superior to the papillary muscles.
6. If LV dysfunction or aneurysm is suspected, make a slow sweep from the AV to the apex.

Short axis view. The two-dimensional transducer should then be rotated 90 degrees to the long axis (Fig. 25-59) to obtain multiple transverse short axis views of the heart at these four levels (Fig. 25-60):

1. Pulmonary valve, right ventricular outflow tract, aorta (A)

   a. Typical sausage-shaped RVOT—PV draped anterior to aorta
   b. Semilunar cusp thickness and mobility
   c. Presence of calcification and/or extraneous echoes in RV or valve areas
   d. Tricuspid valve mobility and thickness
      M-mode: PV

2. Right ventricle, tricuspid valve, aortic cusps, left and right atria (B)

   a. Size of LA and RV
   b. Presence of mass lesions in RA or LA
   c. Mobility and thickness of atrioventricular and semilunar valves
   d. Continuity of intertrial septum
   e. RV wall thickness
   f. Number of cusps with aorta
      M-mode: RVOT, aortic cusps, LA, RV, TV

3. Right ventricle, left ventricular outflow tract, anterior and posterior leaflets of mitral valve (C)

   a. Thickness of LVOT, septum, and PWLV
   b. Size of mitral valve orifice
   c. Presence of mass lesion in LV or RV
   d. Mobility and thickness of MV
   e. Flutter of IVS and/or ALMV
   f. Systolic apposition of MV leaflets
   g. Contractility of IVS and LV
      M-mode: RV, IVS, ALMV, LV, ALMV-PLMV

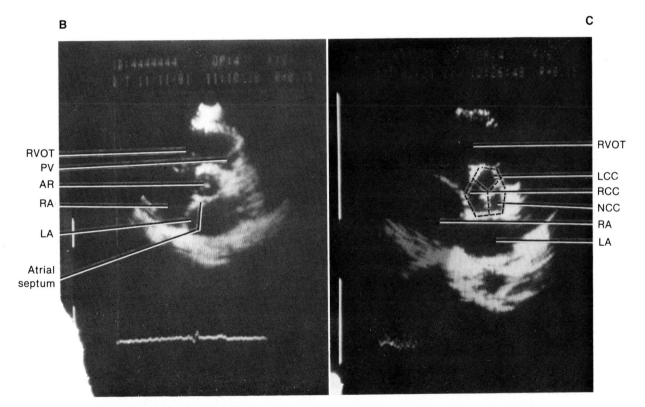

Fig. 25-60, cont'd. B, Short axis view showing the pulmonary valve, right ventricular outflow tract, aortic root, *AR*, right atrium, left atrium, and atrial septum. **C,** Short axis view showing the aortic cusps, right ventricular outflow tract, right atrium, and left atrium.

Continued.

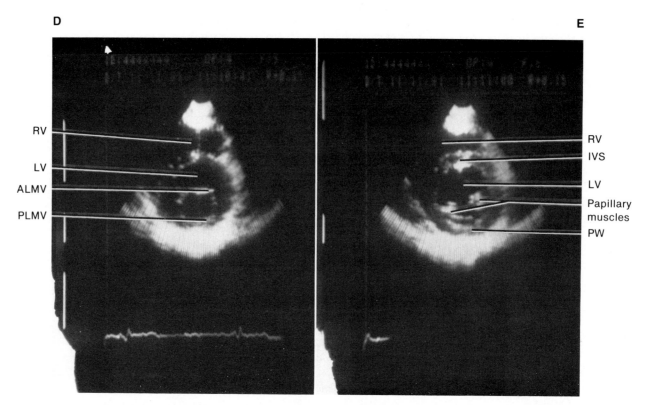

Fig. 25-60, cont'd. D, Short axis view showing the right ventricle, left ventricle, anterior leaflet of mitral valve, and posterior leaflet of mitral valve. E, Short axis view at level of the chordal structures and papillary muscles.

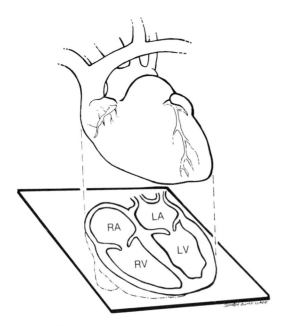

Fig. 25-61. Apical four chamber view.

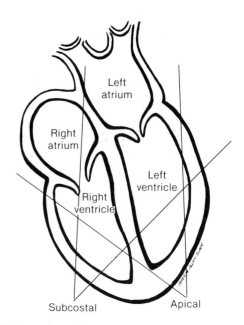

Fig. 25-62. Schematic of the transducer positions for an apical and subcostal view of the four chambers of the heart.

4. Right ventricle, left ventricle, papillary muscles *(D)*

   a. Contractility of IVS and LV walls
   b. Thickness of IVS and PWLV
   c. Size of LV
   d. Presence/absence of mural thrombus
   e. Presence/absence of pericardial fluid, constriction, restriction
   f. Increased echo density in LV wall
   g. Papillary muscles in LV
      M-mode: RV, IVS, chordae tendineae, endocardium, myocardium, epicardium, pericardium; reduce gain and sweep from aorta to mitral to LV

Apical four chamber view (Fig. 25-61). The sonographer should palpate the patient's chest to detect the posterior maximal impulse (PMI) (Fig. 25-62). The transducer should then be directed in a transverse plane at the PMI and angled sharply cephalad to record the four chambers of the heart (Fig. 25-63).

This view is excellent for assessing contractility, relative size of the cardiac chambers, presence of mass lesions, and septal or ventricular hypertrophy. It may also be useful in evaluating the prolapse syndrome or pericardial effusion.

The sonographer observes the following (Fig. 25-63):

1. Size of cardiac chambers
2. Contractility of heart
3. Septal thickness, contractility, and continuity
4. Increased echoes on valve apparatus
5. Presence/absence of flail leaflet
6. Presence/absence of thrombus or mass in chambers
7. Size of LVOT, signs of obstruction

Costal view. This is an alternate approach to obtain the four chambers of the heart. The transducer should be placed in the subxyphoid space and angled sharply toward the patient's left shoulder (Fig. 25-63, *F*).

This approach seems to work best in patients with a flexible abdominal wall (i.e., most pediatric and young patients). It is especially good for visualizing the interatrial septum.

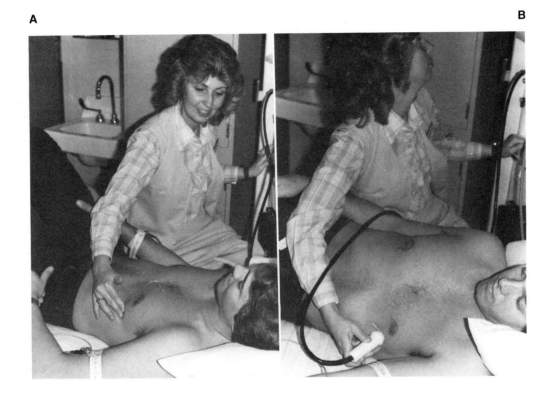

A

B

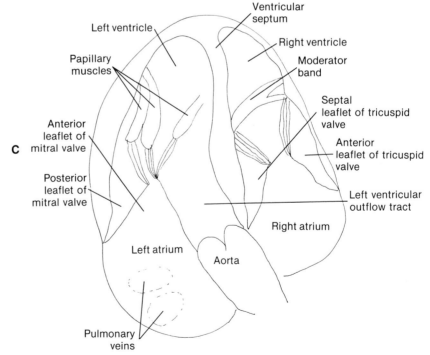

C

Fig. 25-63. A, The cardiac sonographer should palpate the posterior maximal impulse of the patient's heart to place the transducer at this point. **B,** The transducer is directed in a transverse plane at the reversed PMI and angled sharply cephalad to record the four chambers. **C,** Schematic of the apical four chambers. Note the moderator band in the right ventricular cavity, the pulmonary veins in the left atrial cavity, and the papillary muscles and chordal structures in both ventricular cavities. *Continued.*

D

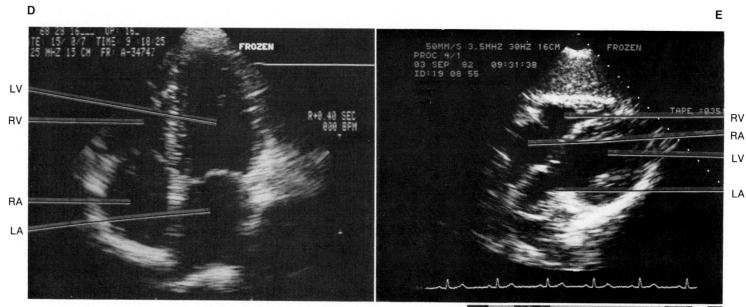

LV

RV

RA

LA

E

RV

RA

LV

LA

Fig. 25-63, cont'd. D, Four chamber view with the transducer in an apical position. **E,** Subcostal or subxyphoid four chamber view. **F,** Transducer position for the four chamber view.

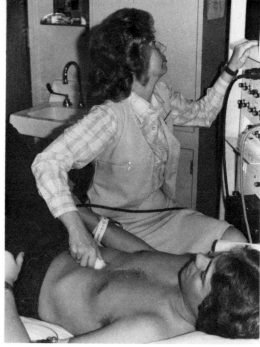

F

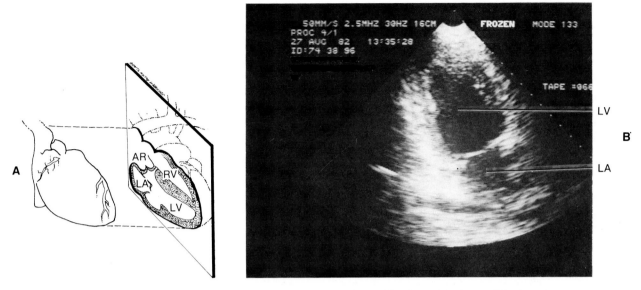

Fig. 25-64. A, Schematic of the apical long axis view of the two chambers of the heart. **B,** Two-dimensional scan of the apical long axis view.

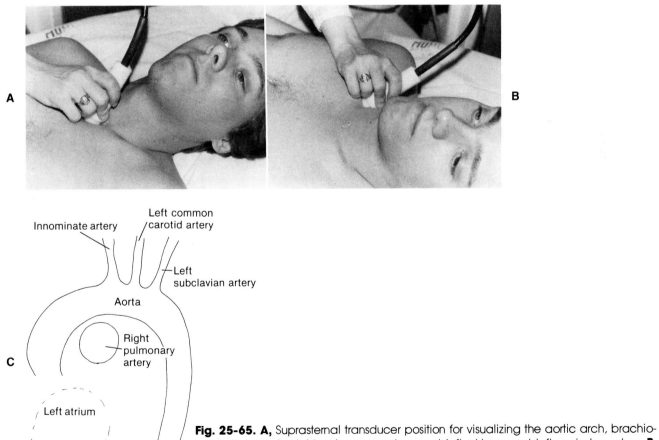

Fig. 25-65. A, Suprasternal transducer position for visualizing the aortic arch, brachiocephalic vessels, right pulmonary artery and left atrium, and left main bronchus. **B,** Alternate transducer position for the suprasternal view. **C,** Schematic of the cardiac structures visualized in the suprasternal view.

Apical long axis view (primarily for adults) (Fig. 25-64). The transducer should then be rotated 90 degrees to obtain a longitudinal view of the LV.

This is an excellent method to observe contractility and thickness and to look for mass lesions in the LV.

Suprasternal view. The transducer should be placed in the suprasternal notch in a transverse plane and angled sharply toward the feet (Fig. 25-65).

The structures visualized are the aortic arch, brachiocephalic vessels, right pulmonary artery, left atrium, and left main bronchus.

The sonographer observes the following:
1. Relative sizes of the arch and RPA
2. Presence/absence of dissection, thrombus, or thickening
3. Coarctation (define discrete tubular hyperplasia)

26 Echocardiographic measurements

The ability to evaluate echographic data has been of great interest to the clinicians and investigators involved in ultrasound techniques. The early pioneers in ultrasound (Feigenbaum, Popp, Gramiak, and Joyner) were able to correlate their ultrasonic data consistently with data from other diagnostic studies to confirm the validity of ultrasonic measurements in echocardiography. To have meaning, the data must be evaluated along with the patient's clinical history and symptoms. Although many laboratories have discontinued certain echocardiographic measurements, we have found the echocardiogram a very useful teaching tool. Instructing students how to evaluate it by using measurements improves their technique and sharpens their skill in echo tracing interpretation. We have also found that "eyeballing" can mislead an inexperienced sonographer to overread or underread a particular study.

Therefore this chapter is devoted to echocardiographic measurements and their explanation. These data have accumulated from the various investigators in the field with specific references to normal values. In addition, an outline of specific diseases and their echocardiographic significance is provided in Table 26-1, on the next page.

To fully evaluate the cardiac patient, we have found it useful to perform the conventional M-mode and real time applications of ultrasound. Thus, when we calculate our measurements, the added dimension of the real time image adds to our understanding of the total picture of cardiac function and contractility. (See report below.)

Calipers facilitate the measurement process and should be used for uniformity and accuracy in data accumulation. The scans and data sheets are then reviewed by the sonographer and physician for final interpretation.

ECHOCARDIOGRAPHY REPORT

Case number _____
interpretation

Height _____ Weight _____
Clinical findings _____
_____
_____

Indicated measurements

Interventricular septum	_____ cm (0.7-1.1 cm)	Ejection time	_____
LV posterior wall	_____ cm (0.7-1.1 cm)	Septal-aortic continuity	_____
Aortic root dimension	_____ cm (2.0-3.7 cm)	Septal motion	_____
Intraaortic cusp spacing	_____ cm (1.3-1.9 cm)	Pericardial effusion	_____
RV cavity	_____ cm (0.7-2.6 cm)	Stroke volume	_____
LV internal dimension(ed)	_____ cm (4.0-5.5 cm)	Ejection fraction	_____ (above 65%)
LV internal dimension(es)	_____ cm (2.5-4.0 cm)		
Left atrial dimension	_____ cm (1.9-4.0 cm)	Cardiac output	_____
Mitral valve amplitude	_____ cm (20-35 mm)		
Mitral valve velocity	_____ cm (70-150 (mm/sec)		

$$V_{cf} = \frac{LVD(ed) - LVD(es)}{LVD(ed) \times LVET} = \underline{\qquad}$$

LV mass _____
Endocardial velocity _____

Prolapse
  ALMV _____
  PLMV _____
  Holosystolic,
    Midsystolic,
    Typical _____
  Suggestive _____
  Possible _____
Suprasternal notch
  Aorta (arch) _____ cm
  Right pulmonary artery _____ cm
  Left atrium (Y axis) _____ cm

Sonographer _____
Physician _____, M.D.

Table 26-1. Echocardiographic structures

Disease	LA	LV	LVO	RV	Mitral valve (anterior and posterior)
MV stenosis	↑			?↑	↓ E-F slope (<35 mm/sec)
					↓ C-E amplitude (severe) No *a* kick (usually) PLMV moves anterior (usually)
MV regurgitation	↑	↑	↑		*e* point touches IVS ↑ C-E amplitude E-F slope >180 mm/sec Flutter ALMV
MV prolapse	↑ (MR)	↑ (MR)	↑ (MR)		Posterior motion in systole (3 to 5 mm)
Aortic insufficiency		↑	↑		↓ E-F slope Flutter of ALMV
Aortic stenosis					↓ E-F slope ? Calcified mitral anulus
CCM	↑	↑	↑	↑	↓ Amplitudes ALMV/PLMV clearly recorded
IHSS or HOCM	?↑ MR		↓		*e* point touches IVS ↓ E-F slope SAM (obstructive)
Vegetations	↑ MR	↑ AI	↑ AI	↑ TR	Multilayered thickening Coarse diastolic flutter (MV veg.)
Normal heart	1.9 to 4.0 cm; 1:1 LA/Ao	4.0 to 5.5 cm	20 to 35 cm	0.7 to 2.6 cm	M shape of ALMV PLMV moves posterior E-F slope 80 to 150 mm/sec C-E amplitude 20 to 35 mm

Code:
MR = Mitral regurgitation
CCM = Concentric cardiomyopathy
IHSS = Idiopathic hypertrophic subaortic stenosis
HOCM = Hypertrophic cardiomyopathy
AI = Aortic insufficiency
TR = Tricuspid regurgitation

Aortic valve	IVS	Posterior heart wall	Other
			Calcification (thickening)
	Hyperdynamic		Prolpase?
			"Hump" in pericardial effusion (pseudo-prolapse)
	↑ Amplitude (may have) ? Flutter IVS		
Calcified walls ↓ Systolic septal wall motion	↑ Thickness	Concentric hypertrophy	Bicuspid (eccentric cusps)
Decreased motion	Thin Poor contracility	Thin Poor contractility	Cardiomegaly; pericardial effusion
Midsystolic closure	>1.8 to 2.0 cm IVS/PHW < 1.3 cm		Pseudo-SAM in hypertension
Coarse diastolic flutter (AR veg.)			Vegetations 2 to 3 mm thick
Box shape Systolic separation 1.5 to 2.6 cm LA index <2.2	0.6 to 1.2 cm IVS/PHW 1.3	1.1 cm	

ALMV   = Anterior leaflet mitral valve
SAM   = Systolic anterior motion
AR   = Aortic root
PHW   = Posterior heart wall
PLMV   = Posterior leaflet mitral valve
LA index = Left atrial size/Body surface area

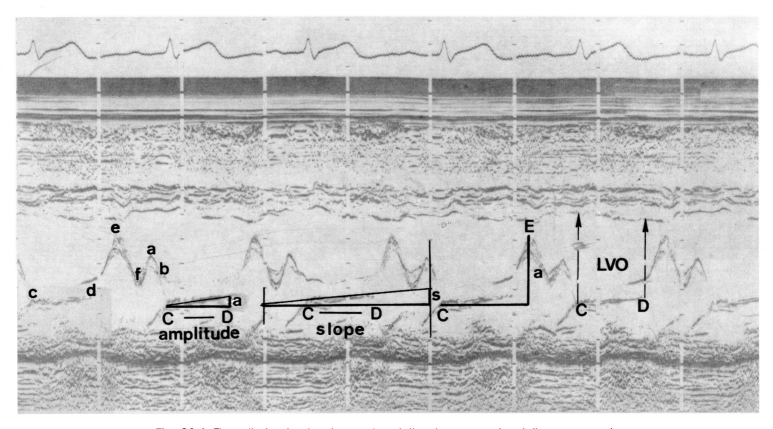

Fig. 26-1. The mitral valve has been given letters to represent systolic components, c and d, and diastolic components, d, e, f, a, b, and c. For an explanation of C-D amplitude *(a)*, C-D slope *(s)*, C-E amplitude *(a)*, and left ventricular outflow tract at C and D, see text.

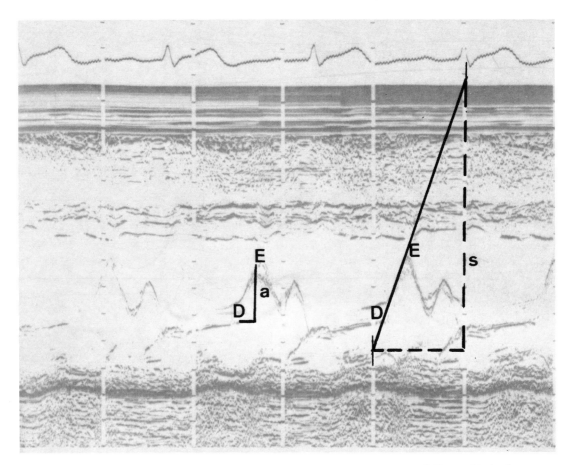

Fig. 26-2. Some laboratories use the D-E amplitude instead of the C-E amplitude for mitral valve excursion. See text for explanation.

MITRAL VALVE

Normal appearance. The anterior and posterior leaflets of the mitral valve are assigned specific letters corresponding to their systolic and diastolic components. The systolic component consists of C and D points.* The diastolic component has E, F, A, and B points. Each letter point coincides with a specific ECG function. The QRS (onset of systole) marks the C point, whereas the T wave coincides with the D point (end of systole). Shortly thereafter (onset of diastole) the E point is shown and the ventricle starts to relax at the F point. The P wave triggers atrial contraction and the A kick is seen. Normally the B point is not identified in patients without elevated end diastolic pressure and occurs just prior to the QRS (Fig. 26-1).

C-D amplitude. This is a measurement from the C point to the D point. It is the closed systolic position during which the valve leaflets move with the mitral anulus.

---

*Throughout Chapters 25 to 35, the references to these letter points along the cardiac cycle are by both lower case and capital letters since both designations are used in the field and authors employ the one more familiar to them.

It normally has little to do with the valve itself and relates to the heart movement. This structure may be an important indicator of a systolic anterior motion (SAM) or mitral valve prolapse (posterior bulging into the atrial cavity) (nl 20 to 30 mm) (Fig. 26-1).

C-E slope. This measurement depicts the rate of movement of the valve leaflets as the anulus moves anteriorly in systole. The slope is measured by extending the line through points C and D and is a time-distance measurement (nl under 35 mm/sec) (Fig. 26-1).

C-E amplitude. This is a measurement from the C point to the E point. It denotes the amplitude at which the mitral valve is opening. The E point is the most anterior excursion (nl 20 to 33 mm) (Fig. 26-1).

LVOT at C point. Measure the left ventricular outflow tract from the left side of the septum to the C point on the mitral valve echo (nl 20 to 33 mm) (Fig. 26-1).

LVOT at D point. Measure from the posterior wall of the septum to the D point on the mitral valve (nl 12 to 33 mm) (Fig. 26-1).

D-E slope. This measurement signifies the

opening movement of the mitral valve in early diastole. The slope is measured by extending the line through points D and E. This may be an indicator of left ventricular failure and elevated end-systolic volume with a decreased D-E slope[2] (nl 240 to 380 mm/sec) (Fig. 26-2).

D-E amplitude. This is a measurement of the maximum excursion of the anterior mitral valve leaflet following early diastolic opening. The measurement is taken from the D point to the E point. It may be an important indicator of mitral regurgitation (nl 17 to 30 mm) (Fig. 26-2).

E-F slope. This measures the rate of motion of the cusp in early diastole and expresses the rate of left atrial emptying. Since a slope is being measured, extend the line connecting the E and F points through 1 second in time. Draw a line from the bottom of the time line (at the point of intersection) and measure the distance along the vertical axis from the end of the completed line to the beginning of the time line (nl 50 to 180 mm/sec) (Fig. 26-3).

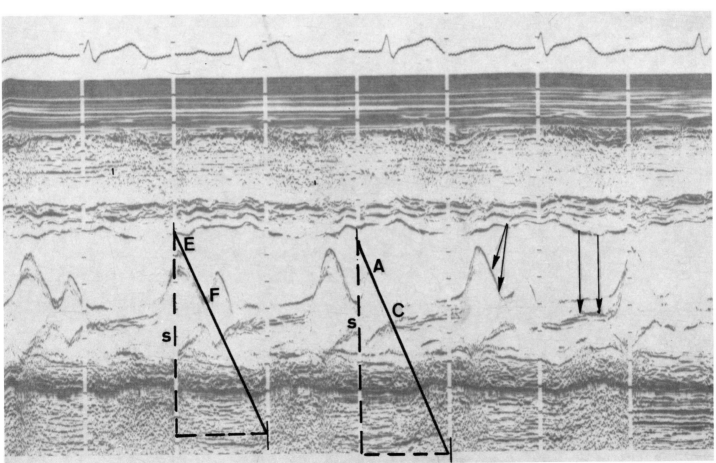

Fig. 26-3. The mitral leaflet should be measured at its greatest excursion. The best excursion is normally below the aorta near the tip of the leaflet (the posterior leaflet may also be seen at this point). In figuring the E-F slope the steepest slope should be measured. See text for explanation of A-C slope, flutter, and SAM.

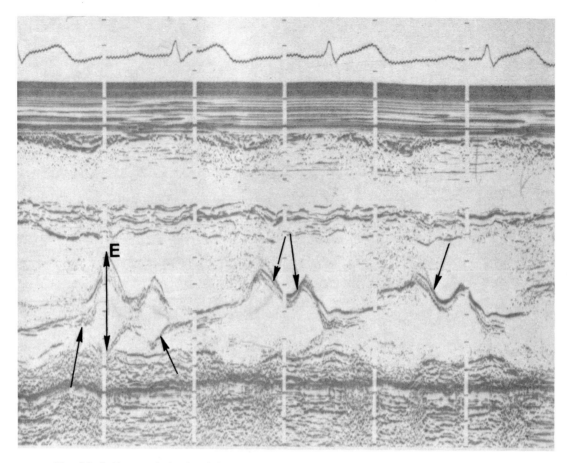

Fig. 26-4. The posterior leaflet is a mirror image of the anterior leaflet in ventricular diastole. The anterior and posterior leaflets should meet in systole at the C and D points. See text for explanation of mitral valve separation, thickening, and multiple echoes (as seen in mitral stenosis).

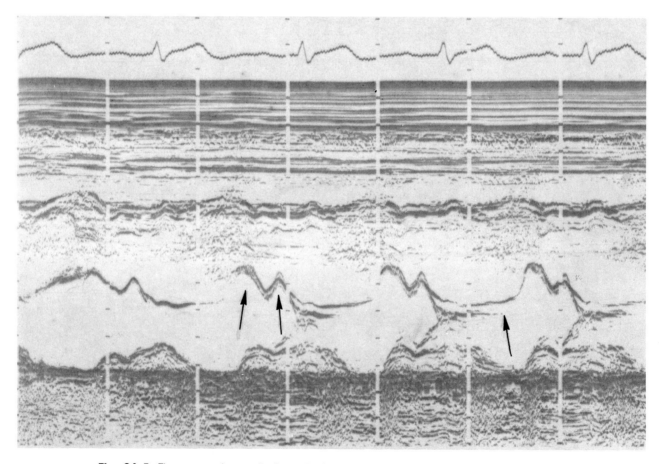

Fig. 26-5. The space beneath the mitral valve's anterior leaflet should be clear of echoes. The systolic segment of the valve should move in an anterior direction.

A-C slope. This depicts the rate of systolic closure of the mitral valve. The measurement is made by extending a slope line through points A and C. A decreased rate of closure may indicate elevated left ventricular end diastolic pressure or poor ventricular performance[2] (nl 350 to 360 mm/sec) (Fig. 26-3).

PR-AC interval. This is a measurement to detect premature closure of the mitral valve (acute aortic insufficiency). It is taken from the beginning of the P wave to the beginning of the Q wave and from the A point to the C point on the mitral valve. The interval is then determined by subtracting the AC from the PR interval. (Time lines of 0.04 sec are used for this calibration; nl less than 0.06 sec.)

Fluttering. Flutter may be seen as a fine oscillation of the anterior mitral leaflet in diastole. It may be secondary to aortic insufficiency, vegetations; or if coarse, it may be due to atrial fibrillation (Fig. 26-3).

Systolic anterior motion (SAM). With this abnormality the anterior mitral leaflet moves anterior after the onset of systole and then returns to its normal position just before diastole. Often it is seen with obstructive hypertrophic cardiomyopathy, and the degree of obstruction is directly related to the size of the SAM (Fig. 26-3).

Multiple echoes. In the absence of calcification, the mitral complex is a thin single reflection (Fig. 26-4).

Thickening. Multiple bright echoes due to fibrosis and/or calcifications may be seen on either the anterior or the posterior leaflet. The degree of thickening or calcification is a function of the amount of multiple echoes seen and may be an indication of a rheumatic process (Fig. 26-4).

Posterior leaflet of mitral valve (PLMV). Designate whether the posterior leaflet moves posteriorly in diastole or anteriorly (as in rheumatic disease, mitral stenosis) (Fig. 26-4).

Posterior bulging. This is indicated when either the anterior or the posterior (or both) leaflets are displaced posteriorly in systole. The normal C-D slope is interrupted by a posterior movement, usually 3 to 5 mm, and is an indication of prolapse[4] (Fig. 26-5).

Space beneath the mitral valve clear. Echoes posterior to the mitral valve in diastole that do not disappear as the gain is decreased are abnormal. If there is an echo-free space in early diastole followed by an increased mass of echoes, this most likely represents a myxoma or tumor (Fig. 26-5).

Amputated E, prominent A. This occurs with elevated left ventricular end diastolic pressure. The E point is diminished, and the A point is accentuated. (It is often seen in gross aortic insufficiency.)

AORTIC ROOT

Dimension. Measure at the end of diastole at the onset of the first rapid deflection of the QRS complex from the leading edge of the anterior aortic root to the leading edge of the posterior aortic root (nl 20 to 37 mm) (Fig. 26-6).

Thickening. Abnormal thickness with an increase in the amount of echoes and/or brightness of the aortic walls are usually due to calcification. A decrease in wall motility may be noted.

Wall amplitude. This is a measurement of the anterior motion of the posterior aortic wall during ventricular systole. It is obtained by drawing a horizontal line between the external boundaries of the posterior aortic wall in diastole and then measuring the maximal vertical distance from this line to the external boundary of the aortic wall during ventricular systole.[1] Decreased values indicate low cardiac output and a reduced stroke volume.[2]

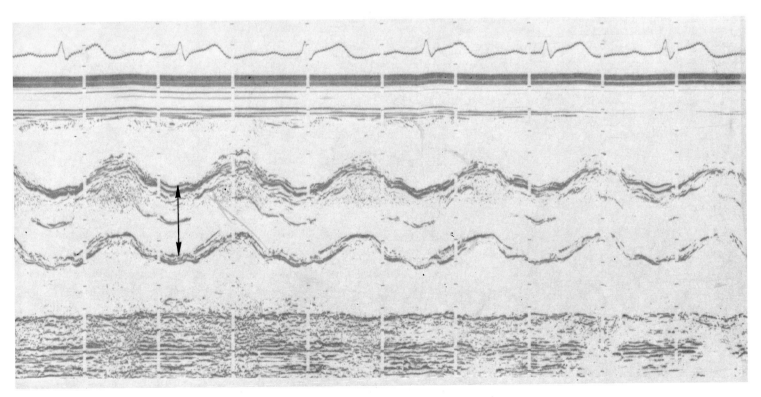

Fig. 26-6. The parallel band of echoes that move anteriorly in systole and posteriorly in diastole delineate the walls of the aorta. The leading edge to leading edge is measured because it is a finite and initial point (according to Popp), and there should be little difficulty separating the walls from the lumen of the aorta.

AORTIC VALVE

Normal appearance. The characteristic feature of the normal valve is the boxlike configuration that presents from the right and noncoronary cusps as they separate in ventricular systole. The closed position in diastole presents as a dominant echo in the middle of the aortic root (Fig. 26-7).

Systolic separation. This is the maximum opening of the coronary cusps during the initial part of ventricular systole. A perpendicular line is drawn from the RCC to the NCC at the opening movement, from leading edge to leading edge at the onset of systole (nl 15 to 26 mm) (Fig. 26-8).

Opening and closing rates. These parameters should be noted as gradual closure of the cusps in systole and may indicate low cardiac output (i.e., congestive failure, cardiomyopathy, or mitral regurgitation) (Fig. 26-8).

Flutter. Flutter may be seen as fine oscillations of either or both of the coronary cusps during opening of the valve in ventricular systole. This is a normal variant of blood flowing through the cusps (Fig. 26-8).

Interrupted opening. This abnormality is seen as a midsystolic closure and reopening of the aortic valve in systole. It is due to a midsystolic obstruction of blood flow as seen in severe IHSS. An abrupt early systolic closure is seen in discrete subaortic stenosis (Fig. 26-8).

Thickening. Thickening of the cusps is seen with calcification or vegetations on the cusps. Vegetations may not hamper the cusp opening, as is seen with aortic calcifications or stenosis.

LEFT ATRIUM

Dimension. The left atrium should be measured at the end of systole so the posterior wall of the aorta to the left atrial wall will be included (nl 19 to 40 mm) (Fig. 26-9).

Left atrium/aortic root ratio. This is the ratio of the atrial dimension taken at end systole to the aortic root dimension taken at end diastole (nl 0.87 to 1.11).

Left atrial index. This is obtained by dividing the left atrial size by the patient's body surface area (nl 12 to 21 mm/sq m).

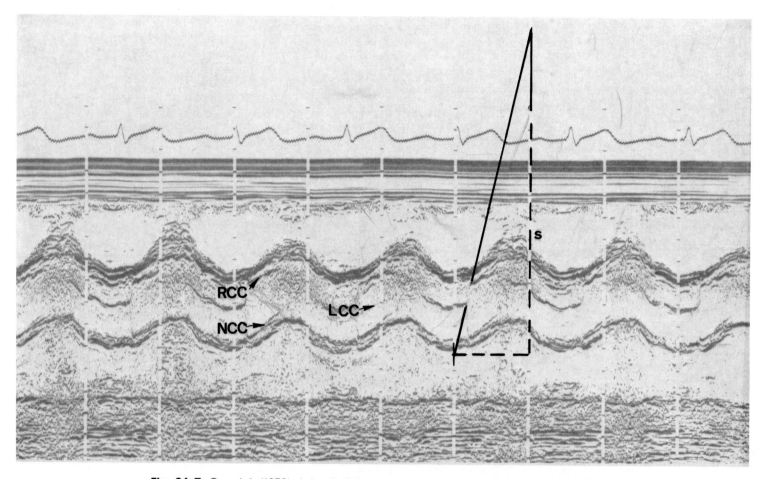

Fig. 26-7. Gramiak (1970) states that the valvular cusps are recognized as thin linear configurations moving to the periphery of the aorta in systole and occupying a mid-aortic position. The right and noncoronary cusps show significant systolic movement in the opposite direction and produce a boxlike configuration. The left coronary cusp is normally not visualized, since it lies at right angles to the sonic beam. See text for systolic opening rate.

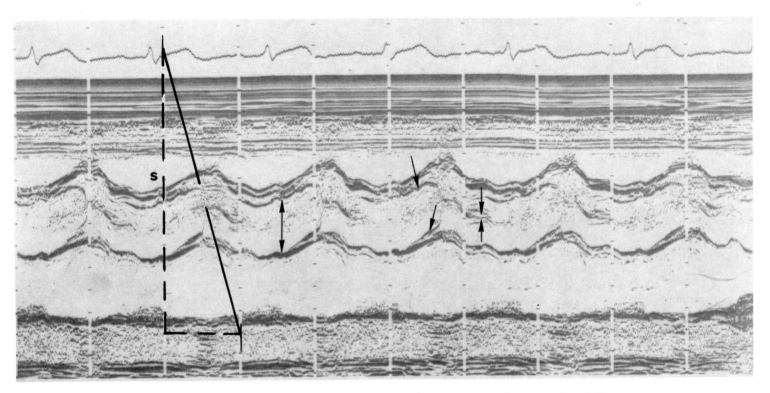

Fig. 26-8. See text for an explanation of systolic closing rate, systolic separation, flutter, thickening, interrupted opening, eccentricity, and coapt signs.

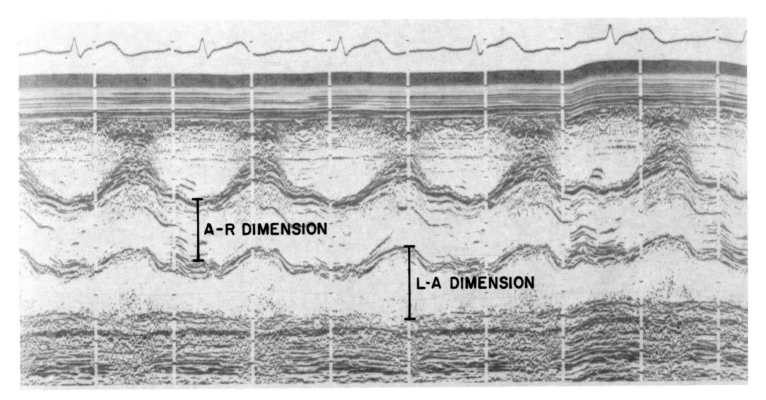

Fig. 26-9. The left atrium is recorded posterior to the aortic root and usually presents as a 1/1 ratio with the aortic root dimension. The measurement of the left atrium includes the anterior edge of the posterior aortic wall. This is a source of error; but if all left atrial dimensions are measured in this fashion, the error will be consistent and constant.

TRICUSPID VALVE

Normal appearance. The anterior leaflet can usually be visualized, at least in part, and moves like the mitral valve. The posterior and septal leaflets are not usually seen (Fig. 26-10).

PR-AC interval. This is a measurement to detect premature closure of the tricuspid valve. A prolonged AC interval is often an indicator of elevated right ventricular end diastolic pressure (nl under 0.06 sec).

E-F slope. This slope is similar to that of the mitral valve. A severe decrease may indicate stenosis (nl 60 to 125 mm/sec).

Posterior echoes. Organized echoes posterior to the anterior leaflet may indicate a tumor mass, vegetations, or a ruptured sinus of Valsalva aneurysm.

Fluttering. Fluttering is caused by fine oscillation of the anterior leaflet in diastole secondary to pulmonary insufficiency.

Thickening. Multiple bright echoes due to fibrosis and/or calcification may be seen on the anterior leaflet and may represent stenosis or vegetations.

PULMONARY VALVE

Normal appearance. Part of the posterior leaflet of the pulmonary valve is visible. The anterior wall of the right ventricle is seen anterior and a characteristic thick mass of echoes (from the pulmonary root) below (Fig. 26-11).

A dip. This presystolic downward motion of the posterior leaflet coincides with the A point of the mitral valve and follows atrial contraction. The measurement is made by drawing a line from the F point to the B point and measuring the distance from the lowest point on the A dip to this line.

An absence of the A dip may indicate pulmonary hypertension or atrial fibrillation. An increase in the dip may indicate pulmonary stenosis. This measurement fluctuates with normal respiration (nl 1 to 8 mm) (Fig. 26-11).

E-F slope. This is similar to the E-F slope of the mitral valve and is measured the same. A flattened or negative slope may be indicative of pulmonary hypertension (nl 6 to 115 mm/sec).

Fluttering. These coarse oscillations of the posterior leaflet occurring with the onset of ventricular systole, and often into early diastole, are indicative of subpulmonary or infundibular stenosis.

Flying W. This sign is seen with a W wave in systole. It is caused by the midsystolic closure of the valve and is often a sign of pulmonary hypertension.

Premature opening. This abnormality is detected by correlating the opening movement of the posterior leaflet with the P wave on the ECG. It occurs with increased pressure from the right ventricle against the pulmonary valve and may be caused by ruptured sinus of Valsalva aneurysm, constrictive pericarditis, or tricuspid insufficiency.

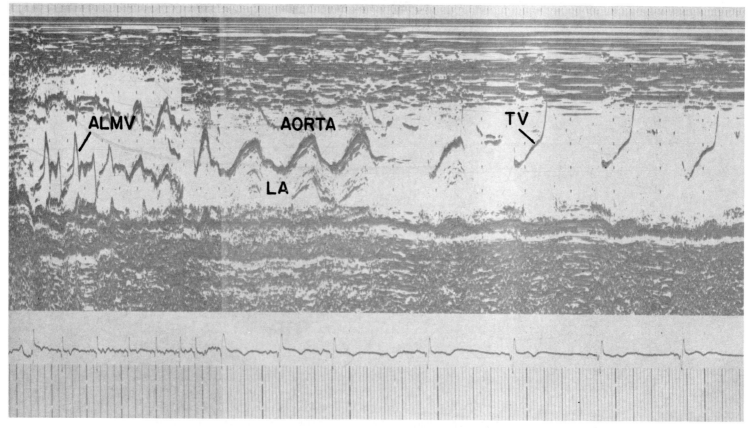

Fig. 26-10. As a sweep is made from the aortic root, medial and inferior, the tricuspid valve should appear at the level of the anterior aortic wall.

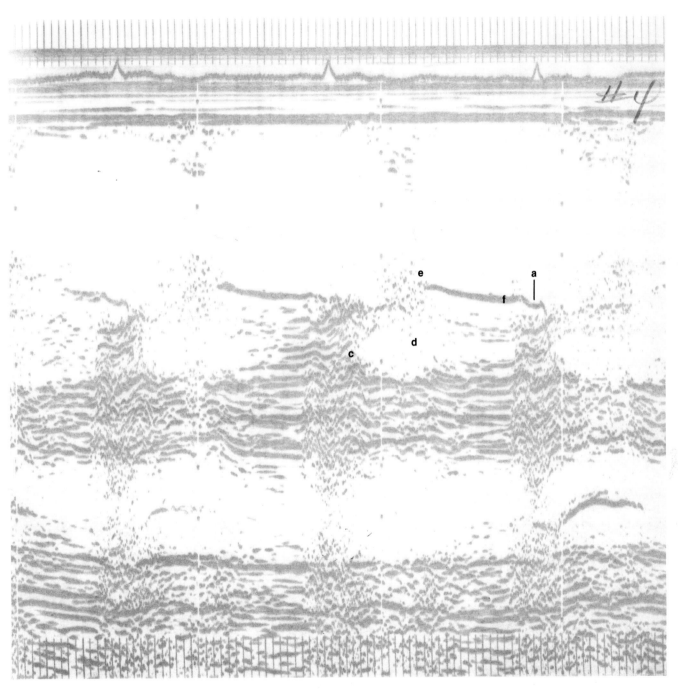

Fig. 26-11. The pulmonary valve is recorded as the beam sweeps laterally from the aortic valve toward the left shoulder.

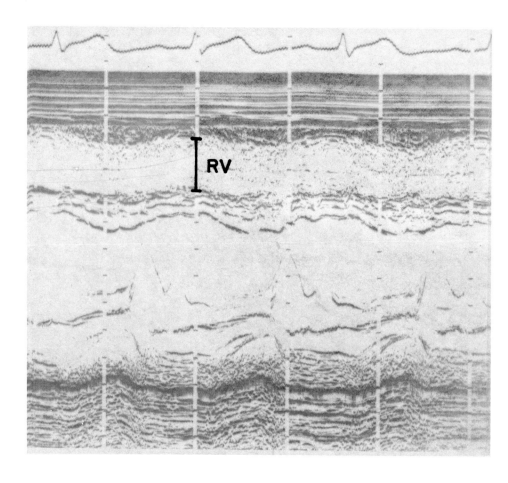

Fig. 26-12. If the right ventricular wall echo cannot be visualized, an estimate of 0.5 cm posterior to the last nonmoving chest wall echo as the location of the right ventricular wall can be made. The right ventricle will appear slightly enlarged as the patient assumes the semidecubitus position because of the tangential angulation of the transducer. Generally, it does not exceed 2.6 cm in either direction in normal subjects.

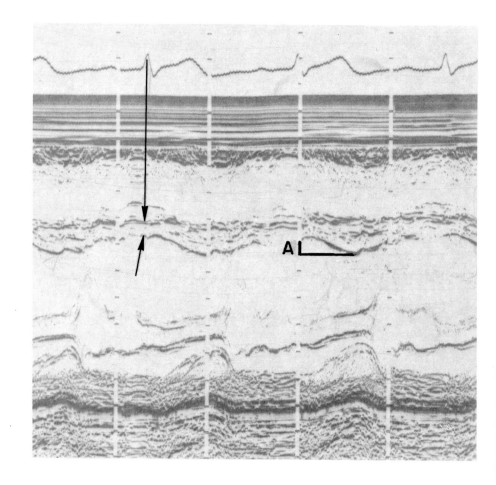

Fig. 26-13. The interventricular septum is identified as two parallel echoes recorded from the right and left sides of the septum. The membranous portion of the septum is continuous with the anterior wall of the aorta. Therefore the basal portion moves anteriorly in systole and posteriorly in diastole. This is paradoxical motion because the septum moves like the left ventricle (which is normal in the basal portion of the septum). The septal motion and measurements are made not at the basal portion but from the muscular septum, which is much thicker than the membranous septum and moves anteriorly in diastole and posteriorly in systole. See text for discussion of septal wall thickness, amplitude, and motion.

RIGHT VENTRICLE

Dimension. This measurement should be made when the right side of the septum and the endocardium of the right ventricular anterior wall are clearly seen (and in the usual plane passing through the left ventricle at the chordal or the mitral valve level depending on the age of the patient).[3] It should also be measured at the onset of the QRS, end diastole (nl supine 7 to 23, decubitus 9 to 26 mm) (Fig. 26-12).

INTERVENTRICULAR SEPTUM

Wall thickness. This is a measurement of the vertical distance from the right to the left ventricular wall at the onset of the QRS. It should be made from leading edge to leading edge. Abnormal thickening may be seen in IHSS or concentric hypertrophy (nl 6 to 11 mm) (Fig. 26-13).

Wall amplitude. This is a measurement of the posterior motion of the left ventricular side of the septum. It is obtained by drawing a horizontal line between the most posterior point of the septum during systole and then measuring the maximal vertical distance from this line to the septum just before the septum moves posteriorly in systole (nl 5 to 12 mm) (Fig. 26-13).

Wall motion. Normally the septum moves posteriorly after the onset of systole (as the posterior wall moves anteriorly). Following is a breakdown of common septal abnormalities:

1. Exaggerated septal motion may indicate hyperdynamic contractility—as seen in aortic or mitral insufficiency, ventricular septal defect, patent ductus arteriosus, increased cardiac output, or coronary artery disease—and implies left ventricular volume overload.
2. Paradoxical septal motion (the septum and posterior wall move anteriorly after the onset of systole) may be caused by left bundle branch block, ventricular aneurysm, atrial septal defect, or pulmonary or tricuspid insufficiency. It is indicative of right ventricular volume overload.
3. Flattened septal motion is suggested when the left side of the septum moves poorly or not at all in systole. This indicates possible left anterior descending coronary artery disease, or it may be due to technical problems connected with patient positioning.

LEFT VENTRICLE

NOTE: Measurements should be made on a tracing that was recorded just inferior to the tips of the mitral leaflets and that includes portions of the chordae. The interventricular septum and three layers of the posterior wall of the left ventricle should be distinct and continuous throughout the cardiac cycle. The technique should involve a sweep with a decrease in gain to visualize the pericardium as separate from the heart wall.

End diastolic dimension. This is a measurement of the maximal left ventricular size in diastole. The vertical distance is measured from the left side of the septum to the endocardial surface of the posterior heart wall at the QRS (end diastole) (nl supine 3.7 to 5.6, lateral 3.5 to 5.7 cm) (Fig. 26-14).

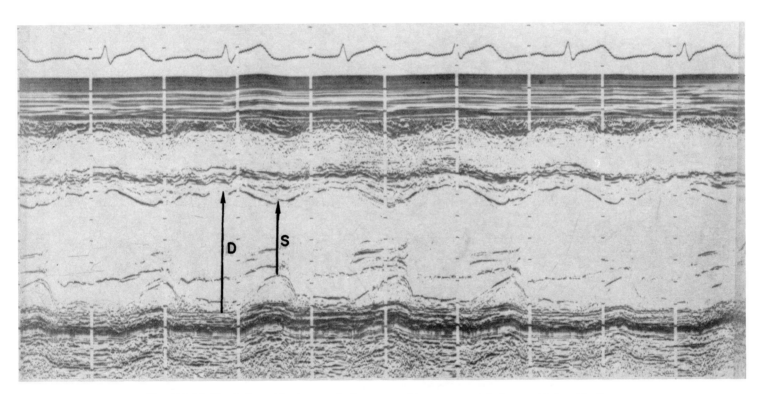

Fig. 26-14. The left ventricular cavity is assessed in a sweep inferior and lateral to the anterior leaflet of the mitral valve. It is important to identify the dense chordae from the endocardial surface of the posterior heart wall for measurement purposes. There seems to be a small twisting motion of the heart at the end of systole and at the onset of diastole. The two heart walls apparently move anteriorly together for a few milliseconds as a result of this twisting motion. The systolic measurement is essentially the same, whether taken at the downward peak of septal motion or the upward peak of posterior endocardial. The only precaution is that this measurement be taken perpendicular. A diagonal connection between the downward peak and the upward peak would result in measurement error.[3]

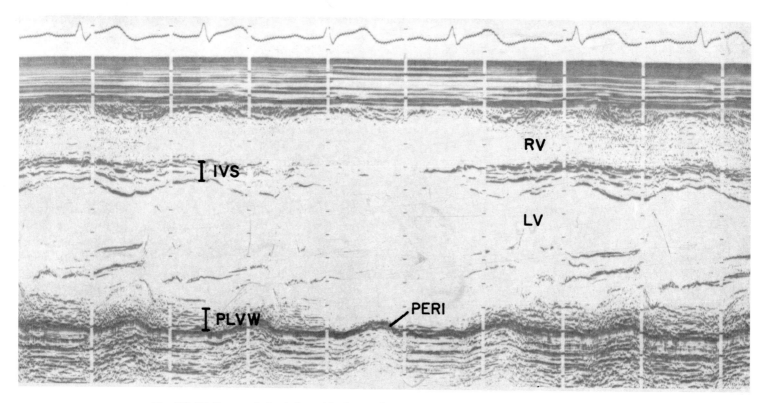

Fig. 26-15. The posterior left ventricular wall should be considered with the septal thickness in evaluations for hypertrophy or thinning of these structures.

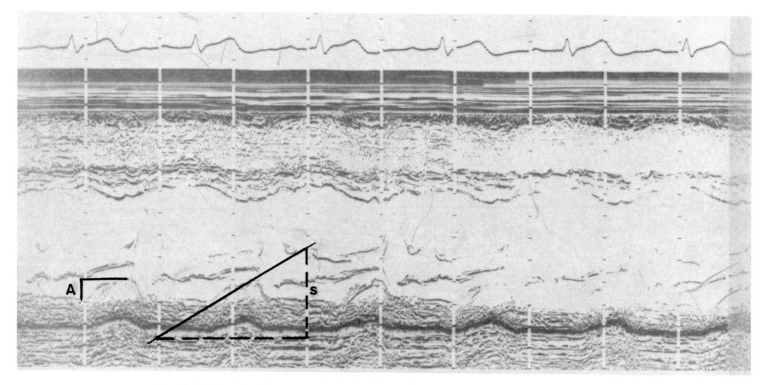

Fig. 26-16. See text for a discussion of posterior left ventricular amplitude and endocardial velocity.

End systolic dimension. This is a measurement of the minimal left ventricular size in systole. The vertical distance is measured from the endocardium to the left side of the septum. The dimension should be measured at the nadir of septal motion in patients whose septal motion is normal. In patients whose septal motion is abnormal or paradoxical, the measurement should be made at the peak of the posterior wall motion (nl 2.2 to 4 cm) (Fig. 26-14).

Wall thickness. This is a measurement of the vertical distance from the epicardium of the posterior wall to the endocardium in end diastole at a point just prior to the presystolic "thinning" of the posterior wall (onset of the QRS) (nl 6 to 11 mm) (Fig. 26-15).

Wall amplitude. This is a measurement of the anterior motion of the posterior wall during systole. It is made by first drawing a horizontal line between the most anterior points of the endocardium in systole and then measuring the maximal vertical distance from this line to the endocardium of the posterior wall at a point just before the free wall begins to move anteriorly in systole (Fig. 26-16).

A reduced wall amplitude may indicate myopathy, coronary artery disease, congestive failure, low cardiac output, or technical problems. Exaggerated wall motion may indicate left ventricular volume overload or coronary artery disease (nl 5 to 14 mm).

Endocardial velocity. This is a measurement of the velocity at which the endocardium of the posterior wall moves. It is made by extending a line from the endocardium in systole to the endocardium in diastole. The slope of this line is measured in millimeters per second (nl 20 to 35 mm/sec) (Fig. 25-16).

IVS/PWLV ratio. This is a ratio of the septal thickness in diastole to the posterior wall thickness in diastole (nl 0.87 to 1.2).

Stroke volume. This is an estimated measurement of the amount of blood ejected from the left ventricle per cardiac cycle. It may be obtained from this formula:

$$SV = EDD^3 - ESD^3$$

Cardiac output. This is an estimated measurement of the amount of blood ejected from the left ventricle per minute in liters.

$$CO = (HR \times SV)/1000$$

HR is heart rate.

Ejection fraction. This is an estimated measurement of the percentage of blood filling the left ventricle in diastole that is ejected in systole.

$$EF = \frac{EDD^3 - ESD^3}{EDD^3} \times 100$$

Left ventricular mass. The mass is a measurement of the weight of the left ventricle and may be determined by

$$LV\ mass = (EDD + IVS\ thickness + PW\ thickness)^3 - EDD^3$$

NOTE: These measurements are made in diastole and are invalid when asymmetric hypertrophy is present.

REFERENCES

1. Clark, R.D.: Case studies in echocardiography, Philadelphia, 1977, W.B. Saunders Co.
2. Feigenbaum, H.: Echocardiography, Philadelphia, 1976, Lea & Febiger.
3. Sahn, D.J., DeMaria, A., Kisslo, J., and Weyman, A.: Recommendations regarding quantitation in M-mode echocardiography: results of a survey of echocardiographic measurements, Circulation **58:**1072, 1978.
4. Williams, R.G., and Tucker, C.R.: Echocardiographic diagnosis of congenital heart disease, Boston, 1977, Little, Brown & Co.

27 Acquired valvular heart disease

Rheumatic fever is probably the primary cause of valvular (valvar) stenosis and regurgitation problems in the heart. It follows an infection caused by group A hemolytic streptococcal bacteria and is actually secondary to the infection. The patient with rheumatic fever becomes hypersensitive to antibodies made by his own system. A continuing reaction develops in all tissues between the streptococcus organism, its poisons, and the antibodies. This constitutes the beginning of rheumatic fever. The interaction between antigens and antibodies keeps the inflammation of rheumatic fever going in many tissues of the body. The inflammation is found in the joints, tissues, brain and heart and under the skin. Masses of these inflamed areas form and heal, but the most dangerous characteristic of the disease is its tendency to leave scar tissue as it heals. Whereas 1 out of 100 individuals will contract rheumatic fever, in only about half of these patients will heart disease develop.

The mitral valve is attacked by the disease in 65% of the patients, the aortic valve in 30%, and the tricuspid and pulmonary valves in less than 5%. During the course of the disease small granules develop on the surface of the affected valve. Healing may be complete, or progressive scarring may develop over time due to the subacute or chronic inflammation.

A pericardial effusion may be detected in the acute phase of the disease; however, echocardiography is not yet sensitive enough to detect the small granular infections on the valve in the early stages. As the scar tissue increases and causes a permanent heart valve deformity, echocardiography may assess the thickness and pliability of the affected valve. Echo may also be sensitive in the detection of thrombus secondary to the rheumatic infection.

Rheumatic fever may cause three forms of carditis: endocarditis, myocarditis, and pericarditis. *Endocarditis* is an acute inflammation that affects the valves and the inner lining of the heart (endocardium). It may involve all the valves or primarily the left-side valves. Small vegetations develop on the affected leaflets, and damage results from the healing of inflamed areas leaving scar tissue and destroying the valve tissue. *Myocarditis* causes the muscles to become weak and balloon outward. Myocardial failure results. *Pericarditis* represents the severest form of the disease, in which large pericardial effusions of serum and fibrin are found in the pericardial space.

The clinical history of a patient who has rheumatic fever may include a streptococcal throat infection with fever, joint tenderness and pain, carditis, chorea (uncontrollable twitching of arms, legs, and face), a skin rash, or subcutaneous nodules.

MITRAL STENOSIS

Obstruction at the mitral valve orifice can be acquired, congenital, or caused by interposition of a tumor mass. This discussion will concentrate on the acquired obstruction of the leaflet secondary to rheumatic fever.

The presence of rheumatic fever may cause several changes to occur on the valve leaflets. These changes will progress with scarring and calcification. The leaflets may be diffusely thickened by fibrous tissue or calcium deposits, or the commissures may be fused. The chordae tendineae may be shortened and fused together. Sometimes the chordae are so retracted that the leaflets appear to insert directly into the posterior papillary muscle. When this occurs, the stenosis is always severe because the interchordal spaces are obliterated. In other cases the chordae inserting into one papillary muscle may be well preserved whereas those inserting into the opposite muscle will be completely fused.

In a normal heart the cross-sectional area of the mitral valve orifice is about 5 sq cm. When stenosis is present in the orifice, this measurement is decreased (Fig. 27-1). Obstruction to the flow of blood from the left atrium into the left ventricle will cause an increase in the left atrial pressure that extends backward into the pulmonary veins, from there into the pulmonary capillaries, and from there into the pulmonary arteries. The resultant condition is pulmonary hypertension, which in turn will lead to pulmonary hypertrophy.

A valve area of 2.5 sq cm represents mild stenosis, whereas an area of 1 sq cm represents moderately severe stenosis.

The amount of calcium in the heart varies considerably with age and sex of the patient. There is apparently more in men than in women, and in older patients than in younger ones.

Echographically the most consistent finding in mitral stenosis is reduction of the E-F slope of the anterior leaflet of the valve; that is, the velocity of the E-F slope measures less than 35 mm/sec (Fig. 27-2). Since the E-F slope is an indicator of the rate of left atrial emptying, in mitral stenosis the decreased slope signifies an obstruction caused by the stenosed orifice.

In addition to the decreased E-F slope, the posterior leaflet moves in the same direction as the anterior leaflet because of commissural fusion (Fig. 27-3). In very mild cases of mitral stenosis with little thickening or calcification, the posterior leaflet may move in its normal posterior position.

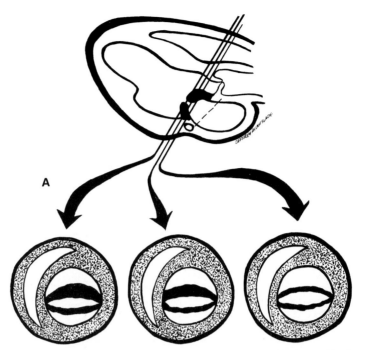

High gain, tip of leaflet   Medium gain, midleaflet   Low gain, base of leaflet

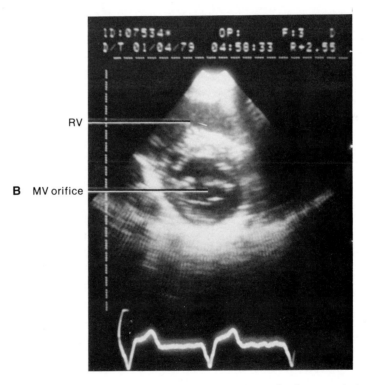

Fig. 27-1. A, Schematic of the long axis and subsequent short axis *(arrows)* of the heart. To obtain a mitral valve area, the mitral orifice should be evaluated at the tips of the leaflets with low-gain settings. **B,** Short axis view of the mitral orifice.

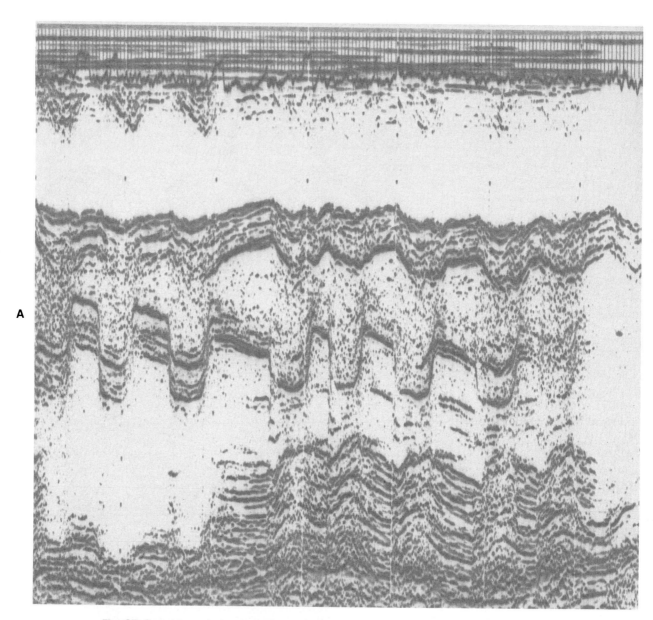

A

Fig. 27-2. A, M-mode tracing of a patient with mitral stenosis. The slope is drawn through the E-F points to assess the velocity of the leaflet in diastole. **B,** The sensitivity should be reduced for assessment of the degree of thickening and calcification present on the leaflet and for more accurate measurements.

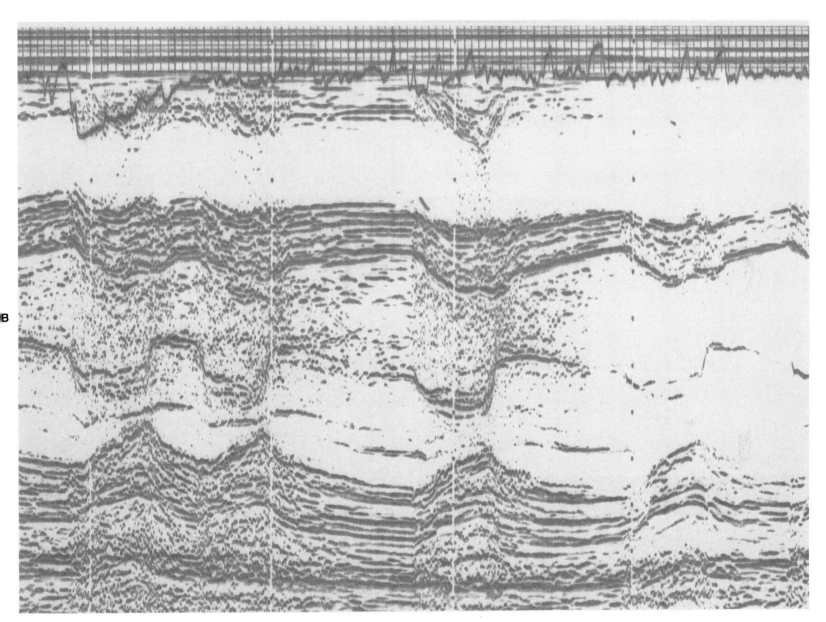

Fig. 27-2, cont'd. For legend see opposite page.

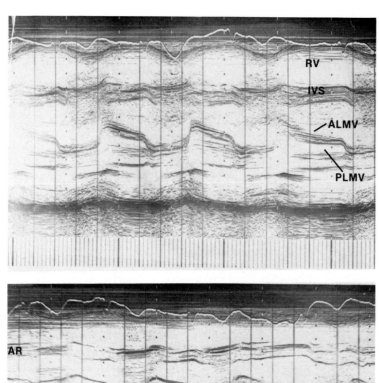

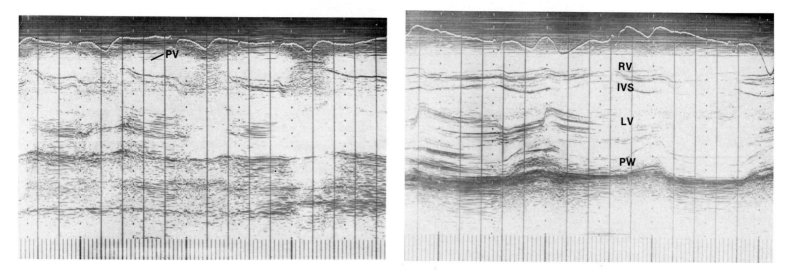

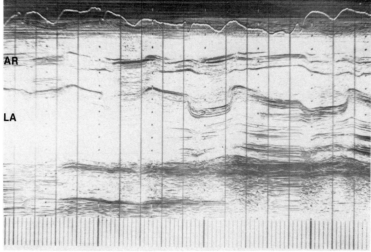

Fig. 27-3. M-mode of a 68-year-old woman with a history of rheumatic heart disease. Evidence of mitral stenosis and regurgitation, with enlarged left atrial and left ventricular chambers. The pulmonary valve shows signs of hypertension.

The amplitude, or C-E excursion, of the valve measures the degree of mobility or restriction of the leaflet (Fig. 27-4). In a heavily calcified valve this amplitude is reduced. To assess the maximum mobility of the valve, the examiner must angle the transducer carefully. When the leaflet is demonstrated, a search is made for its greatest excursion by slight additional angulations of the transducer or by moving the beam up or down an interspace.

Increased echoes on the mitral apparatus indicate thickening or the presence of calcification. The gain settings must be carefully adjusted so calcification can be distinguished from reverberation. When the posterior leaflet is well shown, the sensitivity should be gradually reduced to assess the degree of calcification from the remaining echoes (Fig. 27-5).

In approximately 50% of patients with mitral stenosis, atrial fibrillation develops (Figs. 27-6 and 27-7). This complication is usually serious because there is a loss of atrial contraction. (An atrial contraction may contribute 15% to 20% of left ventricular filling.) The sudden occurrence of this ar-

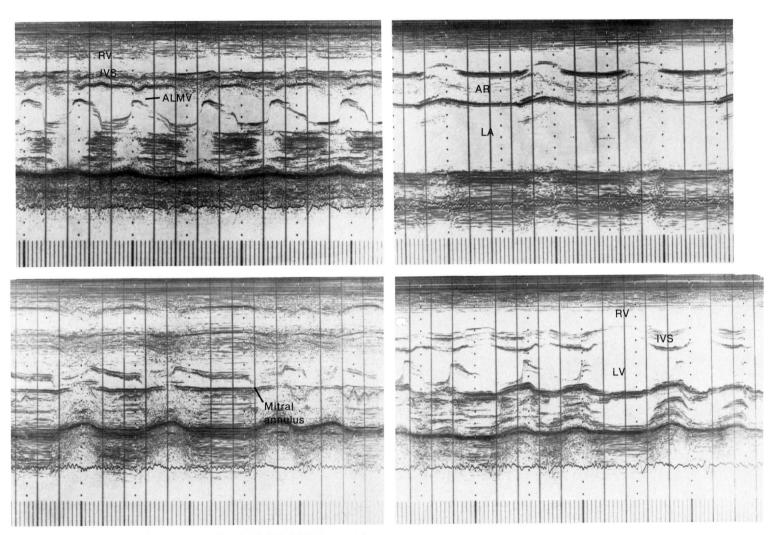

Fig. 27-4. A 49-year-old patient with a history of rheumatic heart disease. She was asymptomatic until a year ago, when she experienced a sudden onset of palpitations, dyspnea, dizziness, and syncope. The echo showed enlarged left ventricular and atrial cavities, calcified mitral anulus, a decreased E-F slope of the mitral valve, and flutter of the posterior leaflet of the mitral valve. Subsequent cardiac catheterization and surgery revealed combined mitral disease and a main chordal rupture with calcific changes in the leaflets and anulus.

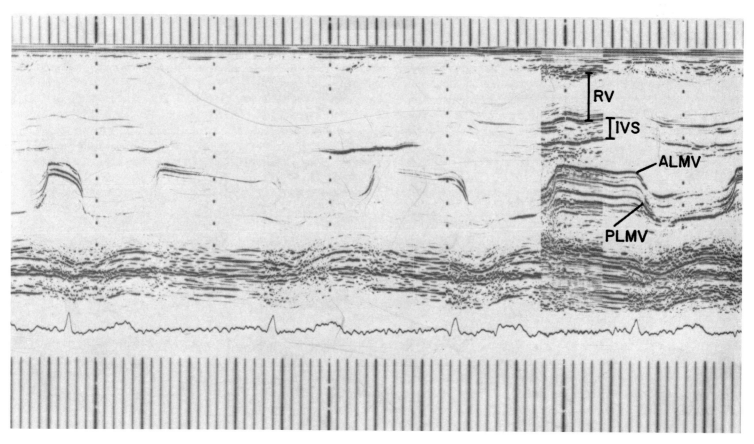

Fig. 27-5. Increased and decreased sensitivities are important in assessing the degree of calcification thickening that a rheumatic valve may have.

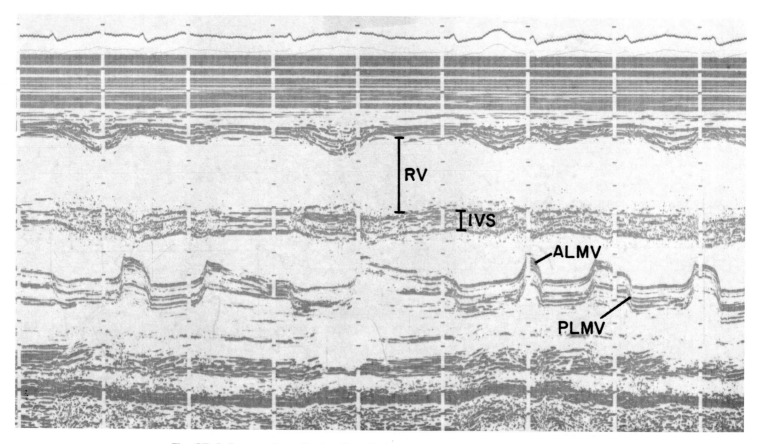

Fig. 27-6. Frequently patients with mitral stenosis will display atrial fibrillation.

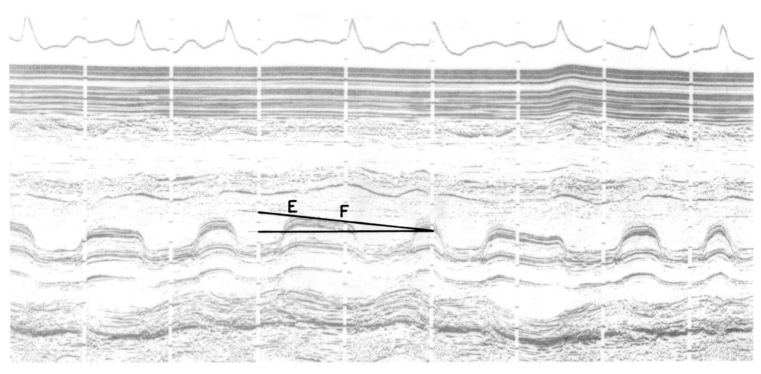

Fig. 27-7. Severe mitral stenosis with calcification. Atrial fibrillation is present, so several mitral complexes should be measured before the E-F slope is determined.

rhythmia, with a rapid ventricular rate response, is often accompanied by pulmonary edema.

Systemic emboli are quite common in patients with mitral stenosis due to the relative stasis and diminished flow from the left atrium to the left ventricle and the inflammatory reaction within the left atrial wall. The stasis and inflammation cause thrombi to form; and when these are dislodged and travel into the systemic circulation, they become emboli.

Real time evaluation. In a study by Kisslo, it was found that patients with E-F slopes of less than 10 mm/sec by M-mode criteria would be considered to have severe mitral stenosis. However, when these patients were evaluated by the short axis real time technique, only two thirds could be expected to have severe mitral stenosis by the criteria of a mitral valve area measuring less than 1.3 sq cm (Fig. 27-8). Kisslo found that for slopes higher than 10 mm/sec the M-mode could not predict the severity of the lesion with any certainty (Fig. 27-9).

Evaluation of the mitral orifice (leaflet pliability, thickening, and restriction of mo-

tion) should be made in two planes, the short and the long axis. The orifice is assessed in the short axis plane first and a planimeter measurement is taken at its narrowest point, near the leaflet tips in diastole (Fig. 27-10). The gain settings are then reduced to eliminate reverberations produced by the fibrosis and thickening. Often the mitral orifice will be found to have an irregular configuration, so care must be taken to record the accurate orifice opening.

Assessment of other cardiac chambers may also help in determining the degree of stenosis or rheumatic involvement. In pure mitral stenosis the left ventricle is of normal size. When mitral insufficiency is coexistent, the left ventricle may enlarge and become hypercontractile with the excess volume load. The left atrium always enlarges in mitral valve disease; however, with combined mitral stenosis and regurgitation it becomes huge, measuring 6 cm or more (Fig. 27-11).

Other factors that can reduce the E-F slope of the mitral valve also may mimic mitral stenosis. Usually this is seen when left ventricular filling is impaired, as with severe LV hypertrophy, aortic stenosis, or pul-

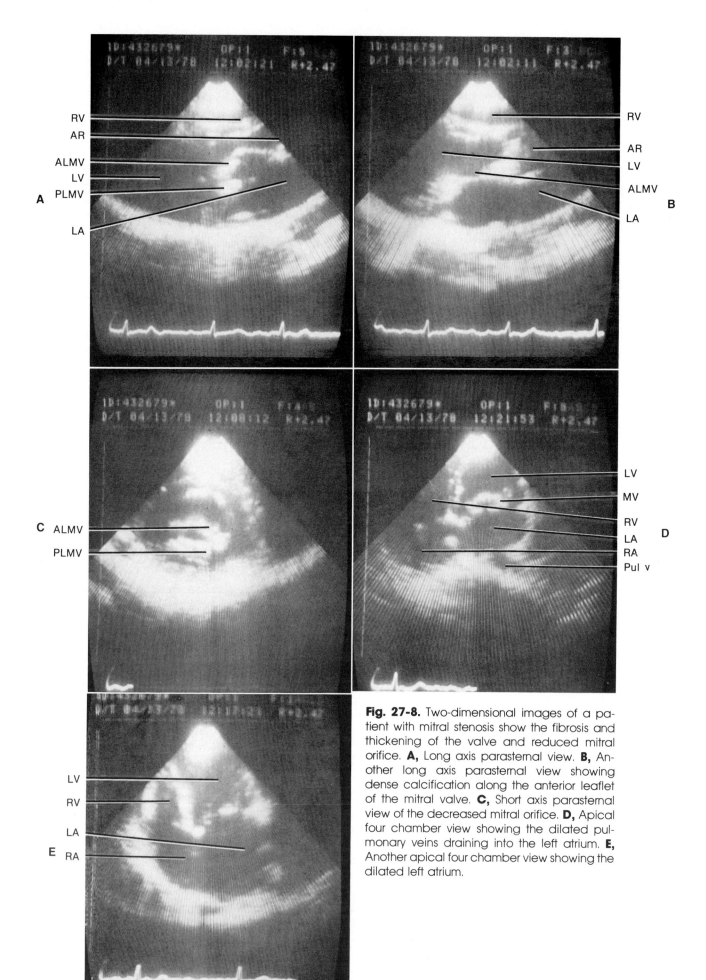

RV
AR
ALMV
LV
PLMV
LA

A

RV
AR
LV
ALMV
LA

B

C ALMV
PLMV

LV
MV
RV
LA
RA
Pul v

D

LV
RV
LA
E RA

Fig. 27-8. Two-dimensional images of a patient with mitral stenosis show the fibrosis and thickening of the valve and reduced mitral orifice. **A,** Long axis parasternal view. **B,** Another long axis parasternal view showing dense calcification along the anterior leaflet of the mitral valve. **C,** Short axis parasternal view of the decreased mitral orifice. **D,** Apical four chamber view showing the dilated pulmonary veins draining into the left atrium. **E,** Another apical four chamber view showing the dilated left atrium.

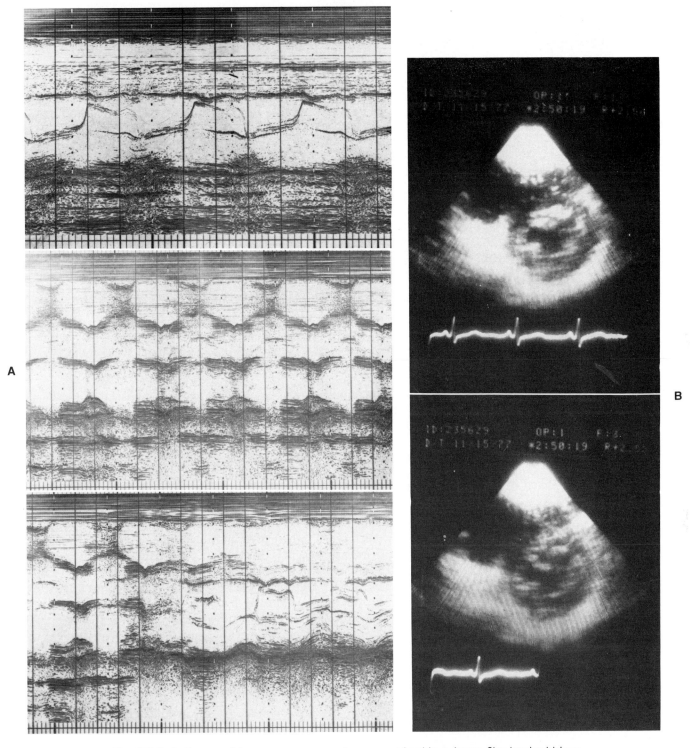

Fig. 27-9. A 41-year-old woman was seen because of ankle edema. She had a history of a pulmonary embolism. Cardiac catheterization showed mild mitral stenosis. The echocardiogram revealed no evidence of left-sided chamber enlargement. **A,** Both leaflets of the mitral apparatus appeared to move normally and were not thickened. The E-F slope and C-E amplitude were decreased. **B,** Two-dimensional short axis parasternal view of the mitral apparatus showing an adequate orifice.

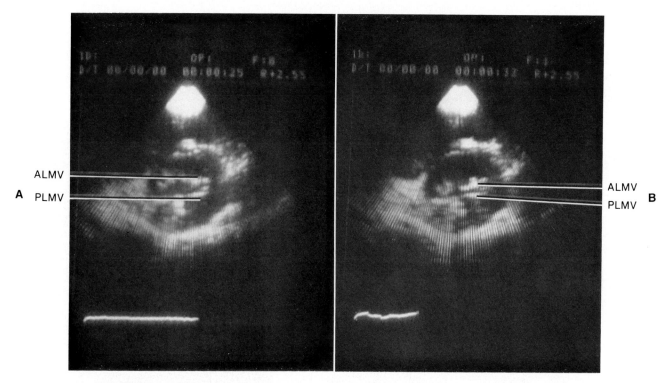

Fig. 27-10. Short axis parasternal views of the mitral apparatus in a middle-aged woman with mitral stenosis and regurgitation. **A,** The leaflets are open in diastole. Some thickening is evident. **B,** In systole the leaflets fail to close, permitting regurgitant flow into the left atrium.

monary hypertension. In these patients there is good amplitude of the valve and no thickening or calcification is present.

Calcification of the mitral anulus can make it difficult to assess the posterior movement of the valve, and one should assess the leaflet both in M-mode and two-dimensionally to separate the posterior leaflet from the calcified anulus (annulus) (Figs. 27-12 to 27-14).

Mitral stenosis is a slowly progressive lesion characterized by narrowing of the orifice so that left atrial pressure rises to maintain adequate filling of the left ventricle.[1] This raised pressure increases the work done by the atrium, which causes hypertrophy and dilation of that chamber. Left atrial hypertension results in pulmonary hypertension, with consequential right ventricular hypertrophy and dilation. The large left atrium is more prone to atrial fibrillation and causes enough stasis in the cavity for thrombi to occur, which may dislodge and travel through the circulation to form systemic emboli.

Decreased mitral valve slope without mitral stenosis. Decreased contractility of the left ventricle can cause a *pseudo* – mitral stenosis, which demonstrates a decreased amplitude and reduced E-F slope of the anterior leaflet of the valve. In such patients the E-F slope usually does not fall below the 35 mm/sec seen in patients with mitral stenosis. The posterior leaflet moves in its

normal posterior direction during diastole.

Aortic stenosis may also cause a reduced mitral slope and amplitude due to the increased pressures within the left ventricle. Further calcification of the mitral anulus may make it difficult to visualize the posterior leaflet, and careful angulation of the transducer should allow the cardiac sonographer to separate the posterior leaflet from the calcification of other structures.

Hypertrophic cardiomyopathy may cause the anterior leaflet to be decreased in diastole. In addition, a systolic anterior motion of the mitral apparatus is seen in the obstructive forms of hypertrophic cardiomyopathy. The posterior leaflet would be unaffected in these patients. There may be some left atrial enlargement secondary to mitral regurgitation.

A left atrial myxoma or other such tumor is another form of obstruction to left atrial flow. The tumor may be small or may completely obstruct the left atrial outflow tract. In patients with a myxoma the tumor is attached to the atrial wall by a pedicle and prolapses into the ventricular chamber after the onset of diastole. It can be distinguished from a severely calcified valve by the early diastolic space that occurs after the onset of diastole before the tumor flops posterior to the mitral apparatus. A heavily calcified valve would show increased echoes throughout the diastolic cycle.

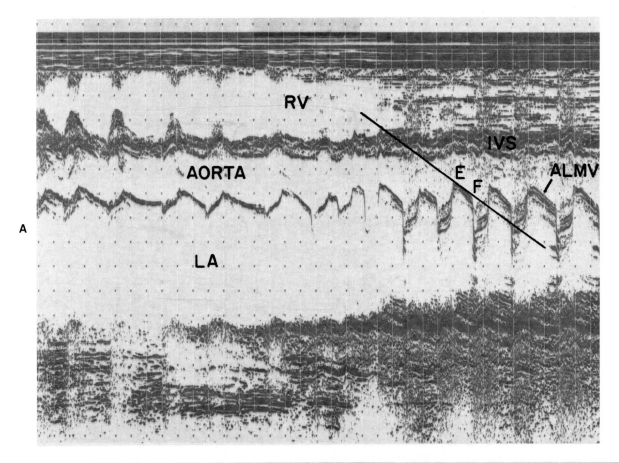

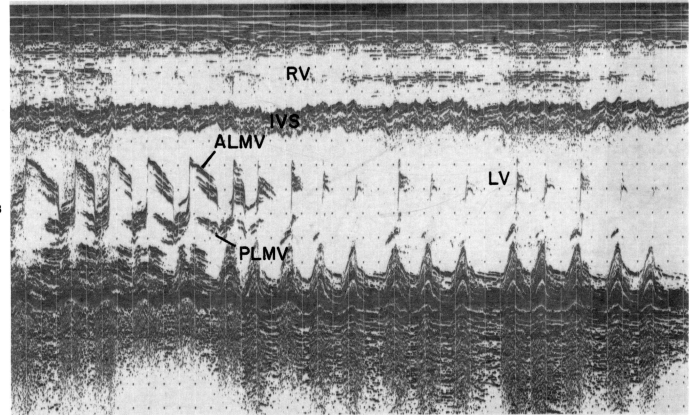

Fig. 27-11. A, Sweep from the aorta to the mitral valve demonstrating an enlarged left atrium, 6 cm, with mitral stenosis and regurgitation. **B,** Sweep into the left ventricle demonstrating an enlarged cavity, 6 cm, indicating that the disease process is chronic.

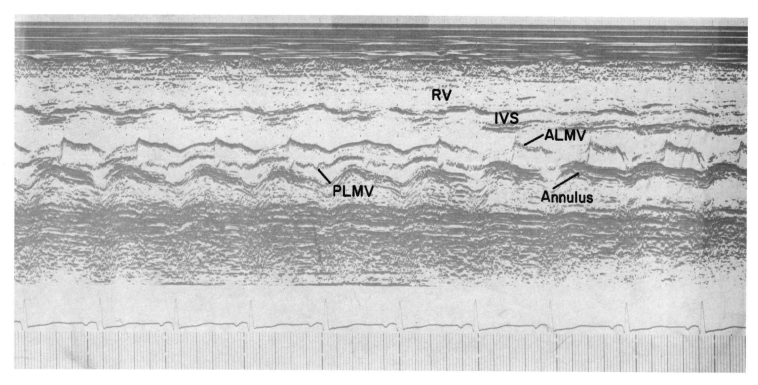

Fig. 27-12. Aortic stenosis and insufficiency can cause the E-F slope of the mitral valve to be reduced. Calcification of the mitral anulus is also shown. Fine flutter of the anterior leaflet is secondary to aortic insufficiency.

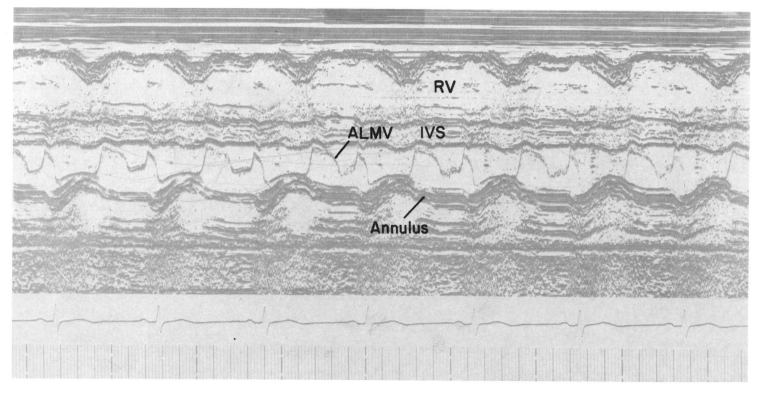

Fig. 27-13. Slightly decreased E-F slope of the anterior leaflet without mitral stenosis and calcification of the mitral anulus extending from the aortic wall calcification.

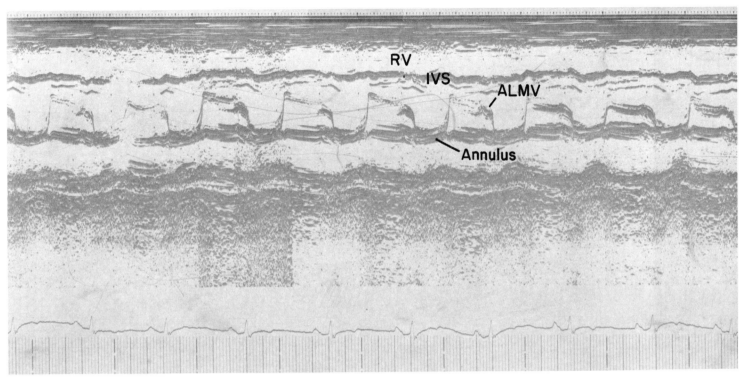

Fig. 27-14. Mild mitral stenosis with calcification of the mitral anulus. The posterior leaflet may be seen to blend anteriorly just above the anulus.

MITRAL REGURGITATION

The inability of the mitral leaflets to close completely or to appose precisely in systole can be due to a variety of lesions. The valve leaflets may be damaged by rheumatic fever, whose effects could cause regurgitation due to leaflet thickening, distortion, and calcification allowing insufficient tissue for opposition or shortening of the chordae tendineae (pulling the cusps into the ventricle). Other causes are a ruptured papillary muscle, mitral valve prolapse, or hypertrophic cardiomyopathy. These conditions may give rise to mitral valve dysfunction and cause regurgitation into the left atrial cavity. Further regurgitation may be due to infective endocarditis, congenital deformity of the valve, increased diameter of the anulus, or rupture of a chorda tendineae.

The magnitude of the leakage is determined by the area of the valve orifice that remains open during systole. The regurgitation of blood into the left atrial cavity causes an increased volume in the left atrium, with a rise in left atrial pressure. This, in turn, causes a stronger atrial contraction (Starling's law) and a longer period of flow. The in-

creased output of the left atrium increases the diastolic volume and pressure in the left ventricular cavity, which leads to dilation and hypertrophy.[1]

Due to the mitral regurgitation the compensation of the left atrium and the left ventricle is achieved by an increased work of both chambers. In an effort to maintain cardiac output, the ejection time of the left ventricle shortens and the peripheral vascular resistance decreases. Such changes enhance the forward flow of blood and diminish the regurgitant jet.

Distinction may be made between acute and chronic forms of mitral regurgitation. In *acute* forms, such as a ruptured chorda tendineae, a sudden rise in left atrial pressure is noted with resulting pulmonary edema. In *chronic* cases there is left ventricular failure with reduced cardiac output and an increased ventricular diastolic pressure. The left ventricular failure may cause right ventricular failure and systemic congestion in the patient.

Echographically patients with rheumatic mitral regurgitation (insufficiency) manifest findings similar to those of patients with mi-

tral stenosis—both have thickening of the leaflet. The left atrial cavity is enlarged (often measuring over 6 cm) (Fig. 27-15). The left ventricle is also enlarged and hypercontractile. Chronic cases will exhibit right ventricular hypertrophy with pulmonary hypertension. The valve should be assessed by both M-mode and two-dimensional techniques.

The C-E amplitude is increased and, due to its wide excursion, may reach the left side of the septum. The E-F slope is very rapid, usually measuring over 180 mm/sec (Fig. 27-16). Often, because of the extreme overload in the left atrial cavity, a fine flutter of the anterior leaflet is seen in the early closure of the diastolic slope (Fig. 27-17). The leaflets may demonstrate a systolic sagging into the left atrium, indicative of prolapse (Fig. 27-18).

The short axis view of the two-dimensional echo is useful in assessing the degree of opening in the systolic segment. In a study by Wann et al.,[2] it was found that large areas of nonclosure of the valve in systole were associated with significant regurgitation. In patients with insignificant regurgitation,

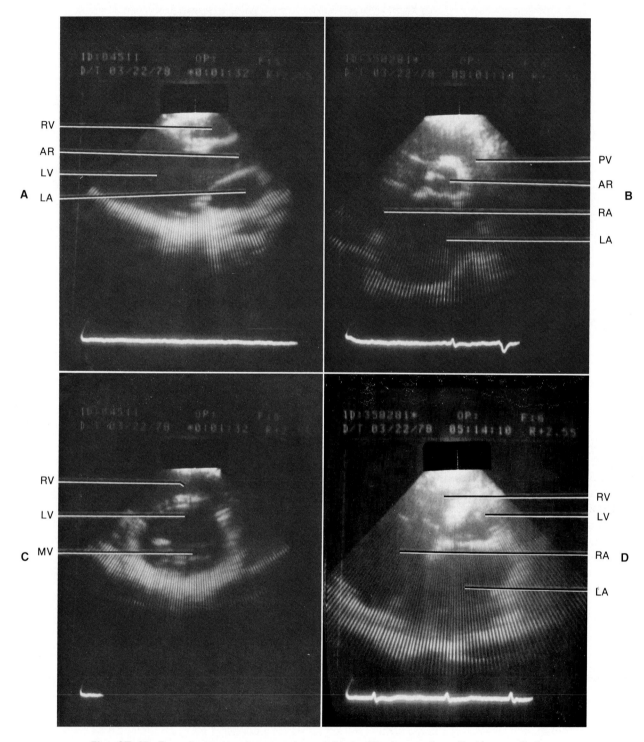

Fig. 27-15. Two-dimensional scan of a patient with rheumatic mitral regurgitation. **A,** Long axis view of the huge left ventricle. **B,** Short axis view of the huge left atrium. **C,** Short axis view of the mitral apparatus floating in the dilated left ventricular cavity. **D,** Apical four chamber view of the dilated atrial cavities.

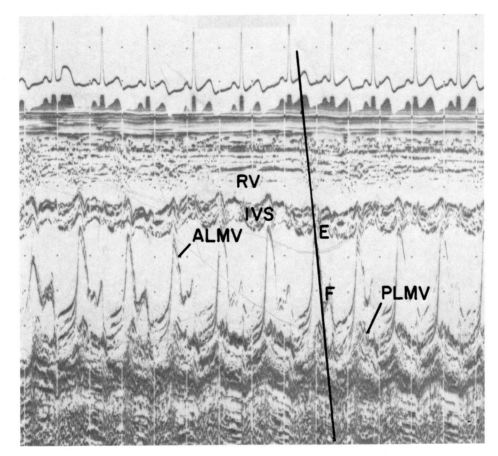

Fig. 27-16. Patient with mitral regurgitation. The E-F slope measures 180 mm/sec.

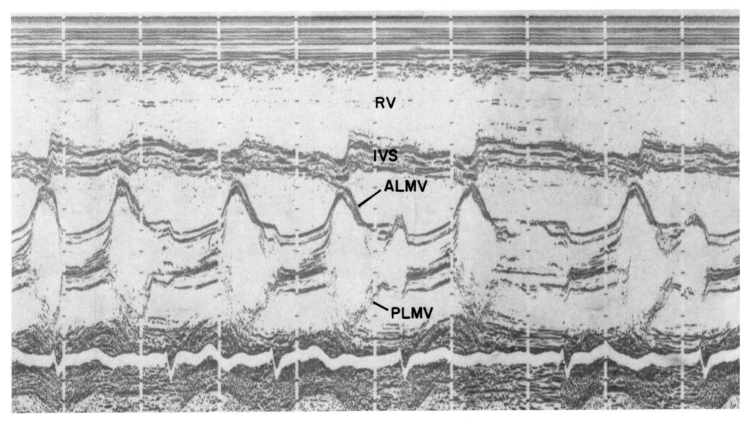

Fig. 27-17. Elderly man with a history of mitral regurgitation. The posterior leaflet moves with the same amplitude as the anterior leaflet. Flutter is shown on the diastolic segment of the posterior leaflet, indicating rupture of the chordae tendineae.

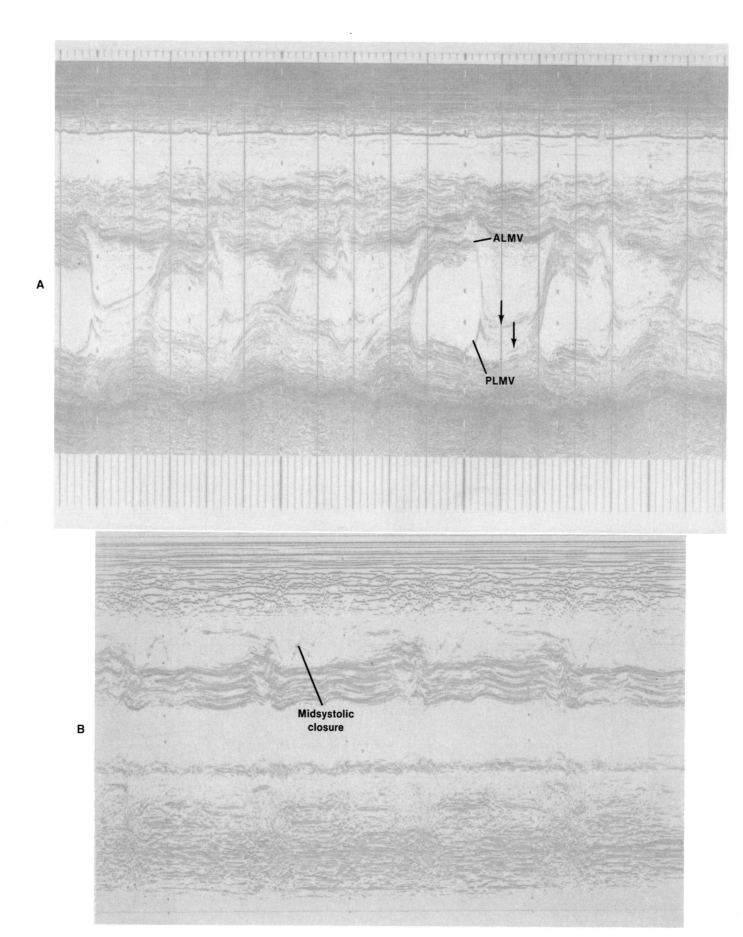

Fig. 27-18. M-mode strips of a patient with severe mitral regurgitation and pulmonary hypertension. **A,** The mitral valve appears thickened, with systolic prolapse. The posterior leaflet moves erratically throughout diastole and represents a ruptured chord. **B,** Midsystolic closure of the pulmonary cusp (flying W sign).

small areas of nonclosure were present at either the medial or the lateral aspect of the valve.

The technique utilized to identify areas of nonclosure involved scanning the leaflet in both long and short axes. The limiting diastolic orifice could be identified as the beam moved superior and inferior. Subsequent stop frames were selected in early systole so the mitral valve closure could be analyzed before caudal movement of the entire valve carried it out of view.

AORTIC STENOSIS

Aortic stenosis will be considered in relation to three entities: isolated stenosis, acquired stenosis, and congenital lesions of the aorta (discussed in Chapter 34).

Isolated aortic stenosis. The most common cause of fatal valvular dysfunction in patients past late adolescence is isolated valvular aortic stenosis. This is nearly always of nonrheumatic origin and commonly represents a congenital malformation. The mitral apparatus is normal in most patients with this condition. In patients under 15 years the aortic valve is either unicuspid or bicuspid. In older patients it is congenitally malformed in 60%.

Acquired aortic stenosis. This is the result of calcification and fibrosis and is generally of two types: that involving a congenitally malformed but initially normally functioning valve and that involving a previously normal valve.

Congenitally malformed valve. Congenital malformations are determined by the number of commissures and cusps. A commissure is the junction between adjacent cusps. Commissures help the cusps to close completely so that no blood can leak through.

There are two types of unicuspid aortic valves. In one the cusp is devoid of lateral attachments to the wall of the aorta, with a centrally located orifice and usually an underlying pulmonary stenosis. In the other the valve orifice is eccentrically located, with one lateral attachment to the aortic wall. (This is often a fatal stenosis found in children under 1 year of age.)

The most frequent malformation of the aortic valve is the presence of only two cusps, or a bicuspid valve. There are two types of bicuspid valves. In the *first* the cusps are located to the right and left with the commissures anterior and posterior. If a raphe or false commissure is present, it always is in the right cusp. A coronary artery arises from behind each cusp. In the *second* type the cusps are located anterior and posterior and the commissures are to the right and left. If a raphe is present, it is always in the anterior cusp and both coronary arteries arise in front of the anterior cusp. Aortic stenosis is the most common complication of this congenital malformation.

Occasionally a tricuspid aortic valve is malformed in such a way that the cusps are of unequal size. The contact of such unequal-sized cusps may lead to focal fibrosis with eventual calcification and stenosis.

Previously normal valve. Acquired aortic stenosis in a normal aortic valve is commonly associated with rheumatic fever. In the normal adult the aortic valve orifice measures 2.5 to 3.5 sq cm. As the valve narrows, the left ventricular pressure becomes higher than the aortic pressure to maintain adequate cardiac output. This increased pressure causes left ventricular hypertrophy. The left ventricle is less distensible than normal, with a resulting higher end diastolic pressure, which causes a higher left atrial pressure because the left atrium must maintain an end systolic pressure as high as the left ventricular end diastolic pressure.[1] Thus left atrial hypertrophy results.

The aortic obstruction is due to calcium deposits, which prevent the cusps from retracting adequately during ventricular systole. The cause of this acquired stenosis in elderly persons has not been ascertained. The wear and tear on the aortic valve probably induce the formation of calcium deposits. Furthermore, it is not uncommon for calcification in the aortic wall to extend into the mitral anulus.

Echographically it is possible to assess calcification and thickness of the aortic wall and cusps (Fig. 27-19). As the aortic root is demonstrated on the M-mode sweep, its motion can be observed swinging forward or anteriorly in systole and moving posteriorly in diastole. A lack of motion indicates the presence of arteriosclerotic heart disease and calcification (Fig. 27-20). The fine echoes from the anterior and posterior aortic walls should have intensities equal to or less than those from the left atrial wall. As the gain is decreased, these wall echoes disappear. In patients with calcification the echoes are very dense and do not disappear as readily when the gain is reduced (Fig. 27-21). As the transducer beam sweeps from the calcified aortic root to the area of the mitral valve, calcification of the mitral anulus will be noted as a thick continuous echo arising from the posterior aortic wall and extending throughout the mitral apparatus.

Normally the anterior and posterior cusps are thin fluttering echoes within the aortic root. With thickening and fibrosis these echoes increase their intensity and lose their characteristic flutter. The wide systolic opening of the cusps diminishes with the degree of calcification (Fig. 27-22). If the valve is severely calcified, the systolic component of the aortic cusp will be difficult to separate from the diastolic since there are so many increased echoes within the aortic root (Fig. 27-23). *Text continued on p. 458.*

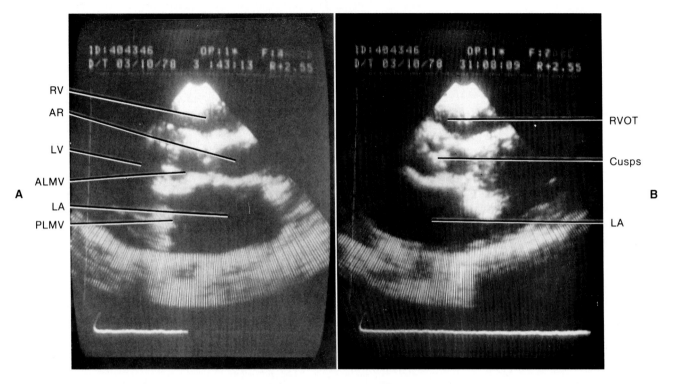

RV
AR
LV
ALMV
LA
PLMV

A

B

RVOT
Cusps
LA

Fig. 27-19. A, Two-dimensional long axis view of a patient with rheumatic heart disease. Calcification on the aortic root and mitral apparatus. **B,** Short axis view of the calcified aortic cusps.

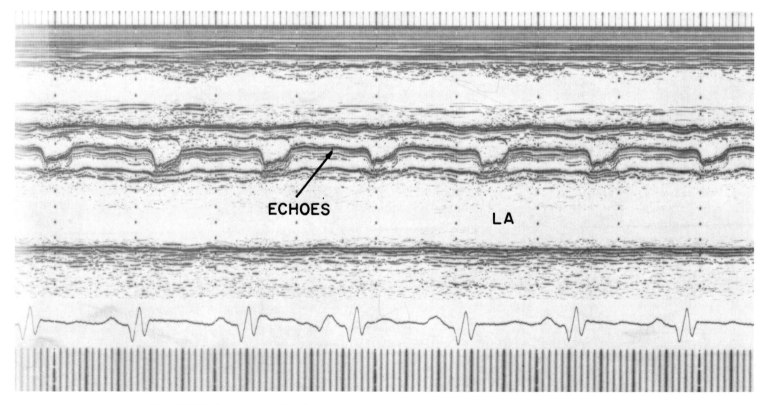

ECHOES

LA

Fig. 27-20. Arteriosclerotic disease and calcification result in decreased motion of the aortic root.

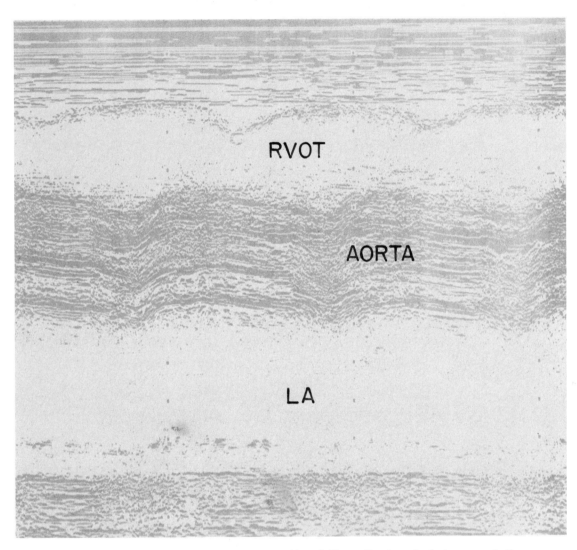

Fig. 27-21. M-mode tracing of a patient with calcific aortic stenosis. A decrease in the gain controls will clean up the aortic echoes so correct measurements can be obtained. The left atrial wall should be maintained in the scan as the gain is reduced on the aortic root.

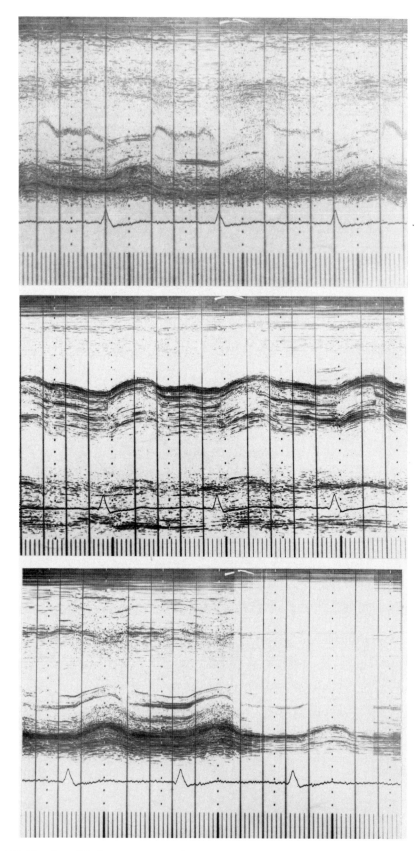

Fig. 27-22. An elderly man presented with increasing dyspnea, orthopnea, and ankle edema. He had rheumatoid arthritis and recurrent congestive heart failure from the cardiomyopathy. The echocardiogram demonstrated flutter on the mitral valve (secondary to aortic insufficiency), calcifications in the aortic root, decreased aortic cusp opening, and a slightly enlarged atrium and ventricle.

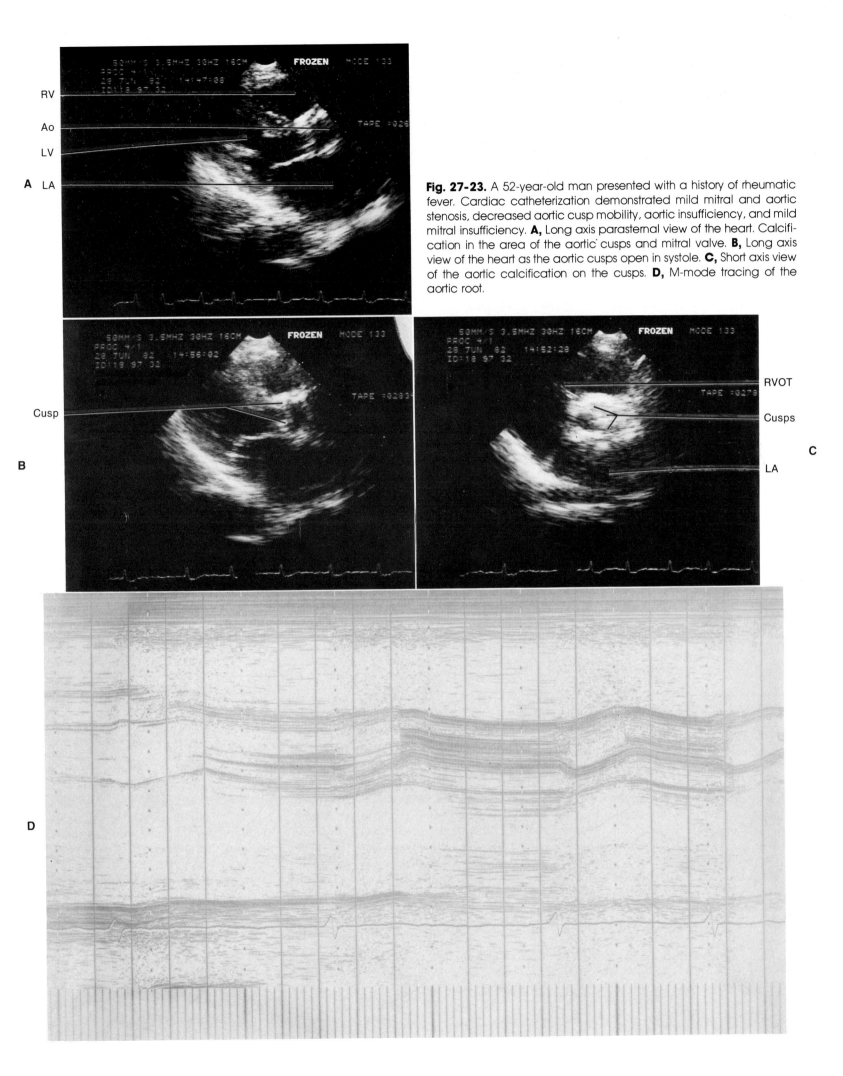

Fig. 27-23. A 52-year-old man presented with a history of rheumatic fever. Cardiac catheterization demonstrated mild mitral and aortic stenosis, decreased aortic cusp mobility, aortic insufficiency, and mild mitral insufficiency. **A,** Long axis parasternal view of the heart. Calcification in the area of the aortic cusps and mitral valve. **B,** Long axis view of the heart as the aortic cusps open in systole. **C,** Short axis view of the aortic calcification on the cusps. **D,** M-mode tracing of the aortic root.

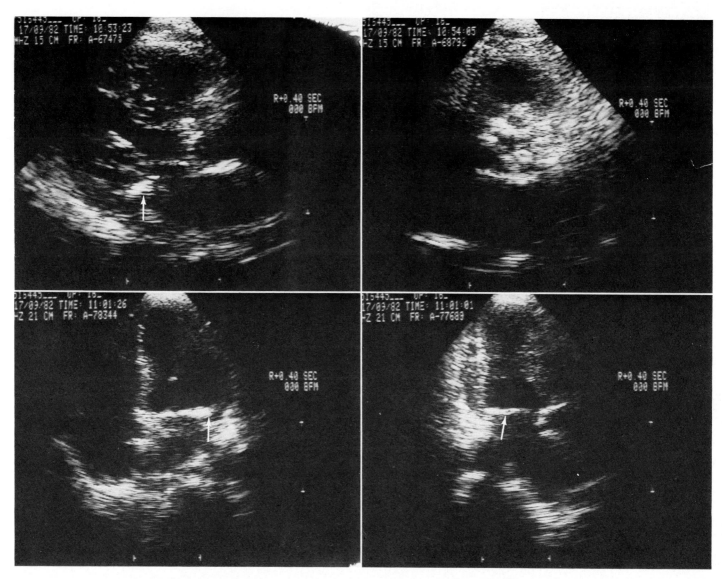

Fig. 27-24. Real time of a patient with aortic stenosis. Increased echoes are shown on the aortic leaflets along with calcification of the mitral anulus (arrows).

Although the mitral valve is often pathologically unaffected by aortic stenosis, changes can be shown on the echo that result from increased pressures in the left ventricle. The amplitude of the mitral valve becomes reduced, and the E-F slope flattens according to the severity of the stenosis. The posterior leaflet of the mitral valve continues its normal posterior motion, and the *a* kick of the anterior leaflet is generally still apparent (Fig. 27-24).

Concentric hypertrophic changes in the left ventricle have also been noted in patients with severe aortic stenosis and increased left ventricular pressure. The left ventricle exhibits decreased contractility with decompensation.

Bicuspid valve. The cusps of the normal aortic valve close concentrically in diastole, whereas those of the bicuspid valve close eccentrically. It is important to record the aortic cusps in various positions to ascertain whether this abnormal condition in the valve is present. It is well known that the beam angulation can cause the normal cusps to appear to close eccentrically. We always evaluate the patient in a supine and left decubitus position and carefully search for the aortic root area to determine the accurate appearance of the aortic cusps.

As the bicuspid valve becomes calcified, ascertaining whether it is normal or bicuspid is difficult because of the increased echoes within the aortic root. The possibility that a valve is bicuspid cannot be ruled out completely by echo; but if the eccentricity is demonstrated, the valve is most likely bicuspid (Fig. 27-25).

The two-dimensional study provides an additional method of evaluating aortic cusp closure. In the short axis view there will be normal cusp motion, simulating an inverted Mercedes-Benz insignia, whereas the bicuspid valve will clearly demonstrate eccentric cusp closure located in the root.

A

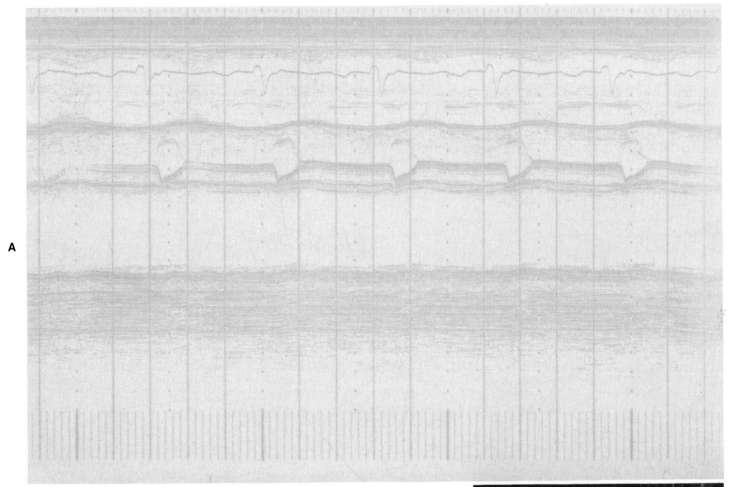

Fig. 27-25. M-mode tracings of a man with a bicuspid aortic valve, decreased mobility of the aortic root, and thickened echoes throughout the aorta. **A,** Flutter on the anterior leaflet of the mitral valve secondary to aortic insufficiency. The left atrium and ventricle are enlarged. **B,** Parasternal short axis of the bicuspid valve illustrating that the valve is domed and opens abnormally.

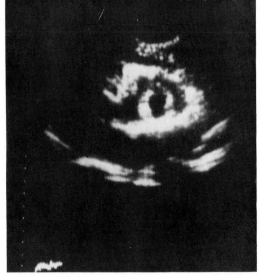

B

Continued.

C

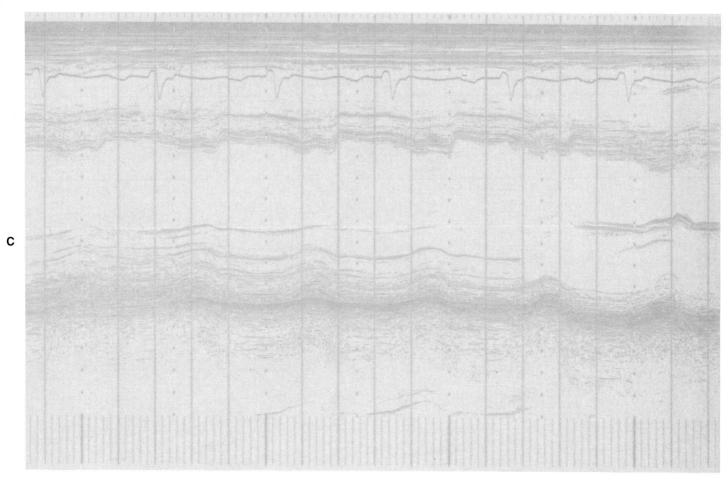

Fig. 27-25, cont'd. C, Dilated left ventricular cavity secondary to aortic insufficiency.

AORTIC INSUFFICIENCY

The causes of aortic insufficiency include rheumatic fever, bacterial endocarditis, syphilis, aneurysm of the ascending aorta, ruptured aortic cusp, myxomatous degeneration of the aortic cusps, and hypertensive dilation of the aortic root.

A number of factors play a role in determining the significance of aortic regurgitation: the size of the diastolic aperture, the compensation and diastolic stretchability of the left ventricle, and the peripheral resistance.

During diastole, if there is aortic valve regurgitation, the left ventricle competes with the peripheral vascular resistance for the blood in the aorta. During systole it must eject whatever extra blood it has received. Critical aortic regurgitation is present when the amount of leak is two to four times the effective cardiac output and the orifice size is 0.3 to 0.7 sq cm.

Rheumatic fever may directly involve the aortic cusps, leaving them shrunken and fibrotic. The aortic insufficiency appears on the anterior leaflet of the mitral valve as fine flutter during diastole (Fig. 27-26). The amplitude and E-F slope of the mitral valve decrease secondary to the increased pressures in the left ventricle (Figs. 27-27 and 27-28). If the mitral apparatus is calcified, the fine flutter will be difficult to detect by echo and may be seen on the left side of the septum.

Left ventricular dilation and hypertrophy will be present in aortic insufficiency, with a hyperdynamic contractile state (Fig. 27-29). Other findings may include dilation of the aortic root (as in cystic medial necrosis, Marfan's syndrome) (Fig. 27-30) and premature closure of the anterior leaflet of the mitral valve secondary to acute aortic insufficiency. In such patients the PR-AC interval would be foreshortened, indicating the rapid increase in left ventricular pressure from the valve leakage (Fig. 27-31).

Text continued on p. 468.

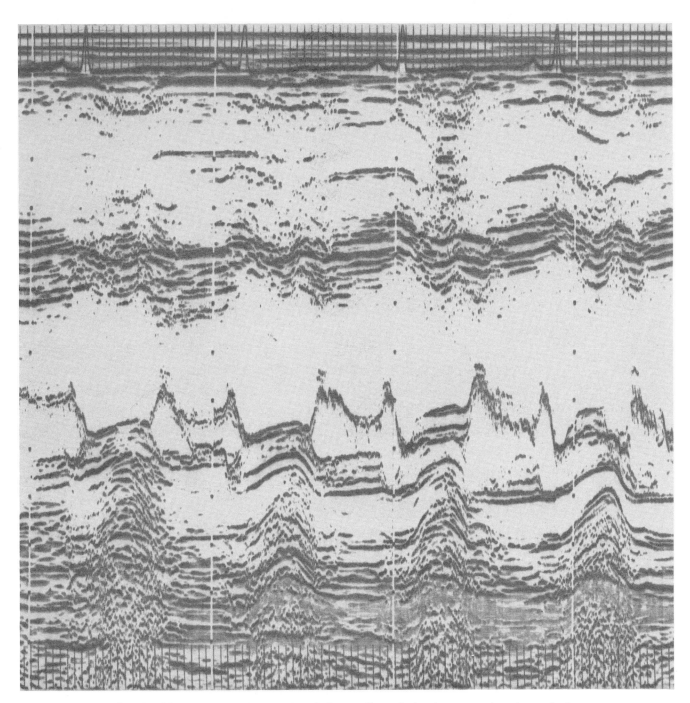

Fig. 27-26. M-mode echo showing flutter on the mitral valve secondary to aortic insufficiency. The cardiac chambers were dilated, with decreased contractility of the septum and posterior wall.

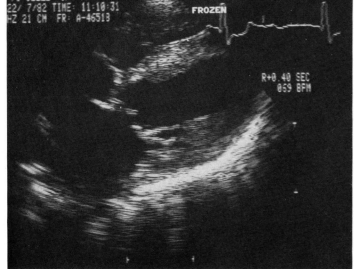

Fig. 27-27. Real time study showing aortic thickening and concentric hypertrophy of the left ventricle. **A,** Parasternal long axis. **B,** Parasternal short axis. **C,** Subxyphoid four chamber.

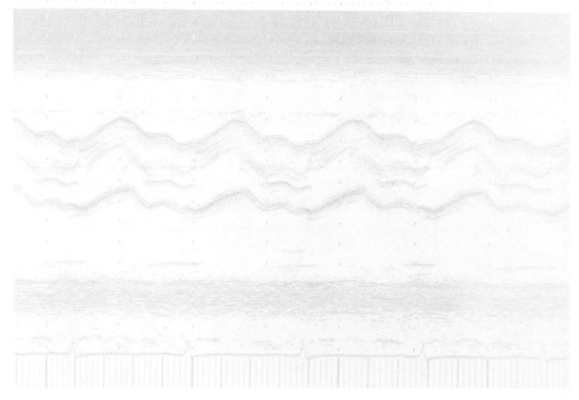

Fig. 27-28. For legend see opposite page.

Fig. 27-28. M-mode tracing of a patient with aortic calcification and insufficiency. Flutter of the mitral leaflet is evident, with concentric hypertrophy of the left ventricle.

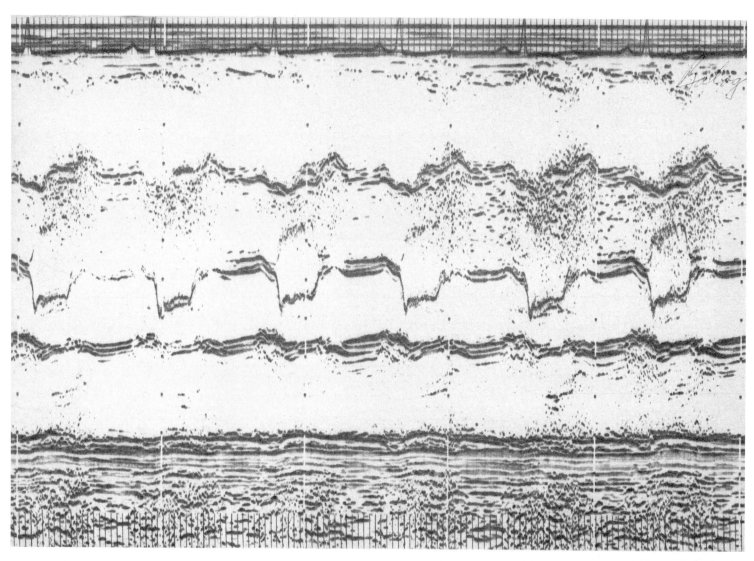

Fig. 27-29. For legend see opposite page.

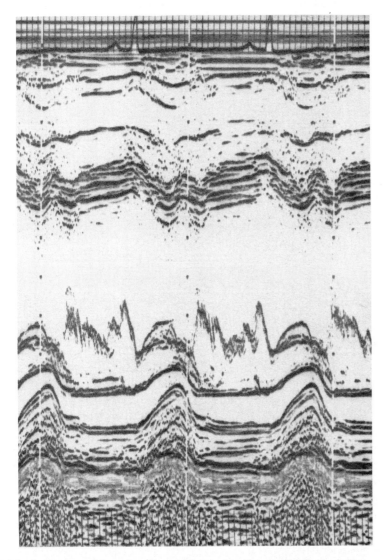

Fig. 27-29. A 58-year-old man with a history of a Grade III/VI diastolic murmur. The M-mode shows a dilated aortic root with severe flutter of the mitral apparatus. There is a pseudo-SAM due to the hypercontractile cardiac status.

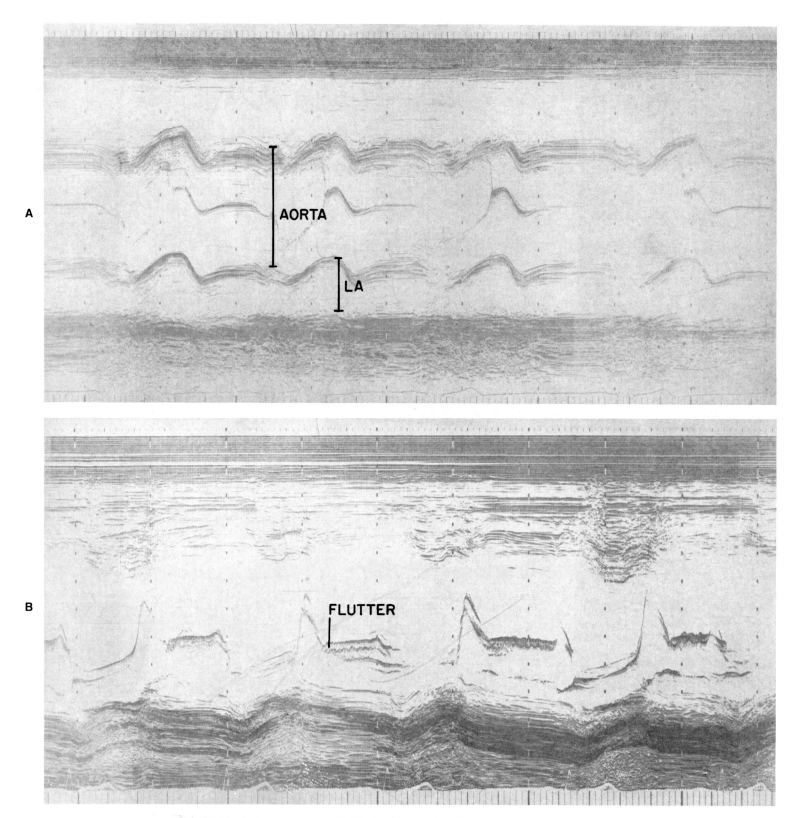

Fig. 27-30. A, A young man with Marfan's syndrome. The M-mode demonstrated an enlarged aortic root. **B,** Flutter of the mitral valve is secondary to the aortic insufficiency.

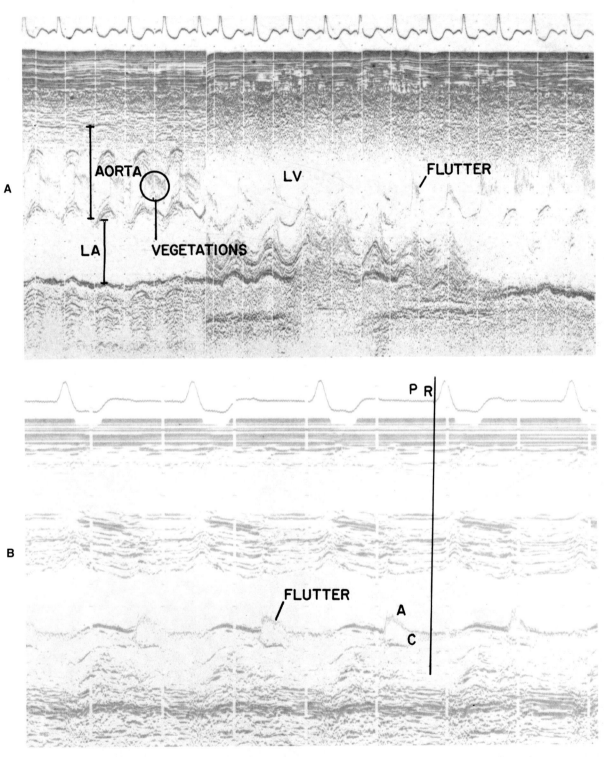

Fig. 27-31. A, Increased echoes in diastole represent vegetations on the aortic valve. Aortic insufficiency, shown on the anterior leaflet of the mitral valve, is caused by destruction of the cusps. **B,** Premature closure of the mitral apparatus representing acute aortic insufficiency.

TRICUSPID STENOSIS AND INSUFFICIENCY

Tricuspid valve disease is usually present in 25% of patients with severe rheumatic heart lesions. However, clinically significant disease is present in only about 5% to 10% of these patients. Because dilation of the right ventricle is a common result of pulmonary hypertension from mitral and aortic valve disease, severe tricuspid incompetence may occur in the absence of a significant valve lesion.

Stenosis. Most cases of tricuspid stenosis are of rheumatic origin, with the mitral and aortic valves being affected first. Other causes are congenital defects, systemic lupus erythematosus, and carcinoid tumors. The stenotic leaflets usually fuse, leaving a roundish hilum in the central area of the leaflets and some degree of incompetence of the valve. Right atrial hypertrophy occurs and cardiac output falls when the right ventricular filling is impaired due to further narrowing of the valve orifice.

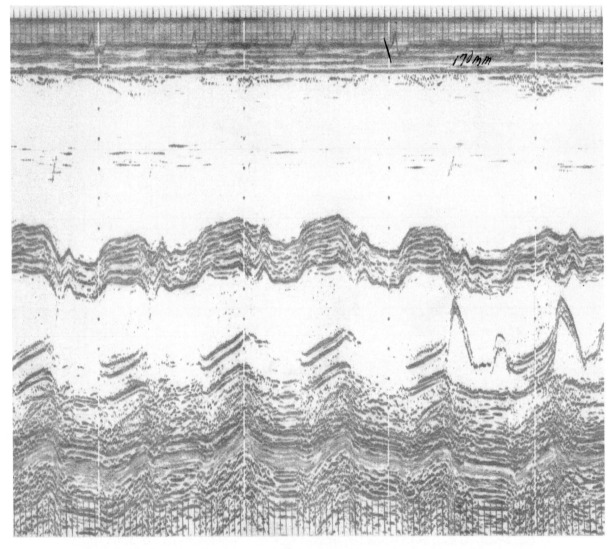

Fig. 27-32. M-mode tracings of a patient with rheumatic heart disease. The tricuspid valve is well seen and appears thickened. The aortic root is thickened, although the cusps open well. A sweep to the left ventricular cavity shows right ventricular dilation and paradoxical septal motion. The patient had tricuspid insufficiency with right ventricular volume overload.

Insufficiency. There are two types of tricuspid insufficiency: functional and organic.

Functional insufficiency is the result of right ventricular failure, which causes right ventricular dilation. This dilation causes the tricuspid ring also to dilate, producing tricuspid valve regurgitation.

Organic regurgitation is caused by rheumatic disease, congenital lesions of Ebstein's disease and endocardial cushion defects, or bacterial endocarditis. The right atrium enlarges with regurgitant flow from the tricuspid valve. Likewise, during diastole the right ventricle receives this blood from the right atrium in addition to that reaching the right atrium from the great veins, causing hypertrophy and dilation. The dilated right side of the heart permits easy visualization of the tricuspid valve echographically (Fig. 27-32).

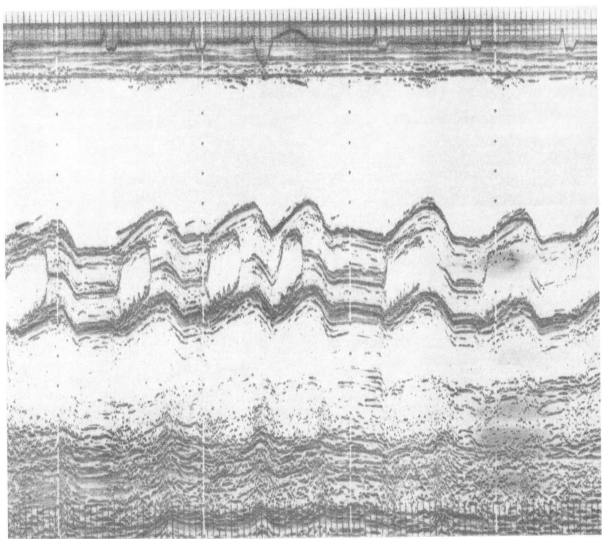

Continued.

Fig. 27-32, cont'd. For legend see opposite page.

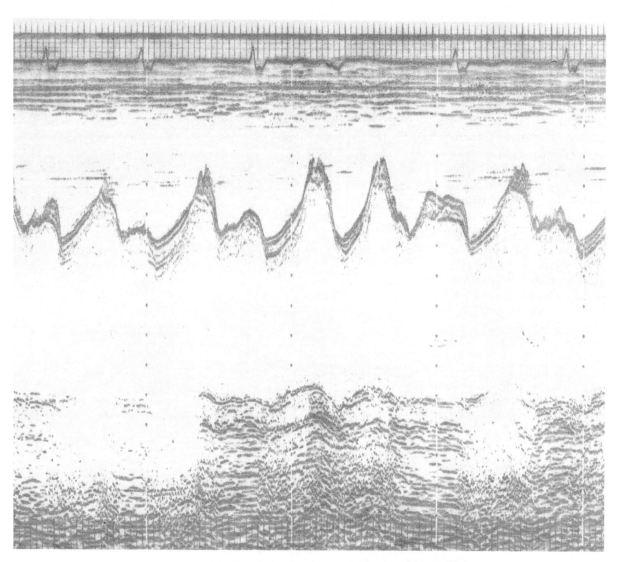

Fig. 27-32, cont'd. For legend see page 468.

The tricuspid leaflet opens and closes as the mitral leaflet does, with no fluttering motion. If fine flutter is noted, there are several possible causes. Pulmonary insufficiency is probably the most common. The regurgitation from the pulmonary valve acts the same as aortic insufficiency does on the mitral apparatus. The backflow of blood strikes the tricuspid leaflet, causing high-frequency flutter.

REFERENCES

1. Bittar, N.: Rheumatic heart disease. Lecture notes for second year medical students, University of Wisconsin, Madison, 1981.
2. Wann, L.S., Feigenbaum, H., Weyman, A.E., et al.: Cross-sectional echocardiographic detection of rheumatic mitral regurgitation, Am. J. Cardiol. **41:**1258, 1978.

28

Other valvular abnormalities

This chapter will concentrate on acquired valvular (valvar) abnormalities—e.g., mitral valve prolapse, rupture of the chordal structures or papillary muscles, papillary muscle dysfunction, calcification of the mitral anulus, supravalvular and subvalvular aortic stenoses, and Marfan's syndrome.

MITRAL VALVE PROLAPSE

The exact cause of prolapse of the mitral valve is a topic of controversy. Numerous studies have been conducted in an effort to relate information about prolapse with other clinical data. One acknowledged condition is a change in the consistency of the leaflet or papillary muscle. Roberts and Henry (1973) reported that a myxomatous degeneration of the mitral apparatus can lead to prolapse of the leaflet. Elongation of the anterior leaflet is a common finding in prolapse and causes the valve to close deep near the posterior heart wall.

Barlow et al. (1963) demonstrated that a midsystolic click and late systolic murmur did, in fact, result from a billowing or prolapse of the mitral leaflet, referred to as Barlow's syndrome. Barlow noted that these particular patients had mitral regurgitation during the latter part of systole. Some patients had unusual anatomic deformities of the mitral valve apparatus characterized by prolapsing in middle to late systole. Other associated conditions included Marfan's syndrome (characteristics: enlarged aortic root, flutter of anterior leaflet of mitral valve, holosystolic prolapse). The cause of such a floppy valve could not be totally explained, but several investigators believed it was a genetic factor.

A high percentage of patients with mitral prolapse have clinical symptoms of chest pain, fatigue, and ventricular arrhythmias at some point in their clinical course. This fact supports the belief that the syndrome of a prolapsed mitral valve is a significant component of left ventricular disease.

The disease frequently is found in young adults and is probably more often discovered with the introduction of echography. The prolapsed leaflet becomes elongated, redundant, and thickened by myxomatous degeneration. The chordae become elongated and thus allow the mitral apparatus to buckle into the left atrium (producing the click on ascultation) (Fig. 28-1). The timing and intensity of the click and murmur (of mitral regurgitation) vary with volume changes of the left ventricle induced by posture changes, Valsalva maneuver, amyl nitrite, or phenylephrine.

The major complications of mitral valve prolapse include mitral regurgitation, spontaneous chordal rupture, increased tendency to develop infective endocarditis, and sudden death.

Echography of the mitral apparatus is very sensitive for prolapse. The systolic posterior displacement of the anterior or posterior leaflet is one of the primary findings in prolapse. Prolapse can occur throughout systole (holosystolic or pansystolic), in midsystole, or in late systole (Figs. 28-2 and 28-3). Normally the C-D segment of the mitral apparatus moves slightly anteriorly in systole. However, in prolapse, the D point sags 2 to 3 mm behind the C point into the left atrial cavity. The midsystolic click coincides with this posterior movement.

The valve may also show several echoes throughout systole and diastole that may represent degeneration, thickening, or redundancy of the leaflet (Fig. 28-4).

The holosystolic or pansystolic bowing of the mitral apparatus was demonstrated by DeMaria et al. (1980) as a collapse of the mitral leaflets to the backwall of the left atrium.

Text continued on p. 477.

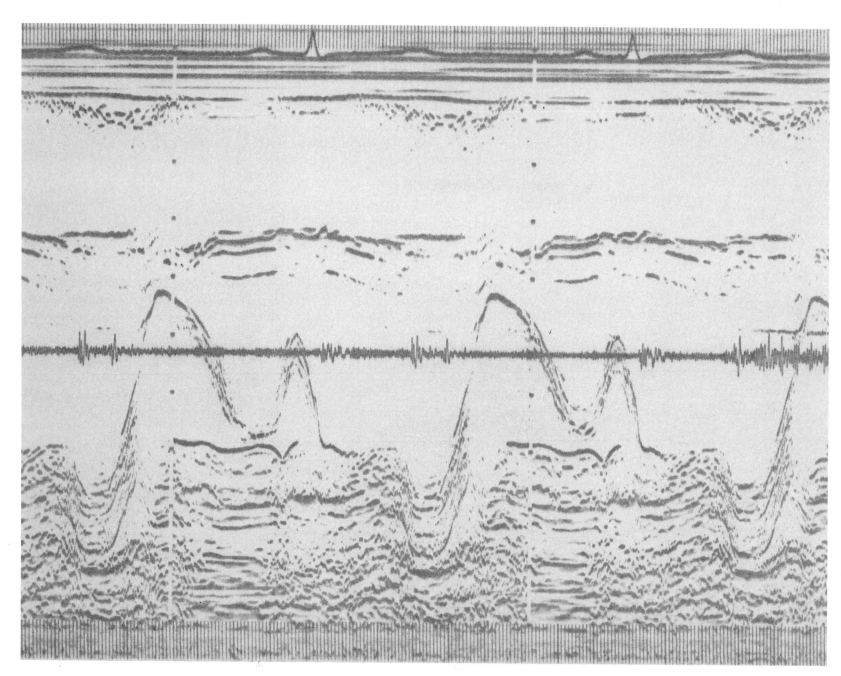

Fig. 28-1. M-mode echocardiogram of a patient with mitral valve prolapse. The phonocardiogram is superimposed to demonstrate the recording of the midsystolic click.

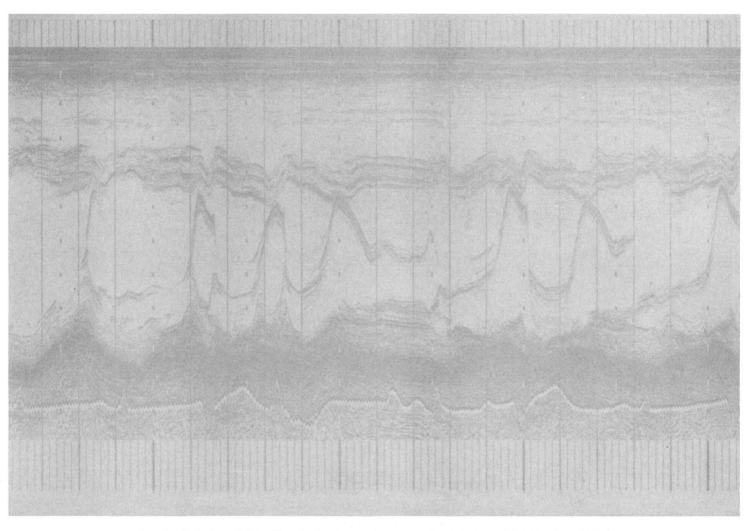

Fig. 28-2. This patient with mitral valve prolapse manifests holosystolic billowing of the anterior and posterior leaflets. There are multiple arrhythmias throughout the recording. Note the increased amplitude of the mitral leaflet, with the E point touching the septum.

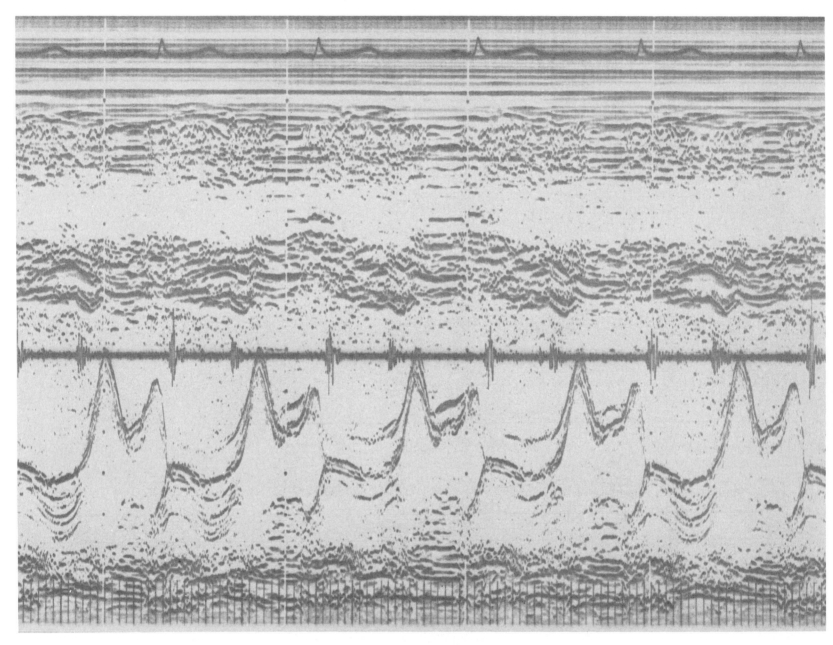

Fig. 28-3. One must be careful to evaluate the true mitral leaflets when looking for prolapse and not be confused by chordal structures that may appear in systole. In this patient the first group of systolic echoes seen is related to chordal structures. If one follows the anterior leaflet through its closure at the C point, the true systolic leaflet may be seen. There is a midsystolic prolapse of both leaflets.

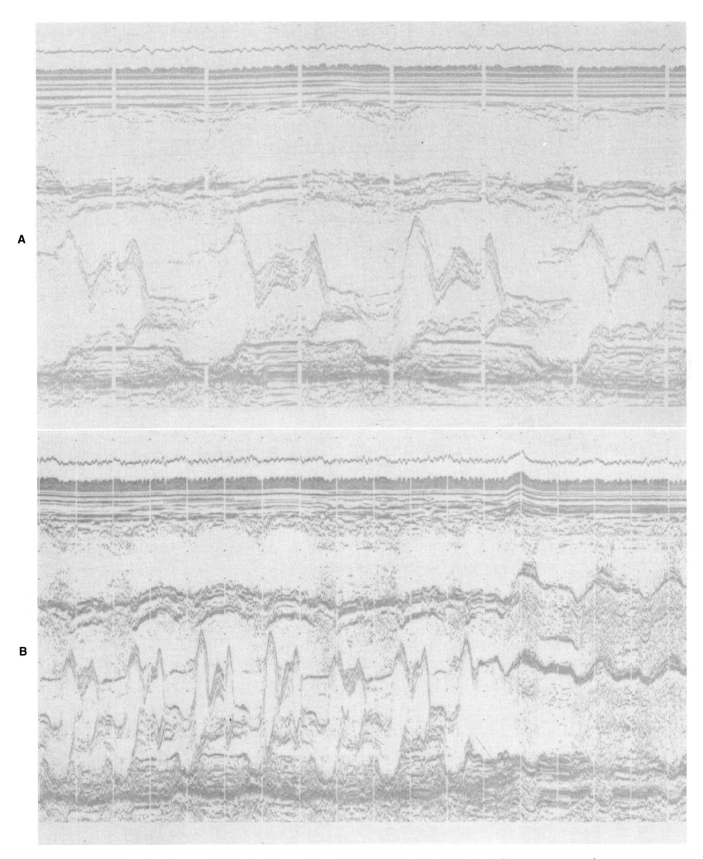

Fig. 28-4. Often a clue to defining the presence of prolapse is the disappearance of systolic echoes as the leaflet prolapses into the left atrium. **A,** A patient with midsystolic prolapse and disappearing echoes in systole. **B,** Mitral-to-aortic sweep. The midsystolic sagging is well seen on both leaflets. The increased echoes in the aorta and left atrium are due to respiration.

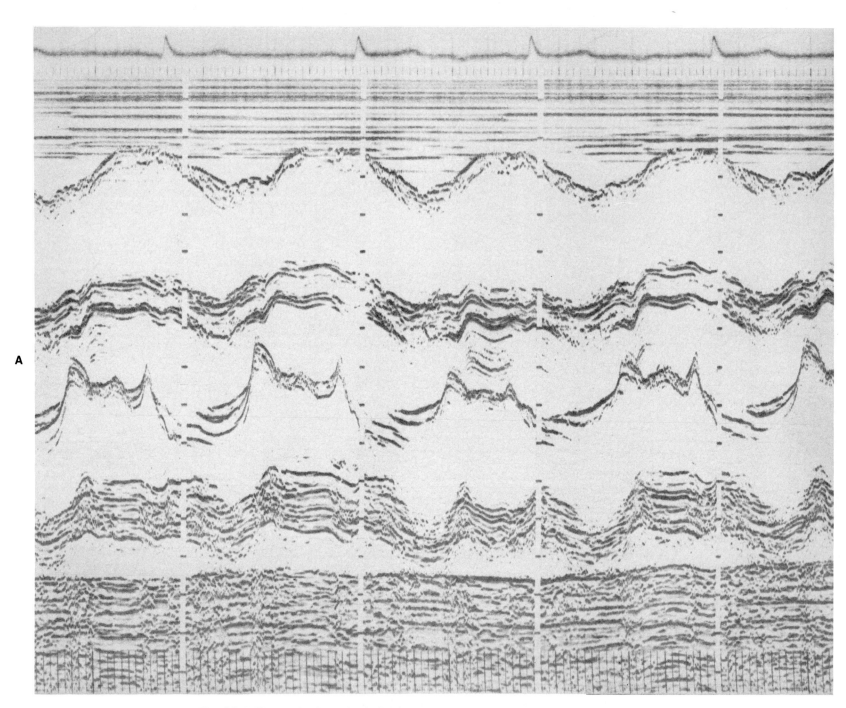

A

Fig. 28-5. The evaluation of mitral valve prolapse should not be made in the presence of pericardial effusion, for the hyperdynamic pattern of the heart may cause a normal valve to prolapse. **A,** Anterior and posterior pericardial effusion. The mitral valve appears to prolapse slightly. **B,** As the mitral valve is better visualized, the prolapse becomes more evident. The scan should be repeated after the effusion has subsided so the mitral apparatus can be evaluated.

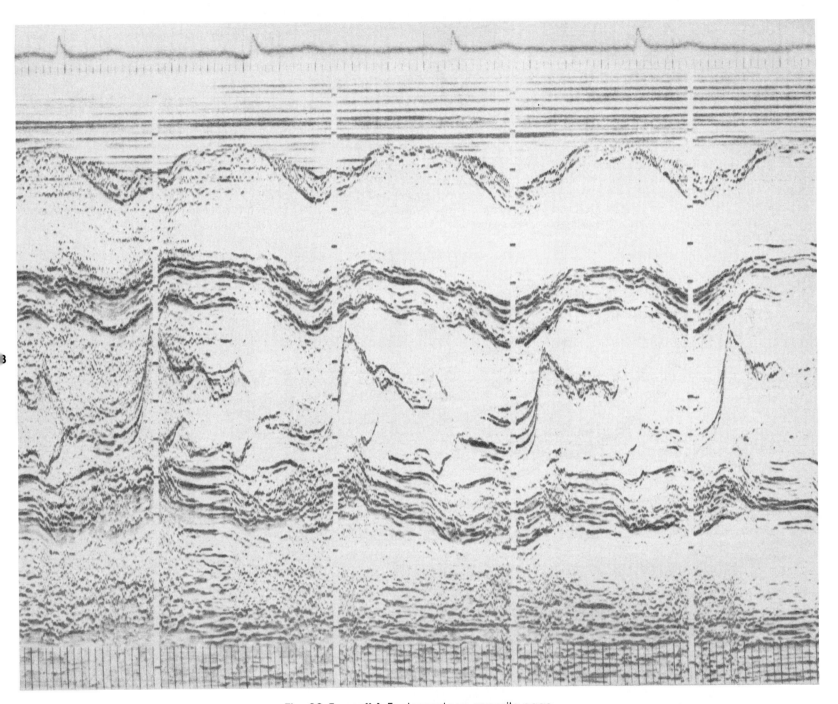

Fig. 28-5, cont'd. For legend see opposite page.

The sonographer should carefully examine the entire mitral apparatus to find the prolapse. If recordings are made at the tip of the leaflets with the beam exiting through the left atrial wall, the abnormal valve movements will more likely be recorded.

The transducer must be perpendicular to the mitral apparatus. If it is too high on the chest and angled down toward the feet, a pseudoprolapse may be projected.

Do not attempt to diagnose a mitral regurgitation from the apparent separation of the leaflet echoes during prolapse. Valves that close tightly may appear to separate when a portion of the leaflet other than the opposed edges are recorded (Fig. 28-5).

The symptoms may be elicited with amyl nitrite or the patient asked to perform a Valsalva maneuver to induce the mitral prolapse. This reduces the left ventricular volume and moves the prolapse earlier into systole. Thus a late prolapse can be moved to a midsystolic prolapse with these maneuvers.

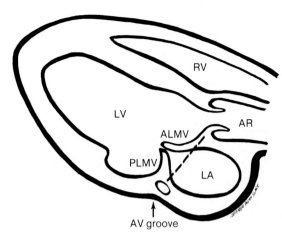

Fig. 28-6. Long axis schematic for evaluating mitral valve prolapse. The anterior and posterior leaflets should not pass beyond the dotted line in a normal closure. *RV*, Right ventricle; *AR*, aortic root; *LV*, left ventricle; *LA*, left atrium; *ALMV*, anterior leaflet of mitral valve; *PLMV*, posterior leaflet of mitral valve; *AV groove*, atrioventricular groove.

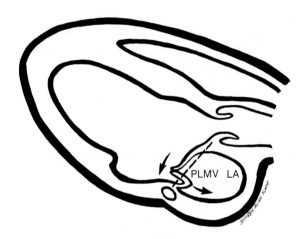

Fig. 28-7. Long axis schematic demonstrating the prolapse of the posterior mitral leaflet into the left atrial cavity.

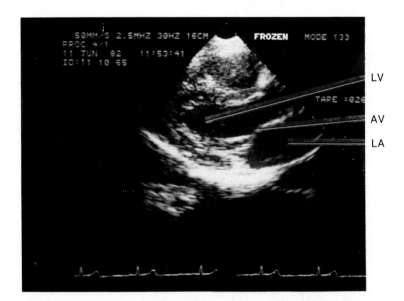

Fig. 28-8. Two-dimensional long axis view of the posterior leaflet as it prolapses into the left atrial cavity.

Another interesting feature of prolapse is that the patient may demonstrate it only when arrhythmias are occurring. If the click-murmur is intermittent, prolapse cannot be demonstrated by echo. One tries to examine the patient as for auscultation—supine, semidecubitus, upright, standing, or squatting—but some patients who present with it in the upright and squatting positions appear completely normal at rest.

Two-dimensional scanning allows a more precise evaluation of mitral prolapse (Fig. 28-6). The long axis and apical four chamber views of the heart provide an opportunity to visualize the mitral apparatus as it prolapses into the left atrial cavity (Figs. 28-7 to 28-9). A more precise evaluation of the posterior leaflet can be made with real time. The amplitude of the leaflets and the structure of the chordae tendineae can be evaluated (Fig. 28-10).

Gilbert (1981) examined patients with angiographically proved prolapse and noted superior movement of the mitral valve apparatus above the mitral ring. Most patients appeared to have a posteriorly located point of coaptation between the anterior and posterior leaflets.

Fraker et al. (1980) reported some degree of unusual systolic "curling" motion of the posterior mitral ring on the adjacent myocardium. In normals the posterior mitral ring moves toward the apex of the left ventricle and slightly anterior in systole. When such curling is seen, the movement of the ring is primarily toward the apex, usually in wide swings between systole and diastole.

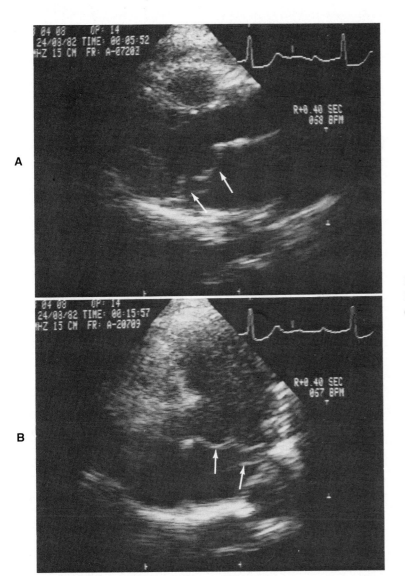

Fig. 28-9. A, Parasternal long axis of both leaflets prolapsing into the left atrium *(arrows).* **B,** Apical four chamber of the prolapsed leaflets *(arrows).*

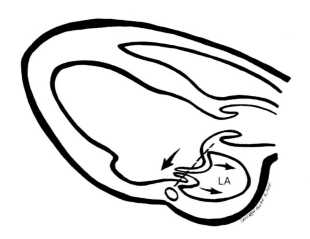

Fig. 28-10. Long axis schematic of both leaflets prolapsing into the left atrium.

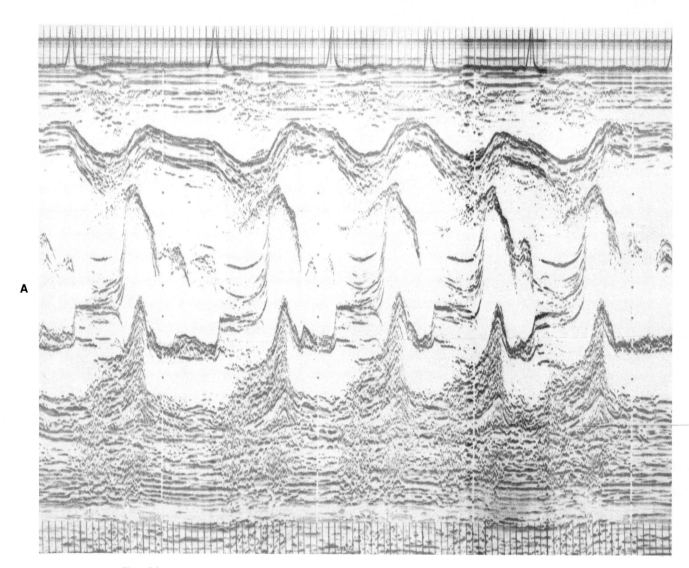

Fig. 28-11. This patient had a chordal rupture, gross mitral regurgitation, and mitral valve prolapse. **A,** M-mode scan at the level of the atrioventricular junction showing the posterior leaflet with a very dynamic AV junction posterior. **B,** As one scans further toward the left atrial cavity, a gross collection of coarse echoes is seen in the area of the posterior leaflet.

FLAIL MITRAL APPARATUS OR PAPILLARY MUSCLE

Rupture of the papillary muscle occurs from a myocardial infarction and death of the papillary muscle or from chest injury. As a result, massive acute mitral regurgitation will occur and if not surgically corrected may result in death.

Rupture of the chordae is not as great an emergency situation, depending on the number and extent of the ruptures. Patients may present with trauma, endocarditis, or idiopathic chordal ruptures.

Clinically there may be signs of chest trauma or recent endocarditis. A gross mitral regurgitation murmur is heard at the apex of the heart. Since the regurgitation is acute, the left atrium will be normal.

Echographic findings may appear as mitral prolapse with a coarse, erratic, and irregular flutter throughout diastole (Fig. 28-11). There may be a systolic dropout, with the flail leaflet dipping far posteriorly and then moving anteriorly with diastole (Figs. 28-12 to 28-14). *Text continued on p. 490.*

B

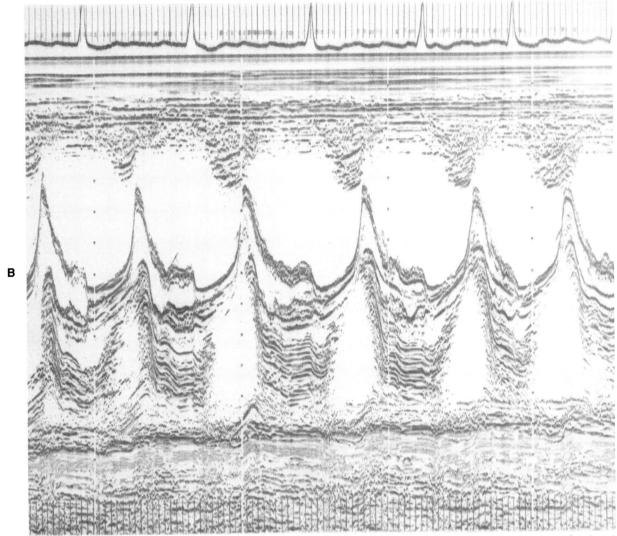

Continued.

Fig. 28-11, cont'd. For legend see opposite page.

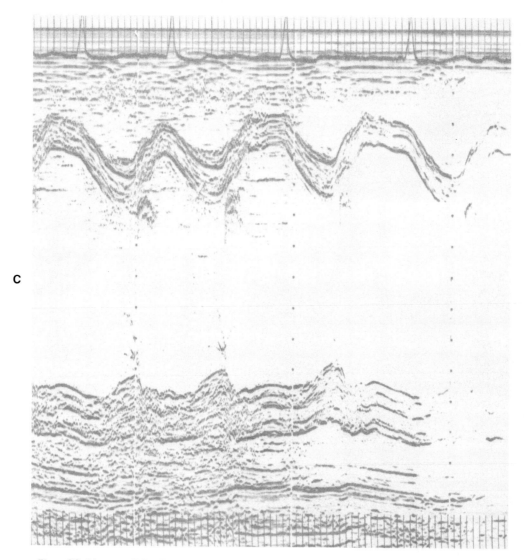

C

Fig. 28-11, cont'd. C, The left ventricular cavity is enlarged, and pericardial effusion is present.

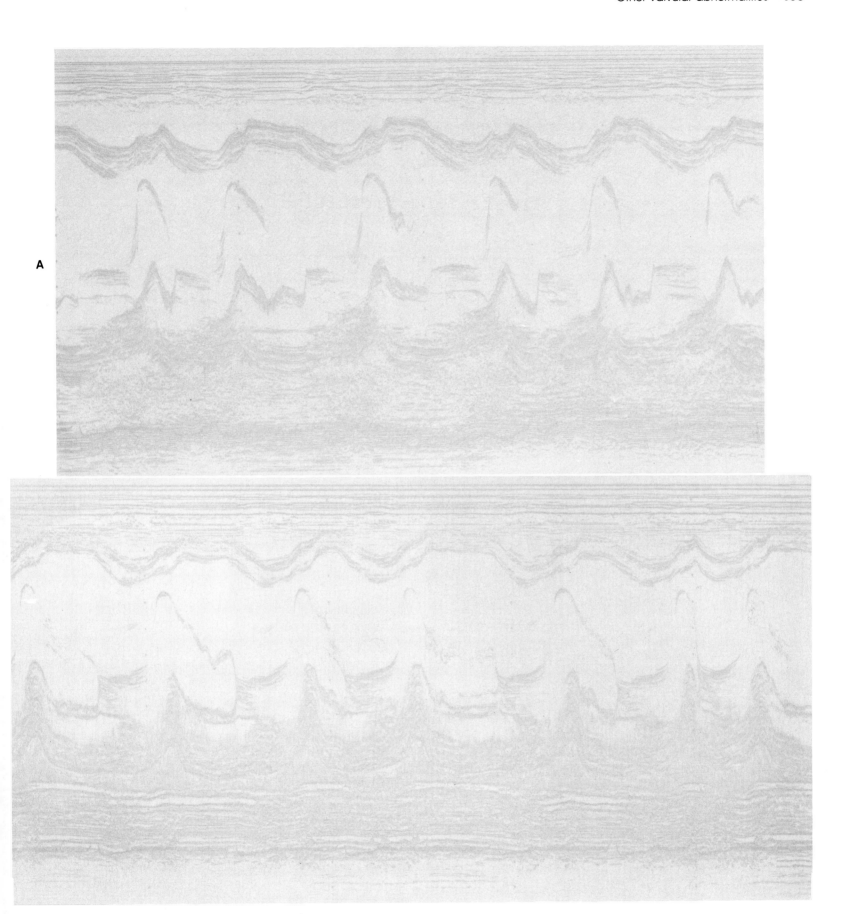

Fig. 28-12. A patient with rheumatic valvular disease. An intensified murmur of mitral regurgitation developed, with congestive heart failure. **A,** M-mode of the anterior and posterior leaflets showing the coarse irregular flutter in the posterior leaflet. **B,** As one sweeps toward the left atrial cavity, the posterior leaflet assumes more of a mass effect secondary to the rupture.

Continued.

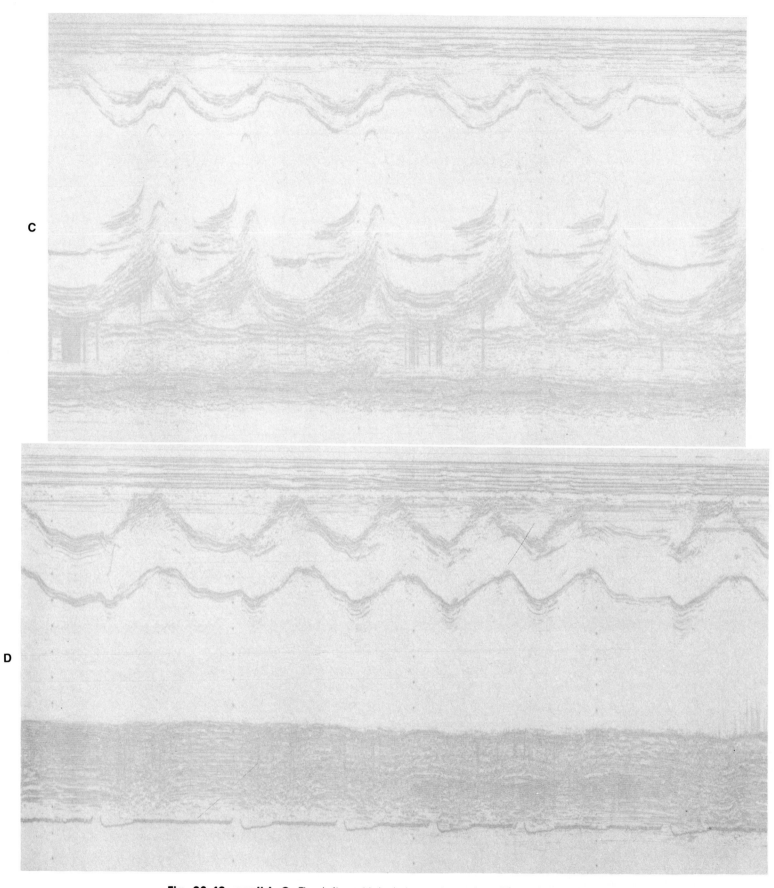

Fig. 28-12, cont'd. C, The left ventricle is hyperdynamic, with posterior pericardial effusion. **D,** An enlarged left atrial cavity is present secondary to the mitral regurgitation.

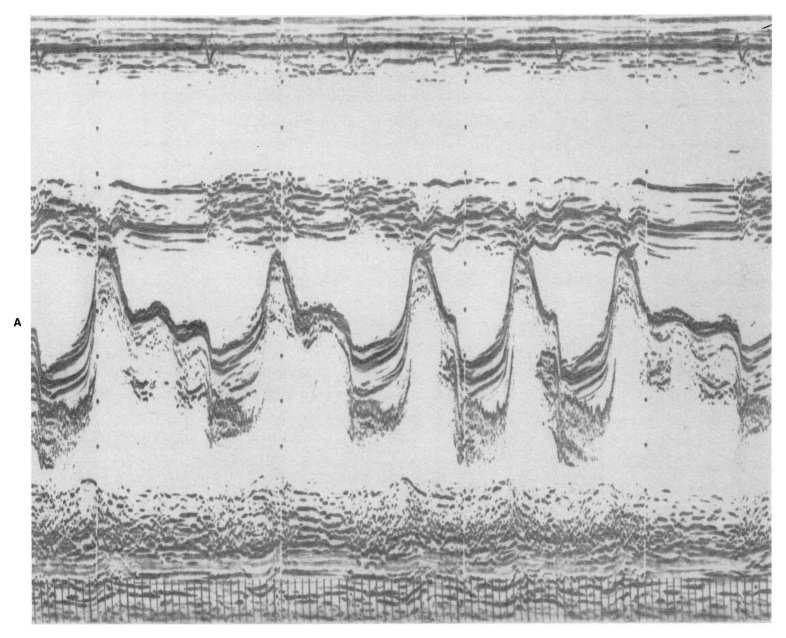

Fig. 28-13. This patient presented with congestive heart failure and a harsh systolic ejection murmur that had increased in intensity from his previous visit. **A,** The systolic segment of the mitral apparatus is very shaggy and shows signs of flutter. Differential would include chordal rupture as well as vegetations.   *Continued.*

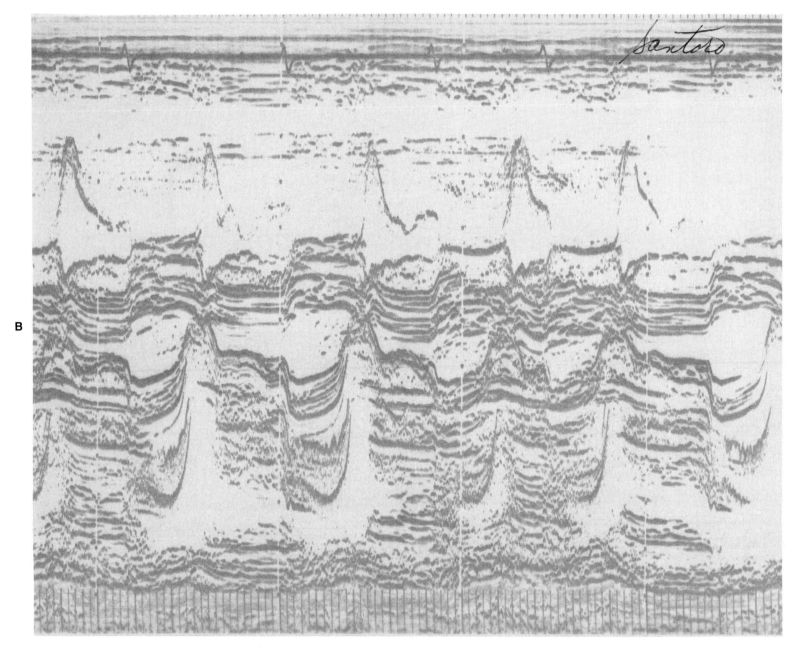

Fig. 28-13, cont'd. B, The right ventricular cavity is enlarged, and the anterior and posterior tricuspid leaflets are well seen. Prolapse of the mitral leaflet is evident with dense echoes in diastole. **C,** A sweep from the aortic root to mitral apparatus demonstrates the erratic flail posterior leaflet simulating a mass.

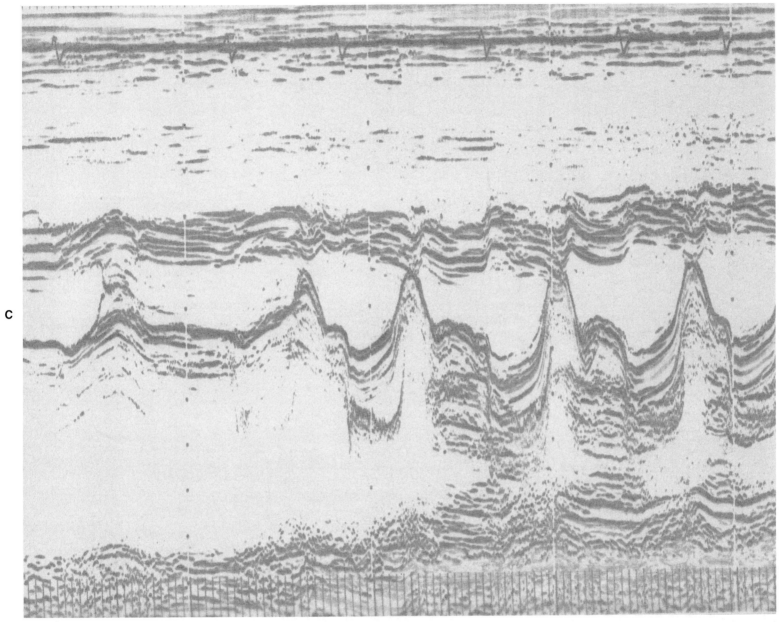

Fig. 28-13, cont'd. For legend see opposite page.

Continued.

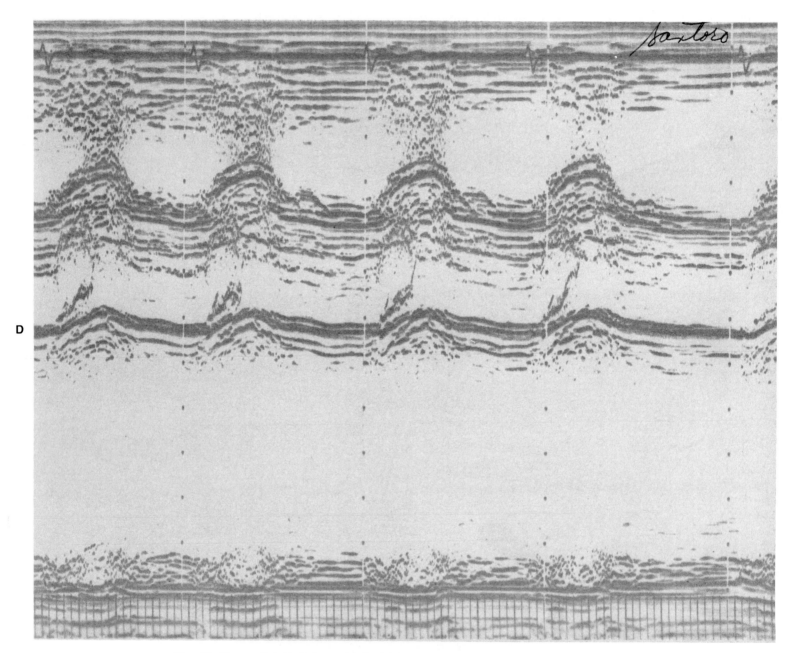

D

Fig. 28-13, cont'd. D, Enlarged left atrial cavity secondary to mitral regurgitation. **E,** The left ventricle is slightly enlarged, with hypercontractility of the posterior wall.

E

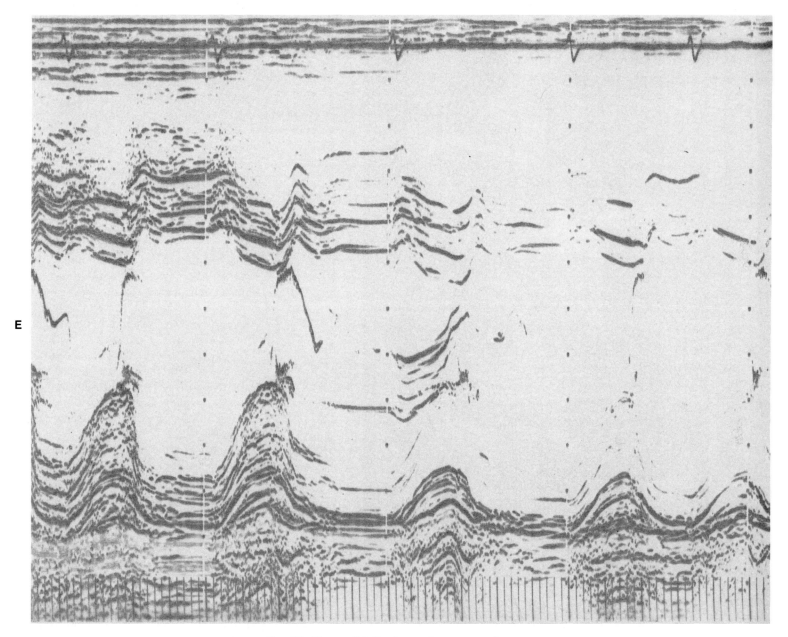

Fig. 28-13, cont'd. For legend see opposite page.

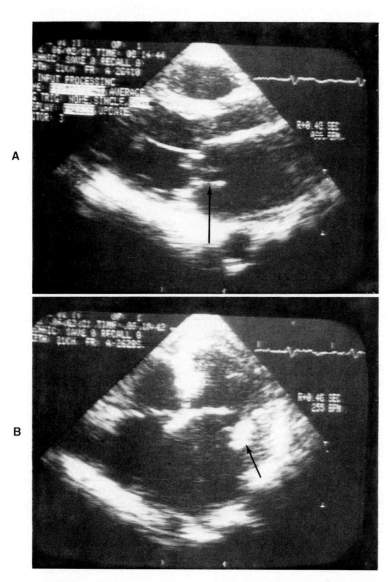

Fig. 28-14. A, Parasternal long axis in systole clearly showing the posterior flail leaflet as it flies into the left atrial cavity *(arrow)*. **B,** Apical four chamber view.

A ruptured chorda tendineae may be seen to fly throughout the mitral valve apparatus and may appear as a pseudo-SAM in systole.

PAPILLARY MUSCLE DYSFUNCTION

Two-dimensional echography may prove to be more useful than M-mode in the diagnosis of papillary muscle dysfunction. Normally in an apical view the mitral leaflets line up in a plane approximately parallel with the mitral anulus. With papillary muscle dysfunction the papillary or adjacent ventricular muscle may be scarred, dyskinetic, or merely dilated; thus the leaflet to which the muscle is attached may not be able to close fully, with resultant incomplete closure of the valve. This finding has been noted in patients with cardiomyopathy and those with ischemic heart disease.

CALCIFIED MITRAL ANULUS (ANNULUS)

Calcification of the mitral anulus appears echographically as a band of very dense, coarse, highly reflective echoes posterior to the mitral valve apparatus. Often the calcification of the anulus will obscure visualization of the posterior mitral leaflet or the endocardial surface of the posterior heart wall (Fig. 28-15).

Care must be taken not to confuse the bright echo of the calcification with that of the posterior heart wall or the echo of the heart wall with that of the pericardium. A false diagnosis of pericardial effusion will not likely be made if careful sweeps from the left atrium to the apex of the heart are performed.

The calcification may extend to other areas of the heart, especially throughout the base. It may extend into both the mitral and the aortic valves, into the root of the aorta, and into the left ventricle (chordae and papillary muscles).

Conditions that are frequently associated with a calcified mitral anulus include calcific aortic stenosis, mitral valve prolapse, and hypertrophic subaortic stenosis. The calcified mitral anulus may impair the normal function of the mitral valve apparatus and frequently produces mitral regurgitation.

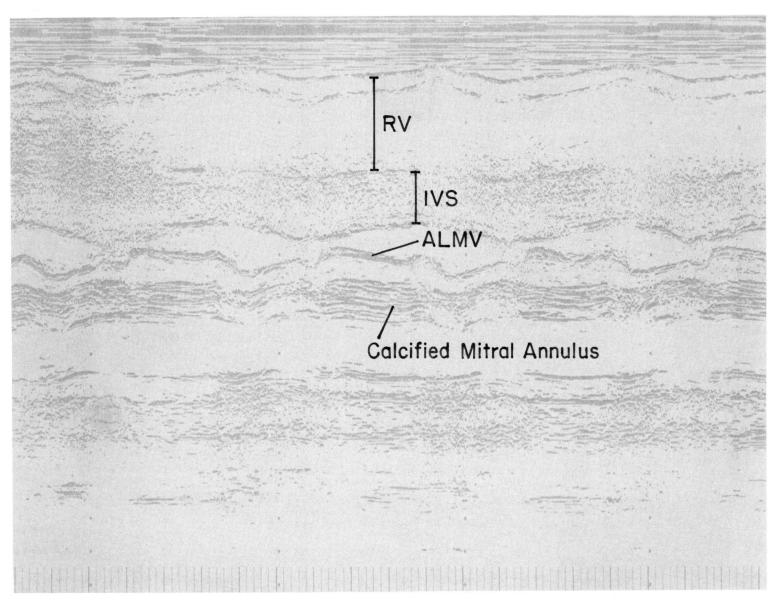

Fig. 28-15. This patient had aortic stenosis and calcification of the mitral anulus. As one sweeps into the left ventricular cavity, the bright calcified anulus obscures visualization of the posterior leaflet and the endocardium. Further angulation and/or alteration in the patient's position allow adequate visualization of the left ventricular cavity.

SUPRAVALVULAR AORTIC STENOSIS

Stenosis above the aortic valve may be a narrow ring, a longer hourglass deformity, or a hypoplasia of the ascending aorta. In a continuous sweep from the aortic root and cusp area to the area above the valve until no aorta can be visualized, the dimension of the valve should become wider, since the beam is transecting the aorta in a tangential plane. However, if this area narrows consistently, supravalvular aortic stenosis is probably present.

SUBVALVULAR AORTIC STENOSIS

The midsystolic closure of the aortic cusps is generally seen in cases of idiopathic hypertrophic subaortic stenosis (IHSS). In cases of IHSS there is a hypertrophied septum with a systolic bulging of the anterior leaflet of the mitral valve. As the left ventricle contracts to eject blood through the outflow tract, this thickened septum and systolic bulge cause the aortic leaflets to close in midsystole. (We have never seen the cusps remain closed throughout systole.) As the obstruction on the anterior leaflet moves away from the septum, the pressure relents in the left ventricle and the blood continues through the aortic cusps. This causes the cusps to reopen in late systole, although not as fully as in early systole (Fig. 28-16). In discrete subaortic stenosis there is no septal hypertrophy or midsystolic obstruction, as seen in IHSS. A piece of tissue shaped like a diaphragm sits below the aortic valve and obstructs the flow from the left ventricle. This causes the aortic cusp to close abruptly in early systole and reopen in late systole.

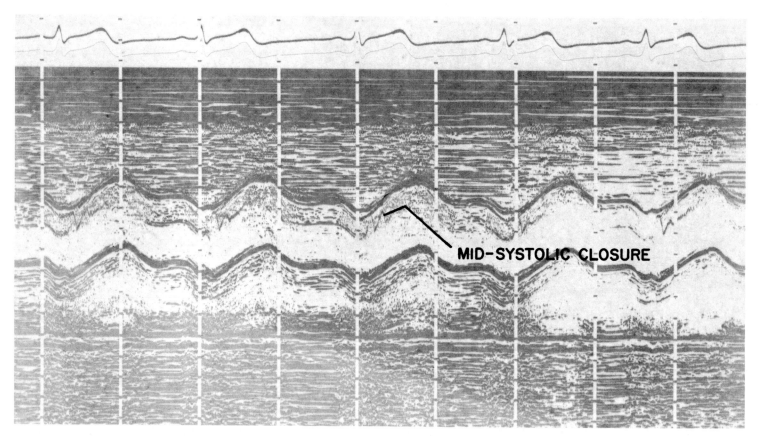

Fig. 28-16. Midsystolic closure of the aortic valve occurs in patients with obstructive hypertrophic cardiomyopathy.

MARFAN'S SYNDROME

Marfan's syndrome is considered a stretch lesion of the valve. The aortic and mitral leaflets stretch and overshoot their normal closing, with resulting mitral or aortic regurgitation. The ascending aorta is also subject to dilation and weakness, which may lead to dissection. Marfan syndrome patients have the following other physical symptoms: long thin fingers, tall stature, double-jointedness, and an abnormal metacarpal index.

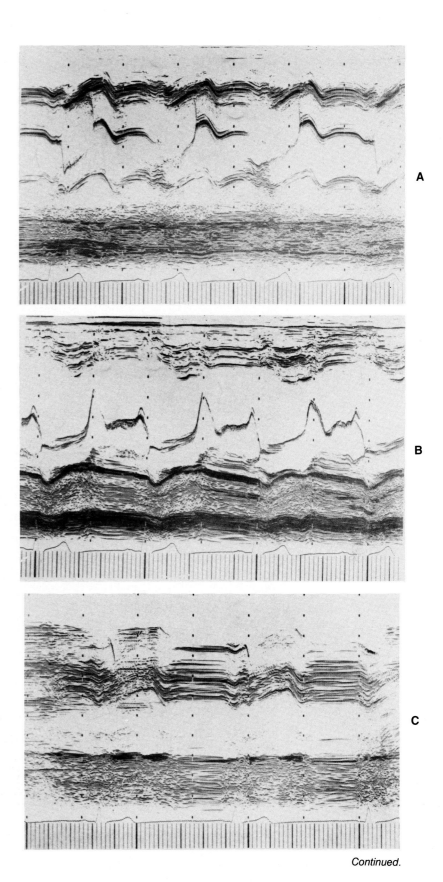

Fig. 28-17. A 23-year-old man with known murmur for 5 years experiencing exertional dyspnea. Auscultation found a prominent apical impulse, a hyperdynamic left ventricle, and an aortic ejection sound with a 3/6 aortic insufficiency murmur. The echo demonstrated a dilated aortic root with minimal flutter of the mitral valve secondary to aortic insufficiency. **A,** Dilated aortic root. **B,** Fine flutter shown on the anterior leaflet of the mitral valve. **C,** Normal pulmonary valve.

Continued.

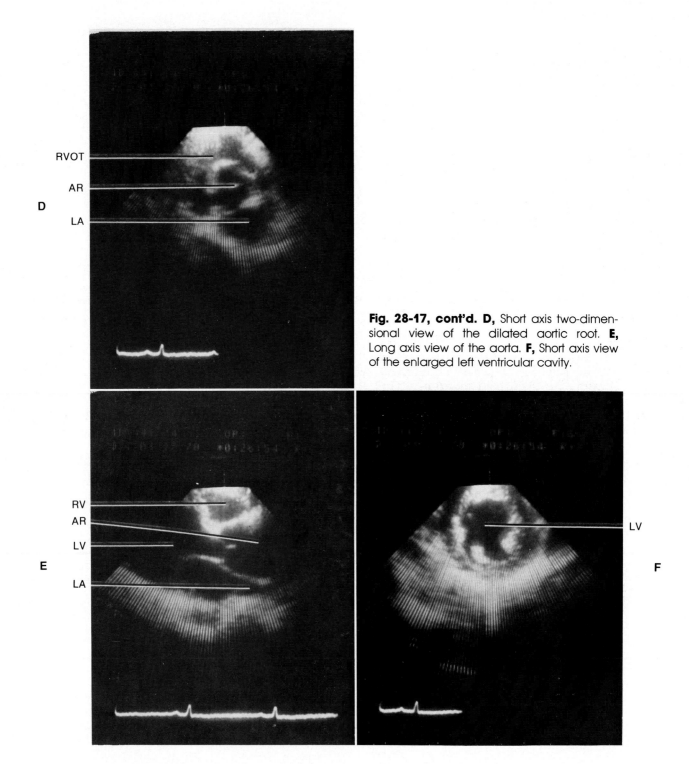

Fig. 28-17, cont'd. **D,** Short axis two-dimensional view of the dilated aortic root. **E,** Long axis view of the aorta. **F,** Short axis view of the enlarged left ventricular cavity.

Patients with the Marfan syndrome display several echographic features. They usually have a huge aortic root with associated aortic insufficiency, shown on the mitral valve as fine flutter (Fig. 28-17). Usually, associated mitral regurgitation is shown with increased amplitude of the anterior leaflet and "spooning" or holosystolic prolapse of both leaflets in systole (Fig. 28-18).

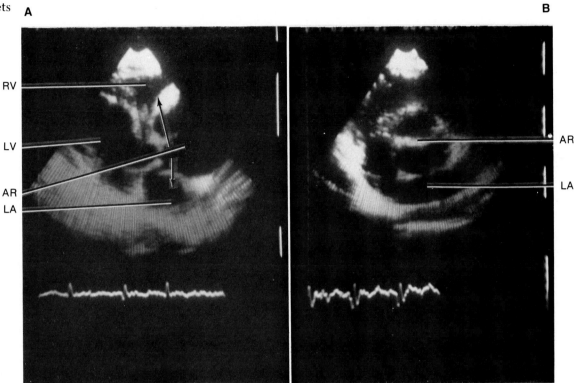

Fig. 28-18. A patient with a markedly dilated aortic root and an aneurysm at the sinus of Valsalva. The left ventricle is enlarged, and there is gross flutter on the anterior leaflet of the mitral valve. The echo alone cannot be used to classify this dilation as due to Marfan's disorder, cystic medial necrosis, or other aneurysm formation. **A,** Two-dimensional long axis view of the dilated aortic root. **B,** Short axis view of the aorta and left atrial cavity. (Courtesy University of Wisconsin, Section of Cardiology.)

29

Cardiomyopathy

When a patient presents with the classic findings of left ventricular failure in the absence of congenital heart disease or hypertension or without abnormalities indicative of disease involving the coronary arteries, heart valves, or pericardium, a presumptive diagnosis of cardiomyopathy is often made.[5]

Cardiomyopathy refers to a heterogeneous group of diseases that have a common abnormality in the structure and/or function of the myocardium.[7] Diseases of the heart that may involve the myocardium (e.g., hypertension, coronary insufficiency, valvular malfunction, or rheumatic heart disease) have been excluded from this discussion.

CLASSIFICATION OF CARDIOMYOPATHIES

Primary cardiomyopathies are divided on the basis of their clinical and hemodynamic features into three types[8]: congestive, hypertrophic, and restrictive (Table 29-1).

Congestive cardiomyopathy consists of a marked destruction of the ventricular myocardium that leads to a dilated left ventricular cavity, a normal or near normal septal and posterior wall thickness, and a diffusely hypokinetic left ventricle resulting in a reduced shortening fraction. Idiopathic congestive cardiomyopathy is a nonspecific diagnosis, and there are no characteristics that differentiate it from other myocardial diseases with a similar end point of congestive failure. Possible causes for the disease include excessive long-term alcohol consumption, ischemic cardiomyopathy, and nutritional deficiencies. Symptoms include dyspnea, chest pain, palpitations, syncope, and emboli. Clinical signs of cardiac hypertrophy and progressive (usually irretractable) heart failure are evident in this disease.

Table 29-1. Echocardiographic findings in the three types of cardiomyopathy

	Con-gestive	Hyper-trophic	Restrictive
LV cavity	I	D or N	N
LV wall thickness	N	I	I
LV contractility	D	I or N	N or D

Modified from DeMaria, A.N., et al.: Am. J. Cardiol. **46:** 1224, 1980.
Code:
LV = Left ventricle
I = Increased
D = Decreased
N = Normal

Restrictive cardiomyopathy is an infiltrative myocardial disease associated with endomyocardial fibrosis, amyloidosis, scleroderma, or hemochromatosis. The left ventricle hypertrophies concentrically but maintains a normal cavity size. Left ventricular filling is impaired, which causes a reduction of left ventricular emptying secondary to a decreased contractile performance.

Hypertrophic cardiomyopathy presents as a thick-walled left ventricular chamber with septal hypertrophy, a reduced or normal left ventricular cavity size, and a marked decrease in contractility of the septum with a normal to hyperkinetic left ventricular contractile pattern. The primary abnormality consists of impaired left ventricular filling frequently accompanied by an obstruction to the left ventricular outflow tract by the mitral valve leaflets in systole.

ETIOLOGIC CLASSIFICATION[5]

Because disease states associated with primary myocardial involvement characteristically result in a specific category of cardiomyopathy, knowing the nature of the process in a patient can enable one to restrict the possible causes[7]:

1. Idiopathic cardiomyopathy
2. Familial cardiomyopathy
3. Endocardial fibroelastosis
4. African endomyocardial fibrosis
5. Postpartum heart disease
6. Alcoholic cardiomyopathy
7. Beer drinker's cardiomyopathy
8. Catecholamine cardiomyopathy
9. Arsenical cardiomyopathy

In patients with congestive cardiomyopathy one should evaluate the possibility of infectious causes, inflammatory processes, toxins (alcohol), skeletal muscle disorders, or myocardial processes associated with pregnancy.

Restrictive cardiomyopathy is most often caused by disorders like amyloidosis, hemochromatosis, and glycogen storage diseases that result in infiltration of the myocardium by foreign substances[7]:

1. Scleroderma
2. Amyloidosis
3. Sarcoidosis
4. Lupus erythematosus
5. Necrotizing arteritis or angiitis
6. Neuromuscular diseases
7. Hurler's syndrome
8. Hemochromatosis
9. Pompe's disease

Hypertrophic cardiomyopathy has been shown to be of genetic origin, being transmitted usually as an autosomal dominant trait.

CONGESTIVE CARDIOMYOPATHY

Generalized cardiac dilation with decreased cardiac output secondary to hypokinesia is characteristic of congestive cardiomyopathy. Clot formation may be found in the ventricular cavity.

There are several distinguishing characteristics of this disease seen on the echocardiogram:

Primary findings
  Dilated cardiac chambers
  Decreased contractility of left ventricle
  Occasional paradoxical septal wall motion
Secondary findings
  Dilated left atrium
  Double-diamond appearance of mitral valve by M-mode
  Altered PR-AC interval, with elevated left ventricular end diastolic pressure
  Decreased excursion of aortic root secondary to low cardiac output

Along with gross cardiac dilation there is decreased amplitude of the mitral valve (Fig. 29-1). In many cases the anterior and posterior leaflets assume the same small amplitude, termed the *double diamond* pattern, by M-mode (Fig. 29-2). This ability to record both leaflets simultaneously is due to the ventricular dilation and slight cardiac rotation. In addition, multiple echoes that arise from the chordal structures are recorded in the systolic and diastolic segments (Fig. 29-3). The systolic segment (C-D) is flattened. The distance from the E point on the anterior leaflet to the interventricular septum (the LVOT) is enlarged (Fig. 29-4). The aortic root motion is decreased, and the cusps do not open as wide secondary to decreased cardiac output (Fig. 29-5). The right-side structures, tricuspid and pulmonary valves, are easily recorded due to the chamber hypertrophy (Figs. 29-6 and 29-7).

Two-dimensional echo can image a greater area of the left ventricular myocardium (Fig. 29-8). Thus it has been useful in distinguishing areas of segmental asynergy from congestive cardiomyopathy in patients with coronary artery disease. It has also provided a means of recognizing left ventricular mural thrombi, which frequently may be associated with congestive cardiomyopathy.

Alcoholic cardiomyopathy

It has been reported that, because of the injurious effects produced by alcohol or its components, alcohol and heart disease may be directly related. Indirectly cardiac problems may result from inadequate diet or lowered resistance. The exact relationship between alcohol and heart disease is as yet unknown; however, an alcoholic history and primary myocardial disease are the basis for the diagnosis of alcoholic cardiomyopathy.

Clinical manifestations of cardiomyopathy are categorized depending on the dominance of either nutritional or toxic effects. Characteristically the nutritional effect shows dilation of the peripheral vascular system with low resistance, dilated veins, edema, and cardiac enlargement. The toxic manifestations are arrhythmias, myocardial hypertrophy, and heart failure.

In an attempt to determine characteristic findings, echocardiograms were obtained in patients with nonischemic cardiomyopathy. The diagnosis was based primarily on radiographic demonstration of cardiac enlargement in the absence of significant occlusive coronary artery disease or valvular disease by arteriography. The study demonstrated an increased size of the left ventricular cavity, in both systole and diastole, with a decreased ejection fraction. The posterior wall of the left ventricle and the septum tended to be thin with decreased mobility. The anterior and posterior leaflets of the mitral valve were readily discernible and demonstrated diminished opening and closing amplitudes. There was generalized cardiac enlargement of all the chambers. These results were compared with those from patients who had ischemic cardiomyopathy in the absence of other disease, and no reliable differentiation was found.

Text continued on p. 505.

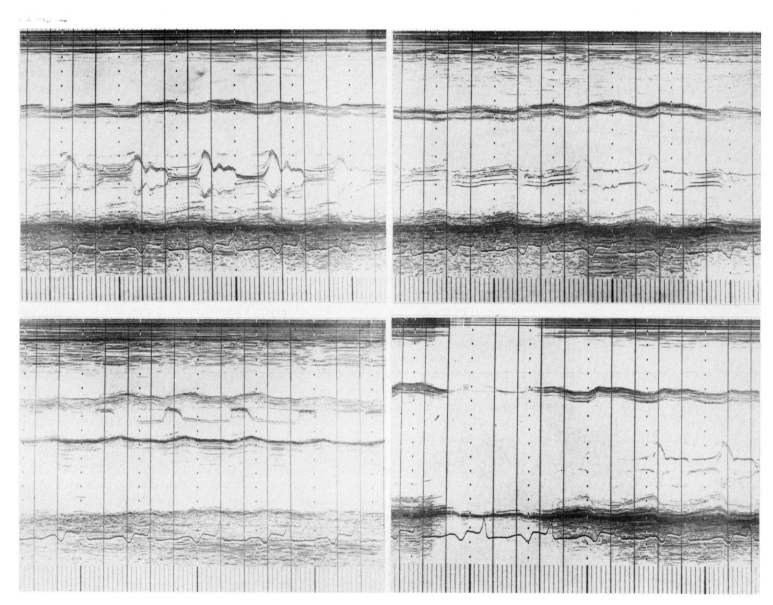

Fig. 29-1. A 35-year-old black who first came to the hospital with the primary complaint of dyspnea on exertion. Cardiac catheterization revealed four chamber cardiac enlargement with elevated pressures. The ventricular contractility was markedly decreased, as were the cardiac output and cardiac index. A history of alcohol abuse most likely gave rise to the congestive cardiomyopathy. The M-mode echocardiogram demonstrated cardiac enlargement with decreased contractility. The septum and posterior wall were thin, and there was increased distance from the E point to the septum.

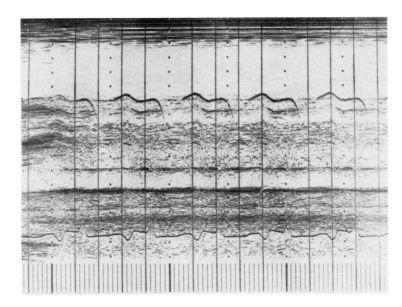

Fig. 29-1, cont'd. For legend see opposite page.

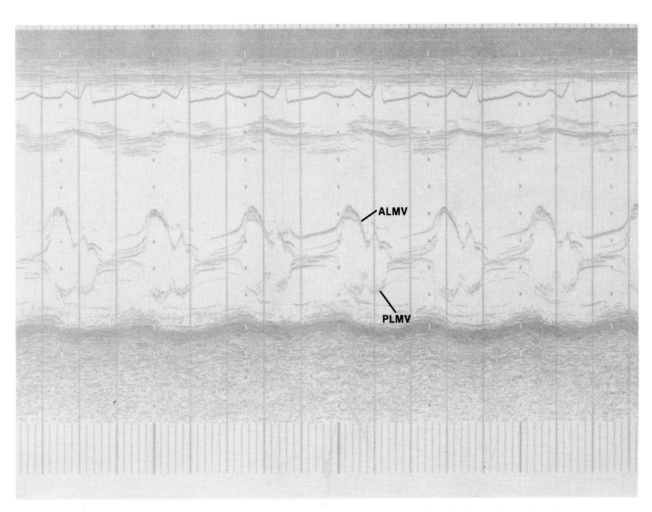

Fig. 29-2. Double diamond appearance of the anterior and posterior mitral valve in a patient with cardiomyopathy.

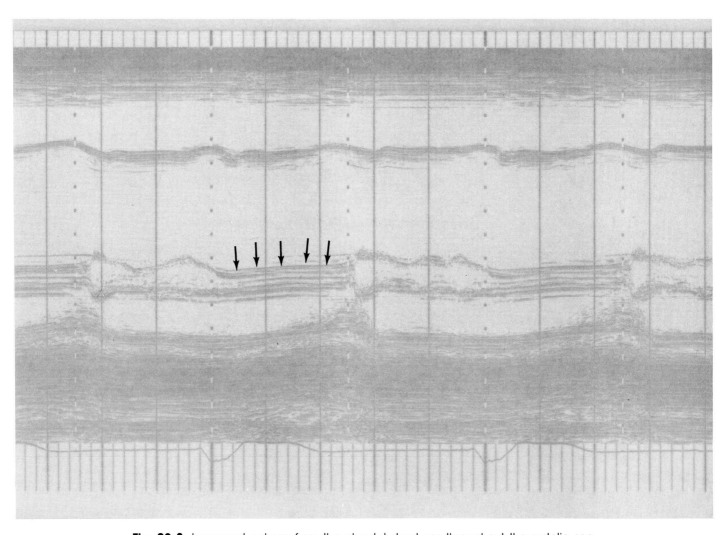

Fig. 29-3. Increased echoes from the chordal structures throughout the systolic segment *(arrows).*

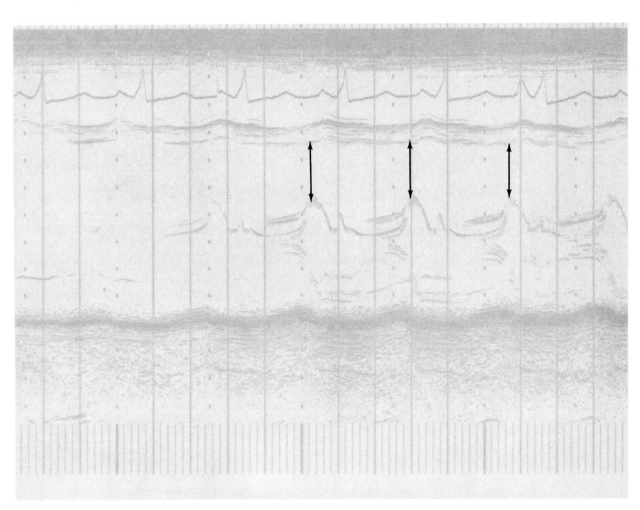

Fig. 29-4. Increased distance from the E point to the interventricular septum.

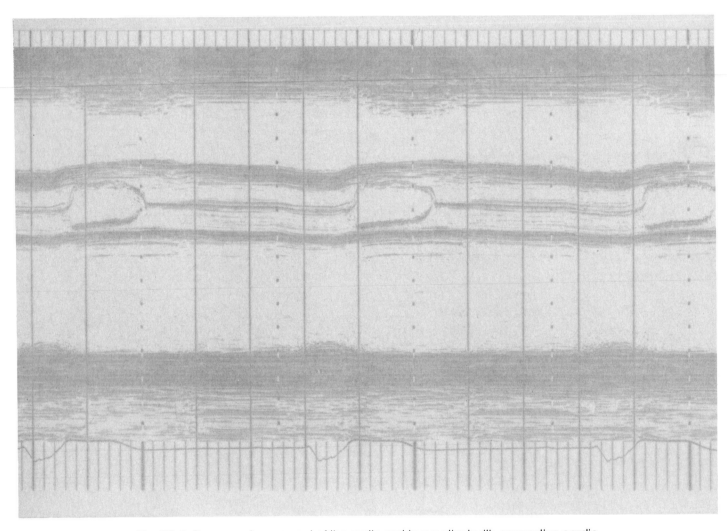

Fig. 29-5. Decreased movement of the aortic root in a patient with congestive cardio-myopathy.

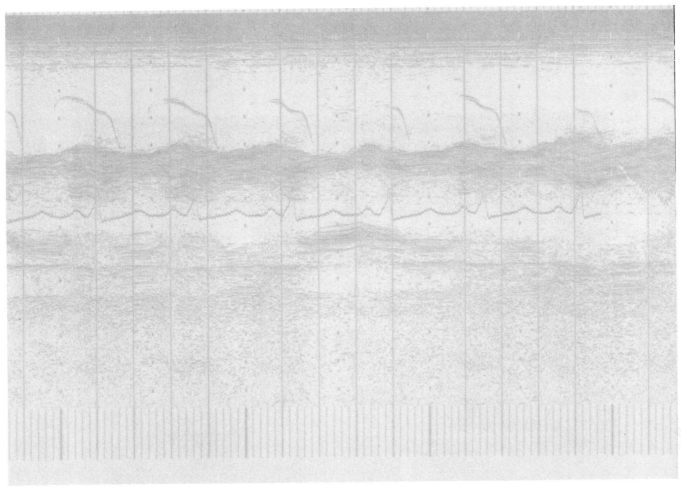

Fig. 29-6. The prominent right side of the heart permits easy visualization of the pulmonary valve.

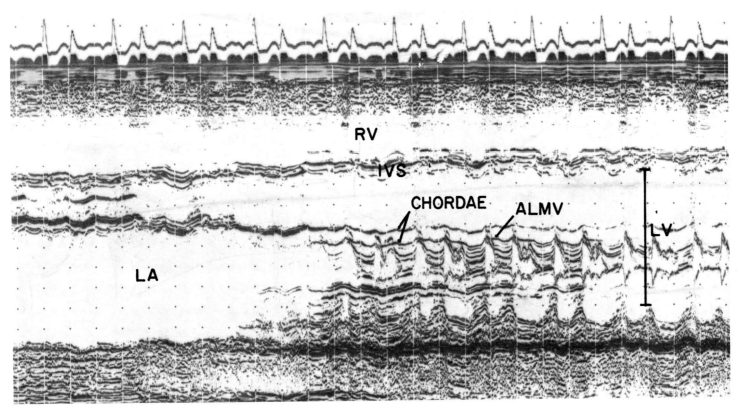

Fig. 29-7. Composite scan from the left atrium to the left ventricle in a patient with end-stage cardiomyopathy. Note the chamber enlargement, double diamond of mitral apparatus, increased echoes in systole, increased distance from the E point to the septum, decreased movement of the aortic root, and decreased septal contractility.

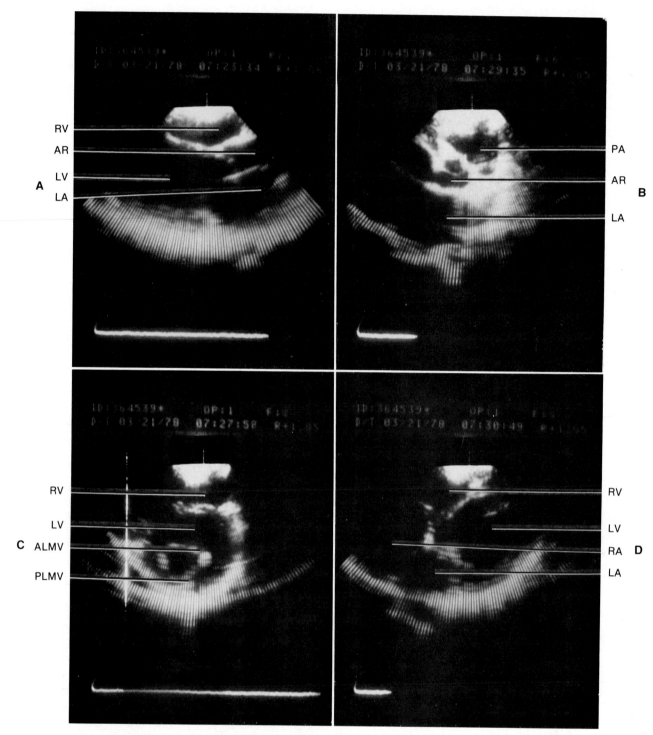

Fig. 29-8. Two-dimensional images of the patient in Fig. 29-7. **A,** Long axis view showing cardiac dilation. **B,** Short axis toward the base of the heart showing prominent pulmonary artery, aorta with cusps, and enlarged left atrium. **C,** Short axis at level of mitral apparatus showing increased distance from the E point to the septum. **D,** Modified apical four chamber of the dilated heart.

RESTRICTIVE CARDIOMYOPATHY

Patients with restrictive cardiomyopathy manifest echographic patterns that are similar to patterns of both congestive and hypertrophic types.[5] The left ventricle is normal unless the myocardium hypertrophies to encroach on the cavity. Wall thickening is symmetric, with the septum and posterior wall equally hypertrophied.

Two-dimensional echo has found its greatest utility in the evaluation of restrictive cardiomyopathy as regards the differentiation from hypertrophic cardiomyopathy and in the demonstration of right ventricular and biatrial involvement in infiltrative processes such as amyloidosis.[5]

HYPERTROPHIC CARDIOMYOPATHY

Asymmetric septal hypertrophy has been reported as hypertrophy of the septum disproportional to the free wall of the left ventricle.[9,10,13] The septum may so bulge that it actually encroaches on the left ventricular outflow tract (Fig. 29-9).

Pathologic evaluation of the septum shows a bizarre arrangement of the muscle fibers characteristic of this condition. The ventricle is small (due to the hypertrophied septum), irregularly shaped, and hyperactive. The posterior wall is much more hyperactive than the poorly contractile septum.

The mitral valve function is altered; there may be signs of mitral regurgitation or obstructive disease, including a systolic anterior motion (SAM).

Clinical findings

The disease is hereditary and has various manifestations. Typical symptoms are murmurs suggestive of obstruction and mitral regurgitation. A fourth heart sound may be present. Other symptoms include dizziness, fainting, fatigue, and chest pain.

Many patients may be asymptomatic, with no obstruction to the outflow tract. Some patients may experience pain, but no obstruction is found. The degree of obstruction depends on the narrowing of the left ventricular outflow tract at the onset of systole.

Other atypical clinical findings may include a nonejection click and murmur (suggestive of mitral prolapse) or chest pain that in many cases tends to simulate coronary artery disease.

The symptoms may be elicited by a Valsalva maneuver or amyl nitrite to increase the degree of obstruction (or intensity of the murmur).

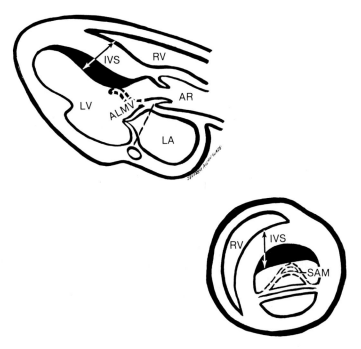

Fig. 29-9. Schematic of septal hypertrophy as it encroaches upon the left ventricular outflow tract.

Echographic findings

One of the most consistent M-mode echographic findings in patients with hypertrophic cardiomyopathy is asymmetric septal hypertrophy or a disproportional thickening of the interventricular septum (1.3 to 1.5 times greater than the left ventricular posterior wall).[5]

Primary echo findings
  Asymmetric septal hypertrophy (ASH)
  Decreased septal wall motion
  Systolic anterior motion (SAM) of mitral valve with or without obstruction
Secondary echo findings
  Midsystolic closure of aortic valve secondary to left ventricular outflow tract (LVOT) obstruction
  Decreased left ventricular diameter
  Increased left atrial size with mitral regurgitation
  Decreased E-F slope of mitral valve secondary to decreased left ventricular compliance

In these patients the sonographer must be careful to measure the true thickness of the septum, especially along the right border (Fig. 29-10). There are many trabeculations along the right septal border and also several echoes from the tricuspid apparatus that can be confused if proper technique is not utilized. Another pitfall in M-mode diagnosis of septal thickness is the problem of not knowing exactly what plane of the septum the beam is traversing. If it is tangential to the septum, a larger diameter will be recorded and a false-abnormal ratio may be created.

Two-dimensional echography has allowed the sonographer a more precise view of the septum and a better opportunity to assess septal thickness and contractility. DeMaria et al.[5] studied a group of patients with ASH and found that most exhibited a gradual increase in septal thickness beginning at the base, reaching its greatest extent in the middle third just at or below the tips of the mitral leaflets, and tapering gradually toward the apex. In addition, these workers found the hypertrophic process to involve the anterior free wall of the left ventricle as well as the interventricular septum in more than half the patients studied.

Recently there have been reports of a change in the acoustic properties of the septal echoes in patients with hypertrophic cardiomyopathy.[4,17] More work will be done in this area as tissue characterization of heart muscle is clinically analyzed and computerized.

The abnormal septum/posterior wall ratio of 1.3:1 is not absolutely diagnostic of ASH. Other problems with this asymmetric abnormality include an inferior myocardial infarction, a maternal diabetic fetal heart,[16] a variety of congenital or acquired anomalies with right ventricular hypertrophy, long-

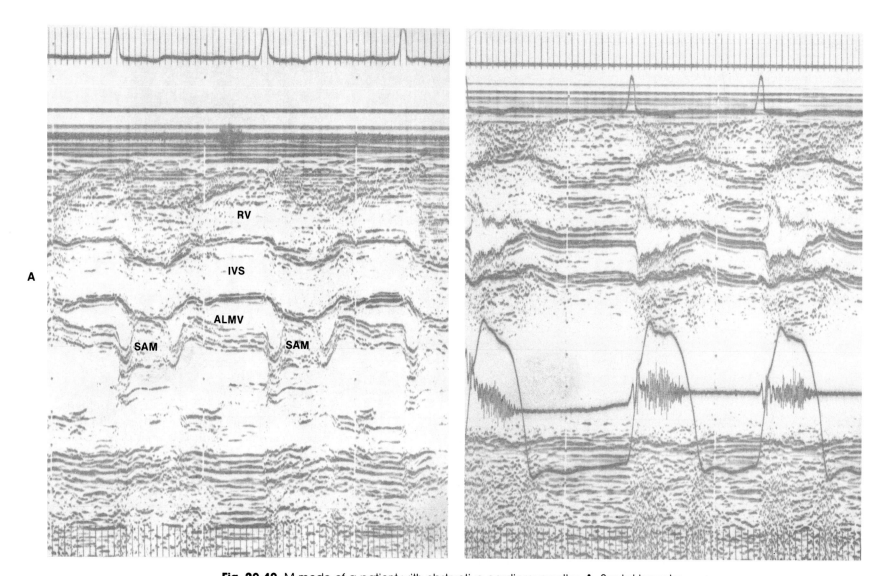

A

Fig. 29-10. M-mode of a patient with obstructive cardiomyopathy. **A,** Septal hypertrophy with complete obstruction to the outflow tract (by SAM). **B,** The aortic root in midsystolic closure of the leaflets secondary to obstruction in the LVOT. **C,** Sweep to the ventricular cavity demonstrating the abnormal septum/posterior wall ratio. A small posterior pericardial effusion, *pce,* is present.

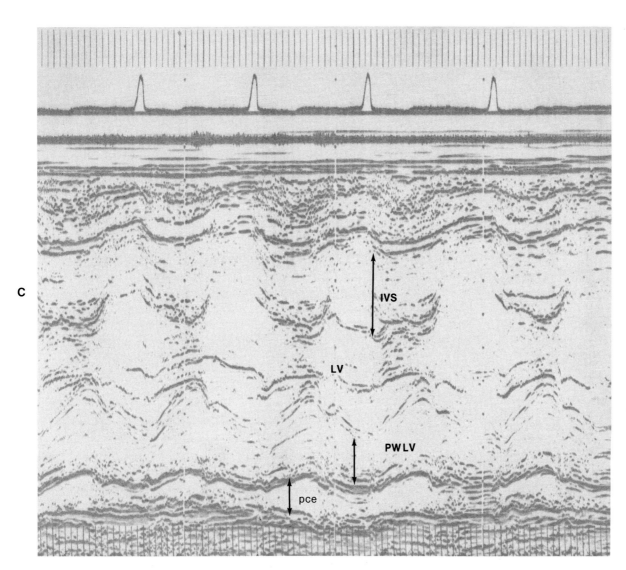

C

Fig. 29-10, cont'd. For legend see opposite page.

standing hypertension (especially in hemodialysis patients),[1] concentric hypertrophy due to pressure overload, and a rare intracardiac tumor that may involve the septum more than the posterior left ventricular wall.[14]

The two-dimensional echo can identify the site of a surgical myotomy and myectomy and can evaluate the amount of septal tissue removed at surgery[17,21] (Fig. 29-11). It also is

useful in performing preoperative and postoperative studies on such patients to evaluate their degree of obstruction and subsequent surgical improvement.

The septal hypertrophy and abnormal contractility of hypertrophic cardiomyopathy may produce an abnormal overall ventricular function.[23] The hypertrophy reduces the left ventricular compliance, and the relaxation and filling patterns are abnormal.[20]

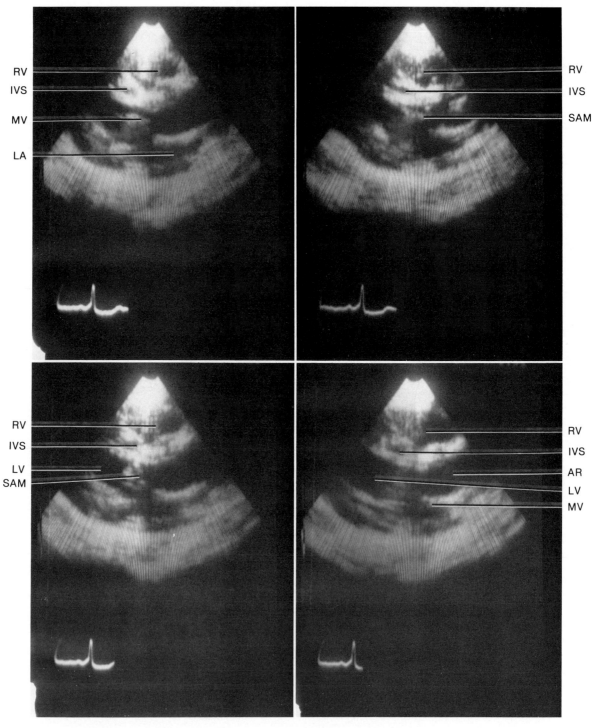

Fig. 29-11. Two-dimensional view of a patient with obstructive hypertrophic cardiomyopathy after myotomy. Long axis views of the left ventricular cavity in various phases of obstruction. The patient still had a prominent SAM following surgery.

Left ventricular outflow obstruction. In hypertrophic cardiomyopathy a common occurrence is dynamic obstruction of the left ventricular outflow tract. In this case the anterior leaflet of the mitral valve moves anteriorly toward the septum shortly after the onset of systole and then returns to its normal position just before the onset of ventricular diastole (Figs. 29-12 and 29-13).

DeMaria et al.[5] reported from their study that the site of anterior motion appears to be heterogeneous. In most cases the two-dimensional echo indicated that the SAM involved the tips of the mitral valve leaflets at the junction of the chordae tendineae as identified by the point of coaptation of the mitral leaflets. The SAM usually also involved the chordae themselves, and in a small minority of cases it appeared to involve the chordae exclusively. The intraventricular obstruction is related to malposition of the papillary muscles, resulting in an anterior displacement of the mitral apparatus that decreases the size of the left ventricular outflow tract and on which is superimposed a marked tethering at the tips of the mitral valve leaflets.[5]

When SAM does touch the septum to a point that it becomes flat, one can be reasonably sure that a high degree of obstruction exists.[12] If the leaflet moves upward and close to the septum and then drops backward without reaching a plateau, a lesser degree of obstruction probably exists.[7]

Technique. To record the abnormal mitral valve SAM, the beam should be directed deep into the left ventricle. The best location is at the edge of the leaflets. Usually the beam is directed through the left ventricular rather than the left atrial wall.

Since the outflow obstruction is classically dynamic, it may not always be present at rest. Thus provocation maneuvers such as Valsalva, amyl nitrite, intravenous isoproterenol, or even a noninvasively induced premature ventricular systole brings out the SAM when it may be absent at rest.

Other conditions reported to be associated with ASH (obstructive) include pericardial effusion and a calcified mitral anulus (Fig. 29-14).

SAM without hypertrophic obstruction. Other causes for a pseudo-SAM may be seen by echo and may be a nonspecific reaction to left ventricular hypertrophy or to any distortion of the ventricular cavity[3] (Fig. 29-15).

Such conditions include transposition of the great arteries, mitral valve prolapse, and newborn infants of diabetic mothers. The SAM is usually due to a floppy chordal structure seen in systole and differs from the normal obstructive SAM in that it does not leave and return to the baseline but floats anterior to the systolic segment of the valve.

Text continued on p. 514.

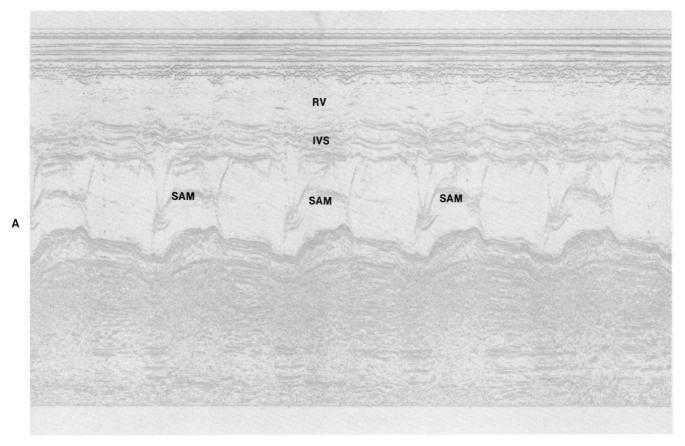

Fig. 29-12. Hypertrophic obstructive cardiomyopathy. **A,** Septal hypertrophy with complete SAM of the chordal structures. *Continued.*

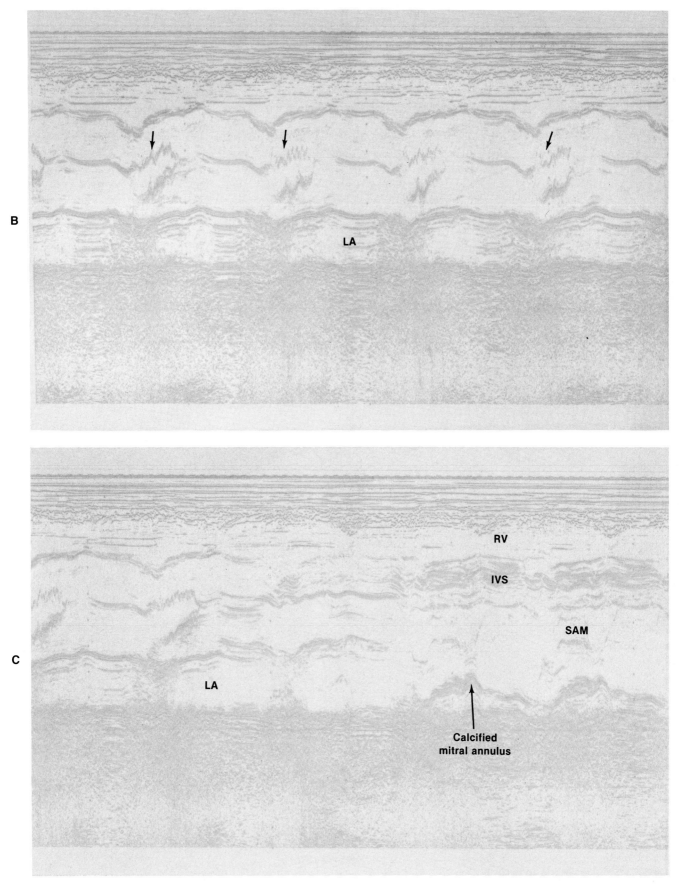

Fig. 29-12, cont'd. B, Midsystolic closure of the aortic cusps. **C,** Calcified mitral anulus (annulus).

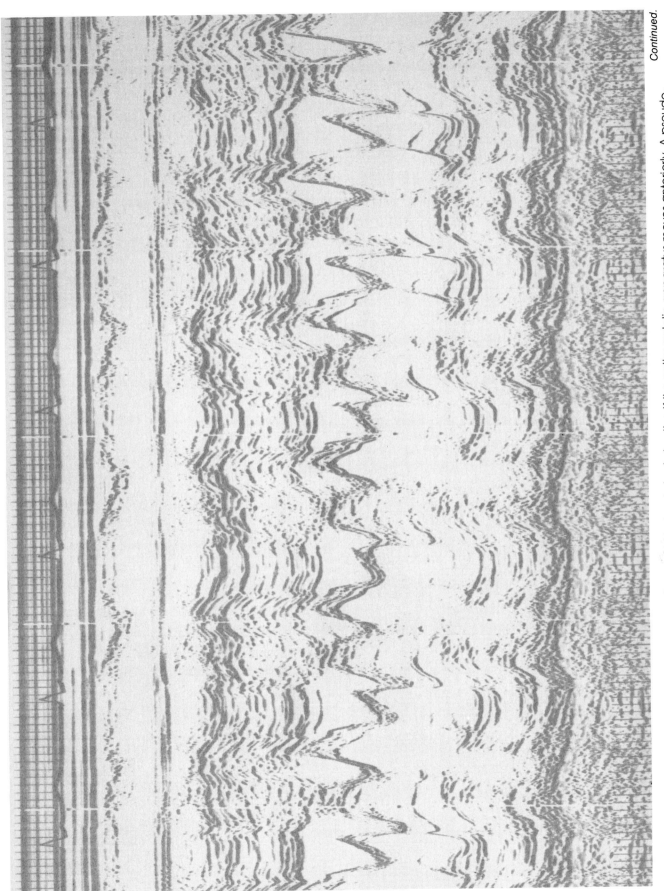

Fig. 29-13. The presence of SAM may be evaluated as truly obstructive if the entire systolic apparatus moves anteriorly. A pseudo-SAM would not assume this pattern.

Continued.

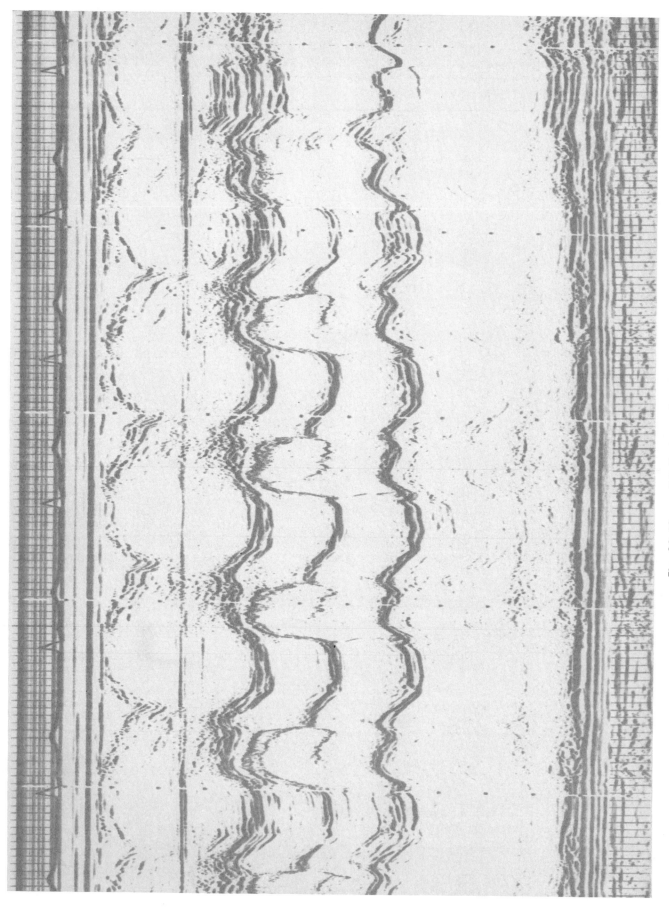

Fig. 29-13, cont'd. For legend see p. 511.

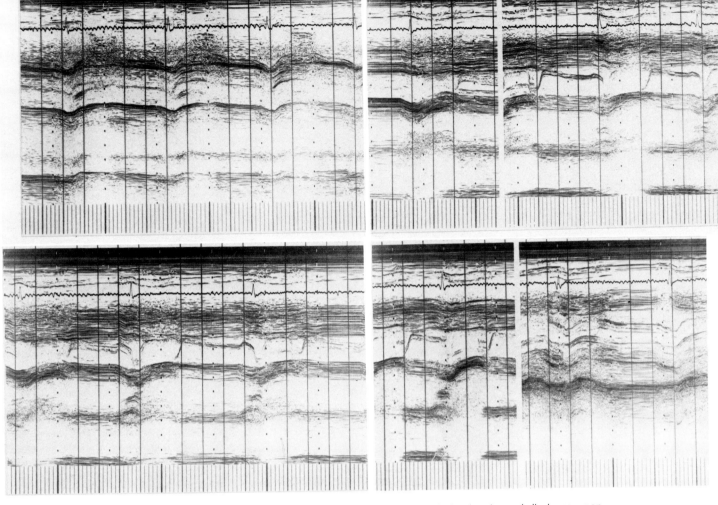

Fig. 29-14. An elderly woman admitted for evaluation of chest pain and dizziness upon exertion. She had a history of rheumatic fever and previous myocardial infarction. Her symptoms had gotten progressively worse. The echocardiogram demonstrated obstructive hypertrophic cardiomyopathy with a calcified mitral anulus.

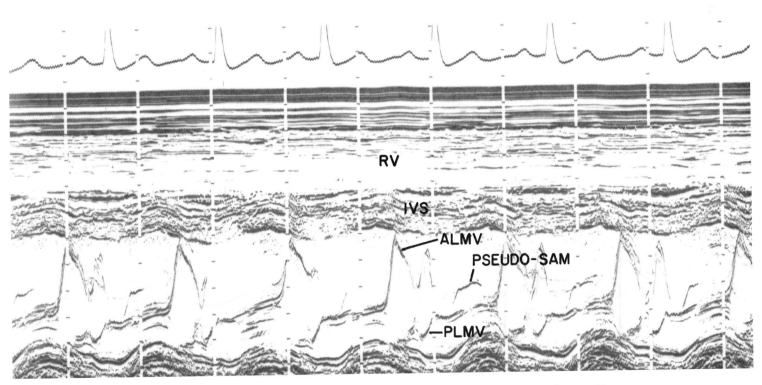

Fig. 29-15. A pseudo-SAM may be seen in a patient who has an anterior prolapse of the posterior leaflet or in whom the chordal apparatus flips in and out of the transducer path. This finding has also been reported in patients with concentric hypertrophy.

SUMMARY

Echocardiography has assumed an important role in the identification of primary myocardial disease. The specific M-mode and two-dimensional characteristics of congestive, restrictive, and hypertrophic cardiomyopathy have been presented. Two-dimensional echo has contributed especially to the classification of hypertrophic cardiomyopathy and has helped distinguish true septal hypertrophy from concentric hypertrophy or artifactual thickening. Additional tissue characterization and computer analysis may aid in further classifying these conditions.

REFERENCES

1. Abbasi, A.S., Slaughter, J.C., and Allen, N.W.: Asymmetric septal hypertrophy in patients on long-term dialysis, Chest **74**:548, 1978.
2. Borer, J.S., Henry, W.L., and Epstein, S.E.: Echocardiographic observations in patients with systemic infiltrative disease involving the heart, Am. J. Cardiol. **39**:184, 1977.
3. Buckley, B.H., and Fortuin, N.J.: Systolic anterior motion of the mitral valve without asymmetric septal hypertrophy, Chest **69**:694, 1976.
4. Clark, C.E., Henry, W.L., and Epstein, S.E.: Familial prevalence and genetic transmission of idiopathic hypertrophic subaortic stenosis, N. Engl. J. Med. **289**:709, 1973.
5. DeMaria, A.N., Bommer, W., Lee, G., et al.: Value and limitations of two-dimensional echocardiography in assessment of cardiomyopathy, Am. J. Cardiol. **46**:1224, 1980.
6. Feigenbaum, H.: Echocardiography, ed. 3, Philadelphia, 1981, Lea & Febiger.
7. Gilbert, E.: Cardiomyopathy. Lecture notes for medical students, University of Wisconsin, Madison, 1981.
8. Gustavson, A., Liedholm, H., and Tylen, U.: Hypertrophic cardiomyopathy: a correlation between echocardiography, angiographic, and hemodynamic findings, Ann. Radiol. (Paris) **20**:419, 1977.
9. Henry, W.L., Clark, C.E., and Epstein, S.E.: Asymmetric septal hypertrophy (ASH): echocardiographic identification of the pathognomonic anatomic abnormality of IHSS, Circulation **47**:225, 1973.
10. Henry, W.L., Clark, C.E., and Epstein, S.E.: Asymmetric septal hypertrophy (ASH): the unifying link in the IHSS disease spectrum. Observations regarding its pathogenesis, pathophysiology, and course, Circulation **47**:827, 1973.
11. Henry, W.L., Clark, C.E., and Glancy, D.L.: Echocardiographic measurement of the LVO gradient in idiopathic hypertrophic subaortic stenosis, N. Engl. J. Med. **288**:989, 1973.
12. Henry, W.L., Clark, C.E., and Griffith, J.M.: Mechanism of LV outflow obstruction in patients with obstructive asymmetric septal hypertrophy, Am. J. Cardiol. **35**:337, 1975.
13. Henry, W.L., Clark, C.E., Roberts, W.C., et al.: Difference in distribution of myocardial abnormalities in patients with obstructive and nonobstructive asymmetric septal hypertrophy (ASH): echocardiographic and gross anatomic findings, Circulation **50**:447, 1974.
14. Isner, J.M., Falcone, M.W., Virmani, R., et al.: Cardiac sarcoma causing ASH and simulating coronary heart disease, Am. J. Med. **66**:1025, 1979.
15. Isshibki, T., Umeda, T., and Machii, K.: Cross-sectional echocardiographic study on the papillary muscles in hypertrophic cardiomyopathy, J. Cardiogr. **8**:631, 1978.
16. Maron, B.J., Verter, J., and Kapur, S.: Disproportionate ventricular septal thickening in the developing normal human heart, Circulation **57**:520, 1978.
17. Martin, R.P., Rakowski, H., French, J., et al.: Idiopathic hypertrophic subaortic stenosis viewed by wide angle, phased array echocardiography, Circulation **59**:1206, 1979.
18. Nanda, N.C., and Gramiak, R.: Clinical echocardiography, St. Louis, 1978, The C.V. Mosby Co.
19. Perloff, J.K.: The cardiomyopathies—current perspectives, Circulation **44**:942, 1971.
20. Sanderson, J.E., Traill, T.A., and St. John Sutton, M.G.: Left ventricular relaxation and filling in hypertrophic cardiomyopathy: an echocardiographic study, Br. Heart J. **40**:596, 1978.
21. Schapira, J.N., Stemple, D.R., Martin, R.P., et al.: Single and two dimensional echocardiographic visualization of the effects of septal myectomy in IHSS, Circulation **58**:850, 1978.
22. Tajik, A.J., Seward, J.B., and Hagler, D.J.: Detailed analysis of hypertrophic obstructive cardiomyopathy by wide-angle two-dimensional sector echocardiography, Am. J. Cardiol. **43**:348, 1979.
23. ten Cate, F.J., Hugenholtz, P.G., and Roelandt, J.: Ultrasound study of dynamic behavior of left ventricle in genetic asymmetric septal hypertrophy, Br. Heart J. **39**:627, 1977.

30 Endocarditis

Endocarditis is an inflammation of the endocardium with superimposed thrombosis, resulting in a grossly visible vegetation. The disease usually involves a heart valve but may also involve mural endocardium and sites of septal defects.

There are four classifications of endocarditis:

1. Rheumatic
2. Infective (bacterial, fungal, rickettsial)
3. Nonbacterial thrombotic
4. Atypical verrucous

This chapter will primarily discuss bacterial endocarditis and its effect on the heart as seen echographically. Two conditions must exist to satisfy the criteria for bacterial endocarditis: (1) There must be a portal of entry for the organism, and (2) there must be conditions suitable for infection.

Suitable circumstances for infection include

a. History of a previous valvulitis (rheumatic, degenerative, idiopathic)
b. Congenital heart lesion (patent ductus arteriosus, ventricular septal defect with endocardial friction, bicuspid aortic valve)
c. Heart surgery (prosthetic valve, septal patch, indwelling catheter)
d. Immunosuppression (treatment of a malignant disease, prolonged use of steroids and antibiotics)
e. Drug addiction

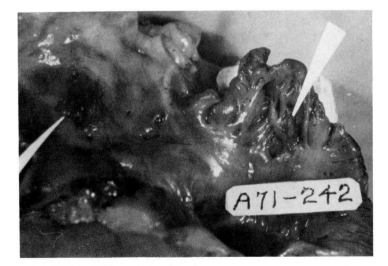

Fig. 30-1. Gross specimen of the tricuspid valve demonstrating bacterial vegetative destruction of the wall and endocardial surface (arrow).

There are two types of infective endocarditis, acute and subacute. *Acute* bacterial endocarditis can occur during a septicemia from organisms such as *Staphylococcus aureus*, *Neisseria gonorrhoeae*, or *Streptococcus pyogenes*. The cardiac valves may be invaded and destroyed by these bacteria. In *subacute* bacterial endocarditis, organisms of a low-grade virulence invade a valve or an area of the endocardium that has been damaged by a previous acquired heart disease such as rheumatic fever or congenital heart defect. The organism can enter the bloodstream as a result of one of several circumstances: dental extraction, apical tooth abscess, diarrhea, osteomyelitis, cardiac surgery, or drug abuse (portal of entry).

Most patients with bacterial endocarditis suffer left heart valvular disease—the aortic valve in 45% of patients, the mitral valve in 35%, and both valves in 19%. The right heart is affected less often—with the tricuspid valve affected more frequently than the pulmonary valve.

PATHOPHYSIOLOGY

The diagnosis of endocarditis is based on clinical findings, the history of predisposing factors, and sustained bacteremia. *Sustained bacteremia* refers to the positive blood cultures obtained from different veins over a short period, and it differentiates bacterial endocarditis from a transient bacteremia (e.g., following the brushing of teeth or a bowel movement).

The presence of pathogens in the bloodstream creates an opportunity for organisms to be deposited on the damaged roughened valves. The organisms are enmeshed in deposits of fibrin and platelets on the endothelium of the valve to form irregular vegetations. These masses may vary in size and shape and become quite large and friable in *Candida* infections (Fig. 30-1). They occur on the downstream side of the damaged valve. The jet effect plays a significant role in the collection of bacteria, on the valves as well as on the chordae tendineae. This effect is related to the insufficiency of one valve, causing a high-pressure source with a low-pressure sink area. The infection usually occurs on the low-pressure side. Thus a patient with aortic insufficiency would have a jet stream from the aortic root into the left ventricle. The stream would flow directly into the chordae tendineae, causing satellite regions of bacterial formation to develop on the chordae*:

Condition	Location of lesion
Coarctation	Downstream wall
Patent ductus arteriosus	Pulmonary artery
A-V fistula	Veins
Aortic insufficiency	Ventricular surface of valves
Mitral insufficiency	Atrial surface of mitral valve
Pulmonary insufficiency	Ventricular surface of pulmonary valve
Tricuspid insufficiency	Atrial surface of tricuspid valve

*From Bittar, N.: Infective endocarditis. Lecture notes for medical students, University of Wisconsin, Madison, 1981.

Sink areas are areas just beyond the point of constriction where forward velocity of the blood is highest and lateral pressure lowest.

Complications of endocarditis may include an aneurysm, perforation, tear, or extensive destruction of the valve. The process may spread to the adjacent mural endocardium or involve the chordae tendineae. The larger more friable vegetations may obstruct the valve orifice or break off to cause large emboli elsewhere in the body.

CLINICAL FEATURES

The common findings in endocarditis are fever, anemia, cardiac murmur, embolic phenomena, splenomegaly, hematuria, nephritis, or elevated rheumatoid factor. The subacute case may present as a fever of unknown origin with only a murmur of anemia. Cardiac findings include changing murmurs (usually over a short period due to the valvular destruction and subsequent regurgitation), cardiac failure, ventricular and muscular involvement (the infection on the aortic valve may spread to the interventricular septum, and an abscess may develop and rupture into the right heart or may interfere with the induction of the cardiac impulse and cause aortic valve block with or without syncope). In addition, there may be a septic abscess of the papillary muscle, with destruction of the mitral ring, or a flail mitral valve apparatus.

ECHOGRAPHIC FINDINGS

The vegetative lesions are of varying size and shape, often pedunculated and rather amorphous. They usually exhibit a distinct motion that is dependent on the motion of the valve. However, if they are very large or pedunculated, they may appear to exhibit motion independent of valvular motion.[1]

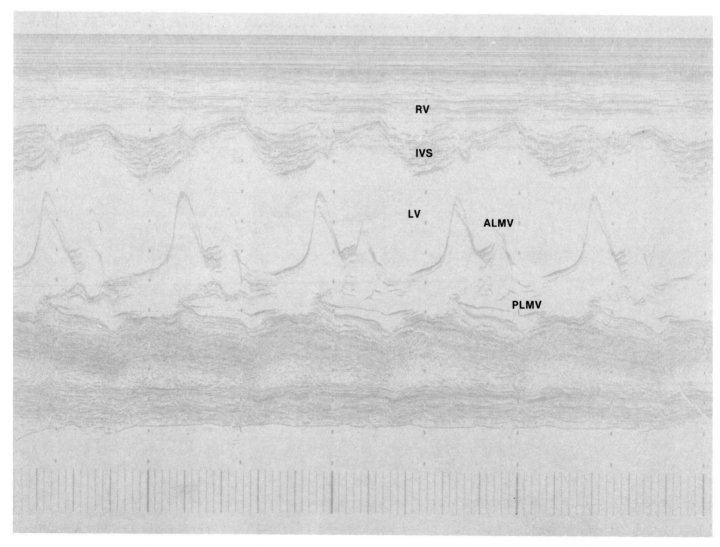

Fig. 30-2. A young patient with aortic vegetations. The shaggy dense echoes are consistently seen in the diastolic period of the aortic cusp closure. Left ventricular enlargement is secondary to aortic insufficiency.

Echographically the vegetative lesions may occur on the leaflet tissue, on the mitral or tricuspid chordae, or on the endocardial surfaces of the ventricular and atrial chambers.

The typical M-mode characteristics of vegetations are shaggy, thick, irregular, bright echoes. The aortic valve may have lesions that appear in systole and/or diastole (Figs. 30-2 and 30-3). The mitral valve may show lesions that originate from the atrial side of either the anterior or the posterior leaflet (Figs. 30-4 and 30-5). Vegetations on the tricuspid valve are usually associated with the anterior leaflet; often there is a mass of echoes somewhat attached to the posterior side of the anterior leaflet (Fig. 30-6). There also may be systolic and/or diastolic flutter. In all valves the vegetations tend not to restrict valvular mobility (Table 30-1).

Text continued on p. 527.

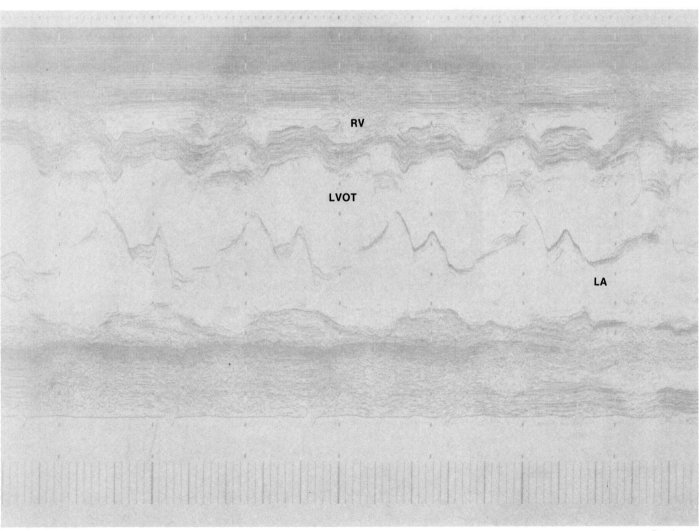

Fig. 30-2, cont'd. For legend see opposite page.

Continued.

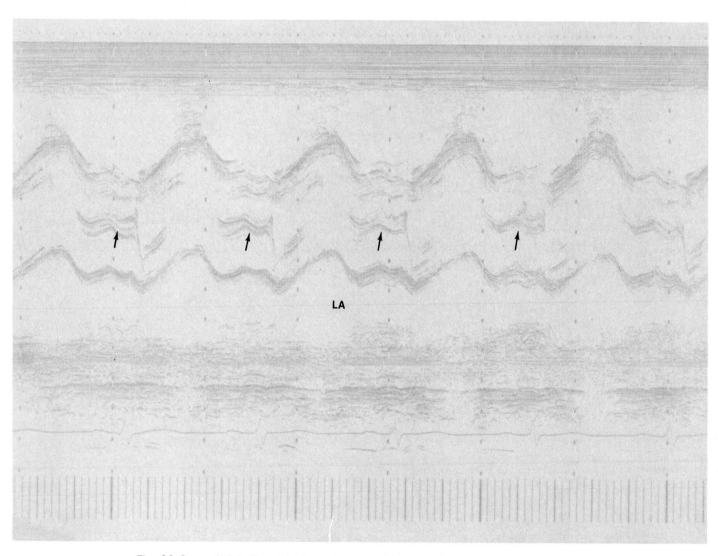

Fig. 30-2, cont'd. Left ventricular enlargement is secondary to aortic insufficiency.

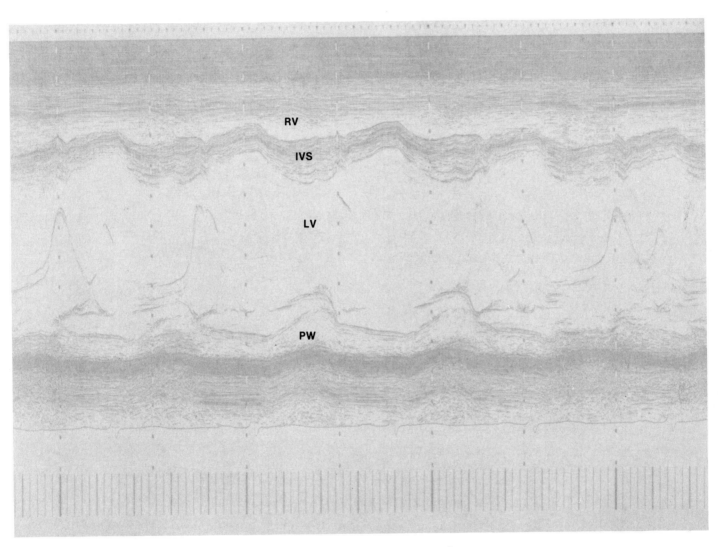

Fig. 30-2, cont'd. For legend see opposite page.

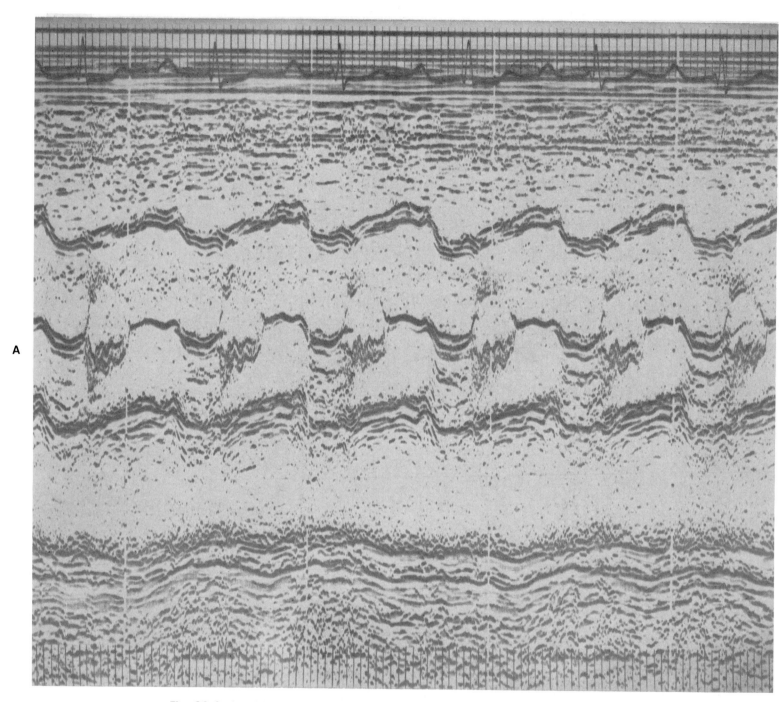

A

Fig. 30-3. An elderly man presented with fever of unknown origin. **A,** Dense echoes were seen throughout areas of the aortic root. It was not certain whether this density was due to calcifications or to a vegetative process. **B,** High-frequency flutter on the anterior leaflet of the mitral valve, due to aortic insufficiency. Combined real time and M-mode evaluation demonstrated a vegetative mass of echoes on the aortic valve. **C,** Parasternal long axis view. **D,** Parasternal short axis of the thickened bicuspid valve *(arrow).*

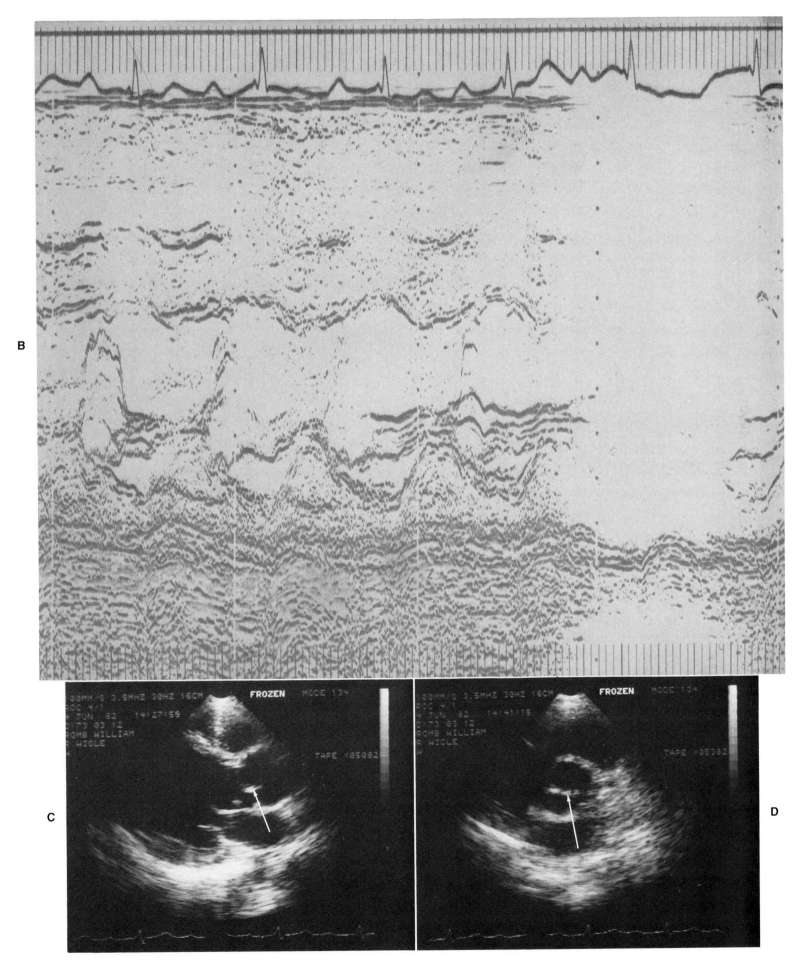

Fig. 30-3, cont'd. For legend see opposite page.

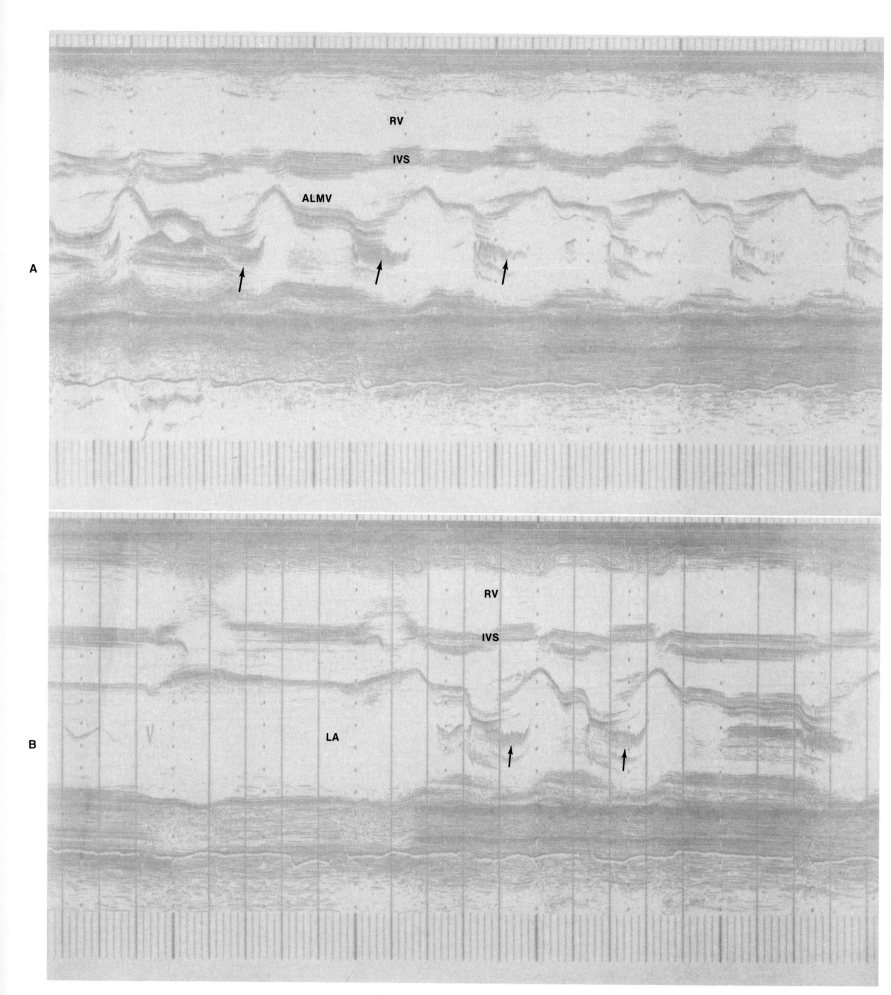

Fig. 30-4. For legend see opposite page.

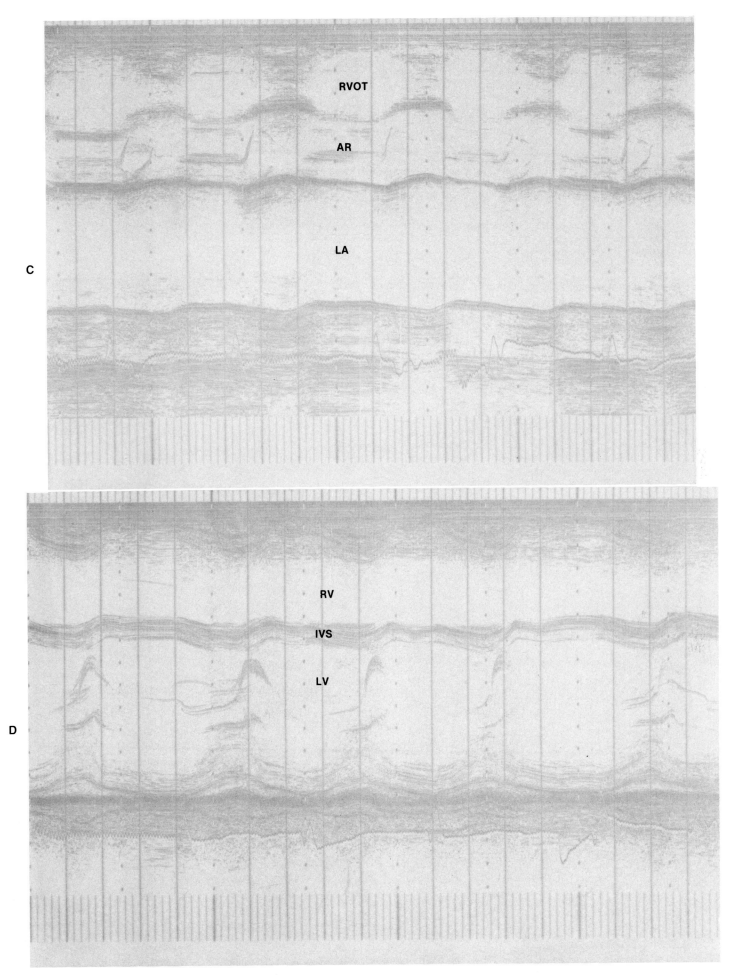

Fig. 30-4. A 29-year-old known drug abuser presented with chills, fever, and seizure episodes. The echocardiogram showed a huge vegetative mass next to the posterior mitral valve. Mitral valve prolapse was evident with left atrial enlargement. **A,** Mitral valve with dense shaggy echoes in the systolic segment *(arrows).* **B,** Sweep from the enlarged left atrium to the mitral valve. **C,** Early closure of the aortic cusps due to mitral regurgitation. **D,** The left ventricular cavity is enlarged. There is also a small posterior pericardial effusion.

Continued.

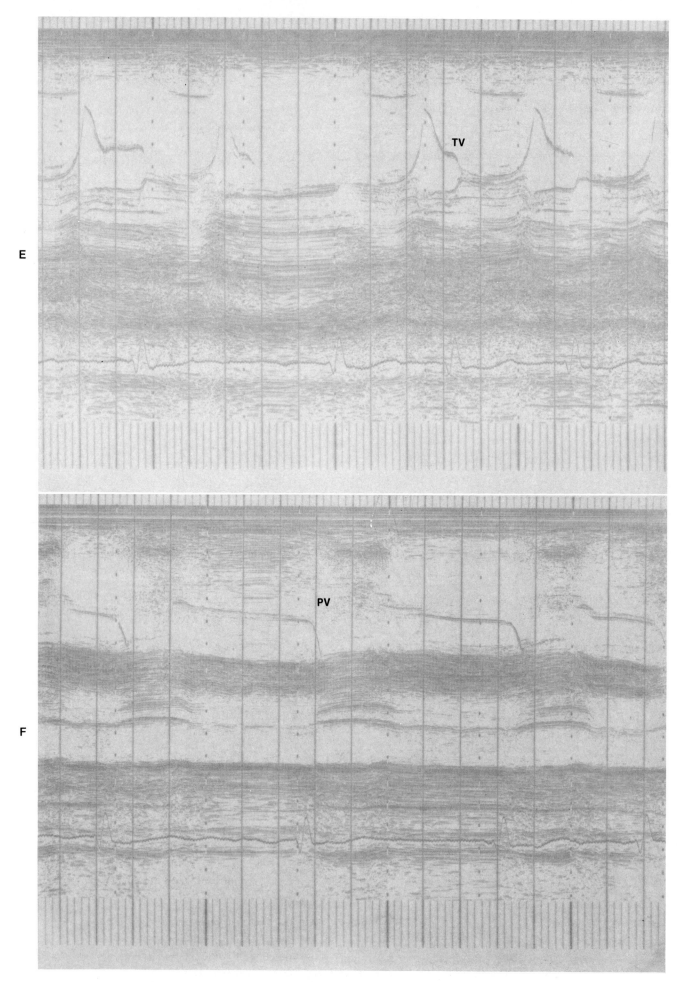

Fig. 30-4, cont'd. E, The right ventricle is slightly dilated, allowing visualization of the anterior and posterior tricuspid valve. **F,** The pulmonary valve shows signs of pulmonary hypertension with a flattened slope and loss of the *a* dip (also called A dip).

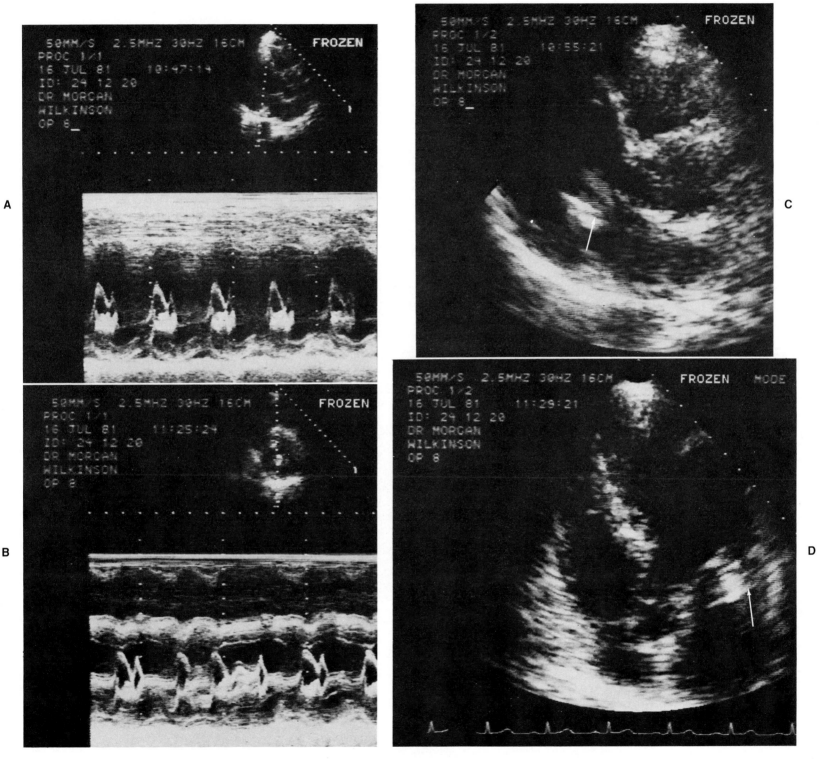

Fig. 30-5. A young woman with a positive blood culture presented for evaluation of her cardiac status. **A** and **B,** M-mode tracings of the mitral valve with a shaggy dense collection of echoes attached to the posterior leaflet. **C,** Parasternal long axis demonstrating the dense collection of echoes *(arrow).* These most likely represent a vegetation. **D,** Apical four chamber of the vegetation *(arrow).*

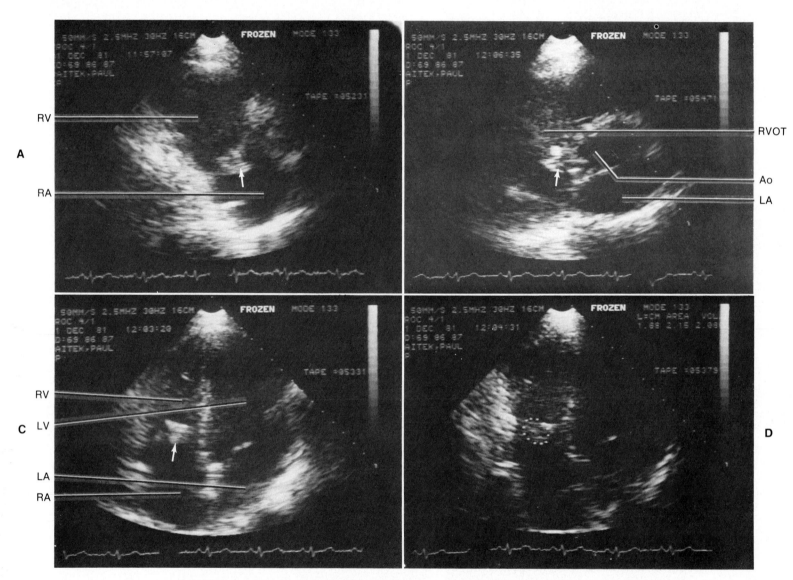

Fig. 30-6. A, Parasternal long axis of the right ventricle, tricuspid valve, and right atrium. Arrow shows a vegetation. **B,** Parasternal short axis view. **C,** Apical four chamber view. **D,** Apical four chamber of a vegetation *(circled).*

Table 30-1. Criteria for echocardiographic diagnosis of endocarditis

Location	Findings
Aortic valve	Shaggy nonuniform thickening in systole or diastole with unrestricted leaflet motion
	Dense shaggy echoes moving across valve and into LVOT
	Flail or ruptured cusps
	Fine diastolic fluttering on ALMV secondary to aortic insufficiency
	Mitral valve preclosure secondary to acute aortic insufficiency
Mitral valve	Thick shaggy echoes attached to or moving behind leaflets demonstrating unrestricted motion
	Systolic flutter of prolapsing segments of mitral valve
	Fuzzy leaflet echoes in left atrial cavity during systole (differentiate from myxoma)
Tricuspid and pulmonary valves	Shaggy thickening of leaflets, demonstrating unrestrictive motion
	Mass of echoes moving with leaflets (dependent motion)
	Rupture of tricuspid chordae
Prosthetic valve	Thick shaggy collection located behind site of attachment of prosthesis to valve ring
	Evidence of severe regurgitation

Indirect signs of endocarditis by echography usually involve rupture of the chordae tendineae to produce a flail leaflet. If posterior leaflet chordal rupture occurs, an early systolic plunge of the leaflet to the posterior left atrial wall will be seen during systole followed by an anterior motion at the onset of diastole. In this case portions of the posterior leaflet may be recorded in the left atrium behind the aorta. Occasionally the flail posterior leaflet will produce multiple diastolic echoes posterior to the anterior leaflet and these may mimic an atrial myxoma.

Other associated abnormalities that can develop during endocarditis are mitral valve preclosure secondary to acute aortic insufficiency, diastolic flutter of the mitral valve secondary to aortic insufficiency, coarse systolic flutter of aortic valve leaflets, localized thickening of the aortic wall secondary to abscess formation, or left ventricular volume overload and hypercontractility.

Questions that must be answered during the echocardiography are whether the abnormal echoes really are vegetations or another disease process that may be mimicking the vegetations and whether the abnormal echoes are real or artifactually produced by incorrect gain settings (Fig. 30-7).

The differential diagnosis should include rheumatic disease of the mitral valve, a flail valve, myxomatous degeneration of the valve, cardiac tumors, and fine fluttering caused by aortic insufficiency.

The two-dimensional echogram permits assessment of the location, size, and morphology of the vegetations. It makes possible examination of both the right and the left sides of the heart for valvular as well as other endocardial involvement (Fig. 30-8). Remember, however, that the lack of a vegetative mass by echo does not rule out bacterial endocarditis. Lesions smaller than 2 mm are difficult to detect by echography. In addition, previous rheumatic heart disease may leave the valves somewhat thickened and thus make it difficult to judge whether the thickening is due to the rheumatic disease or the presence of vegetations on the valves.

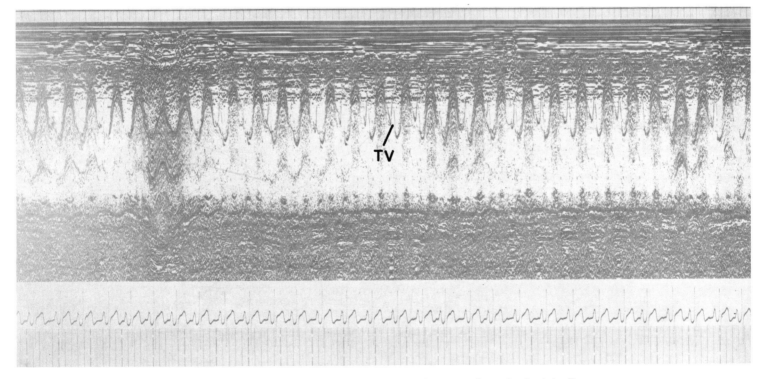

Fig. 30-7. Respiratory echoes can be confusing when seen in early diastole. They appear as equidistant lines at the time of respiration and vary with increased respiratory motion.

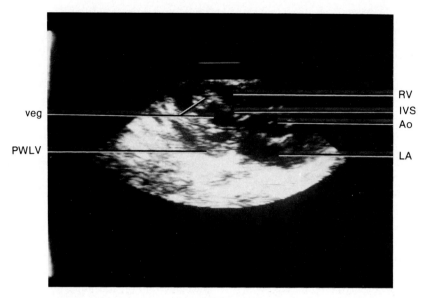

Fig. 30-8. Long axis view in a patient with systemic lupus erythematosus (SLE) and positive blood cultures showing a pedunculated vegetation extending from the ventricular septum. A second vegetation, which was mobile during the cardiac cycle, extends from the papillary muscle. The patient had arterial embolization with gangrene. Both lower extremities were amputated. Neither vegetation was apparent on a subsequent echocardiogram. At postoperative examination, vegetations were adherent to the tricuspid, aortic, and mitral valves and to the walls of the left and right ventricles. It was postulated that these were established Libman-Sacks vegetations associated with SLE to which a second layer of vegetations had become attached.

Other possible sources of error are incorrect equipment settings. If gains are too low, image dropout may occur and the vegetations may actually appear smaller than they really are or may even be missed entirely. On the other hand, excessively high gain settings will cause the image to appear brighter and larger than it really is. The borders may become indistinct and appear to overlap with adjacent valvular tissue, making the echo difficult to interpret.

REFERENCE

1. Martin, R.: Detection of intracardiac masses by cross-sectional echocardiography. In Kisslo, J.A., editor: Two-dimensional echocardiography, New York, 1980, Churchill Livingstone, Inc.

31

Cardiac tumors and thrombi

Cardiac tumors are more frequently metastatic than primary. At autopsy a small percentage of patients will have secondary tumor deposits in the myocardium and pericardium. Metastases from malignant disease elsewhere are 12 times as common as primary tumors of the heart.[1]

Primary tumor. The site of a primary tumor is most often the lung or the breast, which indicates that the tumor is likely to spread locally to involve the heart or pericardium.[3] Metastases seldom affect left ventricular function, although large collections of pericardial fluid may show manifestations of cardiac tamponade.

The most common primary malignant tumors involving the heart are sarcomas of various types. These account for 20% of primary cardiac tumors. The mass usually grows in the right atrium, and death occurs from extension through the wall of the heart into the pericardium rather than from prolapse into the chambers like an atrial myxoma.

Benign tumor. The most common benign cardiac tumor is a myxoma. This comprises 50% of all primary tumors. A myxoma is a polypoid mass of gelatinous tissue usually in the left atrial cavity (Fig. 31-1). It is attached by a pedicle to the fossa ovalis, atrial appendage, or origin of a pulmonary vein.[1] The right atrium is a less common site for atrial myxoma. The right atrial tumor consists of myxomatous tissue with scanty blood vessels and small hemorrhages.[1]

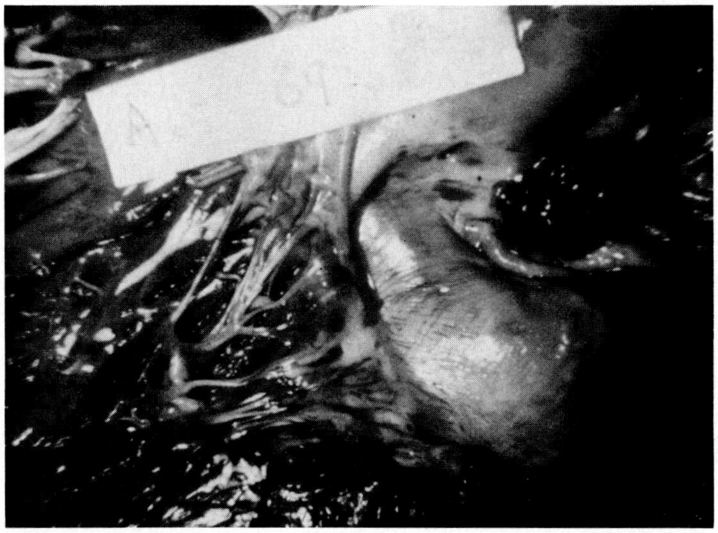

If the myxoma is not totally removed surgically, it may recur. Death can result if fragments of the tumor break off to become systemic or pulmonary emboli.

Other rare cardiac tumors are fibroma, rhabdomyoma, lipoma, and angioma.

CLINICAL FINDINGS

Sarcoma. This tumor presents as malignant pericardial disease that involves retrosternal pain, tachycardia, pulsus paradoxus, raised jugular venous pressure, and an enlarged heart shadow.[1] Death is usually due to cardiac tamponade or cardiac rupture.

Myxoma. The major presenting symptoms of a myxoma are signs of mitral or tricuspid valve obstruction from the tumor's prolapsing into the valve, systemic embolism with possible tumor fragments, chest pain, syncope, and constitutional disturbances (weakness, fatigue, weight loss). In a myxoma the cardiac murmur is often changing, and the tumor plop may be confused with the diastolic rumble of mitral stenosis.

Since the tumor is often pedunculated and mobile, the degree of obstruction to blood flow varies with posture and with hemodynamic events. The patient may have a diastolic murmur in one body position but not in another.

ECHOGRAPHIC EVALUATION OF A CARDIAC MASS

The utilization of two-dimensional echo has aided the diagnosis of cardiac masses. The echo has overcome the narrow or limited field of view seen by M-mode and has proved to be effective in detecting, characterizing, sizing, and locating masses in any of the four cardiac chambers. With two-dimensional echo, images are obtained from multiple transducer positions—long axis, short axis, apical four chamber, and subxyphoid. The cardiac sonographer must be able to differ-

Fig. 31-1. Gross specimen of a left atrial myxoma attached to the left atrial wall.

entiate true lesions from artifacts produced by the instrumentation ("side lobes" by off-axis beams) or from incorrect gain settings. Real mass lesions will remain in the same anatomic position when imaged from different transducer positions, whereas artifacts will disappear[2] (Figs. 31-2 and 31-3).

Small myxomas may be overlooked with M-mode if they do not prolapse through the AV valves or if they are near the base of the atrial cavity. Apical four chamber views allow the sonographer to assess both atrial cavities and interatrial septum to detect the presence of abnormal echoes (Fig. 31-4).

The inferior and superior venae cavae and right atrial cavity may be carefully evaluated for the presence of extension from a primary tumor elsewhere in the body, especially from the kidney.

If only M-mode instrumentation is available, the sonographer should use moderate to high gain settings to image the cardiac structures and perform careful sweeps from the base of the left atrium to the apex of the left ventricle. The absence of a mass formation by M-mode does not exclude the possibility of a cardiac mass. It may be small and out of the way of the beam, or the gain settings may be too low to record its reflective borders (Figs. 31-5 to 31-7).

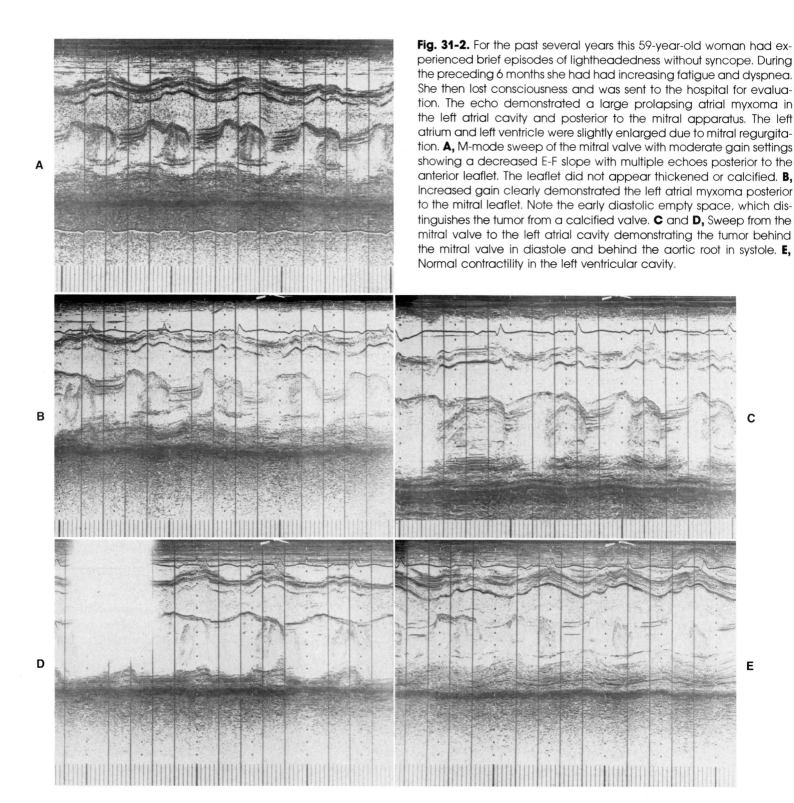

Fig. 31-2. For the past several years this 59-year-old woman had experienced brief episodes of lightheadedness without syncope. During the preceding 6 months she had had increasing fatigue and dyspnea. She then lost consciousness and was sent to the hospital for evaluation. The echo demonstrated a large prolapsing atrial myxoma in the left atrial cavity and posterior to the mitral apparatus. The left atrium and left ventricle were slightly enlarged due to mitral regurgitation. **A,** M-mode sweep of the mitral valve with moderate gain settings showing a decreased E-F slope with multiple echoes posterior to the anterior leaflet. The leaflet did not appear thickened or calcified. **B,** Increased gain clearly demonstrated the left atrial myxoma posterior to the mitral leaflet. Note the early diastolic empty space, which distinguishes the tumor from a calcified valve. **C** and **D,** Sweep from the mitral valve to the left atrial cavity demonstrating the tumor behind the mitral valve in diastole and behind the aortic root in systole. **E,** Normal contractility in the left ventricular cavity.

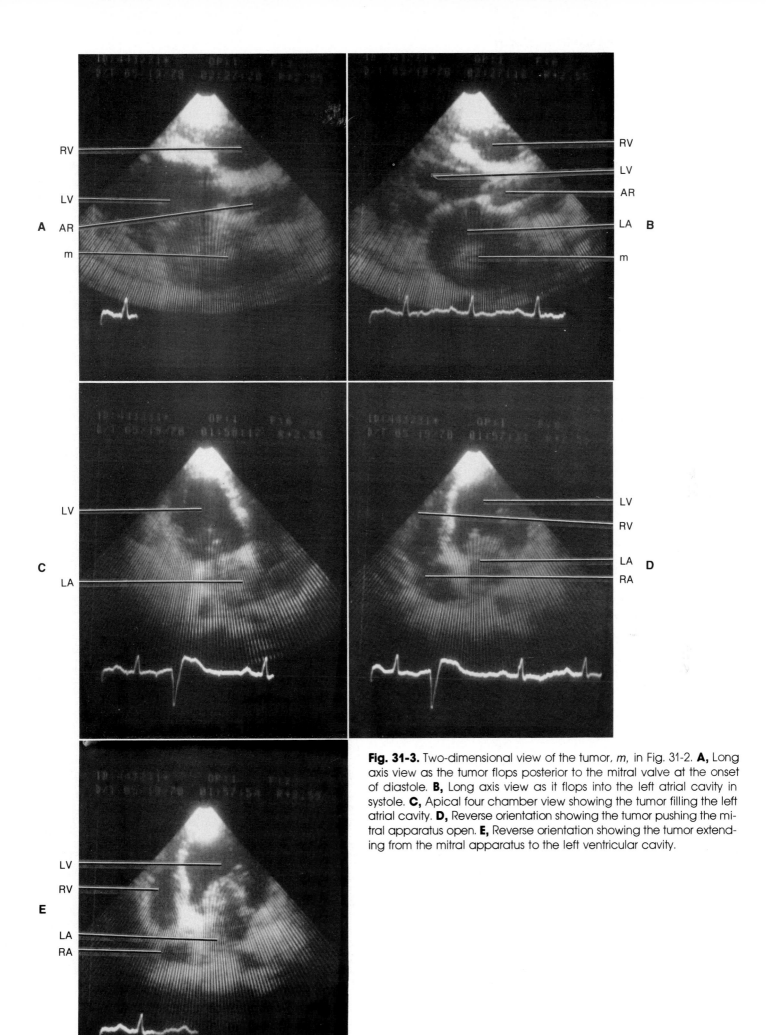

Fig. 31-3. Two-dimensional view of the tumor, *m,* in Fig. 31-2. **A,** Long axis view as the tumor flops posterior to the mitral valve at the onset of diastole. **B,** Long axis view as it flops into the left atrial cavity in systole. **C,** Apical four chamber view showing the tumor filling the left atrial cavity. **D,** Reverse orientation showing the tumor pushing the mitral apparatus open. **E,** Reverse orientation showing the tumor extending from the mitral apparatus to the left ventricular cavity.

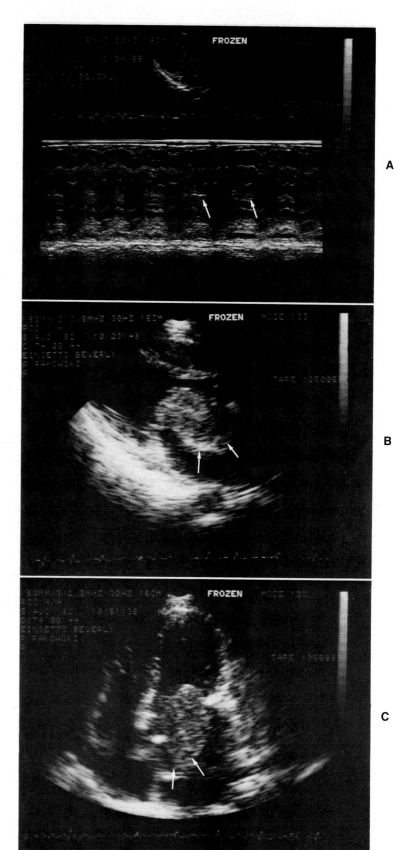

Fig. 31-4. The sonographer must be careful to use adequate gain settings to demonstrate any abnormalities. In **A** the M-mode sweep of the mitral valve shows a decreased E-F slope. As the beam is angled toward the left atrial cavity, the tumor echoes start to appear. Further investigation with the combined real time and M-mode sweep allows the correct gain and transducer position to be used to record the maximum information from the tumor *(arrows)*. **B,** Parasternal long axis view. **C,** Apical four chamber showing the tumor mass flopping from the left atrium into the left ventricle.

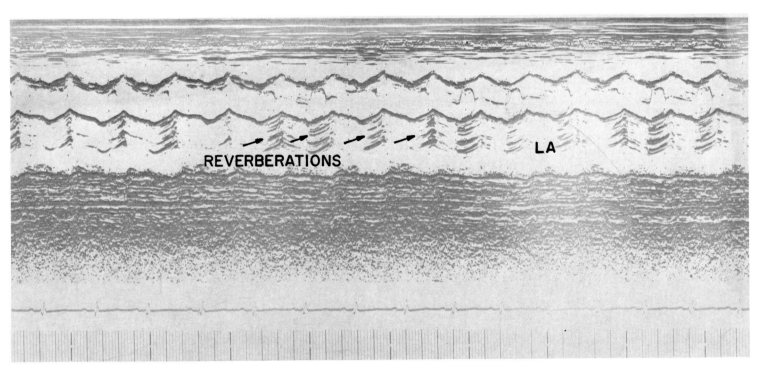

Fig. 31-5. Reverberations within the left atrial cavity may be due to respiration or poor transducer angulation, or to calcification. If careful sweeps are made from the aorta to the mitral valve, these echoes may be further evaluated as to whether they arise from a tumor mass or from artifactual means.

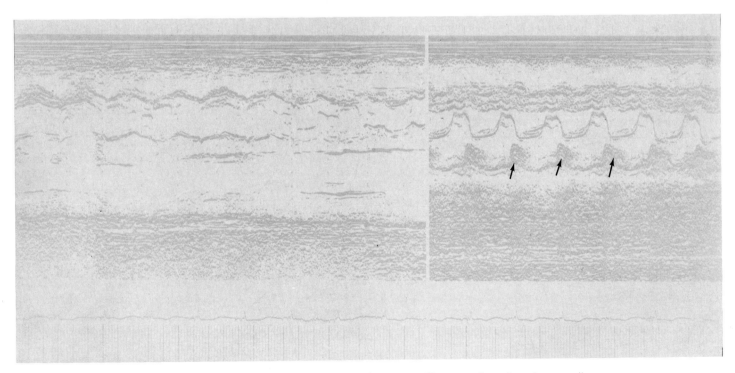

Fig. 31-6. This patient did not have an atrial myxoma. However, there is a dense collection of echoes posterior to the mitral valve in diastole *(arrows)*. These are most likely due to fibrosis or calcification of the mitral apparatus. In addition, the left atrial cavity is enlarged, indicating mitral regurgitation.

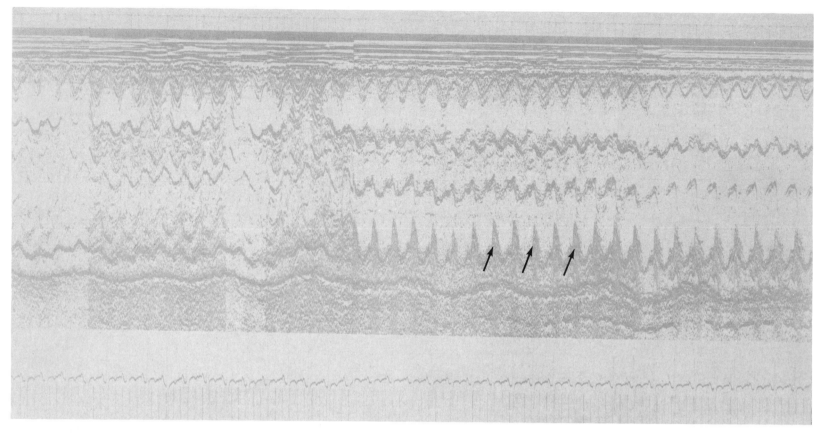

Fig. 31-7. Other forms of tumor masses *(arrows)* may be seen in patients with massive pericardial effusions or hypercontractile hearts.

FORMATION OF THROMBI AND EMBOLI

Thrombi. A thrombosis is the formation, in the blood vessels or the heart, of a blood clot from various elements of flowing blood. After the thrombus forms, part or all of it may break loose to create an embolus that travels downstream to lodge at a peripheral site. The potential consequence of a thrombosis and/or embolism is ischemic necrosis of these peripheral cells and tissue, which is termed *infarction*.

Mural thrombi occur in the lumina of the heart or aorta and attach to one of the walls, usually in the area of infarction. Other sites for mural thrombi are the atrial appendages and left ventricular walls juxtaposed to myocardial infarcts (Fig. 31-8). In the aorta they attach to previously damaged areas (e.g., atherosclerosis or syphilitic aortic aneurysms).

Emboli. An embolism is the occlusion of some part of the cardiovascular system by the impaction of a foreign mass transported to the site through the bloodstream. *Thromboembolism* is the term used for an embolus that is a part or a whole thrombus which has become dislodged and carried downstream to occlude a smaller vessel.

EVALUATION BY TWO-DIMENSIONAL ECHO

The evaluation of left atrial or ventricular thrombi in patients with suspected myocardial infarction or calcific rheumatic heart disease may be performed by two-dimensional echo using the apical and subxyphoid four chamber approach.

The cardiac apex is a frequent location for most ventricular thrombi. This area must be carefully assessed for abnormal masses and separated from large papillary muscles or artifactual masses due to side lobes. It is more difficult to detect all left atrial thrombi; possibly the pressure to which the left atrial thrombi are subjected causes the organizing ventricular thrombi to be firmer and better-reflective targets than the left atrial thrombi, which are not subjected to the same type of pressure.[2]

Martin[2] further states five points to remember in detecting left ventricular thrombi by two-dimensional echo:

1. Left ventricular thrombi are often closely adherent to the endocardial surfaces of the ventricle but have a distinct margin or site of origin from the surrounding endocardial echoes.

2. Whereas the myocardium often appears as a dark structure with bright endocardial surfaces, left ventricular thrombi frequently have a granular appearance quite different from that of the surrounding myocardium.

3. The site of the mass lesion is often near the cardiac apex, so the apical and subxyphoid transducer positions are best for detecting ventricular thrombi.

4. Mural thrombi appear to have a motion synchronous with that of the adjacent ventricular walls.

5. Left ventricular thrombi can arise on a short stalk (adjacent to the akinetic-dyskinetic area) or appear as a large firmly adherent mass of echoes.

Thus echocardiography may prove to be a valuable procedure in the detection of intracardiac masses and thrombi if the sonographer carefully analyzes for the presence or absence of echo return within the cardiac chambers (Fig. 31-9). Care must be taken to separate artifacts produced by side lobes or large papillary muscles from the real intracardiac mass echoes.

Investigation into tissue characterization of echoes within the cardiac chambers is cur-

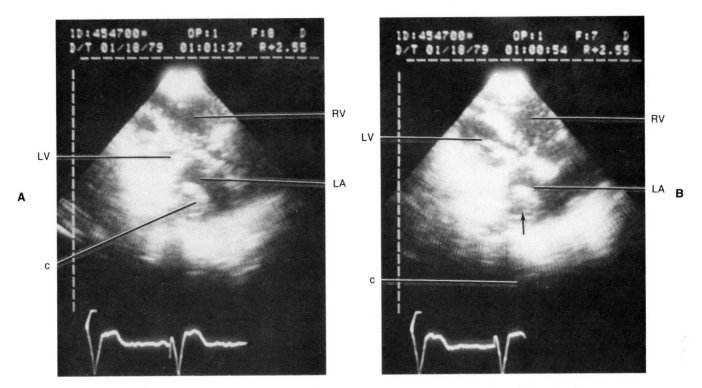

Fig. 31-8. This woman with a history of rheumatic heart disease was found by echo to have severe mitral stenosis with calcification. The right anterior oblique modified four chamber view shows a dense echo formation in the left atrial cavity during diastole, **A.** The tumor does not prolapse posterior to the mitral apparatus in diastole as a myxoma would, **B,** but remains fixed to the atrial wall shortly after systole *(arrow)*. This was a large atrial clot, *c*, secondary to the rheumatic disease.

Fig. 31-9. Apical four chamber view of a tumor in the right ventricular cavity. Note that the tumor is clearly attached to the interventricular septum, with no attachment to the right ventricular free wall or tricuspid valve. Also note the bulging of the interventricular septum toward the left ventricle, caused by tumor growth. *tm,* Tumor mass. (Courtesy H. Rakowski, M.D., Toronto General Hospital.)

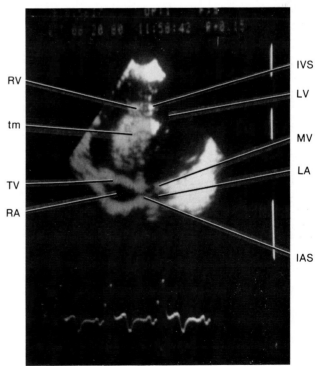
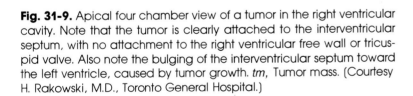

rently being performed in several laboratories, with the objective of making echocardiography an even more specific and sensitive technique.

SUMMARY

Echocardiography has become a useful tool in the evaluation of cardiac masses. The two-dimensional approach has heightened the diagnostic capabilities of sonographers in assessing the size, location, and valvar destruction caused by a mass in the heart cavity. Particular attention to gain settings, transducer position, and clinical findings may further increase these capabilities.

REFERENCES

1. Fleming, J.S., and Braimbridge, M.V.: Lecture notes on cardiology, ed. 2, Oxford, 1967, Blackwell Scientific Publications.
2. Martin, R.P.: Detection of intracardiac mass lesions by cross-section echocardiography. In Kisslo, J.A., editor: Two-dimensional echocardiography, New York, 1980, Churchill Livingstone, Inc.
3. Sokolow, M., and McIlroy, M.B.: Clinical cardiology, Los Altos, Calif., 1977, Lange Medical Publications.

32

Coronary artery disease

Coronary artery disease is any abnormal condition of the coronary arteries that interferes with the delivery of an adequate supply of blood to the structures of the heart. It is the most common cause of heart disease among adults in the United States. Rare types of inflammation of the blood vessels caused by oversensitivity to particular substances and certain types of thickening and hardening of the blood vessel wall may also affect the coronary arteries.

ATHEROSCLEROSIS

There are several causes of coronary artery disease. The most common, and by far the most serious, is *atherosclerosis*—the accumulation of fat in the larger arteries, with narrowing of the lumina of those vessels. This is one particular form of arteriosclerosis that involves the arteries which carry blood to the heart, brain, kidneys, arms, and legs. It is a reversible disease and not necessarily an aging process.

An *atheroma* is a mass of fat that forms on the inside wall of a coronary artery, partly plugging the vessel. It is made up of all the types of fat that normally circulate in the blood (Fig. 32-1).

The presence of an atheroma on the lining of a coronary artery is bad in itself, but worse manifestations follow. Fibrous scar tissue grows into and around the mass of fat, binding it firmly to the wall of the artery. The atheroma, which starts as a soft rubbery mass of fat, ultimately becomes a hard rocklike plaque on the lining of the artery. It may grow to such a size that it blocks the coronary artery completely, as a boulder would dam up a conduit.

A blood clot is very likely to form anyplace in a blood vessel where the blood is partly dammed up. This often happens immediately upstream from an atheroma. When the blood clot has formed, it extends down and sometimes past the original plaque. This is called a *thrombus*. Formation of a thrombus in a coronary artery is *coronary thrombosis*, or stoppage of the artery by a blood clot (Fig. 32-2).

Sometimes there is bleeding in the tissue immediately under the atheroma. The bleeding tends to separate the plaque from the wall of the blood vessel, as if it had been dissected with a knife. The plaque is then lifted out and into the bloodstream and falls across the artery, blocking it completely.

Infection or necrosis of tissue under the atheroma may cause an abscess to form in the wall of the artery immediately under the plaque. This will have the same effect as hemorrhage: the plaque will again be lifted off and block the artery completely.

Heart muscle extracts about four fifths of the oxygen supplied to it in the blood by the coronary arteries. This leaves an extremely small borrowing capacity, or reserve margin, if that blood supply is cut down. The collateral circulation between the coronary arteries is not good. When a coronary artery is blocked, there is death of tissue (Fig. 32-3).

Complications of atherosclerosis

Angina pectoris. Pain arising in the heart muscle is the mildest and earliest clinical symptom of heart disease caused by coronary atheromatosis. It is distress of some type, usually in the chest, brought on by increased heart work. It characteristically appears after physical exertion, large meals, emotional tension, or emotional trauma and is usually relieved by rest or the use of nitroglycerin tablets.

Coronary insufficiency. Myocardial ischemia without infarction is a more severe and prolonged form of disease than angina pectoris. Of the forms of coronary atheromatosis described so far, it can reduce the blood flow to an area of heart muscle to such a degree that the heart muscle actually does not receive enough blood to maintain life. Although there is still blood flow and the coronary artery is not completely blocked, the blood supply to some areas of the myocardium is so far below the requirements of

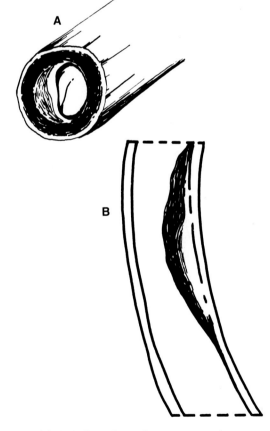

Fig. 32-1. A, End view of a coronary artery partially plugged. Blood flow through this artery would be cut down about 50%. **B,** Drawing of a coronary artery atheroma showing the mass of fat that forms on the wall of the artery and partially blocks the vessel. (From Phibbs, B.: The human heart; a guide to heart disease, ed. 4, St. Louis, 1979, The C.V. Mosby Co.)

□Modified slightly from Griffith, G.C.: Coronary artery disease. In Phibbs, B., editor: The human heart, a guide to heart disease, ed. 3, St. Louis, 1975, The C.V. Mosby Co.

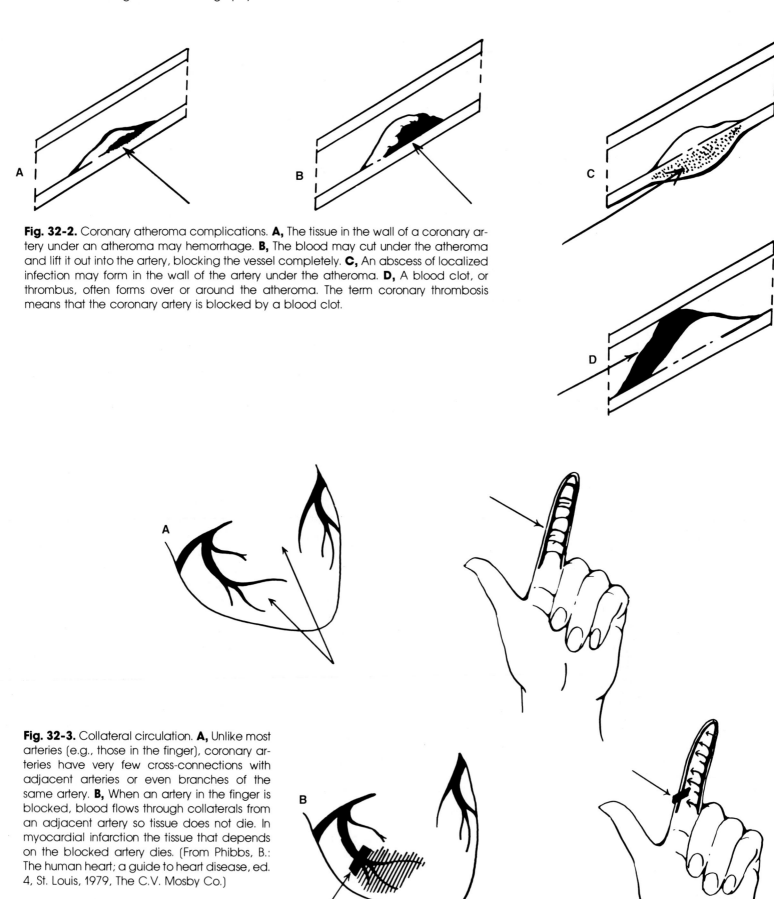

Fig. 32-2. Coronary atheroma complications. **A,** The tissue in the wall of a coronary artery under an atheroma may hemorrhage. **B,** The blood may cut under the atheroma and lift it out into the artery, blocking the vessel completely. **C,** An abscess of localized infection may form in the wall of the artery under the atheroma. **D,** A blood clot, or thrombus, often forms over or around the atheroma. The term coronary thrombosis means that the coronary artery is blocked by a blood clot.

Fig. 32-3. Collateral circulation. **A,** Unlike most arteries (e.g., those in the finger), coronary arteries have very few cross-connections with adjacent arteries or even branches of the same artery. **B,** When an artery in the finger is blocked, blood flows through collaterals from an adjacent artery so tissue does not die. In myocardial infarction the tissue that depends on the blocked artery dies. (From Phibbs, B.: The human heart; a guide to heart disease, ed. 4, St. Louis, 1979, The C.V. Mosby Co.)

the tissues that the cells are actually injured. The cells are not dead, for they can be brought back to normal function; but they do suffer some degree of injury because of their decreased blood supply. This is called the *reversible* disease of the heart muscle produced by coronary atherosclerosis.

The patient often suffers pain, typical of angina pectoris, that is present after rest or after the administration of nitroglycerin tablets.

To summarize, the second most serious type of disease produced by coronary atherosclerosis is prolonged coronary insufficiency or myocardial ischemia without infarction. The word *ischemia* means a lack of adequate blood supply to maintain life in some area of tissue. In other words, an area of the myocardium has not received enough blood supply but it has not actually died since the blood flow, although below the safe level, has not been cut off completely. The word *infarct* signifies that tissue has actually died because of complete blockage of blood flow.

Myocardial infarction. In myocardial infarction an area of tissue dies because its blood supply has been cut off. As a result of coronary artery disease, it often develops in the heart muscle or in the wall of the heart; once the blood supply to the heart muscle has been cut off and the infarct has formed, a certain minimum amount of time is required for the tissue to die and heal with a strong scar formation.

A frequent complication of acute myocardial infarction is an irregularity of the heartbeat or *arrhythmia*. Atrial or ventricular beats may appear. When atrial premature beats become very frequent, they may lead to the rapid forceful heart action called *supraventricular tachycardia* or to a totally irregular heart action called *atrial fibrillation*. The ventricles can also develop similar conditions. A heart block may appear in the conducting system, further complicating the disease.

Another complication is acute congestion of the lungs, known as *pulmonary edema*. This happens when the left side of the heart is so damaged by injury that blood dams up in the ventricle and subsequently in the lungs.

Blood clots are also a hazard. The infarct is frequently caused by the presence of a blood clot in a diseased part of the coronary artery. A mural or wall clot often forms inside the cavity of the left ventricle over the area of the damaged muscle. The prolonged bed rest that goes with the early stages of myocardial infarction produces increased danger of blood clots in the veins of the lower extremities.

ECHOGRAPHIC EVALUATION OF CORONARY ARTERY DISEASE

Wall motion abnormalities. One of the first echographic findings is abnormal wall motion; *hypokinesis* is little movement, *hyperkinesis* overactive movement, *dyskinesis* fragmentary or incomplete movement, and *akinesis* no movement.

The true anterior left ventricular wall may be examined echographically by sliding the transducer in linear fashion toward the left midclavicular line. This allows the sonographer to move off the interventricular septum and record the wall of the left ventricle. When the anterior wall is best seen, there is no right ventricular cavity shown, as there is when the septum is recorded.

Indirect evidence of segmental left ventricular disease may be seen in exaggerated wall motion of the opposing nonischemic area of the left ventricle (Figs. 32-4 and 32-5).

Another indirect clue to the presence of a hypokinetic wall segment is a cloud of intracavitary echoes adjacent to the poorly moving wall.[5] Normally the left ventricular cavity is echo free; but if there are intracavitary echoes, they are uniformly distributed throughout the cavity or appear as a series of straight lines. The echoes frequently accumulate next to a hypokinetic or dyskinetic segment of the ventricle (Figs. 32-6 and 32-7).

Another indirect sign is a prominent, somewhat exaggerated, right ventricular wall motion. It is very unusual for the amplitude of the right ventricular wall echoes to exceed the amplitude of septal motion, except in patients with coronary artery disease.

If the interventricular septal motion is abnormal, there is quite probably a proximal left anterior descending or left main coronary artery obstruction[4,9] (Fig. 32-8). However, normal septal motion in *no* way precludes the possibility of obstruction in these arteries. The septal motion correlates better with the myocardial perfusion of the septum than with anatomic obstructions of the coronary artery.[5]

The two-dimensional echo again offers a better visualization to myocardial contractility than does the M-mode echo. Especially important are the apical four chamber and short axis views in judging wall motion and thickness patterns. Thus the two-dimensional view can record the medial, lateral, and apical portions of the left ventricle.

Wall thickening. Any given segment of the ventricle is influenced in its movement by the adjacent muscle to which it is attached. It may be hypokinetic in one area and be influenced by hyperkinesis in another. Thus by merely looking at wall motion on echo, one usually overestimates the amount of ischemic muscle when looking just for motion abnormalities. A more specific finding for ischemic muscle is the alteration in systolic thickening.[1,6,8,12]

With acute ischemia or infarction one may record systolic thinning, whereby the thickness of the left ventricular wall is greater in diastole than in systole[5] (Figs. 32-9 and 32-10). The affected wall segment exhibits not only the paradoxical motion but also the systolic thinning, which is probably more specific for ischemia. Systolic thinning almost always occurs with a dyskinetic segment and is usually associated with acute myocardial infarction. A decreased or no thickening occurs in both chronic and acute ischemia.[5]

Chronic ischemia will sometimes produce alterations in wall thickness.[4,11]

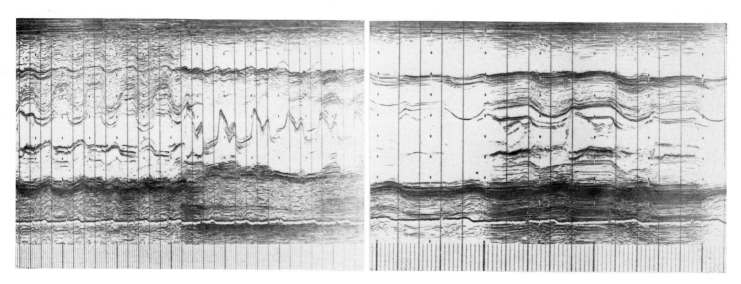

Fig. 32-4. Exaggerated wall motion is seen along the septal segment of the left ventricle.

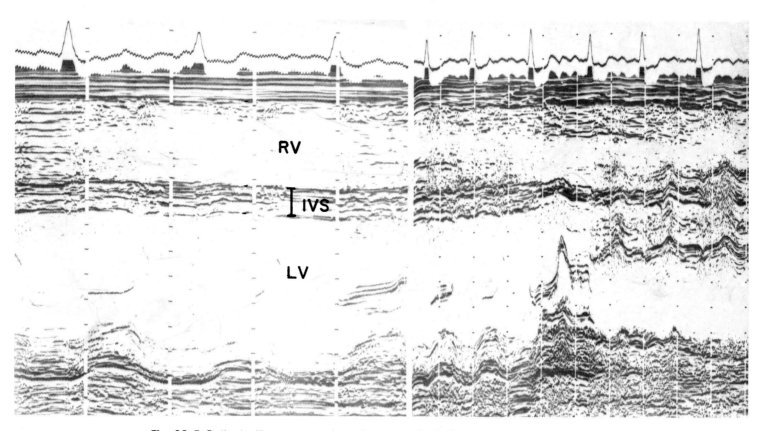

Fig. 32-5. Patient with coronary artery disease and anterior myocardial infarction. Note the flat septal motion with normal posterior wall contractility.

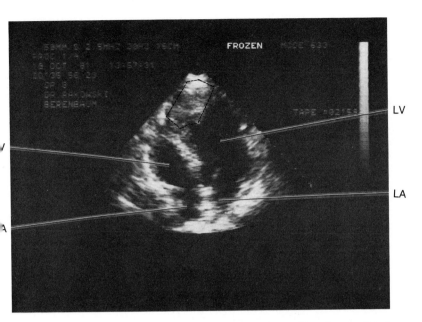

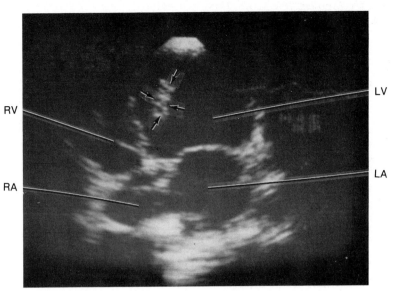

Fig. 32-6. Apical four chamber view in a patient with a large distal septal and apical aneurysm with clot. The areas of sonolucency within the clot represent organized thrombus. The clot is outlined with black lines. (Courtesy H. Rakowski, M.D., Toronto General Hospital.)

Fig. 32-7. Apical four chamber view of a small thrombus *(arrows)* in a patient with cardiomyopathy. All four chambers were enlarged, and there was hypokinesis. (Courtesy H. Rakowski, M.D., Toronto General Hospital.)

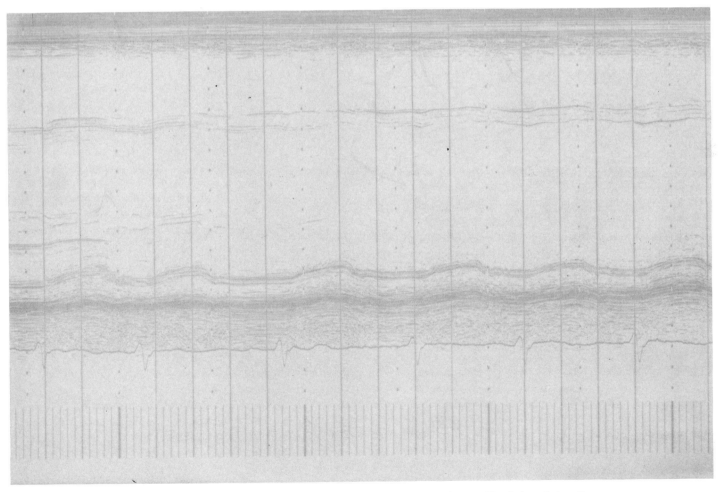

Fig. 32-8. M-mode echo of a patient with coronary artery disease. The flat septal motion indicates that the left anterior or left main coronary artery is obstructed.

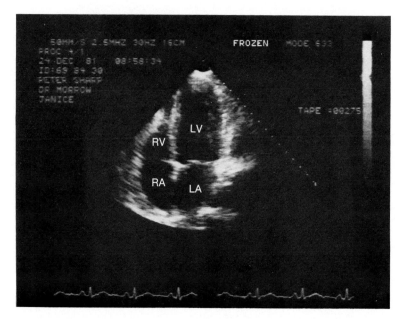

Fig. 32-9. Apical four chamber view in a patient with coronary artery disease. The real time demonstrated akinesis at the apex and along the distal septum and anterolateral wall. (Courtesy H. Rakowski, M.D., Toronto General Hospital.)

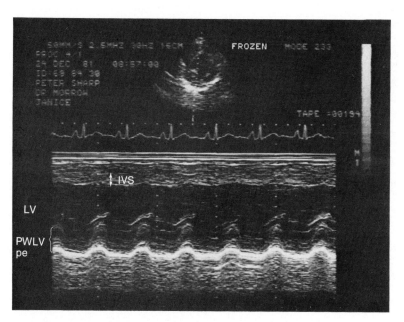

Fig. 32-10. M-mode echocardiogram of the patient in Fig. 32-9 showing a flat septal motion and active posterior heart wall. *pe*, Pericardium. (Courtesy H. Rakowski, M.D., Toronto General Hospital.)

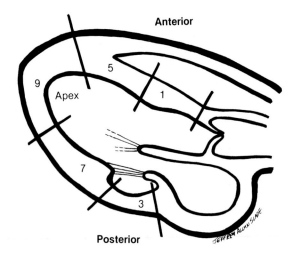

Fig. 32-11. Long axis schematic of the left ventricle. The nine segments of the ventricle are shown along with their corresponding positions in Figs. 32-12 and 32-13. (Modified from Heger, J.J., et al.: Circulation **60:**531, 1979.)

Change in acoustic properties.[5] The healing process of an acute myocardial infarction involves the deposition of collagen and the formation of a scar. These changes produce a decrease in the thickness of the affected wall segment. The second effect, scar formation, is a change in the acoustic properties of the segment. Collagen and scar both change the reflective properties of the wall, although fibrosis is a much stronger reflector of ultrasound than is the normal myocardium.[13]

In efforts to judge wall thickness, motion, and reflective properties, careful technique must be utilized to image the interventricular septum. The entire width and length of the septum must be recorded in the long axis and apical views. The gain setting must be adjusted so the echoes do not appear to be more reflective than they really are.

Quantitation of ischemic muscle. If all the left ventricular segments move abnormally, one can expect to find extensive ischemic damage. However, if no abnormal muscle is recorded, then the damage is considerably less.

In efforts to map out the areas of ischemia in the left ventricle, the cavity has been

divided into a number of areas.[7] The long axis view records the anterior and posterior segments along with the cardiac apex (Fig. 32-11). The short axis view shows the anterior, posterior, medial, and lateral walls of the ventricle (Figs. 32-12 and 32-13). The apical view shows the apex and the medial and lateral walls. If one assumes that each segment is equal in area, the number of abnormal segments can be totaled and the percent surface area or percent mass of the left ventricle that is abnormal can be calculated (Fig. 32-14).

Elevated end diastolic pressure. Patients with coronary artery disease often have high left ventricular end diastolic pressure that is primarily a result of an elevated atrial component of ventricular pressure. Such an alteration in pressure, and possibly to some extent abnormal ventricular contraction, changes the manner in which the mitral valve closes.[10] On the M-mode a notch is recorded between the A and C points* and is termed the B point. This notch may also be a function of poor contractility of the left ventricle (Fig. 32-15).

Ventricular aneurysm. An aneurysm is a common complication of myocardial infarction. If an M-mode strip at slow speed is obtained on a patient with a ventricular an-

---

*Throughout Chapters 25 to 35, the references to these letter points along the cardiac cycle are by both lower case and capital letters. This is because both designations are used in the field and the authors use the one with which they are more familiar.

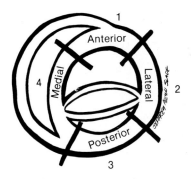

Fig. 32-12. Short axis schematic of the left ventricle at the level of the mitral valve. (Modified from Heger, J.J., et al.: Circulation **60**:531, 1979.)

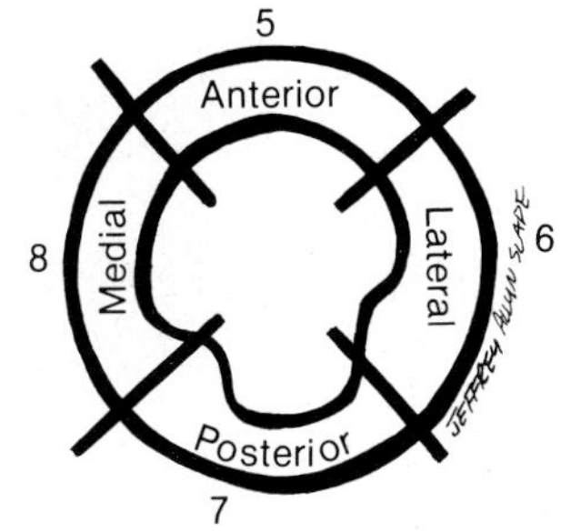

Fig. 32-13. Diagram of the short axis view of the left ventricle at the midventricular level. (Modified from Heger, J.J., et al.: Circulation **60**:531, 1979.)

eurysm, one will see an increase in distance between the left septum and the posterior endocardium as the apex is approached (Fig. 32-16). The two-dimensional echo is probably a better method for examining the left ventricular cavity. Since a common site for aneurysm formation is the apex of the heart, the apical four chamber view is the most sensitive (Fig. 32-17). The aneurysmal dilation can be seen in diastole, with expansion in systole, and may be visible in almost any part of the ventricle.

Some aneurysms are principally the result of lost myocardial tissue rather than of any significant outward bulging of the ventricular wall.

Pseudoaneurysm. This condition occurs when there is a rupture of the free wall of the left ventricle and blood is trapped within the pericardium. An aneurysm develops whose outside wall is the pericardium and clot rather than muscle.

The pseudoaneurysm is illustrated by a large relatively echo-free space beyond the posterior left ventricular epicardium. Pseudoaneurysms have also been observed in which the rupture is in the anterior septal area with a perforation into the pericardial sac. Likewise, septal discontinuity has been reported.[3]

Left ventricular thrombi. The formation of thrombi is another common complication of myocardial infarction. The thrombi occur adjacent to the dyskinetic area, which frequently is dilated. A clot may be recognized on the apical view as an immobile structure or a bright reflector that moves with the cardiac contractions. Further discussion of intracardiac masses is found in Chapter 31.

Other complications. A less common complication of myocardial infarction is rupture of the interventricular septum, which

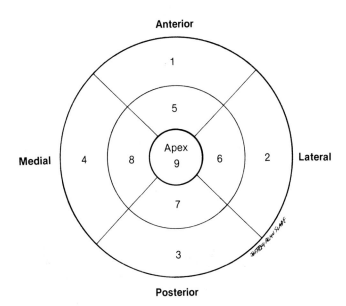

Fig. 32-14. Method of depicting the location of asynergy in acute myocardial infarction. All nine segments are displayed as a series of concentric rings. (Modified from Heger, J.J., et al.: Circulation **60**:531, 1979.)

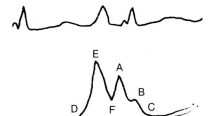

Fig. 32-15. Schematic mitral valve echocardiogram of coronary artery disease with abnormal left ventricular function. The mitral valve closure between *A* and *C* is interrupted, and the A-C interval prolonged. (From Feigenbaum, H.: Echocardiography, ed. 3, Philadelphia, 1981, Lea & Febiger.)

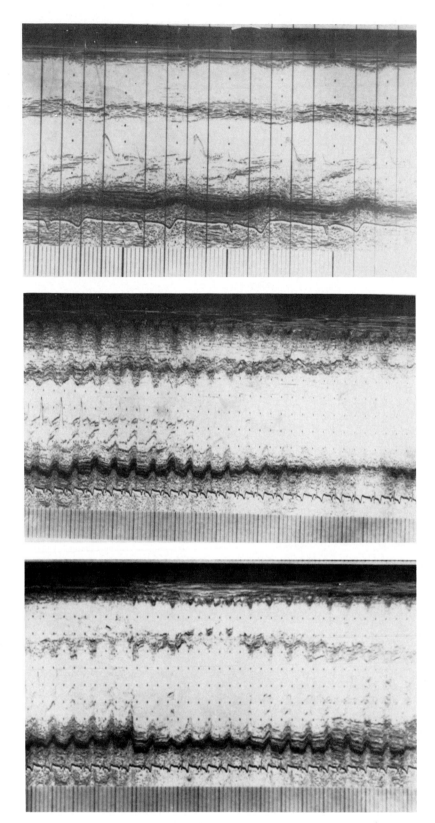

Fig. 32-16. A 32-year-old woman who was on drug therapy for myocardial infarction was sent for cardiac evaluation. The echocardiogram demonstrated decreased contractility of the septum and posterior wall. The septum changed in motion from akinetic to paradoxical. The expansion of the left ventricle was compatible with a small aneurysm of the ventricular wall at the apex.

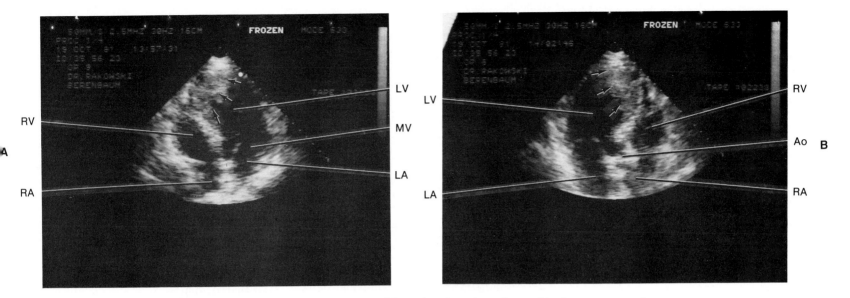

Fig. 32-17. A, Two-dimensional apical four chamber view of a ventricular aneurysm at the apex *(arrows)* and clot. **B,** Modified apical two chamber view.

may extend into the pericardium and produce a pseudoaneurysm.[3] A more common result of a ruptured septum is the communication of blood between the left and right ventricles.[5]

Occasionally the patient will develop a flail mitral leaflet secondary to papillary muscle dysfunction and scarring of the posterior wall of the left ventricle.

REFERENCES

1. Arnett, E.N., Weiss, J.L., and Garrison, J.B.: Quantitative evaluation of regional left ventricular thickening in man by two-dimensional echocardiography, Am. J. Cardiol. **43:**377, 1979. [Abstract.]

2. Corya, B.C.: Echocardiography in ischemic heart disease, Am. J. Med. **63:**10, 1977.

3. Davidson, K.H., Parisi, A.F., Harrington, J.J., et al.: Pseudoaneurysm of the left ventricle: an unusual echocardiographic presentation, Ann. Intern. Med. **86:**430, 1977.

4. Dortimer, A.C., DeJoseph, R.L., Shiroff, R.A., et al.: Distribution of coronary artery disease; prediction by echocardiography, Circulation **54:**724, 1976.

5. Feigenbaum, H., Corya, B.C., Dillon, J.C., et al.: Role of echocardiography in patients with coronary artery disease, Am. J. Cardiol. **37:**775, 1976.

6. Goldstein, S., and Willem de Jong, J.: Changes in left ventricular wall dimension during regional myocardial ischemia, Am. J. Cardiol. **34:**56, 1974.

7. Heger, J.J., Weyman, A.E., Wann, L.S., et al.: Cross-sectional echocardiography in acute myocardial infarction: detection and localization of regional left ventricular asynergy, Circulation **60:**531, 1979.

8. Kerber, R.E., Martins, J.B., and Marcus, M.L.: Effect of acute ischemia, nitroglycerin, and nitroprusside on regional myocardial thickening, stress, and perfusion, Circulation **60:**121, 1979.

9. Kolibash, A.J., Beaver, B.M., Fulkerson, P.K., et al.: The relationship between abnormal echocardiographic septal motion and myocardial perfusion in patients with significant obstruction of the left anterior descending artery, Am. J. Cardiol. **40:**11, 1977.

10. Konecke, L.L., Feigenbaum, H., Chang, S., et al.: Abnormal mitral valve motion in patients with elevated left ventricular diastolic pressures, Circulation **47:**989, 1973.

11. Maron, B.J., Savage, D.D., Clark, C.E., et al.: Prevalence and characteristics of disproportionate ventricular septal thickening in patients with coronary artery disease, Circulation **57:**250, 1978.

12. Motta, J.A., Valdez, R.D., and Popp, R.L.: Septal motion and thickening in significant left anterior descending coronary artery disease, Circulation (suppl. 2)**54:**84, 1976. [Abstract.]

13. Rasmussen, S., Corya, B.C., Feigenbaum, H., et al.: Detection of myocardial scar tissue by M-mode echography, Circulation **57:**230, 1978.

33

Pericardial disease

ANATOMY

The pericardium is a fibroserous sac that contains the heart and the roots of the great vessels. It presents with its base resting on the diaphragm and its narrower upper end enclosing the lower half of the superior vena cava, the greater part of the ascending aorta, and nearly the entire pulmonary trunk (Fig. 33-1). Like the pleura it consists of two distinct sacs, an outer sac called the *fibrous* pericardium and an inner sac (which is invaginated by the heart) called the *serous* pericardium.

The fibrous outer layer is attached superiorly to the great vessels, inferiorly to the diaphragm, anteriorly to the sternum, and posteriorly to the veins behind the left atrium.

The serous pericardium is a membrane that forms a closed sac and has visceral and parietal layers.[7] The visceral layer, EPICARDIUM, covers the heart and is reflected back on itself at the great vessels to form the parietal layer of the pericardium. The parietal layer is continuous with the visceral layer and is closely adherent to the fibrous pericardium. The pericardial space lies between the visceral (epicardium) and the parietal layers (of the serous pericardium) (Fig. 33-2). A small amount of serous fluid (15 to 30 ml) normally is found in this pericardial space.

PHYSIOLOGY[8]

An understanding of the hemodynamics of both the normal and the diseased pericardium is helpful in interpreting the echocardiogram. The potential volume of the pericardium is larger than the actual space occupied by the normal heart in diastole. Distension of the pericardium also occurs, with minimal effects on cardiac function up to a point, and is attributed to the interwoven pattern of elastic fibers. The distension of the pericardium is initially accompanied by stretching of these elastic fibers that is ultimately hindered by the collagen fibers. Pressure-volume studies on the pericardium have shown only a small initial rise with substantial increases in volume. However, beyond a certain point the pressure rises rapidly with small increments in volume and interference with ventricular diastolic size develops.[1]

Surgical removal of the pericardium (pericardiectomy) appears to have no effect on the normal cardiac function.

The pericardium is thought to serve as a protective barrier for the heart when inflammation of the thoracic cavity is present,[6] and it protects the lungs from the trauma of a beating heart. It may also protect the heart from overdilation in hypervolemia and may limit right ventricular filling when the left ventricle is dilated, thus protecting the left ventricle from overload and the lungs from edema.[8]

RECOGNITION OF PERICARDIAL DISEASE

There are three categories of pericardial disease: (1) acute pericarditis, (2) pericardial effusion (with or without tamponade), and (3) chronic constrictive pericarditis. Pericardial disease may be secondary to infection, hypersensitivity (e.g., collagen diseases like rheumatic fever), trauma, metabolic disorders (e.g., myxedema), neoplasm, aortic dissection, myocardial infarction, myocardiopathy, renal disease, radiation therapy, or heart failure.

Acute pericarditis

The characteristic symptom of acute pericarditis is pain (sometimes mimicking that of myocardial infarction). Other symptoms (chills, fever, sweating) will depend on the etiology of the pericarditis. The major sign is cardiac enlargement with a possible pericardial friction rub, which is a scraping sound heard over the heart in the presence of pericardial effusion. The friction rub is produced from the inflamed pericardial layers grating on each other throughout the cardiac cycle.

Other forms of acute pericarditis will be briefly described, but they are not distinguishable histologically by echocardiography:

1. A *fibrinous* or dry pericarditis usually occurs in the presence of a viral infection or rheumatic fever. Deposits of serum and fibrin are seen in the pericardial cavity. Occasionally a small pericardial effusion will be present.
2. A *purulent* pericarditis usually results from a bacterial infection, and the pericardial effusion contains pus. The accumulation of such inflammatory prod-

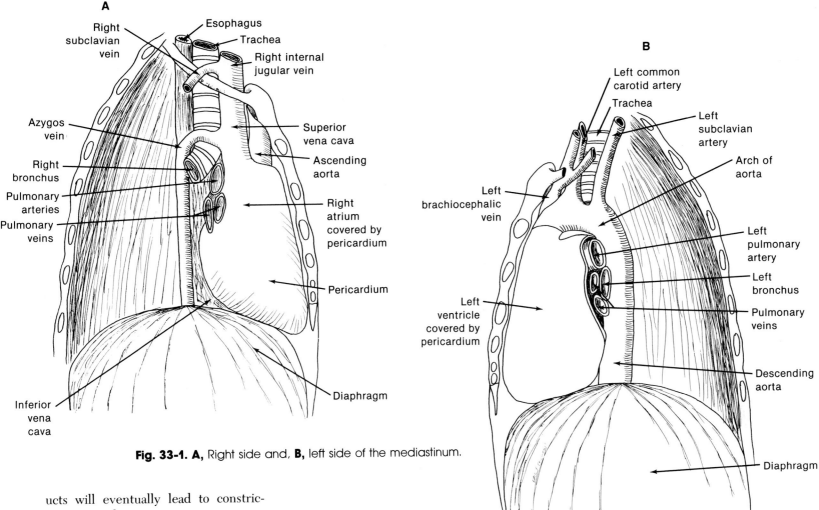

A

Right subclavian vein

Esophagus

Trachea

Right internal jugular vein

Azygos vein

Right bronchus

Pulmonary arteries

Pulmonary veins

Superior vena cava

Ascending aorta

Right atrium covered by pericardium

Pericardium

Inferior vena cava

Diaphragm

B

Left common carotid artery

Trachea

Left subclavian artery

Left brachiocephalic vein

Arch of aorta

Left pulmonary artery

Left bronchus

Left ventricle covered by pericardium

Pulmonary veins

Descending aorta

Diaphragm

Fig. 33-1. A, Right side and, **B,** left side of the mediastinum.

ucts will eventually lead to constrictive pericarditis.

3. A *hemorrhagic* pericarditis is usually caused by a malignancy or injury to the pericardium, and blood is mixed with the inflammatory fluid.

Pericardial effusion

Pericardial effusion is characterized by an enlarged cardiac silhouette and may be confused with cardiac dilation as seen in valvular heart disease or cardiomyopathy. Clinical findings can include distant heart sounds (muffled by the fluid accumulation) and a low-voltage ECG. The speed with which the fluid accumulates largely determines the subsequent clinical manifestations: a rapid accumulation of 200 to 300 ml may lead to tamponade and a shock state from acute cardiac insufficiency, whereas a slower accumulation of 1000 ml may produce no evidence of cardiac insufficiency.

The pericardium is able to adapt to large collections of fluid if permitted to do so over a long time. Cardiac tamponade may result from trauma, a ruptured aneurysm, or pericarditis. With tamponade the systemic venous pressure increases while the arterial pressure decreases, and thus the acute cardiac insufficiency develops.

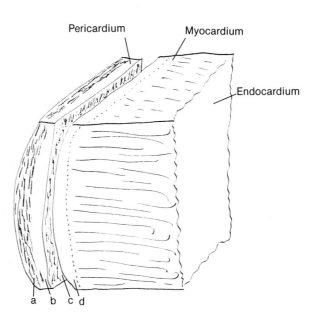

Pericardium

Myocardium

Endocardium

a b c d

Fig. 33-2. The serous pericardium forms a closed sac and has a visceral and parietal component. *a,* Fibrous pericardium; *b,* serous pericardium (parietal layer); *c,* pericardial space; *d,* serous pericardium (visceral layer).

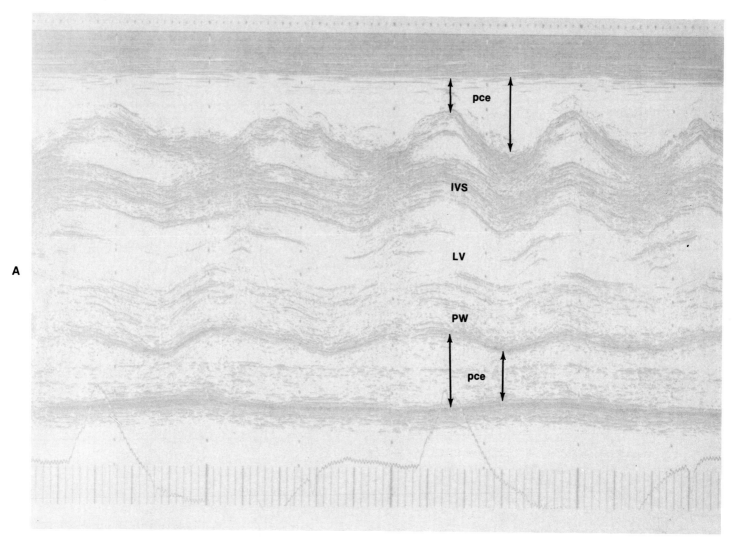

A

Fig. 33-3. A, M-mode scan of the left ventricular cavity showing a large anteroposterior pericardial effusion. The beam was then directed over the ventricular cavity from the subxyphoid approach for ultrasonic guidance in the pericardiocentesis.

Constrictive pericarditis

Constrictive pericarditis is the result of chronic pericardial inflammation and fibrosis caused by an infectious process, neoplasm, or uremia. The disease interferes with cardiac filling and contraction (reduced cardiac output) and leads to chronic congestion in the venous system supplying the right heart and/ or, if the left heart is also involved, pulmonary congestion. The cardiac rate is increased, with a decreased pulse pressure and paradoxical pulse. Signs of congestive heart failure are present, with edema and dyspnea.

Tuberculosis is a common cause of constrictive pericarditis, which develops when there is extension of tuberculosis from the lungs or lymph nodes into the heart. The pericardium becomes shaggy and thickened, with resultant fibrosis and calcification, and the fibrosis may lead to constriction of the normal heart filling or constrictive pericarditis.

Pericardiocentesis

The removal of fluid from the pericardium may serve either a therapeutic or a diagnostic purpose. Needle aspiration of the pericardium is best performed with the patient in a semiupright position, for the fluid tends to gravitate anteriorly and inferolaterally. The apical or subxyphoid approach is generally used. The cardiac sonographer may locate the position of maximum fluid and with a special aspiration transducer guide the physician as the fluid is withdrawn from the pericardial space (Fig. 33-3). The needle may be followed on the A-mode or M-mode so it does not pierce the heart wall.

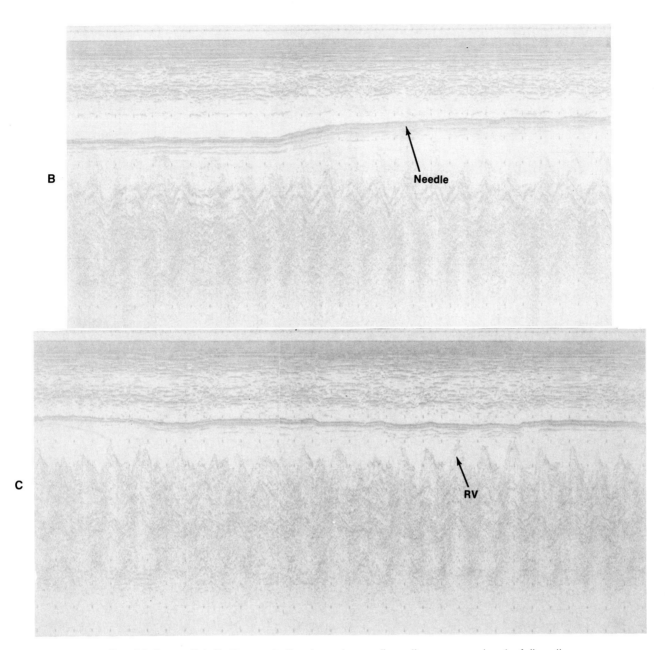

Fig. 33-3, cont'd. B, The aspiration transducer allows the sonographer to follow the needle as it pierces the chest wall. Guidance is given to the physician in an effort to avoid puncturing the ventricular wall. **C,** The fluid has been withdrawn, and the right ventricular wall can be seen much closer to the tip of the needle in this scan. Guidance is given until there is about 10 mm of separation left.

ECHOGRAPHIC EXAMINATION

Echography is the procedure of choice for evaluating pericardial effusion, and a positive diagnosis has been found extremely useful in the clinical management of these patients. If there is ventricular enlargement by physical or radiographic examination, an echo may quickly distinguish that secondary to valvular heart disease or cardiomyopathy from that due to pericardial effusion. Subsequent serial examinations of the patient with pericardial fluid may be made to follow the increase or decrease in fluid accumulation.

The evaluation of a patient with pericardial effusion should be performed carefully and systematically. A routine scan is made to locate the aortic root and left atrium and the mitral apparatus (Fig. 33-4). The transducer beam is then directed inferior and slightly lateral, off the tips of the mitral leaflets, to record the layers of the posterior left ventricular wall and pericardium (Fig. 33-5). The contractions of the ventricle should be followed throughout the cardiac cycle for any compensation or decompensation factors, which may be due to the accumulation of fluid (Fig. 33-6). The pericardial echo reflection is the strongest reflection in the normal heart and thus is easily recognized on the M-mode and two-dimensional recordings as a bright echo reflector. The three layers of the posterior wall (endocardium, myocardium, epicardium) must be defined so these echoes

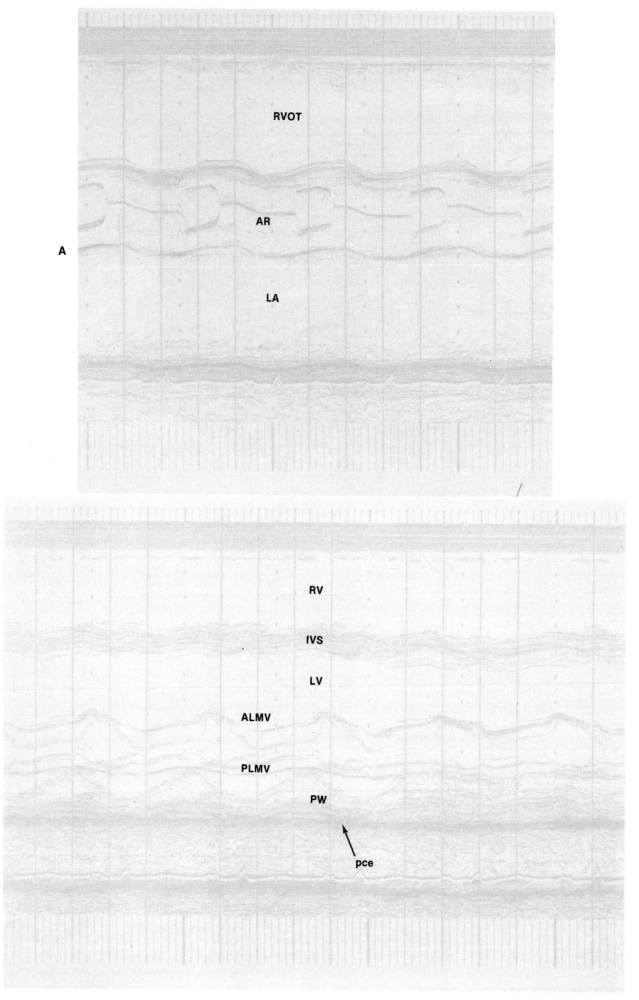

Fig. 33-4. A, M-mode scan over the right ventricular outflow tract, aortic root, and left atrium. **B,** As the beam is directed more perpendicular to the chest wall, the mitral apparatus is seen. There is just the suggestion of a small pericardial effusion, *pce*.

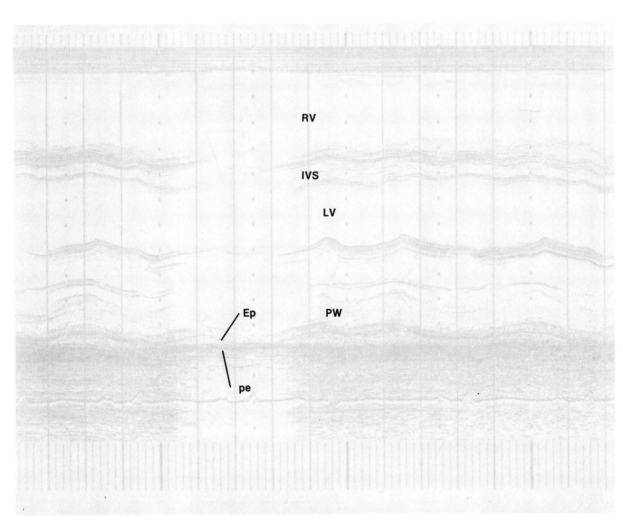

Fig. 33-5. The beam is now directed into the left ventricular cavity to show the posterior heart wall separated from the pericardial echo, *pe*.

can be separated from the pericardial echoes (Fig. 33-7). Various gain settings are used to define the structures. A high gain will allow visualization of the right ventricular wall, septum, posterior layers of the left ventricular wall, and pericardium (Fig. 33-8). As the gain is reduced, the finer less dense echoes of the chordae and endocardium are not recorded. Further reduction in gain allows only the bright pericardial reflection to remain (Fig. 33-9). Thus the sweep from the aortic root through the mitral valve apparatus to the left ventricular cavity must be made while at the same time the gain is increased or decreased to distinguish the presence of fluid separating the epicardium from the pericardium.

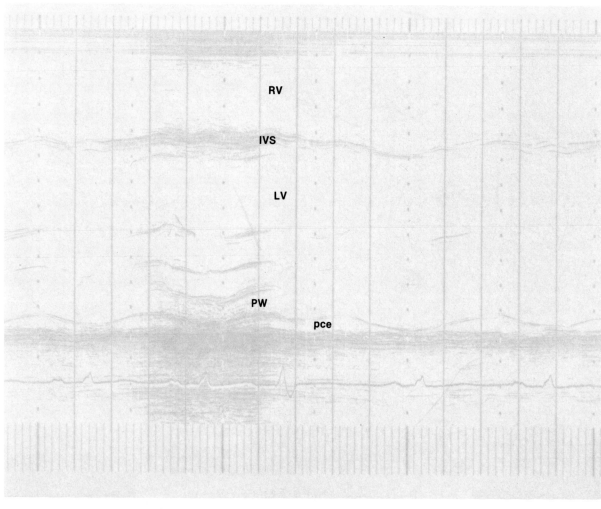

Fig. 33-6. There is decreased contractility of the ventricular cavity, but it is not due to the pericardial effusion. This patient has congestive cardiomyopathy.

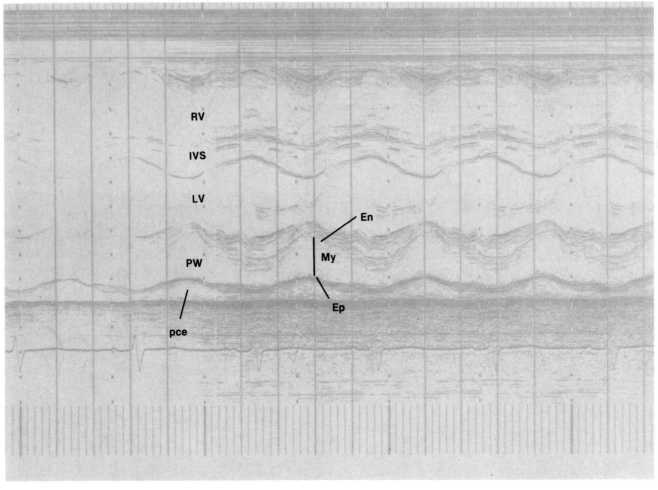

Fig. 33-7. The pericardium must be differentiated from the three layers of the posterior heart wall so the presence of a pericardial effusion can be identified.

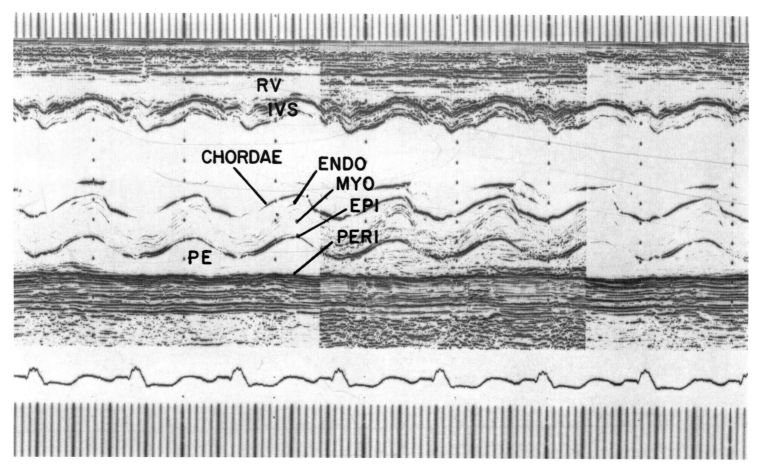

Fig. 33-8. Gain variations may show echoes within an effusion with high gain. A metastatic or hemorrhagic effusion may appear with multiple echoes, but these echoes will persist with decreased gain.

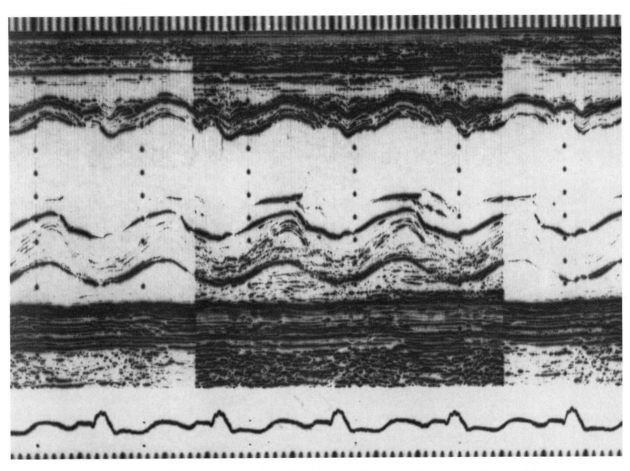

Fig. 33-9. Variations in gain control will allow identification of the pericardium and the separation of the posterior ventricular wall by the effusion.

Pericardial effusion

The echographic diagnosis of pericardial effusion can be very complex if the routine cardiac sweep is not performed. The sonographer must sweep the transducer in an oblique path from the right shoulder to visualize the aorta and left atrium, and to the left hip to visualize the left ventricle and pericardium. Careful observation of the continuity of the left atrial wall with the pericardium must be made. Normally the left atrial wall will be motionless; however, in the presence of a large effusion or in hypercontractile hearts there will be an abrupt anterior movement of the left atrial wall (Fig. 33-10).

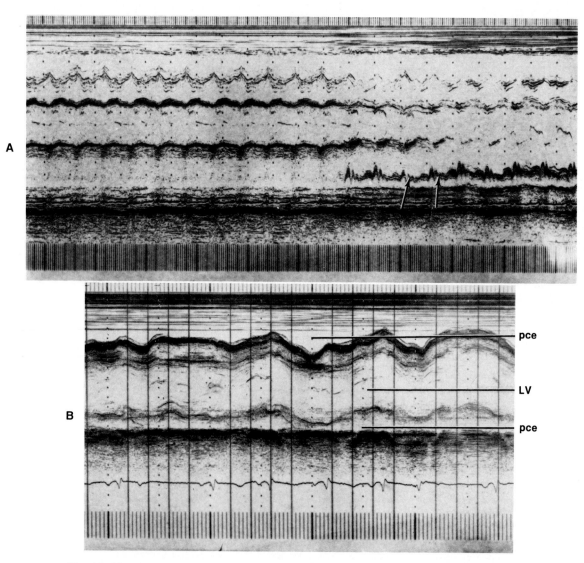

Fig. 33-10. The left atrial wall is motionless in normal patients. In the presence of a large pericardial effusion or hypercontractile states, an abrupt anterior motion of the left atrial wall may be seen. **A,** Sweep from the left atrium to the atrioventricular junction demonstrates the erratic movement of the AV groove *(arrows)*. **B,** As the beam is directed toward the left ventricular cavity, an anteroposterior pericardial effusion is noted.

In pericardial effusion the separation of pericardium from epicardium will cause the cardiac pulsations to be damped by the time they reach the pericardium. Thus one of the more obvious features of an effusion is a nonmobile pericardium, separated from the posterior heart wall by fluid (Fig. 33-11). Sometimes the amount of fluid is so small that these pulsations are transmitted slightly to the pericardium, in which case the sonographer will see diminished motion of the pericardium (Fig. 33-12).

Fluid generally accumulates in the most posterior-dependent area of the heart, accounting for the visualization of posterior effusion before any anterior effusion is seen.

Small effusions may produce an echo-free space behind the epicardium in systole but disappear in diastole (Fig. 33-13). Many echocardiographers prefer to see the separation in diastole before they report a small effusion (Fig. 33-14). A systolic separation of 5 to 10 mm may indicate a small effusion (approximately 100 ml).

Moderate effusions will produce echo-free spaces in systole and diastole in the anterior and posterior pericardial space. Usually a separation of 10 mm in systole means the patient has a moderate-sized effusion (200 to 300 ml) (Fig. 33-15).

A large effusion (500 ml or greater) will exhibit wide spaces anteriorly and posteriorly with a systolic separation of 15 to 20 mm, or more (Fig. 33-16). Such large effusions may seem to be posterior to the left atrium (in the oblique sinus). Erratic motion of the cardiac silhouette may be exhibited in large effusions that go on to cardiac tamponade (Fig. 33-17).

As reported by Nanda and Gramiak,[5] the heart may swing in the pericardial effusion space, with a resultant change in the pattern of wall motion. Normally the right ventricular wall moves posteriorly in systole and anteriorly in diastole. When the heart swings, it may move posteriorly in one cardiac cycle and anteriorly in the next so that it is physically nearer the chest wall with every other beat. This form of cardiac swinging is associated with the phenomenon of electrical alternans (Fig. 33-18).

Cardiac tamponade occurs when the intrapericardial pressure reaches a sufficient level to compromise the filling of the heart. Emergency pericardiocentesis, with or without ultrasound guidance, must be performed to relieve the intrapericardial pressure.

The sonographer should be careful not to evaluate other cardiac structures in the presence of pericardial effusion.[5] The AV valves may exhibit pseudo-SAM (due to chordal structures) or pseudoprolapse patterns (Fig. 33-19). The semilunar valves show late systolic collapse of the aortic valve or systolic notching of the pulmonary valve. The aortic root and interventricular septum and the posterior left ventricular wall may all exhibit abnormal motion. These abnormalities will disappear after the fluid is resorbed. A repeat echo may then be performed so the cardiac structures can be evaluated.

Text continued on p. 564.

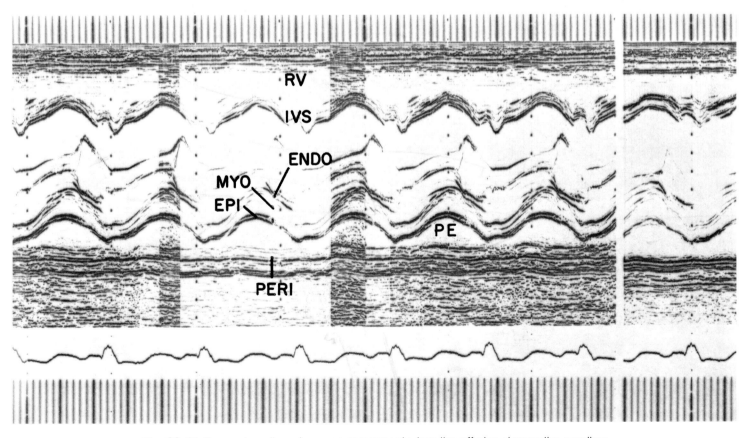

Fig. 33-11. The pericardium shows no movement when the effusion damps the cardiac pulsations.

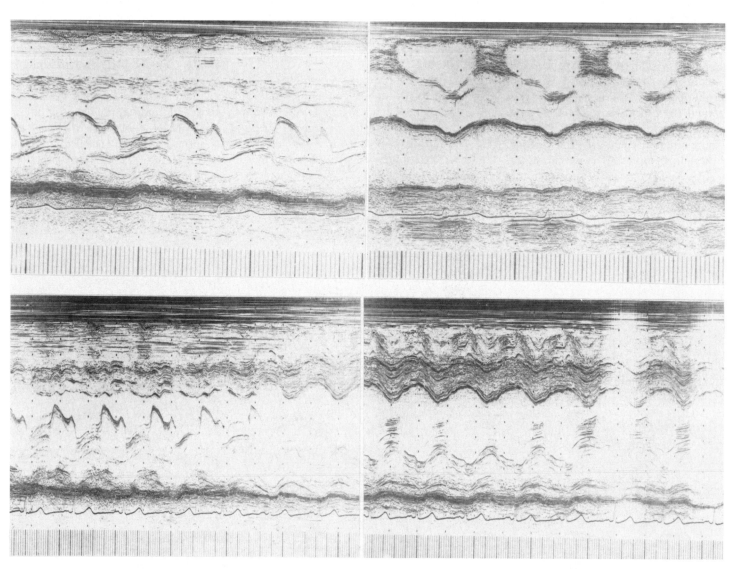

Fig. 33-12. Multiple scans in a young renal patient with a small pericardial effusion. There is some transmitted cardiac pulsation seen in the pericardium.

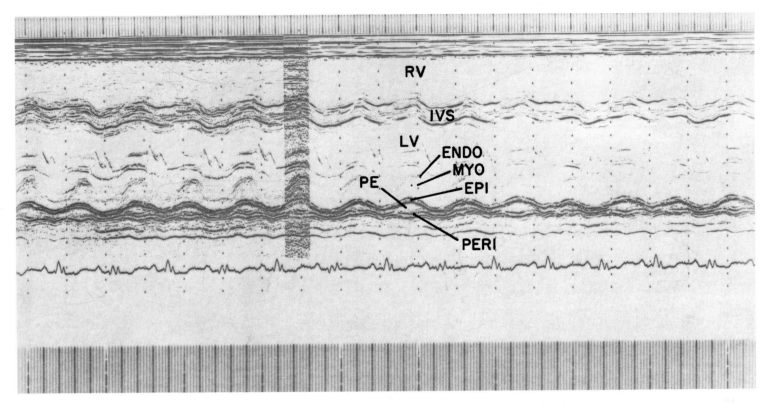

Fig. 33-13. A very small posterior pericardial effusion may produce an echo-free space in systole but disappear in diastole.

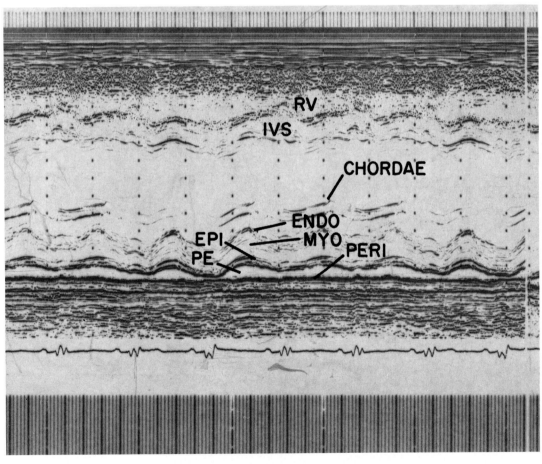

Fig. 33-14. A separation between the epicardium and pericardium along the posterior heart wall indicates that the patient has a small (100 ml or less) effusion.

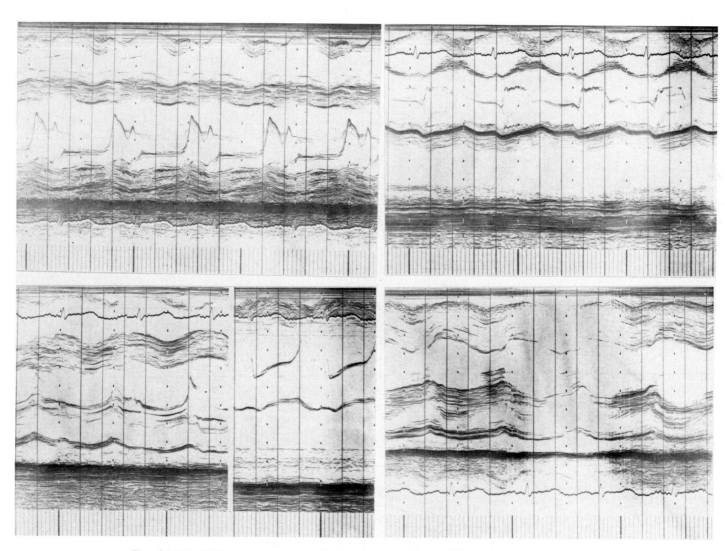

Fig. 33-15. Multiple scans in a middle-aged woman with metastatic carcinoma demonstrate a moderate-sized effusion in the anterior and posterior pericardial sac.

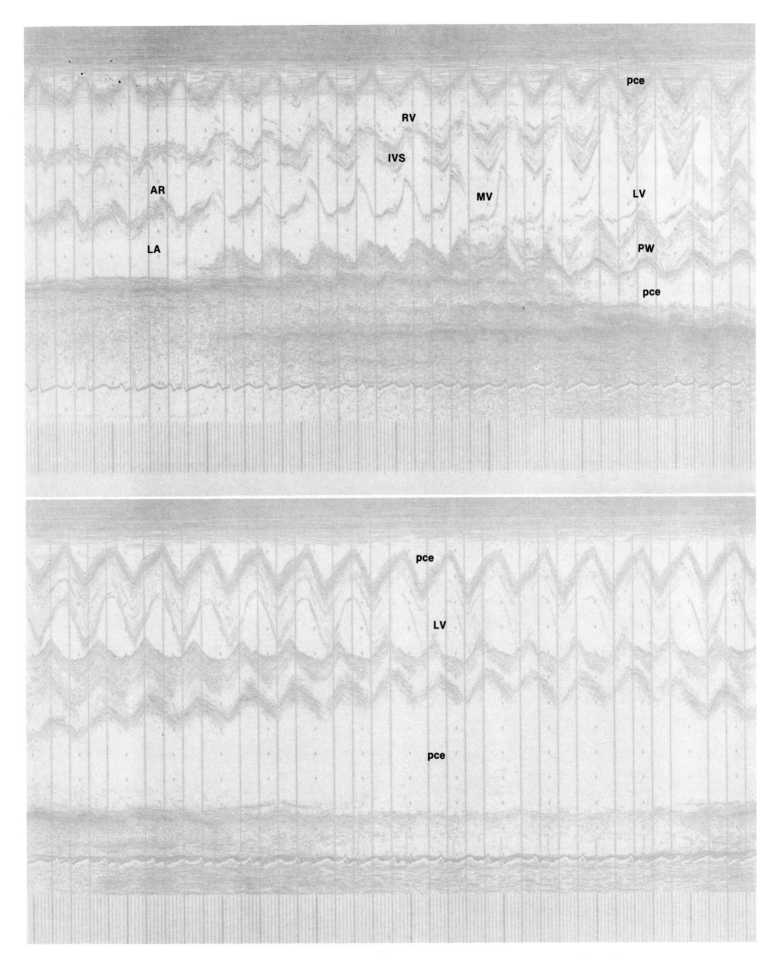

Fig. 33-16. M-mode sweep in a young renal patient in whom a huge pericardial effusion developed without tamponade.

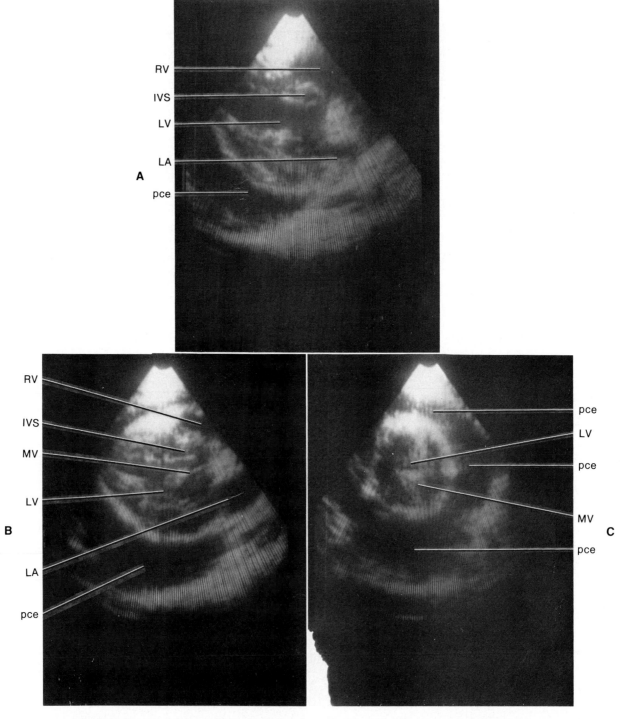

Fig. 33-17. A, Two-dimensional view of the patient in Fig. 33-16. This long axis shows the cardiac structures separated from the pericardium by a huge effusion. **B,** The beam is directed toward the apex of the ventricle to record the maximum amount of effusion. **C,** Short axis of the effusion as it surrounds the ventricular cavity.

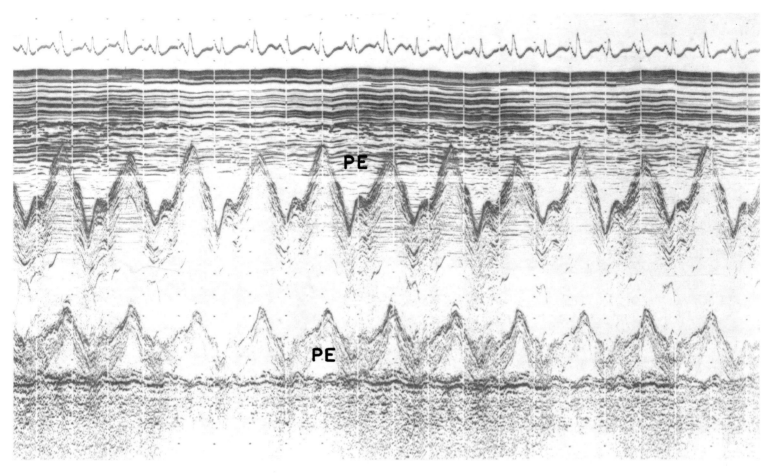

Fig. 33-18. Large anteroposterior pericardial effusion, or swinging heart syndrome, in a patient with cardiac tamponade.

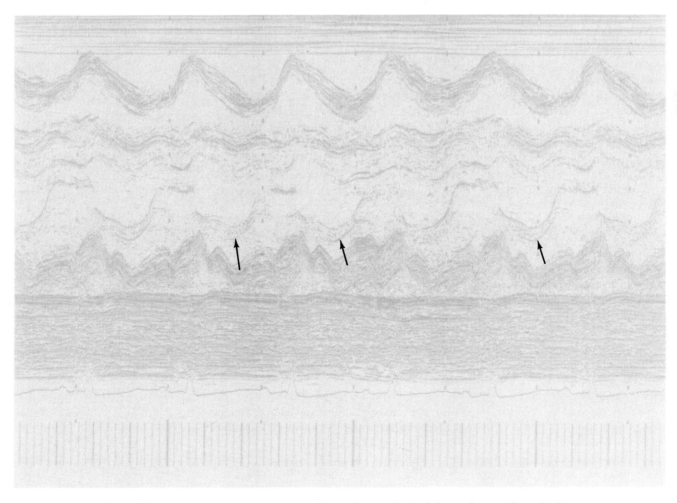

Fig. 33-19. The mitral apparatus should not be evaluated for prolapse, since in the presence of pericardial effusion the hyperdynamic state of the ventricle may cause a pseudoprolapse *(arrows)*.

Differentiation of pericardial effusion from other structures

Occasionally a large echo-free space, representing a pleural effusion, will be detected behind the left ventricle and may be confused with pericardial effusion if one is not careful. A way to distinguish it is to note absence of an echo-free space anterior to the right ventricle: if there is a significant posterior effusion, it will extend into the anterior space as well.

The pleural fluid never extends behind the left atrium, since this chamber lies in the mediastinum and pleural fluid is excluded from that region by the anatomy of the pleural sacs.[5] Confirmation of pleural fluid can be made by placing the transducer along the midaxillary line to show the fluid in the lung.

Haaz et al.[2] utilized the parasternal short axis view to locate the descending thoracic aorta to differentiate pericardial from pleural effusion. In their study patients with an isolated pericardial effusion had an echo-free space between the descending thoracic aorta and the left ventricular posterior wall. Patients with isolated pleural effusion had an echo-free space posterior to the descending aorta. The other group of patients had both a pericardial and a pleural effusion and had echo-free spaces between the descending thoracic aorta and the left ventricular wall and also posterior to the descending aorta. Thus the descending thoracic aorta serves as a valuable landmark in differentiating pericardial from pleural effusions.

Other structures near the atrioventricular groove (i.e., thoracic aorta, pulmonary veins, coronary sulcus) can produce a posterior echo-free space. Again this may be differentiated from an effusion by a careful sweep from the left atrium to the apex of the ventricle. Such structures will appear and disappear quickly as one sweeps to the left ventricular apex.

Anterior separation of the heart wall from the pericardium may be due to subepicardial fat. As one scans toward the apex, the space decreases in size; however, with pericardial effusions the space increases in size toward the apex.

Other lesions (e.g., a pericardial cyst or tumor mass) may lie along the anterior heart wall and mimic an effusion. However, the separation will be seen only anteriorly. If gain settings are slightly increased, some echo fill-in may be evident in the tumor mass.

Another cause for misdiagnosing pericardial effusion is the presence of calcification of the chordal structures or mitral anulus.

When such calcification exists, it makes separating the posterior heart wall layers from the pericardium by M-mode more difficult. However, two-dimensional long, short, and apical views should allow easy assessment for the presence of pericardial effusion.

Constrictive pericarditis

Constrictive pericarditis confines the diastolic expansion of the ventricles, and thus by echo a flattened left ventricular wall is recorded in diastole. There may also be abnormal septal motion.[5] An echo-free space is not identified as in pericardial effusion. Instead, a thickened and calcified pericardium is shown as the gain is reduced.

Martin et al.[4] reported that M-mode tracings were not good for distinguishing fluid loculation or intrapericardial bands. These structures may be better defined by two-dimensional echo. In the presence of intrapericardial bands, absence of positional fluid shifts may suggest fluid loculation.[3] The two-dimensional transducer should be placed in the parasternal, subxyphoid, and apical positions for optimal assessment of pericardial fluid.

In patients with chronic and recurrent pericardial processes, adhesive or fibrinous pericardial bands are more likely to develop and go on to constrictive pericarditis or tamponade.[4]

SUMMARY

Echocardiography may be a safe, reliable, and accurate examination for the detection of pericardial effusion when used in experienced hands. Other structures that can mimic an effusion have been discussed. The sonographer must be able to make several cardiac sweeps from the base of the heart to the apex with varying gain settings to separate the layers of the posterior heart wall from the pericardium.

Normally the pericardial fluid is echo free; however, if it has been bled into or invaded by tumor cells or if it contains pus from a bacterial infection or has postradiation changes, it will not be echo free.

Ultrasound may be utilized for pericardiocentesis to follow the tip of the needle by M-mode or two-dimensional as it enters the pericardial space. Monitoring the withdrawal of fluid is easily done by echo.

The sonographer must be aware of the various pericardial abnormalities and be able to differentiate them from other structures surrounding the cardiac cavity.

REFERENCES

1. Berglund, E., Sarnoff, S.J., and Isaacs, J.P.: Ventricular function. Role of the pericardium in regulation of cardiovascular hemodynamics, Circ. Res. **3:** 133, 1955.
2. Haaz, W.S., Mintz, G.S., Kotler, M.N., et al.: Two-dimensional echographic recognition of the descending thoracic aorta: value in differentiating pericardial from pleural effusions, Am. J. Cardiol. **46:** 739, 1980.
3. Martin, R.P., Rakowski, H., French, J., et al.: Localization of pericardial effusions with wide-angle phased-array echocardiography, Am. J. Cardiol. **42:**904, 1976.
4. Martin, R.P., Rowden, R., Filly, K., et al.: Intrapericardial abnormalities in patients with pericardial effusion, Circulation **61:**568, 1980.
5. Nanda, N.C., and Gramiak, R.: Clinical echocardiography, St. Louis, 1978, The C.V. Mosby Co.
6. Southworth, H., and Stevenson, C.W.: Congenital defects of the pericardium, Arch. Intern. Med. **61:** 223, 1938.
7. Walmsley, R., Watson, H., and Kirklin, J.W.: Clinical anatomy of the heart, New York, 1978, Churchill Livingstone, Inc.
8. Winters, W.L., and Cortes, F.M.: Pericardial disease. In Conn, H.L., and Horwitz, D., editors: Cardiac and vascular diseases, Philadelphia, 1971, Lea & Febiger.

34

Pediatric echocardiography

A. ABIGAIL BROGDEN
JAN EWENKO

The evaluation of the patient with congenital heart disease by echocardiography provides the clinician with specific cardiac spatial information that may be difficult to obtain from other diagnostic tests. An important concept for the cardiac sonographer to remember is to try to assess the heart in relation to what would be found on a normal echogram. Thus first one should assess the number of chambers and valves and their relationship to each other. When the atrioventricular valves are seen, one should assess whether they are normal, overriding, thickened, redundant, cleft, or otherwise deformed. The semilunar cusps should likewise be assessed for their number of cusps, thickness, overriding, doming, or other abnormalities. The chamber size and wall thickness should be evaluated as well as septal defects that may be present. The specific cardiac abnormalities found in congenital cardiac problems will be discussed and examples shown as they relate to pediatric and adult congenital heart conditions.

The pediatric cardiac sonographer deals with children as well as with the complex anatomy associated with their congenital heart defects. Since many visits to the doctor are not generally pleasant, children are often apprehensive when they arrive at the laboratory. Most can be comforted by an explanation of exactly what will happen during the procedure, reassurance that it will not hurt, and the suggestion that it could be fun to see "pictures" of their heart. If the child is not consoled, begin the procedure and try to divert his attention. Since children seem to be very sensitive to sound, such things as mobiles, music boxes, singing, keys, and a variety of rattles and bells may be helpful. For older children, structures can be pointed out on the screen as they appear. Parents can be enlisted to read to the child to keep him occupied. These measures are important, not only to make the task of the cardiac sonographer easier but also to ensure that the child will be as close as possible to a physiologic resting state so measurements can be standaradized.

Patient position. It is important to keep small infants as warm and comfortable as possible. This can be done with a blanket or a warmer. They can be placed entirely on a pillow, which elevates them somewhat as well as allows position changes (e.g., left lateral) with a minimum of disturbance. Dimming the lights and having a bottle or pacifier handy often will help the infant go to sleep. If the infant has been breast fed, holding the pacifier under warm water makes it "more like Mom."

Transducer selection. Since an infant's chest is small and the structures to be visualized are small and anterior, it is important to use a transducer with the best possible resolution. In both M-mode and two-dimensional studies Gutgesell's group[51] has demonstrated that this is best achieved by the use of high-frequency focused transducers. The M-mode transducers available in our laboratory include the following: a 5-MHz 6-mm unfocused transducer, which we use on neonates through toddlers; a 3.5-MHz 6-mm transducer, which we use on preschoolers through young adolescents; a 3.5-MHz quarter-wave transducer, which we use on adolescents through young teenagers; and a 2.25-MHz 13-mm transducer, which we use on older and heavier teenagers. To optimize recording, various transducers are often employed during the study.

Measurements. Measuring sites for infants and small children differ from the standards set by the American Society of Echocardiography (ASE) shown in Fig. 34-1.[77] Since the posterior leaflet of the mitral valve hangs further down in the body of the left ventricle, the minor axis along which the ventricular measurements are made is more accurately represented by a perpendicular dropped in the plane of the posterior leaflet[3] (Fig. 34-2).

Fig. 34-1. Diagrammatic echocardiographic sweep showing, superimposed upon the structures, the recommended criteria for measurement. Diastolic measurements are made at the onset of the QRS complex. Cavities and walls are measured at the level of the chordae below the mitral valve. The illustration and the elliptical inserts, *a* to *e*, illustrate the leading-edge method as well as measurements using the thinnest continuous echo lines. Other abbreviations: *AWRV* anterior wall of right ventricle; *RV*, right ventricle; *LV*, left ventricle; *PWLV*, posterior wall of left ventricle; *S*, septum; *PPM*, papillary muscle; *ALMV, PLMV*, anterior and posterior leaflets of mitral valve; *A, B, C, D, E,* and *F*, points of mitral valve motion; *En*, endocardium; *Ep*, epicardium; *Ao*, aorta. The extra line in insert *b*, which is excluded from the septal measurement, represents a portion of tricuspid valve apparatus. (Modified slightly from Sahn, D.J., et al.: Circulation **58**:1072, 1978. By permission of the American Heart Association, Inc.)

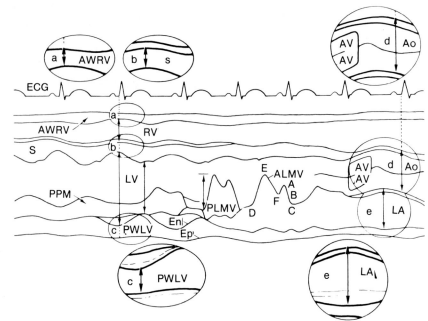

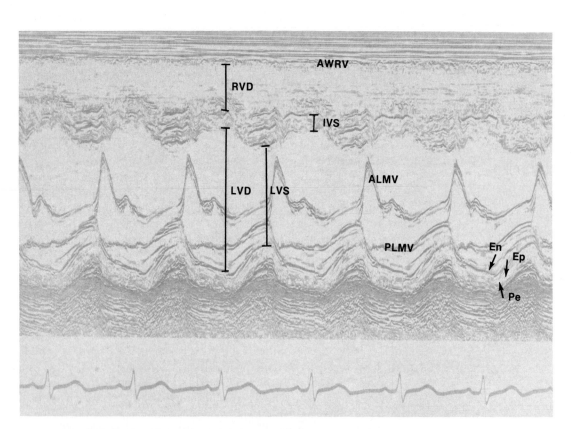

Fig. 34-2. M-mode trace of the systolic and diastolic measurements of the left ventricular cavity. *AWRV,* Anterior wall of right ventricle; *RVD,* right ventricular dimension; *IVS,* interventricular septum; *LVD,* left ventricular dimension (diastole); *LVS,* left ventricular dimension (systole); *ALMV,* anterior leaflet of mitral valve; *En,* endocardium; *Ep,* epicardium; *Pe,* pericardium.

The left and right ventricular chamber dimensions, left and right ventricular wall thickness, and ventricular septal thickness measurements are made at the onset of the QRS complex following the leading edge–to–leading edge recommendations of the ASE. Since poor somatic growth is often associated with heart disease, we evaluate dimensions using graphs from Rogé et al.,[72] which relate them to the patient's body surface area. (See Appendix J.) Special care must be taken to differentiate the right ventricular septal surface from the tricuspid valve apparatus, since there are multiple echoes in the near field due to the proximity of the child's heart to the chest wall. Overestimation of interventricular septal thickness could erroneously indicate right ventricular hypertrophy, left ventricular hypertrophy, or asymmetric septal hypertrophy. The right ventricular septal surface is characterized as the most continuous line that mimics the motion pattern of the left septal surface. Tricuspid lines straighten out and appear more anterior at end diastole. Two instances of tricuspid apparatus riding atop the interventricular septum are shown in Fig. 34-3.

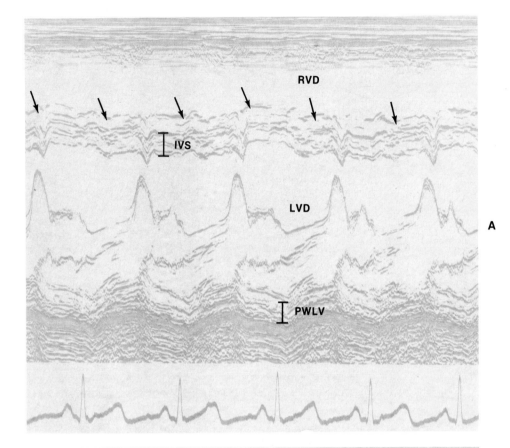

A

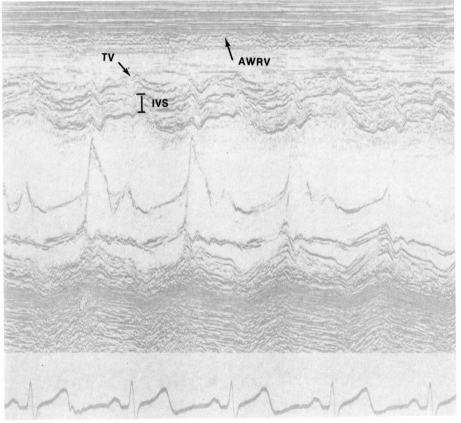

B

Fig. 34-3. A, Normal M-mode trace at the mitral valve level demonstrating the pitfall of tricuspid valve echo seen atop the ventricular septum *(arrows)*. If measured incorrectly, it appears falsely thick. Note that the true interventricular septal measurement and left ventricular posterior wall measurement are 1:1. **B,** Normal M-mode trace of the mitral valve area, with a less apparent tricuspid valve sitting atop the ventricular septal echoes. *RVD,* Right ventricular dimension; *TV,* tricuspid valve; *IVS,* interventricular septum; *LVD,* left ventricular dimension; *PWLV,* posterior wall of left ventricle.

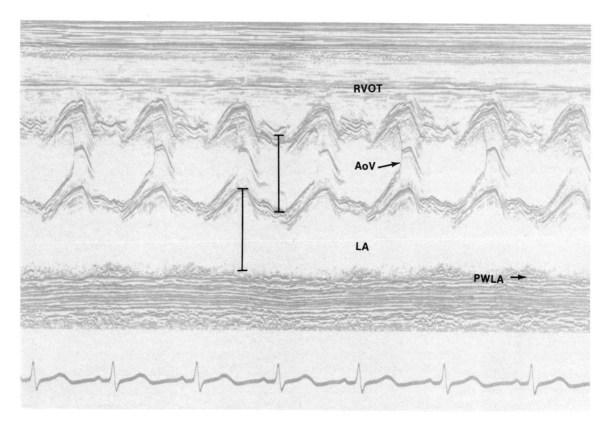

Fig. 34-4. Normal M-mode trace of the aorta and left atrium showing the characteristic left atrial posterior wall motion. Note that the echo beam cuts through both leaflets of the aortic valve. Tricuspid echoes can also be seen atop the anterior wall of the aorta. Standard sites of measurement are shown. *RVOT,* Right ventricular outflow tract; *AoV,* aortic valve; *LA,* left atrium; *PWLA,* posterior wall of left atrium.

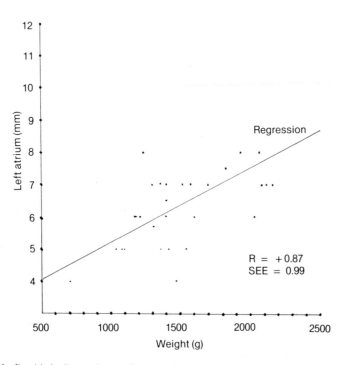

Fig. 34-5. Left atrial dimensions of normal premature infants graphed against their weight in grams. (From Goldberg, S.J., et al.: J. Clin. Ultrasound **5:**161, 1978.)

The left atrial measurement shown in Fig. 34-4 takes on great significance in infants and children, since an increase in the ratio of left atrial to aortic root size (LA/Ao, normally 0.7 to 0.85) is an indicator of a left-to-right shunt. The left atrial size of premature infants must be related to their body weight[29] (Fig. 34-5). Echoes occurring within the left atrium, which could be confused with those from the left atrial posterior wall, have been attributed to entering pulmonary veins or beam width artifacts from the mitral anulus and can be eliminated by decreasing the gain in the area. The true left atrial posterior wall can be identified by its motion as well as its depth. During ventricular systole the left atrial wall moves posteriorly (i.e., away from the transducer) while the ventricular wall moves anteriorly. A sweep from mitral to aortic valve should show the left atrial posterior wall continuous with the endocardium of the left ventricle. A depth measurement from the crystal artifact to each of these structures should normally show them at the same level. In some instances (e.g., sternal retractions with respiratory distress, in which the anteroposterior plane or Z axis is flattened)

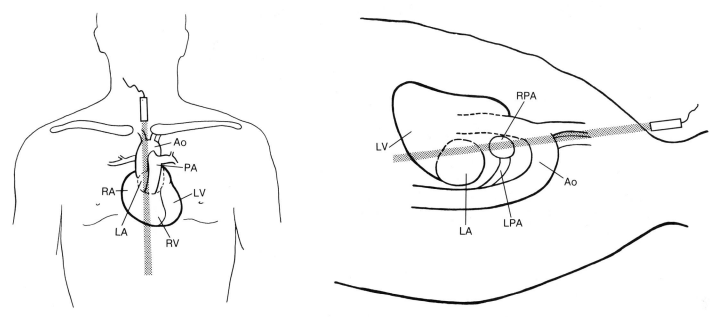

Fig. 34-6. The beam from a transducer placed in the suprasternal notch transects the transverse aortic arch, right pulmonary artery, and left atrium. M-mode dimensions are taken of the arch, right pulmonary artery, and Y axis of the left atrium. (Reproduced with permission from Goldberg, S., et al.: Pediatric and adolescent echocardiography: a handbook, ed. 2, Chicago, 1980, Year Book Medical Publishers, Inc.)

the left atrial dimension may be underestimated. Then the suprasternal notch view, Y axis, cutting through the transverse arch, right pulmonary artery, and left atrium, yields a more representative left atrial dimension[28] (Fig. 34-6). Fig. 34-7 shows an example of each. This view is also helpful in lesions in which an increased pulmonary blood flow may cause dilation of the right pulmonary artery. The transverse aortic arch dimension increases with obstructive lesions, both proximally and distally, as seen with Marfan's and Turner's syndromes. A small transverse aortic arch dimension can help in confirming the diagnosis of hypoplastic left heart syndrome.[4] (See Appendix J for normal transverse aortic arch and right pulmonary artery values based on body surface area.)

Technique. Although the direct M-mode, with its ice pick view, is most helpful in detecting the directional relationship of structures, most of our patients are examined with two-dimensional ultrasound equipment, which shows spatial relationships of the cardiac structures. We use the standardized ASE[41] long axis, apical and subxyphoid four

chamber, and left ventricular short axis views. We also find the high short axis, suprasternal notch, and several subxyphoid views very helpful in delineating the outflows of both ventricles (Fig. 34-8). Their utility is discussed with specific lesions.[14,50,90]

Since the pediatric echocardiographer often deals with complex disease states, we believe it important to have not only as much knowledge as possible of a patient under examination but also a background in embryology, pathology, and anatomy.[62] In addition, the ability to interpret related procedures (e.g., electrocardiogram, chest radiograph, blood studies, cardiac catheterization data, surgical notes, and auscultatory findings) is invaluable. Table 34-1 lists common murmurs and the lesions that are associated with them.

• • •

In pediatric echocardiography one must be aware of technical problems and pitfalls and be prepared for a whole host of anatomies. Objectivity is essential. If objectivity is lost and the anticipated but incorrect diagnosis is made, the error can literally be fatal.

Table 34-1. Common murmurs with their associated lesions

Murmur	Lesion
Holosystolic (pansystolic)	Ventricular septal defect, mitral regurgitation, tricuspid regurgitation
Systolic ejection	Small vsd; flow through semilunar valves (Ao and PA) can be innocent or indicative of stenosis
Late systolic (beginning after 1/3 to 1/2 of systole ± systolic click)	Mitral valve prolapse
Diastolic decrescendo	Aortic insufficiency, pulmonic insufficiency
Middiastolic rumble	Generally indicative of shunt (asd, vsd) greater than 2:1, mitral stenosis, tricuspid stenosis
Continuous	A-V fistula, patent ductus arteriosus

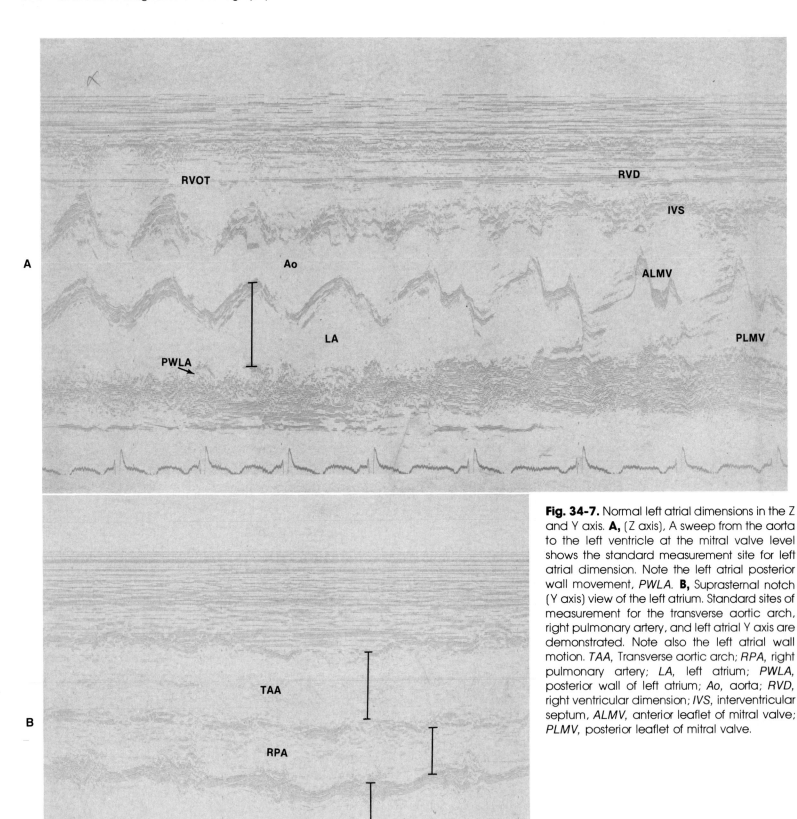

Fig. 34-7. Normal left atrial dimensions in the Z and Y axis. **A,** (Z axis), A sweep from the aorta to the left ventricle at the mitral valve level shows the standard measurement site for left atrial dimension. Note the left atrial posterior wall movement, *PWLA*. **B,** Suprasternal notch (Y axis) view of the left atrium. Standard sites of measurement for the transverse aortic arch, right pulmonary artery, and left atrial Y axis are demonstrated. Note also the left atrial wall motion. *TAA,* Transverse aortic arch; *RPA,* right pulmonary artery; *LA,* left atrium; *PWLA,* posterior wall of left atrium; *Ao,* aorta; *RVD,* right ventricular dimension; *IVS,* interventricular septum, *ALMV,* anterior leaflet of mitral valve; *PLMV,* posterior leaflet of mitral valve.

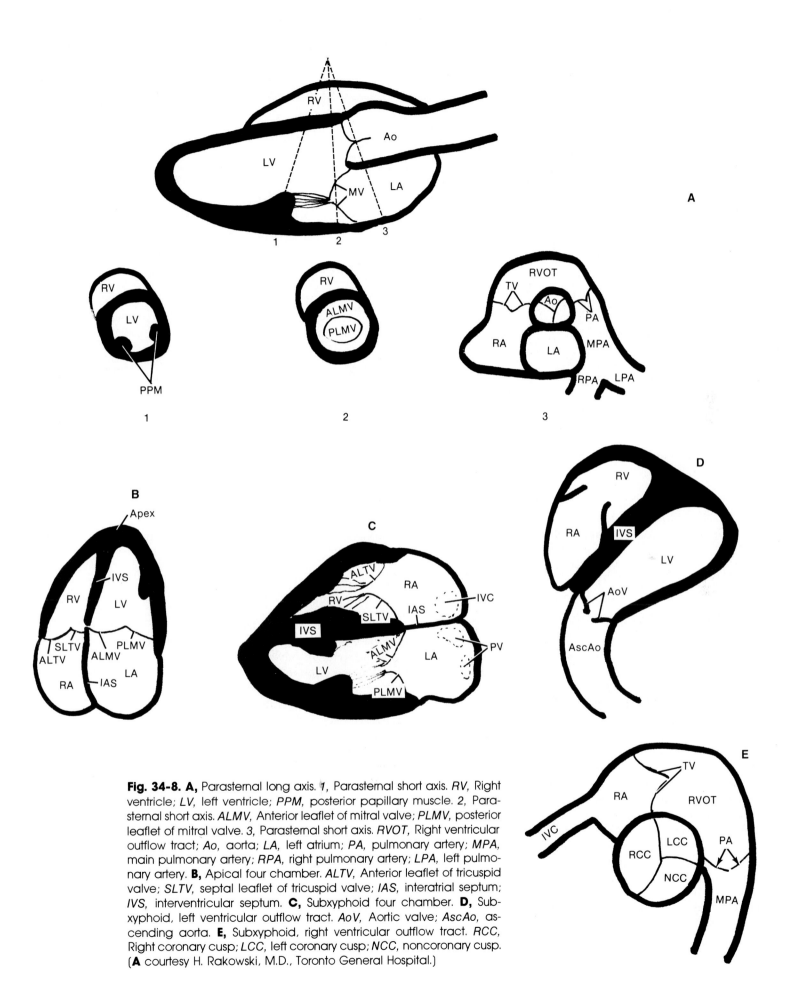

Fig. 34-8. A, Parasternal long axis. **1,** Parasternal short axis. *RV,* Right ventricle; *LV,* left ventricle; *PPM,* posterior papillary muscle. **2,** Parasternal short axis. *ALMV,* Anterior leaflet of mitral valve; *PLMV,* posterior leaflet of mitral valve. **3,** Parasternal short axis. *RVOT,* Right ventricular outflow tract; *Ao,* aorta; *LA,* left atrium; *PA,* pulmonary artery; *MPA,* main pulmonary artery; *RPA,* right pulmonary artery; *LPA,* left pulmonary artery. **B,** Apical four chamber. *ALTV,* Anterior leaflet of tricuspid valve; *SLTV,* septal leaflet of tricuspid valve; *IAS,* interatrial septum; *IVS,* interventricular septum. **C,** Subxyphoid four chamber. **D,** Subxyphoid, left ventricular outflow tract. *AoV,* Aortic valve; *AscAo,* ascending aorta. **E,** Subxyphoid, right ventricular outflow tract. *RCC,* Right coronary cusp; *LCC,* left coronary cusp; *NCC,* noncoronary cusp. (**A** courtesy H. Rakowski, M.D., Toronto General Hospital.)

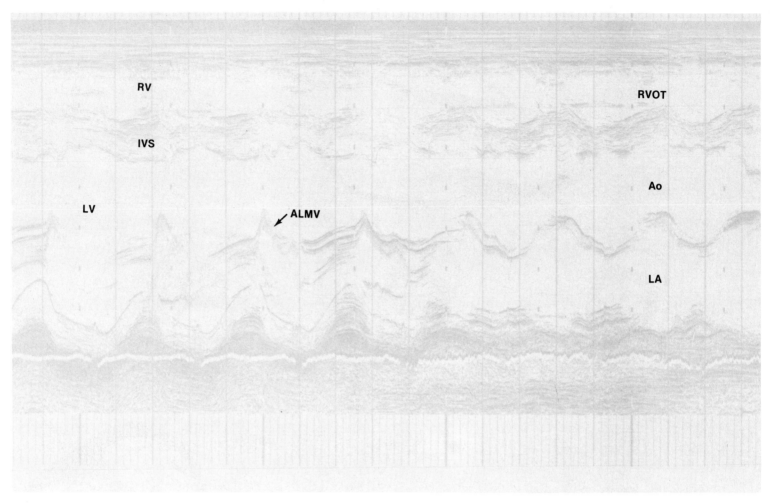

Fig. 34-9. Aorta to mitral valve M-mode scan in a patient with left ventricular volume loading. Note the vigorous contractile pattern of the enlarged left ventricle with normal septal motion.

VENTRICULAR SEPTAL DEFECTS

Approximately 20% of congenital heart patients have a solitary ventricular septal defect (vsd), which makes this defect the most commonly encountered lesion. It is also seen in conjunction with other anomalies.[62] M-mode echocardiography is usually not sensitive enough to pick up ventricular defects, unless they are of considerable size. False signal dropout due to angulation errors can also occur. Increased left atrial and left ventricular size with hypercontractility (i.e., high fractional shortening) suggests left-sided volume loading (Fig. 34-9). Although this may not be apparent with smaller ventricular defects, it is still a useful indicator and is seen in all lesions that cause left ventricular volume loading (e.g., patent ductus arteriosus). Occasionally turbulent flow will cause flutter of the mitral valve leaflets, as seen in Fig. 34-10.

With two-dimensional echo the defect can often be directly visualized. In our experience most are seen in the apical four chamber view just below the AV ring. One must pay particular attention to viewing as much of the septum as possible. This can be done by angling the transducer inferiorly toward the left hip and scanning superiorly toward the right shoulder. At the most superior position the aortic valve in short axis should be visible. Most ventricular septal defects are visualized just as the beam is scanned posteriorly from the aorta and the ventricular septum appears (Fig. 34-11). It is important to remember that small ventricular septal defects often cannot be seen due to beam width artifacts; furthermore, some instruments are better than others at detecting a small ventricular septal defect. High-frequency transducers with good lateral and axial resolution aid in detecting smaller defects. False signal

dropout due to the relatively thin membranous septum should not be confused with a true defect.

High membranous defects are best visualized in the long axis view immediately below the aortic valve. If the defect can be seen in both the four chamber and the long axis views, it is a large communication. Size is difficult to assign to a defect, for the defect may be irregularly shaped and not entirely seen by the echo beam. If the aortic root overrides the ventricular septal defect, more complex forms of congenital heart disease must be considered.

Ventricular septal defects often close spontaneously. The aneurysmal bulge into the right ventricle sometimes associated with this phenomenon can be visualized[88] (Fig. 34-12).

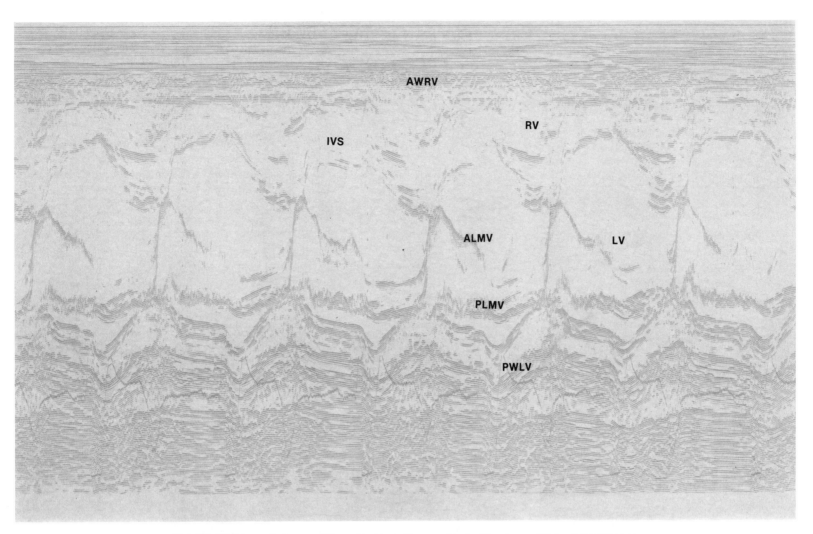

Fig. 34-10. M-mode trace at the mitral level in a patient with a large left-to-right shunt at the ventricular level, demonstrating flutter on both the anterior and the posterior mitral valve leaflets due to the turbulent flow. Note the very hypercontractile interventricular septum. Fractional shortening in this trace was measured at 57%.

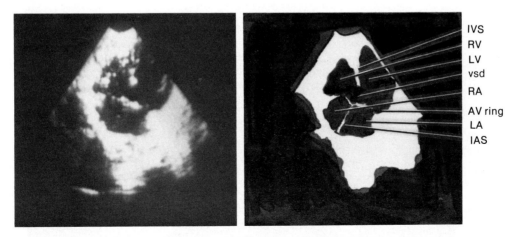

Fig. 34-11. Apical four chamber view demonstrating a break in ventricular septal continuity just below the aortic valve in the membranous septum.

The four chamber view is helpful in detecting muscular ventricular septal defects. Although usually smaller and therefore harder to visualize, these are seen lower in the septum, removed from the AV ring. The same care in scanning as much of the septum as possible should be taken. Occasionally there are multiple "Swiss cheese" defects in this area of the septum that produce false-negatives due to artifact. Moderate to large defects do not pose such a problem and can be detected. Fig. 34-13 illustrates a large muscular ventricular septal defect.

M-mode and two-dimensional contrast echocardiography are used in the confirmation of ventricular septal defects. Fig. 34-14 is an M-mode demonstration of a right-to-left shunt at the ventricular level.[81,82,89,106] The contrast echoes are seen first in the right ventricular cavity and subsequently in the left ventricular cavity above the mitral valve (differentiating this from an atrial level shunt, in which the contrast is seen in the mitral funnel first). Fig. 34-15 is a two-dimensional contrast study in an adolescent with a high membranous ventricular septal defect. A right-to-left shunt produces an echo-free front or negative contrast in the left ventricle.[79,80]

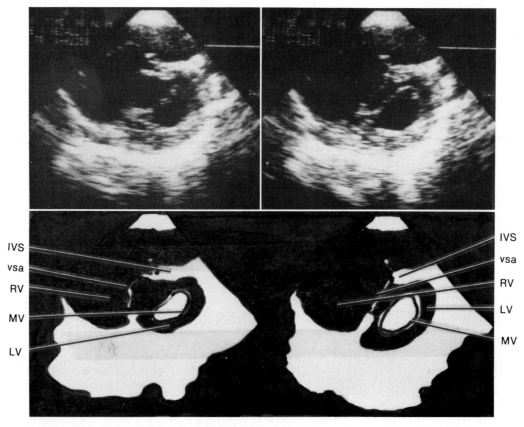

Fig. 34-12. Parasternal short axis views with an accompanying diagram demonstrating a ventricular septal aneurysm, *vsa*.

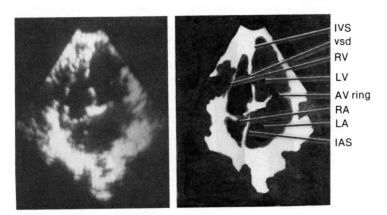

Fig. 34-13. Apical four chamber view demonstrating a ventricular septal defect *vsd*, in the muscular septum removed inferiorly from the AV ring.

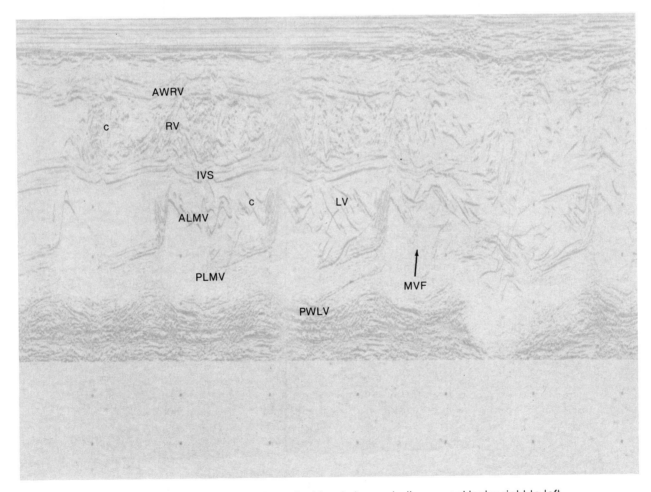

Fig. 34-14. M-mode trace at the mitral level demonstrating a ventricular right-to-left shunt. The contrast initially appears in the right ventricular cavity and in the next complex is seen in the left ventricular cavity above the anterior leaflet of the mitral valve. Note that the contrast is never seen in the funnel of the mitral valve, indicating that the shunt is at the ventricular level and not at the atrial level.

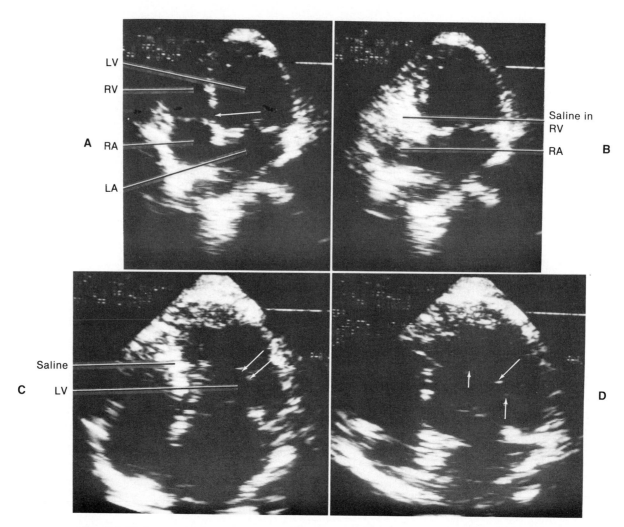

Fig. 34-15. Two-dimensional contrast study in a patient with an apparent membranous ventricular septal defect. **A** shows the break in septal continuity *(arrow)* just before injection. Note the dilated appearance of the left ventricle. **B** shows the saline injection filling the right heart. **C** and **D** show the bubbles *(arrows)* in the left ventricle.

PATENT DUCTUS ARTERIOSUS

Patent ductus arteriosus also produces echocardiographic indications of left ventricular volume loading. Left atrial size[3] and the LA/Ao[30] are often used to assess the size of the left-to-right shunt (Fig. 34-16). Although some authors[74] report being able to visualize the patent ductus arteriosus directly, contrast injection into a well-placed (above the T_4 level in the aortic arch) umbilical artery line still serves as confirmation in premature infants.[5] Injection of echo contrast or the patient's own blood during a suprasternal long axis view produces echoes shunting through a patent ductus arteriosus into the right pulmonary artery.

PULMONARY ARTERY HYPERTENSION

Pulmonary artery hypertension often occurs with ventricular septal defects or patent ductus arteriosus. Several authors have discussed the pulmonary echocardiogram and its inherent difficulties.[65,71,94,97] Since the pulmonary valve is anterior and often hidden behind the aorta, accurate data are technically difficult to derive. In our laboratory we consider the following criteria for establishing the presence or absence of pulmonary artery hypertension: (1) systolic flutter on the posterior pulmonary valve leaflet, with or without (2) a move to early closure; (3) a right ventricular preejection period/ejection time ratio (RVPEP/RVET) of 0.3 or greater; (4) loss of the A wave or dip at atrial systole[45,52,105]; and (5) evidence of right ventricular anterior wall thickening, which is desirable but, given the technical difficulties with measurement, not a necessary criterion. Even with these criteria the reading of pulmonary artery hypertension is open to false-positives and false-negatives.[1,11] Some examples of the pulmonary artery echocardiogram are shown in Figs. 34-17 to 34-20.

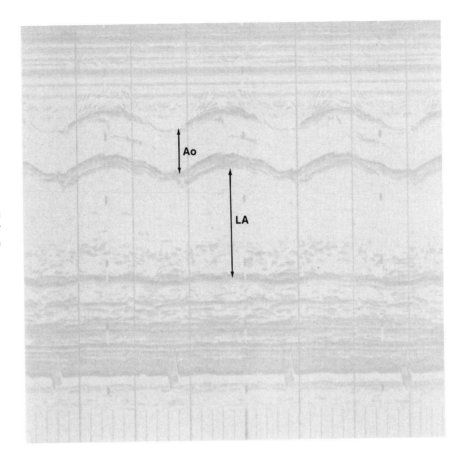

Fig. 34-16. M-mode tracing in a neonate with a patent ductus arteriosus. The aortic root measures 7 mm whereas the left atrium measures 18 mm. The LA / Ao of 2.5 is enlarged.

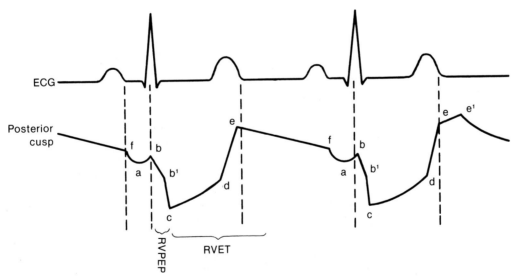

Fig. 34-17. Schematic of a pulmonary valve M-mode echocardiogram showing the normal pattern of its posterior leaflet. *a*, Posterior deflection of the leaflet at atrial systole—the atrial pressure wave following the P wave transiently raises the right ventricular end diastolic pressure above that of the normal pulmonary artery; *b*, onset of ventricular systole; *c*, maximum leaflet opening during ventricular systole; *d*, onset of diastolic closure; *e*, diastolic coaptation point of the leaflet; *f*, onset of atrial contraction.[27] The method for obtaining the ratio right ventricular preejection period to right ventricular ejection time, *RVPEP/RVET*, is shown. The RVPEP is measured from the onset of the QRS complex to the *b* point of the valve. The RVET is measured from this point to closure of the valve, or the *e* point.[28]

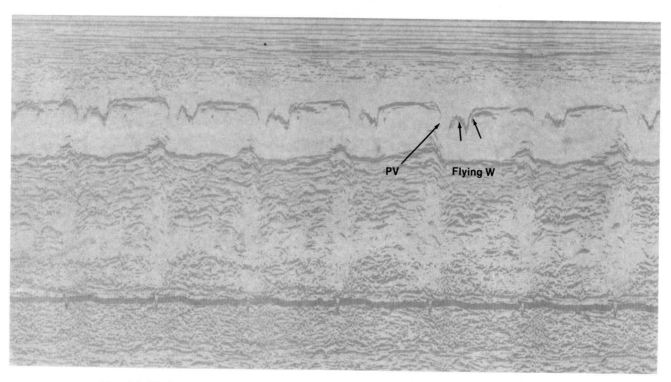

Fig. 34-18. Patent ductus arteriosus. The pulmonary artery pressure measured during cardiac catheterization was at a systemic level of 93/58. Note the flat E-F slope, systolic flutter, premature systolic closure, loss of the A wave, and RVPEP/RVET of 0.41. The classic appearance of the flying W is also evident.

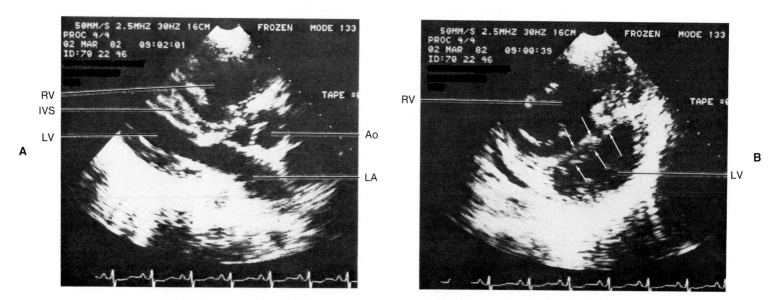

Fig. 34-19. A 20-year-old man with idiopathic pulmonary hypertension. **A,** Parasternal long axis showing the dilated right ventricular cavity and a small left ventricular cavity. **B,** Parasternal short axis showing the flattened septum *(arrows)* secondary to the pulmonary hypertension. **C,** M-mode through the parasternal long axis. **D,** High short axis to show the dilated pulmonary artery and its outflow tract. **E** and **F,** Subxyphoid views of the liver, inferior vena cava, hepatic veins, and right atrium to show the reflux of contrast *(arrows)* throughout the cardiac cycle secondary to tricuspid regurgitation.

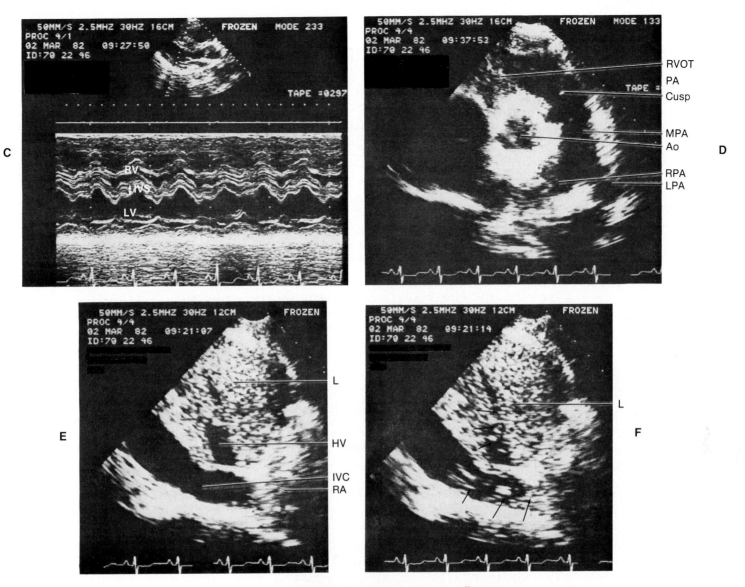

Fig. 34-19, cont'd. For legend see opposite page.

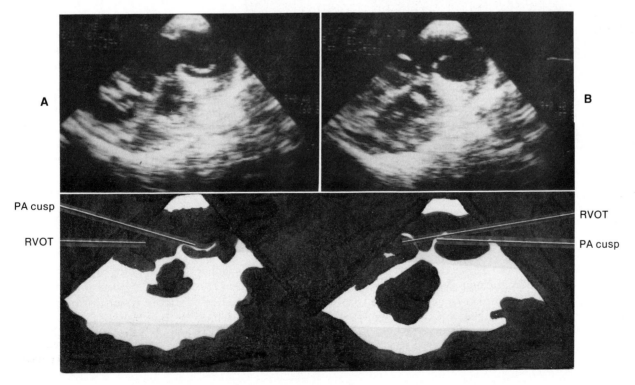

Fig. 34-20. Parasternal short axis of a patient with a domed pulmonary valve — domed back in systole, **A,** and forward in diastole, **B.**

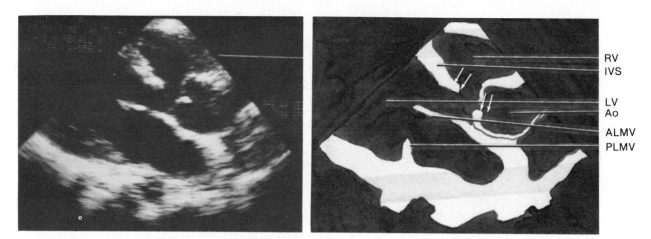

Fig. 34-21. Patient with tetralogy of Fallot. The frame, taken in diastole, shows the aortic override with the interventricular septum meeting the level of the aortic valve *(arrows)*. Note the anterior displacement of the anterior wall of the aorta and the normal-sized left atrium.

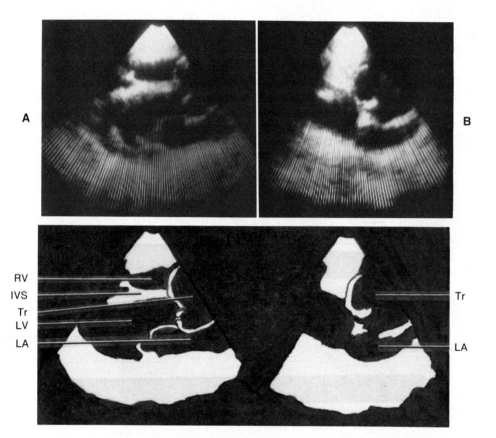

Fig. 34-22. A, Parasternal long axis illustrating multiple valve cusps in a patient with truncus arteriosus. **B,** Parasternal short axis demonstrating a large common vessel with multiple cusps seen in real time.

AORTIC OVERRIDE

The aortic root overrides a ventricular septal defect in tetralogy of Fallot and truncus arteriosus.[6,38,60] Fig. 34-21, from a patient with tetralogy of Fallot, shows a diastolic frame with the ventricular septal echoes at the same level as those from the aortic valve. The systolic frame (not shown) demonstrates

the aortic root's function as an outlet for both left and right ventricles. Tetralogy of Fallot has the following four characteristics: (1) a high membranous ventricular septal defect; (2) a large anteriorly displaced aorta, which overrides the defect; (3) pulmonary stenosis, generally infundibular, whose severity determines the degree of cyanosis apparent clini-

cally; and (4) right ventricular hypertrophy, which develops as a result of the right ventricular outflow tract obstruction. In truncus arteriosus the conal truncus fails to divide, leaving one large vessel with multiple valve leaflets (two to six) overriding a ventricular septal defect (Fig. 34-22) and no right ventricular outflow tract or pulmonary valve. There is increased pulmonary blood flow in types I and II, in which the pulmonary arteries arise from the truncus. Thus the presence or absence of a pulmonary valve is an important differential between tetralogy of Fallot and truncus arteriosus.[19] A subxyphoid view of the right ventricular outflow tract (RVOT) showing a pulmonary valve with fixed infundibular obstruction beneath it is characteristic of tetralogy of Fallot. The subxyphoid RVOT would not be obtainable in truncus arteriosus, but a left ventricular outflow tract (LVOT) scanned superiorly might reveal the pulmonary artery arising from the truncus. A second differential point is that the left atrium is enlarged in truncus arteriosus due to increased flow through the lungs (Fig. 34-23). Tetralogy of Fallot, with its decreased flow to the lungs stemming from RVOT obstruction, should show a normal to small left atrium (Fig. 34-24). Left atrial size, however, must be assessed on the basis of body surface area since the increased aortic dimensions invalidate any LA/Ao. Care must be taken also not to introduce positive or false aortic override by transducer position. If aortic override is apparent from a transducer position high on the chest, change to a transducer position an interspace lower to confirm its existence.[18]

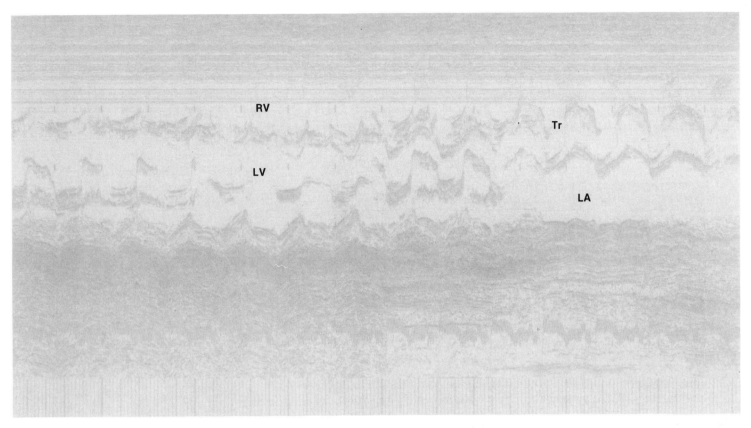

Fig. 34-23. M-mode scan from mitral to truncal valve in a patient with truncus arteriosus. Note the ventricular septal echoes at the same level as the truncal valve; also the anterior displacement of the truncus and the enlarged left atrial dimension. The right ventricular anterior wall is hypercontractile, as are the ventricular septum and the posterior wall.

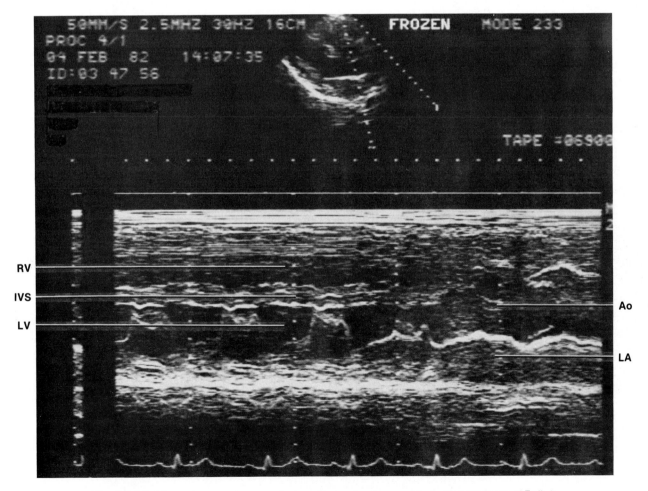

Fig. 34-24. M-mode scan from aorta to mitral valve in a patient with tetralogy of Fallot. The dilated aortic root overrides the ventricular septum. The left atrium is not enlarged.

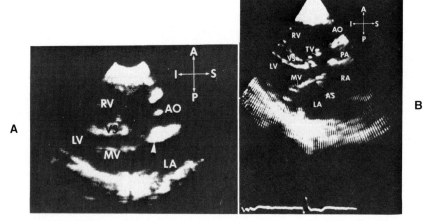

Fig. 34-25. Echocardiographic appearance of a double-outlet right ventricle. **A,** Parasternal long axis showing a posterior aorta displaced anteriorly and separated from the mitral valve by a conus *(arrowhead).* Note that the aorta is almost entirely committed to the right ventricle and that the subaortic ventricular septal defect is the only left ventricular outlet. **B,** Parasternal long axis with the posterior great vessel displaced superiorly and separated from the mitral valve by a conus of elongated dense echoes *(two arrowheads).* If a line is projected superiorly along the plane of the interventricular septum, both great arteries arise anterior to it from the right ventricle. The two great vessels are one on top of the other, with the subpulmonic ventricular septal defect as the only left ventricular outlet. (From Hagler, O.J., et al.: Circulation **63:** 419, 1981. By permission of the American Heart Association, Inc.)

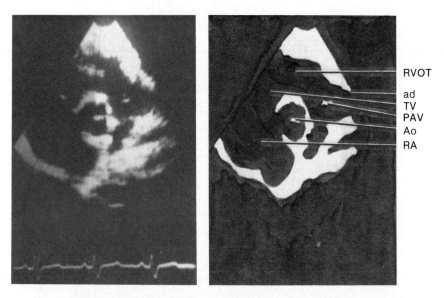

RVOT
ad
TV
PAV
Ao
RA

Fig. 34-26. Postoperative high short axis in a patient with tetralogy of Fallot showing an aneurysmal dilation, *ad,* at the pulmonary valve, *PAV,* due to outflow patch placement.

A posterior great vessel overriding the ventricular septum by 80%, or the ventricular septum and posterior wall of the great vessel appearing at the same level, suggests a diagnosis of double outlet right ventricle (DORV). Echocardiographic characteristics include (1) anterior and superior displacement of the posterior great vessel, due to development of a conus, such that both great arteries arise from the anterior right ventricle; (2) mitral-semilunar valve discontinuity; (3) absence of an LVOT other than through the ventricular septal defect.[39] If the posterior great vessel is displaced anteriorly, the conus may present as a dense area of echoes directly beneath it (Fig. 34-25, *A*). With primarily superior displacement the conus appears as an elongated dense area of echoes between the mitral valve and the posterior great vessel, which in Fig. 34-25, *B,* is the pulmonary artery. The orientation of the great vessels as they arise from the right ventricle varies from normal with a subaortic ventricular septal defect, to dextro- or levotransposed with a subpulmonic (subpulmonary) ventricular septal defect.

The patch closure of ventricular septal defects appears brighter than the surrounding tissue, due to different acoustic impedance of the patch material. Patches are also used to enlarge the RVOT in cases of infundibular obstruction. If the surgeon must extend the patch over a small pulmonary anulus, the pulmonary valve leaflets may float freely in the widened outflow tract (Fig. 34-26).

When the natural outflow tract cannot be widened, an extracardiac conduit containing a porcine valve (Rastelli) is placed from the right ventricle to the pulmonary artery.* Its function can be difficult to assess because of its extreme anterior position and the fact that the thin valve leaflets may be obscured by the acoustic flare off the metal stents on which they are mounted. The views most successful in visualizing the conduit are the high short axis and the long axis scanned superiorly. Peripheral venous contrast injection can confirm the conduit's location for evaluating the amount of flow through it. Since these xenograft valves are prone to calcification in children, follow-up echocardiograms are recommended.[2,78] A valved conduit and ventricular septal patch are also used in patients requiring truncus arteriosus repair, making their postoperative echocardiograms similar to those seen in tetralogy of Fallot.

---

*References 16, 40, 55, 57, 67, 73.

ATRIAL SEPTAL DEFECT

There are three echocardiographic types of atrial septal defect (asd) (1) the secundum type, which occurs in the area of the foramen ovale; (2) the sinus venosus type, located in the most superior portion and usually associated with partial anomalous pulmonary venous drainage; and (3) the primum type, located just above the AV ring and usually associated with a cleft anterior mitral valve leaflet. Since the area of the foramen ovale is thinner than the surrounding atrial tissue, it is prone to signal dropout, particularly in the apical four chamber view.[85] Therefore any break in atrial septal continuity apparent in the apical four chamber view must be confirmed by a subxyphoid view, in which the septum is more perpendicular to the echo beam.[15] Due to beam width artifacts, the edges of the defect may be blunted; and the atrial septum bows toward the atrium receiving the shunt flow (Fig. 34-27). Left-to-right shunting at the atrial level manifests itself on M-mode as right ventricular volume loading, which is characterized by (1) increased excursion of the tricuspid valve, (2) dilation and hypercontractility of the right ventricle, (3) enlargement of the pulmonary artery (*not* pulmonary artery hypertension), and (4) paradoxical septal motion. Septal motion must be evaluated at the chordal level, removed from the hinge point near the aorta, since it can appear paradoxical at this point in normals. Fig. 34-28 shows characteristic right ventricular volume loading at the mitral and chordal levels. Signal dropout in the secundum area, along with M-mode characteristics of right ventricular volume loading, should be present for a definitive diagnosis of a secundum atrial septal defect to be made.

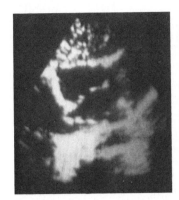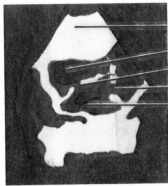

Fig. 34-27. Subxiphoid four chamber showing signal dropout in the secundum region of the interatrial septum. Note the blunting of the edges of the defect, the clear presence of tissue both inferior and superior to the defect, and the bowing of the interatrial septum toward the right atrial cavity.

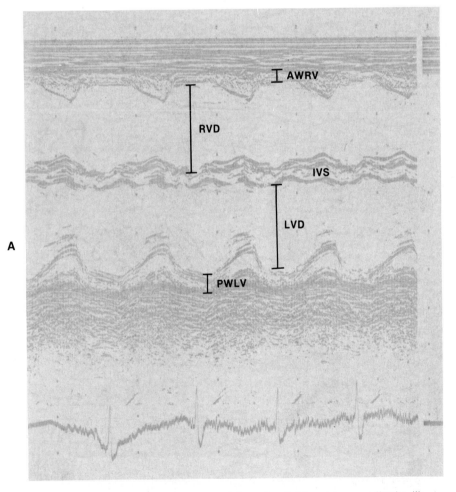

Fig. 34-28. A, M-mode trace at the chordal level in a patient with right ventricular volume loading due to an atrial septal defect. Note the thickened and vigorously contracting right ventricular anterior wall, increased right ventricular dimension, and paradoxical septal motion. *Continued.*

B

Fig. 34-28, cont'd. B is an M-mode trace at the mitral valve level in another patient with right ventricular volume loading due to an atrial septal defect. Once again, note the hyperdynamic and thickened right ventricular anterior wall, increased right ventricular cavity dimensions, and abnormal septal motion.

AWRV

RVD

IVS

ALMV

LVD

PLMV

PWLV

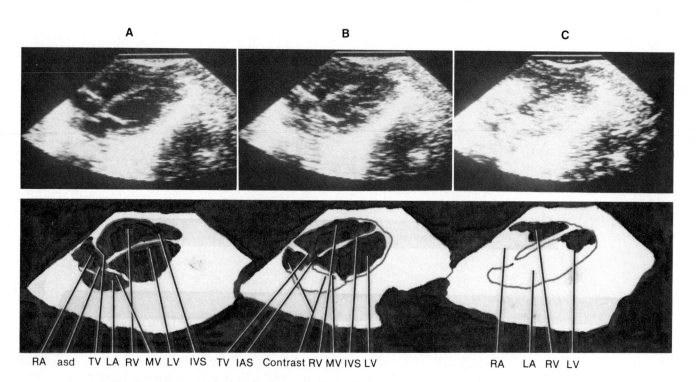

A   B   C

RA   asd   TV LA RV MV LV   IVS   TV IAS Contrast RV MV IVS LV   RA   LA RV LV

Fig. 34-29. Apical four chamber in a patient with a suspected secundum septal defect. A right-to-left shunt is demonstrated with the use of contrast in **A.** A break in the atrial septal continuity is not apparent. **B** shows contrast in both the right and the left atria. **C** demonstrates contrast material in the left side of the heart.

Contrast echo may be extremely helpful in the diagnosis of an atrial septal defect. If the shunt is right to left, direct visualization of contrast appearing in the left atrium from a peripheral venous injection is possible (Fig. 34-29). If the shunt is left to right, negative contrast technique can be used. Injection of contrast in a peripheral vein produces echoes in the right atrium. If there is a left-to-right shunt, a jet of nonopacified blood is seen entering the contrast-filled right atrium as the scan is replayed in slow motion and single frame[103] (Figs. 34-30 to 34-33). Although neither of these techniques is quantitative, both are sensitive enough to pick up shunting from a torn suture line.

Sinus venosus atrial septal defects are technically more difficult to visualize echocardiographically. They lie in the superiormost portion of the atrial septum, too removed from the echo "eye" to be seen. They are most likely to be visualized with the subxyphoid four chamber view (Fig. 34-34). If signs of right ventricular volume loading are present but no signal dropout is detected, a peripheral venous injection showing contrast in the left atrium can be diagnostic. Since partial anomalous pulmonary venous drainage of the right upper pulmonary vein is usually associated with sinus venosus atrial septal defects, it is important to identify the entry site of the pulmonary veins into the left atrium[75] (Fig. 34-35).

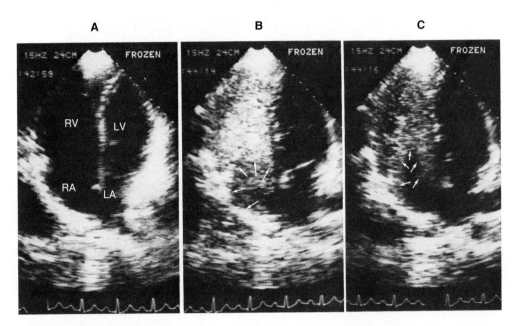

Fig. 34-30. A, Apical four chamber in a patient with an atrial septal defect and an enlarged right ventricle and right atrium. **B,** Saline contrast injection in the right side of the heart. The beginning of a negative contrast effect across the atrial septal defect is present *(arrows)*. **C,** Negative contrast effect *(arrows)* as the blood shunts from left to right.

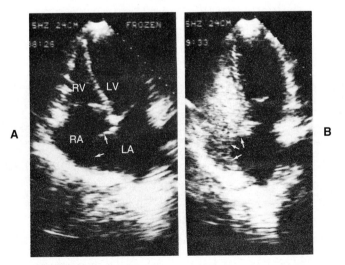

Fig. 34-31. A, Apical four chamber in a patient with an atrial septal aneurysm. **B,** Contrast filling the right heart and outlining the aneurysm *(arrows)*.

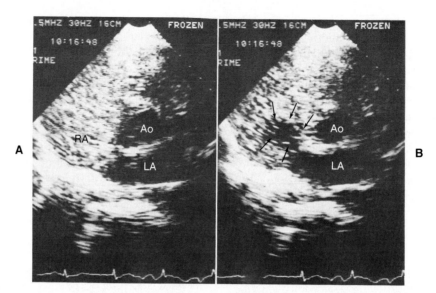

Fig. 34-32. A, Parasternal short axis in a patient with an atrial septal defect. Contrast fills the right side of the heart, delineating the atrial septum. **B,** With careful angling of the transducer cephalad and sweeping to a caudal position, the negative filling can be seen in the right atrium as the blood shunts from left to right *(arrows)*.

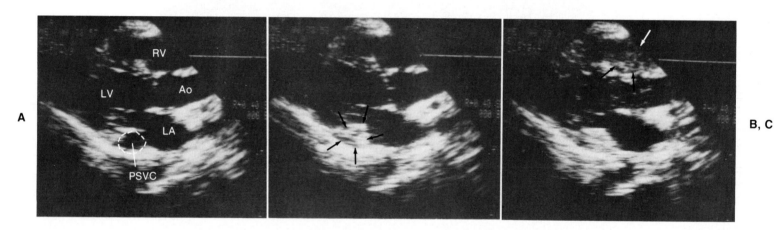

Fig. 34-33. A, Parasternal long axis of a patient with a persistent superior vena cava, *PSVC,* and an atrial septal defect. The PSVC is seen as a circular structure posterior and superior to the mitral anulus along the left atrial wall. **B,** As contrast is injected into the patient's left arm, the dye fills the PSVC *(arrows)* before entering the right ventricle and atrium, **C.**

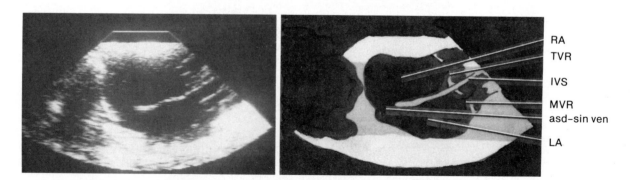

Fig. 34-34. Subxyphoid four chamber demonstrating a sinus venosus–type atrial septal defect. Note the signal dropout in the superiormost portion of the atrial septum. The secundum and primum parts of the septum are intact. *TVR,* tricuspid valve ring.

TOTAL ANOMALOUS PULMONARY VENOUS RETURN

Inability to visualize two pulmonary veins (the right and left upper) entering the left atrium on apical or subxyphoid four chamber views, especially in a cyanotic neonate, suggests total anomalous pulmonary venous return (TAPVR). The pulmonary veins join to form a common vessel or chamber, which then drains into the coronary sinus, superior vena cava, inferior vena cava, or right atrium. The membrane in TAPVR inserts into a more superior portion of the atrial septum than that which is associated with cor triatriatum.[75]

AV CANAL

Ostium primum atrial septal defects (partial AV canal) occur in the lower portion of the atrial septum, just above the AV ring (Fig. 34-36), as a result of failed endocardial cushion development.[105] Failure of the endocardial cushions to fuse leaves the anterior mitral leaflet cleft[12] (Fig. 34-37). Abnormal attachments to the ventricular septum displace the anterior mitral valve leaflet into the left ventricular outflow tract, causing it to open in a superior plane.[37] This abnormal plane of anterior leaflet motion, parallel with rather than perpendicular to the ventricular septum, makes simultaneous recording of both mitral leaflets from the normal transducer position difficult. The echocardiogram shows long diastolic apposition of the anterior leaflet to the interventricular septum, right ventricular volume loading, and multiple mitral echoes due to redundant tissue[104] (Fig. 34-38). A long axis scan with mitral and aortic valves (Fig. 34-39) demonstrates the elongated narrowed left ventricular outflow tract akin to the "gooseneck" deformity seen angiocardiographically.

If the failure of the endocardial cushions to fuse is complete (complete AV canal), a ventricular septal defect and abnormal tricuspid valve are seen in conjunction with a primum atrial septal defect and cleft mitral valve.[9] The ventricular septal defect occurs just below the AV ring and is continuous with the primum atrial septal defect. Paradoxical septal motion is not seen in complete AV canal, because of equalized flow and pressure between the ventricles (Fig. 34-40). Rastelli types A and B are characterized by insertion of the chordae from the cleft mitral valve and tricuspid valve into the crest of the interventricular septum or a right ventricular papillary muscle respectively. Rastelli type C, the most primitive form, has a single undivided, free-floating leaflet stretching across

both ventricles[69] (Fig. 34-41). A sweep from mitral to aortic valve shows the anterior leaflet of the mitral valve swinging through the ventricular septal defect in continuity with the tricuspid valve (Fig. 34-42). The tricuspid valve is said to "cap" the mitral valve. Evaluation of the pulmonary valve for signs of pulmonary artery hypertension is extremely important in AV canal patients, since the right ventricular pressure reaches systemic levels very early.

Postoperative AV canal patients are evaluated for mitral insufficiency and mitral stenosis associated with repair of the cleft anterior mitral leaflet. Mitral insufficiency remains if the repaired anterior leaflet does not coapt evenly with the posterior leaflet. Lack of systolic apposition is demonstrable with a short axis view at the level of the mitral valve.[92] Small to moderate mitral insufficiency is characterized by a single side hole; moderate to large is signified by either one central or two side holes (Fig. 34-37, B) with left atrial enlargement. The sonographer should evaluate the short axis mitral valve orifice to be certain that the dense echo return often seen from the anterior mitral valve leaflet is due to the suture line alone.[56,66,93] Because of its characteristic dense echo return, the patch closure of the defect can be assessed in the four chamber view (Fig. 34-43).

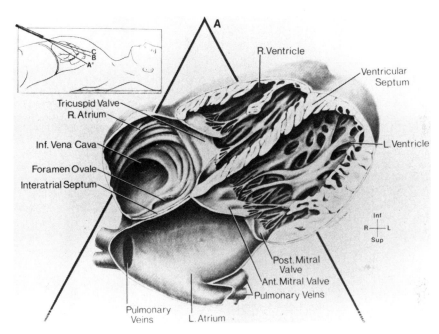

Fig. 34-35. Subxyphoid four chamber along the coronal plane. It corresponds to the most posterior plane, *A*, on the insert. Note especially the insertion sites of the pulmonary veins. (From Sahn, D.J., et al.: Circulation **60:**1317, 1979. By permission of the American Heart Association, Inc.)

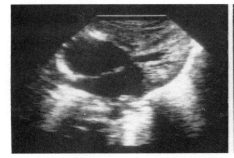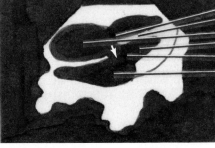

Fig. 34-36. Subxyphoid four chamber in a patient with a primum atrial septal defect, *asd-prim*, demonstrating the break in atrial septal continuity *(arrow)* just above the AV ring in the primum area. Note the blunting of the edge of the defect.

A   B

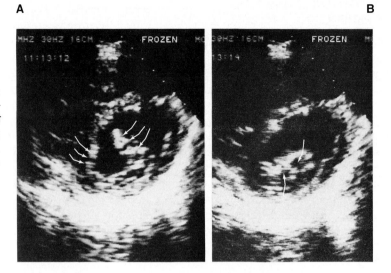

Fig. 34-37. A, Short axis parasternal at the level of the mitral valve in a patient with a cleft mitral valve. There is a break in the normal diastolic curve of the anterior leaflet, with the edges of the cleft leaflet apparent *(arrows)*. The anterior leaflet has two parts—one opening toward the septum, the other toward the lateral wall of the ventricle. **B,** Valve closed in systole. Two small holes *(arrows)* are formed by the two parts of the anterior leaflet.

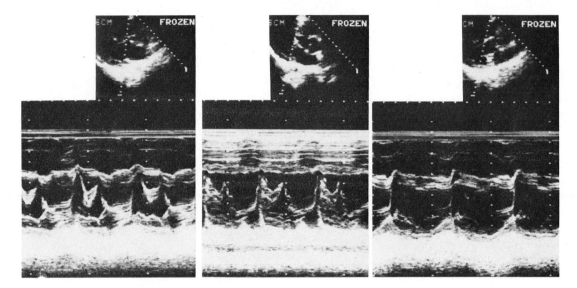

Fig. 34-38. M-mode tracings in a patient with a primum atrial septal defect and cleft mitral valve demonstrating diastolic apposition of the anterior leaflet of the mitral valve to the ventricular septum, echoes off the abnormal mitral valve, and a narrowed left ventricular outflow tract.

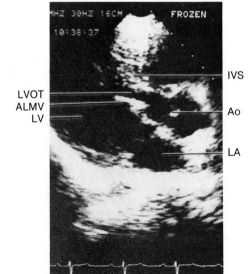

Fig. 34-39. Parasternal long axis of the patient in Fig. 34-38 showing the elongated and narrowed left ventricular outflow tract, *LVOT.*

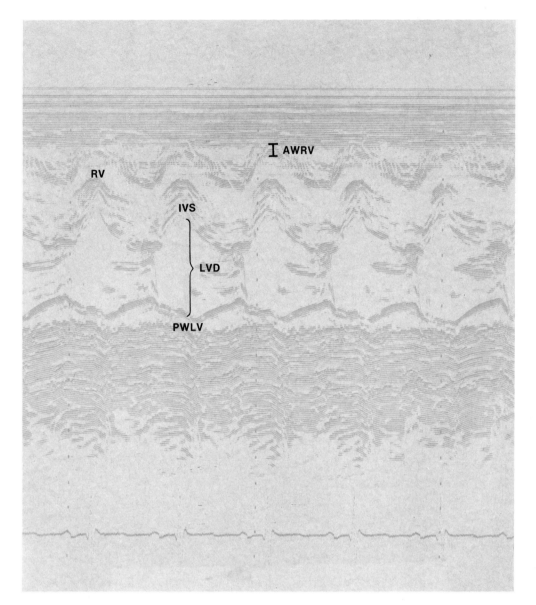

Fig. 34-40. M-mode trace at the chordal level in a patient with an AV canal. Note the normal but hyperdynamic septal motion, demonstrating that right ventricular volume loading is not possible with a complete AV canal. The right ventricular anterior wall is also hyperdynamic.

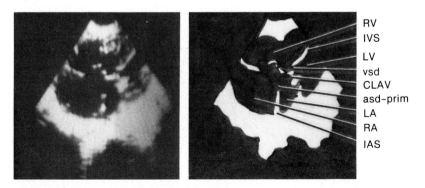

Fig. 34-41. Apical four chamber in a patient with a complete AV canal. The common AV valve leaflet can be seen stretching across the endocardial cushion defect. Note also the blunting at the edges of both defects. *CLAV*, Common leaflet of AV valve.

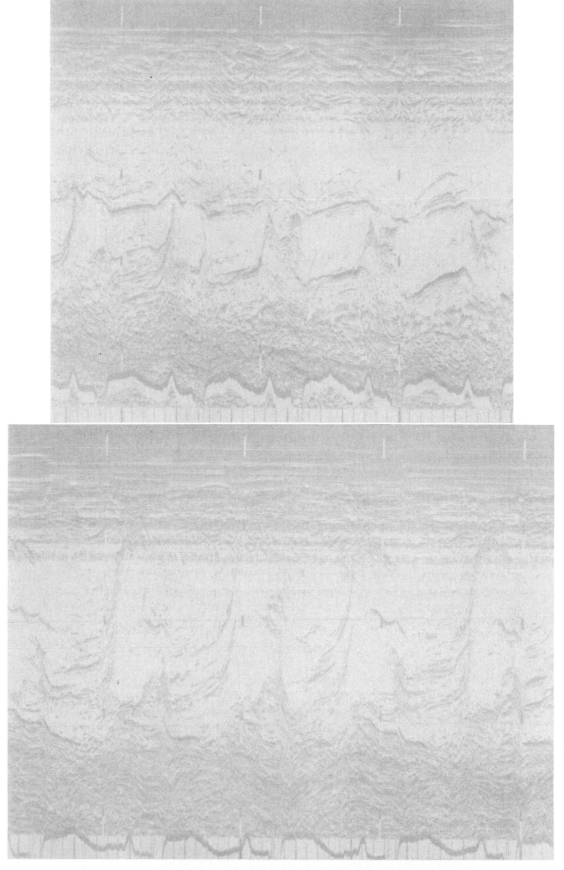

Fig. 34-42. M-mode trace in a patient with a complete endocardial cushion defect. The tricuspid valve caps the mitral valve as the latter "swings" through the ventricular septal defect. Note the multiple echoes off the mitral valve and the diastolic apposition to the septum.

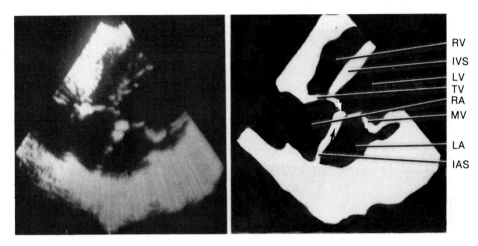

RV
IVS
LV
TV
RA
MV
LA
IAS

Fig. 34-43. Postoperative primum atrial septal defect. Notice the increased echo return from the patch closure of the defect (arrow). The posterior leaflet of the surgically repaired cleft mitral valve is seen dipping superiorly into the left atrial cavity, signifying mitral insufficiency postoperatively.

CYANOTIC CONGENITAL HEART DISEASE

Common causes of cyanosis in the critically ill neonate include tricuspid atresia, Ebstein's malformation, critical pulmonary stenosis or atresia, and dextrotransposition of the great vessels. In tricuspid atresia a dense shelflike membrane is apparent in the four chamber view (Fig. 34-44). Silverman et al.[83] have reported false echoes simulating tricuspid valve motion attributed to this membrane. The only egress from the right atrium is across a patent foramen ovale, or secundum atrial septal defect. If flow is not adequate, an atrial septal defect must be created either in the cardiac catheterization laboratory (balloon septostomy) or surgically (Blalock-Hanlon). Since all the systemic and pulmonary venous return goes through the mitral valve into the left ventricle, a wide-swinging mitral valve and dilated left ventricle are seen by M-mode (Fig. 34-45). The presence or absence of a ventricular septal defect determines the size of the right ventricle, since there is no flow into the sinus or inflow portion. A right ventricular outflow tract of adequate size is essential for surgical correction (Fontan or modified Fontan).[16]

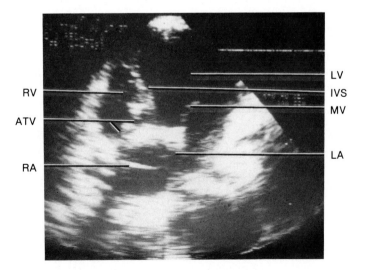

LV
IVS
MV
RV
ATV
LA
RA

Fig. 34-44. Apical four chamber in an adolescent with tricuspid atresia. Note the small right ventricular cavity, the displacement of the interventricular septum to the right due to an enlarged left ventricle, the complete lack of any atrial septum, and the dense echo return from the atretic tricuspid valve, ATV.

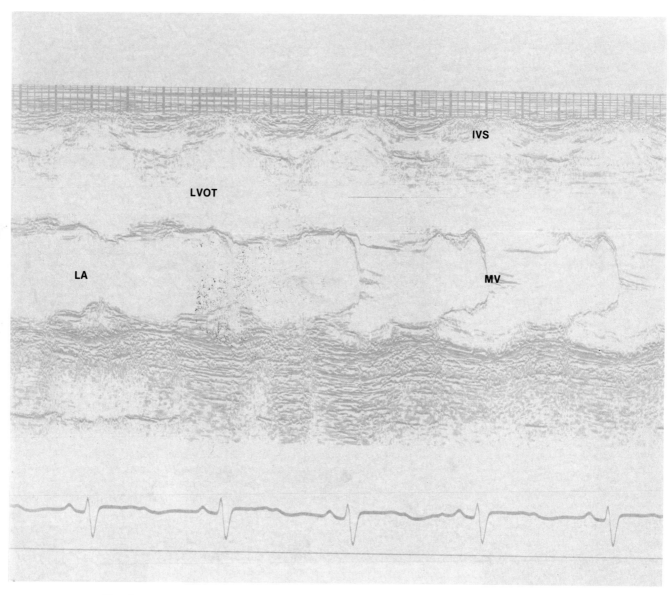

Fig. 34-45. M-mode scan from left ventricular outflow tract to mitral valve in a patient with tricuspid atresia. Note the very anterior placement of the ventricular septum, *IVS*, and the lack of a right ventricular cavity.

EBSTEIN'S MALFORMATION

Ebstein's malformation is a tricuspid abnormality in which one or more of the tricuspid leaflets are displaced inferiorly into the right ventricle. A portion of the right ventricle is atrialized, reducing the functional right ventricle to the apical and outflow regions. The dilated right atrium, which is prone to arrhythmias, can cause the foramen ovale to open, producing a right-to-left shunt. If only the septal leaflet is displaced downward, the anterior leaflet has a characteristic saillike appearance (Fig. 34-46) and should close at least 0.06 second later than the mitral valve.[53] If the whole tricuspid anulus is displaced inferiorly, the leaflets appear foreshortened in the apical four chamber view[24,68] (Fig. 34-47). A high short axis view in both these patients visualized faint leaflets appearing in the right ventricular outflow tract.

CRITICAL PULMONARY STENOSIS

The pulmonary valve cusps are thickened and persist within the lumen throughout systole in severe or critical pulmonary stenosis. Outflow is so restricted that the right ventricle can decompress only back through the tricuspid valve, resulting in right atrial enlargement and subsequent right-to-left shunting across the foramen ovale. The resultant cyanosis is twofold: diminished pulmonary venous return, desaturated even further by the right-to-left atrial shunt. On

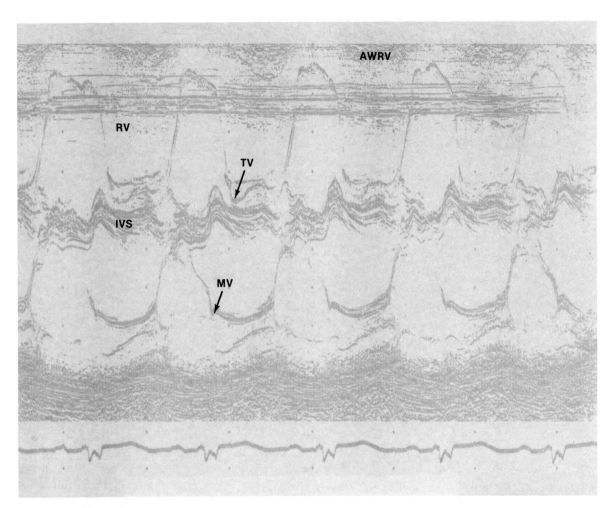

Fig. 34-46. M-mode trace in a patient with Ebstein's anomaly. Note the very wide excursion of the tricuspid valve, the vigorous contraction pattern of the anterior wall of the right ventricle, and the later closure of the tricuspid than of the mitral valve.

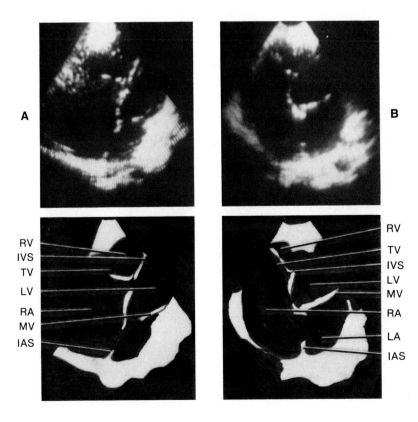

Fig. 34-47. Ebstein's anomaly of the tricuspid valve. **A** is from a patient with a milder form of the anomaly. Note the displacement of the tricuspid valve into the right ventricular cavity, with a large atrialized right ventricle, and the small true right ventricular cavity. **B** is from a patient with a more severe form of the anomaly. Note the even further displacement of the tricuspid valve inferiorly into the right ventricle, with a very large right atrium, and the small right ventricular cavity.

There is false signal dropout of the interatrial septum in both these strips due to a thin foramen ovale.

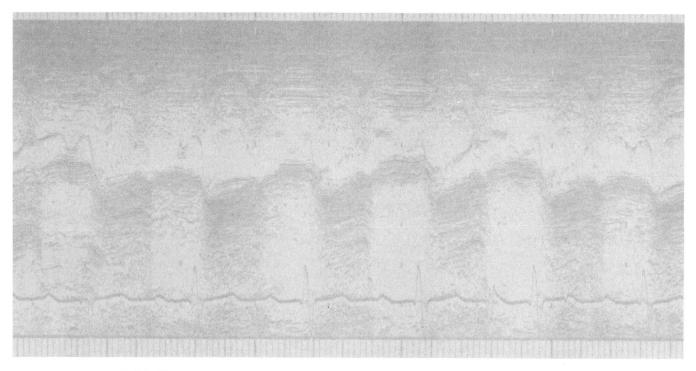

Fig. 34-48. Pulmonary valve tracing from a patient with moderate valvar pulmonary stenosis. The *a* wave measures 8 mm or greater in all of the complexes, and systolic flutter is evident throughout the systolic frame.

the M-mode scan the right ventricular pressure load imposed by the outflow restriction is characterized by thickening of the right ventricular anterior wall and interventricular septum (RVH). Another long-accepted criterion is a markedly accentuated *a* wave on the pulmonary artery valve (Fig. 34-48). This has been proved both insensitive and nonspecific for assessing the degree of obstruction (i.e., absent in patients with significant obstruction, and present for reasons other than severe pulmonary stenosis).[94,96] Significant pulmonary stenosis is best visualized on two-dimensional using the high short axis and subxyphoid RVOT views.[102] If no pulmonary valve cusp motion is apparent, the valve is likely atretic. Unfortunately milder forms of pulmonary stenosis are not as readily detected, and any attempt at quantification of severity is treacherous.

DEXTROTRANSPOSITION OF THE GREAT VESSELS

In dextrotransposition of the great vessels (d-TGV) the truncus septates properly and then spirals in such a manner that the aorta arises from the right ventricle, anterior to and to the right of the pulmonary artery, which arises from the left ventricle (Fig. 34-49). On a normal M-mode scan the pulmonary artery (anterior great vessel) is located by angling the transducer anteriorly toward the patient's left shoulder from a transducer position that reveals the aorta (posterior great vessel). If it is not apparent toward the left shoulder but instead is located by angling toward the right shoulder, a diagnosis of d-TGV should be entertained. Validation of this anterior and rightward location for the anterior great vessel must be obtained by careful notation of transducer position as one scans slowly between the great vessels (in neonates this change may be extremely slight).[32] Simultaneous recording of both great vessels from the same transducer location is another technique proposed by Dillon et al.[22] as an indicator of d-TGV. Little weight should be attached to this finding, however, since it has subsequently been shown to occur in normal neonates.[10] Hirschfeld et al.[46] proposed use of the systolic time interval (STI) for identifying the great vessels in d-TGV. Since the aortic valve faces systemic resistance, it opens later and closes sooner than the pulmonary valve, giving it a greater PEP/ET ratio. On a simultaneous recording of both great vessels it was assumed that the great vessel having the greater STI must be the aorta. The recording of both great vessels must be simultaneous—changes in heart rate, respiratory pattern, or transducer position can introduce variables that invalidate these observations.

This method is also inapplicable in infants whose pulmonary resistance approaches systemic levels.

Contrast echo can be used to aid in the diagnosis of d-transposition. Peripheral venous injection of contrast material should produce echoes in the aorta. M-mode visualization of the transverse aortic arch, right pulmonary artery, and left atrium through the suprasternal notch cut should demonstrate echoes in the transverse aortic arch.[61] If a shunt is present, contrast should subsequently appear in the right pulmonary artery.

Two-dimensional echocardiography eliminates some of the ambiguities associated with M-mode and allows direct visualization of the relationship of the great vessels to each other and to the interventricular septum. Due to right ventricular dilation, both great vessels can be seen superimposed in the long axis view in d-TGV. The posterior great vessel, which normally courses superiorly, arcs posteriorly to the lungs; it can thus be identified as the pulmonary artery (Fig. 34-50). Lateral and inferior angulation of the transducer allows visualization of the pulmonary artery distally.

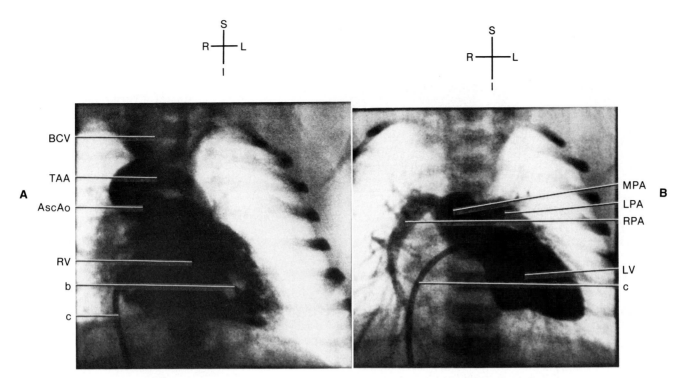

Fig. 34-49. Patient with d-transposition of the great vessels. **A,** Right ventricular injection in the AP projection. The trabecular pattern is recognizable as that of the right ventricle. The aorta clearly comes off this ventricle with no visualization of the pulmonary arteries. **B,** Left ventricular injection in the AP projection. Note the smooth-walled appearance of the left ventricle, with the main pulmonary artery clearly arising from it and the right and left pulmonary branches clearly seen. *c,* Catheter; *b,* balloon; *RV,* right ventricle; *AscAo,* ascending aorta; *TAA,* transverse aortic arch; *BCV,* brachiocephalic vessels.

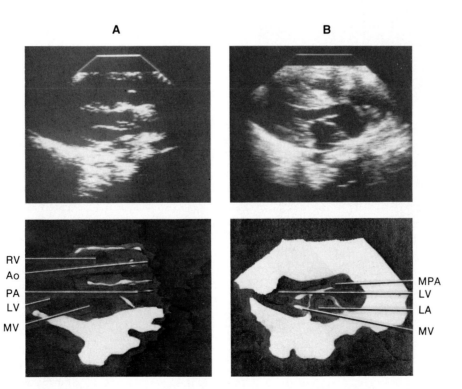

Fig. 34-50. Long axis view representative of transposition of the great vessels. **A** shows both vessels in this diastolic frame one on top of the other. Note the disproportional sizes in the vessels — the anterior great vessel (aorta) is much larger than the posterior great vessel (pulmonary artery). **B** shows the posterior great vessel coursing posteriorly to the lungs, which confirms it as the pulmonary artery.

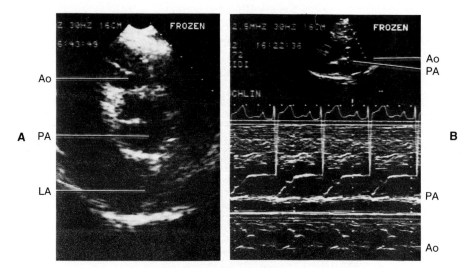

Fig. 34-51. High short axis presentation of transposition of the great vessels. **A** shows the great vessels on top of each other, with the aorta slightly anterior and to the right of the pulmonary artery. **B** is the dual M-mode tracing from these vessels.

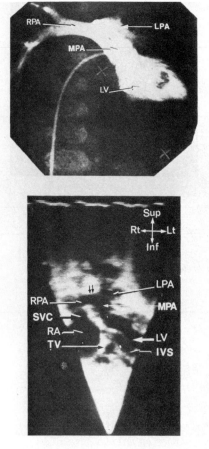

Fig. 34-52. Subxyphoid LVOT view in a patient with d-TGV. The main pulmonary artery arises from the left ventricle and bifurcates into the left and right pulmonary artery branches. Arrows indicate the MPA-RPA junction. (From Bierman, F.Z., et al.: Circulation **60:**1496, 1979. By permission of the American Heart Association, Inc.)

The normal high short axis view with the right ventricular outflow tract wrapping around the aorta has been described by Henry et al.[42] as a "sausage and circle." Since the great vessels are parallel in d-TGV rather than wrapping about each other, they appear as circles (Fig. 34-51). To visualize the anterior great vessel as a *complete* circle, one moves the transducer more cephalad. The vessel remains as a circle, however, because of its natural superior course. Conversely, the pulmonary artery should bifurcate as it passes posterior to the lungs. Caution must be exercised here, for one can produce an apparent posterior great vessel bifurcation in normals by merely manipulating the transducer.

Additional confirmation regarding the dedication of the great vessels to their respective ventricles can be obtained in neonates by using subxyphoid ventricular outflow tract views as described by Bierman and Williams[14] (Fig. 34-52). High-frequency transducers are required to resolve the technical difficulties of visualizing the entire distal portion of each great vessel. In d-TGV one would expect to see the aortic arch, with its brachiocephalic vessels, arising from the right ventricle and the pulmonary artery, with its branches, arising from the left ventricle.

For these critically ill infants with d-TGV to survive, it is essential that communication between the two circuits exist. The patent ductus arteriosus can be pharmacologically kept patent with prostaglandin E_1 until the infant is taken to the cardiac catheterization laboratory, where definitive diagnosis can be made (Fig. 34-53) and an atrial communication created with a balloon septostomy (Fig. 34-54). Should this provide inadequate mixing, an atrial septal defect can be surgically created (Blalock-Hanlon).

The surgical repair of choice in uncomplicated d-transposition of the great vessels is the Mustard procedure. This involves creation of new atria. The blood flow is directed by means of a baffle to the ventricle that feeds the appropriate great vessel; in other words, systemic venous return is directed through the mitral valve to the left ventricle and pulmonary venous return is directed through the tricuspid valve to the right ventricle and out the aorta. The turbulence created by these altered flow paths will create flutter on both AV valves and can be detected by M-mode.[36] Because the right ventricle is carrying the systemic pressure, it will become thick-walled and dilated. The left ventricle may now be relatively smaller (pancaked). The baffle can be seen on the M-

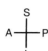

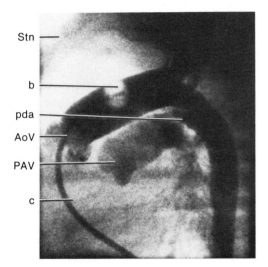

Fig. 34-53. Lateral angiographic projection of an aortic injection in a d-TGV patient. The aorta is clearly anterior to the pulmonary artery, which is filled through the closing patent ductus arteriosus. Notice the narrow pulmonary arterial end of the ductus. *c*, Catheter; *AoV*, aortic valve; *PAV*, pulmonary artery valve; *b*, balloon; *Stn*, sternum; *pda*, patent ductus arteriosus.

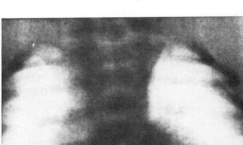

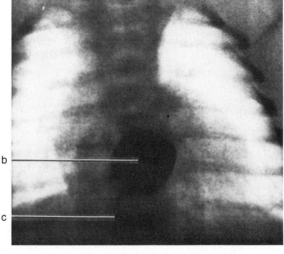

Fig. 34-54. AP projection of a balloon septostomy in a patient with d-TGV. The contrast-filled balloon catheter is shown as it ruptures the atrial septum.

mode scan as a dense line in the left atrium. Similarly it can be detected in the left atrial cavity in the long axis view. It can be seen and evaluated best, however, in the four chamber view. In this view it takes a diagonal course across the atrial cavity and can be seen to move with the cardiac cycle[84] (Fig. 34-55). It is important to scan the baffle as far superiorly as possible in the subxyphoid four chamber view, for obstruction can occur at either the caval-systemic venous atrial junction or the pulmonary vein entry sites.

Some patients with d-TGV have additional lesions that further complicate diagnosis and management. The presence of a vsd necessitates evaluation of the pulmonary valve for signs of pulmonary artery hypertension. The previously described criteria are utilized despite the posterior position of the pulmonary artery. The extent of pulmonary vascular changes secondary to pulmonary artery hypertension determines the timing of definitive repair.

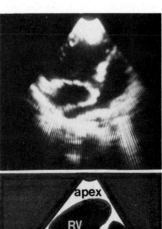
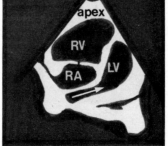

Fig. 34-55. Postoperative apical four chamber in a patient after Mustard's repair of transposition of the great vessels. The baffle is well seen curving through the atrial cavity. (Courtesy H. Rakowski, M.D., Toronto General Hospital.)

Left ventricular outflow obstruction seen in d-TGV is of three types: (1) valvar pulmonary stenosis, (2) fixed subvalvar obstruction, (3) dynamic subvalvar obstruction. Valvar pulmonary stenosis, though left sided, cannot be quantitated except in its most severe form. Fixed subvalvar obstruction, in the form of a membrane, fibromuscular ridge, or tunnel, produces the characteristic move to early closure of the pulmonary valve on M-mode. This pattern is identical to that seen on the aortic valve in left ventricular outflow tract obstruction in normally related great vessels[7,64] (Fig. 34-61). Dynamic left ventricular outflow obstruction, or SAM (systolic anterior motion of the mitral valve), can be present initially but is more commonly first observed following the Mustard repair (Fig. 34-63).

With these additional lesions the surgical repair is more complex. If left ventricular outflow tract obstruction cannot be surgically relieved, a valved conduit bypassing the obstruction is necessary.[70] If a vsd is also present, an internal baffle can be placed to direct the blood flow from the left ventricle through the defect directly to the aorta. A valved conduit is also necessary to direct the systemic venous return to the pulmonary artery.

Postoperative echocardiograms are important in all types of d-TGV. Presence of SAM is a significant finding and should be closely watched with serial echoes. Careful attention must be paid to the left ventricular outflow tract in patients who have undergone surgery to relieve the obstruction, for it can reoccur. Patients who required valved conduits must also be observed serially since calcium deposition on the xenograft conduit is a common finding in children.

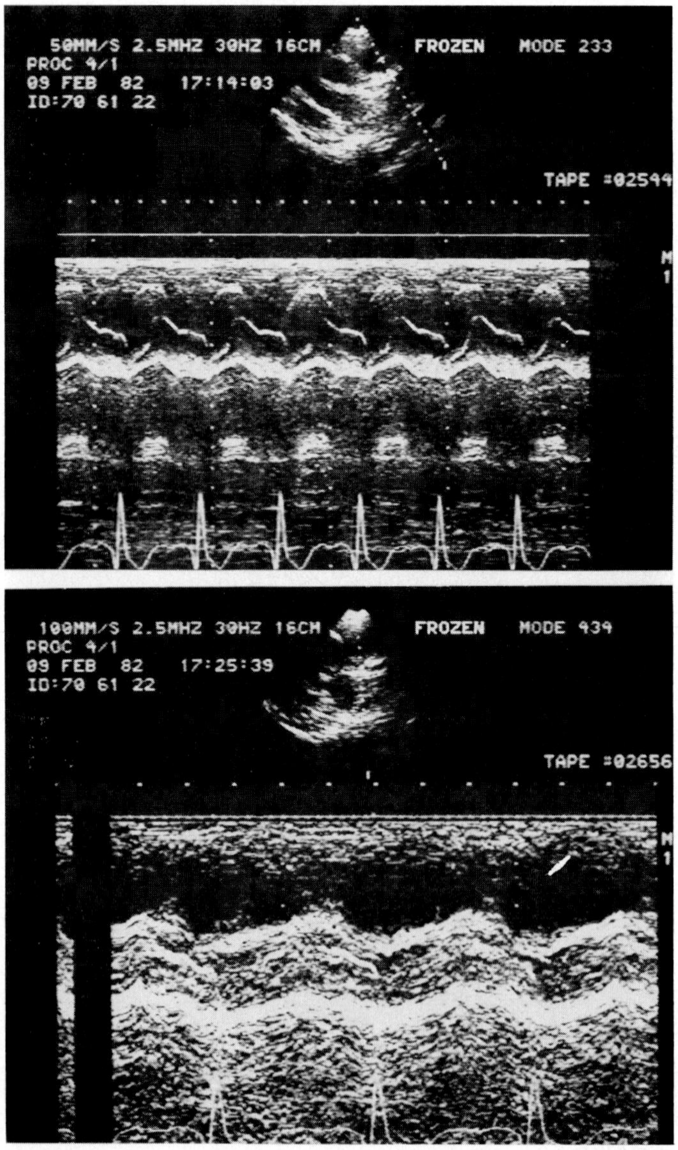

LEVOTRANSPOSITION OF THE GREAT VESSELS

Whenever two circles are visualized in the high short axis view, conal-truncal abnormalities exist. If the anterior great vessel is to the left of the pulmonary artery, levotransposition (l-TGV) must be suspected (Fig. 34-56). The great vessels are transposed, but due to ventricular inversion the circulatory pattern is hemodynamically correct (corrected transposition). Each ventricle keeps its respective AV valve when it inverts. Thus the right atrium empties via the mitral valve into a right-sided morphologic (smooth-walled) left ventricle, which ejects through a posterior pulmonary artery. The left atrium empties via the tricuspid valve into a left-sided heavily trabeculated right ventricle, which ejects through an anterior leftward aorta.[21] Since the crista supraventricularis separates the base of the aorta from the tricuspid valve, continuity is not seen in the long axis view between the left-sided AV valve and the semilunar valve. Visualization of the septal insertion sites of the AV valves in the four chamber view identifies the inverted ventricles. If the tricuspid valve, which inserts into the septum more inferiorly,[43] is on the left side in the four chamber view, that left-sided ventricle is identified as a morphologic right ventricle.[107] Ebstein's malformation of the left-sided tricuspid valve, ventricular septal defect, and pulmonary stenosis are echocardiographic findings commonly associated with l-TGV. Wolff-Parkinson-White syndrome is often seen electrocardiographically.

COARCTATION OF THE AORTA

Coarctation of the aorta classically occurs just distal to the takeoff of the left subclavian artery and can appear as a discrete ridge, membrane, hour-glass, or longer segment of narrowing.[76] It is best visualized from the suprasternal notch (Fig. 34-6). The angle is obtained by propping a pillow or rolled towel under the child's neck so the head rolls back. The transducer is placed in the suprasternal notch and beamed toward the feet to obtain a plane passing between the right nipple and left scapular tip, yielding a long axis view of the suprasternal notch.[87] Angling the beam

Fig. 34-56. M-mode tracing in a patient with l-TGV. The anterior great vessel (aorta), **A,** is to the left of the small posterior vessel (pulmonary artery), **B.**

posteriorly or anteriorly should produce a plane in which the transverse arch and its brachiocephalic vessels, right pulmonary artery, right main bronchus, and descending aorta are visualized. Right- versus left-sided aortic arch differentiation is made by noticing whether the beam passes through the right or left of the sternum as the arch is visualized. Since the arch moves in and out of the field of view during the cardiac cycle, one must monitor several beats in slow motion to be sure the coarctation is not missed. An opposite pitfall is a false narrowing of the lumen produced by beam width artifacts from the walls of the right pulmonary artery and left subclavian artery. If a narrowing is consistent throughout a number of cardiac cycles, one can be relatively confident of the existence of a coarctation. This is demonstrated angiographically in Fig. 34-57. A bicuspid aortic valve often coexists with coarctation whereas a single papillary muscle producing a parachute mitral valve occurs rarely.

Suprasternal notch visualization and measurement of the transverse aortic arch itself can eliminate concern about isthmus hypoplasia between the left carotid and left subclavian arteries, or tubular hypoplasia of the entire arch. A small ascending aorta, as well as an abnormally small aortic arch, proximal to a normal-appearing descending aorta characterizes tubular hypoplasia.

LEFT VENTRICULAR OUTFLOW TRACT OBSTRUCTION

LVOT obstruction can occur at three levels—(1) supravalvar, (2) valvar, (3) subvalvar—and is either fixed or dynamic in nature.[100] Since auscultation often cannot localize either the site or the severity of an LVOT obstruction, two-dimensional echocardiography, with its ability to visualize many planes of the heart, has become very important for qualitative if not quantitative assessment of the condition.

Supravalvar aortic obstruction occurs as a narrowing of the aortic root lumen, from both anterior and posterior walls, just above the level of the aortic valve. It is best visualized in the parasternal long axis view.[95]

M-mode has proved unreliable in the assessment of valvar aortic stenosis, for the ice pick M-mode view may not cut through the tips of the domed aortic valve[30] (Fig. 34-58). Two-dimensional echocardiography, with its ability to visualize the domed aortic leaflets in systole, was used by Weyman et al.[101] to quantitate severity of valvar aortic stenosis in children. (See Appendix J for graph.) These workers compared the ratio of maximum

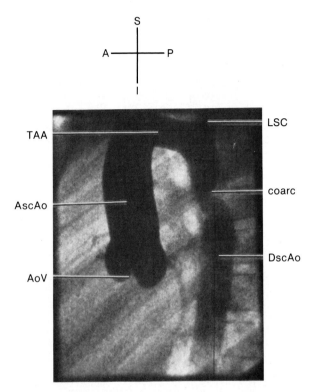

Fig. 34-57. Angiographic demonstration of coarctation of the aorta in the lateral projection. The coaractation occurs in the usual site, just distal to the takeoff of the left subclavian. *AoV,* Aortic valve; *AscAo,* ascending aorta; *TAA,* transverse aortic arch; *LSC,* left subclavian artery; *DscAo,* descending aorta.

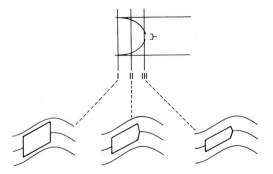

Fig. 34-58. Schematic and M-mode representations of the portions of a domed aortic valve intersected by the M-mode beam. (Reproduced with permission from Goldberg, S., et al.: Pediatric and adolescent echocardiography: a handbook, ed. 2, Chicago, 1980, Year Book Medical Publishers, Inc.)

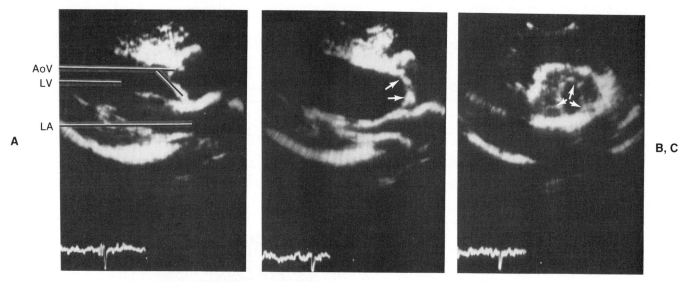

Fig. 34-59. A and **B,** Abnormal diastolic closure configuration in a patient with a domed aortic valve *(arrows).* Note the prominent sagging of the leaflets and the dilation of the aortic root above the valve. **C,** Parasternal short axis of the ovoid aortic cusp opening. The patient had aortic insufficiency without stenosis.

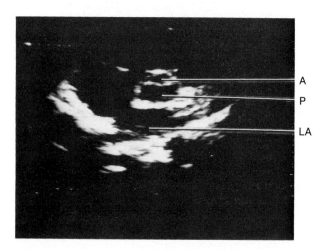

Fig. 34-60. Parasternal short axis showing a bicuspid aortic valve in diastole, with its characteristic single commissure line going straight across the root. The anterior cusp, *A,* is smaller than the posterior cusp, *P.* If a dip in the center of the apparently straight commissure line is seen, a third cusp is probably present.

aortic cusp separation to aortic root diameter against the aortic valve gradients obtained during cardiac catheterization and found that the MAoCS/AoD must be below 0.5 to predict a significant gradient.

Valves that open superiorly into the aortic root, rather than anteriorly and posteriorly, during systole and show a diagonal sagging diastolic closure pattern (Fig. 34-59) warrant more vigorous examination to ensure that significant stenosis is not missed. Dilation of the ascending aorta (poststenotic dilation) is another indicator of obstruction. Parasternal long axis views from the traditional chest position frequently do not visualize the posterior aortic cusp. Changing to a higher-frequency transducer, moving up one or two interspaces, and scanning inferiorly often bring the posterior cusp into view. Since the plane being visualized changes during the cardiac cycle, several cycles must be examined in an area of the tape where both valve cusps are visible. Care must be taken to measure the maximum aortic cusp separation at the tip of the valve dome, just as the T wave of the electrocardiogram is being inscribed. Significant gradients have been discovered echocardiographically in children even before changes occurred in the resting electrocardiogram. These children are referred for cardiac catheterization.

The MAoCS/AoD technique is not applicable to all patients with stenotic aortic valves. Increased echo return from calcified leaflets results in an artificially small maximum aortic cusp separation. The aortic orifice in postoperative patients has been difficult to evaluate reliably. A dilated aortic root (found in Marfan's and Turner's syndromes) invalidates this technique since it makes the denominator artificially large. Because surgical results and long-term prognosis are better with tricuspid than bicuspid aortic valves, it is important to visualize the number of cusps present in the high short axis view of the aortic root. The aortic valve cusps are generally evident in a short axis scan from the level of the mitral valve just as the root becomes visible. If they are not apparent there, an apical four chamber view scanned anteriorly will many times bring them into view.

An eccentric diastolic closure line (eccentricity index of 1.3 or more) was the accepted M-mode indicator for bicuspid aortic valve.[63] However, since the two-dimensional echocardiogram allows visualization of the commissure lines in the high short axis view, it has become apparent that many valves labeled bicuspid by an M-mode study are actually tricuspid. A bicuspid valve and its schematic representation are shown in Fig. 34-60.[8] The characteristic short axis diastolic single commissure line is often located eccentrically within the root. The long axis diastolic closure line can also be located eccentrically.

Subvalvar aortic stenosis is an uncommon type of LVOT obstruction. It can occur as a discrete ridge or membrane, a diffuse long tunnel involvement, or a dynamic obstruction due to systolic motion of the anterior leaflet of the mitral valve. All of these are delineated in the long axis view, in which a commonly seen characteristic is premature closure of the aortic valve (Fig. 34-61). The anterior leaflet of the aortic valve demonstrates this most often. Since a pressure load causes muscular hypertrophy, the left ventricular posterior wall and interventricular septum are generally thickened and hyperdynamic. Fig. 34-62 shows a patient with discrete subaortic obstruction protruding from the septal-aortic junction, with an additional ventricular septal component. Membranous subaortic obstructions can be difficult to visualize either by M-mode or two-dimensionally.[99] Dynamic LVOT obstruction with systolic anterior motion of the anterior leaflet of the mitral valve (or SAM) is demonstrated in Fig. 34-63, from a child with dextrotransposition of the great vessels after resection of a fibromuscular ridge. In this child one form of LVOT obstruction was masked by another and became evident only after the first was removed. The mitral valve should be examined for SAM only in the plane of the posterior leaflet of the mitral valve, since a pseudo-SAM can be produced by catching a portion of the aortic ring. SAM is most often associated with the asymmetric septal hypertrophy of idiopathic hypertrophic subaortic stenosis (IHSS). Such septa often exhibit a ground glass appearance due to the different or varying acoustic impedances of the abnormal tissue.

Hypoplastic left heart syndrome represents the most severe form of LVOT obstruction.[25] Whether due to severe tubular hypoplasia of the arch, severe aortic stenosis, or aortic atresia, the left-sided chambers are diminutive and poorly contractile. When the aortic root of an infant measures 6 mm or less, hypoplastic left heart syndrome must be differentiated from severe aortic stenosis (Fig. 34-64). Aortic stenosis may be surgically correctible whereas hypoplastic left heart syndrome is invariably fatal. With severe aortic stenosis a tiny mobile valve is seen within the aortic root. Care must be taken when the left ventricular cavity is very small or absent to avoid mistaking the tricuspid valve for the mitral valve. Depth measurements from the crystal artifact to the valve level can aid in this diagnosis.

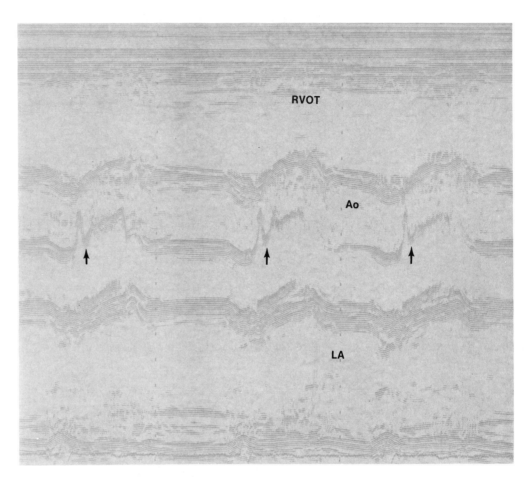

Fig. 34-61. M-mode trace in a patient with subvalvar aortic stenosis. Early closure of the valve is well seen *(arrows)*.

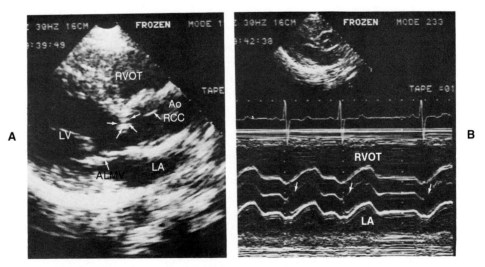

Fig. 34-62. Long axis parasternal in a patient with subaortic obstruction *(arrows)*. **A,** Reduced orifice of the left ventricular outflow tract due to a thickened ridge in the interventricular septum just below the aortic valve. **B,** M-mode of the early systolic notching of the aortic valve. Other frames showed a SAM of the mitral valve.

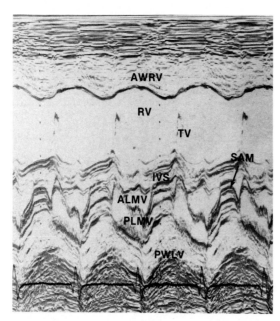

Fig. 34-63. M-mode trace at the mitral valve level in a patient with transposition of the great vessels and dynamic left ventricular outflow tract obstruction. Note the thick-appearing right ventricular anterior wall, *AWRV*, and the dilated right ventricular cavity with wide excursion of the tricuspid valve. There is a marked degree of systolic anterior motion by the anterior leaflet of the mitral valve, *ALMV*. Also note the multiple echoes of the mitral valve and the relatively small left ventricular cavity.

LEFT VENTRICULAR INFLOW TRACT OBSTRUCTION

LVIT obstruction may be due to severe mitral stenosis, mitral valve atresia, parachute mitral valve, supravalvar mitral ring, or cor triatriatum.

In congenital mitral stenosis the traditional decreased E-F slope may not be apparent. Cases of significant mitral stenosis exhibit diastolic anterior motion of the posterior mitral valve leaflet and diastolic flutter of the valve.[23] The left atrial dimension is usually large, and signs of pulmonary artery hypertension may be present. M-mode and two-dimensional configurations in patients with congenital mitral stenosis, documented at cardiac catheterization, are shown in Fig. 34-65.[66] A mitral valve orifice can be planimetered from the short axis view.[56]

Parachute mitral valve is a form of mitral stenosis, often associated with coarctation of the aorta, in which all chordae insert into a single papillary muscle. Two-dimensional echocardiography affords a striking demonstration of the single papillary muscle in short axis compared to the normal pair of papillary muscles.

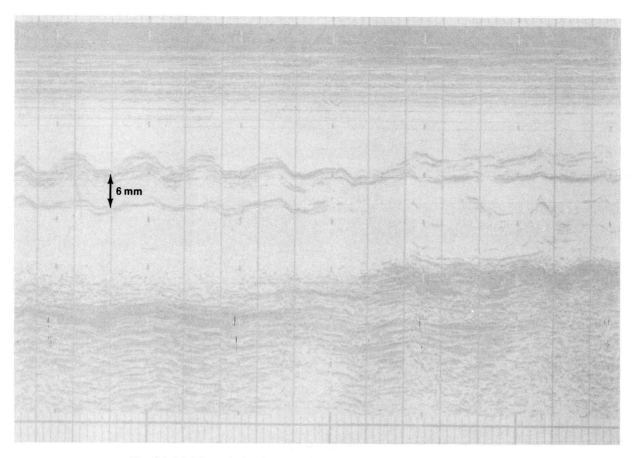

Fig. 34-64. M-mode tracing in a patient with coarctation of the aorta and aortic stenosis. The aortic root measured 6 mm.

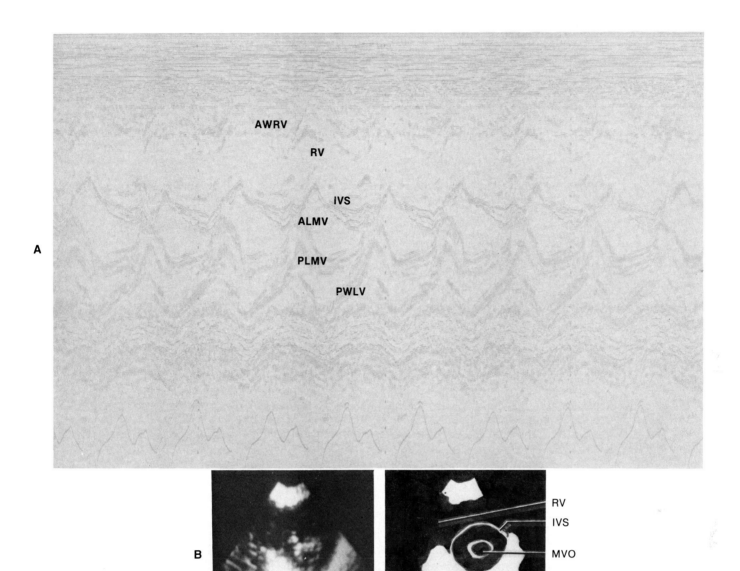

Fig. 34-65. Congenital mitral stenosis. **A** is an M-mode scan demonstrating the abnormal mitral valve, which is thick and has multiple echoes, and anterior movement of the posterior leaflet in diastole. The E-F slope is not markedly diminished, as is found in adult-acquired mitral stenosis. The heart is hypercontractile. At cardiac catheterization this patient was found to have a 14-mm gradient across the mitral valve. **B,** from another patient with congenital mitral stenosis, is a short axis view of the mitral valve's maximum diastolic orifice. Note the enlarged right ventricular cavity and the very reduced orifice of the thickened valve. The mitral valve orifice was estimated echocardiographically to be 0.61 sq cm. At cardiac catheterization this patient had a gradient of 28 mm Hg across the valve (with an A wave of 45 and a V wave of 40) and a mean of 35 mm Hg in the left atrium (with a left ventricular end diastolic pressure of 17). At autopsy the mitral valve was found to be cleft with its leaflets opaque, firm, and markedly thickened. The circumference of the mitral valve orifice was 3 cm. The papillary muscles were markedly hypertrophied, with obliteration of the chordae tendineae; and the left ventricular posterior wall was also markedly hypertrophied, with a thickness of 1.7 cm.

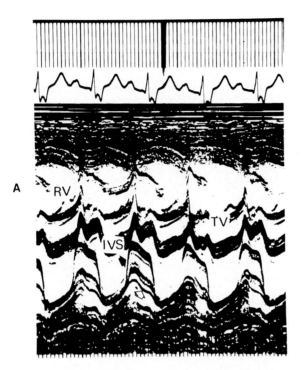
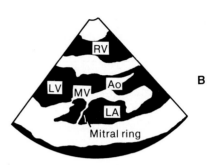

Fig. 34-66. A is from a patient with a supravalvar mitral ring, mitral stenosis, and tetralogy of Fallot. The dark and light arrows represent the anterior and posterior mitral valve leaflets respectively, and the dense echo between them is thought to be from the supravalvar mitral ring. **B** is a parasternal long axis schematic of a patient with a supravalvar mitral ring. A membrane is seen in the left atrium, just above the mitral ring. It extends to the right to the primum area of the interatrial septum and to the left to the lateral left atrial wall. (**A** from LaCorte, M., et al.: Circulation **54**:562, 1976, **B** from Snider, R.A., et al.: Circulation **61**:898, 1980. By permission of the American Heart Association, Inc.)

Supravalvar rings, membranes, and cor triatriatum all divide the left atrium to various degrees, obstructing flow into the left ventricle.[49,86] In cor triatriatum a distinct chamber within the left atrium receives the pulmonary venous blood flow and has only limited egress to the mitral valve area. It may be visualized as a dense echo within the left atrium just beneath the aortic root and mitral valve anulus or, alternatively, just above the true left atrial wall. Mitral valve motion may be normal since the obstructing chamber is removed from the valve area. Low gain settings and maximal damping must be used so the dense structural echo can be distinguished from artifact. With supravalvar rings, however, proximity to the mitral valve leaflets often produces multiple echoes within the mitral valve funnel (Fig. 34-66).

CARDIOMYOPATHY

Occasionally we study infants who have congestive or hypertrophic cardiomyopathy. The congestive cardiomyopathies seen in our laboratory have been attributed to viral myocarditis, endocardial fibroelastosis, or in one family a systemic carnitine deficiency. In myocarditis the left ventricle is dilated and poorly contractile, with an increased distance between the mitral valve's E point and the ventricular septum, which is indicative of left ventricular dysfunction[20] (Fig. 34-67). Serial studies as the myocarditis resolves demonstrate normalization of left ventricular size and function. Fig. 34-68, illustrates the left atrial and left ventricular changes that occurred in the patient with systemic carnitine deficiency during carnitine replacement therapy.[91]

Infants of diabetic mothers exhibit a transient form of hypertrophic cardiomyopathy. Resultant ventricular septal hypertrophy and SAM can produce subaortic obstruction.[33] Early closure of the aortic valve in systole can be observed by M-mode. This obstructive cardiomyopathy usually resolves by 6 months of age.[35,54]

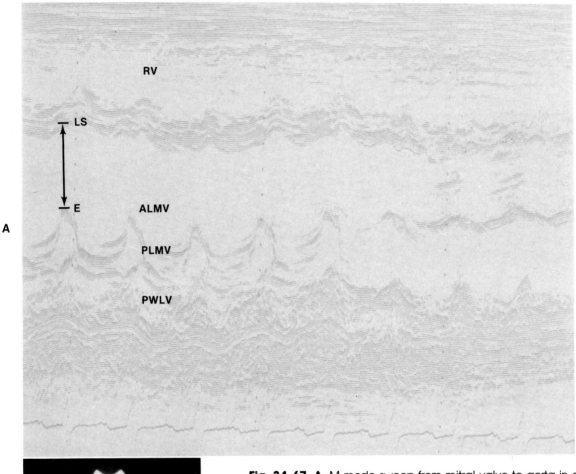

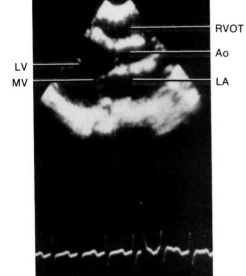

Fig. 34-67. A, M-mode sweep from mitral valve to aorta in a patient with viral myocarditis. Note the markedly enlarged ventricular cavity, with poor excursion of interventricular septum and posterior wall. The E point septal separation is markedly increased, with a measurement of 17 mm. Fractional shortening of this ventricle is 12%, also markedly abnormal. *LS,* Left side of the ventricular septum; *E,* E point of the anterior mitral valve leaflet. **B,** Long axis diastolic view again demonstrating the markedly dilated left ventricular cavity. Note: The references to the letter points along the cardiac cycle are by both lower case and capital letters. This is because both designations are used in the field and the authors use the one with which they are more familiar.

Cardiac Feature	Before Therapy		After Therapy		
			At 2 Wk	At 2½ Mo	At 6 Mo
Right ventricle	1.6	(50)	1.0 (25)	1.5 (50)	1.7 (60)
Left atrial dimension	3.2	(80)	2.8 (55)	2.3 (40)	2.2 (25)
Septum	0.9	(90)	0.9 (90)	0.9 (90)	1.0 (90)
Left ventricular posterior wall	1.1	(>90)	0.8 (75)	0.9 (85)	0.9 (85)
Left ventricle					
Systole	4.3	(>90)	4.5 (>90)	3.3 (85)	2.8 (60)
Diastole	5.3	(90)	5.6 (>90)	4.5 (70)	4.2 (50)
% myocardial fractional shortening	19		19	27	34

*Dimensions are expressed in centimeters; figures in parentheses denote percentile for body-surface area.

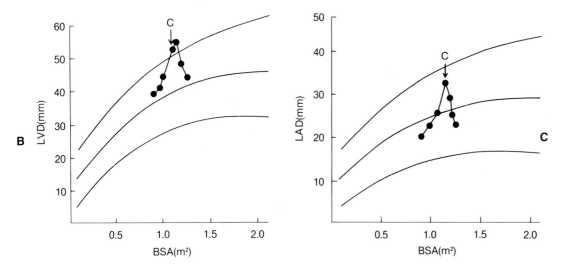

Fig. 34-68. **A** is a table of echocardiographic measurements of cardiac structures obtained 2 weeks, 2½ months, and 6 months after initiation of carnitine replacement therapy. **B** is a graph comparing the left ventricular end diastolic dimension, *LVD*, with body surface area, *BSA*. The carnitine starting point is marked by *c*. Note that the diameter decreases to near normal levels. **C** is a graph comparing left atrial dimensions, *LAD*, to body surface area.

MUCOCUTANEOUS LYMPH NODE SYNDROME

Weyman et al.[98] have been using cross-sectional echocardiography to visualize the coronary arteries in coronary artery disease. However, the increase in mucocutaneous lymph node syndrome cases, whose major cause of death is myocardial infarction related to coronary artery aneurysm, has sparked interest in cross-sectional detection of coronary artery aneurysms in children. Mucocutaneous lymph node syndrome (MLNS), first described by Kawasaki in 1967[47] and again in 1974,[48] is often referred to as "Kawasaki disease." Several authors[27,31,58] have now reported its incidence in the United States. Others[26,44,109] offer technical advice on visual-ization of this lesion, which occurs in approximately 20% to 30% of patients with clinical features of MLNS.[31] Often these aneurysms are quite large and therefore fairly easy to detect echocardiographically.

OTHER ANOMALIES

Occasionally the pediatric echocardiographer encounters very rare or very complex heart disease, which provides a tremendous challenge and may require hours of concentrated effort. Malposition and/or malrotation of the heart usually indicate complex disease states. These factors complicate the echocardiographic examination, making conventional views difficult to obtain and interpret. For example, if the heart is found in the right chest, one must perform transducer manipulations in mirror image (the plane must be rotated approximately 90 degrees). The heart may not be mirror-image dextrocardia, but this will standardize the echo examination and make interpretation somewhat easier. It is important to keep in mind that dextrocardia does not necessarily indicate any intracardiac abnormality.

An abnormal relationship between the interventricular septal plane and the rest of the cardiac structures in which the ventricular septum is perpendicular to the atrial septum is a manifestation of complex anatomy. Often the great vessels and their origins cannot be identified. Subsequent cardiac catheterization in these ambiguous cases has revealed superoinferior ventricular malrotation, as described by Van Praagh et al.[308] in 1980.

Structures that prove difficult to locate may be totally absent in primitive hearts. Cor biloculare has a single atrium, a single AV valve, and a single ventricle. If both AV valves are present and empty into one ventricle, the heart is termed a *double-inlet* ventricle. If it has an outflow chamber, it is termed a *single* ventricle. Differentiation of a single or common ventricle from a large ventricular septal defect is essential for consideration of surgical repair. This can be done by observing the filling pattern of the ventricle in four chamber view during a peripheral venous contrast injection. A phenomenon to be ruled out if the contrast study reveals a large ventricular septal defect is straddling or displacement of the AV valve[13] (Fig. 34-69).

CONCLUSION

Pediatric echocardiography allows a biologically safe noninvasive method of obtaining data that were impossible to obtain in the past. In many cases the echo examination affords a better picture of anatomic relationships and disease states than does any other diagnostic tool available to the clinician. However, there are inherent limitations and pitfalls in this technique: overinterpretation and underinterpretation can be misleading and dangerous. Conclusions must not be drawn without sufficient data. Good background knowledge in all aspects of congenital heart disease will help to alleviate these problems and draw one toward a valid conclusion.

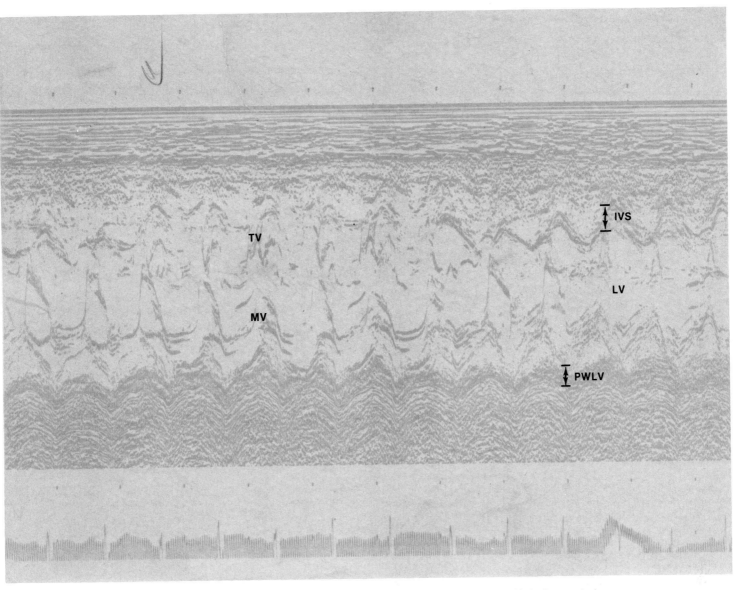

Fig. 34-69. M-mode trace in a patient with a straddling tricuspid valve. Note the posterior displacement of the tricuspid valve below the level of the interventricular septum, the flutter on the tricuspid valve, and the small right ventricular dimension anterior to the interventricular septum.

REFERENCES

1. Acquatella, H., Schiller, N.B., Sharpe, D.N., and Chagterjee, K.: Lack of correlation between echocardiographic pulmonary valve morphology and simultaneous pulmonary artery pressure, Am. J. Cardiol. **43:**946, 1979.
2. Alam, M., Madrazo, A.C., and Magilligan, D.J.: M-mode and two-dimensional echocardiographic features of porcine valve dysfunction, Am. J. Cardiol. **43:**502, 1979.
3. Allen, H.D., Goldberg, S.J., and Sahn, D.J.: Workbook in pediatric echocardiography, Chicago, 1978, Year Book Medical Publishers, Inc.
4. Allen, H.D., Goldberg, S.J., Sahn, D.J., et al.: Suprasternal notch echocardiography: assessment of its clinical utility in pediatric cardiology, Circulation **55:**605, 1977. [Preprint.]
5. Allen, H.D., Sahn, D.J., and Goldberg, S.J.: New serial contrast technique for assessment of left to right shunting patent ductus arteriosus in the neonate, Am. J. Cardiol. **41:**288, 1978.
6. Assad-Morell, J.L., Seward, J.B., Tajik, A.J., et al.: Echophonocardiographic and contrast studies in conditions associated with systemic arterial trunk overriding the ventricular septum: truncus arteriosus, tetralogy of Fallot, and pulmonary atresia with ventricular septal defect, Circulation **53:**663, 1976.
7. Aziz, K.U., Paul, M.H., and Muster, A.J.: Echocardiographic assessment of left ventricular outflow tract in d-transposition of the great arteries, Am. J. Cardiol. **41:**543, 1978.
8. Bansol, R.C., Tajik, A.J., Seward, J.B., and Offord, K.P.: Feasibility of detailed two-dimensional echocardiographic examination in adults—prospective study of 200 patients, Mayo Clin. Proc. **55:**291, 1980.
9. Bass, J.L., Bessinger, F.B., and Lawrence, C.: Echocardiographic differentiation of partial and complete atrioventricular canal, Circulation **57:**1144, 1978.
10. Bass, N.M., Roche, A.H.G., Brandt, P.N.T., and Neutze, J.M.: Echocardiography in assessment of infants with complete d-transposition of the great arteries, Br. Heart J. **40:**1165, 1978.
11. Bauman, W., Wann, S.L., Childress, R., et al.: Midsystolic notching of the pulmonary valve in the absence of pulmonary hypertension, Am. J. Cardiol. **43:**1049, 1979.
12. Beppu, S., Nimura, Y., Sakokibara, H., et al.: Mitral cleft in ostium primum atrial septal defect assessed by cross-sectional echocardiography, Circulation **62:**1099, 1980.
13. Bharati, S., McAllister, H.A., Jr., and Lev, M.: Straddling and displaced atrioventricular orifices and valves, Circulation **60:**673, 1979.
14. Bierman, F.Z., and Williams, R.G.: Prospective

diagnosis of d-transposition of the great arteries in neonates by subxyphoid two-dimensional echocardiography, Circulation **60**:1496, 1979.

15. Bierman, F.Z., and Williams, R.G.: Subxyphoid two-dimensional imaging of the interatrial septum in infants and neonates with congenital heart disease, Circulation **60**:80, 1979.

16. Bowman, F.O., Jr., Hancock, W.D., and Maim, J.R.: A valve-containing Dacron prosthesis; its use in restoring pulmonary artery–right ventricular continuity, Arch. Surg. **107**:724, 1973.

17. Brown, J.S., Billmeier, G.J., Jr., Cox, F., et al.: Mucocutaneous lymph node syndrome in the continental United States, J. Pediatr. **88**:81, 1976.

18. Chang, S.: M-mode echocardiographic techniques and pattern recognition, Philadelphia, 1976, Lea & Febiger.

19. Chung, K.J., Alexson, C.G., Manning, J.A., and Gramiak, R.: Echocardiography in truncus arteriosus: the value of pulmonic valve detection, Circulation **48**:281, 1973.

20. D'Cruz, I.A., Lalmalani, G.G., Sambasivan, V., et al.: The superiority of mitral E point–ventricular septum separation to other echocardiographic indicators of left ventricular performance, Clin. Cardiol. **2**:140, 1979.

21. de la Cruz, M.V., Anselmi, G., Cisneros, F., et al.: An embryologic explanation for the corrected transposition of the great vessels. Additional description of the main anatomic features of this malformation and its varieties, Am. Heart J. **57**:104, 1959.

22. Dillon, J.C., Feigenbaum, H., Konecke, L.L., et al.: Echocardiographic manifestations of d-transposition of the great vessels, Am. J. Cardiol. **32**:74, 1973.

23. Driscoll, D.J., Gutgesell, H.P., and McNamara, D.G.: Echocardiographic feature of congenital mitral stenosis, Am. J. Cardiol. **42**:250, 1978.

24. Farooki, Z.Q., Henry, J.G., and Green, E.W.: Echocardiographic spectrum of Ebstein's anomaly of the tricuspid valve, Circulation **53**:63, 1976.

25. Farooki, Z.Q., Henry, J.G., and Green, E.W.: Echocardiographic spectrum of the hypoplastic left heart syndrome, Am. J. Cardiol. **38**:337, 1976.

26. Fujiwara, H., and Hamashima, Y.: Pathology of the heart in Kawasaki disease, Pediatrics **61**:100, 1978.

27. Fukushige, J., Nihill, M.R., and McNamara, D.G.: Spectrum of cardiovascular lesions in mucocutaneous lymph node syndrome: analysis of eight cases, Am. J. Cardiol. **45**:98, 1980.

28. Goldberg, S.J.: Suprasternal ultrasonography, J.A.M.A. **215**:245, 1971.

29. Goldberg, S.J., Allen, H.D., and Sahn, D.J.: Echocardiographic detection and management of patient ductus arteriosus in neonates with respiratory distress syndrome: a two and one-half year prospective study, J. Clin. Ultrasound **5**:161, 1978.

30. Goldberg, S.J., Allen, H.D., and Sahn, D.J.: Pediatric and adolescent echocardiography: a handbook, ed. 2, Chicago, 1980, Year Book Medical Publishers, Inc.

31. Goldsmith, R.W., Gribetz, D., and Strauss, L.: Mucocutaneous lymph node syndrome in the continental United States, Pediatrics **57**:431, 1976.

32. Gramiak, R., Chung, K.J., Nanda, N., et al.: Echocardiographic diagnosis of transposition of the great vessels, Radiology **106**:187, 1973.

33. Gutgesell, H.P., Mullins, C.E., Gillett, P.C., et al.: Transient hypertrophic subaortic stenosis in infants of diabetic mothers, J. Pediatr. **89**:120, 1976.

34. Gutgesell, H.P., and Raquet, M.: Atlas of pediatric echocardiography, New York, 1978, Harper & Rowe, Publishers.

35. Gutgesell, H.P., Speer, M.E., and Rosenberg, H.S.: Characterization of the cardiomyopathy in infants of diabetic mothers, Circulation **61**:441, 1980.

36. Hagler, D.J., Tajik, A.J., and Ritter, D.G.: Fluttering of atrioventricular valves in patients with d-transposition of the great arteries after Mustard operation: an echocardiographic observation, Mayo Clin. Proc. **50**:69, 1975.

37. Hagler, D.J., Tajik, A.J., Seward, J.B., et al.: Real-time wide-angle sector echocardiography: atrioventricular canal defects, Circulation **59**:140, 1979.

38. Hagler, D.J., Tajik, A.J., Seward, J.B., et al.: Wide-angle two-dimensional echocardiographic profiles of conotruncal abnormalities, Mayo Clin. Proc. **55**:73, 1980.

39. Hagler, D.J., Tajik, A.J., Seward, J.B., et al.: Double outlet right ventricle: wide-angle two-dimensional echocardiographic observations, Circulation **63**:419, 1981.

40. Heck, H.A., Schieken, R.M., Lauer, R.M., et al.: Conduit repair for complex congenital heart disease. Late follow-up, J. Thorac. Cardiovasc. Surg. **75**:806, 1978.

41. Henry, W.A., DeMaria, A., Gramiak, R., et al.: Report of the American Society of Echocardiography Committee on Nomenclature and Standards in Two-dimensional Echocardiography, Circulation **62**:212, 1980.

42. Henry, W.L., Maron, B.J., and Griffith, J.M.: Cross-sectional echocardiography in the diagnosis of congenital heart disease: identification of the relation of the ventricles and great arteries, Circulation **56**:267, 1977.

43. Henry, W.L., Sahn, D.J., Griffith, J.M., et al.: Evaluation of atrioventricular morphology in congenital heart disease by real-time cross-sectional echocardiography, Circulation **52**(suppl. 2):120, 1975. [Abstract.]

44. Hiraishi, S., Yashiro, K., and Kusano, S.: Noninvasive visualization of coronary artery aneurysms in infants and children with mucocutaneous lymph node syndrome with two-dimensional echocardiography, Am. J. Cardiol. **43**:1225, 1979.

45. Hirschfeld, S., Meyer, R., Schwartz, D.C., et al.: The echocardiographic assessment of pulmonary artery pressure and pulmonary vascular resistance, Circulation **52**:642, 1975.

46. Hirschfeld, S., Meyer, R., Schwartz, D.C., et al.: Measurement of right and left ventricular systolic time intervals by echocardiography, Circulation **51**:304, 1975.

47. Kawasaki, T.: Mucocutaneous lymph node syndrome: clinical observation in 50 cases, Jpn. J. Allerg. **16**:178, 1967.

48. Kawasaki, T., Kosaki, F., Okawa, S., et al.: A new infantile acute febrile mucocutaneous lymph node syndrome (MLNS) prevailing in Japan, Pediatrics **54**:271, 1974.

49. La Corte, M., Harada, K., and Williams, R.G.: Echocardiographic features of congenital left ventricular inflow obstruction, Circulation **54**:562, 1976.

50. Lange, L.W., Sahn, D.J., Allen, H.D., and Goldberg, S.J.: Subxyphoid cross-sectional echocardiography in infants and children with congenital heart disease, Circulation **59**:513, 1979.

51. Latson, L.A., Cheatham, J.P., and Gutgesell, H.P.: Resolution and accuracy in two-dimensional echocardiography, Am. J. Cardiol. **48**:106, 1981.

52. Lew, W., and Karliner, J.S.: Assessment of pulmonary valve echogram in normal subjects and in patients with pulmonary arterial hypertension, Br. Heart J. **42**:147, 1979.

53. Lundstrom, N.R.: Echocardiography in the diagnosis of Ebstein's anomaly of the tricuspid valve, Circulation **47**:597, 1973.

54. Mace, S., Hirschfeld, S.S., Riggs, T., et al.: Echocardiographic abnormalities in infants of diabetic mothers, J. Pediatr. **95**:1013, 1979.

55. Martin, R.P., French, J.W., and Popp, R.L.: Clinical utility of two-dimensional electrocardiography in patients with bioprosthetic valves, Adv. Cardiol. **24**:294, 1980.

56. Martin, R.P., Rakowski, H., Kleiman, J.H., et al.: Reliability and reproducibility of two-dimensional echocardiographic measurement of the stenotic mitral valve orifice area, Am. J. Cardiol. **43**:569, 1979.

57. McGoon, D.C., Rastelli, G.C., and Ongley, P.A.: An operation for the correction of truncus arteriosus, J.A.M.A. **205**:59, 1968.

58. Melish, M.E., Hicks, R.M., and Larsen, E.J.: Mucocutaneous lymph node syndrome in the United States, Am. J. Dis. Child. **130**:599, 1976.

59. Meyer, R.A.: Pediatric echocardiogarphy, Philadelphia, 1977, Lea & Febiger.

60. Morris, D.C., Felner, J.M., Schlant, R.C., and Franch, R.H.: Echocardiographic diagnosis of tetralogy of Fallot, Am. J. Cardiol. **36**:908, 1975.

61. Mortera, C., Hunter, S., Terry, G., and Tynan, M.: Echocardiography of primitive ventricles, Br. Heart J. **39**:847, 1977.

62. Moss, A.J., et al.: Heart disease in infants, children, and adolescents, ed. 2, Baltimore, 1977, The Williams & Wilkins Co.

63. Nanda, N.C., Gramiak, R., Manning, J., et al.: Echocardiographic recognition of the congenital bicuspid aortic valve, Circulation **49**:870, 1974.

64. Nanda, N.C., Gramiak, R., Manning, J.A., et al.: Echocardiographic features of subpulmonic obstruction in dextrotransposition of the great vessels, Circulation **51**:515, 1975.

65. Nanda, N.C., Gramiak, R., Robinson, T.L., and Shah, P.M.: Echocardiographic evaluation of pulmonary hypertension, Circulation **50**:575, 1974.

66. Nichol, P.M., Gilbert, B.W., and Kisslo, J.A.: Two-dimensional echocardiographic assessment of mitral stenosis, Circulation **55**:120, 1977.

67. Norwood, W.I., Freed, M.D., and Rocchini, A.P.: Experience with valve conduits for repair of congenital cardiac lesions, Ann. Thorac. Surg. **24**:223, 1977.

68. Ports, T.A., Silverman, N.H., and Schiller, N.B.: Two-dimensional echocardiographic assessment of Ebstein's anomaly, Circulation **58**:336, 1978.

69. Rastelli, G., Kirklin, J.W., and Kinkaid, O.W.: Angiocardiography of persistent common atrioventricular canal, Mayo Clin. Proc. **42**:200, 1967.

70. Rastelli, G.C., Wallace, R.B., and Ongley, P.A.: Complete repair of transposition of the great arteries with pulmonary stenosis. A review and report of a case corrected by using a new surgical technique, Circulation **39**:83, 1969.

71. Riggs, T., Hirschfeld, S., Borkat, G., et al.: Assessment of the pulmonary vascular bed by echocardiographic right ventricular systolic time intervals, Circulation **57**:939, 1978.

72. Rogé, C.L.L., Silverman, N.H., Hart, P.A., and Ray, R.M.: Cardiac structure growth pattern deter-

mined by echocardiography, Circulation **57**:285, 1978.

73. Ross, D.N., and Somerville, J.: Correction of pulmonary atresia with a homograft aortic valve, Lancet **2**:1446, 1966.

74. Sahn, D.J., and Allen, H.D.: Real-time cross-sectional echocardiography imaging and measurement of the patent ductus arteriosus in infants and children, Circulation **58**:343, 1978.

75. Sahn, D.J., Allen, H.D., Lange, L.W., and Goldberg, S.J.: Cross-sectional echocardiographic diagnosis of the sites of total anomalous pulmonary venous drainage, Circulation **60**:1317, 1979.

76. Sahn, D.J., Allen, H.D., MacDonald, G., and Goldberg, S.J.: Real-time cross-sectional echocardiographic diagnosis of coarctation of the aorta—a prospective study of echocardiographic-angiographic correlations, Circulation **56**:762, 1977.

77. Sahn, D.J., DeMaria, A., Kisslo, J., and Weyman, A.—Committee on M-Mode Standardization of the American Society of Echocardiography: Recommendations regarding quantitation in M-mode echocardiography: results of a survey of echocardiographic measurements, Circulation **58**:1072, 1978.

78. Schapira, J.N., Martin, R.P., Fowles, R.E., et al.: Two-dimensional echocardiogarphic assessment of patients with bioprosthetic valves, Am. J. Cardiol. **43**:510, 1979.

79. Serruys, P.W., Van Den Brand, M., Hugenholz, P.G., and Roelandt, J.: Intracardiac right-to-left shunts demonstrated by two-dimensional echocardiography after peripheral vein injection, Br. Heart J. **42**:429, 1979.

80. Serwer, G.A., Armstrong, B.E., Anderson, P.A.W., et al.: Use of contrast echocardiography for evaluation of right ventricular hemodynamics in the presence of ventricular septal defects, Circulation **58**:327, 1978.

81. Seward, J.B., Tajik, A.J., Hagler, D.J., and Ritter, D.G.: Peripheral venous contrast echocardiography, Am. J. Cardiol. **39**:202, 1977.

82. Seward, J.B., Tajik, A.J., Spangler, J.G., and Ritter, D.G.: Echocardiographic contrast studies—initial experience, Mayo Clin. Proc. **50**:163, 1975.

83. Silverman, N.H., Payot, M., and Stanger, P.: Simulated tricuspid valve echoes in tricuspid atresia, Am. Heart J. **95**:761, 1978.

84. Silverman, N.H., Payot, M., Stanger, P., and Rudolph, A.M.: The echocardiographic profile of patients after Mustard's operation, Circulation **58**:1083, 1978.

85. Silverman, N.H., and Schiller, N.B.: Apex echocardiography: a two-dimensional technique for evaluation of congenital heart disease, Circulation **57**:503, 1978.

86. Snider, A.R., Rogé, C.L.L., Schiller, N.H., and Silverman, N.H.: Congenital left ventricle inflow obstructions evaluated by two-dimensional echocardiography, Circulation **61**:848, 1980.

87. Snider, A.R., and Silverman, N.H.: Suprasternal notch echocardiography: two-dimensional technique for evaluating congenital heart disease, Circulation **63**:165, 1981.

88. Snider, A.R., Silverman, N.H., Schiller, N.B., and Ports, T.A.: Echocardiographic evaluation of ventricular septal aneurysms, Circulation **59**:290, 1979.

89. Tajik, A.J., and Seward, J.B.: Contrast echocardiography, Cardiol. Clin. 9(2):317, 1978.

90. Tajik, A.J., Seward, J.B., Hagler, D.J., et al.: Two-dimensional real-time ultrasonic imaging of the heart and great vessels: technique, image orientation, structure identification, and validation, Mayo Clin. Proc. **53**:271, 1978.

91. Tripp, M.E., Katcher, M.L., Peters, H.A., et al.: Systemic carnitine deficiency presenting as familial endocardial fibroelastosis—a treatable cardiomyopathy, N. Engl. J. Med. **305**:385, 1981.

92. Wann, L.S., Feigenbaum, H., Weyman, A.E., and Dillon, J.C.: Cross-sectional echocardiographic detection of rheumatic mitral regurgitation, Am. J. Cardiol. **41**:1258, 1978.

93. Wann, L.S., Weyman, A.E., Feigenbaum, H., et al.: Determination of mitral valve area by cross-sectional echocardiography, Ann. Intern. Med. **88**:337, 1978.

94. Weyman, A.E.: Pulmonary valve echo motion in clinical practice, Am. J. Med. **62**:843, 1977.

95. Weyman, A.E., Caldwell, R.L., Hurwitz, R.A., et al.: Cross-sectional echocardiographic characterization of aortic obstruction. 1. Supravalvular aortic stenosis and aortic hypoplasia, Circulation **57**:491, 1978.

96. Weyman, A.E., Dillon, J.C., Feigenbaum, H., and Chang, S.: Echocardiographic patterns of pulmonary valve motion in valvular pulmonic stenosis, Am. J. Cardiol. **34**:544, 1974.

97. Weyman, A.E., Dillon, J.L., Feigenbaum, H., and Chang, S.: Echocardiographic patterns of pulmonic valve motion with pulmonary hypertension, Circulation **50**:905, 1974.

98. Weyman, A.E., Feigenbaum, H., Dillon, J.C., et al.: Noninvasive visualization of the left main coronary artery by cross-sectional echocardiography, Circulation **54**:169, 1976.

99. Weyman, A.E., Feigenbaum, H., Hurwitz, R.F., et al.: Cross-sectional echocardiography in evaluating patients with discrete subaortic stenosis, Am. J. Cardiol. **37**:358, 1976.

100. Weyman, A.E., Feigenbaum, H., Hurwitz, R.A., et al.: Localization of left ventricular outflow obstruction by cross-sectional echocardiography, Am. J. Cardiol. **40**:33, 1976.

101. Weyman, A.E., Feigenbaum, H., Hurwitz, R.A., et al.: Cross-sectional echocardiographic assessment of the severity of aortic stenosis in children, Circulation **55**:773, 1977.

102. Weyman, A.E., Hurwitz, R.A., Girod, D.A., et al.: Cross-sectional echocardiographic visualization of the stenotic pulmonary valve, Circulation **56**:769, 1977.

103. Weyman, A.E., Wann, L.S., Caldwell, R.L., et al.: Negative contrast echocardiography: a new method for detecting left-to-right shunts, Circulation **59**:498, 1979.

104. Williams, R.G., and Rudd, M.: Echocardiographic features of endocardial cushion defects, Circulation **49**:418, 1974.

105. Williams, R.G., and Tucker, C.R.: Echocardiographic diagnosis of congenital heart disease, Boston, 1977, Little, Brown and Co.

106. Valdes-Cruz, L.M., Pieroni, D.R., Roland, J.M.A., and Varghese, P.J.: Echocardiographic detection of intracardiac right-to-left shunts following peripheral vein injections, Circulation **54**:558, 1976.

107. Van Mierop, L.H.S., Alley, R.D., Kausel, H.W., and Stranahan, A.: Ebstein's malformation of the left atrioventricular valve in corrected transposition with subpulmonary stenosis and ventricular septal defect, Am. J. Cardiol. **8**:270, 1961.

108. Van Praagh, R., and Takao, A.: Etiology and morphogenesis of congenital heart disease, Mt. Kisco, N.Y., 1980, Futura Publishing Co.

109. Yoshikawa, S., Yanagihara, K., Owaki, T., et al.: Cross-sectional echocardiographic diagnosis of coronary artery aneurysms in patients with the mucocutaneous lymph node syndrome, Circulation **59**:133, 1979.

35

Prosthetic valves

Our laboratory has had experience with three basic types of prosthetic valves—the cage with ball (Starr-Edwards), the cage with disk (Beall), and the tilting disk or hinge (Björk-Shiley) (Fig. 35-1). It is important for the echographer to know the type of prosthetic valve in use for adequate recording of its most perpendicular axis.

There are three basic parts to each type of valve—the disk or ball, the strut or cage, and the sewing ring or seating of the valve (the upper and lower round attachment of the valve). Any of these components is subject to changes. The Starr-Edwards ball is composed of silicon and is subject to ball variance or a grooving irregularity. This ball variance is not seen in Teflon disk valves. Some of the valves are cloth covered and not as subject to thrombus formation.

The incidence of thrombosis with good anticoagulation is 30%. The upper and lower seating is frequently subject to thrombosis, which in turn narrows the valve. The lower-seating thrombosis interferes with closure of the valve and eventually can lead to regurgitation. In addition to these problems with thrombosis, the sutures around the area of the valve can come loose, causing regurgitation.

The evaluation of defects in the valve is sometimes quite difficult. Most patients are asymptomatic. Some demonstrate signs of fatigue. Some go into congestive heart failure because of a sticking poppet. Embolism to various organs may be seen as a result of thrombus formation on the valve. Bacterial endocarditis is one complication of prosthetic valves, because the malfunctioning valve is a seedbed for bacteria.

The disk and hinge valves can be used interchangeably in the aorta and mitral valve by reversing their positions. During auscultation the valves should make two noises during one cycle. At the onset of systole the mitral valve should have a closing click whereas the aortic valve should have an opening click. Likewise, during diastole the mitral valve should have an opening click and the aortic a closing click. With the valve in the aortic area there is normally a slight gradient. In the mitral area there is a small gradient as the blood flows from a low pressure to a high pressure, giving rise to the middiastolic murmur. The various valves have different intensities in their opening and closing clicks. For example, a Björk-Shiley prosthesis has a soft opening and loud closing.

The presence of a systolic murmur in the mitral valve area is abnormal and is frequently attributed to a paravalvar leak. If there is a clot inside the cage, it causes the valve to close improperly and regurgitation is the inevitable result.

Phonocardiography has become an important aid in assessing prosthetic valve function. In the aortic valve the onset of systole should give a loud S_1, and the onset of diastole should give a soft S_2. In the mitral valve area the soft S_1 coincides with systole whereas diastole gives a loud S_2. The duration of these sounds can also be measured. Usually, the S_2 distance is fixed and does not change with diastole. In the mitral valve area, thrombus can increase the duration of the aortic and mitral valve openings. Thus phonocardiography can assess (1) the presence or absence of valve sounds, (2) muffled or attenuated click, (3) timing of the S_2 opening click and the QS interval, and (4) the ratio of aortic

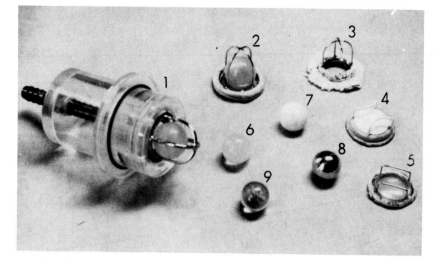

Fig. 35-1. Plastic chamber with a 3M Starr-Edwards valve, 1. Other valves are model 6100 Starr-Edwards valve, 2, specially modified Starr-Edwards cage, 3, Beall mitral prosthesis, 4, Björk-Shiley mitral prosthesis, 5, nonradiopaque Silastic rubber, 6, radiopaque Silastic rubber, 7, Stellite metal, 8, and glass, 9. Glass is not used clinically. (From Gramiak, R., and Waag, R.: Cardiac ultrasound, St. Louis, 1975, The C.V. Mosby Co.)

closing to aortic opening click (this ratio may indicate ball variance caused by poppet swelling or the appearance of a clot around the ball).

Other studies helpful in assessing prosthetic function are chest radiography, fluoroscopy, angiography, and echography.

Chest radiography can determine cardiac enlargement or position of the prosthesis. Fluoroscopy is helpful if there is a detachment of the valve or a paravalvar leak causing the valve to tilt in the mitral position (i.e., into the LA). In the aortic valve, movement is usually very dramatic; and if there is a problem, side-to-side "flipping" of the valve can be recorded.

Angiography can detect leakage; but since there is a slight degree of regurgitation with the prosthesis, it may be more difficult. Diagnostic regurgitation is physiologic in the mitral valve area. In pathologic regurgitation the dye will be seen to go into the ventricle during systole.

Echography has proved to be a useful technique in the assessment of valve function because of the strong reflecting interface between the artificial valve and the surrounding structures. The exact model and size of the prosthesis are noted prior to recording the valve. If the examiner is not careful, only the supporting structures of the cage may be recorded without disk or ball movement. By angling the transducer so the beam is more perpendicular to the prosthesis, one can record the proper echoes (Fig. 35-2). This transducer angle is critical in the assessment of valvar motion and excursion. The motion of the prosthesis is determined by valve characteristics and the entire cardiac structure. To provide the most accurate assessment of valve function, recordings should be made shortly after surgery (5 to 7 days) and followed at specified time intervals (3 months, 6 months, etc.).

MITRAL VALVE

The best mitral recording will clearly record the valve opening and closure and most closely approximate the valve's normal excursion. Disk or hinge valves can generally be recorded in their usual mitral position (Fig. 35-3). However, it may be necessary to locate Starr-Edwards valves on the chest x-ray film for proper transducer angulation (Fig. 35-4). Often the examiner must move to the apex of the heart and angle the transducer severely cephalad to record the valve at its most perpendicular angle. Simultaneous phonocardiograms can be added to most echographic equipment and will help in measuring the

interval of aortic valve closure to mitral valve opening.

The actual thrombus formation is difficult to distinguish by echo, but the altered valve motion may be recorded. Sometimes there is a delay in the valve opening, or there is no opening at all during some cycles. Decreased amplitude of valve opening must be assessed with the transducer in various angles to ascertain the maximum excursion. Because of the intense echo reflection of the valve apparatus, there often appear to be large clumps or ring-down echoes behind the open valve. This should not be confused with thrombus and usually can be eliminated by slight transducer angulations or a reduction in the sensitivity of the equipment.

Johnson (1975) described the actual measurement of the older type of ball valve by echo and has multiple charts available for analysis of individual tracings. He also discovered that the Starr-Edwards ball was made of Silastic rubber, a slower sound-conduction material. Thus, when recordings are made from such a valve, it appears that the posterior edge of the ball is actually beyond its posterior cage (Fig. 35-5). A correction factor of 0.64 can be applied to the measurement of the ball diameter to adjust for this factor.

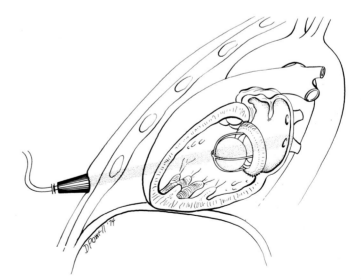

Fig. 35-2. Diagram depicting the location of the transducer on the anterior chest wall in a patient with a mitral prosthetic ball valve. The beam is perpendicular to the longitudinal axis of the valve. The ball opens toward the transducer during diastole. (From Gramiak, R., and Waag, R.: Cardiac ultrasound, St. Louis, 1975, The C.V. Mosby Co.)

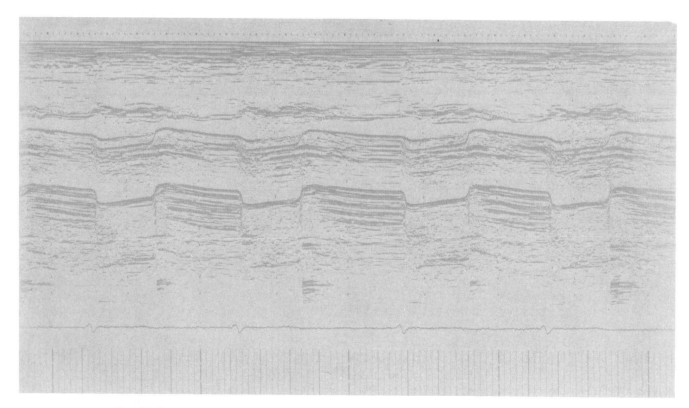

Fig. 35-3. Echographic example of a prosthetic disk type of valve in the mitral valve position.

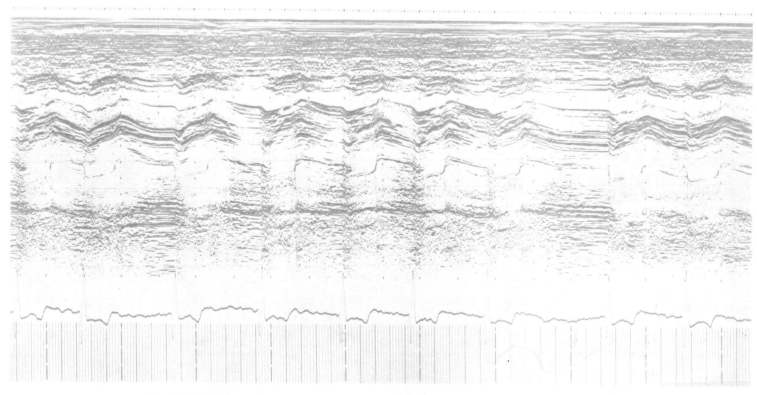

Fig. 35-4. Echographic example of a normal prosthetic Starr-Edwards valve in the mitral valve position. In this patient continuity is seen between the aortic root, interventricular septum, and mitral valve. Because of the unusual angulation that one must use to record the echoes at a perpendicular angle, this continuity is usually not possible when a prosthetic valve is in place.

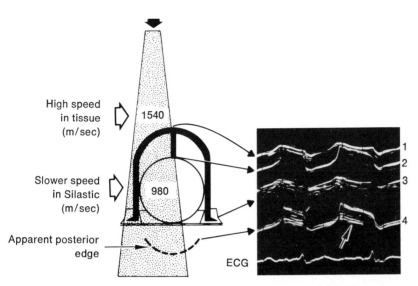

Fig. 35-5. *Left*, Schematic showing the sound beam traversing a Starr-Edwards ball valve. Sound travels at a slower speed through Silastic rubber than through body tissue. Because the oscilloscope is calibrated for the faster speed, the diameter of the ball seems to be greater than it actually is. *Right*, Echocardiogram from a patient with a Starr-Edwards mitral valve. Traces *1* to *4* are apex, anterior surface of the ball, suture ring, and posterior surface of the ball. Arrow points to the suture ring as seen through the ball in diastole. (From Gramiak, R., and Waag, R.: Cardiac ultrasound, St. Louis, 1975, The C.V. Mosby Co.)

AORTIC VALVE

Usually, because of its surgical position, the aortic valve is more difficult to assess. Often it is difficult to observe the poppet motion in a perpendicular path. Various angles of the transducer are used to record the greatest amplitude (Fig. 35-6).

As in the mitral valve, a loss of motion may represent thrombus formation (Figs. 35-7 and 35-8). Many prostheses are associated with aortic regurgitation. In this case the echographic changes are shown on the anterior leaflet of the mitral valve as fine flutter during diastole or premature closure caused by acute aortic regurgitation.

Changes can also be noted in the motion of the interventricular septum. Both normal and paradoxical septal motions have been noted in postsurgical patients. Whether the paradoxical motion is the result of superimposed tricuspid insufficiency, some effect of the prosthetic valve, or surgery on left ventricular dynamics has not been ascertained (Johnson, 1975). However, it has been noted in serial evaluation of patients with a paradoxical septum that the development of normal septal motion and an inappropriately large stroke volume are highly suggestive of a mitral or possibly aortic paraprosthetic or intraprosthetic leak.

Pericardial effusion is not an uncommon finding in post–valvar surgery patients and may be serially followed by echography.

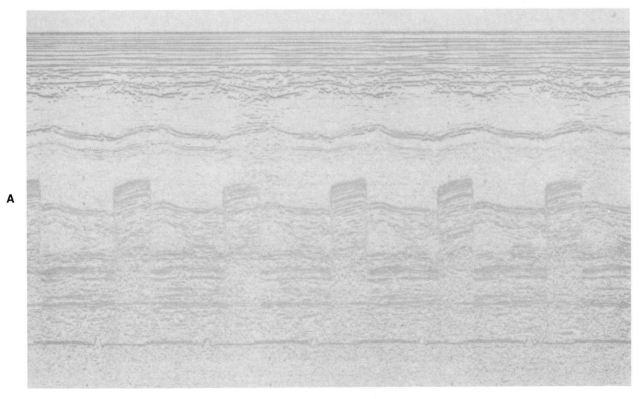

Fig. 35-6. This patient has an aortic valve disk prosthesis. **A,** The disk appears to be functioning well. *Continued.*

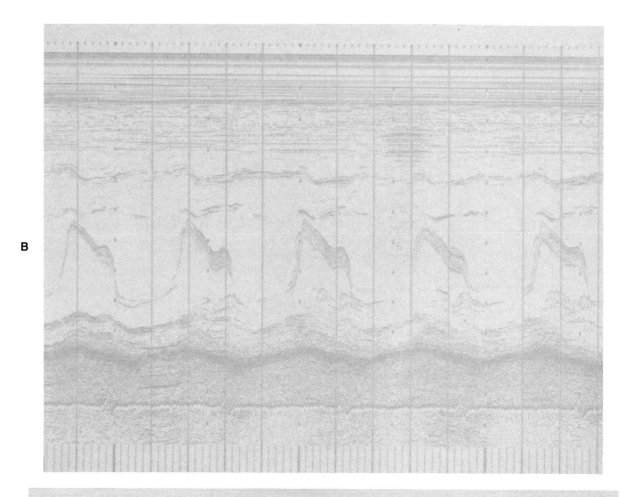

B

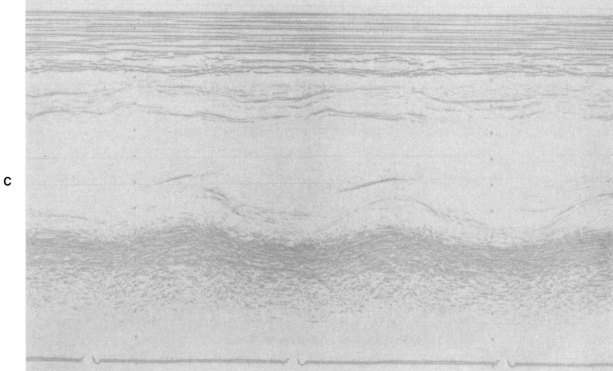

C

Fig. 35-6, cont'd. B, Thickening and flutter on the anterior leaflet of the mitral valve could be due to aortic insufficiency, bacterial endocarditis, or previous rheumatic heart disease. There is normal closure of the mitral valve, which rules out the possibility of acute aortic insufficiency. **C,** The interventricular septum has returned to normal in this 8-year postsurgical patient.

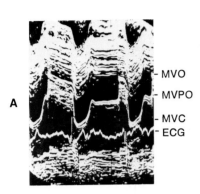
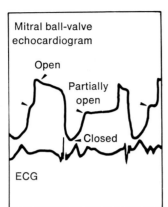

A

- MVO
- MVPO
- MVC
- ECG

Mitral ball-valve
echocardiogram

Open

Partially
open

Closed

ECG

Fig. 35-7. Echocardiogram from a malfunctioning Smeloff-Cutter mitral valve. The posterior ball surface is visualized. **A,** Note the marked delay in the opening of the ball. **B,** The ball fails to open at all. (From Belenkie, I., et al.: Am. Heart J. **86:**399, 1973.)

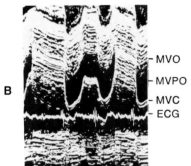
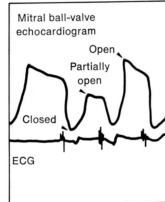

B

- MVO
- MVPO
- MVC
- ECG

Mitral ball-valve
echocardiogram

Open

Partially
open

Closed

ECG

A   **B**

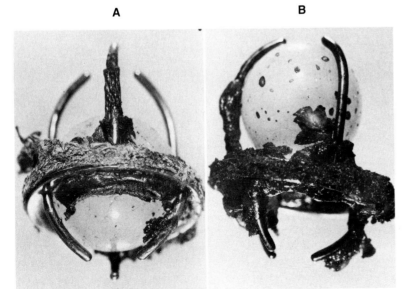

Fig. 35-8. Surgical specimen of a Smeloff-Cutter valve from the patient in Fig. 35-7. The thrombus was found to extend into the orifice of the suture ring, which hampered normal movement of the ball and resulted in the ball's sticking in a partially open position. The valve is shown in partially open, **A,** and open, **B,** positions. (From Belenkie, I., et al.: Am. Heart J. **86:**399, 1973.)

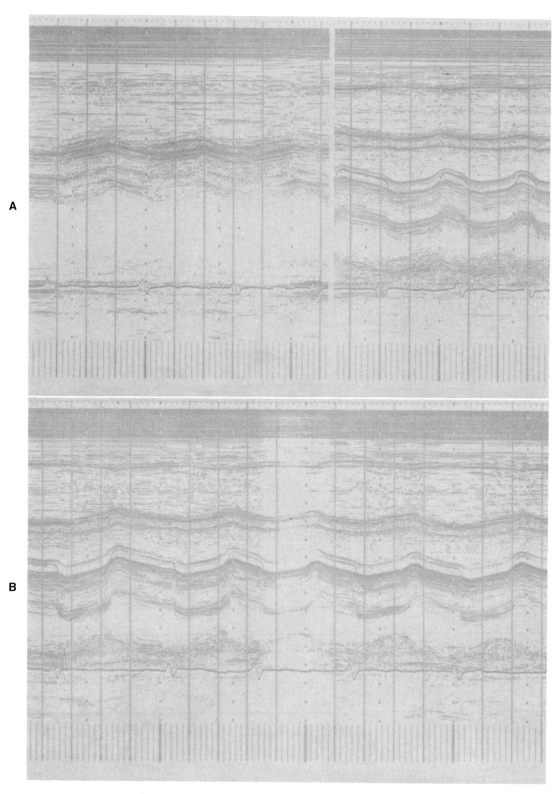

Fig. 35-9. This patient had a double prosthesis. A Beall disk was replaced in the mitral valve area, and a Starr-Edwards valve in the aortic area. There were no abnormalities on either prosthetic valve. The left atrium was slightly enlarged. Paradoxical septal motion was noted from the postsurgical state. **A,** The aortic prosthesis is shown on the left, with the mitral disk prosthesis on the right. It is extremely difficult to sweep from the prosthetic aortic valve to the prosthetic mitral valve. **B,** Mitral disk prosthesis.

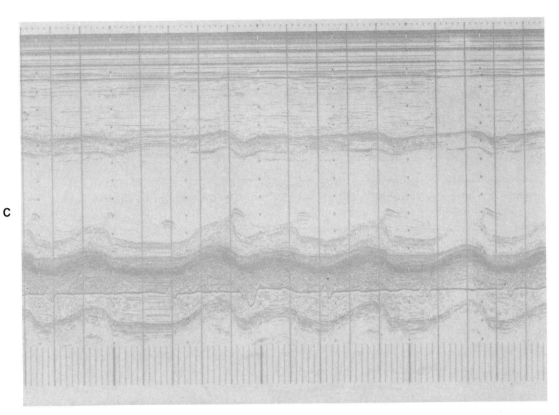

TRICUSPID VALVE

It is often confusing to evaluate patients with two or three prosthetic valves, and careful examination must be done to separate each (Fig. 35-9). With routine cardiac sweeps the transducer may record the individual valves to help the sonographer evaluate the most perpendicular axis. Then the transducer can be moved to the tricuspid area or to the apex of the heart for recording maximum amplitudes of the valves (Fig. 35-10).

Fig. 35-9, cont'd. C, Left ventricle with abnormal interventricular septal motion.

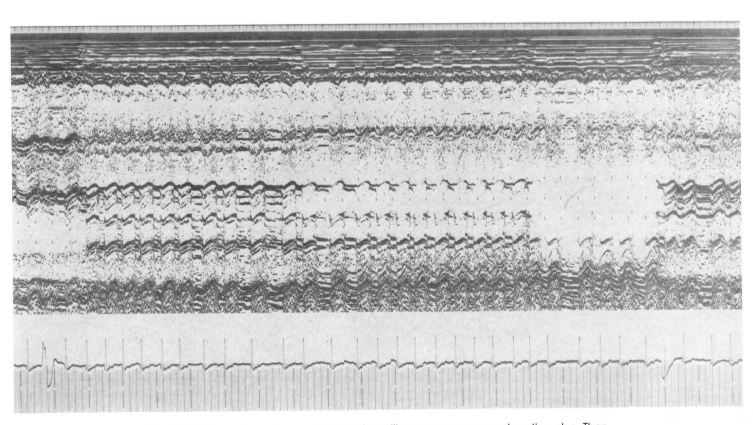

Fig. 35-10. Sometimes the prosthetic valve will appear as a normal aortic valve. Then, to obtain the opening and closing movements of the artificial valve, the examiner must be certain that the beam is perpendicular to the valve.

The diagnostic sonographer

The diagnostic sonographer is a skilled person qualified by academic and clinical training to provide patient services using diagnostic ultrasound under the supervision of a physician or osteopath responsible for the use and interpretation of ultrasound procedures. The sonographer may be involved with the patients of the physician in any medical setting for which the physician is responsible.

EDUCATION

Individuals admitted for training should have completed high school or the equivalent and should have post-secondary education in the following areas: medical ethics, medical terminology, clinical anatomy and physiology, medical orientation and administration, nursing procedures, general human anatomy, and elementary physics. Individuals in the allied health field of nuclear medicine or radiologic technology are good applicants for diagnostic ultrasound, since they already possess imaging capabilities. Cardiopulmonary technologists and cardiac catheterization technologists have proved to be capable candidates for the echocardiology section of ultrasound.

PERSONAL QUALIFICATIONS

Individuals should be mature, responsible, and able to use initiative and independent judgment when necessary. They should have a high standard of medical ethics and empathy with the patient.

Sonographers must have the ability to establish and maintain effective working relationships with patients, employees, physicians, and the general public. They should be capable of working without supervision within the guidelines set by department heads.

Self-motivation to maintain an increasing level of understanding and knowledge of the field and new procedures is necessary for the development of the sonographer.

SKILLS

The sonographer should have a high degree of technical aptitude with an in-depth knowledge of anatomy and physiology. An ability to improvise the standard of procedure when necessary is essential. The sonographer must be able to supervise the work activities of the backup technologist and ancillary personnel.

Knowledge of ultrasound techniques should be thorough. The number of procedures known will depend on the sonographer's particular interests, background, and training. The general sonographer should have current knowledge of neurology, cardiology, and abdominal, obstetric, and gynecologic applications. In addition, this person must have the ability to deal effectively with patients and to act quickly in an emergency.

A complete knowledge and understanding of the complex instrumentation used to extract the finest-quality performance from the equipment is necessary.

The ability to deviate from normal techniques when necessary and to develop new and better techniques to keep the department up to date is also the responsibility of the sonographer and the physician.

DUTIES

Sonographer I*

Qualifications. High school graduate and 2 years of allied health background in an AMA-accredited program.

Performance of diagnostic ultrasound procedures

1. Check the physician's requisition for complete information on the procedure requested; refer any questions to the ultrasound physician before performing the procedure.
2. Review the patient's chart to obtain pertinent clinical history, correlative test results, and laboratory data.
3. Position the patient for examination, explain the procedure, and give neces-

---

*The roman numeral designates level of training.

sary instructions for carrying out the procedure.

4. Perform emergency examinations in the department or at the bedside with physician supervision.

Operation of diagnostic ultrasound equipment

1. Operate ultrasound equipment with a knowledge of A-mode, M-mode, B-mode, Doppler, and real time techniques.
2. Select the proper transducer frequency and diameter for performance of the examination.
3. Utilize ancillary devices (oscilloscopes, cameras [Polaroid and multiformat], videorecorders) to obtain a permanent record of the examination.
4. Maintain quality control of the equipment.

Interpretation of ultrasound procedures

1. Recognize the significance of all structures that are visualized on the oscillosope.
2. Be able to differentiate artifacts from anatomic/pathologic structures and to recognize equipment limitations.
3. Be capable of recognizing a diagnostic quality scan.
4. Possess a knowledge of anatomy and physiology and be able to relate this to the ultrasound examination.

Professional development

1. Read journals and attend local symposiums to keep abreast of new techniques.
2. Review the pathology, surgery, and delivery reports to follow the patient's progress and provide a means of reviewing the accuracy of ultrasound examinations.
3. Periodically review anatomy, physiology, and pathology as related to ultrasonics.
4. Maintain ethical working relationships and good rapport with all referring physicians, hospital staff, and commercial agencies.

Administrative responsibilities

1. Maintain supplies for the service or room assigned.
2. Maintain cleanliness of the equipment and a general orderliness of the area assigned.
3. Obtain x-ray film folders from the file room, inscribe the x-ray and ultrasound film folders with the appropriate data, and record the examination performed on a file card.
4. Make copies of teaching or research cases as needed.

Sonographer II

Qualifications. Two years' allied health background in an AMA-approved program or 2 years of college. One year in diagnostic ultrasound (either a formal program or 18 months' equivalent experience). Must be ARDMS eligible.

Performance of diagnostic ultrasound procedures

1. Check the physician's requisition for complete information on the procedure requested; refer any questions to the ultrasound physician before performing procedure.
2. Consult with the referring physician regarding the patient's medical history and the appropriate ultrasound procedure required.
3. Review the patient's chart to obtain pertinent clinical history, correlative test results, and laboratory data.
4. Position the patient for examination, explain the procedure, and give necessary instructions for carrying out the procedure.
5. Be able to deviate from normal techniques when necessary and to develop better techniques to keep the department up to date.
6. Perform emergency examinations in the department or at the bedside with physician supervision.

Operation of diagnostic ultrasound equipment

1. Operate ultrasound equipment with an in-depth knowledge of A-mode, M-mode, B-mode (analog and digital), Doppler, and real time techniques.
2. Select the proper transducer frequency and diameter for performance of the examination.
3. Utilize ancillary devices (oscilloscopes, cameras [Polaroid and multiformat], videorecorders) to obtain a permanent record of the examination.
4. Maintain quality control of the equipment.
5. Calibrate ultrasound and photographic equipment when necessary.

Interpretation of ultrasound procedures

1. Recognize the significance of all structures that are visualized on the oscilloscope.
2. Be able to differentiate artifacts from anatomic/pathologic structures and to recognize electronic equipment limitations.
3. Possess a high degree of technical expertise, with an in-depth knowledge of anatomy and physiology, and be able to

improve standard procedures to enhance diagnostic results when needed.

4. Be capable of recognizing a diagnostic scan and rendering an initial interpretation to the referring physician as reported by the staff sonologist.
5. Maintain ethical working relationships and good rapport with all referring physicians, hospital staff, and commercial agencies.

Research in and development of ultrasound techniques

1. Evaluate new products and equipment for future use.
2. Read journals and attend annual conventions, seminars, and symposiums to keep abreast of new techniques.
3. Review the pathology, surgery, and delivery reports to follow the patient's progress and provide a means of reviewing the accuracy of ultrasound examinations.
4. Continuously review anatomy and physiology and the effect of disease processes with relation to ultrasonics.

Coordination of administrative responsibilities

1. Maintain supplies for the service or room assigned.
2. Obtain x-ray film folders from the file room, inscribe the x-ray and ultrasound film folders with the appropriate data, and record the examination performed on a file card.
3. Record interesting cases for teaching or research purposes.
4. Make copies of teaching or research cases as needed.

Sonographer III

Qualifications. Two years' allied health background in an AMA-accreditated program or 2 years of college. Two years' experience/training in diagnostic ultrasound. Must have ARDMS in at least two specialty areas (i.e., abdomen, obstetrics, Doppler, or cardiology).

Performance of diagnostic ultrasound procedures

1. Check the physician's requisition for complete information on the procedure requested; refer any questions to the ultrasound physician (sonologist) before performing the procedure.
2. Consult with the referring physician regarding the patient's medical history and the appropriate ultrasound procedure required.
3. Review the patient's chart to obtain pertinent clinical history, correlative

test results, and laboratory data as they apply to the ultrasound examination.

4. Position the patient for examination, explain the procedure, and give necessary instructions for carrying out the procedure.

5. Be able to deviate from normal techniques when necessary and to develop better techniques to keep the department up to date.

6. Perform emergency examinations in the department or at the bedside without physician supervision.

Operation of diagnostic ultrasound equipment

1. Operate ultrasound equipment with an in-depth knowledge of A-mode, M-mode, and B-mode (analog and digital), Doppler, and real time techniques.

2. Select the proper transducer frequency and diameter for performance of the examination.

3. Utilize ancillary devices (oscilloscopes, cameras [Polaroid and multiformat] videorecorders) to obtain a permanent record of the examination.

4. Maintain quality control of the equipment. Record results on a regular basis.

5. Calibrate ultrasound and photographic equipment when necessary.

Interpretation of ultrasound procedures

1. Recognize the significance of all structures that are visualized on the oscilloscope.

2. Be able to differentiate artifacts from anatomic/pathologic structures and recognize electronic equipment limitations.

3. Possess a high degree of technical expertise, with an in-depth knowledge of anatomy and physiology, and be able to improve standard procedures when needed.

4. Be capable of recognizing a diagnostic scan and rendering an initial interpretation to the referring physician as reported by the staff sonologist.

5. Establish and maintain ethical working relationships and good rapport with all referring physicians, hospital staff, and commercial companies.

Research in and development of ultrasound techniques

1. Evaluate new products and equipment for possible future use.

2. Research, develop, and formulate new techniques for ultrasound procedures.

3. Read journals and attend annual conventions, seminars, and symposiums to keep abreast of new techniques.

4. Review the pathology, surgery, and delivery reports to follow the patient's progress and provide a means of reviewing the accuracy of ultrasound examinations.

5. Continuously review anatomy and physiology and the effect of disease processes with relation to ultrasonics.

Coordination of administrative responsibilities

1. Maintain a procedures manual.

2. Secure and maintain supplies for the service or room assigned.

3. Keeps records on all service calls for equipment and what service was done.

4. Obtain x-ray film folders from the file room, inscribe the x-ray and ultrasound film folders with the appropriate data, and record the examination performed on a file card.

5. Record interesting cases for teaching or research purposes.

6. Make copies of teaching or research cases as needed.

Instruction and supervision of clinical experience for ultrasound students and radiologic technology students

1. Teach the techniques and applications of ultrasound to students, visiting sonographers, and physicians, residents, and fellows.

2. Provide impromptu explanations and demonstrations for visitors and students.

Sonographer IV, Chief

Qualifications. High school graduate and 2 years' allied health background in an AMA-accredited program or 2 years of college. Three years' experience/training in diagnostic ultrasound. Must have ARDMS in at least three speciality areas (i.e., abdomen, obstetrics, Doppler, or cardiology). Should have extensive experience with available ultrasound equipment in terms of product evaluation, troubleshooting, and quality control. Must be mature and responsible, able to use initiative and independent judgment when necessary, and capable of working without supervision within guidelines established by the director of the division. Self-motivation with regard to increasing one's level of understanding and knowledge of the field is important, as is a background that will qualify one to teach diagnostic ultrasound.

In addition to the duties of Sonographer III, the Sonographer IV candidate is responsible for coordinating the activities of the sonologic staff and ancillary personnel and, under the supervision of the director of ultrasound, performing administrative duties of supervision within the division.

Coordination of staff within the ultrasound division

1. Act as coordinating bond for all staff sonographers assigned within the division of ultrasound.

2. Maintain the quality of performance of sonographers as related to skills and duties.

3. Mediate problems relative to staffing, morale, scheduling, salary adjustments, discipline, and other actions regarding personnel.

4. Act as consultant in hiring, promoting, or terminating employees.

5. Assume responsibilities for patient flow and all other matters pertaining to patient care within the division.

6. Ensure patient and employee safety.

Operation of diagnostic ultrasound equipment

1. Have a knowledge of the correct operation of all divisional equipment, accessories, and procedures (as listed for Sonographer III).

2. Be able to diagnose basic equipment malfunction, communicate with service personnel, and maintain service records.

Coordination of administrative responsibilities

1. Review monthly budget reports for accuracy and report discrepancies.

2. Maintain files on revenue analysis and expenditures, trend reports, and storehouse charges.

3. Secure supplies for the division.

4. Recommend action necessary for improvement of the overall quality of the department.

5. Assume responsibilities for public relations in intrahospital dealings.

Supervision

The sonographer is under the supervision of the director of diagnostic ultrasound. Working under personal initiative to achieve quality work after initial assignments are received, the sonographer may also supervise other staff sonographers with less experience, students of ultrasound, visiting sonographers and physicians, or visiting house staff, medical students, and fellows.

Line of promotion

The larger medical centers with diagnostic ultrasound programs have a more extensive staff than do community hospital laboratories. The former program may have a staff consisting of an educational coordinator, a clinical coordinator, staff instructors, and staff sonographers specializing in neurology, cardiology, and B-scan techniques. The smaller departments may have one of three sonographers sharing the duties of the department.

Performance

The number of cases a sonographer can perform in a day depends on the type of examination ordered; for example, abdominal and cardiac cases may take longer than an obstetric case. Although there is usually a protocol established for each examination, the sonographer may take additional views of the area of interest for a more accurate diagnostic interpretation by the physician. Because of the anatomic and acoustic properties of each patient, it is difficult to place a rigid time factor for each examination performed. The experienced sonographer, in most cases, should be able to perform an average of 10 to 12 cases a day.

The approximate time (in minutes) required to complete each ultrasound study is as follows:

Echocardiography, complete: 30 to 45
Doppler: 40 to 60
Abdominal: 20 to 40
Renal: 15 to 30
Gynecologic: 15 to 30
Obstetric: 10 to 15
Thyroid: 15 to 20

Of course, the number of patients a sonographer can examine depends on ancillary personnel to aid in the function of the ultrasound department. Escort service for the patient, secretarial assistance for the mounting, labeling, and sorting of scans, and telephone assistance for appointments and reports are necessary to increase the number of patients whom the sonographer is able to examine daily.

AVAILABILITY

The director of the ultrasound laboratory should determine whether 24-hour service is necessary for quality patient care. If it is deemed necessary, the sonographer and physician should provide adequate technical and interpretive skills.

CURRICULUM

The structure of the curriculum for individuals meeting the entrance requirements should be based on a minimum of a calendar year (12 months) of full-time study. This is to provide didactic content of appropriate scope and depth as well as clinical experiences of sufficient variety and quantity to ensure adequate opportunity to acquire the needed knowledge and skills.

The subject matter for a 1-year program would include introduction to basic physics, ultrasound applications of physics and biologic safety, laboratory experiments, instrumentation, biometrics, cross-sectional anatomy, pathology, physiology, cardiology, clinical medicine, differential diagnosis, comparison of other diagnostic modalities, ultrasonic techniques, interpretation, and journal review, research, and clinical experience.

CONTINUING EDUCATION

The sonographer should maintain an active interest in the field of ultrasound. A current library of ultrasound textbooks, videotapes, slide series, and journals should be maintained in the laboratory as a reference for updating current techniques and interpretations. The sonographer should be encouraged to attend local and regional ultrasound seminars. Attendance at the national ultrasound and echocardiography meetings is important for the sonographer to keep abreast of current developments in the field. Experts in ultrasound should be encouraged to visit particular laboratories if special techniques are newly employed.

Guidelines for establishing an educational program

I became interested in educational programs while I was at the University of California–San Diego in the late 1960s. The early stages of sonography offered no formal education for physicians or sonographers; and as a result numerous short-term courses, seminars, and lecture series were devised to stimulate the growth of ultrasound. I organized several 12-week seminars through the continuing education department at UCSD and discovered that there was an overwhelming quest for education in diagnostic ultrasound that was not yet met on a national basis.

My first real experience in hospital-based formal education was in Philadelphia with Barry Goldberg. We began with three students for a 6-month period and gradually built the program to 14 students for a 1-year period.

The contents of Appendix B reveals the experience I have had over the past 7 years in establishing a hospital-based program in sonography. To maintain a program that is viable year after year, one must meet and overcome several obstacles. Support must be gained from the hospital administrator, department chairman, medical director of the program, technical staff in the department, other departments within the hospital through which the students should rotate, clinical affiliates, and the students themselves.

We have found it very efficient to render all our lecture notes in either outline or text form so that transparencies and copies can be made for the students. We then use the overhead projector in the lecture room and the students are able to follow along with their own copy, making additional notes as the discussion proceeds.

Likewise, the lesson plan can utilize slides or other teaching aids. (In case the lecture has been given by another individual, the material will be ready and class will not have to be cancelled.)

STAGE I

When you have decided to start a program in diagnostic medical sonography, you should consider several things:

1. Do you have a *medical director* who is really interested in an educational program and willing to spend a great deal of time teaching the students? The medical director should have thoughts on education similar to yours (so the program will be effective), should be able to lecture to students and spend time in readout sessions, should provide a stimulus for various student projects, and should be supportive of the program in terms of the entire department's needs.

2. Do you have a *hospital administrator* who is enthusiastic toward starting a program?

3. Do you have a *department administrator* who is enthusiastic about the program? This is extremely important as regards the purchasing of new equipment and teaching aids (audiovisual, phantoms, etc.) or the funding of special projects that may be called for.

4. Is your *clinical staff* in sonography supportive of students? Does it understand exactly your feelings toward having students in the department? Are the members good instructors (can they teach clinical concepts to the students)?

5. What *subject areas* do you plan to cover in your program? Do you have communicative access to other departments (cardiology, ophthalmology, obstetrics, etc.) if necessary to provide adequate experience for the students?

6. Are there *other hospitals* nearby through which the students may rotate for different viewpoints and broader clinical experience?
7. What is your *source of students?* Is there a need for educated sonographers in your area? Are there other hospitals that already offer formal education in sonography?

STAGE II

Your next step is to become familiar with the teaching facilities that your hospital has to offer. Ideally a hospital connected with a larger university or a medical school will offer more teaching aids than will a small community hospital.

First, search the library for
Research material
Audiovisual material and equipment
Individual teaching carrels
Journal accessibility
Then, locate possible lecturers:
Medical school
Medical physics
Specialty departments
Residents
Ph.D. candidates
Finally, contact other departments:
Cardiology
Pediatrics
Ophthalmology
Obstetrics
Oncology
Vascular surgery
Medical physics
You may receive a tremendous amount of support from departments other than your own. Most people involved with sonography are eager to educate others and are very enthusiastic about a program in the specialty.

STAGE III

Now you should have a fairly accurate impression as to the type of program you can offer and the kind of support you will receive from your own department as well as the rest of the hospital. The previous two stages may take some time to establish if you are new to the hospital. If you have been an employee for a few years, you should be familiar with all the politics and personalities within the hospital and thus be able to plan your program fairly easily.

A curriculum should be established. I use the *SDMS Educational Outline* as my starting point and build from that.

In our own program we include
Physics
Anatomy (gross and cross-sectional)

Pathology
Physiology
Clinical medicine (differential diagnosis, comparison with other modalities)
Cardiology
Abdomen, retroperitoneal
Obstetrics and gynecology
Superficial structures
Doppler
Breast
Ultrasonic techniques
Ultrasound interpretation
Teaching file, museum cases
Journal club
Research papers
Clinical experience
When you have decided which subjects to offer, you may decide what teaching aids you have and what you should purchase for the program.
Videotapes
Slide sets
Library books
Other teaching aids we have found to be very effective are
Local ultrasound meetings
Visiting physicians/sonographers
Outside seminars
Affiliate hospitals
Field trips (other hospitals, commercial companies)
Commercial teaching aids (lecturers, videotapes)
You will have to decide how many students you can handle with your present equipment, staff, and classroom facilities. We generally plan on one student per piece of equipment (contact scan/real time or M-mode/real time). If you have a large classroom, you may find it beneficial to open your lectures to more students. For example, we offer our affiliate hospitals the opportunity to send their personnel for the lecture series at no charge in return for letting our students rotate through their department. This has proved very effective—it promotes good will and good education in the ultrasound community, which in turn benefits the patient. We also allow students to audit the courses for a reduced tuition if they are able to receive their clinical experience at some other institution.

STAGE IV

Publicity about the program
Brochure
Advertisements—*SDMS Newsletter*, *Journal of Clinical Ultrasound*
Word of mouth spreads very quickly

STAGE V

In the selection of students we try to make a decision at least 6 months before the starting date; this lets students prepare for the 1-year program without salary. We require a nonrefundable tuition of $100 (which is applied to the tuition) upon acceptance into the program.

It is difficult to make a general statement about the type of student selected. I have found that some radiology students do very well if they have been in a program that stressed anatomy, pathology, and differential diagnosis in their training. I have also found students with a 4-year degree doing extremely well in sonography regardless of their major course of study. Individuals with a particular interest in photography seem to succeed in sonography.

Our selection of students is based upon several items: grade point average, previous medical background, interest and level of knowledge of the field of ultrasound, letters of recommendation, previous work experience, personal reasons for entering the ultrasound field. It is important to choose a student who has a high scholastic average, for the workload in a comprehensive program is very extensive.

ESTABLISHING A DIAGNOSTIC ULTRASOUND EDUCATIONAL PROGRAM

Since the 1970s, interest in ultrasound has risen geometrically, causing an acute shortage of educated sonographers and physicians. This demand has been the impetus for the extensive development of training facilities.

The Society of Diagnostic Medical Sonographers and several leading medical institutions have developed extensive programs in diagnostic ultrasound. These programs have evolved through the cooperative efforts of physicians and sonographers dedicated to quality education in ultrasound. Much of the material has been revised through the experience of the program directors. It is through these revisions that the following guidelines ae presented to institutions interested in establishing such an educational program.

Admission requirements

The sonographer is a unique member of the allied health field, working closely with the physician to reach a diagnosis through the use of ultrasound. Qualifications and duties of the sonographer have already been discussed; therefore it will suffice to reemphasize the responsibility and clinical exposure that the sonographer must have to be an asset to the clinician. Thus it was decided at our institution not to admit students directly from high school but instead to admit only students who had completed a 2-year allied health program or 2 years of undergraduate work.

Institutions

The ideal location for such programs has been within the confines of the medical center, hospital, clinic, or busy physician's office. Junior and senior colleges and universities have had success establishing ultrasound programs when working in conjunction with an active medical center.

Some institutions will work cooperatively to offer a total program to students. Thus specialized hospitals performing echocardiograms, obstetric care, etc. could be attended on a rotating basis for the students' learning experiences. If carefully structured and monitored, this rotating program could be effective in providing students with several technical outlooks during their training period.

Number of students

The number of students selected for each program should be proportional to the size of the ultrasound staff and should not exceed a ratio of 3:1. Ideally two students to each sonographer allows a more in-depth clinical exposure.

Length of the program

Because ultrasound encompasses so many aspects, a general program in diagnostic ultrasound should be a minimum of 1 year. Shorter programs have been attempted, without success. The 6-month program does not allow sufficient didactic and clinical exposure to the field.

Instructors

Instructors should be qualified in their respective areas of ultrasound. It is recommended that they have completed a formal training program in ultrasound and possess clinical experience beyond training.

The *Registry for Diagnostic Medical Sonographers* should be taken by the instructors to measure their competence on a national level. The physicians involved in the program likewise should have undergone formal training either through short courses or in their residency or fellowship program. It is generally agreed that physicians should spend a minimum of 3 months to an ideal of 1 year in ultrasound prior to entering the teaching profession.

If the program has at least six students, the staff may be composed of a director of ultrasound and staff physicians with specialty areas in anatomy, neurology, cardiology, abdominal and renal studies, and obstetrics and gynecology. A physicist who specializes in acoustic energy or ultrasound is highly recommended. The staff of sonographers should include an educational coordinator, chief sonographer, and staff sonographers with specialty areas in neurology, cardiology, abdominal and renal studies, and obstetrics and gynecology. These staff members may overlap in some areas; but as the program expands, the staff specialty areas should also develop.

Tuition

Fees should be kept at a minimum (i.e., only to support the program). When tuition is being established, outside speakers and additional teaching equipment such as audiovisual aids, library facilities, and phantoms should be considered as part of the operating budget.

Recommended program

Physics is an important part of ultrasound, and care should be taken to choose a physicist with experience in acoustic properties or ultrasound modalities. The course should consist of an introduction to the basic laws of physics, followed by a concentrated approach in ultrasound physics, including biologic safety. Laboratory experiments should be used to emphasize lecture material further—with concentration on transducer construction, testing and evaluation, frequency change effects, etc. A thorough understanding of ultrasound equipment is necessary so the operation of such machinery will be done correctly and well. An understanding of biometrics and statistical analysis may be beneficial in the research-directed program.

Anatomic relationships are the core of the ultrasound examination; therefore this subject cannot be overemphasized. We have found it particularly useful to begin with gross anatomy and then proceed to cross-sectional and sagittal relationships. Our anatomist has sectioned two cadavers, one in the sagittal plane and the other in the transverse plane, and has had these sections mounted in plastic containers for use in the classroom. Additional instruction in embryology will give the students a better understanding of anatomic anomalies, defects, and variations that appear in the developmental process.

Pathology provides the sonographer with an insight into the ultrasonic visualization of disease. Gross pathology is probably the most helpful to the sonographer. This class may be held in the surgical pathology classroom or may be illustrated by slides of gross pathologic specimens and their sections. Actually feeling the consistency of cystic masses versus solid tumors enables the sonographer to gain a better understanding of the scans to be performed.

Physiology should be a prerequisite to the program so the subject may be presented in more depth in specialized areas of neurology, cardiology, and specific organ function.

The sonographer needs to have an understanding of various aspects of *clinical medicine* as related to ultrasound. We have found it useful to be able to evaluate the patients' clinical symptoms and history prior to performing the examination. This eliminates unnecessary scanning time if an initial differential diagnosis is made prior to the study. After the study is completed, the sonographer should have at hand an initial preliminary reading with differentials to be presented to the physician. The other diagnostic modalities will provide a better understanding of the final diagnosis.

Cardiology lectures may be offered in electrocardiography, phonocardiography, vector cardiography, carotid and jugular pulse tracings, cardiac catheterization, cardiac disease processes, and congenital anomalies. Attendance at joint conferences between cardiology and ultrasound personnel to evaluate echocardiograms should be encouraged. In addition, the clinical cardiology conference presents the total history, diagnostic evaluation, interpretation, and discussion of the cardiac patient.

Ultrasonic techniques include scanning protocol and procedures necessary to perform an adequate examination. This should be combined with clinical experience and ultrasonic interpretation.

Journal review of current articles enables the student to stay abreast of current developments and gain an insight into investigative research and data collection for use in their own particular research projects.

FORMAT FOR THE ANALYSIS OF A MEDICAL ARTICLE

Journal (complete title, volume, page, date)

_____

Author _____
Title of article _____
Summarize the article:

Define the terminology used in the article:

Write three questions and answers that pertain to the article:

Ultrasound equipment

Sufficient equipment should be available for the students to gain clinical competence in the ultrasound examination. Each student should be able to spend at least 60% to 75% of the daily allotted time physically learning the "art" of scanning. State-of-the-art equipment should be available for the training center. Ideally it will include commercially different gray scale, real time, A-mode, M-mode, and Doppler equipment. Optional equipment may include the pulsed Doppler, ophthalmologic instruments, and a computerized water-path scanner.

Teaching aids

Attendance at weekly *cardiac conferences* is beneficial to the students involved in echocardiography. These conferences are generally of two types. A clinical cardiac conference involves clinical case presentations of two or more patients. Patient symptoms, history, and results of ECG, vector, phonocardiography, treadmill, echocardiography, cardiac catheterization, and surgical evaluation are presented. The other type of cardiac conference is more didactic, involving specific cardiac subjects including invasive and noninvasive cardiac procedures.

Additional teaching aids should be used throughout the program. Attendance at *outside courses* and *seminars* provides exposure to current new developments in ultrasound. *Visiting physicians and sonographers* often add to the educational program by relating personal experience with ultrasound techniques and problems. Review of problem cases with these visitors is sometimes a beneficial exercise. New techniques may also be adopted or tried experimentally as the result of such visits.

Local society meetings may be educationally stimulating to the training programs. Guest speakers and case presentations provide continuing challenge in this field. Many regions now have specialized local meetings, and thus echocardiography may be discussed exclusively or in combination with other ultrasound modalities.

Currently there are video slide sets, videotapes, and cassette tapes available from the known experts in ultrasound. These should be a supplementary part of the ultrasound program.

Library facilities should include all current books, journals, and reprints on diagnostic ultrasound. Students should be encouraged to read as much material as they can during their educational exposure. Journals can routinely be assigned to certain students. Each student should be required to copy the pertinent ultrasound articles for reference and discussion in the weekly or bimonthly journal club review. This exposes students to current literature in a uniform manner and encourages them to read and selectively interpret the available information.

Research assignments are an important part of the students' training. The first project should be a review of the literature and/or cases on a particular subject of the student's choice. This paper will be critiqued by and discussed among the other students. The second project should consist of research

in which the student actually evaluates one particular aspect of ultrasound. Thus scanning techniques, artifacts, patient data and evaluation, and a review of the pertinent literature are included in this paper.

RESEARCH PAPER FORMAT

Each student will be responsible for completing two research papers during the 1-year program.

The first should be more of a review-type paper that concentrates on a particular subject of the student's choice—e.g., "The Renal Transplant," "Common Artifacts Encountered in Sonography," "Gallbladder Disease," "Vascular Aneurysms."

The second paper should be a research-oriented approach concentrating again on a particular subject with accumulated data compiled by the student to include sonograms, clinical history, and surgical and laboratory results—e.g., "The Sonographic Appearance of Renal Transplant Rejection," "The Echogenicity of the Normal Pancreas," "Patterns of Liver Disease."

For both papers the following format should be utilized:
1. Title page
2. Table of contents
3. Abstract
4. Contents
   Introduction
   Anatomy
   Physiology
   Laboratory data
   Pathology
   Ultrasound patterns and differential diagnoses
   Summary
5. Annotated bibliography
   Should include 10 to 15 current articles (after 1975) and 4 or 5 textbooks

Some laboratories may find field trips to other laboratories useful. This exposes the students to new or different techniques available to the ultrasonographer. Trips to manufacturers of equipment or transducers may promote understanding and appreciation of ultrasound devices.

Of course, interdepartmental exposure to other diagnostic modalities should be incorporated if the students' acquaintance with these modalities is limited. Thus exposure to cardiac catheterization, phonocardiography, treadmill electrocardiography, cardiac clinic, radiology, and nuclear medicine will add to their understanding of the echographic procedure.

Echocardiographic measurements and normal values (adult)

Table C-1. Adult normal values

	cm
Body surface area	1.45 to 2.22
Right ventricular dimension (flat)	0.7 to 2.3
Right ventricular dimension (left lateral)	0.9 to 2.6
Left ventricular internal dimension (flat)	3.7 to 5.6
Left ventricular internal dimension (left lateral)	3.5 to 5.7
Posterior left ventricular wall thickness	0.6 to 1.1
Posterior left ventricular wall amplitude	0.9 to 1.4
Interventricular septal thickness	0.6 to 1.1
Interventricular septal amplitude	0.3 to 0.8
Left atrial dimension	1.9 to 4.0
Aortic root dimension	2.0 to 3.7
Aortic cusp separation	1.5 to 2.6
Mean rate of circumferential shortening (Vcf)	1.02 to 1.94 circ./sec

From Feigenbaum, H.: Echocardiography, ed. 3, Philadelphia, 1981, Lea & Febiger.

Table C-2. Adult normal values corrected for body surface area

	cm/sq m
Right ventricular dimension/sq m (flat)	0.4 to 1.4
Right ventricular dimension/sq m (left lateral)	0.4 to 1.4
Left ventricular internal dimension/sq m (flat)	2.1 to 3.2
Left ventricular internal dimension/sq m (left lateral)	1.9 to 3.2
Left atrial dimension/sq m	1.2 to 2.2
Aortic root/sq m	1.2 to 2.2

From Feigenbaum, H.: Echocardiography, ed. 3, Philadelphia, 1981, Lea & Febiger.

Sine and cosine functions

(Chapter 1)

The sine and cosine are trigonometric functions used quite often in acoustics and descriptions of wave phenomena. They are defined with the use of the right triangle (Fig. D-1). Let a, b, and c be the sides of this triangle, as shown. For angle B

$$\sin B \equiv \frac{b}{c}$$

$$\cos B \equiv \frac{a}{c}$$

(The notation $\equiv$ means "is defined as.")
It is easy to see that for a small angle (e.g., angle B) which is nearly 0 degrees side B is also very small and sin B is nearly 0. If angle B is small, side a is almost equal to side c. It follows then that the cosine for a very small angle is nearly 1. Similarly, as angle B approaches 90 degrees, sin B goes to 1 and cos B goes to 0.

A graph of cos B and sin B when angle B is between 0 and 90 degrees appears in Fig. D-2. Obviously such a graph could be carried farther, but the point probably has been made.

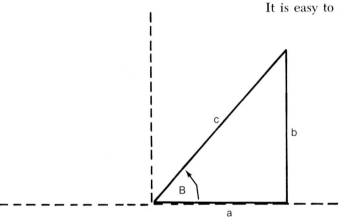

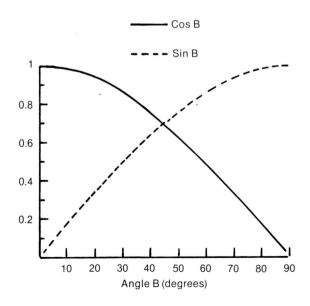

Exponential notation and pulse-echo response profiles

(Chapter 2)

USE OF EXPONENTIAL NOTATION

Although perhaps not necessary for a cursory understanding of the material, liberal use of exponentials is made in the examples worked out in the text. It is suggested that the student who wishes more than a brief review of this material consult a textbook on college mathematics.

A quantity is usually expressed in scientific notation as a number between 1 and 10 multiplied by 10 raised to the correct power.

$$25 = 2.5 \times 10^1$$
$$693 = 6.93 \times 10^2$$
$$3200 = 3.2 \times 10^3$$
$$6{,}000{,}000 = 6 \times 10^6$$
$$0.25 = 2.5 \times 10^{-1}$$
$$0.003 = 3 \times 10^{-3}$$
$$0.00042 = 4.2 \times 10^{-4}$$

In adding or subtracting two numbers expressed with this notation, it is necessary to express both numbers as the same power of 10 first and then carry on with the operation. Thus

$$1.75 \times 10^6 - 3 \times 10^5$$
$$= 1.75 \times 10^6 - 0.3 \times 10^6$$
$$= (1.75 - 0.3) \times 10^6$$
$$= 1.45 \times 10^6$$

$$0.23 + 4.1 \times 10^{-2}$$
$$= 23 \times 10^{-2} + 4.1 \times 10^{-2}$$
$$= (23 + 4.1) \times 10^{-2}$$
$$= 27.1 \times 10^{-2}$$
$$= 2.71 \times 10^{-1}$$

To multiply or divide numbers expressed as 10 to a power, use the formula

$$\frac{a \times 10^m}{b \times 10^n} = \frac{a}{b} \times 10^{m-n}$$

$$(a \times 10^m) \times (b \times 10^n) = (a \times b) \times 10^{m+n}$$

This means that exponential values are *subtracted* from each other when you divide and *added* to each other when you multiply.

PULSE-ECHO RESPONSE PROFILES

One way to demonstrate the beam pattern from an ultrasound transducer is to obtain pulse-echo response profiles at different distances from the face of the probe. The technique is illustrated in Fig. E-1. Either spherical reflectors or rod reflectors are positioned at different distances from the transducer. The transducer is scanned across each reflector and the echo amplitude is measured versus the distance from the reflector to the beam axis. The resulting curves of echo amplitude versus distance from the reflector to the beam axis are referred to as *pulse-echo response profiles,* a term that accurately describes their method of production.

Several examples of pulse-echo response profiles are presented in Figs. E-2 to E-5. These data are specifically for transducers that are used with manual scanning instruments employed in abdominal imaging (see Chapter 3). However, the size, frequency, and focusing characteristics also are common to many automatic scanners that mechanically sweep the transducer beam.

Fig. E-2 presents a set of pulse-echo response profiles for a 3.5-MHz 13-mm diameter focused transducer. Each curve corresponds to a different axial distance from the transducer, the distances being labeled (in centimeters) directly beneath the curve. At each distance the echo signal from the reflector is quite small when the reflector is near the periphery of the beam, reaches a maximum value (usually when the reflector is directly along the beam axis), and then decreases magnitude as the reflector–to–beam axis distance increases. The relative width of each profile can be inferred by using the 1-cm scale marker on the figure. At the 3-cm axial distance we see evidence of near-field effects, with the double peak in the

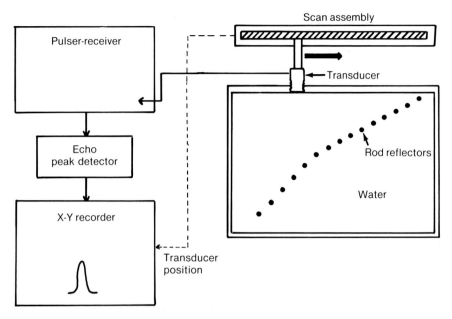

Fig. E-1. Technique used for obtaining pulse-echo response profiles from ultrasonic transducers.

3.5-MHz, 13-mm diameter, focused

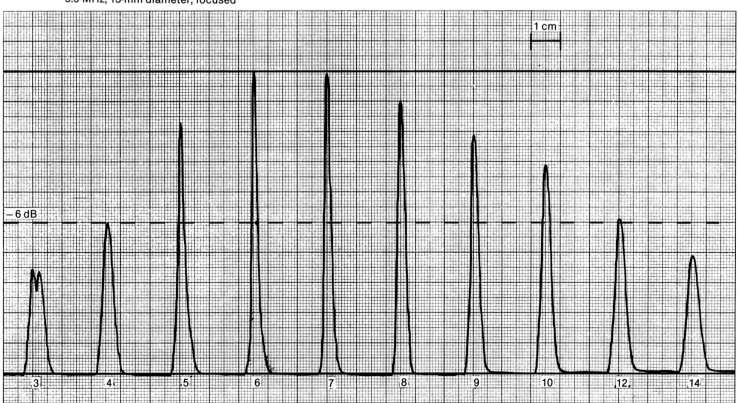

Fig. E-2. Pulse-echo response profiles at different depths for a 3.5-MHz 13-mm diameter transducer. Bottom numbers are centimeters of waterpath. (Courtesy K.B. Aerotech, Lewistown, Pa.)

3.5-MHz, 19-mm diameter, focused

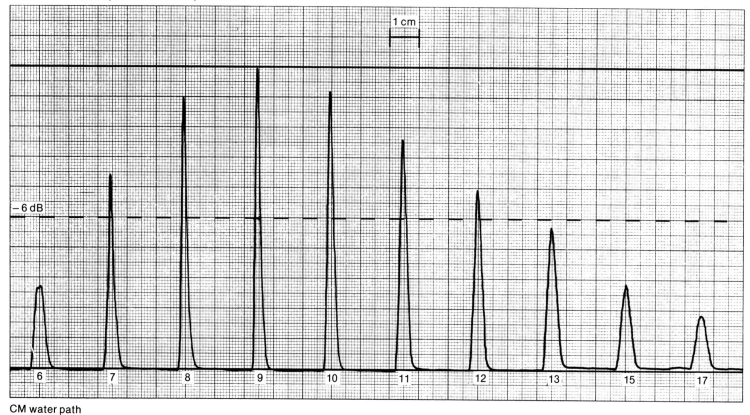

CM water path

Fig. E-3. Pulse-echo response profiles at different depths for a 3.5-MHz 19-mm diameter transducer. Bottom numbers are centimeters of waterpath. (Courtesy K.B. Aerotech, Lewistown, Pa.)

5.0-MHz, 19-mm diameter, focused

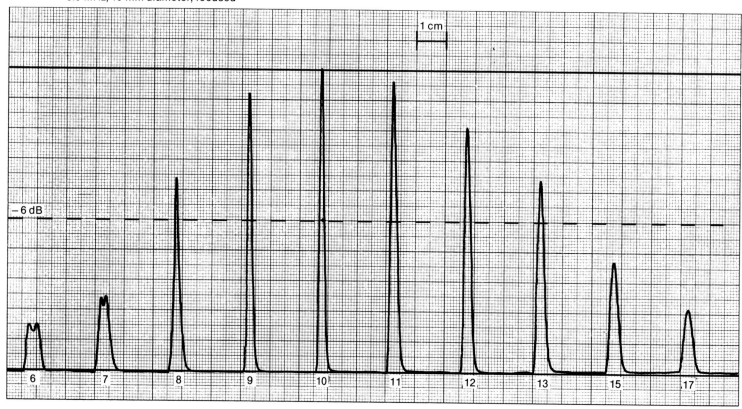

Fig. E-4. Pulse-echo response profiles at different depths for a 5.0-MHz 19-mm diameter transducer. Bottom numbers are centimeters of waterpath. (Courtesy K.B. Aerotech, Lewistown, Pa.)

response profile. Minima and maxima such as these are not evident in any of the response profiles beyond the 3-cm depth. At the *pulse-echo focal distance* the axial response is usually maximal for the entire set of profiles* and the width of the profile (measured at, say, the half-amplitude points) is minimal. The pulse-echo focal distance for this transducer is approximately 6 cm.

If one were doing a study using a 3.5-MHz probe, this 13-mm diameter transducer would be suitable for structures situated down to about an 8-cm depth from the skin surface. For studies in which the region of interest is 8 cm and deeper the larger-diameter, 19-mm, 3.5-MHz transducer would

probably be better suited (Fig. E-3). For a given frequency, larger-diameter transducers generally can be focused in a way that yields narrower beam patterns at greater depths than can smaller-diameter probes. Close comparison of Figs. E-2 and E-3 will bear this out.

Beam profiles for two other transducers are presented in Figs. E-4 and E-5. With the 5.0-MHz 19-mm diameter transducer (Fig. E-4) near field minima and maxima extend as far as the 7-cm deep profile. Notice that beyond 7 cm this probe provides a very narrow beam. It would be superior for imaging deep structures, except for the significantly higher beam attenuation in soft tissues at 5 MHz. The 2.25-MHz 19-mm diameter probe's chief advantage appears to be its ability to penetrate large distances in soft tissue. Pulse-echo response profiles for the latter transducer are given in Fig. E-5.

---

*If significant sound beam attenuation takes place, this would not necessarily be the case. However, at low ultrasound frequencies, attenuation in water has a negligible effect on these profiles. Beam profiles in tissue have somewhat different characteristics from those presented here. (See Bom et al.[1] and Iinuma et al.[3])

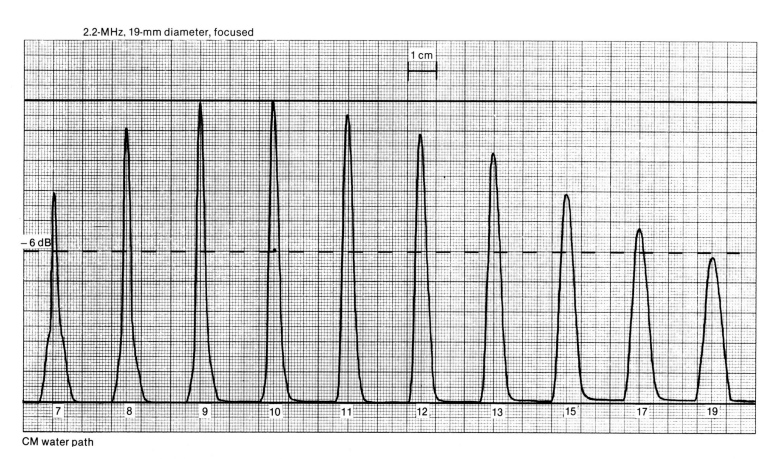

2.2-MHz, 19-mm diameter, focused

1 cm

−6 dB

7   8   9   10   11   12   13   15   17   19

CM water path

Fig. E-5. Pulse-echo response profiles at different depths for a 2.2-MHz 6-mm diameter transducer. Bottom numbers are centimeters of waterpath. (Courtesy K.B. Aerotech, Lewistown, Pa.)

Summary of important units

(Chapter 3)

The metric units commonly used in an ultrasound study are as follows:

Length	meters	m
Mass	kilograms	kg
Time	seconds	sec
Speed	meters/second	m/sec
Period	inverse seconds	sec^{-1}
Area	square meters or meters squared	sq m, m^2
Volume	cubic meters or meters cubed	cu m, m^3
Frequency	cycles per second (hertz)	cps Hz
Density	kilograms per cubic meter	kg/m^3
Impedance	kilograms per square meter per second	$kg/m^2/sec$
Attenuation	decibels	dB
Attenuation coefficient	decibels per centimeter	dB/cm
Power	watts	W
Intensity	watts per square meter	W/m^2
Amplifier gain	decibels	dB

Following are the more commonly used metric system conversions:

Prefix	Meaning	Abbreviation
micro	10^{-6}	μ
milli	10^{-3}	m
centi	10^{-2}	c
deci	10^{-1}	d
kilo	10^{3}	k
Mega	10^{6}	M

Ultrasound scanner performance evaluation

(Chapter 6)

Table G-1 presents acoustic power and intensity data for various classes of diagnostic ultrasound instruments. These data were obtained from Dick (1980), and they represent results taken for a number of instruments in each class. Every entry is provided in the form of a range, which includes the lowest and the highest values obtained among different instruments. On instruments whose power and intensity can be varied, the authors quoted the values obtained when instrument settings were adjusted to produce the maximum value.

Several observations on these data are presented:

1. For each class of equipment a fairly broad range of powers and intensities is apparent. This may be a result of the use of different-frequency transducers and different performance capabilities. Often instruments capable of producing high power and intensity values have output power controls that can substantially reduce the power and intensity from the maximum values quoted.

2. For pulsed instruments the instantaneous peak intensity, I(IP), may exceed the time average intensity, I(TA), by a factor of 1000.

3. On some peripheral vascular Doppler instruments it appears necessary to use high spatial peak–time average intensities, I(SPTA), exceeding, for example, 100 mW/sq cm. This stresses the importance of the instrument operator's being aware of the intensities produced by the equipment used so that such instruments are not used for purposes other than those for which they were designed. It also stresses the importance of sonographer's following the suggested steps in utilizing the minimal acoustic exposure necessary to acquire the desired diagnostic information.

Table G-1. Ranges of exposure levels from diagnostic ultrasound systems

Class of equipment	Acoustic power (mW)	I(SATA) at transducer (mW/sq cm)	I(SPTA) (mW/sq cm)	I(SPIP) (W/sq cm)
Manual compound scanner	0.5-20	0.4-10	10-170	2-1700
M-mode	0.5-20	0.4-10	10-100	2-600
Ophthalmic A-mode and B-mode	0.6-1	0.3-5	20-34	Not available
Pulsed Doppler (peripheral vascular)	6-10	87-175	350-700	Not available
CW Doppler (obstetric, portable)	1-18	0.2-7	0.6-20	Not applicable

From Dick, D: In Fullerton, G., and Zagzebski, J., editors: Medical physics of CT and ultrasound, New York, 1980, AAPM.

UNIVERSITY OF WISCONSIN
SCANNER PERFORMANCE EVALUATION WORKSHEET

Scanner identification _____ Transducer _____ Date _____

_____ _____ MHz, _____ mm, no. _____ Sonographer _____

Phantom or test object _____

1. Depth calibration (20 cm f₀V)
   Distance between end targets of Column A   Vertical markers _____ cm
                                                     Horizontal markers _____ cm

2. Digital calipers (20 cm f₀V)
   Distance between end targets of Column A   _____ cm
   Distance between end targets of Row B   _____ cm

3. B-scan position registration accuracy (20 cm f₀V)
   Maximum separation between centers of displayed echo   _____ cm
   images of single target

4. Sensitivity check
   Maximum depth of visualization of parenchymal echoes   _____ cm
   from phantom

5. −20 dB axial resolution
   Depth of target group _____
   Minimum target separation resolved   _____ mm

6. Photography check (leave image on scan converter)
   Detection of weakly scattered texture   _____ OK _____ Poor
   Contrast between high-level echo signals   _____ OK _____ Poor

Obstetric parameters

(Chapter 22)

Table H-1. Tolerance limits for fetal volume as a quadratic function of weeks of gestation*

Weeks (fetal/menstrual)	Tolerance (ml)						
	2.5%	5.0%	10%	50%	90%	95%	97.5%
18/20	517	647	797	812	827	977	1107
19/21	502	635	789	912	1036	1190	1322
20/22	507	644	801	1020	1238	1395	1533
21/23	536	675	836	1134	1432	1593	1732
22/24	589	731	895	1256	1616	1780	1922
23/25	667	813	981	1384	1788	1956	2101
24/26	771	920	1091	1520	1949	2120	2269
25/27	895	1046	1221	1663	2105	2280	2431
26/28	1033	1187	1364	1813	2262	2439	2593
27/29	1179	1335	1516	1970	2425	2605	2762
28/30	1329	1488	1672	2134	2597	2781	2940
29/31	1483	1645	1832	2306	2780	2967	3129
30/32	1642	1806	1996	2485	2973	3163	3327
31/33	1806	1973	2165	2670	3175	3367	3535
32/34	1980	2149	2345	2863	3381	3577	3746
33/35	2171	2343	2541	3062	3585	3783	3955
34/36	2384	2558	2759	3270	3781	3982	4156
35/37	2623	2800	3004	3484	3965	4169	4346
36/38	2887	3067	3273	3705	4138	4345	4524
37/39	3175	3357	3566	3934	4302	4511	4693
38/40	3484	3668	3880	4170	4459	4671	4855
39/41	3812	4000	4215	4412	4610	4825	5011

From Levine, S.C., et al.: J. Clin. Ultrasound **7:**21, 1979.
*Intrauterine volume measurements are expressed as percentile categories for fetal and menstrual ages.

Table H-2. Fetal age percentile values for biparietal diameter*

BPD	5	10	25	50	75	80	95	BPD	5	10	25	50	75	80	95	BPD	5	10	25	50	75	80	95
3.5	17+	17	16+	16	16−	16−	15+	5.5	24	24−	23	22+	22−	21+	21−	7.5	32	32−	30−	29−	28+	28−	26+
3.6	18	17+	17	16+	16	16	15+	5.6	24	24−	23+	23−	22	22−	21	7.6	33−	32	30	29	28+	28	27−
3.7	19	18	18	17−	16	16	16	5.7	24+	24	24−	23	22+	22+	21+	7.7	33	32	30+	30−	29−	38+	27
3.8	19	18+	18+	17	16+	16+	16	5.8	25−	24+	24	23+	23−	23−	21+	7.8	33	32+	31−	30	29−	29−	27+
3.9	19+	19	18+	17+	17−	17−	16	5.9	25	25−	24+	24−	23	23−	22−	7.9	33+	33	31+	30+	29	29	28−
4.0	19+	19	19−	18−	17	17−	16	6.0	25+	25	25−	24	23	23	22−	8.0	34	33+	32	31−	29+	29+	28
4.1	19+	19	19−	18	17+	17+	16	6.1	26−	25+	25	24+	23+	23+	22	8.1	34+	34	32+	31	30−	30−	28+
4.2	20−	19+	19	18+	17+	17+	16+	6.2	26	26−	25+	25−	24	23+	22+	8.2	35	35−	33−	31+	30	30	29−
4.3	20	20−	19+	19−	18−	18−	17−	6.3	26+	26	26−	25	24	24	23−	8.3	36−	35	33	32	31	30+	29
4.4	20+	20	20−	19	18+	18	17	6.4	27−	26+	26	25+	24+	24+	23+	8.4	36	37−	33+	32+	31	31−	29
4.5	21−	20+	20	19+	19−	18	17+	6.5	27+	27	26+	26−	25	25	24−	8.5	36+	36−	34−	33	31+	31	29+
4.6	21	21−	20+	20−	19	18+	18−	6.6	28−	27+	27−	26	25+	25+	24−	8.6	36+	36−	34	33+	31+	31	29+
4.7	21+	21	21−	20	19+	19	18	6.7	28	28−	27	26+	26−	26−	24	8.7	37−	36	35−	34	32−	31+	30−
4.8	21+	21	21	20+	20−	19+	18+	6.8	28+	28	27+	27−	26	26−	24+	8.8	37	36+	35+	34+	32	32−	30
4.9	22−	21+	21+	21−	20	19+	19−	6.9	29	28+	28−	27	26+	26+	25−	8.9	38−	37	36	35+	33	32+	31
5.0	22	22	22−	21	20+	20−	19	7.0	29+	29−	28	27+	27−	26+	25−	9.0	38+	37+	37−	36−	33+	33	32−
5.1	22+	22	22−	21+	20+	20	19+	7.1	30	30−	28+	28−	27	27−	25+	9.1	39−	38−	37	36+	34	34	32−
5.2	23−	22+	22	22−	21−	20+	20−	7.2	31−	30−	29−	28−	27+	27	25+	9.2	39	39−	37+	36+	35	35	33
5.3	23	23−	22+	22−	21	21−	20	7.3	31	30	29	28	28−	27+	26−	9.3	39+	39−	38−	37−	35	35	34−
5.4	24−	23+	23−	22	21+	21+	20+	7.4	32−	31	29+	28+	28−	27+	26	9.4	40−	39	38	37	36−	35	34+
																9.5	40	39+	38+	37+	36	35	35−

From Sabbagha, R. E., et al.: Am. J. Obstet. Gynecol. **126:**485, 1976.

+ = 1 to 3 days.

− = 1 to 3 days.

Table H-3. Sonar crown-rump measurements*

Fetal maturity (wk + da)	Corrected regression analysis (mm) (mean values)	Fetal maturity (wk + da)	Corrected regression analysis (mm) (mean values)
4 + 2	5.5	8 + 2	33.2
4 + 3	6.1	8 + 3	34.6
4 + 4	6.8	8 + 4	36.0
4 + 5	7.5	8 + 5	37.4
4 + 6	8.1	8 + 6	38.9
5 + 0	8.9	9 + 0	40.4
5 + 1	9.6	9 + 1	41.9
5 + 2	10.4	9 + 2	43.5
5 + 3	11.2	9 + 3	45.1
5 + 4	12.0	9 + 4	46.7
5 + 5	12.9	9 + 5	48.3
5 + 6	13.8	9 + 6	50.0
6 + 0	14.7	10 + 0	51.7
6 + 1	15.7	10 + 1	53.4
6 + 2	16.6	10 + 2	55.2
6 + 3	17.6	10 + 3	57.0
6 + 4	18.7	10 + 4	58.8
6 + 5	19.7	10 + 5	60.6
6 + 6	20.8	10 + 6	62.5
7 + 0	21.9	11 + 0	64.3
7 + 1	23.1	11 + 1	66.3
7 + 2	24.2	11 + 2	68.2
7 + 3	25.4	11 + 3	70.2
7 + 4	26.7	11 + 4	72.2
7 + 5	27.9	11 + 5	74.2
7 + 6	29.2	11 + 6	76.3
8 + 0	30.5	12 + 0	78.3

From Robinson, H.P., and Fleming, J.E.E.: Br. J. Obstet. Gynaecol. **82:**702, 1975.

*Expressed as ±2 SD limits and 4.7 days for one measurement or ±2.7 days for the average of three independent CRL values.

Table H-4. Biparietal diameter at level of third ventricle versus menstrual age

BPD (mm)	Menstrual age (wk since LNMP)
28	14
31	15
34	16
37	17
40	18
44	19
47	20
50	21
53	22
56	23
59	24
62	25
65	26
67	27
69	28
73	29
75	30
78	31
80	32
82	33
84	34
86	35
88	36
90	37
92	38
94	39
95	40

From Shepherd, M., and Filly, R.A.: J. Ultrasound Med. (In Press.)

Table H-5. Mean and lower confidence limits of femoral lengths in fetuses

BPD	Mean	Lower	BPD	Mean	Lower
27	15	12	51	39	33
28	16	13	51	39	33
29	17	14	51	39	33
30	18	15	52	40	34
31	19	16	53	41	35
32	20	17	54	42	36
33	21	18	55	43	37
34	22	19	56	44	38
35	23	19	56	44	38
36	24	20	57	45	38
37	25	21	58	46	39
38	26	22	59	47	40
39	27	23	60	48	41
40	28	24	61	49	42
40	28	24	62	50	43
41	29	25	63	51	44
42	30	26	63	51	44
43	31	26	63	51	44
43	31	26	64	52	45
44	32	27	65	53	45
45	33	28	66	54	46
45	33	28	67	55	47
46	34	29	67	55	47
47	35	30	68	56	48
48	36	31	69	57	49
48	36	31	70	58	50
48	36	31	71	59	51
49	37	32	72	60	51
49	37	32	73	61	52
50	38	32	74	62	53
50	38	32	75	63	54
50	38	32	76	64	55
			77	65	56

From Filly, R.A., et al.: Radiology **138:**653, 1981.

Examples of Doppler cases, waveforms, spectral analysis, and carotid sonograms

(Chapter 23)

ARTERIAL DOPPLER STUDIES

Case 1. Normal right leg, mild iliac and severe superficial femoral occlusion in left leg (Fig. I-1)

History. This 63-year-old woman, long troubled by circulation problems, had undergone a left femoral-popliteal embolectomy in 1974. The symptoms of claudication were in the left leg only, and they progressed until 1981. At the time of examination she was having constant calf cramping and rest pain, with no relief obtained during rest or activity. She also had heel pain with reddening and scaling of the toes. She was not having any difficulties in the right leg.

Examination. The right ankle/brachial ratio is 1.07; the left 0.28, in the danger zone.

On the right are shown normal femoral, popliteal, posterior tibial, and dorsal pedal tracings. Both brachial artery tracings are also normal (pressures 140/80). There are normal pressure gradient intervals in the posterior tibial artery, which was used since the ankle pressure there was higher than in the dorsalis pedis. (The difference of more than 40 mm Hg between the low thigh segment and the calf segment is due to the cuff's having slipped over the patella.)

On the left the femoral signal is losing components, which signifies mild disease in the femoral-iliac area. A tracing made midway along the thigh at the superficial femoral shows blunting of the first and loss of the second component, with a corresponding loss of dynamics. The popliteal signal is even more diminished, implying severe obstruction. Posterior tibial artery flow on this side was absent. Finally, a weak dorsalis pedis waveform is seen. The pressures are correspondingly low, with the high thigh pressure suggesting occlusion of the iliac and a drop between the low thigh and calf segments confirming the superficial femoral disease.

The patient was admitted, and a femoral-popliteal graft was implanted on the left. Flow improved, and she was able to resume some normal activity.

Right femoral artery

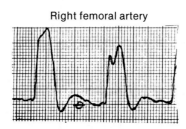

Right popliteal artery

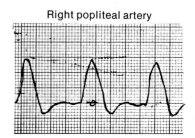

Right brachial artery
140/80

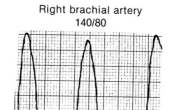

Right ankle/brachial index

$$\frac{150}{140} = 1.07$$

Right posterior tibial artery

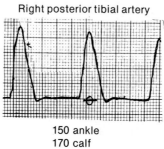

Right dorsal pedal artery

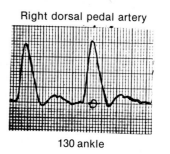

150 ankle
170 calf
220 low thigh
220 high thigh

130 ankle

Left superficial femoral artery
(midthigh)

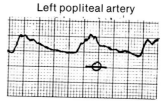

Left brachial artery
140/80

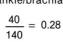

Left ankle/brachial index

$$\frac{40}{140} = 0.28$$

Left femoral artery

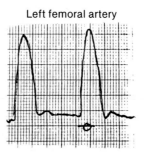

No
posterior
tibial
signal

Left popliteal artery

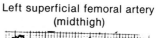
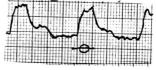

Left dorsal pedal artery

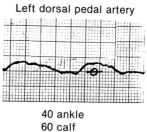

40 ankle
60 calf
100 low thigh
140 high thigh

Fig. I-1

Case 2. Normal lower extremities, left pudendal artery occlusion (Fig. I-2)

History. This 39-year-old man complained of lop-sided erections, with the left side of the penis remaining flaccid but normal erectile qualities on the right. No equality had been obtained at any time for 1 year. He had no claudication symptoms.

Examination. The ankle/brachial index was 1.08 bilaterally; the penile-brachial indices 1.28 on the right and 0.61 on the left.

Normal brachial artery signals were obtained, with a pressure of 130/80 on the right and 120/80 on the left. Normal femoral, popliteal, and posterior tibial signals were also obtained. There may or may not have been anterior tibial disease, for the dorsalis pedis signals were not well heard. In light of the other tracings, the dorsal pedal signals were not considered abnormal. Normal pressure gradients were obtained bilaterally.

The penile study showed normal antegrade flow in the right cavernosal artery, with a pressure of 180. The left cavernosal, however, showed some diminishing of the second component and a pressure of only 80. This implied a left internal iliac or pudendal artery stenosis.

It is not known whether any surgical correction was performed.

Right brachial artery 130/80
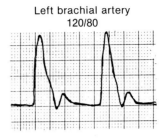

Left brachial artery 120/80
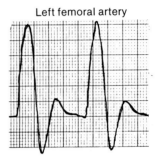

Right femoral artery
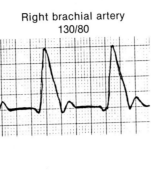

Left femoral artery
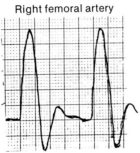

Right popliteal artery
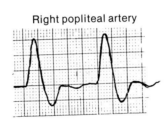

Left popliteal artery
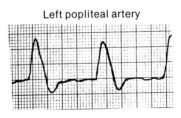

140 ankle
130 calf
180 low thigh
170 high thigh

Right dorsal pedal artery
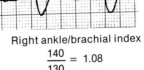

Left dorsal pedal artery
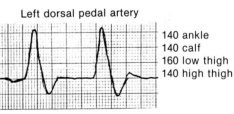

140 ankle
140 calf
160 low thigh
140 high thigh

Right ankle/brachial index
$$\frac{140}{130} = 1.08$$

Both posterior tibials inaudible

Left ankle/brachial index
$$\frac{140}{130} = 1.08$$

Right cavernosal artery 180
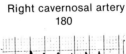

Left cavernosal artery 80
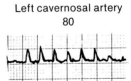

Right penile/brachial index
$$\frac{180}{130} = 1.28$$

Left penile/brachial index
$$\frac{80}{130} = 0.61$$

Fig. I-2

Case 3. Normal left arm, abnormal right arm with extensive arteriovenous fistulas (Fig. I-3)

History. This 40-year-old woman had a history of congenital A-V fistulas of the right subclavian, brachial, and radial artery-vein systems. She had also had congestive heart failure in 1973 because of the flow problems. A macrofistular area was repaired at the elbow level in 1978.

At the time of this examination she had had intermittent pain and swelling in the right hand for 2 weeks. The right arm itself was swollen, with dilated and tortuous superficial varices, and large purplish green blotches on the right chest, shoulder, and arm. The hand at the base of the thumb was greatly swollen, and the patient could move the fingers only weakly. Amputation had been declined.

Examination. The right forearm/brachial index was 1.00, the left 0.92.

On the left side characteristic normal tracings can be seen at the brachial, subclavian, vertebral, axillary, radial, and ulnar arteries. The compression responses show normal flow through the left palmar arch.

On the right side the brachial shows a prominent signal indicative of obstruction and turbulence. The subclavian signal also shows proximal venous connections reducing the flow. The vertebral shows a subclavian steal present, regardless of the normal blood pressure in the arm. The axillary artery also has a turbulent signal, showing flow problems. The radial arterial signal was turbulent and difficult to interpret, for reversed flow in the accompanying vein possibly prevented normal flow to the hand. Compression of the ulnar artery resulted in retrograde flow in the artery, implying a prominent A-V connection. The ulnar signal also indicated flow discrepancies, with high-pitched turbulence present. Compression of the radial artery occluded the A-V fistula and resulted in resumption of normal flow through the ulnar artery segment.

At surgery the radial artery was ligated and the A-V fistula and palmar arch injected and blocked with Ivalon sponge solution. The patient's symptoms subsided, and she was released.

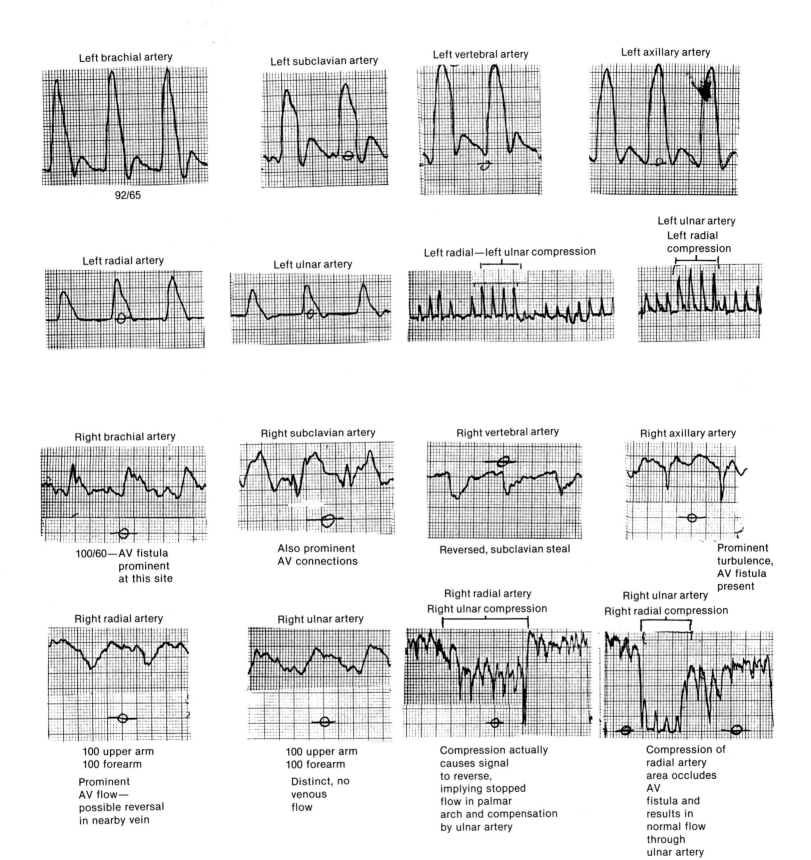

Left brachial artery
92/65

Left subclavian artery

Left vertebral artery

Left axillary artery

Left radial artery

Left ulnar artery

Left radial—left ulnar compression

Left ulnar artery
Left radial compression

Right brachial artery
100/60—AV fistula prominent at this site

Right subclavian artery
Also prominent AV connections

Right vertebral artery
Reversed, subclavian steal

Right axillary artery
Prominent turbulence, AV fistula present

Right radial artery
100 upper arm
100 forearm

Prominent AV flow— possible reversal in nearby vein

Right ulnar artery
100 upper arm
100 forearm

Distinct, no venous flow

Right radial artery
Right ulnar compression
Compression actually causes signal to reverse, implying stopped flow in palmar arch and compensation by ulnar artery

Right ulnar artery
Right radial compression
Compression of radial artery area occludes AV fistula and results in normal flow through ulnar artery

Fig. I-3

VENOUS DOPPLER STUDIES

Case 4. Normal responses and flow in right leg, abnormal responses in left leg (Fig. I-4)

History. This 23-year-old woman was admitted to the hospital with left leg pain and swelling of 2 weeks' duration. She had recently had hepatitis. There was marked tenderness of the calf and thigh but no red streaking. Thrombophlebitis was suspected.

Examination

The right leg showed normal responses and qualities at the posterior tibial, popliteal, and femoral veins.

The left leg had phasic flow at the posterior tibial, with normal responses. At the popliteal, superficial femoral, and femoral sites, however, there was definite continuous flow with only a vague hint of phasicity. Valsalva maneuvers did not stop the flow as they did in the right leg. Iliofemoral thrombophlebitis and valvular incompetence were implied by these findings and confirmed by a subsequent venogram.

The patient was given anticoagulant therapy, which resolved the problem and dissolved the thrombus. Illustrated in Fig. I-4 are typical normal and abnormal responses in the lower limb.

Normal femoral vein signal

Inspiration   Distal compression—thigh   Distal compression—calf   Proximal compression   Release

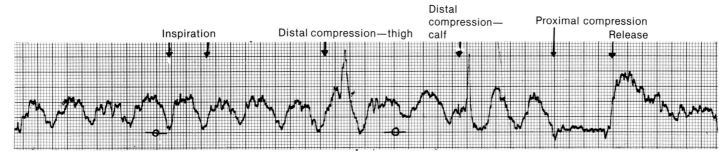

Normal popliteal vein signal

Valsalva (cardiac cycle comes through)
Release

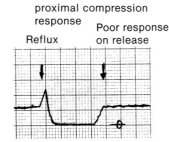

Inspiration   Inspiration   Valsalva Release   Distal compression

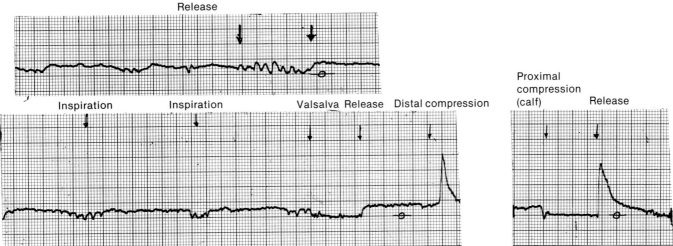

Proximal
compression
(calf)   Release

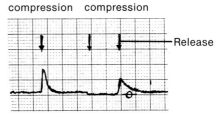

Normal posterior tibial vein signal ————————— Posterior tibial vein

Continuous signal

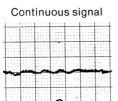

Abnormal
proximal compression
response
Reflux   Poor response
on release

Diminished augmentation

Distal   Proximal
compression   compression

Release

Normal responses in nonspontaneous
posterior tibial vein

Distal   Proximal
compression compression
Release

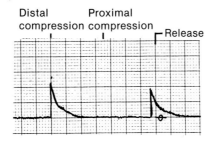

Fig. I-4

Case 5. Bilateral venous insufficiency (elephantiasis)

History. This 28-year-old woman had bilaterally swollen legs, with the left much larger than the right. She was physically rather petite, which made the leg enlargement more striking.

She had had many problems related to lymph nodes and had undergone a hysterectomy at age 16. Her left leg began to swell at age 18; her right leg at age 20. She found walking difficult and had constant pain from the tightness of the legs. The physician's main concern was to rule out venous problems versus lymphedema-elephantiasis.

Examination. Abnormal continuous flow was found at all sites in both legs. Augmentation responses were also abnormal at all sites above the posterior tibial veins.

The right leg had weak posterior tibial flow, with increased flow from the popliteal site up. The left leg had weak flow from the posterior tibial to the superficial femoral, with an increased signal heard midway in the superficial femoral. Flow seemed to slow in the femoral vein area. The valves were incompetent bilaterally. Bilateral iliac vein insufficiency was suggested.

A venogram was made and showed relatively normal flow through the right iliac vein. The left common iliac vein was severely compromised by a mass compressing the area, which caused turbulent flow in the inferior vena cava and massive backing up of flow in the legs. The ureters were also dilated because of the mass, which was of lymphatic origin.

The mass was nonoperable, but the inferior vena cava was ligated. This brought some relief of the symptoms; however, the lymphatic elephantiasis remained.

Case 6. Normal upper extremity venous flow — postoperative examination (Fig. I-5)

History. This 68-year-old woman was admitted for a mass felt in the right supraclavicular fossa, which was suspected to be a thrombosed subclavian artery aneurysm. The patient went to surgery, but the mass was found to be a subclavian *vein* aneurysm involving the external jugular and three adjacent veins. It was thrombosed, but fortunately was off one wall of the subclavian vein and did not involve the entire circumference of the vein. It was resected, and the four involved branches were ligated. Determination of flow was performed postoperatively.

Examination. Normal waveforms with normal phasicity, pulsatility, and augmentation maneuvers are shown. The internal jugular was checked to ensure that proximal flow was normal. There was a normal response to the Valsalva maneuver.

Right
brachial vein
Forearm compression

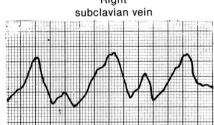

Right axillary vein
Forearm/Upper arm compression
Valsalva Release

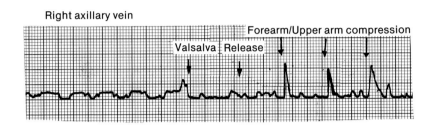

Right
subclavian vein

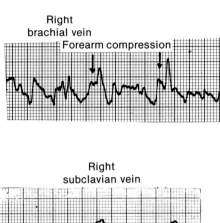

Right basilic vein (arrows indicate
percussions)

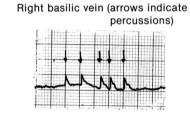

Right
internal
jugular
vein
Valsalva
Release

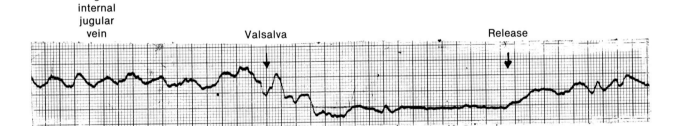

Left brachial vein
Valsalva Release
(artery)

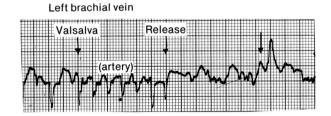

Left axillary vein
Forearm compression

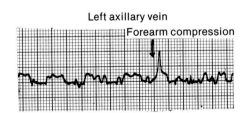

Fig. I-5

CEREBROVASCULAR STUDIES

Case 7. Normal carotid examination with subclavian steal syndrome (Fig. 1-6)

History. This 56-year-old man was admitted for evaluation of intermittent dizziness, left arm numbness and fatigue, and amaurosis fugax episodes in the right eye. He described the amaurosis spells as "having a shade come down over my vision." They lasted from 2 to 6 minutes each.

Examination

On the right side, normal signals were obtained in the brachial artery; and a blood pressure of 160/80 was present. Normal signals were found in the common carotid, bifurcation, vertebral, facial, and temporal arteries. The bifurcation signal was roughened in sound, which implied that an occlusion may have been present. The ophthalmic test showed normal frontal and supraorbital flow, with normal responses to bilateral compressions, except for those in the right infraorbital artery. Here the frontal signal was reversed with compression, despite normal responses at the other compression sites. This could be explained only by the presence of intracranial collaterals.

The left side had an abnormal left brachial artery signal, implying occlusion or stenosis higher up in the system. A blood pressure of 130/70 was obtained, and with the reduced waveform implied the existence of a subclavian steal. Subsequent examination of the left vertebral artery showed strong retrograde flow, verifying the steal. Normal signals were obtained from all other sites. The ophthalmic test showed normal frontal and supraorbital flow with normal compression responses.

A carotid sonographic examination showed 50% stenosis of the right internal carotid artery and 20% stenosis of the left. An arteriogram was subsequently performed, and it confirmed the lesions in the carotid arteries and verified the subclavian artery occlusion and the vertebral steal.

A carotid-subclavian bypass was surgically installed, and the patient was released.

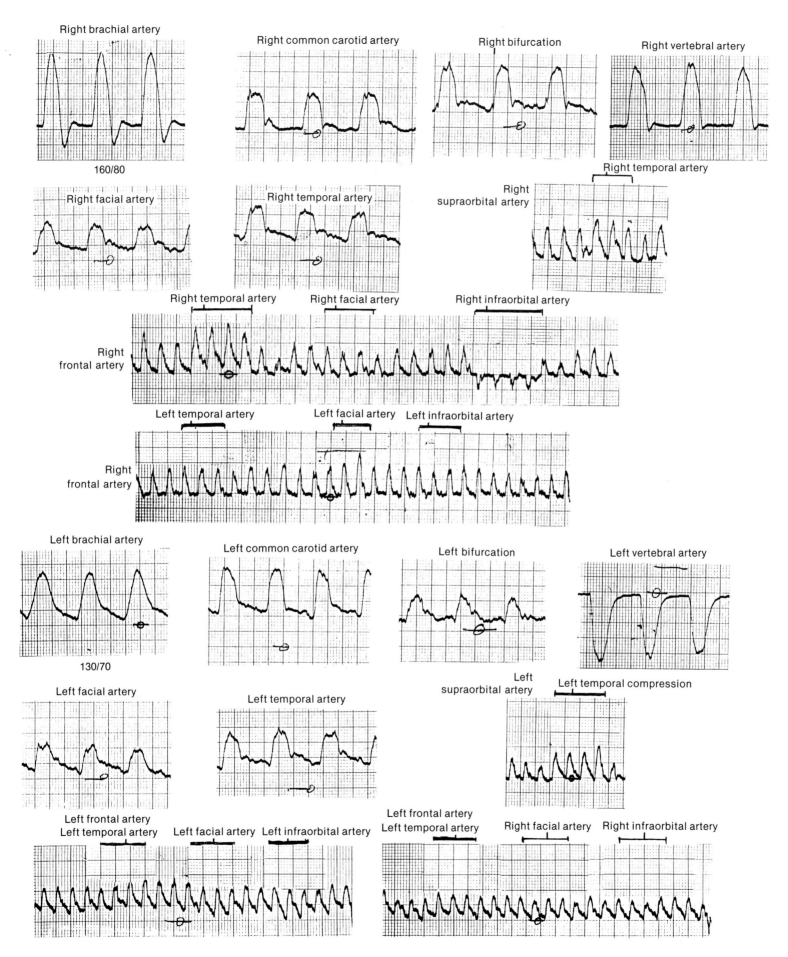

Fig. I-6

Case 8. Total right carotid occlusion, partial left carotid stenosis, and left subclavian steal (Fig. I-7)

History. This 56-year-old woman was admitted for a possible coronary artery bypass operation. She had a long history of vascular disease and mitral insufficiency. She also complained of occasional dizziness and had numbness of three fingers of the right hand since an earlier cardiac catheterization. She had bilateral bruits in the carotids, and surgery was to be performed or cancelled depending on the results of the Doppler examination and carotid sonography.

Examination

On the right side a normal brachial signal with a pressure of 190/100 was obtained. The common carotid artery at the clavicle had abnormally low, practically nonexistent, flow; and the signal at the bifurcation was barely more than a thump. The right vertebral had normal but reduced antegrade flow. The facial artery signal was also reduced. The right temporal artery was actually *reversed*, implying severe collateral compensation. The ophthalmic test showed retrograde flow in the frontal artery, which was not affected by right-sided compressions. Compression of the left temporal, however, caused resumption of antegrade flow in the right frontal, suggesting contralateral collateralization from the left temporal. The other compressions had no effect. In regard to the apparent occlusion of the right common, it was thought that the frontal flow's becoming antegrade was caused by circle of Willis collateral supplies.

The left side was next examined. The left brachial artery signal was reduced and significant of subclavian stenosis and vertebral steal. A reduced antegrade vertebral signal was seen; however, postocclusive hyperemia caused a flow reversal within 10 seconds, verifying the steal. A much more normal-looking common carotid signal was noted; but throughout the carotid there was roughening of the sound quality, implying flow problems. Bifurcation, facial, and temporal signals were of normal pattern, with some increase in flow in the temporal artery. The ophthalmic test showed an antegrade but decreased frontal signal, which increased markedly with left facial compression. All other compressions were normal. Neither right nor left supraorbital arteries were audible.

Carotid sonography showed a thrombus occluding the right common, internal, and external carotids from the middle of the common carotid up, with a partly congealed clot floating free and moving up and down with each cardiac cycle in the low common carotid. The left side had scattered areas of plaque partly occluding the bulb and internal carotid. (See Case 13 for selected examples of this case.)

An arteriogram was obtained, and confirmed the level and extent of the occlusion in the right carotid. The right vertebral flow reduction was caused by a stenosis at the takeoff of the vessel. A severe stenosis of the left internal carotid was also shown, as was a confirmation of the left subclavian obstruction and subclavian steal.

The patient was observed for 3 months until the loose "bouncing" clot had congealed. At that time the patient was readmitted and had another arteriogram which showed some collateralization that filled the external carotid. The patient was taken to surgery, and a combination right carotid endarterectomy and mitral commisurotomy and repair were performed. The patient recovered and was released.

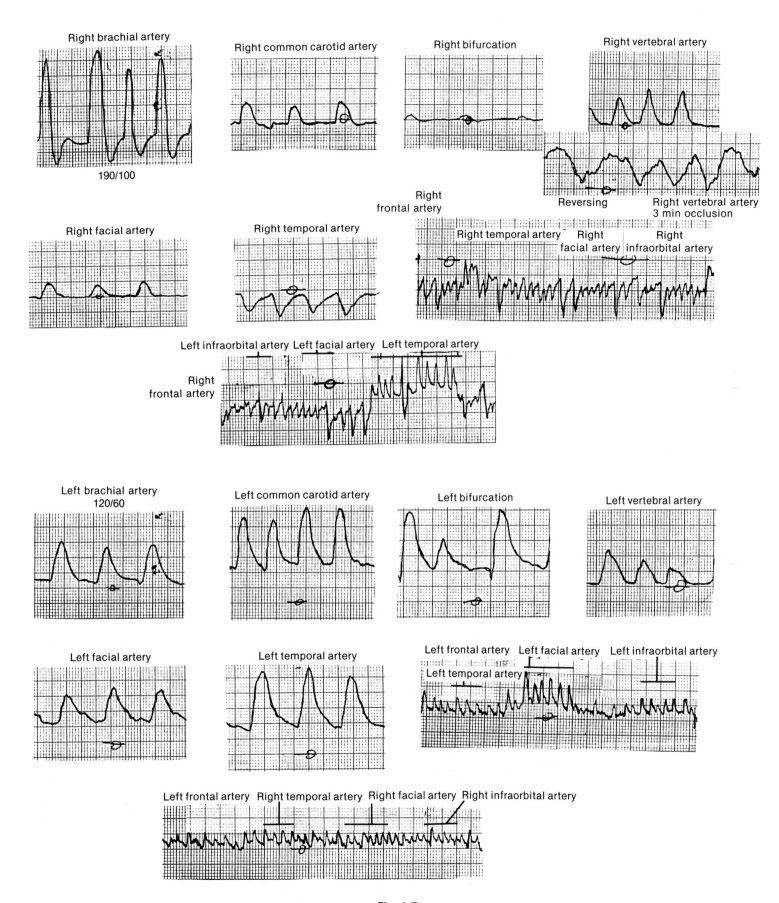

Right brachial artery
190/100

Right common carotid artery

Right bifurcation

Right vertebral artery

Reversing   Right vertebral artery
3 min occlusion

Right facial artery

Right temporal artery

Right frontal artery

Right temporal artery   Right facial artery   Right infraorbital artery

Left infraorbital artery   Left facial artery   Left temporal artery

Right frontal artery

Left brachial artery
120/60

Left common carotid artery

Left bifurcation

Left vertebral artery

Left facial artery

Left temporal artery

Left frontal artery   Left facial artery   Left infraorbital artery

Left temporal artery

Left frontal artery   Right temporal artery   Right facial artery   Right infraorbital artery

Fig. I-7

SPECTRALLY ANALYZED DOPPLER WAVEFORMS

Case 9. Normal brachial and carotid arteries and branches (Fig. I-8, *A*). Note the high concentration of blood flow near the upper frequencies. The systolic window is present but is not well seen because of some fill-in by random frequencies. Note also the strong clearly defined envelope. The short spike seen between the systolic and diastolic components corresponds to the second, normally reversed, component in a normal triphasic Doppler waveform. Due to the nondirectional nature of the analyzer used for these examples, the waveform appears on the positive side of the baseline. The lines at regular intervals indicate 1-kHz frequency levels, for the scale is set to the 5-kHz range. The value of the scale lines changes with the setting of the frequency scales.

The following four signals represent normal tracings from a 24-year-old man:

B, Normal common carotid signal. Note the window, the prominent systolic frequencies, the distinct envelope, and the high flow velocity typical of the carotid system. The dicrotic notch between the systolic and diastolic components is readily evident. The scale is set to 10 kHz on this and the next three images to facilitate comparison.

C, Another normal common carotid signal, illustrating the use of the frequency-measuring cursor. The cursor line can be moved to the peak frequency point and the frequency value read out as 6 kHz.

D, Normal internal carotid signal. The characteristic envelope shape and flow pattern are seen, as is the relatively clear window sign.

E, Normal external carotid signal. The flow, decelerating rapidly, drops nearly to the baseline. The window sign is clearly evident.

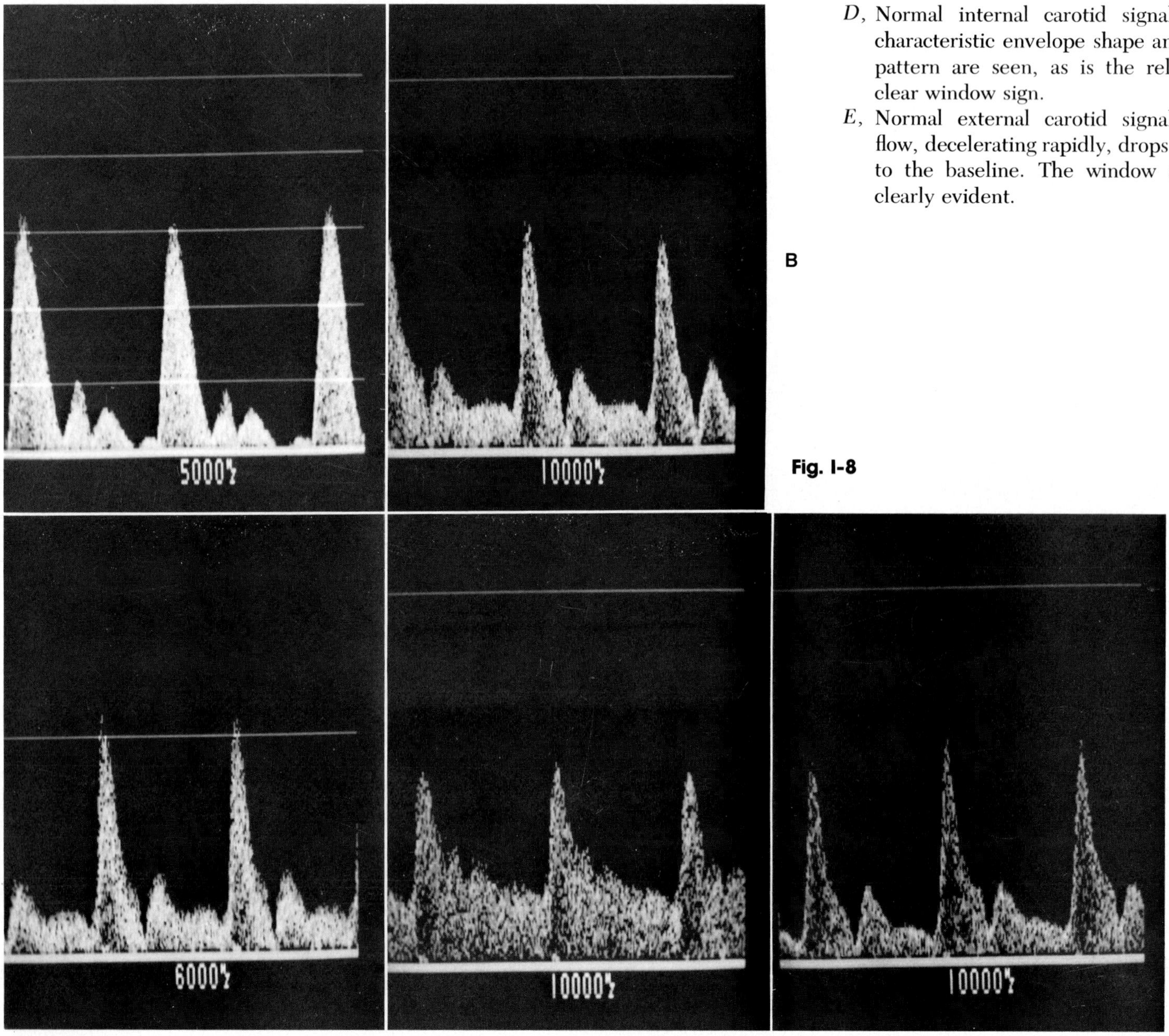

Fig. I-8

Case 10. Abnormal carotid waveforms and correlative sonograms (Fig. I-9). These waveforms and images are from a 70-year-old woman who complained of a sudden onset of right leg discomfort and near paralysis of the extremity from the hip down. She also complained of pain and cramping in the limb, with some numbness of the leg below the knee. Her left leg gave her no difficulties. Distal extremity pulses were nonpalpable. She had prominent carotid bruits, the left louder than the right, but denied dizziness, syncope, and other cerebral symptoms. She was referred for a Doppler examination of the lower extremities and the carotid system. Flow in the right leg was within normal limits but in the left leg was diminished, suggesting a CVA or TIA as the source of the right leg paralysis and discomfort.

The following examples are real time sonographic images of this woman's left carotid showing the stenoses within. (For an explanation of typical carotid image characteristics and interpretations, see Case 11.) They are included here so the reader can more easily locate the areas where the spectral signals were obtained and directly compare the degree of luminal reduction with the resulting flow patterns. In all the following images the head of the patient is oriented toward the bottom of the longitudinal sections and the medial side of the body toward the bottom of the transverse sections:

A, Midportion of the common carotid artery. Note the gray soft tissue plaque areas on the superficial and deep walls of the artery.

B, Transverse section across the center of the area in A showing the vessel with the plaque and the stenosed lumen.

C and D, Carotid bulb, bifurcation, and internal and external carotid arteries. A large, circumferential, complex plaque is obstructing both the internal and the external carotids about 80%. Shadowing is seen from the calcified portion of the lesion. C shows part of the circumferential plaque on the lateral wall of the bulb more clearly.

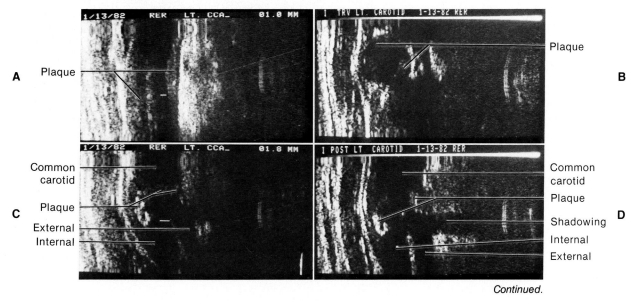

Continued.

Fig. I-9

E, Transverse image of the bulb area just below the bifurcation. Note the irregular circumferential plaque lining the artery, of which only a small section could be visualized in the longitudinal views.

F, Transverse view showing the internal carotid artery at its origin. Note the obstructive plaque on the superficial wall (also shown in C and D) and the reduced size of the remaining lumen.

Fig. I-9, G to M, is a series of spectrally analyzed Doppler flow signals of this artery recorded at various levels to show the changes that occurred along the course of the vessel. The scale factors (5, 10, and 20 kHz) are shown at the bottom of each photograph.

G, Tracing taken midway in the common carotid, at approximately the center of the stenotic area. Note that the envelope has begun to take on a ragged appearance and that the window is nearly filled in. The frequencies are fairly evenly distributed, which signifies a moderate stenosis.

H, Signal obtained from the bulb area across the stenotic region. Note the blunting of the waveform and the short clear area signifying some turbulence. The window is absent, and the envelope is still ragged. A strained, burbling sound was heard at this site.

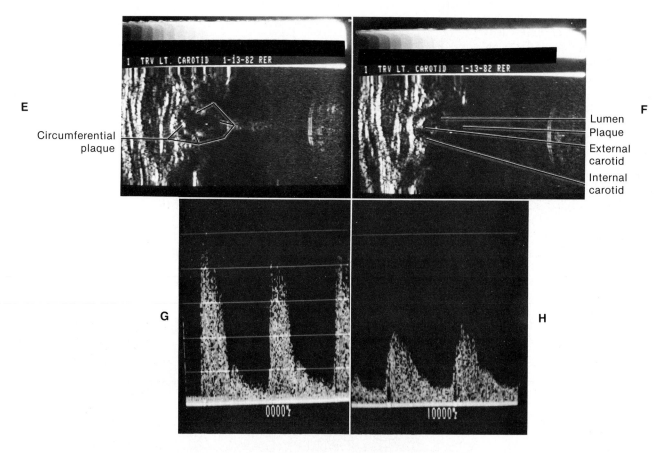

E

Circumferential plaque

F

Lumen
Plaque
External carotid
Internal carotid

G

H

Fig. I-9, cont'd.

I, Signal obtained immediately distal to the stenosis at the base of the internal carotid and typical of the jet effect. Note the concentration of frequencies at the baseline, indicative of turbulence, along with the extremely high peak, which could barely be shown at the 20-kHz scale setting. A harsh, strained, hissing sound was heard here.

J, Signal obtained more distally from the stenosis, away from the jet area. Flow is markedly reduced (see the 5-kHz scale), with a disrupted envelope and turbulence still present.

K, Signal taken along the clear well-preserved distal internal carotid. The disrupted envelope and lower-frequency intensities are still evident. The window reappears, but the flow is still uneven. A low-pitched, almost normal, but roughened sound was heard here.

L, Signal of the external carotid immediately distal to the stenotic plaque at its origin. Though the artery is not obstructed enough to give a jet effect, turbulence is still present (as evidenced by the baseline concentration). The roughened envelope and reduced overall frequencies suggest a proximal stenosis. A high-pitched wheezing sound was heard here.

M, Signal obtained along the clear distal external carotid. Most of the normal waveform features reappear; however, note the widely distributed frequencies and ragged envelope. Some baseline concentrations are still evident. A strained sound was again heard but was a bit smoother overall.

The examinations were interpreted as significant of carotid disease. Frontal artery flow was antegrade, implying enough flow compensation to maintain pressure despite the better than 80% stenosis found by carotid sonography and both arch and digital subtraction arteriography. By all these modalities the plaque was considered ulcerated. The patient had no further problems, and surgery was postponed pending observation.

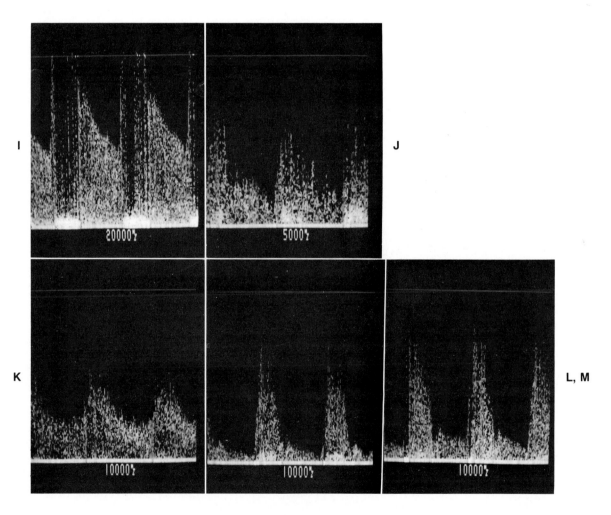

Fig. I-9, cont'd.

CAROTID REAL TIME SONOGRAPHY

Case 11. Normal carotid sonographic images (Fig. I-10). These examples are from a 20-year-old man who complained of headaches. The individual scans are labeled as to the normal structures and positions.

A, Normal anterior view of the common carotid. The walls and intima are well seen.

B, Normal lateral view of the bifurcation area, showing the carotid bulb and the internal and external carotid arteries. The jugular vein is anterior.

C, Normal transverse view of the middle common carotid. The medial side is to the top of the screen.

D, Normal transverse view at the bifurcation point showing the figure-8 where the individual vessels join the bulb.

E, Normal transverse view showing the appearance of the internal and external carotids above the bifurcation.

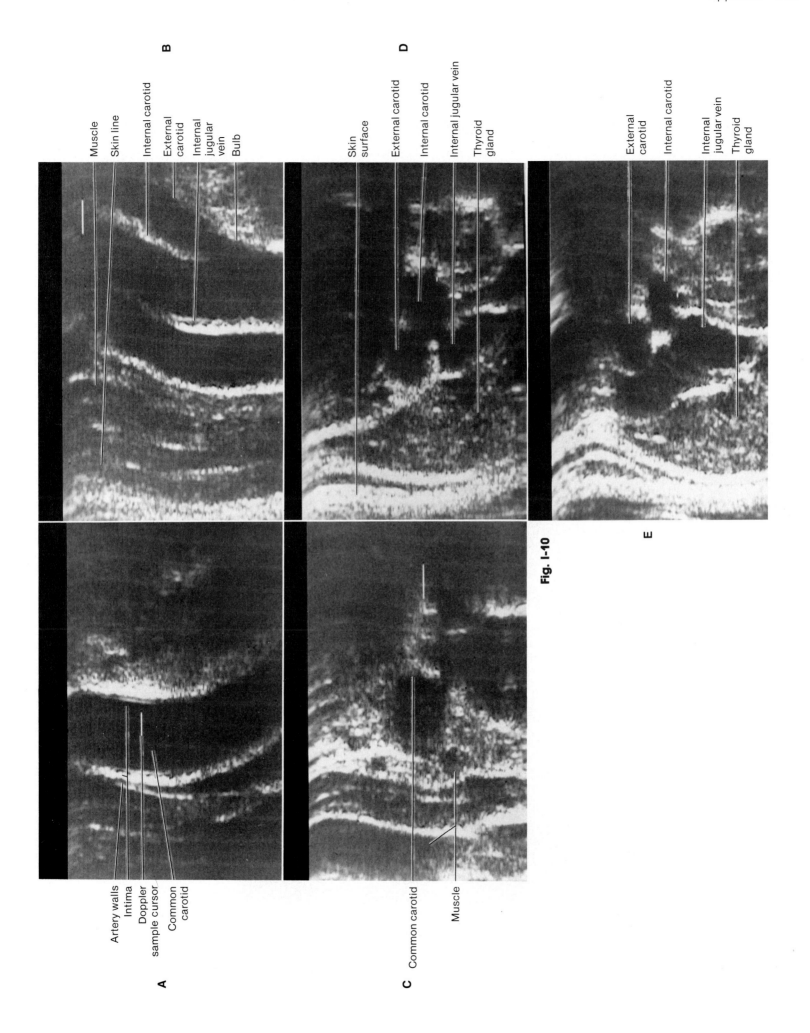

Muscle
Skin line
Internal carotid
External carotid
Internal jugular vein
Bulb

B

Skin surface
External carotid
Internal carotid
Internal jugular vein
Thyroid gland

D

External carotid
Internal carotid
Internal jugular vein
Thyroid gland

E

Artery walls
Intima
Doppler sample cursor
Common carotid

A

Common carotid

Muscle

C

Fig. I-10

Case 12. Abnormal carotid sonographic images and disease appearances (Fig. I-11). These examples are from various cases. The patient's head is to the bottom of the screen in both examples.

A, Appearance of calcified plaque, here seen on the superficial wall of the carotid. Note the dropout behind the lesion.

B, Appearance of irregular soft plaque in the bulb area. Some calcified plaque is also visible.

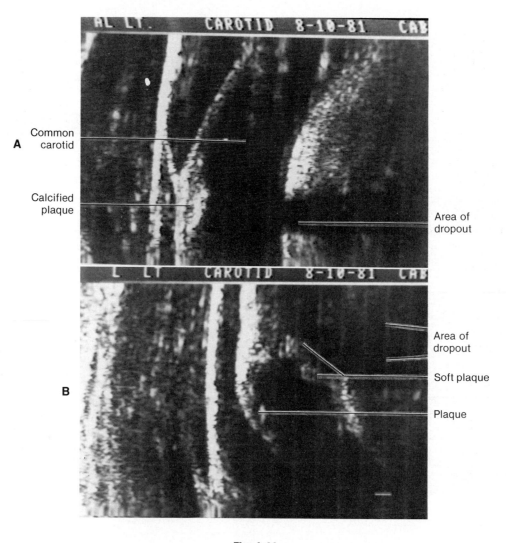

Fig. I-11

Case 13. Total carotid occlusion secondary to thrombus in the common, internal, and external carotid arteries — partial internal carotid occlusion (Fig. I-12)

History. The history for this patient can be found in Case 8, along with the patient's Doppler examination and surgical procedures.

Examination

A, Lateral view of the right common carotid artery low in the neck. The thrombus, which "bounces" up and down with each cardiac beat, is shown. This thrombus was completely free and unattached to the walls. Above this, the proximal portion of the congealed thrombus lining the carotid is shown. The intima is clearly seen, showing the thrombus to be separate and not a thickened part of the intima.

B, Anterior view taken just above the previous image. A much more extensive view of the thrombus is seen, as is a clear area on the deep wall that had minimal flow. This clear area was sealed off just below the bulb.

C, Lateral view showing the bulb and bifurcation. The same mass of gray echoes fills the entire lumen. Doppler examination here gave an absent signal.

D, Anterior view, giving a better perspective of the filled-in external carotid and bulb.

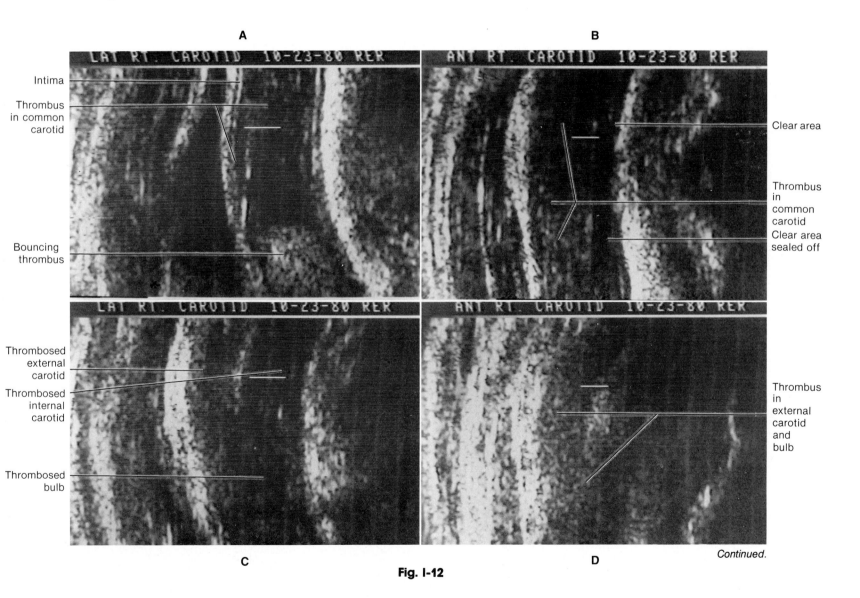

Fig. I-12

Continued.

In the following series of transverse views, levels have been chosen to correspond best with the longitudinal images.

E, View low in the common carotid, showing the transverse appearance of the moving thrombus caught in a freeze-frame image.

F, View of the area of the carotid just above the area with the moving plaque, showing the irregular edges of the thrombus and the decreased lumen.

G, Area of the bulb, just below the bifurcation. The bulb is entirely filled in with echoes. No Doppler signals could be heard.

H, Appearance of the internal and external carotid arteries. Once again, they too are filled in, which corresponds with the findings in the long-axis images. No Doppler flow signals could be obtained.

The left side was also diseased and gives good examples of severe disease in the bulb and internal and external carotid arteries. Reference to the Doppler tracings mentioned earlier may be of aid in understanding flow correlations. In all the views on the left side the patient's head now inverts to the *bottom* of the image. All directions will be given in respect to the patient's actual position and not the position of the structure in the image unless otherwise stated.

I, Anterior view of the left common carotid. Areas of plaque and intimal thickening are readily seen.

J, Posterior view of the area of the bulb and external carotid. Highly stenotic soft plaque can be seen on both the superficial and deep walls, with the superficial plaque extending into the origin of the external carotid.

K, Lateral view shows the internal carotid. Plaque areas can again be seen on both walls, extending partly up into the internal carotid. The dark area between the plaque sites is the actual lumen that remains unobstructed.

The two transverse views are oriented so that the medial side of the body is to the bottom of the image.

L, Common carotid just below the bulb. The areas of circumferential plaque are easily seen, corresponding with the areas seen in the long-axis views.

M, Transverse view of the bulb, showing the occluded appearance of the bulb area, as the circumferential soft plaque surrounds the lumen. This is a cross section through the widest area of bulb plaque; the lumen tended to widen superior to the bulb, as can be seen in the long-axis views.

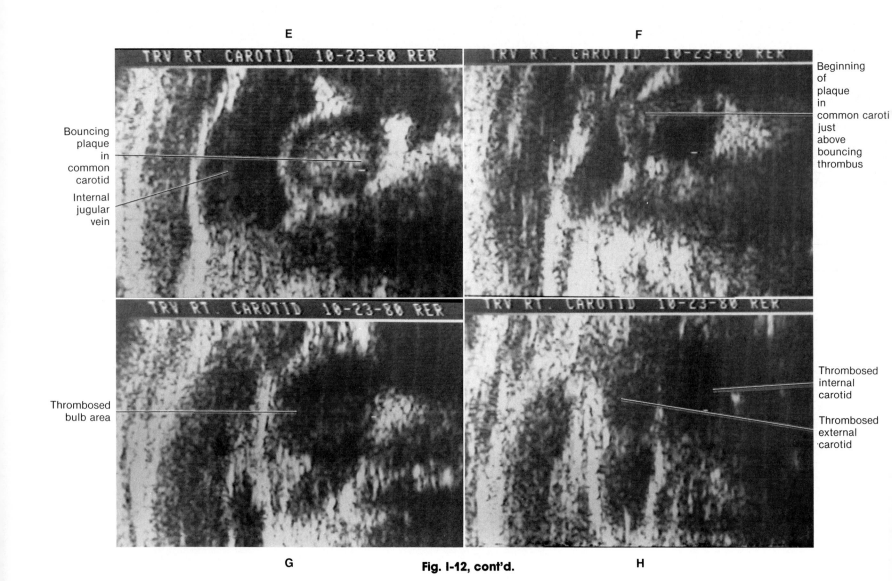

Fig. I-12, cont'd.

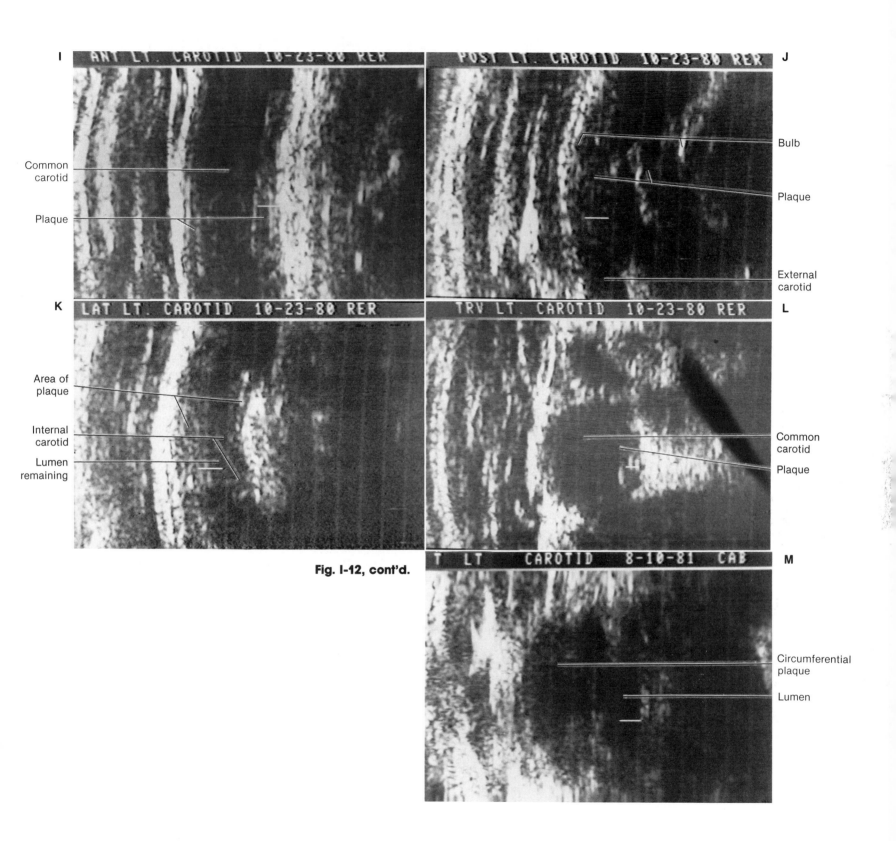

Fig. I-12, cont'd.

Pediatric cardiac structure growth patterns
(Chapter 34)

Rogé et al.[2] used M-mode echocardiography to measure the dimensions of the ventricular walls and cavities, great vessels, and left atrium and atrioventricular valve excursions in 93 children and infants without heart disease. The data were analyzed by relating each dimension (in millimeters) to body surface area (in square meters) and the 90% tolerance limits were calculated (Fig. J-1).

METHOD OF MEASURING

The peak of the R wave on the electrocardiogram was used to measure right ventricular anterior wall thickness (AWRVD), left ventricular posterior wall thickness (PWLVD), right and left ventricular cavity diastolic dimensions (RVDD and LVDD), interventricular septal thickness (IVSD), and mitral valve excursion (MVE). The measurements were obtained at the level of the posterior mitral leaflet in end diastole.

Left ventricular end systolic dimensions were measured at the peak upward motion of the posterior left ventricular endocardium. Right ventricular anterior wall thickness was obtained by proper selection of transducer and careful anterior gain control. The right

ventricular-septal and left ventricular-septal interfaces were defined by proper damping and reject control. Anterior mitral leaflet excursion was measured from the D point vertically to the E point at maximal excursion. The left atrium and aorta were measured on a continuous sweep from the left ventricle. Left atrial systolic dimensions (LASD) were measured at the largest distance between the anterior aspect of the left atrial posterior wall and the inner aortic posterior wall. Aortic end diastolic diameter (AoD) was measured at the beginning of the QRS complex, and end systolic diameter (AoS) at the same point used for measuring the left atrium. The aorta was measured from the anterior surface of the anterior root echo to the anterior surface of the posterior root echo.

The pulmonary artery diameter (PAD) was measured at the onset of the QRS complex, whenever possible, or when the anterior echo moved parallel with the posterior pulmonary root at any point in the cardiac cycle. The maximum excursion of the anterior leaflet of the tricuspid valve (ALTVE) was measured the same way as for the mitral valve.

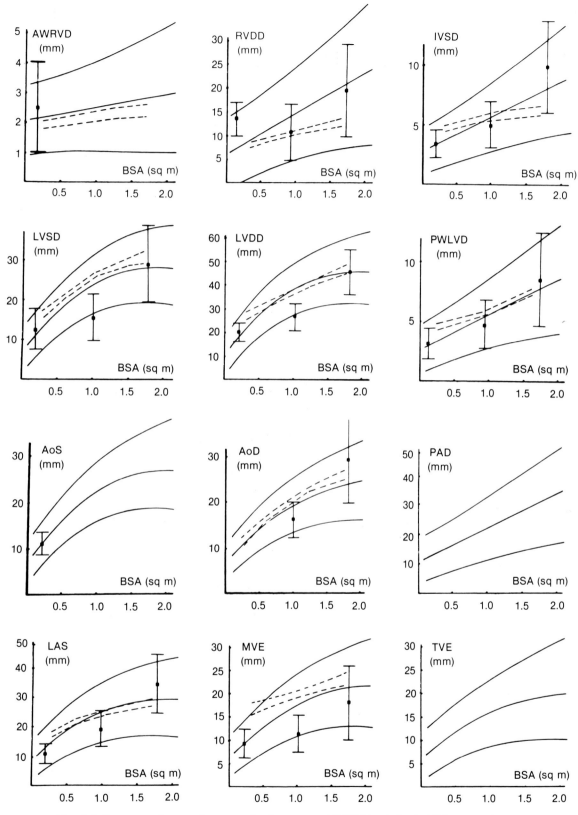

Fig. J-1. The normal range for neonates (mean and 2 S.D.) is plotted at 0.2 sq m, whereas normal adult data and the corrected values per square meter BSA are shown at 1.73 and 1 sq m respectively. The inner growth curves (broken lines) are the fifth and ninety-fifth percentile limits of the data from Epstein et al.[1] The outer heavy lines are the 90% tolerance lines of Rogé et al.[2]

NORMAL VALUES FOR THE TRANSVERSE AORTIC ARCH AND RIGHT PULMONARY ARTERY

The suprasternal view provides visualization of the aortic arch and right pulmonary artery. These normal values are presented in Fig. J-2.

AORTIC VALVE GRADIENT

Weyman et al. presented the relationship of peak systolic gradient to the ratio of maximum aortic cusp separation to aortic root diameter (Fig. J-3).

REFERENCES

1. Epstein, M.L., Goldberg, S.J., Allen, H.D., et al.: Great vessel, cardiac chamber, and wall growth patterns in normal children, Circulation **51**:1124, 1975.
2. Rogé, C.L.L., Silverman, N.H., Hart, P.A., and Ray, R.M.: Cardiac structure growth pattern determined by echocardiography, Circulation **57**:285, 1978.

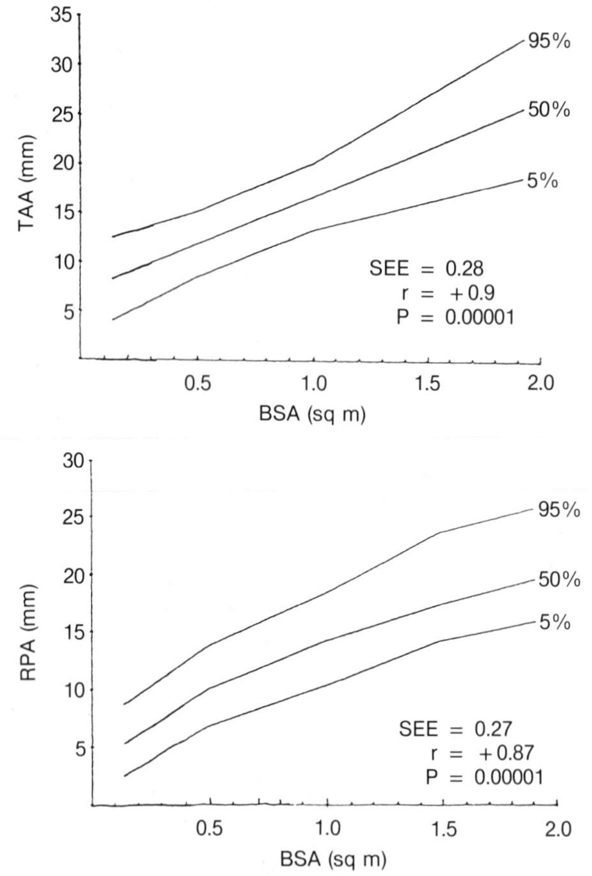

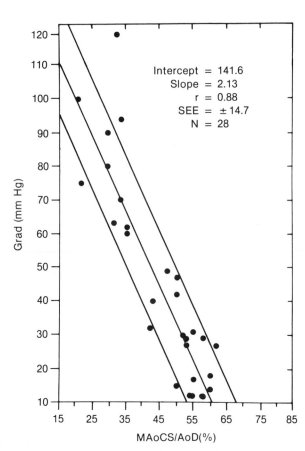

Fig. J-2. Normal values for transverse aortic arch (TAA) and right pulmonary artery (RPA) dimensions based on body surface area (BSA). (From Allen, H.D., Goldberg, S.J., Sahn, D.J., et al.: Circulation **55**:605, 1977. By permission of the American Heart Association, Inc.)

Fig. J-3. Aortic valve gradient. Relationship of the peak systolic gradient (mm Hg) to the ratio of maximum aortic cusp separation to aortic root diameter (mm). MAoCS is expressed as a percentage of AoD. (Modified slightly from Weyman, A.E., Feigenbaum, H., Hurwitz, R.A., et al.: Circulation **55**:773, 1977. By permission of the American Heart Association, Inc.)

Bibliography

PHYSICS OF DIAGNOSTIC ULTRASOUND

Goldstein, A.: Range ambiguities in real-time ultrasound, J. Clin. Ultrasound 9:85, 1981.

Morgan, C.L., Trought, W.S., Clark, W.M., et al.: Principles and applications of a dynamically focused array real time ultrasound system, J. Clin. Ultrasound 6:385, 1978.

Schwenker, R.P.: Film selection for computed tomography and ultrasound video imaging. In Haus, A.G., editor: The physics of medical imaging, 1979, AAPM.

Winsberg, F.: Real-time scanners: a review, Med. Ultrasound 3:99, 1979.

CROSS-SECTIONAL ANATOMY

Anderson, P.D.: Clinical anatomy and physiology for allied health sciences, Philadelphia, 1976, W.B. Saunders Co.

Clemente, C.D.: Anatomy: a regional atlas of the human body, Philadelphia, 1975, Lea & Febiger.

Crafts, R.C.: A textbook of human anatomy, New York, 1979, John Wiley & Sons, Inc.

Hollinshead, W.H.: Textbook of anatomy, ed. 3, New York, 1974, Harper & Row Publishers.

Lyons, E.A.: A color atlas of sectional anatomy chest, abdomen, and pelvis, St. Louis, 1978, The C.V. Mosby Co.

Sauerland, E., and Sauerland, B.A.T.: Human anatomical dissections. Laboratory exercises for the health professions, Baltimore, 1980, The Williams & Wilkins Co.

Snell, R.S.: Clinical anatomy for medical students, Boston, 1973, Little Brown & Co.

Thompson, J.S.: Core textbook of anatomy, Philadelphia, 1977, J.B. Lippincott Co.

VASCULAR STRUCTURES

Anderson, .P.D.: Clinical anatomy and physiology for allied health sciences, Philadelphia, 1976, W.B. Saunders Co.

Athey, P.A., and Tamez, L.: Lateral decubitus position for demonstration of the aortic bifurcation, J. Clin. Ultrasound 7:154, 1979.

Carlsen, E.N., and Filly, R.A.: Newer ultrasonographic anatomy in the upper abdomen. I. The portal and hepatic venous anatomy, J. Clin. Ultrasound 4:85, 1976.

Filly, R.A., and Goldberg, B.B.: Abnormal vessels. In Abdominal gray scale ultrasonography, New York, 1977, John Wiley & Sons, Inc.

Filly, R.A., and Goldberg, B.B.: Normal vessels. In Abdominal gray scale ultrasonography, New York, 1977, John Wiley & Sons, Inc.

Goldberg, B.B., Ostrum, B.J., and Isard, H.J.: Ultrasonic aortography, J.A.M.A. 198:353, 1966.

Gooding, G.A.W.: Ultrasonography of the iliac arteries, Radiology 135:161, 1980.

Gooding, G.A.W., and Effeney, D.J.: Ultrasound of femoral artery aneurysms, A.J.R. 134:477, 1980.

Isikoff, M.B., and Hill, M.C.: Sonography of the renal arteries; left lateral decubitus position, A.J.R. 134: 1177, 1980.

Leopold, G.R.: Ultrasonic abdominal aortography, Radiology 96:9, 1970.

Leopold, G.R., Goldberger, L., and Bernstein, E.: Ultrasonic detection and evaluation of abdominal aortic aneurysms, Surgery 72:939, 1972.

Taylor, K.J.W.: Ultrasonic investigation of inferior vena-caval obstruction, Br. J. Radiol. 48:1024, 1975.

Winsberg, F., and Cole, C.M.: Continuous ultrasound visualization of the pulsating abdominal aorta, Radiology 103:455, 1972.

LIVER

Albarelli, J.N., and Springer, G.E.: A technical approach to evaluating the jaundiced patient, Semin. Ultrasound 1:96, 1980.

Bree, R.L., and Silver, T.M.: Differential diagnosis of hypoechoic and anechoic masses with gray scale sonography: new observations, J. Clin. Ultrasound 7:249, 1979.

Broderick, T.W., Gosink, B.B., Menuck, L., et al.: Echographic and radionuclide detection of hepatoma, Radiology 135:149, 1980.

Callen, P.W.: Letter to editor, J. Clin. Ultrasound 7: 81, 1979.

Callen, P.W., Filly, R.A., and DeMartini, W.J.: The left portal vein: a possible source of confusion on ultrasonograms, Radiology 130:205, 1979.

Filly, R.A., and Carlsen, E.N.: Newer ultrasonographic anatomy in the upper abdomen. 2. The major systemic veins and arteries, with a special note on localization of the pancreas, J. Clin. Ultrasound 4:91, 1976.

Filly, R.A., and Laing, F.C.: Anatomic variation of portal venous anatomy in the porta hepatis: ultrasonographic evaluation, J. Clin. Ultrasound 6:83, 1978.

Gosink, B.B., and Leymaster, C.E.: Ultrasonic determination of hepatomegaly, J. Clin. Ultrasound 9:37, 1981.

Green, B., and Goldstein, H.M.: Hepatic ultrasonography. In Sarti, D.A., and Sample, W.F., editors: Diagnostic ultrasound, Boston, 1980, G.K. Hall & Co.

Hillman, B.J., D'Orsi, C.J., Smith, E.H., et al.: Ultrasonic appearance of the falciform ligament, A.J.R. 132:205, 1979.

Ingis, D.A.: Pathophysiology of jaundice—a primer, Semin. Ultrasound 1:143, 1980.

Joseph, A.E.A., Dewbury, K.C., and McGuire, P.G.: Ultrasound in the detection of chronic liver disease, Br. J. Radiol. 52:184, 1979.

Kamin, P.D., Bernadino, M.E., and Green, B.: Ultrasound manifestations of hepatocellular carcinoma, Radiology 131:459, 1979.

Kane, R.A.: Ultrasonographic anatomy of the liver and biliary tree, Semin. Ultrasound 1:87, 1980.

Kuni, C., Johnson, M., and Holmes, J.: Polycystic liver disease, J. Clin. Ultrasound 6:332, 1978.

Leopold, G.R.: Ultrasonography of jaundice, Radiol. Clin. North Am., vol. 17, no. 1, 1979.

Leyton, B., Halpern, S., Leopold, G.R., and Hagen, S.L.: Correlation of ultrasound and colloid Scintiscan studies of normal and diseased liver,

Marks, W.M., Filly, R.A., and Callen, P.W.: Ultrasonic anatomy of the liver: a review with new applications, J. Clin. Ultrasound 7:137, 1979.

Miller, E.I., and Thomas, R.H.: Portal vein invasion

663

demonstrated by ultrasound, J. Clin. Ultrasound 7:57, 1979.

Monroe, L.S., Leopold, G.R., Brown, J.W., et al.: The ultrasonic scan in the management of amebic hepatic abscess, Digest. Dis. 16:523, 1971.

Neiman, H.L.: Hepatocellular causes of jaundice, Semin. Ultrasound 1:118, 1980.

Netter, F., The digestive system. Vol. 3. Liver, gallbladder, and pancreas, Summit, N.J., 1972, Ciba Pharmaceutical Co.

Prando, A., Goldstein, H.M., Bernardino, M.E., et al.: Ultrasonic pseudolesions of the liver, Radiology 130: 403, 1979.

Sample, W.F.: Normal abdominal anatomy defined by gray scale ultrasound, Radiol. Clin. North Am., vol. 17, no. 1, 1979.

Sample, W.F., Sarti, D.A., Goldstein, L.I., et al.: Gray scale ultrasonography of the jaundiced patient, Radiology 128:719, 1978.

Scheible, W., Gosink, B.B., and Leopold, G.R.: Gray scale echographic patterns of hepatic metastatic disease, A.J.R. 129:983-987, 1977.

Scott, W.W., Sanders, R.C., and Siegelman, S.S.: Irregular fatty infiltration of the liver, A.J.R. 135:67, 1980.

Shwker, T.H., Moran, B., and Linzer, M.: B-scan echo-amplitude measurement in patients with diffuse infiltrative liver disease, J. Clin. Ultrasound 9:293, 1981.

Sones, P.J., and Torres, W.E.: Normal ultrasonic appearance of the ligamentum teres and falciform ligament, J. Clin. Ultrasound 6:392, 1978.

Spiegel, R.M., King, D.L., and Green, W.M.: Ultrasonography of primary cysts of the liver, A.J.R. 131: 235, 1978.

Sukov, R.J., Cohen, L.J., and Sample, W.F.: Sonography of hepatic amebic abscesses, A.J.R. 134:911, 1980.

Taylor, K.J.W., editor: Diagnostic ultrasound in gastrointestinal disease, Clin. Diagn. Ultrasound, vol. 1, 1979.

Weaver, R.M., Goldstein, H.M., Green, B., et al.: Gray scale ultrasonographic evaluation of hepatic cystic disease, A.J.R. 130:849, 1978.

Weill, F., Eisenscher, A., Aucant, D., et al.: Ultrasonic study of venous patterns in the right hypochrondrium: an anatomical approach to differential diagnosis of obstructive jaundice, J. Clin. Ultrasound 3:23, 1979.

Wooten, W.B., Green, B., and Goldstein, H.M.: Ultrasonography of necrotic hepatic metastases, Radiology 128:447, 1978.

GALLBLADDER AND THE BILIARY SYSTEM

Albarelli, J.N., and Springer, G.E.: A technical approach to evaluating the jaundiced patient, Semin. Ultrasound, vol. 1, no. 2, 1980.

Arger, P.H.: Obstructive jaundice of malignant origin, Semin. Ultrasound, vol. 1, no. 2, 1980.

Behan, M., and Kazam, E.: Sonography of the common bile duct: value of the right anterior oblique view, A.J.R. 130:701, 1978.

Buschi, A.J., Brenbridge, N.A.G., Cochrane, J.A., et al.: A further observation on gallbladder debris, J. Clin. Ultrasound 7:152, 1979.

Glancy, J.J., Goddard, J., and Pearson, D.E.: In vitro demonstration of cholesterol crystals' high echogenicity relative to protein particles, J. Clin. Ultrasound 8:27, 1980.

Harbin, W., and Ferrucci, J.T.: Nonoperative management of malignant biliary obstruction: a radiographic alternative, A.J.R. 135:103, 1980.

Ingis, D.A.: Pathophysiology of jaundice, Semin. Ultrasound, vol. 1, no. 2, 1980.

Kane, R.A.: Ultrasonographic anatomy of the liver and biliary tree, Semin. Ultrasound, vol. 1, no. 2, 1980.

Kane, R.A.: Ultrasonographic diagnosis of gangrenous cholecystitis and empyema of the gallbladder, Radiology 134:191, 1980.

Krook, P.M., Allen, F.H., Bush, W.H., et al.: Comparison of real time cholecystosonography and oral cholecystography, Radiology 135:145, 1980.

Leopold, G.R., Amberg, J., Gosink, B.B., et al.: Gray scale ultrasonic cholecystography: a comparison with conventional radiographic techniques, Radiology 121: 445, 1976.

Mindell, J.J., and Ring, B.A.: Gallbladder wall thickening: ultrasonic findings, Radiology 133:699, 1979.

Sample, W.F., Sarti, D.A., Goldstein, L.I., et al.: Grey scale ultrasonography of the jaundiced patient, Radiology 128:719, 1978.

Scheske, G.A., Cooperberg, P.L., Cohen, M.M., et al.: Dynamic changes in caliber of the major bile ducts related to obstruction, Radiology 135:215, 1980.

Sukov, R.J., Sample, W.F., Sarti, D.A., et al.: Cholecystosonography—the junctional fold, Radiology 133: 435, 1979.

Taylor, K.J.W., and Rosenfield, A.T.: Grey scale ultrasonography in the differential diagnosis of jaundice, Arch. Surg. 112:820, 1977.

Weeks, L.E., McCune, B.R., Martin, J.F., et al.: Unusual echographic appearance of a Courvoisier gallbladder, J. Clin. Ultrasound 5:341, 1977.

Weinstein, D.P., Weinstein, B.J., and Brodmerkel, G.J., Ultrasonography of biliary tract dilatation without jaundice, A.J.R. 132:729, 1979.

Yum, H.Y., Fink, A.H. Sonographic findings in primary carcinoma of the gallbladder, Radiology 134:693, 1980.

Zeman, R., Taylor, K.J.W., Burrell, M.I., et al.: Ultrasound demonstration of anicteric dilatation of the biliary tree, Radiology 134:689, 1980.

PANCREAS

Andrew, W.K., Hons, B.C., and Goudie, E.: A method of visualizing and documenting lesions by diagnostic ultrasound, Br. J. Radiol. 50:882, 1977.

Arger, P.H., Mulhern, C.B., Bonavita, J.A., et al.: Analysis of pancreatic sonography in suspected pancreatic disease, J. Clin. Ultrasound 7:91, 1979.

Burrell, M., Gold, J., Simeone, J., et al.: Liquefactive necrosis of the pancreas, Radiology 135:157, 1980.

Carroll, B., and Sample, W.F.: Pancreatic cystadenocarcinoma; CT body scan and gray scale ultrasound appearance, A.J.R. 131:339, 1978.

Cotton, P.B., Lees, W.R., Vallon, A.G., et al.: Gray scale ultrasonography and endoscopic pancreatography in pancreatic diagnosis, Radiology 134:453, 1980.

Eisenscher, A., and Weill, F.: Ultrasonic visualization of Wirsung's duct: dream or reality? J. Clin. Ultrasound 7:41, 1979.

Ferrucci, J.T.: Radiology of the pancreas. 1976 Sonography and ductography, Radiol. Clin. North Am. 14: 543, 1976.

Filly, R.A., and Carlsen, E.: Newer ultrasonic anatomy in the upper abdomen. II. The major systemic veins and arteries, with a special note on localization of the pancreas, J. Clin. Ultrasound 4:91, 1976.

Filly, R.A., and Freimanis, A.K.: Echographic diagnosis of pancreatic lesions, Radiology 96:575, 1970.

Filly, R.A., and London, S.S.: The normal pancreas: acoustic characteristics and frequency of imaging, J. Clin. Ultrasound 7:121, 1979.

Garrett, W.J., Kossoff, G., and Carpenter, D.A.: Gray scale compound scan echography of the normal upper abdomen, J. Clin. Ultrasound 3:199, 1975.

Gerzof, S.G., Robbins, A.H., Birkett, D.H., et al.: Percutaneous catheter drainage of abdominal abscesses guided by ultrasound and CT, A.J.R. 133:1, 1979.

Gold, J., Rosenfield, A.T., Sostman, D., et al.: Non-functioning islet cell tumors of the pancreas, A.J.R. 131:715, 1978.

Goldberg, B.B.: Ultrasound in the diagnosis of intra-abdominal hemorrhage and pseudocyst. In Clearfield, H.R., editor: Gastrointestinal emergencies, New York, 1976, Grune & Stratton, Inc.

Goldstein, H.M., and Katragadda, C.S.: Prone view ultrasonography for pancreatic tail neoplasms, A.J.R. 131:231, 1978.

Gooding, G.A.W.: Pseudocyst of the pancreas with mediastinal extension: an ultrasonographic demonstration, J. Clin. Ultrasound 5:121, 1977.

Gosink, B.B., and Leopold, G.R.: The dilated pancreatic duct: ultrasonic evaluation, Radiology 126:475, 1978.

Grose-Brown, M., Mitchell, M.A., and Hagen-Ansert, S.L.: Echographic noninvasive clinical assessment of the upper abdomen using various contrast media in the stomach, Med. Ultrasound 3:60, 1979.

Hagen-Ansert, S.L., and Manich, B.: Echographic visualization of normal pancreatic tissue patterns, Med. Ultrasound 1:11, 1977.

Hassani, S.N., Smulewicz, J.J., and Bard, R.: Pattern of pancreatic carcinoma by real time and gray scale ultrasonography, Appl. Radiol., September-October, 1977.

Kovac, A., Zali, M.R., and Geshner, J.: False aneurysm of the superior mesenteric artery—a complication of pancreatitis, Br. J. Radiol. 52:836, 1979.

Laing, F.C., Gooding, G.A.W., Brown, T., and Leopold, G.R.: Atypical pseudocysts of the pancreas: an ultrasonographic evaluation, J. Clin. Ultrasound 7:27, 1979.

Lawson, T.L.: Sensitivity of pancreatic ultrasonography in the detection of pancreatic disease, Radiology 128:733, 1978.

Leopold, G.: Pancreatic echography: a new dimension in the diagnosis of pseudocyst, Radiology 104:365, 1972.

Leopold, G.R., Berk, R.N., and Reinke, R.T.: Echographic-radiological documentation of spontaneous rupture of a pancreatic pseudocyst into the duodenum, Radiology 120:699, 1972.

Macmahon, H., Bowie, J.D., and Beezhold, C.: Erect scanning of pancreas using a gastric window, A.J.R. 132:587, 1979.

Marks, W.M., Filly, R.A., and Callen, P.W.: Ultrasonic evaluation of normal pancreatic echogenicity and its relationship to fat deposition, Radiology 137:475, 1980.

Ohto, M., Sastome, N., Saisho, H., et al.: Real time sonography of the pancreatic duct, A.J.R. 134:647, 1980.

Raymond, H.W., and Zwiebel, W.J., editors: The pancreas, Semin. Ultrasound, vol. 1, no. 3, 1980.

Sample, W.F.: Techniques for improved delineation of normal anatomy of the upper abdomen and high retroperitoneum with grey scale ultrasound, Radiology 124:197, 1977.

Sample, W.F., Po, J.B., Gray, R.K., and Cahill, P.J.: Gray scale ultrasonography techniques in pancreatic scanning, Appl. Radiol., p. 63, September-October, 1975.

Sarti, D.A.: Rapid development and spontaneous regression of pancreatic pseudocysts documented by ultrasound, Radiology **125:**789, 1977.

Slovis, T.L., Vonberg, V.J., and Mikelic, V.: Sonography in the diagnosis and management of pancreatic pseudocysts and effusions in childhood, Radiology **135:**153, 1980.

Smith, E.H., Bartrum, R.J., and Chang, Y.C.: Ultrasonically guided percutaneous aspiration biopsy of the pancreas, Radiology **112:**737, 1974.

Sokoloff, J., et al.: Pitfalls in the echographic evaluation of pancreatic disease, J. Clin. Ultrasound 2:321, 1974.

Warren, P.S., Garrett, W.J., Kosoff, G.: The liquid-filled stomach: an ultrasonic window to the upper abdomen, J. Clin. Ultrasound 6:295, 1978.

Weighall, S.L., Wolfman, N.T., and Watson, N.: The fluid-filled stomach: a new sonic window, J. Clin. Ultrasound 7:353, 1979.

Weinstein, B.J., Weinstein, D.P., and Brodmerkel, G.J.: Ultrasonography of pancreatic lithiasis, Radiology **134:**185, 1980.

Weinstein, D.P., and Weinstein, B.J.: Ultrasonic demonstration of the pancreatic duct, Radiology **130:**729, 1979.

Wright, C.H., Maklad, F., and Rosenthal, S.: Grey scale ultrasonic characteristics of carcinoma of the pancreas, Br. J. Radiol. **52:**281, 1979.

KIDNEYS

Arger, P.H., Mulhern, C.B., Pollack, H.M., et al.: Ultrasonic assessment of renal transitional cell carcinoma, A.J.R. **132:**407, 1979.

Bree, R.L., and Silver, T.M.: Differential diagnosis of hypoechoic and anechoic masses with gray scale sonography; new observations, J. Clin. Ultrasound 7:249, 1979.

Brown, J.M.: The ultrasound approach to the urographically nonvisualizing kidney, Semin. Ultrasound 11:44, 1981.

Elyaderani, M.K., and Gabriele, O.F.: Ultrasound of renal masses, Semin. Ultrasound 11:21, 1981.

Finberg, H.: Renal ultrasound: anatomy and technique, Semin. Ultrasound 11:7, 1981.

Goldberg, B.B., and Pollack, H.M.: Ultrasonically guided renal cyst aspiration, J. Urol. **109:**5, 1973.

Goldberg, B.B., and Ziskin, M.C.: Echo patterns with an aspiration ultrasonic transducer, Invest. Radiol. 8:78, 1973.

Goldstein, H.M., Green, B., and Weaver, R.M., Ultrasonic detection of renal tumor extension into the IVC, A.J.R. **130:**1083, 1978.

Kay, C.J., Rosenfield, A.J., and Armm, J.M.: Gray-scale ultrasonography in the evaluation of renal trauma, Radiology **134:**461, 1980.

Lawson, T.L., McClennan, B.L., and Shirkhoda, A.: Adult polycystic disease: ultrasonographic and computed tomographic appearance, J. Clin. Ultrasound 6:297, October, 1978.

Lee, J.K.T., McClennan, B.L., Melson, G.L., and Stanley, R.J.: Acute focal bacterial nephritis: emphasis on gray scale sonography and computed tomography, A.J.R. **135:**87, 1980.

Lewis, E., and Ritchie, W.G.M.: A simple ultrasonic method for assessing renal size, J. Clin. Ultrasound 8:417, 1980.

Maklad, N.F., Chuang, V.P., Doust, B.D., et al.: Ultrasonic characterization of solid renal lesions: echographic, angiographic, and pathologic correlation, Radiology **123:**733, 1977.

McDonald, D.G.: The complete echographic evaluation of solid renal masses, J. Clin. Ultrasound 6:402, 1978.

Morin, M.E., and Baker, D.A.: The influence of hydration and bladder distention on the sonographic diagnosis of hydronephrosis, J. Clin. Ultrasound 7:192, 1979.

Pollack, H.M., Arger, P.H., Goldberg, B.B., et al.: Ultrasonic detection of nonopaque renal calculi, Radiology **127:**233, 1978.

Ralls, P.W., and Halls, J.: Hydronephrosis, renal cystic disease, and renal parenchymal disease, Semin. Ultrasound 11:49, 1981.

Ralls, P., Esensten, M.L., Boger, D., and Halls, J.M.: Severe hydronephrosis and severe renal cystic disease: ultrasonic differentiation, A.J.R. **134:**473, 1980.

Resnick, M.I., and Sanders, R.C.: Ultrasound in urology, Baltimore, 1979, The Williams & Wilkins Co.

Rosenfield, A.T., Glickman, M.G., and Hodson, J.: Diagnostic imaging in renal disease, New York, 1979, Appleton-Century-Crofts.

Rosenfield, A.T., Taylor, K.J.W., Crade, M., and DeGraaf, C.S.: Anatomy and pathology of the kidney by gray scale ultrasound, Radiology **128:**737, 1978.

Rosenfield, A.T., Taylor, K.J.W., Dembner, A.G., and Jacobson, P.: Ultrasound of renal sinus: new observations, A.J.R. **133:**441, 1979.

Sanders, R.C.: Renal ultrasound, Radiol. Clin. North Am., vol. 13, no. 3, 1975.

Sanders, R.C., Scott, W., Conrad, M.R., and Kuhn, J.: The sonographic pattern of infantile polycystic disease, Ultrasound Med. 4:251, 1977.

Scheible, W., Ellenbogen, P.H., Leopold, G.R., et al.: Lipomatous tumors of the kidney and adrenal: apparent echographic specificity, Radiology **129:**153, 1978.

Scheible, W., and Talner, L.B.: Gray scale ultrasound and the genitourinary tract: a review of clinical applications, Radiol. Clin. North Am. 17:281, 1979.

Talmont, C.: Renal ultrasonography. In Taylor, K., et al., editors: Manual of ultrasonography, New York, 1980, Churchill Livingstone, Inc.

RENAL TRANSPLANT

Alley, K., and Geelhoed, G.W.: The use of ultrasonography and renal scanning in renal transplant patients, Am. Surg. 46:55, 1980. (General information on transplant abnormalities.)

Anthony, C.P., and Thibodeau, G.A.: Textbook of anatomy and physiology, ed. 10, St. Louis, 1979, The C.V. Mosby Co. (General information on kidney anatomy and physiology.)

Bartrum, R., Jr., Smith, E., D'Orsi, C., and Tilney, L.: Evaluation of renal transplants with ultrasound, Radiology **118:**405, 1976. (Covers all aspects of transplant abnormalities.)

Brenbridge, A.N., Buschi, A., Cochrane, J.A., and Lees, R.: Renal emphysema of the transplanted kidney: sonographic appearance, A.J.R. **132:**656, 1978. (Emphysema correlation with abscess ultrasound findings.)

Chabner, C.E.: The language of medicine, Philadelphia, 1976, W.B. Saunders Co. (General information on kidney anatomy and function.)

Conrad, M., Dickerman, R., Love, I., et al.: New observations in renal transplants using ultrasound, A.J.R. **131:**851, 1978. (Renal rejection with ultrasound.)

Cook, J., III, Rosenfield, A., and Taylor, K.: Ultrasonic demonstration of intrarenal anatomy, A.J.R. **129:**831, 1977. (Renal anatomy sonographically.)

Goldberg, B.B., Kotler, M.N., Ziskin, M.C., and Waxham, R.: Diagnostic uses of ultrasound, New York, 1975, Grune & Stratton, Inc. (General information on ultrasound characteristics.)

Guttmann, R.G.: Renal transplantation. 1, N. Engl. J. Med. **301:**975, 1979. (Excellent information on pretransplant procedings.)

Guttmann, R.G.: Renal transplantation. 2, N. Engl. J. Med. **301:**1038, 1979. (Excellent information on transplant procedure and posttransplant abnormalities.)

Hillman, B., Birnholz, J., and Busch, G.: Correlation of echographic and histologic findings in suspected renal allograft rejection, Radiology **132:**673, 1979. (Good information on histologic correlation of rejection with ultrasound.)

Hricak, H., Pereyra, L.T., and Eyler, W.: Evaluation of acute post-transplant renal failure by ultrasound, Radiology **133:**443, 1979. (Good explanation of ATN with ultrasound.)

Hricak, H., Pereyra, L.T., Eyler, W., et al.: The role of ultrasound in the diagnosis of kidney allograft rejection, Radiology **132:**667, 1979. (General information on rejection with ultrasound.)

Koehler, P.R., Kanemoto, H., and Maxwell, J.G.: Ultrasonic B-scanning in the diagnosis of complications in renal transplant patients, Radiology **119:**661, 1976. (General information on ultrasound with kidney transplant abnormalities.)

Kurtz, A., Rubin, C., Cole-Beught, C.B., et al.: Ultrasound evaluation of renal transplant, J.A.M.A. **243:**2429, 1980. (Excellent article on ultrasound of renal transplant.)

LaMasters, D., Katzberg, R.W., Confer, D., and Slaysman, M.: Ureteropelvic fibrosis in renal transplants: radiographic manifestations, A.J.R. **135:**79, 1980. (Good information on fibrosis with obstruction.)

Makland, N., Wright, C., and Rosenthal, S.: Gray scale ultrasonic appearances of renal transplant rejection, Radiology **131:**711, 1979. (Excellent article on ultrasound findings of rejection.)

Netter, F.H.: Kidneys, ureters, and urinary bladder, vol. 16, Ciba collection of medical illustrations, Summit, N.J., 1975 Ciba. (Excellent information on and illustrations of kidney anatomy, physiology, and transplant procedures.)

Raymond, H.W.: Fundamentals of abdominal sonography—a teaching approach, New York, 1979, Grune & Stratton, Inc. (Good information on sonographic appearance of kidney.)

Rosenfield, A.: Ultrasonography in renal transplantation. No. 2. Genitourinary ultrasonography, Clin. Diagn. Ultrasound, vol. 12, 1979. (Excellent information on kidney transplant ultrasound findings.)

Rosenfield, A., Glickman, M., and Hodson, J.: Diagnostic imaging in renal disease, New York, 1979, Appleton-Century-Crofts. (Good information on transplant sonographic appearances and abnormalities. Nuclear medicine explanation of principles and characteristics excellent.)

Sanders, B.M., and Roger, C.: Renal ultrasound, Radiol. Clin. North Am. **13:**417, 1975. (General information on kidney and transplant abnormalities.)

Sarti, D.A., and Sample, W.F.: Diagnostic ultrasound, text and cases, Boston, 1980, G.K. Hall Co. (Sonographic appearance of the kidney transplant.)

Singh, A., and Cohen, W.N.: Renal allograft rejection: sonography and scintigraphy, A.J.R. **135:**73, 1980. (Good correlation of ATN and rejection with radionuclide scanning and ultrasound.)

Weller, J.M.: Fundamentals of nephrology, New York, 1979, Harper & Row, Publishers. (General information.)

ADRENAL GLANDS

Bernardino, M.E., Goldstein, H.M., and Green, B.: Gray scale ultrasonography of adrenal neoplasms, A.J.R. **130**:741, 1978.

Birnholz, J.C.: Ultrasound imaging of adrenal mass lesions, Radiology **109**:163, 1973.

Davidson, J.D., Morley, P., Hurley, G.D., et al.: Adrenal venography and ultrasound in the investigation of the adrenal gland: an analysis of 58 cases, Br. J. Radiol. **48**:535, 1975.

Forsythe, J.R., Gosink, B.B., and Leopold, G.R.: Ultrasound in the evaluation of adrenal metastases, J. Clin. Ultrasound **5**:31, 1977.

Madayag, M., Bosniak, M.A., Beranbaum, E., et al.: Renal and suprarenal pseudotumors caused by variations of the spleen, Radiology **105**:43, 1972.

Pond, J.D., and Haber, K.: Echography: a new approach to the diagnosis of adrenal hemorrhage of the newborn, J. Can. Assoc. Radiol. **27**:40, 1976.

SPLEEN

Asher, W.M., Parvin, S., Virgilio, R.W., et al.: Echographic evaluation of splenic injury after blunt trauma, Radiology **118**:411, 1976.

Bhimji, S.D., Cooperberg, P.K., Naiman, S., et al.: Ultrasound diagnosis of splenic cysts, Radiology **122**:787, 1977.

Carlsen, E.N.: Liver, gallbladder, and spleen (R.D. Sanders, editor), Radiol. Clin. North Am., p. 554, 1975.

Crafts, R.C.: A textbook of human anatomy, ed. 2, New York, 1979, John Wiley & Sons, Inc.

Gooding, G.A.W.: The ultrasonic and CT appearance of splenic lobulations: a consideration in the ultrasonic differential of masses adjacent to the left kidney, Radiology **126**:719, 1978.

Green, B., Bree, R.D., Goldstein, H.M., et al.: Gray scale ultrasound evaluation of hepatic neoplasms: patterns and correlations, Radiology **124**:203, 1977.

Harell, G.S., Breiman, R.S., Glatstein, E.J., et al.: Computed tomography of the abdomen in the malignant lymphomas, Radiol. Clin. North Am. **15**:391, 1977.

Hollinshead, W.H.: Textbook of anatomy ed. 3, New York, 1974, Harper & Row, Publishers.

Rasmussen, S.N., Christensen, B.E., Holm, H.H., et al.: Spleen volume determination by ultrasonic scanning, Scand. J. Haematol. **10**:298, 1973.

Shirkhoda, A., McCartney, W.H., Staab, E.V., and Mittelstaedt, C.A.: Imaging of the spleen: a proposed algorithm, A.J.R. **135**:195, 1980.

Snell, R.S.: Clinical anatomy for medical students, Boston, 1973, Little, Brown & Co.

Talmont, C.A.: Spleen. In Taylor, K., et al., editors: Manual of ultrasonography, New York, 1980, Churchill Livingstone, Inc.

Thompson, I.S.: Core textbook of anatomy, Philadelphia, 1977, J.B. Lippincott Co.

Vicary, F.R., and Souhami, R.L.: Case reports. Ultrasound and Hodgkin's disease of the spleen, Br. J. Radiol. **50**:521, 1977.

RETROPERITONEUM

Brascho, D.J., Durant, J.R., and Green, L.E.: The accuracy of retroperitoneal ultrasonography in Hodgkin's disease and non-Hodgkin's lymphoma, Radiology **125**:485, 1977.

Bree, R.L., and Green, B.: The gray scale sonographic appearance of intra-abdominal mesenchymal sarcomas, Radiology **128**:193, 1978.

Doust, B.D., Quiroz, F., and Stewart, J.M.: Ultrasonic distinction of abscesses from other intra-abdominal fluid collections, Radiology **125**:213, 1977.

Filly, R.A., Marglin, S., and Castellino, R.A.: The ultrasonographic spectrum of abdominal and pelvic Hodgkin's disease and non-Hodgkin's lymphoma, Cancer **38**:2143, 1976.

Harbin, W.P., Wittenberg, J., Ferrucci, J.T., et al.: Fallibility of exploratory laparotomy in detection of hepatic and retroperitoneal masses, A.J.R. **135**:115, 1980.

Hillman, B.J., and Haber, K.: Echographic characteristics of malignant lymph nodes, J. Clin. Ultrasound **8**:213, 1980.

Kaftori, J.K., Rosenberger, A., Pollack, S., et al.: Rectus sheath hematoma: ultrasonographic diagnosis, A.J.R. **128**:283, 1977.

Laing, F.C., and Jacobs, R.P.: Value of ultrasonography in the detection of retroperitoneal inflammatory masses, Radiology **123**:169, 1972.

McCullough, D.L., and Leopold, G.R.: Diagnosis of retroperitoneal fluid collections by ultrasonography: a series of surgically proved cases, J. Urol. **115**:656, 1976.

Rochester, D., Bowie, J.D., and Kunzmann, A.: Ultrasound in the staging of lymphoma, Radiology **124**:483, 1977.

Smith, E.H., and Bartrum, R.J.: Ultrasonically guided percutaneous aspiration of abscesses, A.J.R. **122**:308, 1974.

HIGH-RESOLUTION ULTRASONOGRAPHY OF SUPERFICIAL STRUCTURES

Albert, N.E.: Testicular ultrasound for trauma, J. Urol. **124**:558, 1980.

Anson, B.J.: Morris' human anatomy, ed. 12, New York, 1966, McGraw-Hill Book Co.

Baker, C.R.F.: Complications and management of methods of dialysis access for renal failure, Am. Surg. **42**:859, 1976.

Basmajian, J.V.: Primary anatomy, ed. 5, Baltimore, 1964, The Williams & Wilkins Co.

Blum, M., Passalaque, A.M., Sackler, J.P., et al.: Thyroid echography of subacute thyroiditis, Radiology **125**:795, 1977.

Blumhagen J.D., and Coombs, J.B.: Ultrasound in the diagnosis of hypertrophic pyloric stenosis, J. Clin. Ultrasound **9**:289, 1981.

Crocker, E.F., Bautovich, G.J., and Jellins, J.: Grayscale echographic visualization of a parathyroid adenoma, Radiology **126**:233, 1978.

Davies, A.G.: Thyroid physiology, Br. Med. J. **2**:206, 1972.

Edis, A.J.: Surgical treatment for thyroid cancer, Surg. Clin. North Am. **57**:533, 1977.

Favus, M.J., Schneider, A.B., Stachura, M.E., et al.: Thyroid cancer occurring as a late consequence of head-and-neck irradiation, N. Engl. J. Med. **294**:1019, 1976.

Forsham, P.H.: Endocrine system and selected metabolic diseases, ed. 3, Summit, N.J., 1974, Ciba Pharmaceutical Co.

Frigolette, F.D., Birnholz, J.C., Driscoll, S.G.: Ultrasound diagnosis of cystic hygroma, Am. J. Obstet. Gynecol. **136**:962, 1980.

Guyton, A.C.: Function of the human body, ed. 3, Philadelphia, 1969, W.B. Saunders Co.

Haimou, M., Baez, A., Neff, M., et al.: Complications of arteriovenous fistulas for hemodialysis, Arch. Surg. **110**:708, 1975.

Haimou, M., and Jacobson, J.H.: Experience with the modified bovine arterial heterograft in peripheral vascular reconstruction and vascular access for hemodialysis, Ann. Surg. **180**:291, 1974.

Hammill, F.S., Johnston, C.G., Collins, G.M., et al.: A critical appraisal of the changing approaches to vascular access for chronic hemodialysis, Dial. Transpl. **19**:325, 1980.

Kangarloo, H., and Sample, W.F.: Ultrasound of the pediatric abdomen and pelvis, Chicago, 1980, Year Book Medical Publishers, Inc.

Leopold, G.: Ultrasonography of superficially located structures, Radiol. Clin. North Am. **18**:161, 1980.

Leopold, G., Woo, V.C., Scheible, R.W., et al.: High-resolution ultrasonography of scrotal pathology, Radiology **131**:719, 1979.

Massry, S., and Sellers, A.: Clinical aspects of uremia and dialysis, Springfield, Ill., 1976, Charles C Thomas, Publisher.

Miller, F.N., Jr.: Pathology, ed. 3, Boston, 1978, Little, Brown & Co.

Miskin, M., Rosen, I.B., and Walfish, P.G.: Ultrasonography of the thyroid gland, Radiol. Clin. North Am. **13**:479, 1975.

Oakes, D.D., Spees, E.D., Light, J.A., et al.: A three-year experience using modified bovine arterial heterografts for vascular access in patients requiring hemodialysis, Ann. Surg. **187**:423, 1978.

O'Brien, W.F., Cefalo, R.C., and Bair, D.B.: Ultrasonic diagnosis of fetal cystic hygroma, Am. J. Obstet. Gynecol. **138**:464, 1980.

Oppenheimen, E.: Reproductive system, ed. 5, Summit, N.J., 1974, Ciba Pharmaceutical Co.

ReMine, W.H., and McConahey, W.M.: Management of thyroid nodules, Surg. Clin. North Am. **57**:523, 1977.

Robbins, S.L., and Lotran, R.S.: Pathologic basis of disease, ed. 2, Philadelphia, 1979, W.B. Saunders Co.

Rohr, M.S., Browder, W., Freutz, G.D., et al.: Arteriovenous fistulas for long-term dialysis, Arch. Surg. **113**:153, 1978.

Sackler, J.P., Passalaque, A.M., Blum, M., et al.: A spectrum of diseases of the thyroid as imaged by gray scale water bath sonography, Radiology **125**:467, 1977.

Sample, W.F., Gottesman, J.E., Skinner, D.G., et al.: Gray scale ultrasound of the scrotum, Radiology **127**:225, 1978.

Sample, W.F., Mitchell, S.P., and Bledsoe, R.C.: Parathyroid ultrasonography, Radiology **127**:485, 1978.

Scheible, F.W., and Leopold, G.R.: Diagnostic imaging in head and neck disease: current applications of ultrasound, Head Neck Surg. **1**:1, 1978.

Scheible, F.W., Leopold, G.R., Woo, V.L., et al.: High-resolution real-time ultrasonography of thyroid nodules, Radiology **133**:413, 1979.

Scheible, W.: Pediatric applications of high resolution real time ultrasonography, Clin. Diagn. Ultrasound, 1981.

Scheible, W., Deutsch, A.L., and Leopold, G.R.: Parathyroid adenoma: accuracy of preoperative localization by high resolution real-time ultrasonography, J. Clin. Ultrasound. **9**:325, 1981.

Scheible, W., Skram, C., and Leopold, G.R.: High-resolution real-time sonography of hemodialysis vascular access complications, A.J.R. **134**:1173, 1980.

Spencer, R., Brown, M.C., and Annis, D.: Ultrasonic scanning of the thyroid gland as a guide to the treatment of the clinically solitary nodule, Br. J. Surg. **64**:841, 1977.

Tellis, V.A., Kohlberg, W.I., Bhat, D.J., et al.: Expanded polytetrafluoroethylene graft fistula for chronic hemodialysis, Am. Surg. **189**:101, 1979.

Walfish, P.G., Hazain, E., Strawbridge, H.T.G., et al.: A prospective study of combined ultrasonography and needle aspiration biopsy in the assessment of the hypofunctioning thyroid nodule, Surgery **82:**474, 1977.

Young, L.W.: Radiology case of the month, Am. J. Dis. Child. **134:**311, 1980.

BREAST

Abramson, D.J.: The needle biopsy in diagnosis of breast masses, Breast, vol. 7, no. 2, 1981.

American Cancer Society: 1981 Cancer facts and figures, New York, 1981, The Society.

Baum, G.: The detection of breast tumors by ultrasound methods. In Radiologic and other biophysical methods in tumor diagnosis, Chicago, 1975, Year Book Medical Publishers, Inc.

Baum, G.: Ultrasonographic examination of the breast. In Fundamentals of medical ultrasonography, New York, 1975, G.P. Putnam's Sons.

Baum, G.: Ultrasound mammography, Radiology **122:**199, 1977.

Baum, G.: Curent status of ultrasound mammography. In White, D., and Lyons, E.A., editors: Ultrasound in medicine, vol. 4, New York, 1978, Plenum Publishing Corp.

Calderson, D., Vilkomerson, D., Mezrich, R., et al.: Differences in the attenuation of ultrasound by normal, benign, and malignant breast tissue, J. Clin. Ultrasound **4:**249, 1976.

Cole-Beuglet, C.M.: Criteria for benign breast lesions. Lecture for Breast imaging conference, Las Vegas, 1981.

Cole-Beuglet, C., and Beique, R.A.: Continuous ultrasound B-scanning of palpable breast masses, Radiology **117:**123, 1975.

Ezo, M.E.: Tissue compression for the optimization of images in water-path breast scanning, Med. Ultrasound, October 1981.

Fry, W.J., Leichner, G.H., Okuyama, D., et al.: Ultrasound visualization system employing new scanning and presentation methods, J. Acoust. Soc. Am. **44**(5): 1325, 1968.

Griffths, K.: Ulrasound examination of the breast, Med. Ultrasound **2**:(3)13, 1978.

Harper, P., and Kelly-Fry, E.: Combined use of mammography and ultrasound visualization using a laboratory-modified commercial breast scanner to improve differential diagnosis. Proceedings, 23rd annual meeting of AIUM, San Diego, 1978.

Harper, P., and Kelly-Fry, E.: Ultrasound visualization of the breast in symptomatic patients, Radiology **137:**465, 1980.

Jellins, J., and Kossoff, G.: Velocity compensation in water coupled breast echography, Ultrasonics **11:**223, 1973.

Jellins, J., Kossoff, G., Buddee, F.W., et al.: Ultrasonic visualization of the breast, Med. J. Aust. **1:**305, 1971.

Jellins, J., Kossoff, G., Reeve, T.S., et al.: Ultrasonic grey scale visualization of breast disease, Ultrasound Med. Biol. **1:**393, 1975.

Kelly-Fry, E.: The use of ultrasound methods to detect changes in breast tissue which precede the formation of a malignant tumor. In Kessler, L.W., Jr., editor: Acoustical holography, vol. 7, New York, 1977, Plenum Publishing Corp.

Kelly-Fry, E., Fry, F.J., and Gardner, G.W.: Recommendations for widespread application of ultrasound visualization techniques for examination of the female breast. In White, D., and Brown, R.E., editors: Ultrasound in medicine, vol. 3A, New York, 1977, Plenum Publishing Corp.

Kelly-Fry, E., Fry, F.J., Sanghvi, N.T., et al.: A combined clinical and research approach to the problem of ultrasound visualization of breast. In White, D., editor: Ultrasound in medicine, vol. 1, New York, 1975, Plenum Publishing Corp.

Kelly-Fry, E., Harper, P., and Gardner, G.W.: Possible misdiagnosis of sound-attenuating breast masses as detected by ultrasound visualization techniques, and solutions to this problem. Proceedings, 23rd annual meeting of AIUM, San Diego, 1978.

Kelly-Fry, E., Sanghvi, N.T., Fry, F.J., et al.: Determination of alterations of phase angle of ultrasound transmitted through a malignant breast tumor: a preliminary investigation. In White, D., and Lyons, E.A., editors: Ultrasound in medicine, vol. 4, New York, 1978, Plenum Publishing Corp.

Kobayashi, T.: Review. Ultrasonic diagnosis of breast cancer, Ultrasound Med. Biol. **1:**383, 1975.

Kobayashi, T.: Gray-scale echography for breast cancer, Radiology **122:**207, 1977.

Kobayashi, T.: Grey scale echography for early breast cancer. In White, D., and Brown, R.E., editors: Ultrasound in medicine, vol. 3A, New York, 1977, Plenum Publishing Corp.

Kobayshi, T., Takatani, O., Hattori, N., et al.: Differential diagnosis of breast tumors, Cancer **33:**940, 1974.

Kossoff, G., Kelly-Fry, E., and Jellins, J.: Average velocity of ultrasound in the human female breast, J. Acoust. Soc. Am. **53:**1730, 1973.

Leis, H.P., Jr.: Diagnosis and treatment of breast lesions, Flushing, N.Y., 1970, Medical Examinations Publishing Co.

Pilnik, S., and Leis, H.P., Jr.: Clinical diagnosis of breast lesions. In Gallager, H.S., et al., The breast, St. Louis, 1978, The C.V. Mosby Co.

Pilnik, S., and Leis, H.P., Jr.: Nipple discharge. In Gallager, H.S., et al., editors: The breast, St. Louis, 1978, The C.V. Mosby Co.

Rubin, C.S., Jurtz, A.B., Goldberg, B.B., et al.: Ultrasound mammographic parenchymal patterns: a preliminary report, Radiology **130:**515, 1979.

Urban, J.A., and Adair, E.F.: Sclerosing adenomatosis, Cancer **2:**625, 1949.

Wagai, T., and Tsutsumi, M.: Mass screening of breast cancer by grey scale serial echography. In White D., and Brown, R.E., editors: Ultrasound in medicine, vol. 3A, New York, 1977, Plenum Publishing Corp.

Wagai, T., and Tsutsumi, M.: Ultrasound examination of the breast. In Logan, W.W., editor: Breast carcinoma: the radiologist's expanded role, New York, 1977, John Wiley & Sons, Inc.

GYNECOLOGIC ULTRASOUND

Bowie, J.D.: Ultrasound in gynecology. In Sabbagha R.E., editor: Diagnostic ultrasound applied to obstetrics and gynecology, New York, 1980, Harper & Row, Publishers.

Brown, T.W., Filly, R.A., Laing, F.C., and Barton, J.: Analysis of ultrasonographic criteria in the evaluation for ectopic pregnancy, A.J.R. **131:**967, 1978.

Callen, P.W., DeMartini, W.J., and Filly, R.A.: The central uterine cavity echo: a useful anatomic sign in the ultrasonographic evaluation of the female pelvis, Radiology **131:**187, 1979.

Callen, P.W., Filly, R.A., and Munyer, T.P.: Intrauterine contraceptive devices: evaluation by sonography, A.J.R. **135:**797, 1980.

Cochrane, W.J.: The value of ultrasound in the management of intrauterine devices. In Sanders, R.C., and James, A.E., Jr., editors: Ultrasonography in obstetrics and gynecology, ed. 2, New York, 1980, Appleton-Century-Crofts.

deSantos, L.A., and Goldstein, H.M.: Ultrasonography in tumors arising from the spine and bony pelvis, A.J.R. **129:**1061, 1977.

Fleischer, A.C., James, A.E., Jr., Millis, J.B., and Julian, C.: Differential diagnosis of pelvic masses by gray scale sonography, A.J.R. **131:**469, 1978.

Fleischer, A.C., Julian, C., and James, A.E., Jr.: Principles of differential diagnosis of pelvic masses by sonography. In Sanders, R.C., and James, A.E., Jr., editors: Ultrasonography in obstetrics and gynecology, ed. 2, New York, 1980, Appleton-Century-Crofts.

Green, B.: Pelvic ultrasonography. In Sarti, D.A., and Sample, W.F., editors: Diagnostic ultrasound; text and cases, Boston, 1980, G.K. Hall & Co.

Guttman, I.P., Jr.: In search of the elusive benign cystic ovarian teratoma: application of the ultrasound "tip of the iceberg" sign, J. Clin. Ultrasound **6:**403, 1977.

Hackeloer, B.J., and Dabelstein, S.N.: Ovarian imaging by ultrasound: an attempt to define a reference plane, J. Clin. Ultrasound **8:**497, 1980.

Hall, D.A., Hann, L.E., Ferrucci, J.T., et al.: Sonographic morphology of the normal menstrual cycle, Radiology **133:**185, 1979.

Haller, J.O., Schneider, M., Kassner, E.G., et al.: Ultrasonography in pediatric gynecology and obstetrics, A.J.R. **128:**423, 1977.

Haney, A.F., and Trought, W.S.: Paraovarian cysts resembling a filled urinary blader, J. Clin. Ultrasound **6:**53, 1978.

Lawson, T.: Diagnosis of gynecologic pelvic masses by gray scale ultrasonography: an analysis of specificity and accuracy, A.J.R. **128:**1003, 1977.

Marks, W.M., Filly, R.A., Callen, P.W., and Laing, F.C.: The decidual cast of ectopic pregnancy: a confusing ultrasonographic appearance, Radiology **133:**451, 1979.

Morley, P., and Barnett, W.: Use in ultrasound in diagnosis of pelvic masses, Br. J. Radiol. **43:**602, 1970.

Rochester, D., Levin, B., Bowie, J.D., and Kunmann, A.: Ultrasonic appearance of the Krukenberg tumor, A.J.R. **129:**919, 1977.

Rubin, C., Kurtz, A.B., and Goldberg, B.B.: Water enema: a new ultrasound technique in defining pelvic anatomy, J. Clin. Ultrasound **6:**28, 1978.

Sample, W.F.: Pelvic inflammatory disease and endometriosis. In Sanders, R.C., and James, A.E., Jr., editors: Ultrasonography in obstetrics and gynecology, ed. 2, New York, 1980, Appleton-Century-Crofts.

Sandler, M.A., and Karo, J.J.: The spectrum of ultrasonic findings in endometriosis, Radiology **127:**229, 1978.

Sample, W.F., Lippe, B.M., and Gyepes, M.T.: Gray-scale ultrasonography of the normal female pelvis, Radiology **125:**455, 1977.

VonMisky, L.: Sonographic study of uterine fibromyomas. In Sanders, R.C., and James, A.E., Jr., editors: Ultrasonography in obstetrics and gynecology, New York, 1977, Appleton-Century-Crofts.

Walsh, J.W., Taylor, K.J., and Rosenfield, A.T.: Gray-scale ultrasonography in the diagnosis of endometriosis and adenomyosis, A.J.R. **132:**87, 1979.

Walsh, J.W., Taylor, K.W., Wasson, J.F., et al.: Gray-scale ultrasound in 204 proved gynecologic masses: accuracy and specific diagnostic criteria, Radiology **130:**391, 1979.

Wilson, D.A., Stacy, T.M., and Smith, E.I.: Ultrasound diagnosis of hydrocolpos and hydrometrocolpos, Radiology **128:**451, 1978.

Zemlyn, S.: Comparison of pelvic ultrasonography and pneumography for ovarian size, J. Clin. Ultrasound **2:**331, 1974.

OBSTETRIC ULTRASOUND

Cooperberg, P.L., Chow, T., Kite, V., and Austin, S.: Biparietal diameter: a comparison of real-time and conventional B-scan techniques, J. Clin. Ultrasound 4:421, 1976.

Donald, I., Morley, P., and Barnett, E.: The diagnosis of blighted ovum by sonar, Br. J. Obstet. Gynaecol. 79:304, 1972.

Fisher, C.C., Garrett, W., and Kossoff, G.: Placental aging monitored by gray-scale echography, Am. J. Obstet. Gynecol. 124:483, 1976.

Grossman, M., Fisherman, E., and German, J.: Sonographic findings in gastrochisis, J. Clin. Ultrasound 6:143, 1978.

CARDIAC ANATOMIC AND PHYSIOLOGIC RELATIONSHIPS

Anderson, P.D.: Clinical anatomy and physiology for allied health sciences, Philadelphia, 1976, W.B. Saunders Co.

Clemente, C.D.: Anatomy, a regional atlas of the human body, Philadelphia, 1975, Lea & Febiger.

Crafts, R.C.: A textbook of human anatomy, New York, 1979, John Wiley & Sons, Inc.

DeBakey, M., and Gotto, A.: The living heart, New York, 1977, Grosset & Dunlap, Inc.

Green, J.H.: Basic clinical physiology, New York, 1969, Oxford University Press, Inc.

Hollinshead, W.H.: Textbook of anatomy, New York, 1979, Harper & Row, Publishers.

Introduction to medical sciences for clinical practice. A self-instructional/tutorial curriculum. Physician's assistant program, Bowman Gray School of Medicine (Winston-Salem, North Carolina), Chicago, 1976, Year Book Medical Publishers, Inc.

Snell, R.S.: Clinical anatomy for medical students, Boston, 1973, Little, Brown & Co.

Sokolow, M., and McIlroy, M.B.: Clinical cardiology, Lange Medical Publications, 1977, Los Altos, Calif.

Tilkian, A.G., and Conover, M.B.: Understanding heart sounds and murmurs, Philadelphia, 1979, W.B. Saunders Co.

ECHOCARDIOGRAPHIC TECHNIQUES AND EVALUATION

Allen, H., Goldberg, S., Sahn, D., et al.: Suprasternal notch echocardiography: assessment of its clinical utility in pediatric cardiology, Circulation 55:605, 1977.

Borer, J.S., Henry, W.L., and Epstein, S.E.: Echocardiographic observations in patients with systemic infiltrative disease involving the heart, Am. J. Cardiol. 39:184, 1977.

Cooper, R., and Leopold, G.: Diagnostic ultrasound in cardiology, Med. Ann. D.C. 41:748, 1972.

Cortina, A., and Lopez-Bescos, L.: Ultrasonics in cardiology, Rev. Esp. Cardiol. 26:15, 1973.

DeMaria, A.N., Neumann, A., Schubart, P.J., et al.: Systemic correlation of cardiac chamber size and ventricular performance determined with echocardiography and alterations in heart rate in normal persons, Am. J. Cardiol. 43:1, 1979.

Dillon, J., and Feigenbaum, H.: Echocardiography, J. Indiana State Med. Assoc. 67:104, 1974.

Feigenbaum, H.: Clinical applications of echocardiography, Prog. Cardiovasc. Dis. 14:531, 1972.

Feigenbaum, H.: Echocardiography, Philadelphia, 1972, Lea & Febiger.

Feigenbaum, H.: Echocardiography. Cardiovascular review, World Med. News, 1973.

Feigenbaum, H.: Newer aspects of echocardiography, Circulation 47:833, 1973.

Feigenbaum, H.: Ultrasound as a clinical tool in valvular heart disease, Cardiovasc. Clin. 5:219, 1973.

Feigenbaum, H.: Educational problems in echocardiography, Am. J. Cardiol. 34:741, 1974. [Editorial.]

Feigenbaum, H.: Hazards of echocardiographic interpretation, N. Engl. J. Med. 289:1311, 1974. [Editorial.]

Feigenbaum, H., Dillon, J., and Chang, S.: Recent developments in echocardiography. In Russek, H.I., editor: New horizons in cardiovascular practice, Baltimore, 1975, University Park Press.

Friedman, W.F., et al.: A review: newer, noninvasive cardiac diagnostic methods, Washington, D.C., 1977, International Pediatric Research Foundation.

Gehrke, J.: Critical appraisal of one- and two-dimensional echo in hypertrophic cardiomyopathy, Ann. Radiol. 20:409, 1977.

Gehrke, J.: M-mode and real time B-scan diagnostic criteria and pitfalls in right ventricular volume overloads, Z. Kardiol. 66(8):429, 1977. [English abstract.]

Gehrke, J., et al.: Non-invasive left ventricular volume determination by two-dimensional echo, Br. Heart J. 37(9):911, 1976.

Gilbert, B.W., et al.: Mitral valve prolapse, two-dimensional echo and angiographic correlation, Circulation 54:716, 1976.

Gilbert, B.W., et al.: Two-dimensional echo assessment of vegetative endocarditis, Circulation 55:346, 1977.

Goldberg, B.B.: Suprasternal ultrasonography, J.A.M.A. 215:245, 1972.

Goldberg, S., Allen, H., and Sahn, D.: Pediatric and adolescent echocardiography: a handbook, Chicago, 1975, Year Book Medical Publishers, Inc.

Goldschlager, S., et al.: Right atrial myxoma with right to left shunt and polycythemia presenting as congenital heart disease, Am. J. Cardiol. 30:82, 1972.

Gramiak, R.: Cardiac ultrasonography. A review of current applications, Radiol. Clin. North Am. 9:469, 1971.

Gramiak, R.: Echocardiography, J.A.M.A. 229:1009, 1974.

Gramiak, R., Shah, P., and Kramer, D.: Ultrasound cardiography: contrast studies in anatomy and function, Radiology 92:939, 1969.

Gramiak, R., et al.: Report of the inter-society commission for heart disease resources. Optimal resources for ultrasonic examination of the heart, J. Clin. Ultrasound 3:2, 1975.

Harbold, N., Jr., and Gau, G.: Echocardiographic diagnosis of right atrial myxoma, Mayo Clin. Proc. 48:284, 1973.

Henry, W.L., DeMaria, A., Gramiak, R., et al.: Report of the American Society of Echocardiography Committee on Nomenclature and Standards in Two-dimensional Echocardiography, 62:212, 1980.

Henry, W.L., Ware, J., Gardin, J.M., et al.: Echocardiographic measurements in normal subjects; growth-related changes that occur between infancy and early childhood, Circulation 57:278, 1978.

Houston, A.B., et al.: Two-dimensional echo with wide-angle (60-degree) sector scanner, 39:1071, 1977.

Houston, A.B., et al.: Two-dimensional sector scanner echocardiography in cyanotic congenital heart disease, Br. Heart J. 39:1076, 1977.

Kambe, T., et al.: Clinical application of high speed B-mode echo, J. Clin. Ultrasound 5:202, 1977.

Kerber, R.: Errors in performance and interpretation of echocardiograms, J. Clin. Ultrasound 1:330, 1973.

Kerber, R., Kioschos, J., and Lauer, R.: Use of an ultrasonic contrast method in the diagnosis of valvular regurgitation and intracardiac shunts, Am. J. Cardiol. 34:722, 1974.

Kisslo, J., et al: A phased array ultrasound system for cardiac imaging. Ultrasonics in medicine, Excerpta Medica, no. 363, p. 67, 1975.

Kisslo, J., et al.: Cardiac imaging using a phased array ultrasound system. Clinical technique and application, Circulation 53:262, 1976.

Kisslo, J.A., et al.: Clinical results of real time ultrasonic scanning of the heart using a phased array system, Yale J. Biol. Med. 50:355, 1977.

Kisslo, J.A., et al.: A comparison of real time, two-dimensional echo and cineangiography in detecting left ventricular asynergy, Circulation 55(1):134, 1977.

Kisslo, J.A., et al.: Dynamic cardiac imaging using a focused, phased array ultrasound system, Am. J. Med. 63(1):61, 1977.

Kossof, G.: Principles of two-dimensional echo and real time imaging, Med. J. Aust. 1(1 suppl.):8, 1977.

Kossof, G., et al.: Cross-sectional visualization of the normal heart by the UI Octoson, J. Clin. Ultrasound 6:3, 1978.

Lange, L.W., Sahn, D.J., Allen, H.D., and Goldberg, S.J.: The utility of subxiphoid cross-sectional echocardiography in infants and children with congenital heart disease, 59:513, 1979.

Lappe, D.L., et al.: A two-dimensional echo diagnosis of left atrial myxomas, Chest 74(1):55, 1978.

Lieppe, W., et al.: Two-dimensional findings in atrial septal defect, Circulation 56:447, 1977.

Ligtvoet, C., Vogel, J., and van Egmond, F.: Direct conversion of real-time two-dimensional echocardiographic images, Ultrasonics 15:89, 1977.

Martin, R.P., et al.: Reliability and reproducibility of two dimensional echocardiographic measurement of the stenotic mitral valve orifice area, Am. J. Cardiol. 43:560, 1979.

Matsumoto, M., et al.: Three-dimensional echocardiograms and two-dimensional echocardiographic images at desired planes by a computerized system, Ultrasound Med. Biol. 3(2-3):163, 1977.

Matsumoto, M., et al.: Use of kymo–two-dimensional echoaortocardiography for the diagnosis of aortic root dissection and mycotic aneurysm of the aortic root, Ultrasound Med. Biol. 3(2-3):153, 1977.

Matsumoto, M., et al.: A two-dimensional echoaortocardiographic approach to dissecting aneurysms of the aorta to prevent false positive diagnosis, Radiology 127:491, 1978.

Mintz, G.S., et al.: Two-dimensional echo recognition of ruptured chordae tendineae, Circulation 57:244, 1978.

Nichol, P.M., et al.: Two-dimensional echo assessment of mitral stenosis, Circulation 55:120, 1977.

Nishimura, K., et al.: Real time observation of cardiac movement and structures in congenital and acquired heart diseases employing high-speed ultrasonocardiotomography, Am. Heart J. 92:340, 1976.

Pai, A.L., Cahill, N.S., Dubroff, R.J., et al.: Digital computer analysis of M-scan echocardiograms, J. Clin. Ultrasound 4:173, 1976.

Pederson, J.F.: An ultrasonic multitransducer scanner for real time heart imaging, J. Clin. Ultrasound 5:11, 1977.

Popp, R.L., et al.: Cardiac anatomy viewed systematically with two-dimensional echocardiography, Chest 75:579, 1979.

Ports, T.A., et al.: Two-dimensional echo assessment of Ebstein's anomaly, Circulation 58:336, 1978.

Roberts, W.C.: Valvular, subvalvular, and supravalvular aortic stenosis: morphologic features, Cardiovasc. Clin. 5:98, 1973.

Robinson, E.P., et al.: Recognition of left ventricular borders using two-dimensional echo imaging, Comput. Biomed. Res. 9(3):247, 1976.

Roeland, J., et al.: Ultrasonic two-dimensional analysis of the mitral valve. In Kalmanson, D., editor: The mitral valve, Acton, Mass., 1976, Publishing Science Group.

Rossen, R.M., Goodman, D.J., Ingham, R.E., and Popp, R.L.: Ventricular systolic septal thickening and excursion in idiopathic hypertrophic subaortic stenosis, N. Engl. J. Med. 291:1317, 1974.

Rourke, T., Asinger, R.W., Mikell, F.L., et al.: Sector echocardiographic technique: a systematic approach, Med. Ultrasound 3:51, 1979.

Sahn, D.J., et al.: The comparative utilities of real time cross-sectional echo imaging systems for the diagnosis of complex congenital heart diseases, Am. J. Med. 63(1):50, 1977.

Sahn, D.J., et al.: Real time cross-sectional echo diagnosis of coarctation of the aorta, a prospective study of echo-angiographic correlations, Circulation 56: 762, 1977.

Sahn, D.J., DeMaria, A., Kisslo, J., and Weyman, A.: Recommendations regarding quantitation in M-mode echocardiography; results of a survey of echocardiographic measurements, Circulation 58:1072, 1978.

Sahn, D.J., et al.: Real time cross-sectional echo imaging and measurement of the patent ductus arteriosus in infants and children, Circulation 58:327, 1978.

Schieken, R.M., and Kerber, R.E.: Echocardiographic abnormalities in acute rheumatic fever, Am. J. Cardiol. 38:458, 1976.

Serruys, P.W., et al.: Bidimensional real time echo visualization of a ventricular right to left shunt following peripheral vein injection, Eur. J. Cardiol. 6(2): 99, 1977.

Shah, P.: IHSS—HOCM—MSS—ASH? Circulation 51:577, 1975. [Editorial.]

Shah, P., et al.: Role of echocardiography in diagnostic and hemodynamic assessment of hypertrophic subaortic stenosis, Circulation 44:891, 1971.

Shah, P., et al.: Echocardiographic assessment of the effects of surgery and propranolol on the dynamics of outflow obstruction and hyperpranolol on the dynamics of outflow obstruction and hypertrophic subaortic stenosis, Circulation 45:516, 1972.

Shaw, A., et al.: A real time two-dimensional ultrasonic scanner for clinical use, Ultrasonics 14(1):35, 1976.

Silverman, N.H., and Schiller, N.B.: Apex echocardiography. A two-dimensional technique for evaluating congenital heart disease, Circulation 57:503, 1978.

Stack, R., and Kisslo, J.: Evaluation of the left ventricle with two-dimensional echocardiography, Am. J. Cardiol. 46:1117, 1980.

Tajik, A.J., et al.: A two-dimensional real time ultrasonic imaging of the heart and great vessels. Technique, image orientation, structure, identification, and validation, Mayo Clin. Proc. 53:271, 1978.

Tomoda, H., et al.: An experience in clinical application of real time two-dimensional echo, Jpn. Heart J. 17(4):437, 1976.

Vogel, J.A., et al.: Processing equipment for two-dimensional echo data, Ultrasound Med. Biol. 2(3):171, 1976.

Von Ramm, O.T., et al.: Cardiac imaging using a phased array ultrasound system. System design, Circulation 53:258, 1976.

Weyman, A., et al.: Cross-sectional echocardiography in evaluating patients with discrete subaortic stenosis, Am. J. Cardiol. 37:358, 1976.

Weyman, A., et al.: Mechanism of abnormal septal motion in patients with right ventricular volume overload, a cross-sectional echocardiographic study, Circulation 54:179, 1976.

Weaver, W.F., et al.: Mid-diastolic aortic valve opening

in severe acute aortic regurgitation, Circulation 55: 145, 1977.

Wilcken, D.E., et al.: The clinical applications of two-dimensional echo, Med. J. Aust. 1(1 suppl.):8, 1977.

Winkle, R., Goodman, D., and Popp, R.: Simultaneous echocardiographic-phonocardiographic recordings at rest and during amyl nitrite administration in patients with mitral valve prolapse, Circulation 51:522, 1975.

Winsberg, F., and Mercer, E.: Echocardiography in combined valve disease, Radiology 105:405, 1972.

Mitral valve

Abbasi, A.S., MacAlpin, R.N., Eber, L.M., et al.: Echocardiographic diagnosis of idiopathic hypertrophic cardiomyopathy without outflow obstruction, Circulation 46:897, 1972.

Barlow, J.B., Pocock, W.A., Marchand, P., and Denny, M.: The significance of late systolic murmurs, Am. Heart J. 66:443, 1963.

Bolton, M.R., Jr., King, J.F., Polumbo, R.A., et al.: The effects of operation on the echocardiographic features of idiopathic subaortic stenosis, Circulation 50:897, 1974.

Botvinick, E.H., Schiller, N.B., Wickramasekaren, R., et al.: Echocardiographic demonstration of early mitral valve closure in severe aortic insufficiency. Its clinical implications, Circulation 51:836, 1975.

Burgess, J., Clark, R., Kamigaki, M., et al.: Echocardiographic findings in different types of mitral regurgitation, Circulation 48:97, 1973.

Chung, K., Manning, J., and Gramiak, R.: Echocardiography in coexisting hypertrophic subaortic stenosis and fixed left ventricular outflow obstruction, Circulation 49:673, 1974.

Craige, E., and Fortuin, J.: Studies on mitral valve motion in the presence of the Austin-Flint murmur, Trans. Am. Clin. Climatol. Assoc. 83:209, 1972.

DeMaria, A.N., King, J.F., Bogren, H.G., et al.: The variable spectrum of echocardiographic manifestations of the mitral valve prolapse syndrome, Circulation 50:33, 1974.

DeMaria, A., Lies, J.E., King, J.F., et al.: Echographic assessment of atrial transport, mitral movement, and ventricular performance following electroversion of supraventricular arrhythmias, Circulation 51:273, 1975.

Dillon, J.C., Feigenbaum, H., Konecke, L.L., et al.: Echocardiographic manifestations of valvular vegetations, Am. Heart J. 86:698, 1973.

Dillon, J.C., Haine, C.L., Chang, S., et al.: Use of echocardiography in patients with prolapsed mitral valve, Circulation 43:503, 1971.

Dodd, M., and Wilcken, D.: Echocardiography in left atrial myxoma: relation to the findings in mitral stenosis, Aust. N.Z. J. Med. 2:124, 1972.

Duchak, J.M., Jr., Chang, S., and Feigenbaum, H.: The posterior mitral valve echo and the echocardiographic diagnosis of mitral stenosis, Am. J. Cardiol. 29:628, 1972.

Finegan, R., and Harrison, D.: Diagnosis of left atrial myxoma by echocardiography, N. Engl. J. Med. 282: 1022, 1970.

Flaherty, J., Livengood, S., and Fortuin, N.: Atypical posterior leaflet motion in echocardiogram in mitral stenosis, Am. J. Cardiol. 35:675, 1975.

Fortuin, N., and Craige, E.: Echocardiographic studies of genesis of mitral diastolic murmurs, Br. Heart J. 35:75, 1973.

Goodman, D., Harrison, D., and Popp, R.: Echocardiographic features of primary pulmonary hypertension, Am. Heart J. 86:847, 1973.

Goodman, D., Harrison, D., and Popp, R.: Echocardio-

graphic features of primary pulmonary hypertension, Am. J. Cardiol. 33:438, 1974.

Gramiak, R., and Waag, R.C.: Cardiac ultrasound, St. Louis, 1975, The C.V. Mosby Co.

Henry, W.L., Clark, C.E., Glancy, D.L., et al.: Echocardiographic measurement of the left ventricular outflow gradient in idiopathic hypertrophic subaortic stenosis, N. Engl. J. Med. 288:989, 1973.

Hernberg, J., Weiss, B., and Keegan, A.: The ultrasonic recording of aortic valve motion, Radiology 94: 361, 1970.

Johnson, A., Lonky, S., and Carleton, R.: Combined hypertrophic subaortic stenosis and calcific aortic valvular stenosis, Am. J. Cardiol. 35:706, 1975.

Johnson, M.L., Holmes, J.H., Spangler, R.D., et al.: Usefulness of echocardiography in patients undergoing mitral valve surgery, J. Thorac. Cardiovasc. Surg. 64:922, 1972.

Johnson, M.L., et al.: Echocardiographic diagnosis of a left atrial myxoma found attached to the free left atrial wall, J. Clin. Ultrasound 1:75, 1973.

Kamigaki, M., and Goldschlager, N.: Echocardiographic analysis of mitral valve motion in atrial septal defect, Am. J. Cardiol. 30:343, 1972.

Kerber, R., Kelly, D., Jr., and Gutenkauf, C.: Left atrial myxoma. Demonstrated by stop-action cardiac ultrasonography, Am. J. Cardiol. 34:838, 1974.

King, J.F., DeMaria, A.N., Miller, R.R., et al.: Markedly abnormal mitral valve motion without simultaneous interventricular pressure gradient due to uneven mitral-septum contact in idiopathic hypertrophic subaortic stenosis, Am. J. Cardiol. 34:360, 1974.

Konecke, L.L., Feigenbaum, H., Chang, S., et al.: Abnormal mitral valve motion in patients with elevated left ventricular diastolic pressures, Circulation 47:989, 1973.

Levisman, J.A., and Abbasi, A.S.: Abnormal motion of the mitral valve with pericardial effusion: pseudoprolapse of the mitral valve, Am. Heart J. 91:18, 1976.

Lortscher, R.H., Toews, W.H., Nora, J.J., et al.: Left atrial myxoma presenting as rheumatic fever, Chest 66:302, 1974.

Markiewicz, W., Stoner, J., London, E., et al.: Effect of transducer placement on echocardiographic mitral valve systolic motion, Eur. J. Cardiol. 4:359, 1976.

Meyer, J.F., Frank, M.J., Goldberg, S., and Cheng, T.O.: Systolic mitral flutter, an echocardiographic clue to the diagnosis of ruptured chordae tendineae, Am. Heart J. 93:3, 1977.

Nanda, N.C., Gramiak, R., Shah, P.M., et al.: Echocardiography in the diagnosis of idiopathic hypertrophic subaortic stenosis coexisting with aortic valve disease, Circulation 50:752, 1974.

Nanda, N.C., Gramiak, R., Shah, P.M., et al.: Mitral commissurotomy versus replacement: preoperative evaluation by echocardiography, Circulation 51:263, 1975.

Nasser, W.K., Davis, R.H., Dillon, J.C., et al.: Atrial myxoma. I. Clinical and pathologic features in nine cases, Am. Heart J. 83:694, 1972.

Nasser, W., et al.: Atrial myxoma. 2. Phonocardiographic, echocardiographic, hemodynamic, and angiographic features in nine cases, Am. Heart J. 83: 810, 1972.

Nichol, P.M., Gilbert, B.W., and Kisslo, J.A.: Two-dimensional echocardiographic assessment of mitral stenosis, Circulation 55:120, 1977.

Parisi, A., and Milton, B.: Relation of mitral valve closure to the first heart sound in man: echocardiographic and phonocardiographic assessment, Am. J. Cardiol. 32:779, 1973.

Popp, R., and Levine, R.: Left atrial mass simulating cardiomyopathy, J. Clin. Ultrasound 1:96, 1973.

Popp, R., et al.: Echocardiographic abnormalities in the mitral valve prolapse syndrome, Circulation **49**:428, 1974.

Pridie, R.B., Beham, R., and Oakley, C.M.: Echocardiography of the mitral valve in aortic valve disease, Br. Heart J. **33**:296, 1971.

Quinones, M., et al.: Reduction in the rate of diastolic descent of the mitral valve echogram in patients with altered left ventricular diastolic pressure-volume relations, Circulation **49**:246, 1974.

Rubenstein, J., et al.: The echocardiographic determination of mitral valve opening and closure: correlation with hemodynamic studies in man, Circulation **51**:98, 1975.

Shah, P., et al.: Role of echocardiography in diagnostic and hemodynamic assessment of hypertrophic subaortic stenosis, Circulation **44**:891, 1971.

Shah, P., et al.: Echocardiographic assessment of the effects of surgery and propranolol on the dynamics of outflow obstruction and hypertrophic subaortic stenosis, Circulation **45**:516, 1972.

Spangler, R.D., Johnson, M.L., Holmes, J.H., et al.: Echocardiographic demonstration of bacterial vegetations in active infective endocarditis, J. Clin. Ultrasound **1**:126, 1973.

Spangler, R., and Okin, T.: Echocardiographic demonstration of left atrial thrombus, Chest **67**:716, 1975.

Sweatman, T., et al.: Echocardiographic diagnosis of mitral regurgitation due to ruptured chordae tendineae, Circulation **46**:580, 1972.

Aorta and left atrium

Brown, O., Harrison, D., and Popp, R.: An improved method for echographic detection of left atrial enlargement, Circulation **50**:58, 1974.

Chang, S., Clements, S., and Chang, J.: Aortic stenosis: echocardiographic cuspi separation and surgical description of aortic valve in 22 patients, Am. J. Cardiol. **39**:499, 1977.

Cooperberg, P., Mercer, E.N., Mulder, D.S., et al.: Rupture of a sinus Valsalva aneurysm. Report of a case diagnosed preoperatively by echocardiography, Radiology **113**:171, 1974.

DeMaria, A.N., King, J.F., Salel, A.F., et al.: Echography and phonography of acute aortic regurgitation in bacterial endocarditis, Ann. Intern. Med. **82**:329, 1975.

Feizi, O., Symons, C., and Yacoub, M.: Echocardiography of the aortic valve. Studies of normal aortic valve, aortic stenosis, aortic regurgitation and mixed aortic valve disease, Br. Heart J. **36**:341, 1974.

Francis, G.S., et al.: Echocardiographic criteria of normal left atrial size in adults, Cathet. Cardiovasc. Diagn. **2**:69, 1976.

Glasser, S.: Late mitral valve opening in aortic regurgitation, Chest **70**:70, 1976.

Goldberg, B.: Suprasternal ultrasonography, J.A.M.A. **215**:245, 1971.

Gottlieb, S., Khuddus, S.A., Balooki, H., et al.: Echocardiographic diagnosis of aortic valve vegetations in candida endocarditis, Circulation **50**:826, 1974.

Gramiak, R., and Shah, P.: Echocardiography of the aortic root, Invest. Radiol. **3**:356, 1968.

Gramiak, R., and Shah, P.: Echocardiography of the normal and diseased aortic valve, Radiology **96**:1, 1970.

Henry, W.L., Morganroth, J., Pearlman, A.S., et al.: Relation between echocardiographically determined left atrial size and atrial fibrillation, Circulation **53**:273, 1976.

Hirata, T., Wolfe, S.B., Popp, R.L., et al.: Estimation of left atrial size using ultrasound, Am. Heart J. **78**:43, 1969.

Hirschfeld, D.S., and Schiller, N.: Localization of aortic valve vegetations by echocardiography, Circulation **53**:280, 1976.

Johnson, A.D., Alpert, J.S., Francis, G.S., et al.: Assessment of left ventricular function in severe aortic regurgitation, Circulation **54**:975, 1976.

Johnson, M.L., Warren, S.G., Waugh, R.A., et al.: Echocardiography of the aortic valve in non-rheumatic left ventricular outflow tract lesions, Radiology **112**:677, 1974.

Kelly, D., Wulfsberg, E., and Rowe, R.: Discrete subaortic stenosis, Circulation **46**:309, 1972.

Kronzon, I., and Mehta, S.: Giant left atrium, Chest **65**:677, 1974.

Martinez, E., Burch, G., and Giles, T.: Echocardiographic diagnosis of vegetative aortic bacterial endocarditis, Am. J. Cardiol. **34**:845, 1974.

Millward, D., Robinson, N., and Craige, E.: Dissecting aortic aneurysm diagnosed by echocardiography in a patient with rupture of the aneurysm into the right atrium, Am. J. Cardiol. **30**:427, 1972.

Nanda, N.C., Gramiak, R., Manning, J., et al.: Echocardiographic recognition of the congenital bicuspid aortic valve, Circulation **49**:870, 1974.

Nanda, N., Gramiak, R., and Shah, P.: Diagnosis of aortic root dissection by echocardiography, Circulation **48**:506, 1973.

Nanda, N.C., Gramiak, R., Shah, P.M., et al.: Echocardiography in the diagnosis of idiopathic hypertrophic subaortic stenosis coexisting with aortic valve disease, Circulation **50**:752, 1974.

Petsas, A.A., Gottlieb, S., Kingsley, B., et al.: Echocardiographic diagnosis of left atrial myxoma, Br. Heart J. **37**:627, 1976.

Popp, R.L., Silverman, J.F., French, J.W., et al.: Echocardiographic findings in discrete subvalvular aortic stenosis, Circulation **49**:226, 1974.

Pratt, R.C., Parisi, A.F., Harrington, J.J., et al.: The influence of left ventricular stroke volume on aortic root motion: an echocardiographic study, Circulation **53**:947, 1976.

Rothbaum, D.A., Dillon, J.C., Chang, S., et al.: Echocardiographic manifestations of right sinus of Valsalva aneurysm, Circulation **49**:768, 1974.

Spangler, R.D., Johnson, M.L., Holmes, J.H., et al.: Echocardiographic demonstration of bacterial vegetations in active infective endocarditis, J. Clin. Ultrasound **1**:126, 1973.

Strunk, B.L., Fitzgerald, J.W., Lipton, M., et al.: The posterior aortic wall echocardiogram, its relationship to left atrial volume change, Circulation **54**:744, 1976.

TenCate, F., et al.: Dimensions and volumes of left atrium and ventricle determined by single beam echocardiography, Br. Heart J. **36**:737, 1974.

Vredevoe, L., Creekmore, S., and Schiller, N.: The measurement of systolic time intervals by echocardiography, J. Clin. Ultrasound **2**:99, 1974.

Weyman, A.E., Feigenbaum, H., Dillon, J.C., et al.: Noninvasive visualization of the left main coronary artery by cross-sectional echocardiography, Circulation **54**:179, 1976.

Winsberg, F., and Goldman, H.: Echo pattern of cardiac posterior wall, Invest. Radiol. **4**:173, 1969.

Tricuspid valve

Ainsworth, R.P., Hartmann, A.F., Aker, U., and Schad, N.: Tricuspid valve prolapse with late systolic tricuspid insufficiency, Radiology **107**:309, 1973.

Chandraratna, P., et al.: Echocardiographic detection of tricuspid valve prolapse, Circulation **51**:823, 1975.

Gooch, A.S., Maranhao, V., Scampardones, G., et al.: Prolapse of both mitral and tricuspid leaflets in systolic murmur-click syndrome, N. Engl. J. Med. **287**:1218, 1972.

Green, E., Agruss, N., and Adolph, R.: Right-sided Austin-Flint murmur: documentation of intracardiac phonocardiography, echocardiography and postmortem findings, Am. J. Cardiol. **32**:370, 1973.

Hagan, A., Sahn, D.J., and Friedman, W.F.: Cross-sectional echocardiographic features of Ebstein's malformation, Circulation **50**(suppl. 3):17, 1974. [Abstract.]

Lundstrom, N.: Echocardiography in the diagnosis of Ebstein's anomaly of the tricuspid valve, Circulation **47**:597, 1973.

Nanda, N., Gramiak, R., and Manning, J.: Echocardiography of the tricuspid valve in congenital left ventricular-right atrial communication, Circulation **51**:268, 1975.

Seides, S.F., DeJoseph, R.I., Brown, A.E., and Damato, A.N.: Echocardiographic findings in isolated, surgically created tricuspid insufficiency, Am. J. Cardiol. **35**:679, 1975.

Tavel, M.E., Baugh, D., Fisch, C., and Feigenbaum, H.: Opening snap of the tricuspid valve in atrial septal defect: a phonocardiographic and reflected ultrasound study of sounds in relationship to movements of the tricuspid valve, Am. Heart J. **80**:550, 1970.

Waxler, E.B., Kawai, N., and Kasparian, H.: Right atrial myxoma: echocardiographic, phonocardiographic and hemodynamic signs, Am. Heart J. **83**:251, 1972.

Wolfe, S.B., Popp, R.L., and Feigenbaum, H.: Diagnosis of atrial tumors by ultrasound, Circulation **39**:615, 1969.

Pulmonary valves

Chung, K.J., Alexson, C.G., Manning, J.A., and Gramiak, R.: Echocardiography in truncus arteriosus: the value of pulmonic valve detection, Circulation **48**:281, 1973.

Goldberg, S., Allen, H., and Sahn, D.: Pediatric echocardiography, Chicago, 1974, Year Book Medical Publishers, Inc.

Goodman, D., Harrison, D., and Popp, R.: Echocardiographic features of primary pulmonary hypertension, Am. J. Cardiol. **33**:438, 1974.

Gramiak, R., Nanda, N.C., and Shah, P.M.: Echocardiographic detection of the pulmonary valve, Radiology **102**:153, 1972.

Nanda, N., et al.: Evaluation of pulmonary hypertension by echocardiography, J. Clin. Ultrasound **1**:225, 1973.

Nanda, N.C., Gramiak, R., Robinson, T.I., and Shah, P.M.: Echocardiographic evaluation of pulmonary hypertension, Circulation **50**:575, 1974.

Nanda, N., et al.: Echocardiographic evaluation of pulmonary hypertension, Circulation **50**:575, 1974.

Wann, L.S., et al.: Premature pulmoanry valve opening, Circulation **55**:128, 1977.

Weyman, A.E., Dillon, J.C., Feigenbaum, H., and Chang, S.: Echocardiographic patterns of pulmonary valve motion in valvular pulmonary stenosis, Am. J. Cardiol. **34**:644, 1974.

Weyman, A.E., Dillon, J.C., Feigenbaum, H., and Chang, S.: Echocardiographic patterns of pulmonic valve motion with pulmonary hypertension, Circulation **50**:905, 1974.

Weyman, A.E., Dillon, J.C., Feigenbaum, H., and Chang, S.: Echocardiographic differentiation of infundibular from valvular pulmonary stenosis, Am. J. Cardiol. **36**:21, 1975.

Weyman, A.E., Dillon, J.C., Feigenbaum, H., and Chang, S.: Premature pulmonic valve opening following sinus of Valsalva aneurysm rupture into the right atrium, Circulation **51**:556, 1975.

Right ventricle

Brown, O.R., Harrison, D.C., and Popp, R.I.: Echocardiography study of right ventricular hypertension producing asymmetrical septal hypertrophy, Circulation 48(suppl. IV):47, 1973. [Abstract.]

DeMaria, A.N., Vismara, I.A., Miller, R.R., Neumann, A., et al.: Unusual echocardiographic manifestations of right and left heart myxomas, Am. J. Med. **59**:713, 1975.

Diamond, M.A., Dillon, J.C., Haine, C.L., et al.: Echocardiographic features of atrial septal defect, Circulation **43**:129, 1971.

Henry, W.L., Clark, C.E., and Epstein, S.E.: Asymmetric septal hypertrophy (ASH): the unifying link in the IHSS disease spectrum, Circulation **47**:827, 1973.

Popp, R.L., Wolfe, S.B., Hirata, T., and Feigenbaum, H.: Estimation of right and left ventricular size by ultrasound. A study of the echoes from the interventricular septum, Am. J. Cardiol. **24**:523, 1969.

Interventricular septum and interatrial septum

Abbasi, A., et al.: Echocardiographic diagnosis of idiopathic hypertrophic cardiomyopathy without outflow obstruction, Circulation **46**:897, 1972.

Cohen, M.V., et al.: B-scan ultrasonography in idiopathic hypertrophic subaortic stenosis, Br. Heart J. **37**:1976.

Devereux, R.B., and Reichek, N.: Echocardiographic determination of left ventricular mass in man. Anatomic validation of the method, Circulation **55**:613, 1977.

Dillon, J., et al.: Cross-sectional echocardiographic examination of the interatrial septum, Circulation **55**:115, 1977.

Epstein, S.E., Henry, W.L., Clark, C.E., et al.: Asymmetric septal hypertrophy, Ann. Intern. Med. **81**: 650, 1974.

Henry, W.L., Clark, C.E., and Epstein, S.E.: Asymmetric septal hypertrophy: echocardiographic identification of the pathognomonic anatomic abnormality of IHSS, Circulation **47**:225, 1973.

Henry, W.L., Clark, C.E., and Epstein, S.E.: Asymmetric septal hypertrophy (ASH): the unifying link in the IHSS disease spectrum, Circulation **47**:827, 1973.

Henry, W.L., Clark, C.E., Roberts, W.C., et al.: Difference in distribution of myocardial abnormalities in patients with obstructive and nonobstructive asymmetric septal hypertrophy (ASH): echocardiographic and gross anatomic findings, Circulation **50**: 447, 1974.

Kerber, R., et al.: Effects of acute coronary occlusion on the motion and perfusion of the normal and ischemic interventricular septum, Circulation **54**:928, 1976.

Kerin, N., et al.: Ventricular septal defect complicating acute myocardial infarction, Chest **70**:560, 1976.

King, J.F., DeMaria, A.N., Miller, R.R., et al.: Markedly abnormal mitral valve motion without simultaneous intraventricular pressure gradient due to uneven mitral-septal contact in idiopathic hypertrophic subaortic stenosis, Am. J. Cardiol. **34**:360, 1974.

Nanda, N.C., Gramiak, R., Shah, P.M., et al.: Echocardiography in the diagnosis of idiopathic hypertrophic subaortic stenosis co-existing with aortic valve disease, Circulation **50**:752, 1974.

Popp, R.L., and Harrison, D.C.: Ultrasound in the diagnosis and evaluation of therapy of idiopathic hypertrophic subaortic stenosis, Circulation **40**:905, 1969.

Pridie, R., and Oakley, C.: Mechanism of mitral regurgitation in hypertrophic obstructive cardiomyopathy, Br. Heart J. **32**:203, 1970.

Left ventricle

Abbasi, A., et al.: Paradoxical motion of interventricular septum in LBBB, Circulation **49**:423, 1974.

Bergeron, G.A., Cohen, M.V., Teichholz, L.F., and Gorlin, R.: Echocardiographic analysis of mitral valve motion after acute myocardial infarction, Circulation **51**:82, 1975.

Burch, G.E., Giles, T.D., and Martinez, E.: Echocardiographic detection of abnormal motion of the interventricular septum in ischemic cardiomyopathy, Am. J. Med. **57**:293, 1974.

Chang, S., and Feigenbaum, H.: Subxiphoid echocardiography, J. Clin. Ultrasound **1**:14, 1973.

Chang, S., Feigenbaum, H., and Dillon, J.: Condensed M-mode echocardiographic scan of the asymmetrical left ventricle, Chest **68**:93, 1975.

Chang, S., Feigenbaum, H., and Dillon, J.: Subxyphoid echocardiography: a review, Chest **68**:233, 1975.

Corya, B.C., Feigenbaum, H., Rasmussen, S., and Black, M.J.: Anterior left ventricle wall echoes in coronary artery disease: linear scarring with a single element transducer, Am. J. Cardiol. **34**:652, 1974.

Diamond, M., et al.: Echocardiographic features of atrial septal defect, Circulation **43**:129, 1974.

Dillon, J., Chang, S., and Feigenbaum, H.: Echocardiographic manifestations of left bundle branch block, Circulation **49**:876, 1974.

Fortuin, N., et al.: Determinations of left ventricular volumes by ultrasound, Circulation **44**:575, 1971.

Goldstein, S., and Willem de Jong, J.: Changes in left ventricular wall dimension during regional myocardial ischemia, Am. J. Cardiol. **34**:56, 1974.

Gramiak, R., and Nanda, N.: Echocardiographic diagnosis of ostium primum septal defect, Circulation **45** (suppl. 2):46, 1972.

Hagan, A., et al.: Ultrasound evaluation of systolic anterior septal motion in patients with and without right ventricular volume overload, Circulation **50**:248, 1974.

Henning, H., Schelbert, H., Crawford, M.H., et al.: Left ventricular performance assessed by radionuclide angiocardiography and echocardiography in patients with previous myocardial infarction, Circulation **52**:1069, 1975.

Karliner, J., et al.: Mean velocity of fiber shortening: a simplified measure of left ventricular myocardial contractility, Circulation **44**:323, 1971.

Kerber, R.E., and Abboud, F.M.: Echocardiographic detection of regional myocardial infarction: an experimental study, Circulation **48**:997, 1973.

Kraunz, R., and Kennedy, J.: Ultrasonic determination of left ventricular wall motion in normal man. Studies at rest and after exercise, Am. Heart J. **79**:36, 1970.

Kraunz, R., and Ryan, T.: Ultrasound measurements of ventricular wall motion following administration of vasoactivity drugs, Am. J. Cardiol. **27**:464, 1971.

Kreamer, R., Kerber, R., and Abbound, F.: Ventricular aneurysm: use of echocardiography, J. Clin. Ultrasound **1**:60, 1973.

Layton, C., et al.: Assessment of left ventricular filling and compliance using an ultrasound technique, Br. Heart J. **35**:559, 1973.

Levitsky, S., and Merchani, F.: Non-invasive methods of measuring myocardial contractility, Surg. Annu. **5**:205, 1973.

Ludbrook, P., Karliner, J.S., London, A., et al.: Posterior wall velocity: an unreliable index of total left ventricular performance in patients with coronary artery disease, Am. J. Cardiol. **33**:475, 1974.

Ludbrook, P., Karliner, J.S., Paterson, K., et al.: Comparison of ultrasound and cineangiographic measurements of left ventricular performance in patients with and without wall motion abnormalities, Br. Heart J. **35**:1026, 1973.

McDonald, I.: Assessment of myocardial function by echocardiography, Adv. Cardiol. **12**:221, 1974.

McLaurin, I., et al.: A new technique for the study of left ventricular pressure-volume relations in man, Circulation **48**:56, 1973.

Morganroth, J., et al.: Comparative left ventricular dimensions in trained athletes, Ann. Intern. Med. **82**:521, 1975.

Payvandi, M., et al.: Echocardiography in congenital and acquired absence of the pericardium. An echocardiographic mimic of right ventricular volume overload, Circulation **53**:86, 1976.

Pombo, J., et al.: Comparison of stroke volume and cardiac output determination by ultrasound and dye dilution in acute myocardial infarction, Am. J. Cardiol. **27**:630, 1971.

Pombo, J., Troy, B., and Russell, R., Jr.: Left ventricular volumes and ejection fraction by echocardiography, Circulation **43**:480, 1971.

Popp, R., et al.: Ultrasonic cardiac echography for determining stroke volume and valvular regurgitation, Circulation **41**:493, 1970.

Popp, R., et al.: Sources of error in calculation of left ventricular volumes by echography, Am. J. Cardiol. **31**:152, 1973.

Popp, R., et al.: Effect of transducer placement on echocardiographic measurement of left ventricular dimensions, Am. J. Cardiol. **35**:537, 1975.

Ratshin, R., Rackley, C., and Russell, R.: Serial evaluation of left ventricular volumes and posterior wall movement in the acute phase of myocardial infarction using diagnostic ultrasound, Am. J. Cardiol. **29**:286, 1972.

Ratshin, R., Rackley, C., and Russell, R.L.: Determination of left ventricular preload and afterload by quantitative echocardiography in man, Circ. Res. **34**: 711, 1974.

Ratshin, R., et al.: Quantitative echocardiography: correlations with ventricular volumes by angiography in patients with coronary artery disease with and without wall motion abnormalities, Circulation 48(suppl. 4): 48, 1973.

Ratshin, R., et al.: The accuracy of ventricular volume analysis by quantitative echocardiography in patients with coronary artery disease with and without wall motion abnormalities, Am. J. Cardiol. **33**:164, 1974.

Redwood, D., Henry, W., and Epstein, S.: Evaluation of the ability of echocardiography to measure acute alterations in left ventricular volume, Circulation **50**:901, 1974.

Stack, R., et al.: Left ventricular performance in coronary artery disease evaluated with systolic time intervals and echocardiography, Am. J. Cardiol. **37**:331, 1976.

Weyman, S., et al.: Localization of left ventricular outflow obstruction by cross-sectional echocardiography, Am. J. Med. **60**:33, 1976.

ECHOCARDIOGRAPHIC MEASUREMENTS

Burgess, J., et al.: Echocardiographic findings in different types of mitral regurgitation, Circulation **48**: 97, 1973.

Chang, S.: M-mode echocardiographic techniques and pattern recognition, Philadelphia, 1976, Lea & Febiger.

ACQUIRED VALVULAR HEART DISEASE

Abbasi, A.S., Allen, M.W., DeCristofaro, D., et al.: Detection and estimation of the degree of mitral regurgitation by range-gated pulsed Doppler echocardiography, Circulation **61**:143, 1980.

Clark, R.D., Korcuska, K., and Cohn, K.: Serial echocardiographic evaluation of left ventricular function in valvular disease, including reproducibility guidelines for serial studies, Circulation **62**:564, 1980.

Cope, G.D., Kisslo, J.A., Johnson, M.L., et al.: A reassessment of the echocardiogram in mitral stenosis, Circulation **52**:664, 1975.

Cunha, C.P., Guiliani, E.R., Fuster, V., et al.: Preoperative M-mode echocardiography as a predictor of surgical results in chronic aortic insufficiency, J. Thorac. Cardiovasc. Surg. **79**:256, 1980.

DeMaria, A.N., Bommer, W., Joye, J., et al.: Value and limitations of cross-sectional echocardiography of the aortic valve in the diagnosis and quantification of valvular aortic stenosis, Circulation **62**:304, 1980.

Henry, W.L., Griffth, J.M., Michaelis, L.L., et al.: Measurement of mitral orifice area in patients with mitral valve disease by real time, two-dimensional echocardiography, Circulation **51**:827, 1975.

Kotler, M.N., Mintz, G.S., Parry, W.R., et al.: M-mode and two dimensional echocardiography in mitral and aortic regurgitation: pre- and postoperative evaluation of volume overload of the left ventricle, Am. J. Cardiol. **46**:1144, 1980.

Levisman, J.A., Abassi, A.S., and Pearce, M.L.: Posterior mitral leaflet motion in mitral stenosis, Circulation **51**:511, 1975.

Naito, M., Morganroth, J., Mardelli, T.J., et al.: Rheumatic mitral stenosis: cross-sectional echocardiographic analysis, Am. Heart J. **100**:34, 1980.

Nichol, P.M., Gilber, B.W., and Kisslo, J.A.: Two-dimensional echocardiographic assessment of mitral stenosis, Circulation **55**:120, 1977.

Popp, R.L., Rubenson, D.S., Tucker, C.R., et al.: Echocardiography: M-mode and two-dimensional methods, Ann. Intern. Med. **93**:844, 1980.

Wise, J.R.: Echocardiographic evaluation of mitral stenosis using diastolic posterior left ventricular wall motion, Circulation **61**:1037, 1980.

OTHER VALVULAR ABNORMALITIES

DeMaria, A.N., King, J.F., Bogren, H.C., et al.: The variable spectrum of echocardiographic manifestations of the mitral valve prolapse syndrome, Circulation **50**:33, 1974.

Feigenbaum, H.: Echocardiography, ed. 3, Philadelphia, 1981, Lea & Febiger.

Fraker, T.D., Johnson, M.L., and Kisslo, J.A.: Echocardiographic diagnosis of mitral valve disease. In Kisslo, J.A., editor: Two-dimensional echocardiography, New York, 1980, Churchill Livingstone, Inc.

Gilbert, B.W., Schatz, R.A., vonRamm, O.T., et al.: Mitral valve prolapse: two-dimensional echocardiographic and angiographic correlation, Circulation **54**:716, 1976.

Godley, R.W., Rogers, E.W., Wann, L.S., et al.: Relation of incomplete mitral leaflet closure to the site of dyssynergy in patients with papillary muscle dysfunction, Circulation **60**(suppl. 2):204, 1979. [Abstract.]

Godley, R.W., Weyman, A.E., Feigenbaum, H., et al.: Patterns of mitral leaflet motion in patients with probable papillary muscle dysfunction, Am. J. Cardiol. **43**:411, 1979. [Abstract.]

Kronzon, I., and Glassman, E.: Mitral ring calcification in idiopathic hypertrophic subaortic stenosis, Am. J. Cardiol. **42**:60, 1978.

McLean, J., Felner, J.M., Whipple, R., et al.: The echocardiographic association of mitral valve prolapse and mitral annulus calcification, Clin. Cardiol. **2**:220, 1979.

Nanda, N.C., and Gramiak, R.: Clinical echocardiography, St. Louis, 1978, The C.V. Mosby Co.

Winkle, R.A., Lopes, M.G., Popp, R.L., et al.: Life-threatening arrhythmias in the mitral valve prolapse syndrome, Am. J. Med. **60**:961, 1976.

ENDOCARDITIS

Berger, M., Delfin, L.A., Jelveh, M., et al.: Two-dimensional echocardiographic findings in right-sided infective endocarditis, Circulation **61**:855, 1980.

Estevez, C.M., Dillon, J.C., Walker, P.D., et al.: Echocardiographic manifestations of aortic cusp rupture in a myxomatous aortic valve, Chest **69**:685, 1976.

Gilbert, E.: Infective endocarditis. Lecture notes for second year medical students, University of Wisconsin, 1981.

Gottlieb, S., Khuddus, S.A., Balooki, H., et al.: Echocardiographic diagnosis of aortic valve vegetations in Candida endocarditis, Circulation **50**:826, 1974.

Hirschfeld, D.S., and Schiller, N.: Localization of aortic valve vegetations by echocardiography, Circulation **53**:280, 1976.

Kleiner, J.P., Brundage, B.H., Ports, T.A., et al.: Echocardiographic manifestation of flail right and non-coronary aortic valve leaflets, Chest **74**:301, 1978.

Kramer, N., Gill, S., Patel, R., et al.: Pulmonary valve vegetations detected by echocardiography, Am. J. Cardiol. **39**:1064, 1977.

Martin, R., Meltzer, R.S., Chia, B.L., et al.: Clinical utility of two-dimensional echocardiography in infective endocarditis, Am. J. Cardiol. **46**:379, 1980.

Martinex, E.C., Burch, G.E., and Giles, T.D.: Echocardiographic diagnosis of vegetative aortic bacterial endocarditis, Am. J. Cardiol. **34**:845, 1974.

Ramirez, J., Guardiola, J., and Flowers, N.C.: Echocardiographic diagnosis of ruptured aortic valve leaflets in bacterial endocarditis, Circulation **57**:634, 1978.

Roy, P., Tajik, A.J., Giuliani, E.R., et al.: Spectrum of echocardiographic findings in bacterial endocarditis, Circulation **53**:474, 1976.

Rubenson, D.S., Tucker, C.R., Stinson, E.B., et al.: The use of echocardiography in diagnosing culture-negative endocarditis, Circulation **64**:641, 1981.

Wray, T.M.: Echocardiographic manifestations of flail aortic valve leaflets in bacterial endocarditis, Circulation **51**:832, 1975.

CARDIAC TUMORS AND THROMBI

DeMaria, A.N., Bommer, W., Neumann, A., et al.: Left ventricular thrombi identified by cross-sectional echocardiography, Ann. Intern. Med. **90**:14, 1979.

Martin, R.P., Rakowski, H., Kleiman, J.H., et al.: Ultrasonic sector scanning as an alternative or adjunct to cardiac angiography, Am. J. Cardiol. **19**:278, 1977. [Abstract.]

Meller, J., Teichholz, L.E., Pichard, A.O., et al.: Left ventricular myxoma: echocardiographic diagnosis and review of the literature, Am. J. Med. **63**:816, 1977.

Nanda, N.C., Barold, S.S., Gramiak, R., et al.: Echocardiographic features of right ventricular outflow tumor prolapsing into the pulmonary artery, Am. J. Cardiol. **40**:272, 1977.

Popp, R.L., and Harrison, D.C.: Ultrasound in the diagnosis of atrial tumor, Ann. Intern. Med. **71**:785, 1969.

Ports, T.A., Cogan, J., Schiller, N.B., et al.: Echocardiography of left ventricular masses, Circulation **58**:528, 1978.

Ports, T.A., Schiller, N.B., and Strunk, B.L.: Echocardiography of right ventricular tumors, Circulation **56**:439, 1977.

Seward, J.B., Gura, G.M., Hagler, D.J., et al.: Evaluation of M-mode echocardiography and wide-angle two-dimensional sector echocardiography in the diagnosis of intracardiac masses, Circulation **58**(suppl. 2): 234, 1978. [Abstract.]

Spangler, R.D., and Okin, J.T.: Echocardiographic demonstration of a left atrial thrombus, Chest **67**: 716, 1975.

CORONARY ARTERY DISEASE

Bain, C., Willett, W., Hennekens, C.H., et al.: Use of postmenopausal hormones and risk of myocardial infarction, Circulation **64**:42, 1981.

Fleming, J.S., and Brainbridge, M.V.: Lecture notes on cardiology, Oxford University, 1975.

Gaasch, W.H., and Bernard, S.A.: The effect of acute changes in coronary blood flow on left ventricular end-diastolic wall thickness, Circulation **56**:593, 1977.

Gordon, M.S., editor: Self-assessment in clinical cardiology, Chicago, 1976, Year Book Medical Publishers, Inc.

Mintz, G.S., Victor, M.F., Kotler, M.N., et al.: Two-dimensional echocardiographic identification of surgically correctable complications of acute myocardial infarction, Circulation **64**:91, 1981.

Morganroth, J., Chen, C.C., David, D., et al.: Exercise cross-sectional echocardiographic diagnosis of coronary artery disease, Am. J. Cardiol. **47**:20, 1981.

Nanda, N.C., and Gramiak, R.: Clinical echocardiography, St. Louis, 1978, The C.V. Mosby Co.

Rogers, E.W., Feigenbaum, H., Weyman, A.E., et al.: Possible detection of atherosclerotic coronary calcification by two-dimensional echocardiography, Circulation **62**:1046, 1980.

Shine, K.I., Fogelman, A.M., Kattus, A.A., et al.: Pathophysiology of myocardial infarction, Ann. Intern. Med. **87**:75, 1977.

Sokolow, M., and McIlroy, M.B.: Clinical cardiology, Los Altos, Calif., 1977, Lange Medical Publications.

Wann, L.S., Faris, J.V., Childress, R.H., et al.: Exercise cross-sectional echocardiography in ischemic heart disease, Circulation **60**:1300, 1979.

Weiss, J.L., Bulkley, B.H., Hutchins, G.M., et al.: Two-dimensional echocardiographic recognition of myocardial injury in man. Comparison with post-mortem studies, Circulation **63**:401, 1981.

Weyman, A.E., Feigenbaum, H., Dillon, J.C., et al.: Non-invasive visualization of the left main coronary artery by cross-sectional echo, Circulation **54**:169, 1976.

Weyman, A.E., Peskoe, S.M., Williams, E.S., et al.: Detection of left ventricular aneurysms by cross-sectional echography, Circulation **54**:936, 1976.

PERICARDIAL DISEASE

Chandraratna, P.A.N., and Aronow, W.S.: Detection of pericardial metastases by cross-sectional echocardiography, Circulation **63**:197, 1981.

Feigenbaum, H.: Echocardiographic diagnosis of pericardial effusion, Am. J. Cardiol. **26**:475, 1970.

Hancock, E.W.: Subacute effusive-constrictive pericarditis, Circulation **43**:183, 1971.

Horowitz, M.S., Schultz, C.S., Stinson, E.B., et al.: Sensitivity and specificity of echocardiographic diagnosis of pericardial effusion, Circulation **50**:239, 1974.

Klein, J.J., and Segal, B.L.: Pericardial effusion diagnosed by reflected ultrasound, Am. J. Cardiol. **22:** 57, 1968.

Lemire, F., Tajik, A.J., Giuliani, E.R., et al.: Further echocardiographic observations in pericardial effusions, Mayo Clin. Proc. **51:**13, 1976.

Lin, T.K., Stech, S.M., Eckert, W.G., et al.: Pericardial angiosarcoma simulating pericardial effusion by echocardiography, Chest **73:**881, 1978.

Millman, A., Meller, J., Motro, M., et al.: Pericardial tumor or fibrosis mimicking pericardial effusion by echocardiography, Ann. Intern. Med. **86:**434, 1977.

Ratshin, R.A., Smith, M., and Hood, W.P.: Possible false-positive diagnosis of pericardial effusion by echocardiography in the presence of a large left atrium, Chest **64:**112, 1974.

Schnittger, I., Bowden, R.E., Abrams, J., et al.: Echocardiography: pericardial thickening and constrictive pericarditis, Am. J. Cardiol. **42:**388, 1978.

Tajik, A.J.: Echocardiography in pericardial effusion, Am. J. Med. **63:**29, 1977.

PEDIATRIC ECHOCARDIOGRAPHY

Caldwell, R.L., et al.: Right ventricular outflow tract assessment by cross-sectional echocardiography in tetralogy of Fallot, Circulation **59:**395, 1979.

Chesler, E., Joffe, H.S., Beck, W., and Schrire, V.: Echocardiographic recognition of mitral-semilunar valve discontinuity: an aid to the diagnosis of origin of both great vessels from the right ventricle, Circulation **43:**725, 1971.

Chesler, E., Joffee, H.S., Vecht, R., et al.: Ultrasound cardiography in single ventricle and the hypoplastic left and right heart syndromes, Circulation **42:**123, 1970.

Diamond, M.A., Dillon, J.C., Haine, C.L., et al.: Echocardiographic features of atrial septal defect, Circulation **43:**129, 1971.

Dillon, J.C., Weyman, A.E., Feigenbaum, H., et al.: Cross-sectional echocardiographic examination of the interatrial septum, Circulation **55:**115, 1977.

DiSessa, T.G., Hagan, A.D., Pope, C., et al.: Two-dimensional echocardiographic characteristics of double outlet right ventricle, Am. J. Cardiol. **44:**1146, 1979.

Fraker, T.D., Harris, P.J., Behar, V.S., and Kisslo, J.A.: Detection of exclusion of interatrial shunts by two-dimensional echocardiography and peripheral venous injection, Circulation **59:**379, 1979.

French, J.W., and Popp, R.: Variability of echocardiographic discontinuity in double outlet right ventricle and truncus arteriosus, Circulation **51:**848, 1975.

Hagler, D.J., Tajik, A.J., Seward, J.B., et al.: Wide-angle two-dimensional echocardiographic profiles of conotruncal abnormalities, Mayo Clin. Proc. **55:**73, 1980.

Lange, L.W., Sahn, D.J., Allen, H.D., and Goldberg, S.J.: Subxyphoid cross-sectional echocardiography in infants and children with congenital heart disease, Circulation **59:**513, 1979.

Meltzer, R.S., Tickner, E.G., Sahines, T.P., and Popp,

R.L.: The source of ultrasound contrast effect, J. Clin. Ultrasound **8:**121, 1980.

Meyer, R.A., and Kaplan, S.: Echocardiography in the diagnosis of hypoplasia of the left or right ventricles in the neonate, Circulation **46:**55, 1972.

Meyer, R.A., Schwartz, D.C., Benzing, G., and Kaplan, S.: Ventricular septum in right ventricular volume overload: an echocardiographic study, Am. J. Cardiol. **30:**349, 1972.

Orsmond, G.S., Ruttenberg, H.D., Bessinger, F.B., and Moller, J.H.: Echocardiographic features of total anomalous pulmonary venous connection to the coronary sinus, Am. J. Cardiol. **41:**597, 1978.

Paquet, M., and Gutgesell, H.: Echocardiographic features of total anomalous pulmonary venous connection, Circulation **51:**599, 1975.

Pieroni, D.R., Homcy, E., and Freedom, R.M.: Echocardiography in atrioventricular canal defect: a clinical spectrum, Am. J. Cardiol. **35:**54, 1975.

Radtke, W.E., Tajik, A.J., Gau, G.T., et al.: Atrial septal defect: echocardiographic observations, Ann. Intern. Med. **84:**246, 1976.

Seward, J.B., Tajik, A.J., Hagler, D.J., and Ritter, D.G.: Echocardiographic spectrum of tricuspid atresia, Mayo Clin. Proc. **53:**100, 1978.

Silverman, N.H., Snider, A.R., and Rudolph, A.M.: Evaluation of pulmonary hypertension by M-mode echocardiography in children with ventricular septal defects, Circulation **61:**1125, 1980.

Tajik, A.J., Gau, G.T., Ritter, D.J., and Schattenberg, T.T.: Echocardiographic pattern of right ventricular diastolic volume overload in children, Circulation **46:** 36, 1972.

Vick, G.W., III, and Serwer, G.A.: Echocardiographic evaluation of the postoperative tetralogy of Fallot patient, Circulation **58:**842, 1978.

Weyman, A.E., Wann, S., Feigenbaum, H., and Dillon, J.C.: Mechanism of abnormal septal motion in patients with right ventricular volume overload—a cross-sectional echocardiographic study, Circulation **54:**179, 1976.

Williams, R.G., and Tucker, C.R.: Echocardiographic diagnosis of congenital heart disease, Boston, 1977, Little, Brown & Co.

PROSTHETIC VALVES

Alderman, E.L., Rytand, D.A., Crow, R.S., et al.: Normal and prosthetic atrioventricular valve motion in atrial flutter, Circulation **45:**1206, 1972.

Assad-Morell, J., et al.: Malfunctioning tricuspid valve prosthesis. Clinical, phonocardiographic, echocardiographic and surgical findings, Mayo Clin. Proc. **42:**443, 1974.

Belenkie, I., Carr, M., Schlant, R.C., et al.: Malfunction of a Cutter-Smeloff mitral ball valve prosthesis: diagnosis by phonocardiography and echocardiography, Am. Heart J. **86:**399, 1973.

Brodie, B.R., Grossman, W., McLaurin, L., et al.: Diagnosis of prosthetic mitral valve malfunction with combined echo-phonocardiography, Circulation **53:** 93, 1976.

Burgraff, G.W., and Craige, E.: Echocardiographic studies of left ventricular wall motion and dimensions after valvular heart surgery, Am. J. Cardiol. **35:**473, 1975.

Douglas, J., and Williams, G.: Echocardiographic evaluation of the Björk-Shiley prosthetic valve, Circulation **50:**52, 1974.

Gold, H., and Hertz, L.: Death caused by fracture of Beall mitral prosthesis, Am. J. Cardiol. **34:**371, 1974.

Horowitz, M., Goodman, D., and Popp, R.: Echocardiographic diagnosis of calcific stenosis of a stented aortic homograft in the mitral position, J. Clin. Ultrasound **2:**179, 1974.

Johnson, M.L.: Echocardiographic evaluation of prosthetic heart valves. In Gramiak, R., and Waag, R.C., editors: Cardiac ultrasound, St. Louis, 1975, The C.V. Mosby Co.

Johnson, M.L., Holmes, J.H., and Paton, B.C.: Echocardiographic determination of mitral disc valve excursion, Circulation **47:**1274, 1973.

Johnson, M.L., Paton, B.C., and Holmes, J.H.: Ultrasonic evaluation of prosthetic valve motion, Circulation **41**(suppl. 2):3, 1970.

Miller, H., Gibson, D., and Stephens, J.: Role of echocardiography and phonocardiography in the diagnosis of mitral paraprosthetic regurgitation with Starr-Edwards prostheses, Br. Heart J. **35:**1217, 1973.

Miller, H., Stephens, J., and Gibson, D.: Echocardiographic features of mitral Starr-Edwards paraprosthetic regurgitation, Br. Heart J. **35:**560, 1973.

Nanda, N.C., Gramiak, R., and Shah, P.M.: Diagnosis of aortic root dissection by echocardiography, Circulation **48:**506, 1973.

Nanda, N.C., Gramiak, R., Shah, P.M., and DeWeese, J.A.: Mitral commissurotomy versus replacement: preoperative evaluation by echocardiography, Circulation **51:**263, 1975.

Popp, R., and Carmichael, B.: Cardiac echography in the diagnosis of prosthetic mitral valve malfunction, Circulation **44:**33, 1971.

Siggers, D.C., Srivongse, S.A., and Deuchar, D.: Analysis of dynamics of mitral Starr-Edwards valve prosthesis using reflected ultrasound, Br. Heart J. **33:**401, 1971.

Smith, R.A., et al.: Non-invasive diagnostic evaluation of the normal Beall mitral prosthesis, Cathet. Cardiovasc. Diagn. **2:**289, 1976.

Srivastava, T.N., et al.: Echocardiographic diagnosis of a stuck Björk-Shiley aortic valve prosthesis, Chest **70:**94, 1976.

Willerson, J.T., Kastor, J.A., Dinsmore, R.E., et al.: Non-invasive assessment of prosthetic mitral paravalvular and intravalvular regurgitation, Br. Heart J. **34:**561, 1972.

Yoshikawa, J., Owaki, T., Kato, H., and Tanaka, K.: Abnormal motion of interventricular septum of patients with prosthetic valve. In White, D., editor: Ultrasound in medicine, New York, 1975, Plenum Publishing Corporation.

Index